The Foot

The Foot

EDITED BY

Basil Helal MCh (Orth), FRCS, FRCS (Edin)
Consultant Orthopaedic Surgeon to The London Hospital,
The Royal National Orthopaedic Hospital and Enfield Group of Hospitals

Derek Wilson MBBS, FRCS
Consultant Orthopaedic Surgeon, The Royal Free Hospital, London

VOLUME 2

CHURCHILL LIVINGSTONE
EDINBURGH LONDON MELBOURNE AND NEW YORK 1988

CHURCHILL LIVINGSTONE
Medical Division of Longman Group UK Limited

Distributed in the United States of America by
Churchill Livingstone Inc., 1560 Broadway, New York,
N.Y. 10036, and by associated companies, branches
and representatives throughout the world.

First published 1988

ISBN 0 443 029814 (2 volumes)

British Library Cataloguing in Publication Data
The Foot.
1. Foot——Wounds and injuries
I. Helal, Basil II. Wilson, Derek
617'.585 RD781

Library of Congress Cataloging in Publication Data
The Foot.
Includes index.
1. Foot——Surgery. 2. Foot——Diseases. 3. Foot.
I. Helal, Basil. II. Wilson, Derek. [DNLM: 1. Foot——
surgery. 2. Foot Diseases——therapy. WE 880 P6858]
RD563.F635 1988 617'.585 87-23838

Printed and bound in Great Britain by
William Clowes Limited, Beccles and London

Preface

The foot is an orthopaedic 'Cinderella'. It has received scant attention in comparison to more proximal parts.

The foot accepts as much load as the hip or knee and indeed some of its smaller joints accept even more per unit area and its disorders can produce as much pain and disability as these joints. Biomechanically it is an immensely complex zone with its torque convertor function and the impetus it has to provide in walking and running.

Foot surgery was commonly relegated to the end of an operating list and often left to the most junior member of the surgical team. This trend has left a wake of painful, ruined feet — the blight of so many lives.

It is in relatively recent times that the foot has become the focus of organized scientific study and under the stimulus of foot societies and publications devoted to the subject there has been an explosion of new knowledge.

We have brought together a group of authors who have made important contributions in this field and who are in our opinion the most authoritative sources for their subdivisions of the subject.

By comparison with the foot the bibliography of the hand is enormous, a fact which does not in fact reflect their relative importance. Wood Jones, who wrote classic books on both the hand and the foot, writes 'Zoologists describing the anthropoids have named the human subspecies Bimanus .... That a ridiculously simple and primitive appendage such as the hand should be thus lauded is illogical .... Man's foot is all his own. It is unlike any other foot. It is the most distinctly human part of the whole of his anatomical make up. It is a human specialization ... it is his hallmark and so long as Man has been Man and as long as he remains Man, it is by his feet that he will be known from all other members of the animal kingdom .... It is his feet which confer upon Man his only real distinction and provide his only valid claim to human status'.

The British Orthopaedic Foot Surgery Society was convened at The London Hospital in 1978 and was soon affiliated to the International Society (Société International du Médecin et Chirurgie du Pied (CIP). The Society has flourished and grown and in 1985 became affiliated with the British Orthopaedic Association. Thus in Britain, as elsewhere, there is a rapidly expanding interest in the foot and a great input of new knowledge and world wide communication of expertise.

We are grateful to our authors for the standards they have maintained and to our folk at home for putting up with the paper chaos and the disruption of many hours of family life; we sincerely hope they will all find the end result worthwhile. We hope also that this book will act as the glass slipper for the 'Cinderella' foot and elevate it to the position of importance that it deserves.

London, 1988 B.H. and D.W.

Contributors

B. G. Andrews MBBS, FRCS, MRCS, LRCP
Consultant Orthopaedic Surgeon,
Westminster and Queen Mary's Hospitals,
London;
Honorary Consultant,
Limb Fitting Centre;
Member of the Court of Examiners,
Royal College of Surgeons.

Barbara M. Ansell CBE, MD, FRCS, FRCP
Head,
Division of Rheumatology,
Clinical Research Centre,
Northwick Park Hospital, Harrow;
Consultant Rheumatologist,
Wexham Park Hospital, Slough, Berkshire.

Colin G. Barnes BSc, MBBS, FRCP
Consultant Rheumatologist,
The London Hospital.

Edward H. Bates MBBS(Sydney), FRCS,
FRACS
Visiting Orthopaedic Surgeon,
Prince of Wales Children's Hospital, Randwick,
NSW, Australia.

Alexander Benjamin MBBS, FRCS
Honorary Consultant,
West and Mid Hertfordshire Group of Hospitals.

S. C. Chen BA(Tech), FRCS
Consultant Orthopaedic Surgeon,
Enfield Group of Hospitals, Middlesex.

Wui K. Chung FRACS
Visiting Orthopaedic (Paediatric) Surgeon,
Prince of Wales Children's Hospital, Sydney;
Visiting Orthopaedic Surgeon, Nepean Hospital,
NSW, Australia.

Andrea Cracchiolo III MD
Professor of Orthopaedic Surgery,
University of California, Los Angeles, USA.

H. L. F. Currey M Med(Cape Town) FRCP
Professor of Rheumatology and Director,
Bone and Joint Research Unit,
The London Hospital Medical College.

B. Martina Daly MB, MRCP
Consultant Dermatologist,
Burnley General Hospital, Burnley, Lancashire.

Michael Devas MChir, FRCS
Professor of Orthopaedics (Retired),
Universiti Sains, Penang, Malaysia, and Royal
East Sussex Hospital, Hastings.

Thomas Duckworth MB, ChB, BSc, FRCS
Professor of Orthopaedic Surgery,
University of Sheffield;
Honorary Consultant Orthopaedic Surgeon,
Sheffield Health Authority.

Geoffrey R. Fisk MBBS, FRCS, FRCS(Edin)
Honorary Consultant Orthopaedic Surgeon,
Harlow Group of Hospitals, Essex;
Professor of the Royal College of Surgeons of
England.

J. M. Fitton MBE, MB, FRCS
Consultant Orthopaedic Surgeon (Retired),
St. James's University Hospital, Leeds.

John Foulston BA, MSc, MChS
Honorary Principal Scientist,
Diabetic Department,
King's College Hospital;
Visiting Lecturer,
Chelsea School of Chiropody, London.

J. D. Frame FRCS
Registrar in Plastic Surgery,
Mount Vernon Hospital, Northwood, Middlesex.

Barry E. Francis SRCh, FPodA, MChS
Chiropodist,
North Middlesex Hospital;
Examiner to Podiatry Association;
Honorary Podiatrist,
British Olympic Association.

E. N. Glick MB, ChB, FRCP, DPhysMed
Consultant in Rheumatology and Rehabilitation,
Enfield District Hospitals, Middlesex.

Ian Goldie MD
Professor and Chairman, Department of Orthopaedic Surgery,
Karolinska Institute, Stockholm, Sweden.

Paul P. Griffin MD
Chief of Staff,
Shriners Hospitals for Crippled Children,
Chicago, Illinois, USA.

Hamilton Hall MD, FRCS(C)
Associate Professor,
Faculty of Medicine, University of Toronto, Canada;
Staff Orthopedic Surgeon,
Women's College Hospital and Orthopedic and Arthritic Hospital;
Orthopedic Consultant to National Ballet of Canada.

Douglas H. Harrison MB, BS, FRCS
Consultant Plastic Surgeon,
Regional Plastic and Jaw Surgery Centre,
Mount Vernon Hospital, Northwood, Middlesex.

Basil Helal MCh(Orth), FRCS, FRCS(Edin)
Consultant Orthopaedic Surgeon, The London Hospital, The Royal National Orthopaedic Hospital, London, and Enfield Group of Hospitals, Middlesex.

J. Anthony Herring MD
Associate Professor of Orthopedic Surgery,
University of Texas Health Science Center;
Chief of Staff,
Texas Scottish Rite Hospital, Dallas, Texas, USA.

David Hirschowitz MB, ChB, FRCS
Consultant Orthopaedic Surgeon,
North West Hertfordshire District Health Authority.

Geoffrey Hooper MSc, FRCS
Consultant Orthopaedic Surgeon, Princess Margaret Rose Orthopaedic Hospital, Edinburgh.

Sean P. F. Hughes MS, FRCS(Edin Orth), FRCS(Edin), FRCS, FRCSI
Professor of Orthopaedic Surgery,
University of Edinburgh.

C. G. Iwegbu MD, MChOrth, FRCS(Edin), FRCS(Glas), FWACS, FICS
Senior Lecturer and Consultant in Orthopaedic and Accident Surgery,
Ahmadu Bello University Teaching Hospital, Zaria, Nigeria.

J. P. Jackson MBBS(Lond), FRCS
Emeritus Surgeon,
Harlow Wood Orthopaedic Hospital and the Nottingham Hospitals;
Clinical Lecturer,
University of Nottingham.

John Edwin Jellis OBE, FRCS
Consultant Orthopaedic Surgeon,
University Teaching Hospital, Lusaka, Zambia;
Honorary Lecturer,
University of Zambia.

Kenneth A. Johnson MD
Associate Professor of Orthopedics,
Mayo Medical School;
Consultant, Department of Orthopedics,
Mayo Clinic and Mayo Foundation, Rochester, Minnesota, USA.

Charles E. Johnston II MD
Assistant Professor of Orthopedic Surgery,
University of Texas Health Science Center, Dallas;
Staff Orthopedist,
Texas Scottish Rite Hospital, Dallas, Texas, USA.

J. B. King FRCS, MBBS, LRCP
Senior Lecturer in Trauma and Orthopaedic Surgery, and Director of the Diploma Course in Sports Medicine,
The London Hospital Medical College;
Consultant Trauma and Orthopaedic Surgeon,

Tower Hamlets Health Authority and Newham Health Authority.

John Kirkup FRCS, DHM
Consultant Surgeon,
Bath and Wessex Orthopaedic Hospital;
Archivist,
British Orthopaedic Association.

B. Levack MBBS, FRCS
Senior Registrar,
Department of Orthopaedic Surgery,
The London Hospital, Whitechapel, and Black Notley Hospital, Braintree, Essex.

Jenny Lewis BSc, PhD

Lowell Dean Lutter MD
Staff Physician,
St. Anthony Sports Medicine Clinic and
St. Anthony Orthopedic Clinic, St. Paul, Minnesota;
Chief of Staff,
Gillette Children's Hospital, Minnesota, USA.

Gordon E. MacLellan FRCS
Consultant Orthopaedic Surgeon,
Oldchurch Hospital, Romford, Essex.

Roger A. Mann MD
Associate Clinical Professor,
University of California, San Francisco, USA.

Bernard F. Meggitt MA, FRCS
Consultant Orthopaedic Surgeon,
Addenbrooke's Hospital, Cambridge;
Associate Lecturer,
University of Cambridge.

George Murdoch MB, ChB, FRCS(Edin)
Emeritus Professor of Orthopaedic Surgery,
University of Dundee;
Visiting Professor,
University of Strathclyde, Glasgow.

A. C. Nicol BSc, PhD
Lecturer,
Bioengineering Unit,
University of Strathclyde, Glasgow.

K. I. Nissen MD, FRCS
Formerly Surgeon,
The Royal National Orthopaedic Hospital, London.

Sureshwar Pandey MBBS(Hons), FICS(Chicago), MS(General Surgery), FIAMS, MS(Orth. Surg.), FACS(USA)
Professor and Chief of Orthopaedic Surgery, Traumatology, Rehabilitation and Paraplegia Services,
Rajendra Medical College and Hospital,
University of Ranchi;
Director,
GNH Handicapped Children and Ram Janam Sulakshana Artificial Limb Center, Ranchi;
Visiting Professor,
Universities of Teikyo, Osaka, Tokyo, Adelaide and Flinders;
Senior Consultant,
Ram Janam Sulakshana Institute of Orthopaedics, Ranchi, India.

J. P. Paul BSc, PhD, CEng, FIMechE, FISPO, cFBOA, FRSE
Professor and Head of Bioengineering Unit,
University of Strathclyde, Glasgow.

Hugh Phillips FRCS
Consultant Orthopaedic Surgeon,
Norfolk and Norwich Hospital, Norwich.

Paul F. Plattner MD
Resident in Orthopedics,
Mayo Graduate School of Medicine, Rochester, Minnesota, USA.

Robert William Povey (Air Commodore Retired), MBBS, FRCS(Eng)
Late CADE Professor of Surgery, Royal College of Surgeons, London;
Late Consultant Advisor in Orthopaedic Surgery, Royal Air Force.

Frank Rand MD
Assistant in Orthopedics,
Children's Hospital, Boston, Massachusetts, USA.

P. A. Revell PhD, MRCPath
Senior Lecturer in Histopathology;
Honorary Consultant Pathologist,
The London Hospital Medical College.

Colin P. Reynolds MB, BS, DObst, RCOG, DMRD, FRCR
Consultant Radiologist,

The London Hospital, The London Clinic, and The Royal Masonic Hospital, London.

D. Ruano-Gil MD
Chairman of the Department of Human Anatomy, Faculty of Medicine, Barcelona, Spain;
Member of the Royal Academy of Medicine.

G. James Sammarco MD, FACS
Associate Clinical Professor,
Department of Orthopaedic Surgery,
University of Cincinnati Medical Center;
Director of the Foot and Ankle Center, Good Samaritan Hospital;
Director of the Clinic for Performing Arts, Cincinnati, Ohio, USA.

Pierce Scranton MD
Assistant Clinical Professor,
University of Washington, USA.

Sam Shuster MB, PhD, FRCP
Professor of Dermatology,
University of Newcastle upon Tyne.

Brian C. Sommerlad MBBS, FRCS
Consultant Plastic Surgeon,
The London Hospital, and St. Andrew's Hospital, Billericay, Essex.

William J. Stripp MBE, FCR
Formerly Superintendent Radiographer (Retired),
The Royal National Orthopaedic Hospital, London.

David Stuart MB, FRCS(Edin)
Consultant Orthopaedic Surgeon,
Nairobi Hospital, Kenya.

Malcolm Swann FRCS
Consultant Orthopaedic Surgeon,
Wexham Park Hospital, Slough and Heatherwood Hospital, Ascot.

N. P. Thomas BSc, MBBS, FRCS
Consultant Orthopaedic Surgeon,
Lord Mayor Treloar Hospital, Alton, and Basingstoke District Hospital, Hampshire.

Russell H. Tuttle BSc, MA, PhD
Professor,
Department of Anthropology, Committee on Evolutionary Biology, The Morris Fishbein Center for the Study of the History of Science and Medicine, and the College,
The University of Chicago, Illinois, USA;
Affiliate Scientist in Behavioral Biology,
Yerkes Regional Primate Research Center,
Emory University, Atlanta, Georgia, USA.

Valente Valenti MD
Orthopedic Surgeon,
Collège International de Médecine et Chirurgie du Pied, Rome, Italy.

Antonio Viladot MD
Professor of Orthopaedic Surgery,
Universidad Autónoma de Barcelona;
President of the Sociedad Española de Cirugia Ortopédica y Traumatología;
Chief of Service,
Cirugía del Aparato Locomotor del Hospital de San Rafael, Barcelona, Spain.

Geoffrey Walker MB, FRCS
Honorary Senior Lecturer,
St. George's Hospital Medical School, London;
Orthopaedic Surgeon,
Queen Mary's Hospital for Children, Carshalton, Surrey.

Michael Ward CBE, MD, FRCS
Consultant Surgeon,
St. Andrew's Hospital, and Newham District General Hospital, London;
Lecturer in Surgery,
London Hospital Medical College.

William Waugh MA, MChir, FRCS
Professor Emeritus,
Orthopaedic and Accident Surgery,
University of Nottingham.

Derek W. Wilson MBBS, FRCS
Consultant Orthopaedic Surgeon,
The Royal Free Hospital, London.

J. N. Wilson ChM, FRCS
Consulting Orthopaedic Surgeon,
Royal National Orthopaedic Hospital, and National Hospital for Nervous Diseases, London.

C. B. Wynn Parry MBE, MA, DM, FRCP, FRCS
Director of Rehabilitation,
Royal National Orthopaedic Hospitals, London.

Contents

VOLUME 2

Paul Plattner and Kenneth Johnson

Tendons and bursae

INTRODUCTION

Tendon injuries about the foot and ankle are much less common than ligament sprains in this area, but they are not as rare as generally supposed (Gilcreest 1933, McMaster 1933, Haldeman & Soto-Hall 1935, Conwell & Alldredge 1937, Lipscomb 1950, Lipscomb & Kelly 1955, Anzel et al 1959, Griffiths 1965, Nicholas 1974, Scheller et al 1980, Wicks et al 1980, Floyd et al 1983). This chapter will focus on only the extrinsic tendons that cross the ankle. The literature is reviewed in regard to the cause, type, classification, anatomic distribution of and pathological changes associated with tendon injuries. Problems that specifically affect the Achilles tendon, tibialis posterior tendon, peroneal tendons, extensor tendons about the foot and ankle, and flexor hallucis longus tendon are also addressed.

ANATOMY OF TENDONS

Eleven extrinsic muscles whose tendons cross the ankle originate in the leg (Fig. 29.1). Except for the Achilles and plantaris tendons, all have true synovial sheaths along part of their extent (Hartmann 1981, Sarrafian 1983).

Anteriorly, the main extensors of the foot are the tibialis anterior, the extensor hallucis longus, the extensor digitorum longus, and the peroneus tertius. These tendons pass under a tight osteofibrous canal formed by the superior and inferior extensor retinacula.

Medially at the ankle, the tibialis posterior, flexor digitorum longus, and flexor hallucis longus each lie in separate compartments behind the malleolus deep to the flexor retinaculum. The medial malleolus serves as a pulley for the tibialis posterior and flexor digitorum longus, and the posterior process of the talus and the sustentaculum tali of the calcaneus provide fulcrums for the flexor hallucis longus.

Behind the lateral malleolus in the same compartment lie the peroneus brevis and the peroneus longus. These tendons are restrained by the superior and inferior peroneal retinacula. The lateral malleolus (peroneal sulcus) serves as a pulley for both the peroneus brevis and the peroneus longus. As the peroneus longus courses distally, it also has a fulcrum at the peroneal trochlea (tubercle) of the calcaneus and another on the undersurface of the cuboid bone.

Posteriorly, the Achilles and plantaris tendons insert onto the posteroinferior surface of the calcaneus. The tendons are separated from the superior aspect of the calcaneus by a bursa, from the deep flexors by the deep transverse fascia, and from the skin by loose areolar tissue.

AETIOLOGY OF INJURIES TO MUSCLES AND TENDONS (Gilcreest 1933, McMaster 1933, Haldeman & Soto-Hall 1935, Conwell & Alldredge 1937)

Many factors may be responsible for muscle and tendon dysfunction (Gilcreest 1933, Jahss 1982b) (Table 29.1). Most injuries are probably caused by a combination of these factors.

A classification of injury is also important, and the scheme modified from Haldeman & Soto-Hall (1935), based on causative factors, contributing forces, and relative frequency is most helpful (Table 29.2).

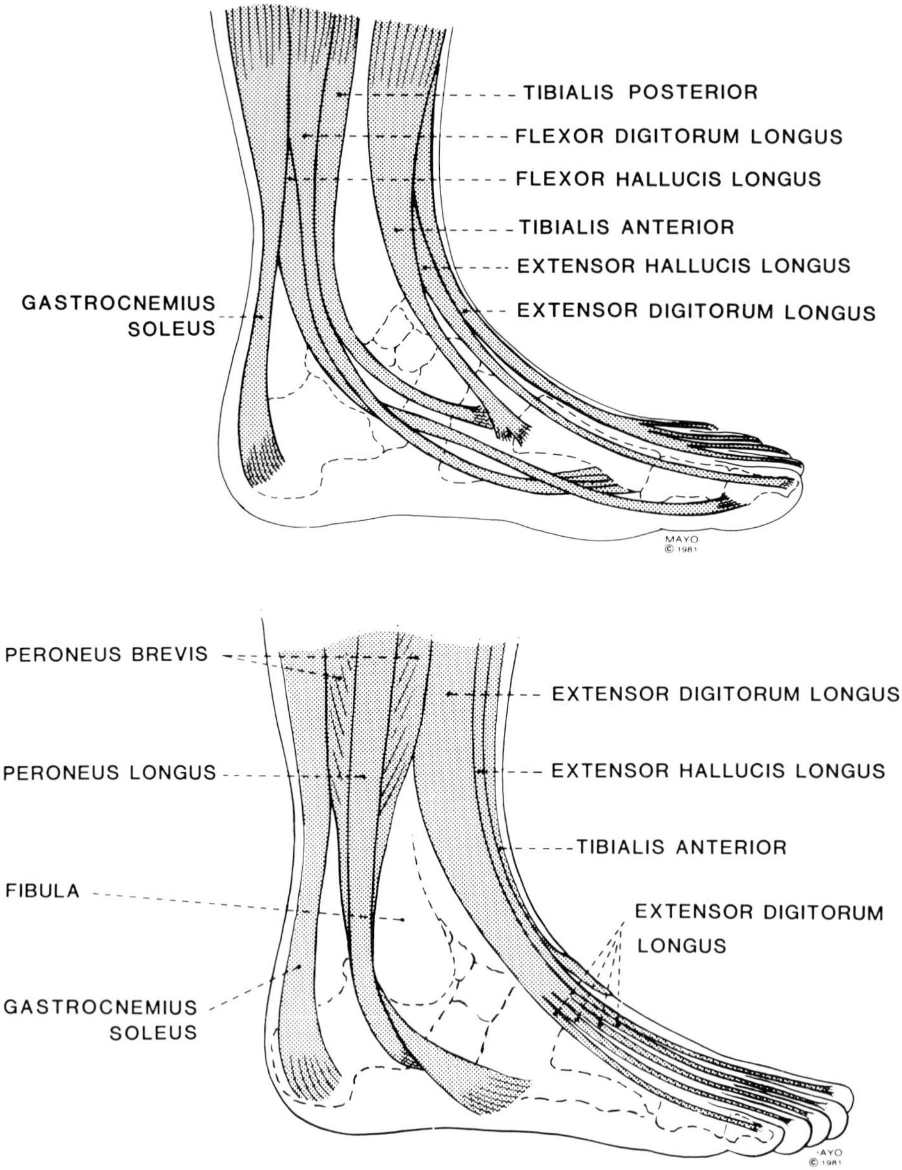

Fig. 29.1 Extrinsic muscles of foot. A: Medial view. B: Lateral view. (By permission of Mayo Foundation)

In the broadest sense, tendons may become inflamed (so-called tendinitis), rupture, and sublux or dislocate.

PATHOLOGY OF INJURIES TO MUSCLES AND TENDONS

A knowledge of the anatomy and physiology of tendons, tendon sheaths, and bursae is necessary for a clear concept of inflammatory processes involving these structures (Schatzker & Brånemark 1969, Hartmann 1981, Jahss 1982b).

A tendon is connective tissue composed of closely packed collagen fibres and protein-mucopolysaccharide. These components are elaborated by the tenocyte and grouped together in bundles surrounded by a woven mesh of loose connective tissue, the endotenon. All of these bundles make up

Table 29.1 Causes of muscle and tendon dysfunction

Aging and degeneration
Pathological changes
Peritendinitis
Nonspecific
Arthritic
Infectious
Neoplastic
Myositis
Calcinosis
Vascular
Bony changes
Fractures
Rough bone
Spurs/exostoses
Tethering
Partial constriction
Trigger toes, tarsal tunnel
Peroneal constriction with fractured os calcis
Complete tethering
Incarceration
Adhesive, including check rein deformity
Contractures
Occupation
Fatigue/stress
Trauma
Direct
Indirect
Iatrogenic conditions
Congenital conditions

the tendon, which is also surrounded by a fine connective tissue sheath, the epitenon (peritenon), which is continuous with the endotenon. The paratenon is loose, fatty areolar tissue that surrounds the entire tendon. In areas where the tendon is subjected to increased local pressure or friction, the paratenon is replaced by a synovial sheath or bursa. For the most part, true synovial sheaths are found only in the distal portions of the upper and lower extremities, especially where tendons lie contiguous to joints and motion is the chief function. The mesotenon, called 'vinculum' in some areas, is a specialized mesentery-like structure on the non-friction side of the tendons that carries blood vessels.

A tendon receives its blood supply at the musculotendinous junction, at the tendo-osseous junction, and along its length by means of the paratenon, mesotenon, and tendon sheath. These specialized structures are responsible for most of the segmental blood supply to the majority of tendons (Lagergren & Lindholm 1958–1959, Schatzker & Brånemark 1969, Stein & Luekens 1976a).

A standard sequence of histological changes occur after a tendon injury. The inflammatory process is

Table 29.2 Classification of muscle and tendon injuries

Direct injury
Laceration (open wound)
Blow or crush (closed wound)
Indirect injury
Stretching force applied to contracting muscle
Unusually forceful contraction
Spontaneous rupture (partial or complete)
Post-traumatic
Single injury (catastrophic failure)
Repetitive injury (fatigue failure)
Pathological (disease of tendon)
Degenerative
Dislocation/subluxation of tendons
Acute
Chronic
Iatrogenic (corticosteroids?) (Kleinman & Gross 1983)

the response of the body to tissue injury involving neurological, vascular, humoral, and cellular reactions within the site of injury. The factors that influence the characteristics of this inflammatory response depend on the intensity and duration of insult, the type of injury (for example, mechanical, bacterial, chemical, or immunological), the amount of cell degeneration and death (which ultimately influence the extent and progress of the inflammatory response), and the kinds of cells and tissues involved.

Inflammation is usually designated as acute or chronic according to its duration and the type of cells that predominate in the inflamed tissue. In acute inflammation, the dominant histological changes are vascular and exudative with the emigration and accumulation of leukocytes. Chronic inflammation is characterized by proliferative changes as tissue attempts repair and healing. The undifferentiated connective tissue that is formed may have changes of mucoid, fatty, hyaline, myxoid, or fibrinoid degeneration, cartilage metaplasia, calcification, or bone metaplasia (Arner et al 1958–1959, Lipscomb & Wakim 1961a, 1961b, Davidsson & Salo 1969, Fisher & Woods 1970, Burry & Pool 1973, Fox et al 1975, Clancy et al 1976, Puddu et al 1976, Gould & Korson 1980, Trevino et al 1981, Clancy 1982). Arner et al (1958–1959b, 1959) described this orderly sequence of histological changes in their classification of healing after rupture of the Achilles tendon (Table 29.3).

Recently, Clancy et al (1976, 1982) used clinical findings to classify the inflammatory response as acute, subacute, or chronic on the basis of temporal

Table 29.3 Sequential changes of tendon healing

Stage	Histological change	Time (days)
I	Sparse inflammatory cellular infiltrate	0–1
II	Diffuse infiltration of leukocytes	1–4
III	Abundant granulation tissue	4–14
IV	Formation of undifferentiated connective tissue	>14

considerations, as follows: acute, symptoms present for less than 2 weeks; subacute, symptoms present for longer than 2 weeks but less than 6 weeks; and chronic, symptoms present for 6 weeks or longer.

The local signs of the inflammatory process, calor, rubor, tumour, and dolor, have remained unchanged since they were first described by Celsus in the 1st century AD. The orthopaedic surgeon is interested in minimizing the concept of functiolaesa (loss of function), which Galen described in the 2nd century AD.

Peritendinitis

There is much confusion in the literature regarding the proper terminology for inflammation about tendons (Lipscomb 1942, 1944, 1950, Lapidus & Seidenstein 1950, Griffiths 1952, Lapidus 1953, Hauser 1956, Clancy 1982). Puddu et al (1976) argued that the connective tissue of tendons is dense and fibrous with little inherent vascularity and therefore it is not predisposed to inflammatory processes. Hence, they thought that use of the term 'tendinitis' was inappropriate. Inflammatory processes can take place in the vascular peritendinous tissue. Lipscomb (1950) defined 'paratendinitis' as an inflammatory process about tendons or portions of tendons that possess no sheath and used 'tenosynovitis' to refer to inflammatory processes about tendons with sheaths. He used 'peritendinitis' as an inclusive term to denote either tenosynovitis or paratendinitis. Puddu et al (1976) introduced the term 'tendinosis', which they defined as degenerative lesions in tendon tissue with no evidence of alteration of the peritenon. Therefore, tendon disease could be manifested by pure peritendinitis, peritendinitis with tendinosis, or tendinosis alone. Peritendinitis with tendinosis or tendinosis alone may eventually result in rupture. For purposes of this discussion, the classification in Table 29.4 is preferred.

Inflammatory processes involving tendons about the ankle are more common than is generally believed. Lipscomb (1950) analysed 651 cases of nonspecific peritendinitis at the Mayo Clinic, Minnesota, between 1935 and 1948. He described various types of peritendinitis (Table 29.5). 48% of his cases involved the forearm, wrist, and hand, 36% involved the ankle and foot, and 6% involved the long head of the biceps. The anatomic distribution of the involved tendons in the lower extremity was as follows: tibialis anterior, 24%; Achilles tendon, 20%; tibialis posterior, 16%; peroneals, 16%; and others, 24%.

The distribution and type of injuries that are occurring are changing as more people participate in jogging as a sport. Brody (1980) stated that 30% of the running-associated injuries he treated involved the knee, 20% involved the Achilles tendon, 15% were shin splints and stress fractures, and 10% were plantar fasciitis.

Rupture

McMaster's (1933) classic experiments with the tendons of rabbits showed that rupture does not occur when a normal muscle-tendon system is subjected to severe strain. Rupture occurred at one of four sites: tendon insertion into bone, musculotendinous junction, muscle belly, or tendon origin from bone. Approximately half of the fibres of a tendon had to be severed to permit immediate rupture when subjected to severe strain. Even when 75% of the fibres were severed, normal activity did not cause rupture. He concluded that true rupture of normal tendon does not occur and that rupture can take place only through diseased tendon substance.

Table 29.4 Classification of tendon inflammation

Peritendinitis: an inflammatory process involving peritendinous structures
- Paratendinitis: no synovial sheath
- Tenosynovitis: synovial sheath

Peritendinitis with tendinosis: inflammatory process involving peritendinous structures with degenerative lesion of tendon tissue

Tendinosis: asymptomatic degenerative process of tendon tissue without inflammation

Table 29.5 Types of peritendinitis

Nonspecific:	Infectious:
Stenosing	Suppurative
Crepitans	Nonsuppurative
Hypertrophica	Tuberculous
Serosa chronica	Fungal
	Syphilitic
Arthritic:	Gonococcal
Hypertrophic	Neoplastic:
Rheumatoid	
Sarcoid	Xanthomatous
Gout	Lipomatous
Reiter's syndrome	Haemangiomatous
Collagen-vascular disease	Neurofibromatous
Scleroderma	

Data from Lipscomb (1950)

When disease is mild, microscopic changes are minimal. More extensive inflammation may lead to gross thickening of the peritendinous sheath and enlargement and fraying of tendon. The final event in this process may result in a degenerated, fibrotic tendon that ultimately ruptures. Clancy et al (1976, 1982) classified these chronic inflammatory changes as interstitial microscopic failure, central necrosis, frank partial rupture, and acute complete rupture.

Microscopic damage to portions of the vascular supply of the tendon substance is likely an important factor in pathological ruptures (Lagergren & Lindholm 1958–1959, Schatzker & Brånemark 1969). Other factors such as aging, degeneration, and recurrent microtrauma are also contributory (Davidsson & Salo 1969). Clancy et al (1976, 1982) thought that repetitive mechanical stress results in disruption of the collagen fibrils and that subsequent chronic inflammatory changes permanently alter the capacity of fibroblasts to synthesize collagen; a vicious cycle is set up, and rupture finally ensues.

Anzel et al (1959) analysed 1014 disruptions of muscles or tendons in 781 patients from 1945 to 1954 at the Mayo Clinic. They found an incidence of approximately 70 disruptions per 100,000 patients per year. The upper extremity was involved six times more often than the lower extremity. The average age of the patients was 40.5 years. Males were affected more often than females for each type of injury.

Of the 1014 disruptions, approximately 60% were due to lacerations and 40% were due to all other causes (direct closed injury, stress rupture, and 'normal' activity). The anatomic distribution of the 143 injuries to the lower extremity is shown in Table 29.6.

As has been shown, tendon lesions about the foot are quite common but often present diagnostic problems. Swelling about a tendon may result from various pathologic conditions and even masquerade as neoplasm. Many times these 'pseudotumours' are unsuspected ruptures caused by underlying tendinosis and associated peritendinitis (Webster 1968, Jahss 1972, 1974, Fitzgerald & Coventry 1980). With increased awareness and recognition, the diagnosis of peritendinitis, rupture, and dislocation or subluxation will be more obvious.

BURSAE

Synovial bursae are potential spaces with a secretory endothelial-type lining. These bursae are usually associated with joint cavities and are present at birth. They function to reduce friction and are usually located between the skin and bony projections (superficial or subcutaneous) and between tendons and prominences over which they must move (deep or subfascial) (Kaplan & Ferguson 1937, Cherry & Ghormley 1941, Bywaters 1965).

Adventitial bursae are acquired and form in unusual locations after birth in response to repeated trauma (friction) to soft tissue over a bony prominence. They are most often subcutaneous or superficial. These bursae have no true endothelial lining but rather seem to be a myxomatous or mucoid change of connective tissue. When a well

Table 29.6 Location of 143 tendon disruptions in the lower extremity

Muscle/tendon	No.	(%)
Quadriceps	54	(38)
Achilles tendon	22	(15)
Triceps surae	21	(15)
Extensors of toes	16	(11)
Tibialis anterior	10	(7)
Tibialis posterior	3	(2)
Flexor hallucis longus	3	(2)
Peroneus longus	2	(1.5)
Peroneus tertius	2	(1.5)
Others	10	(7)
Total	143	100

Modified from Anzel et al (1959)

formed cyst is present, histological study usually shows flattened fibroblastic cells rather than the secretory endothelial cells of synovial bursae (Kaplan & Ferguson 1937, Buck et al 1943, Kuhns 1943).

Jahss (1982b) classified bursae according to location and type (Table 29.7). Sarrafian (1983) and Hartmann (1981) provided excellent anatomic depictions and descriptions of the numerous bursae about the foot.

Bywaters (1965) stated that synovial bursae were a neglected class of anatomic structures of considerable importance 'subject to the same ills that joints are heir to'. This statement is probably most true for bursae about the foot and ankle, where Roberts (1929a, 1929b) believed that bursitis was a neglected cause of disability. Affliction of the various bursae about the foot was amply described in the early literature (Hertzler 1926, Roberts 1929a, 1929b) but seems less well recognized in recent publications.

BURSITIS

Various classifications of bursitis based on cause have appeared in the literature. Meyerding (1938) thought that bursitis could be classified as acute or chronic, traumatic or infectious, syphilitic, gouty, or malignant. He also mentioned tuberculosis, gonorrhea, and rheumatism as aetiologic factors. Jones (1930) noted that when bursae become distended they are called bursal cysts or hygromas. Cherry & Ghormley (1941) modified and expanded on Meyerding's classification for further clarity. Jahss (1982b) also outlined a simple, workable classification of pathological bursae (Table 29.8).

Any bursa about the foot can become inflamed by the mechanisms described above. Probably the most common cause of chronic bursitis about the foot and ankle is increased pressure or friction over a bony area that leads to an adventitial bursa. Ill-fitting shoes often result in such a finding. Recently, this condition was referred to eponymically as 'last bursitis' (Layfer 1980). The bony prominences and tendons in and about the calcaneus, malleoli, metatarsophalangeal and interphalangeal joints, and dorsal and plantar surfaces of the foot are particularly susceptible to this condition. In most instances, symptomatic relief can be obtained by removing the pressure. Nonoperative means usually consist of modifications of footwear, such as a wider and deeper toe box, stretching the shoe at localized areas, softer heel counters, or various foot orthoses and pads.

Table 29.7 Types of bursae

Anatomic
Subfascial
Between tendon and bone
Between tendon or muscle and bony prominence
Between tendons
Between tendons and ligaments
Subcutaneous
Adventitial
Usually subcutaneous

Table 29.8 Classification of bursal irritation

Noninflammatory
Pressure-induced
Traumatic
Spontaneous
Inflammatory
Gout
Rheumatoid arthritis
Suppurative
Calcified or ossified

Aspiration of an inflamed bursa may sometimes be helpful in decompressing the area and ruling out metabolic, rheumatoid, or infectious causes (Nielson 1921, Patterson & Darrach 1937, Meyerding 1938, Sarma 1940). Corticosteroids can be injected locally when not contraindicated (such as in cases of sepsis) (Altman 1966, Helfand et al 1971).

Surgical measures usually relieve pressure by removing underlying exostoses or bony prominences or correcting an underlying deformity. An example of such a procedure is removal of the medial eminence and correction of the metatarsus primus varus with a metatarsal osteotomy for bursal inflammation of a hallux valgus deformity. These measures are usually performed only after failure of nonoperative methods.

Two bursal areas about the foot deserve special mention because the literature deals with them most extensively: bursa associated with the insertion of the Achilles tendon into the calcaneus and intermetatarsal bursa.

Bursitis at the posterior part of the heel

Anatomy (Hartmann 1981, Sarrafian 1983)

Two separate bursae flank the Achilles tendon at its insertion: the superficial, subcutaneous bursa of the Achilles tendon and the deep, subfascial, retrocalcaneal bursa. The former is an adventitial bursa that forms in response to chronic trauma. This bursa lies superficial to the insertion of the Achilles tendon and is frequently, although not always, present. The deep, subfascial, retrocalcaneal bursa is a synovial-lined structure that is constantly present; it is situated between the posterosuperior end of the calcaneus and the deep surface of the Achilles tendon.

Achilles tendon bursitis and retrocalcaneal bursitis

The clinical entity that manifests as irritation at the posterosuperior aspect of the heel may have various causes and has been variously referred to in the literature (Table 29.9).

It is important to distinguish anatomically between inflammatory lesions involving the subcutaneous and subfascial bursal structures at the insertion of the Achilles tendon (bursitis) and those of the peritendinous lining of the Achilles tendon (peritendinitis).

If the superficial, subcutaneous, adventitial bursa of the Achilles tendon is inflamed, tenderness will be palpable directly over the calcaneus at the tendon insertion. A noticeable bursal thickening may be present over the bony prominence lateral to the tendon attachment. This condition has been referred to as a 'pump bump' by some authors. Women are affected more often than men (Keck & Kelly 1965, Dickinson et al 1966). The formation of superficial bursitis of the Achilles tendon seems to be related to mechanical factors (that is, chronic irritation from friction between the shoe and a prominence of the posterosuperior aspect of the calcaneus). This superficial adventitial bursitis of the Achilles tendon is more common than deep, subfascial, retrocalcaneal bursitis (Keck & Kelly 1965).

If the deep, subfascial, synovial, retrocalcaneal bursa is inflamed, tenderness is less well located but is usually palpable anterior (deep) to the tendon. Men are affected more often than women (Keck & Kelly 1965). Because of the synovial origin of this bursa, inflammation may be a prodrome of rheumatoid arthritis or one of its variants, such as Reiter's syndrome (Bywaters 1954, Keck & Kelly 1965, Brahms 1967, Palmer 1970, Weston 1970, Pavlov et al 1982, Canoso et al 1984, Heneghan & Pavlov 1984). Lateral radiographs of the calcaneus must be critically assessed for the presence of erosions suggestive of an inflammatory articular disorder. No conclusive evidence implicates a prominence of the superior portion of the calcaneal tuberosity as a major factor in producing retrocalcaneal bursitis (Keck & Kelly 1965).

Numerous authors have postulated that a prominent posterosuperior surface of the calcaneus may be a factor predisposing to bursal inflammation at the insertion of the Achilles tendon (Haglund 1928, Zadek 1939, Fowler & Philip 1945, Nisbet 1954, Steffensen & Evensen 1958, Fuglsang & Torup 1961, Keck & Kelly 1965, Dickinson et al 1966, Miller & Buhr 1969, Ruch 1974, Pavlov et al 1982, Heneghan & Pavlov 1984) (Fig. 29.2). This condition is particularly exacerbated by wearing high-heeled shoes or shoes with a closely contoured, rigid heel counter. Various angles, ratios, or other radiographic relationships, such as the parallel pitch

Table 29.9 Terms used for inflammation of heel bursae in the literature

Achillodynia (Albert 1893, Haglund 1928, Bywaters 1965)
Albert's disease (Albert 1893, White 1913)
Retrocalcanean bursitis (White 1913, Nielson 1921, Keck & Kelly 1965)
Bursitis retrocalcanea Achilli (Steffensen & Evensen 1958)
Bursitis retrocalcanearis (Fuglsang & Torup 1961)
Inflammation of the deep calcaneal bursa (Hertzler 1923)
Bursitis of the posterior part of the heel (Keck & Kelly 1965)
Bursitis Achillea (Haglund 1928)
Achillobursitis (Zadek 1939)
Tendo-Achillis bursitis (Nisbet, 1954, Keck & Kelly 1965, Dickinson et al 1966)
Winter heel (Nisbet 1954)
Pump bumps (Dickinson et al 1966, Miller & Buhr 1969, Ruch 1974, Pavlov et al 1982)
Prow-beak deformity (Ruch 1974)
High prow heels (Miller & Buhr 1969)
Heel tuberosities (Brahms 1967)
Haglund's disease, syndrome (Haglund 1928, Ruch 1974, Berlin et al 1982, Pavlov et al 1982, Heneghan & Pavlov 1984)
Sever's disease (apophysitis of the os calcis) (Sever 1912, Ferguson & Gingrich 1957)
Knobbly heels (Miller & Buhr 1969)
Calcaneus altus (Miller & Buhr 1969)
Cucumber heels (Miller & Buhr 1969)

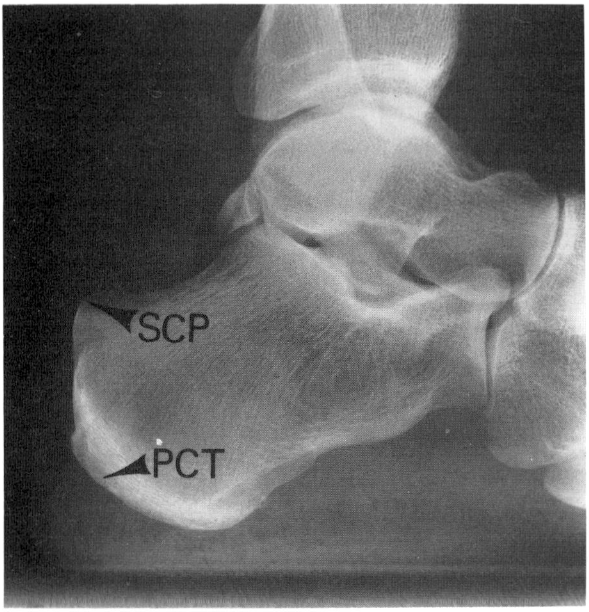

Fig. 29.2 Radiograph of posterior calcaneus shows superior calcaneal prominence (*SCP*) and posterior calcaneal tuberosity (*PCT*)

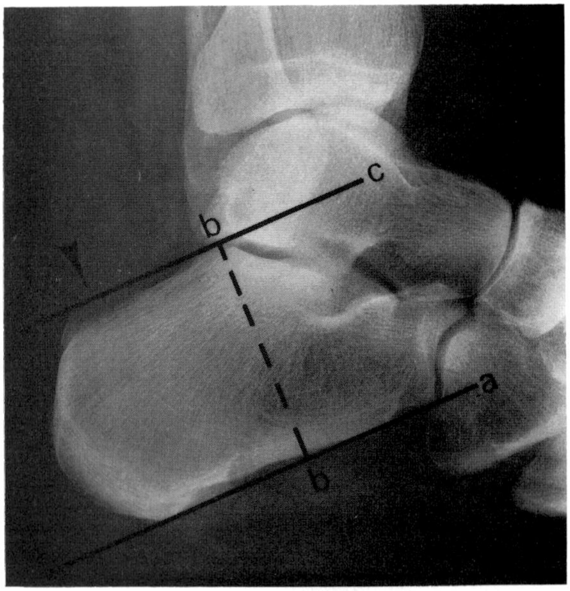

Fig. 29.3 Parallel pitch line of Pavlov (c–b) is derived from inferior calcaneal pitch line (a–b). When superior calcaneal prominence (*arrowhead*) is superior to line c–b, a predisposition to retrocalcaneal bursitis is thought to exist

line of Pavlov (Fig. 29.3), have been presented and are said to correlate with bursal abnormalities (Fowler & Philip 1945, Ferguson & Gingrich 1957, Steffensen & Evensen 1958, Pavlov et al 1982, Heneghan & Pavlov 1984).

Pavlov et al (1982) and Heneghan & Pavlov (1984) radiographically characterized Haglund's syndrome by the presence of four features: retrocalcaneal bursitis, Achilles peritendinitis, superficial bursitis of Achilles tendon (pump bump), and cortically intact but prominent bursal projection of the posterosuperior aspect of the calcaneus, as seen on lateral radiographs. Although all four of these conditions may coexist, this situation is not uniformly the case.

Treatment

When superficial bursitis of the Achilles tendon is associated with a prominence of the superior part of the tuberosity of the calcaneus and is unresponsive to conservative (nonoperative) measures, excision of the prominence may be necessary (Haglund 1928, Zadek 1939, Fowler & Philip 1945, Nisbet 1954, Steffensen & Evensen 1958, Fuglsang & Torup 1961, Keck & Kelly 1965, Dickinson et al 1966, Miller & Buhr 1969, Ruch 1974, Berlin et al 1982, Jones & James 1984). Keck & Kelly (1965) were cautious about recommending surgical resection of a calcaneal prominence in cases of retrocalcaneal bursitis because they thought that the bursitis may be a forerunner of rheumatoid arthritis. Injection of corticosteroids into the deep bursa, heel elevation, rest, and nonsteroidal anti-inflammatory drugs often provide relief. Occasionally, surgical extirpation of the bursa is necessary (Ippolito & Ricciardi-Pollini 1984).

When operation is indicated, two basic types have been described. Haglund (1928) recommended resection of the most prominent portion of the posterosuperior aspect of the calcaneus. This procedure can be combined with removal of the superficial or deep bursa. Zadek (1939) described a dorsally-based wedge resection of the calcaneus in order to leave the posterior surface of the calcaneus intact. The surgical method for the posterior calcaneus may be either a medial or a lateral para-Achilles tendon approach or a direct posterior approach through the Achilles tendon, as described by Fowler & Philip (1945). The foot is usually splinted for 2 to 4 weeks in a walking cast until healing is complete (Fig. 29.4).

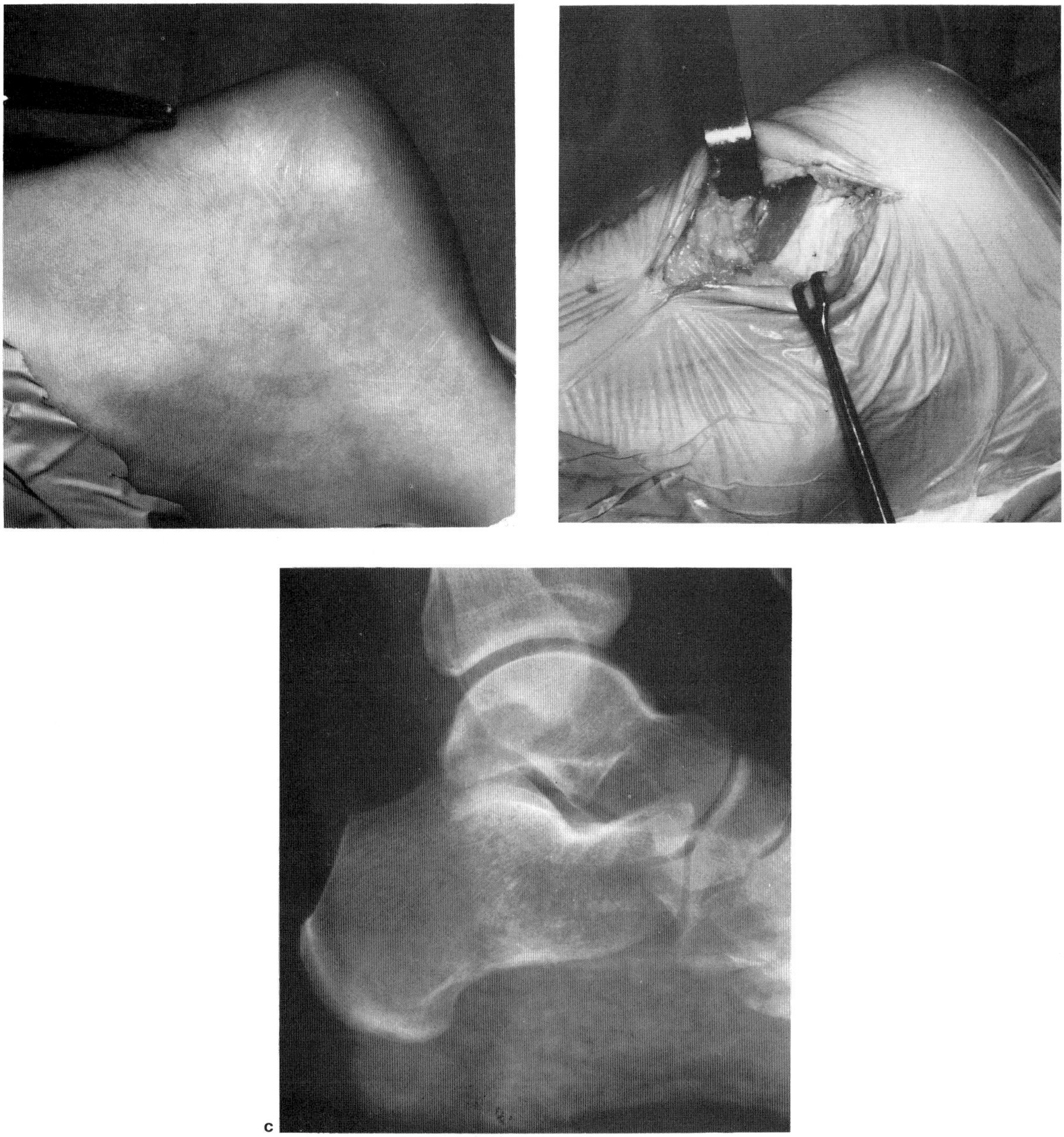

Fig. 29.4 A: Inflammation secondary to pressure over posterosuperior prominence of calcaneus. B: Lateral view shows area of resection of posterosuperior aspect of calcaneus. C: Radiograph shows area of resection of superior calcaneal prominence

Bursitis associated with intermetatarsophalangeal bursae (Bossley & Cairney 1980, Hartmann 1981, Sarrafian 1983)

Anatomy texts do not devote much attention to the bursae associated with the web spaces of the foot. The intermetatarsophalangeal bursa lies between the metatarsophalangeal joints and is dorsal to the transverse metatarsal ligament, whereas the neurovascular bundle lies plantar to the ligament and courses dorsally as it passes distally to the end of the ligament. Bursae in web spaces one, two, and three are constant, whereas the bursa in the fourth web space is missing in 80% of cases, according to Hartmann (1981). Bossley & Cairney (1980), in a cadaveric and clinical study, found that the intermetatarsal bursa in the second and third web spaces extended 1 cm distally to the transverse metatarsal ligament, whereas it lay at the same level as the distal margin of the transverse ligament in the fourth web space.

Intermetatarsal bursitis

Inflammation of the intermetatarsophalangeal bursa from any cause can be a source of pain in the forefoot in the region of the metatarsal heads. Classic Morton's metatarsalgia is often described as a clinical syndrome of pain under the metatarsal heads that often radiates to the toes and is sometimes associated with numbness (Scranton 1980). Symptoms are often exacerbated by walking in close-fitting shoes and are lessened when walking barefoot.

As pointed out by Bossley & Cairney (1980), because of the close proximity of the plantar digital nerve and the intermetatarsal bursa in the second and third web spaces, the classic symptoms of Morton's metatarsalgia could be caused not only by a neuroma but also by an intermetatarsophalangeal bursitis with pressure on a normal nerve.

Bursal swelling can often be detected clinically and radiographically by divergence of the toes bordering the affected web space (Shephard 1975). Lateral compression of the metatarsal heads squeezes the inflamed bursa, reproduces pain, and may cause a click. Because the intermetatarsophalangeal bursa is of synovial origin, its inflammation may be one of the first manifestations of rheumatoid arthritis in the foot (Palmer 1970, Shephard 1975). Radiographs should be closely inspected for any evidence of erosions of the metatarsophalangeal heads. The intermetatarsophalangeal bursae in patients with rheumatoid arthritis is often thick-walled with lymphocytic infiltration, villous proliferation, fibrinoid necrosis, and the presence of 'rice bodies' (Jones 1930, Shephard 1975, Bossley & Cairney 1980).

Injection of hydrocortisone into the bursa often gives relief. Occasionally, surgical extirpation of the bursa is necessary.

ACHILLES TENDON

The Achilles tendon (Fig. 29.5) will serve as the prototype for discussing peritendinitis and rupture. These two pathological processes can affect any tendon about the ankle. The peroneal tendons will serve as the prototype for discussing subluxation and dislocation, processes that seem to affect these tendons most often.

Peritendinitis and rupture

Pain in the Achilles tendon is a common problem, especially in runners (Snook 1972, Clancy et al 1976, Gould & Korson 1980, Kvist & Kvist 1980, Leach et al 1981, Ljungqvist & Eriksson 1982). Disease of the Achilles tendon is likely to be a spectrum of manifestations on a continuum from peritendinitis to tendinosis to rupture (Clancy et al 1976, Puddu et al 1976, Gould & Korson 1980, Leach et al 1981, Clancy 1982). It is important to distinguish among bursitis at the posterior part of the heel, Achilles peritendinitis, and Achilles peritendinitis with tendinosis and partial rupture. The distinction between Achilles peritendinitis and Achilles peritendinitis with tendinosis and partial rupture is not always easy, but it is important if one is to prevent partial rupture from becoming complete (Ljungqvist 1968, Snook 1972, Puddu et al 1976, Clancy et al 1976, Gillström & Ljungqvist 1978, Denstad & Roaas 1979, Gould & Korson 1980, Kvist & Kvist 1980, Leach et al 1981, Skeoch 1981, Clancy 1982, Ljungqvist & Eriksson 1982).

The diagnosis of acute, complete rupture should not be difficult because the history is very characteristic. However, most published series estimate that the diagnosis of complete rupture is missed in 20% to 25% of cases (Lawrence et al 1955, Arner & Lindholm 1959, Ralston & Schmidt 1971, Nillius et al 1976). The diagnosis is missed because complete rupture, although not rare, is unfamiliar to many physicians. A patient may tend to minimize the symptoms after the acute pain of the initial 'snap' has subsided. Some active plantar flexion is maintained because of the combined action of the peroneus longus, tibialis posterior, and long toe flexors, and the loss of true gastrocnemius-soleus action on plantar flexion may be missed. If a patient presents late, swelling and haemorrhage into the site

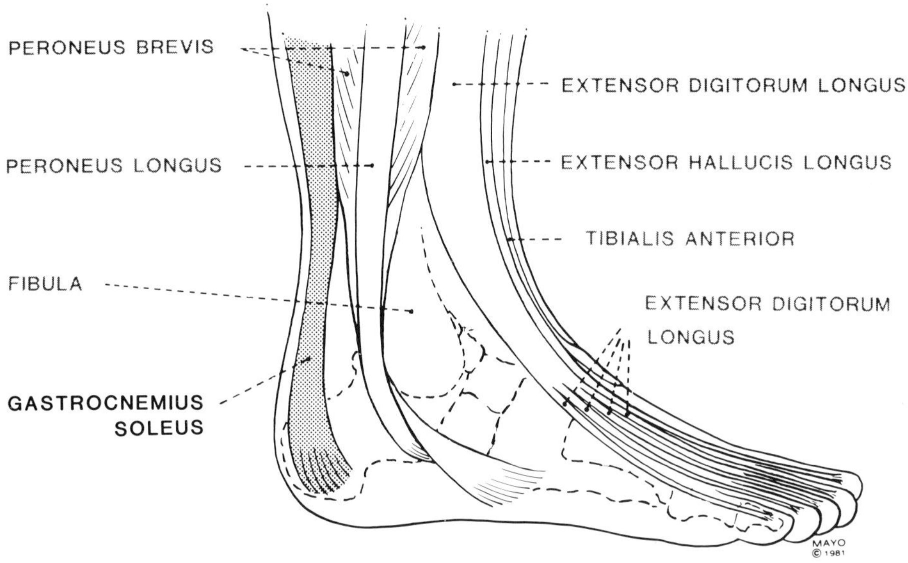

Fig. 29.5 Lateral view of Achilles tendon from gastrocnemius-soleus muscle complex. (By permission of Mayo Foundation)

of disruption may obscure the discontinuity in the tendon (Lawrence et al 1955, Hooker 1963, Ralston & Schmidt 1971). The rupture usually occurs 2 to 6 cm proximal to the insertion of the Achilles tendon, where vascularity has been shown to be decreased (Håstad et al 1958–1959, Lagergren & Lindholm 1958–1959) (Fig. 29.6). As the rupture becomes chronic, the defect in the tendon becomes more difficult to palpate, but irregularity of the tendon can often be noted. Weakness in plantar flexion is the one constant finding due to lengthening of the tendon. Table 29.10 summarizes some of the differentiating findings of peritendinitis, partial rupture, and complete rupture.

The Thompson calf 'squeeze test' is very useful for the diagnosis of complete rupture (Thompson 1962, Thompson & Doherty 1962). If the calf muscles are squeezed just distal to their maximal girth, the foot invariably flexes plantarly unless the soleus is detached from the Achilles tendon. A positive reaction, then, is no plantar movement of the foot, which indicates the complete rupture of the heel cord. Recently, a 'needle test' for complete rupture of the Achilles tendon was also described, and it seems to be more sensitive than the squeeze test (O'Brien 1984).

Some authors have suggested that a lateral radiograph or xerogram of the soft tissue may reveal subtle findings. Arner et al reviewed the previous reports on the radiographic diagnosis of Achilles tendon rupture, including those of Kager and Toygar, and they also analysed the reliability of those techniques (Arner et al 1958–1959a). In 1939, Kager described what has been called Kager's

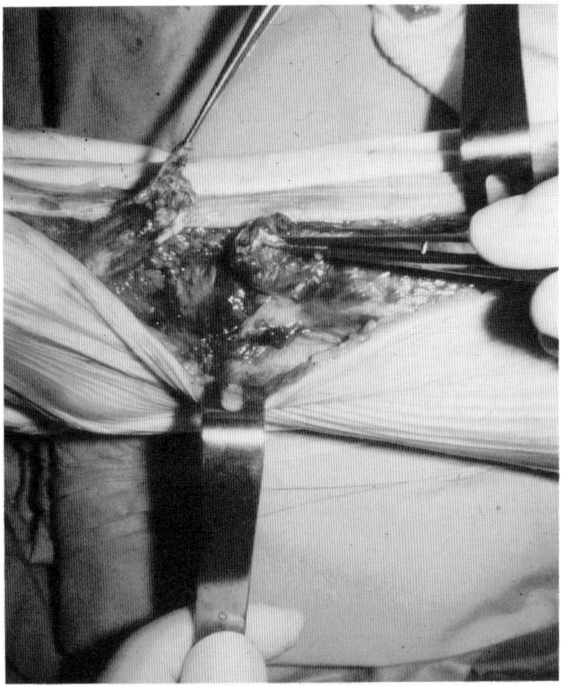

Fig. 29.6 Typical acute, complete tear of Achilles tendon

Table 29.10 Differentiating factors of peritendinitis, peritendinitis with tendinosis and partial rupture, and tendinosis with acute, complete rupture

Factor	Peritendinitis	Peritendinitis with tendinosis and partial rupture	Tendinosis with acute, complete rupture
Symptoms	Acute	Subacute, chronic	Immediate
Audible snap	No	Maybe	Yes
Weakness	Yes	Yes	Yes
Limp	Yes	Yes	Yes
Swelling	Yes	Yes	Yes
Tenderness	Yes	Yes	Yes
Defect in tendon	No	Maybe	Yes
Crepitus	Maybe	Maybe	No
Passive dorsiflexion	Decreased	Decreased	Increased
Thompson test	Negative	Negative	Positive
Atrophy	No	Yes	Proximal calf belly retraction
Ability to stand on tiptoe	Probably	Possibly	No

triangle. This space is filled with fatty tissue bounded by the margins of the Achilles tendon, the calcaneus, and the deep flexors. When the Achilles tendon is ruptured, the triangle loses its regular configuration. In 1947, Toygar suggested the value of measuring the angle of the posterior skin surface as visualized on the roentgenogram because the ends of the tendon are displaced anteriorly after rupture; the angle becomes 130°–150°. This angle and the decrease of Kager's triangle were considered virtually diagnostic by Toygar.

In their series of 39 patients, however, Arner et al found that deformation of Kager's triangle was very nonspecific and that Toygar's sign rarely was positive. Ultrasonography, bursography, electromyography, and computed tomography may be helpful for the diagnosis of partial ruptures (Ljungqvist & Eriksson 1982). However, other authors have not found these tests as useful and consider roentgenographic studies as only of secondary importance to physical examination for the diagnosis of Achilles tendon rupture (Hattrup & Johnson 1985).

Treatment

Peritendinitis. The initial treatment of inflammatory lesions should be nonoperative (Table 29.11).

Operation is generally indicated only in a patient who is unresponsive to nonoperative treatment for several weeks to months (Snook 1972, Clancy et al 1976, Denstad & Roaas 1979, Kvist & Kvist 1980, Lea 1981, Leach et al 1981, Skeoch 1981, Clancy 1982). Surgical treatment usually consists of exploration and excision of the diseased peritendinous structures and resection of any diseased or degenerated tissue. The latter method may require some form of surgical reconstruction of the tendon.

Rupture. More than 400 articles have been published about rupture of the Achilles tendon (Barfred 1973). A great area of controversy is the

Table 29.11 Types of nonoperative treatment of peritendinitis

- Patient education
  - Proper warm-up, cool down
  - Reduction or cessation of athletic activity
    - No running on hills
    - No interval training
    - Avoid training on hard surfaces
- Proper equipment
  - Good running shoes (flexible, cushioned soles)
  - Orthoses (heel lifts, University of California — Biomechanics Laboratory [UCBL] inserts, inlays)
- Physical therapy
  - Massage
  - Stretching exercises
  - Ultrasound, heat, ice
- Immobilization
  - Taping
  - Crutches
  - Casting
- Medication
  - Nonsteroidal anti-inflammatory drugs
  - Corticosteroid injections? (Kleinman & Gross 1983)

proper treatment of this condition (*Lancet* Editorial, 1973). Some investigators favour surgical repair and postoperative casting (Jessing & Hansen 1975, Inglis et al 1976, Percy & Conochie 1978, Jacobs et al 1978, Schedl & Fasol 1979, Scott et al 1979, Edna 1980, Rubin & Wilson 1980, Leach 1982), and others favour casting alone (Lea & Smith 1968, 1972, Gillies & Chalmers 1970, Nistor 1976, 1981, Stein & Luekens 1976a, 1976b, Lea 1981). For years, casting in an equinus position to minimize tension at the site of injury was the accepted treatment; now, this approach has come into question. Häggmark & Eriksson (1979) described selective atrophy of the soleus muscle if tension is not kept on the musculotendinous unit during healing.

Proponents of closed treatment state that the underlying reason for the success of this method is the ability of the Achilles tendon to reconstitute itself when severed. This trait has been shown both experimentally and clinically (Lipscomb & Wakim 1961a, 1961b, Saunders et al 1978, Lennox et al 1980, Taylor 1981). They also claim that the functional differences in strength, power, and endurance are not statistically significant between patients treated operatively and those treated nonoperatively (Lea & Smith 1972, Lea 1981, Nistor 1981). The nonoperative approach avoids the risks of anaesthesia and the complications of open operation. Nistor (1981) reviewed 25 reports, with a total of 2,647 ruptures, in which surgical complications were recorded. The following major complications were noted: fistulas, 3%; necrosis of skin and tendon, 2%; rerupture, 2%; and deep infection, 1%. Minor complications — haematoma, superficial infection, granulomas, and skin adhesions — occurred in 5% of the cases. Although rare, death from pulmonary embolus has been reported after surgical repair (Arner & Lindholm 1959). The major drawback of the closed technique is a reportedly higher incidence of rerupture and questionably inferior dynametric data (Inglis et al 1976, Jacobs et al 1978, Shields et al 1978, Scott et al 1979, Edna 1980, Brown et al 1981, Nistor 1981, Taylor 1981).

The nonoperative technique is uncomplicated (Lea & Smith 1968, 1972, Lea 1981). It consists of gravity equinus casting for 8 to 12 weeks with cast changes at monthly intervals to gradually increase the amount of dorsiflexion. Casting is followed by heel elevations and possibly a double upright ankle-foot orthosis with a stop at the neutral position for an additional 4 to 8 weeks (Taylor 1981).

Advocates of open surgical treatment have a sound biomechanical rationale for this approach. An immediate repair that allows closure of the gap will keep the musculotendinous unit at its proper physiological length:tension ratio (Ma & Griffith 1977, 1981). Theoretically, this treatment should provide optimal strength, power, and endurance. The site of repair may also have greater mechanical strength than the scar tissue that forms if the gap is not closed. This added strength should ultimately lead to a decreased rate of rupture. The advantages of operation in patients with a delay in diagnosis are less clear (Lennox et al 1980). Often, the gap cannot be closed without lengthening the tendon (Abraham & Pankovich 1975, Fish 1982). Therefore, in such cases, the biomechanical advantage of immediate repair is lost. Rather than performing a repair procedure in such cases, one is sometimes faced with a rather difficult reconstruction to close the gap (Bosworth 1956, Arner & Lindholm 1959, Lindholm 1959, Bugg & Boyd 1968, Goldman et al 1969, Teuffer 1974, Quigley & Scheller 1980, Taylor 1981). The literature abounds with methods of repair (Lynn 1966, Ma & Griffith 1977, 1981, Schedl & Fasol 1979, Cetti & Christensen 1983) and reconstruction (Bosworth 1956, Arner & Lindholm 1959, Lindholm 1959, Bugg & Boyd 1968, Goldman et al 1969, Teuffer 1974, Abraham & Pankovich 1975, Quigley & Scheller 1980, Taylor 1981, Fish 1982). For acute, complete injuries, direct suturing with buried stitches is preferred if surgical treatment is selected. For the reconstruction, a lengthening of the tendon at the musculotendinous junction in a V-Y manner, resection of the diseased tendon, and direct suturing seem most reasonable. After operation, the immobilization is similar to that used for the nonoperative approach.

To date, the best study assessing the results of surgical and nonsurgical treatment of rupture of the Achilles tendon is that by Nistor (1981). This study was prospective and randomized and therefore avoided a bias in selecting which patients would receive a particular type of treatment. Nistor concluded that nonoperative treatment offers advantages over operative treatment (Table 29.12).

The ultimate decision as to which form of treatment is used must be individualized and

Table 29.12 Considerations in the choice of treatment of acute rupture of the Achilles tendon

Consideration	Type of treatment	
	Nonoperative (casting alone)	Operative (operation and casting)
Morbidity	Decreased	Increased
Surgical risk	None	Increased
Hospital stay (cost)	Decreased	Increased
Dynametric data	Inferior	Superior
Rerupture	10%	2%
Compliance with rehabilitation	Less	More

depends on the physician, the patient, and the circumstances. Probably, the persons who benefit most from operative treatment are high performance athletes.

TIBIALIS POSTERIOR TENDON

Anatomy

The tibialis posterior (Fig. 29.7) arises from all except the lowest part of the posterior surface of the interosseous membrane, from the upper lateral part of the posterior surface of the tibia, and from the upper two-thirds of the medial surface of the fibula. The tendon passes in front of the flexor digitorum longus muscle in the lower one-fourth of the leg and then behind the medial malleolus under the flexor retinaculum, and it is the most anteromedial structure behind the malleolus. It passes through the groove of the medial malleolus across the deltoid ligament and under the plantar calcaneonavicular ligament, and inserts into the tuberosity of the navicular bone and the underside of the cuneiform bone and to the bases of the second, third, and fourth metatarsals. One expansion passes backwards to the sustentaculum tali. The sheath of this tendon is 7 to 9 cm long and extends about 6 cm above the malleolus.

By virtue of its lever arm length from the axis of the talocalcaneal joint and its muscle strength, this muscle-tendon unit is the main dynamic stabilizer of the hindfoot against valgus (eversion) deformity (Fig. 29.8). A tear of the tibialis posterior tendon therefore imposes excessive stress on the static ligament-bone hindfoot constraints. With loss of the muscle power, the soft tissue gradually elongates and pain develops.

Rupture

Clinical features

In 1936, Kulowski first mentioned tenosynovitis of the sheath of the tibialis posterior tendon. This condition was also noted by Lipscomb (1950), who stated that it occurred in about 16% of cases of

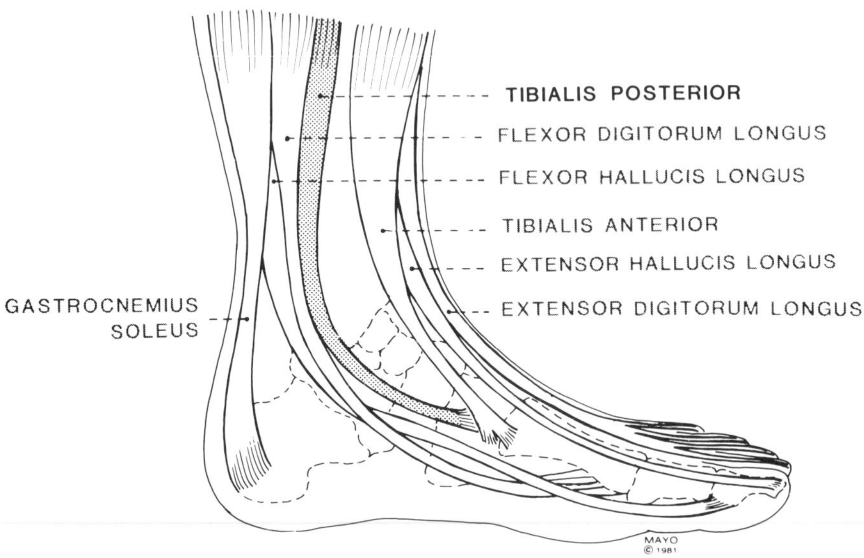

Fig. 29.7 Relationship of tibialis posterior tendon to other tendons on medial aspect of ankle. (By permission of Mayo Foundation)

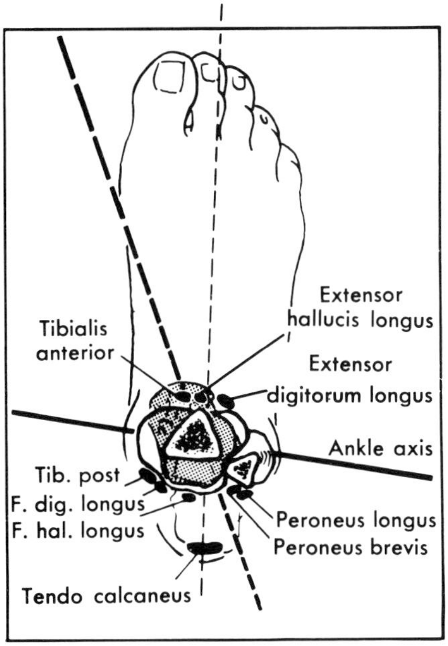

Fig. 29.8 Relationship of extrinsic tendon of foot to ankle axis (solid line) and subtalar axis (dashed line). dig. = digitorum; F. = flexor; hal. = hallucis. (From Mann 1985 By permission of the publisher)

tenosynovitis and peritendinitis of the feet and ankles. Other sporadic reports have appeared in the literature (Ghormley & Spear 1953, Fowler 1955, Williams 1963, Cozen 1965, Langenskiöld 1967, Norris & Mankin 1978, Lipsman et al 1980, Trevino et al 1981, Fredenburg et al 1983).

Rupture of the tibialis posterior tendon is a cause of the painful acquired flatfoot deformity in adults (Goldner et al 1974, Henceroth & Deyerle 1982, Gould 1983, Mann 1983, Mueller 1984, Mann & Thompson 1985). Although rupture of the tibialis posterior tendon has been described previously, the frequency of this problem has become more evident in recent years (Kulowski 1936, Key 1953, Williams 1963, Langenskiöld 1967, Kettelkamp & Alexander 1969, Goldner et al 1974, Trevino et al 1981, Jahss 1982a, Mann & Specht 1982, Johnson 1983, Mann & Thompson 1985). This deformity is commonly described as being traumatic (Giblin 1980, De Zwart & Davidson 1983), degenerative, or spontaneous in origin (Henceroth & Deyerle 1982). Possibly a combination (Kettelkamp & Alexander 1969) of all three factors results in the disruption. The peritendinitis that has been described (Kulowski 1936, Lipscomb 1950, Key 1953, Langenskiöld 1967, Trevino et al 1981) may be a secondary reaction to a tendon tear. Another possibility is that deformity causes tenosynovitis (Cozen 1965).

The history, symptoms, and signs of rupture of the tibialis posterior tendon are so typical that, once understood, they allow the correct diagnosis to be made readily.

Prior acute trauma of a substantial degree usually *cannot* be recalled by a patient. Instead, with minimal or no trauma, the deformity of the foot gradually begins to evolve and becomes painful. A predilection for females is evident, and patients are most often older than 40 years.

Pain and tenderness are present but are only mild to moderate in degree. Early, tenderness along the course of the tendon from just distal to the medial malleolus to its infranavicular insertion may predominate. The pain is not incapacitating; rather, it is a chronic medial weight-bearing ache that limits activities. Later, as the deformity progresses to the foot, the discomfort also commonly involves the lateral tarsal region.

Swelling just medial to the hindfoot will be present early; it is most evident when viewed posteriorly and compared with the noninvolved foot (Fig. 29.9).

Deformity, however, is the hallmark of the rupture of the tibialis posterior tendon and gradually increases over a few months to years. The concurrent development of hindfoot valgus and forefoot abduction produces the so-called flatfoot. The hindfoot valgus, which can be mild to marked, is best evaluated from the posterior view. Although best appreciated from a frontal view, the presence of forefoot abduction can be suspected and clinically quantitated from the posterior view by being aware of the too-many-toes sign (Fig. 29.10) (that is, when a patient faces directly away from the observer, too many toes will be visible lateral to the patient's heel area when forefoot abduction is present). Quantitation is based on the number of toes that are seen.

Loss of function of the tibialis posterior tendon is best evaluated by using the single heel-rise test. The tendon must be used to bring the hindfoot into a locked, stable varus position. This position is necessary before the patient can easily rise up on the ball of the foot with the power of the gastrocnemius-soleus muscle. The single heel-rise test on the affected side is positive when, with an attempt to go

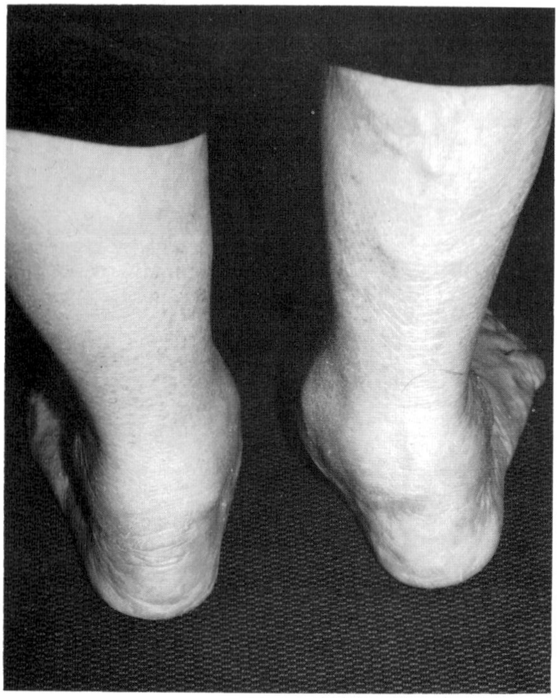

Fig. 29.9 Swelling of sheath of tibialis posterior tendon is evident on right foot just inferior to medial malleolus. (From Johnson K A 1983. By permission of J B Lippincott)

up on the ball of the affected foot with the contralateral foot raised, the hindfoot does not assume a stable varus position and only with difficulty can the heel be even slightly raised off the ground (Fig. 29.11).

Radiographic findings

Routine lateral and anteroposterior radiographic views of the foot will show pronounced changes in cases of rupture of the tibialis posterior tendon. As the head and neck of the talus rotate medially and inferiorly off the calcaneus, the forefoot distal to the talus deviates laterally. Thus, the talocalcaneal angle is increased, and a break at the talonavicular articulation is seen on a lateral view (Fig. 29.12). From an anteroposterior view, an increase of the talocalcaneal angle is evident, and subluxation at the talonavicular articulation is present (Fig. 29.13).

Treatment

As with many musculoskeletal conditions, rupture of the tibialis posterior tendon can be treated nonoperatively or operatively.

Nonoperative. Rest provided by crutches or a cast, anti-inflammatory agents, or shoe modifications such as inserts or heel and sole lifts may all be used to palliate tears of the tibialis posterior tendon. Probably the only nonoperative method that would not be indicated is an injection of corticosteroids into the tendon itself. In fact, however, these 'noninvasive' means provide only 'nonrelief'.

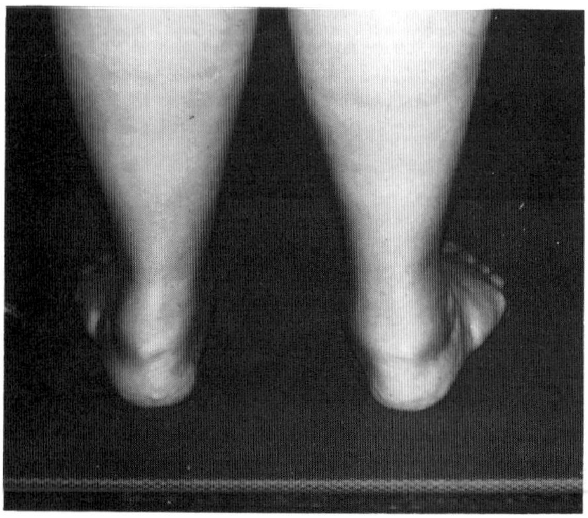

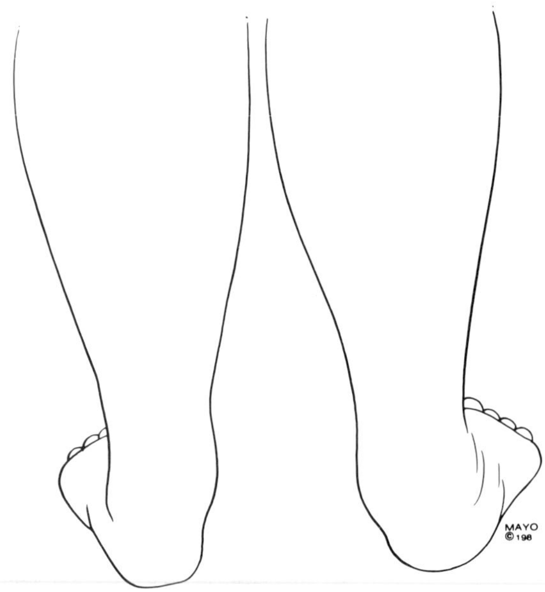

Fig. 29.10 A: Asymmetry is demonstrated by too-many-toes sign (four) lateral to heel on right compared with left (two). (From Johnson 1983. By permission of J B Lippincott). B: Line diagram shows too-many-toes sign

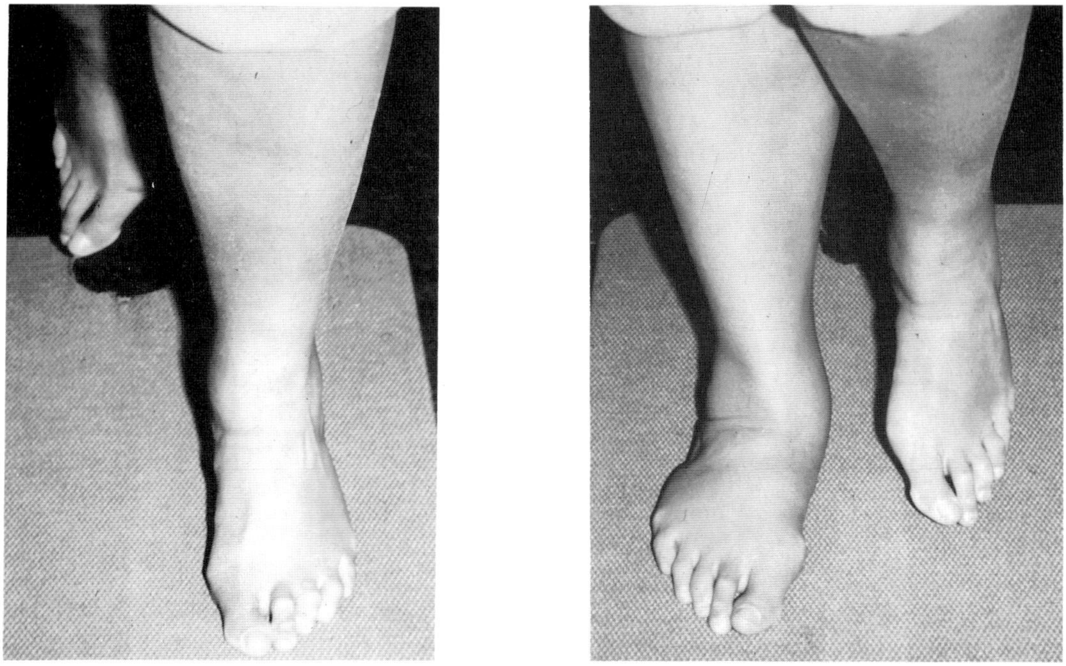

Fig. 29.11 Single heel-rise test. A: Patient is easily able to rise up on normal forefoot. B: Patient is unable to rise up on forefoot with rupture of tibialis posterior tendon. (From Johnson 1983. By permission of J B Lippincott)

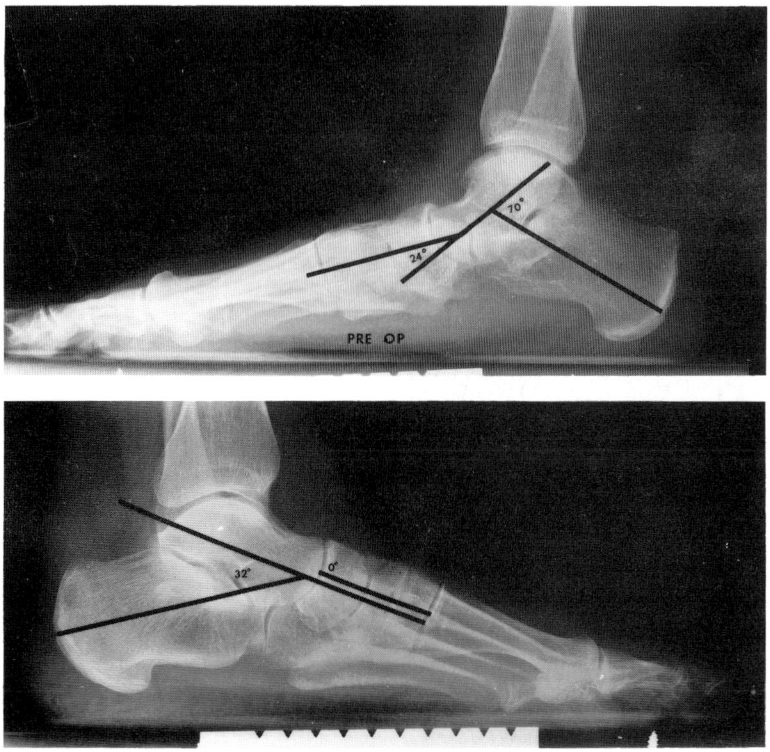

Fig. 29.12 A: Increased talocalcaneal angle (70°) and talonavicular angle (24°) with rupture of tibialis posterior tendon. B: Normal talocalcaneal and talonavicular relationships. (From Johnson 1983. By permission of J B Lippincott)

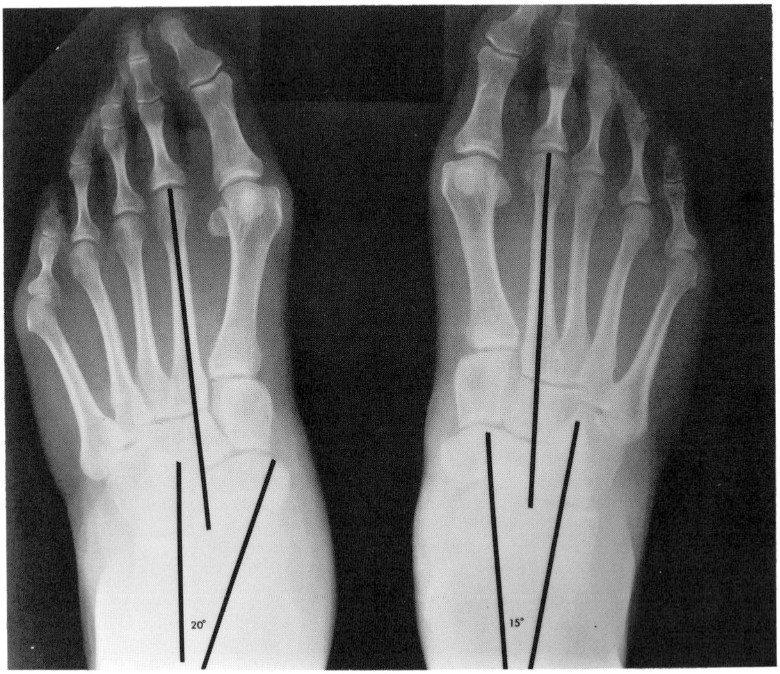

Fig. 29.13 With rupture of left tibialis posterior tendon, note that hindfoot talocalcaneal angle is increased and line of second metatarsal of forefoot is deviated laterally. (From Johnson 1983. By permission of J B Lippincott)

Factors such as advanced age, other medical problems, a low level of activity, and only minimal discomfort may frequently make a nonoperative approach the most prudent.

Operative. If chronic synovitis is present and the tendon is not disrupted, then only a tenosynovectomy and sheath division may be necessary (Goldner & Irwin 1949, Cozen 1965, Langenskiöld 1967, Wrenn 1975). In the more frequent situation in which restoration of the function of the tendon or foot alignment (or both) is thought to be indicated, the operative procedure depends on the site and the extent of the tear, the duration and the severity of the deformity, and some nebulous factors such as the expectations of the patient and physician. Four discrete surgical procedures are currently used.

An end-to-end suture (Fig. 29.14) can be used when the tear involves a relatively short portion of the tendon, usually just distal to the medial malleolus (Goldner et al 1974). This procedure allows restoration of the proper tendon length and function. When a tendon such as the tibialis posterior has a short excursion, even 1 or 2 cm of elongation will cause a functional deficit.

If the tear involves the tendon insertion to the underside of the navicular bone, then a reattachment (Goldner et al 1974) (Fig. 29.15) through a drill hole would be most appropriate. During surgical exposure of the tendon, the surgeon may find an apparently intact tendon. If, however, the exposure is carried distally to the navicular attachment, the separation from the bone can almost invariably be seen. It is this tear that is best treated with reattachment.

Most commonly, however, the tear will involve a long segment of degenerated tendon that cannot be brought together. In such cases, the gap can be bridged by tendon transfer (Fig. 29.16) (Key 1953, Fowler 1955, Kettelkamp & Alexander 1969). Because of its size, strength, and availability, the flexor digitorum longus is used. The segment of affected tendon is bridged, and function is restored. The flexor digitorum longus can be either attached distally by a tenodesis to healthy tibialis posterior tendon or inserted directly into bone at the undersurface of the navicular bone through a drill hole. The last step of tenodesis of the distal stump of the flexor digitorum longus to the adjacent flexor

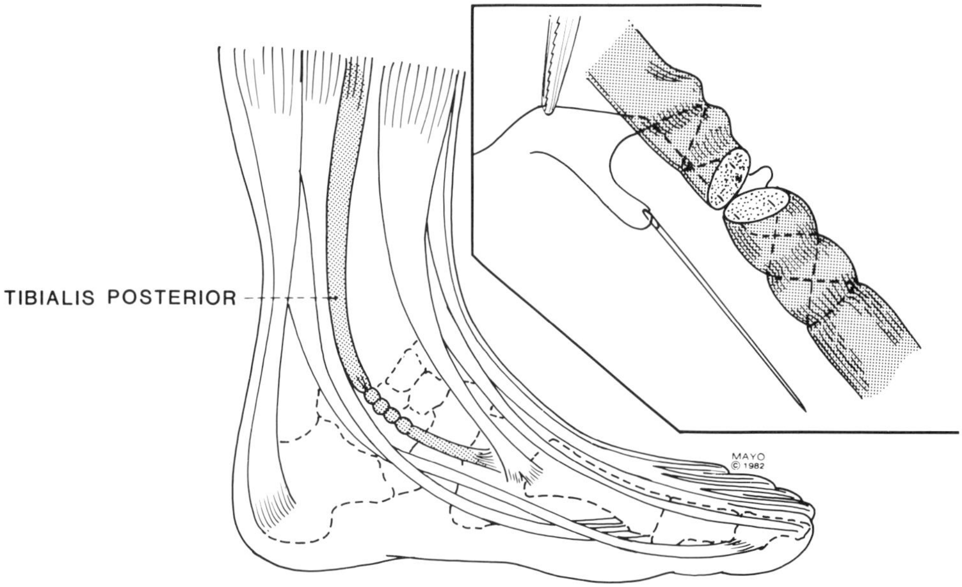

Fig. 29.14 End-to-end suture for interstitial tear of tibialis posterior tendon. (By permission of Mayo Foundation)

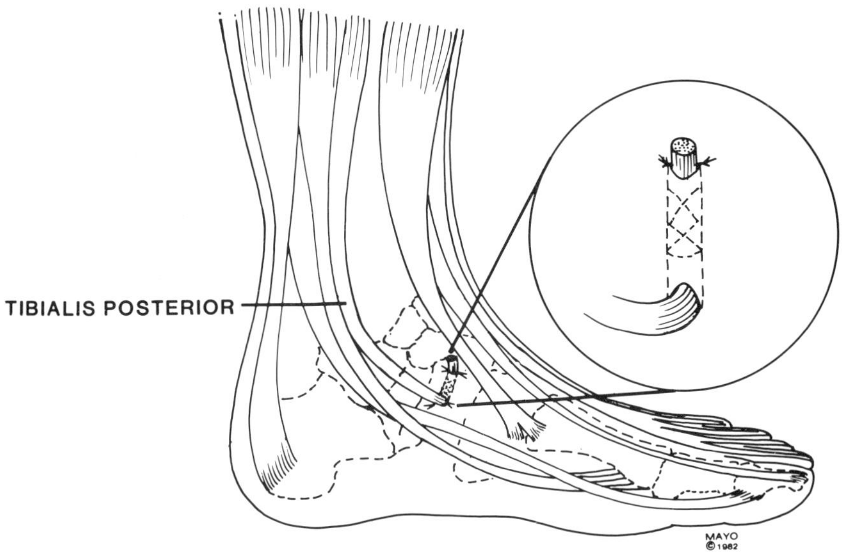

Fig. 29.15 Reattachment of tear of tibialis posterior tendon from its insertion at undersurface of navicular bone. (By permission of Mayo Foundation)

hallucis longus is optional because lesser toe flexion will be provided to a degree by the intact flexor digitorum brevis and perhaps by the quadratus plantae as well as other intrinsic muscles of the foot.

When the foot deformity is severe, supporting tissues are stretched, and secondary degenerative arthritic changes are evident, an arthrodesis (Fig. 29.17) is the only reasonable surgical procedure. The 'triple' arthrodesis, which involves the talonavicular, calcaneocuboid, and talocalcaneal joints, has been the traditional operative treatment of hindfoot deformity. In neglected rupture of the tibialis posterior tendon, however, the main deformity is rotation of the head and neck of the talus off the

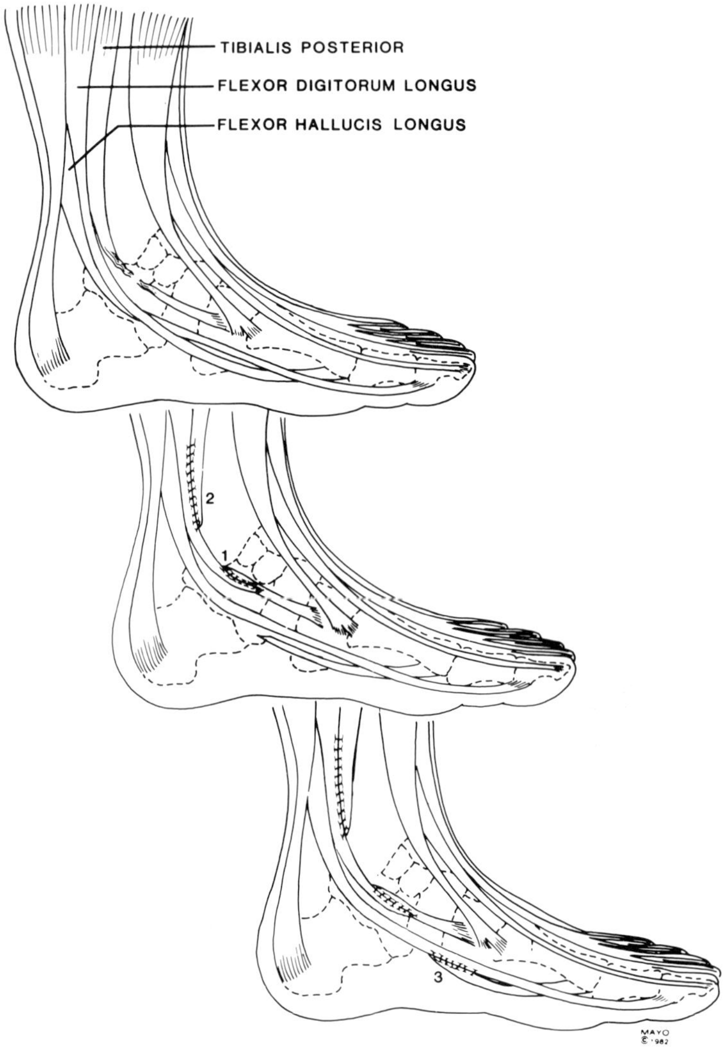

Fig. 29.16 Interposition of flexor digitorum longus tendon for extensive tear of tibialis posterior tendon. (By permission of Mayo Foundation)

calcaneus medially and inferiorly. Because of this, the anatomic alignment can be restored with only a talocalcaneal arthrodesis, and the talonavicular and calcaneocuboid joints are spared.

If surgical treatment is elected, the specific procedure used will depend on the anatomic presentation of the tendon deficit.

PERONEAL TENDONS

Reports in the literature of peroneal involvement with peritendinitis, rupture, and dislocation are sparse. Peritendinitis and traumatic dislocation are thought to be more common than recognized, and spontaneous rupture is rare. All of these entities may be a cause for persistent lateral ankle pain and swelling, which are most commonly thought to be residuals of disruption of the lateral ligaments and ankle instability.

Anatomy

The tendons of the peroneus longus and brevis (Fig. 29.18) enter a common synovial sheath 4 cm proximal to the lateral malleolus. They pass under

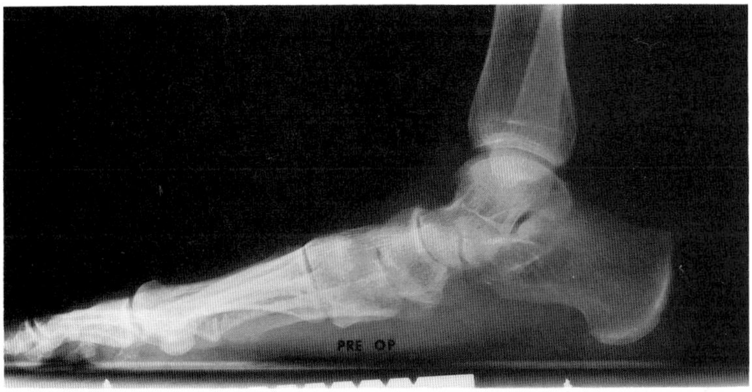

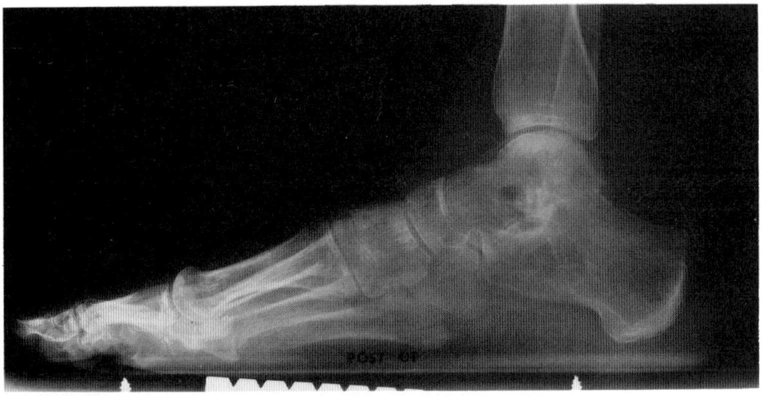

Fig. 29.17 A: Deformity of foot as a result of old tear of tibialis posterior tendon. B: Subtalar arthrodesis was used to realign hindfoot. (From Johnson 1983. By permission of J B Lippincott)

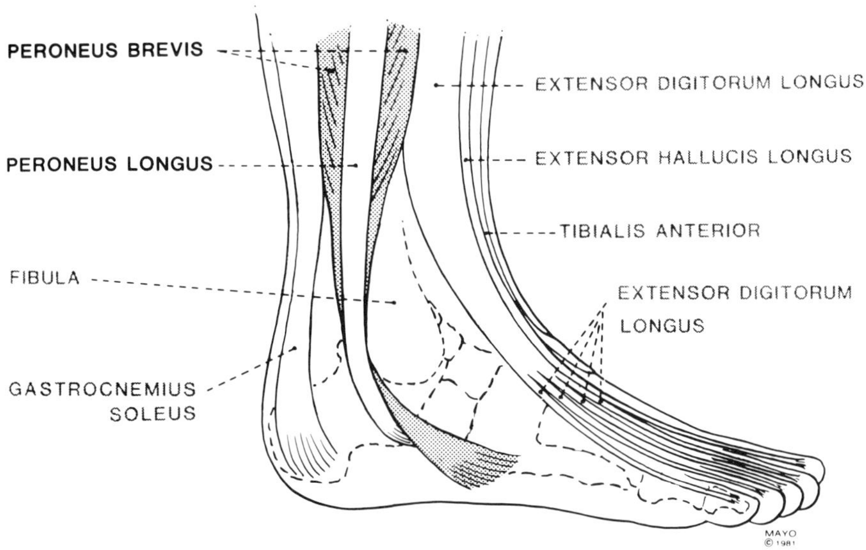

Fig. 29.18 Peroneal tendons on lateral aspect of foot. (By permission of Mayo Foundation)

the superior retinaculum and behind the lateral malleolus within this common sheath. A fibro-osseous tunnel restrains these tendons posterior to the lateral malleolus. The most important restraining anatomic structure proximally is the superior retinaculum. Also present distally along the posterior lip of the lateral malleolus is a fibrocartilaginous ridge (Marti 1977). The retro-malleolar sulcus was described in detail by Edwards (1928); in 82% of cases it is very shallow, and 18% of cases have no well formed sulcus.

Proximal to the peroneal trochlea of the calcaneus, the tendons enter separate sheaths. Each sheath is covered by the inferior retinaculum, an extension of the cruciate crural ligament, at the level of the peroneal trochlea. The sheath about the peroneus brevis extends to within 1 cm of the insertion of the tendon into the tuberosity at the base of the fifth metatarsal. The other sheath, enveloping the tendon of the peroneus longus as it passes from the plantar aspect of the peroneal trochlea, ends as it glides to the undersurface of the cuboid. A second sheath envelops the peroneus longus as it emerges from the canal formed by the long plantar ligament and cuboid groove.

Peritendinitis

Several articles have addressed nonspecific and post-traumatic peroneal tenosynovitis (Burman 1953, Parvin & Ford 1956, Webster 1968, Fitzgerald & Coventry 1980, Trevino et al 1981). The most common type of tenosynovitis is stenosing. The peroneal tendon may become stenosed at three anatomic sites (Burman 1953): posterior to the lateral malleolus (peroneal sulcus), at the peroneal trochlea (tubercle) of the calcaneus, and at the undersurface of the cuboid bone.

Trauma has been the major factor attributed to precipitating tenosynovitis about the peroneal tendon sheath. Lateral malleolar fractures and inversion ankle injuries, direct trauma to the peroneal tubercle, and calcaneal fractures with or without calcaneofibular impingement of the peroneal tendon sheaths (Isbister 1974a, 1974b) have been associated with stenosing tenosynovitis. Burman (1956) also believed that a congenitally enlarged peroneal tubercle or a sesamoid bone in the peroneus longus could be inciting factors. In addition, he thought that nontraumatic acquired lesions such as compressive tenosynovitis or tenosynovitis as a manifestation of arthritis were possible aetiological factors.

Clinical features

Pain and swelling inferior to the lateral malleolus with point tenderness over the peroneal tendons at the inferior peroneal retinaculum are suggestive of peritendinitis. Symptoms are exacerbated by forced plantar flexion and inversion. A patient may relate a history of increased pain when walking barefoot or on rough terrain. Physical examination reveals an antalgic gait, limitation of subtalar motion, and point tenderness. The diagnosis of peroneal peritendinitis is enhanced if the pain is relieved by injections of a local anaesthetic into the tendon sheath. Peroneal tenography may show either complete block or constriction of the sheath at the inferior peroneal retinaculum (Fitzgerald & Coventry 1980, Teng et al 1984). Pseudotumour formation of the peroneal tendons may also be visible at the level of the inferior peroneal retinaculum. This finding should not be confused, however, with enlargement of the peroneus longus distally by the os peroneum.

Treatment

Treatment options are similar to those outlined for the Achilles tendon. Nonoperative measures consist of rest, anti-inflammatory agents, stretching exercises, physical therapy, and possibly injections of corticosteroids. A medial heel wedge, custom-fabricated foot orthosis, or shoes with a rocker-bottom sole and cushioned heel may diminish calcaneofibular impingement of the peroneal tendon sheath. If these measures are unsuccessful, surgical exploration and tenolysis may be advisable. Subtalar arthrodesis is recommended if significant degenerative changes exist at the subtalar joint.

Rupture

Closed, subcutaneous rupture of one or both of the peroneal tendons is rare but has been reported (Burman 1956, Evans 1966, Munk & Davis 1977, Abraham & Stirnaman 1979, Tehranzadeh et al 1984) (Fig. 29.19). Initially, in most case reports the

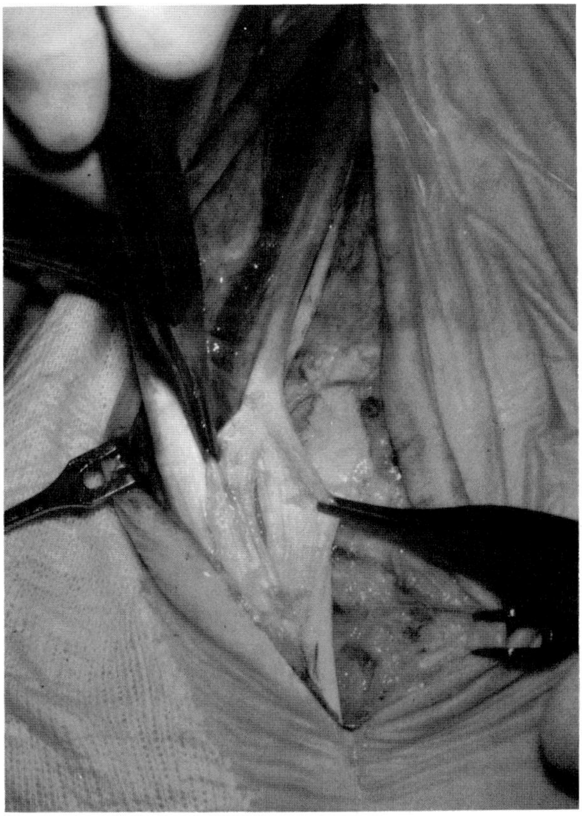

Fig. 29.19 Longitudinal tear of peroneus brevis tendon where it changes direction inferior to lateral malleolus

patients have been treated nonoperatively with the measures outlined above, including casting for 6 to 8 weeks. Because the chronic lateral ankle pain and swelling persisted despite an adequate trial of nonoperative treatment, surgical intervention was suggested for a presumed diagnosis of chronic lateral ligamentous instability or tenosynovitis of the peroneal sheath. In each case, either a partial or complete rupture of the peroneal tendon(s) was discovered with pathological changes suggestive of peritendinitis or tendinosis or both. It is interesting to speculate about how and why these tendons tend to develop longitudinal tears as they change direction around soft tissue or, more commonly, bony fulcrums. One idea is that the tendon does not compensate for the difference in the distance travelled in the outer compared with the inner tendon sides and therefore tears.

Surgical repair consisted of tenolysis, excision of the diseased tendon tissue and end-to-end repair, if possible, or tenodesis of the peroneus longus and brevis tendons. Follow-up revealed satisfactory results.

These reports emphasize the importance of considering peritendinitis and rupture of the peroneal tendons in the differential diagnosis of any patient with chronic lateral ankle pain.

Traumatic dislocation

Dislocation of tendons about the ankle is uncommon. Although traumatic dislocation of the posterior tibial tendon is rare (Larsen & Lauridsen 1984), this injury may be more common in the peroneal tendons than is recognized. It is most often associated with various athletic activities, most commonly skiing, soccer, and ice-skating and less commonly basketball or football (Murr 1961, Stover & Bryan 1962, Sarmiento & Wolf 1975, Marti 1977, Zoellner & Clancy 1979, McLennan 1980, Savastano 1980, Cohen et al 1983).

Peroneal dislocation may be classified as acute or chronic. Acute injuries are often unrecognized as anterior dislocations of the peroneal tendons and are misdiagnosed as 'ankle sprains', especially if a patient is not examined when the tendons are dislocated or if the physician is unaware of suggestive findings if the tendons have already returned to their retromalleolar groove. Because the acute injury is often undiagnosed, lack of adequate treatment may result in chronic dislocations. Most of the literature deals with operations designed to treat patients with chronic dislocations (Kelly 1920, Jones 1932, Miller 1967, Sarmiento & Wolf 1975, Zoellner & Clancy 1979, Arrowsmith et al 1983, Pöll & Duijfjes 1984, Pozo & Jackson 1984, Mann 1986).

Classification

In 1976, Eckert & Davis reported their surgical experience with 73 acute anterior dislocations of the peroneal tendon with injury to the peroneal retinaculum. Three gradations of injury were recognized (Table 29.13).

Certain anatomic variants have been suggested to predispose the peroneal tendons to subluxation or dislocation (Stover & Bryan 1962). These variants include absence of the posterior fibular groove (11% of cases), convex surface to the posterior fibula (7%

Table 29.13 Gradations of dislocations of the peroneal tendon

Grade	Characteristic
I	Retinaculum separated from lateral malleolus and fibrocartilaginous ridge (51% of cases)
II	Retinaculum and fibrocartilaginous ridge elevated from lateral malleolus (33% of cases)
III	Small chip fracture of the lateral malleolus avulsed along with the fibrocartilaginous ridge and retinaculum (16% of cases)

of cases), and laxity (either congenital or acquired) of the retinaculum (Edwards 1928).

In Edwards' study (1928), 82% of the 178 fibulas that were examined had a groove present, but it was usually very shallow — 2–3 mm in the dry, clean bone.

Clinical features

Most authors believe that this injury is the result of sudden, forceful, passive dorsiflexion of the inverted foot with reflex contraction of the peroneal tendons and plantar flexors (Murr 1961, Stover & Bryan 1962, Eckert & Davis 1976). During skiing, this injury occurs if the ski tips dig in and the skier falls forward by deceleration. Escalas et al (1980) believed that the forceful contraction of the peroneal tendons as a skier digs the inner border of the ski into the snow when making turns also enhanced the risk of dislocating these tendons.

A history of a snapping sensation accompanied by pain in the posterolateral ankle is usually given (Eckert & Davis 1976). Characteristic swelling and tenderness occur posterior and superior to the lateral malleolus (Murr 1961, Eckert & Davis 1976, Escalas et al 1980, McLennan 1980, Savastano 1980, Arrowsmith et al 1983). The more common ankle sprain involving the anterior talofibular ligament manifests with swelling more distal and anterior to the lateral malleolus. Injury to the posterior talofibular ligament may elicit point tenderness similar to that of an acute dislocation. Stressing the retinaculum by eliciting dorsiflexion against resistance with the foot in plantar flexion and eversion causes retromalleolar pain and may result in dislocation. The findings of a grade III injury and a rim avulsion fracture of the lateral malleolus are considered pathognomonic of tendon dislocation (Mortiz 1959, Murr 1961, Stover & Bryan 1962). Of course, lateral ankle instability must be considered in the differential diagnosis for any patient with significant lateral ankle trauma, and stress views to determine the presence of talar tilt must be obtained when indicated. Peroneal tenograms may show leakage of the contrast dye anteriorly. Computed tomography has also been reported to be of value for the evaluation of peroneal tendon dislocation (Szczukowski et al 1983). In the final assessment, however, unless the dislocation is seen when the patient is first examined or can be reproduced on examination, the diagnosis of acute anterior dislocation is uncertain and is only suspected.

Chronic dislocation of the peroneal tendons should present less diagnostic difficulty. The history of a sense of uneasiness, giving way, or snapping at the ankle, especially when walking on uneven ground, is highly suggestive. Retinacular structures that are lax secondary to recurrent dislocations should be discernible on physical examination. Observation of the opposite uninjured ankle is helpful.

Treatment

Nonoperative treatment of the acute injury is controversial (Stover & Bryan 1962, Eckert & Davis 1976, Marti 1977, Escalas et al 1980, McLennan 1980, Savastano 1980, Arrowsmith et al 1983). Strapping techniques or well-moulded, non-weightbearing casts for 5 to 6 weeks are the usual methods used. The rationale behind this therapy is that holding the tendons reduced in an anatomic position heals the superior peroneal retinaculum by scarring. The ankle is placed in mild plantar flexion to relax the tendons.

Stover & Bryan (1962) reported the results in 19 patients with acute injuries. Five of the 19 patients treated with non-weightbearing casts had excellent results and no evidence of recurrent dislocation. Ten patients were treated with strapping techniques. Follow-up data were obtained for nine of these patients; six had recurrent dislocation, and four of the six had subsequent operations. They concluded that a well-moulded, non-weightbearing cast for 5 to 6 weeks was the initial treatment of choice. They thought that elastic strapping techniques were inadequate, especially if followed by early weight bearing.

Eckert & Davis (1976) stated that their experiences with closed treatment were disappointing. Hence, they treat all acute injuries operatively. They believe that if a lesion is determined to be grade I, closed treatment may be adequate.

McLennan (1980) reported the results in a mixed series of acute and chronic dislocations. He concluded that the morbidity associated with nonoperative treatment is minimal and that this approach may be satisfactory in most cases (56%). He thought operative treatment may be indicated for acute injuries in athletes. Nonoperative treatment seemed effective in cases that demonstrated stability against dislocation after an acute injury.

Most authors believe that recurrent, symptomatic, documented peroneal dislocations should be treated operatively (Kelly 1920, Jones 1932, Murr 1961, Miller 1967, Sarmiento & Wolf 1975, Zoellner & Clancy 1979, McLennan 1980, Arrowsmith et al 1983). Operation consists of soft tissue procedures to reconstruct the peroneal retinaculum, bony procedures to reconstruct the peroneal retinaculum, bony procedures to deepen the retromalleolar groove, or a combination of the soft tissue and bony procedures.

One criticism of the soft tissue and bony procedures raised by many investigators is that they use normal structures or alter the normal bony architecture, perhaps to their detriment, in order to accomplish the goal of preventing recurrent subluxation-dislocation.

Several of these methods as described in the English literature are summarized in Table 29.14.

EXTENSOR TENDONS OF THE FOOT AND ANKLE

Peritendinitis

There are few reports of peritendinitis affecting the extensor tendons about the dorsum of the foot (Fig. 29.20). In Lipscomb's review (1950), the tibialis anterior tendon was the most frequently involved, and the extensor digitorum longus was often affected. Tenosynovitis of these tendons is thought to be secondary to irritations by shoes, boots, or skis. Rest, modification of footwear that impinges on the dorsum of the foot, and physical therapy usually suffice for treatment. Incision of the synovial sheath in front of the ankle is necessary only occasionally.

Table 29.14 Types of surgical treatment of dislocations of the peroneal tendons, as described in the literature

Type of procedure	Reference	Description
Bony	Kelly (1920)	Bone block (lateral malleolus osteotomy)
	Zoellner & Clancy (1979)	Groove deepening with osteoperiosteal flap (as described by F F Thompson)
	Pöll & Duijfjes (1984)	Calcaneofibular ligament mobilized with bone block from calcaneus
	Pozo & Jackson (1984)	Calcaneofibular ligament mobilized by osteotomizing lateral malleolus
	Mann (1986)	Sliding graft (lateral malleolus as described by H L DuVries)
Soft tissue	Jones (1932)	Achilles tendon sling
	Miller (1967)	Plantaris tendon sling
	Sarmiento & Wolf (1975)	Calcaneofibular ligament sling
	Arrowsmith et al (1983)	Peroneus brevis sling

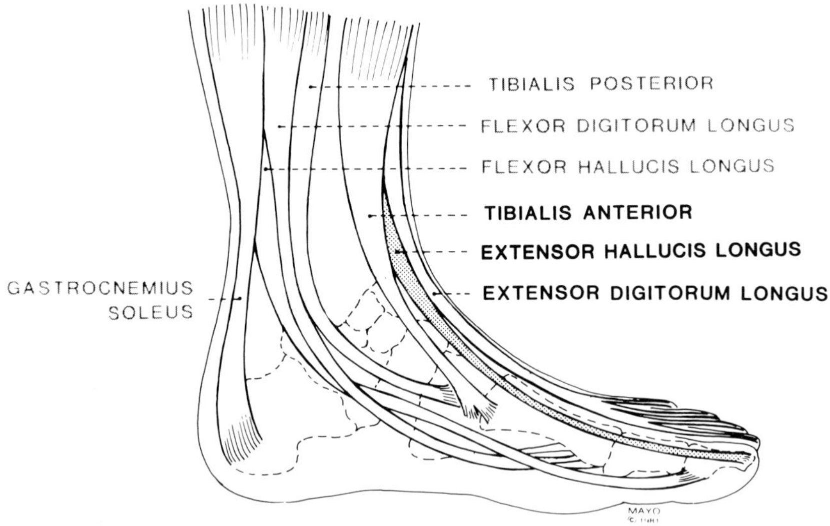

Fig. 29.20 Extensor tendons that can be affected by disruption. (By permission of Mayo Foundation)

Rupture

Disruption of the extensor tendons about the dorsum of the foot and ankle is an infrequent injury, usually the result of an open wound or laceration (Lipscomb & Kelly 1955, Anzel et al 1959, Griffiths 1965, Floyd et al 1983). Closed subcutaneous rupture has been reported in the tibialis anterior tendon and extensor hallucis longus tendon (Fig. 29.21), but this condition is much less frequent than the open lacerations involving the extensor tendons.

Tibialis anterior tendon

Less than 20 reports of closed subcutaneous rupture of the tibialis anterior tendon have appeared in the literature (Burman 1934, 1943, Lapidus 1941, Moberg 1947, Mensor & Ordway 1953, Moskowitz 1971, Meyn 1975, Dooley et al 1980). The patients have almost always been males who are older than 45 years. Rupture usually occurs after minimal or insignificant trauma that consists of forced plantar flexion against actively contracting dorsiflexors.

Clinical features. A patient often presents with weakness of the ankle and swelling about the dorsum of the foot and ankle. If a patient presents late the pain is minimal, and the patient is left with a minor degree of footdrop. Three cases of rupture of the tibialis anterior tendon have been reported in which the patient was thought to have an underlying neurological lesion: a peroneal palsy in two cases and an acute L-5 radiculopathy in one case (Moskowitz 1971, Meyn 1975).

Active dorsiflexion of the ankle may produce some eversion, and attempted inversion is weak. Discontinuity of the tendon may reveal a gap with no signs of a palpable tendon distally.

Treatment. The literature seems to favour surgical reattachment of closed rupture of the tibialis anterior tendon if a patient is active and presents within 3 to 4 months after injury (Mensor & Ordway 1953, Dooley et a! 1980). In patients who are treated nonoperatively, the tendon usually scars down more proximally and results in less ankle motion in dorsiflexion and less strength. However, in elderly patients who lead sedentary lives, the gait is almost always functionally normal and nonoperative treatment is thus justified (Meyn 1975, Dooley et al 1980).

Extensor hallucis longus and extensor digitorum longus

Incidence. In 1959, Anzel et al reported the incidence of tendon and muscle disruptions in a large series of patients examined at the Mayo Clinic. Disruptions of the toe extensors occurred in 16 patients and accounted for 11% of the 143 injuries to the lower extremity (see Table 29.6). All of these

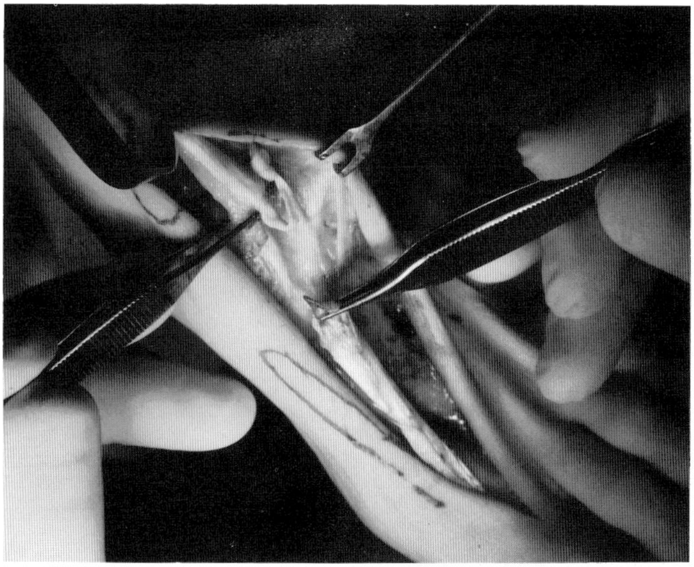

Fig. 29.21 Closed rupture of extensor hallucis longus because of prolonged pressure of ski boot

injuries were open lacerations. Griffiths (1965) described 20 patients with tendon injuries about the ankle. Nine patients had involvement of the extensor hallucis longus or extensor digitorum longus; only one patient had a closed disruption secondary to erosion by rheumatoid tissue. Floyd et al (1983) recently published a retrospective review of 80 patients with open injuries of various tendons about the foot and ankle. Of the 46 patients for whom follow-up data were obtained, 13 had laceration of the extensor hallucis longus and 8 had lacerations of the extensor digitorum longus. Few reports have documented closed subcutaneous rupture or dislocation of the extensor hallucis longus or extensor digitorum longus (Sim & DeWeerd 1977, Akhtar & Levine 1980).

Treatment. Generally, an aggressive surgical approach is advocated for open lacerations of tendons about the foot, especially in children (Lipscomb & Kelly 1955, Griffiths 1965, Wicks et al 1980, Floyd et al 1983). This treatment includes thorough debridement and exploration to define the extent of the injury followed by anatomic restoration whenever possible. Griffiths (1965) alluded to the well-known tendency of the extensor tendons for spontaneous repair after tenotomy for clawtoe deformity. He therefore suggested that formal repair of the extensor hallucis longus may be unnecessary. This view is also shared by Wicks et al (1980). Floyd et al (1983), however, concluded that firm recommendations against repair of any specific tendon could not be supported by the literature and recommended surgical repair of both the extensor hallucis longus and the extensor digitorum longus, when possible. A turndown technique is possible if substance loss has occurred (Fig. 29.22).

FLEXOR HALLUCIS LONGUS

Several reports about lacerations of the flexor hallucis longus have been published, but until recently only a few reports have concerned other problems that affect this tendon (Reinherz 1984). The consensus regarding lacerations of the flexor hallucis longus is that they should be repaired primarily (Frenette & Jackson 1977, Yancey 1977, Wicks et al 1980, Floyd et al 1983). Frenette & Jackson (1977) also suggested that if both the flexor hallucis brevis and the flexor hallucis longus were divided and the proximal portion of the latter could not be retrieved, the distal stump of the flexor hallucis longus should be sutured into the flexor hallucis brevis. Two articles have described closed ruptures of the flexor hallucis longus. This event is distinctly uncommon. Sammarco & Miller (1979)

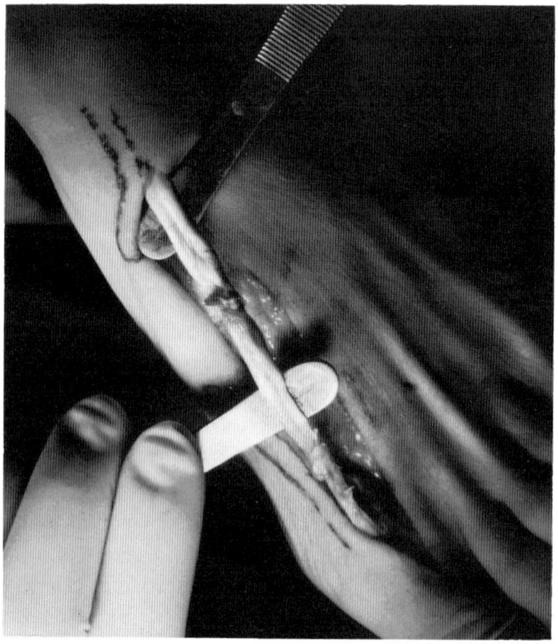

Fig. 29.22 Turndown of portion of extensor hallucis longus to span gap

described two cases of partial rupture of the central fibres of the flexor hallucis longus in classical ballet dancers, and Krackow (1980) described one case of an acute, complete, traumatic rupture of the flexor hallucis longus in combination with a rupture of the Achilles tendon in a patient injured in a diving accident; all three cases were surgically repaired.

Stenosing tenosynovitis

Recently, several reports have described stenosing tenosynovitis of the flexor hallucis longus (Sammarco & Miller 1979, Gould 1981, Hamilton 1982, McCarroll et al 1983, Tudisco & Puddu 1984). Stenosing tenosynovitis occurs most often when a tendon with its surrounding peritendinous structures passes through or around a restricted fibro-osseous space. In the flexor hallucis longus, stenosis has been reported to occur at three anatomic sites: 1) within the flexor tendon sheath behind the medial malleolus, 2) at the fibro-osseous tunnel on the posterior aspect of the talus between the medial and lateral tubercles and 3) distally as the tendon passes through the sesamoid bones and inserts into the terminal phalanx of the great toe. As a result of stenosis at both of these sites, 'triggering' can occur in the great toe.

Stenosis at the posteromedial ankle

Aetiology

Stenosis at the posterior process of the talus or sustentaculum tali of the calcaneus may result from fractures in this region, but it more commonly has been associated with ballet dancers (Sammarco & Miller 1979, Hamilton 1982) who, because of the unnatural position of the foot and ankle when in the pointe position, develop a tenosynovitis at the posteromedial ankle. McCarroll et al (1983) reported triggering of the great toe caused by entrapment of the flexor hallucis longus tendon within the flexor tendon sheath posterior to the medial malleolus.

Clinical features

The symptoms may be similar to those described for posterior tibial peritendinitis. Pain, swelling, tenderness, and crepitus may be present behind the medial malleolus. Triggering and locking of the great toe associated with a pop or snap in the posteromedial aspect of the ankle as the foot is brought into plantar flexion and the hallux is actively flexed are diagnostic of stenosing tenosynovitis of the flexor hallucis longus. If pain is present on forced plantar flexion of the foot and ankle, one must consider posterior impingement or block of the ankle joint caused by an os trigonum, a large posterior tubercle of the talus or prominence on the posterior part of the os calcis (Hamilton 1982, Howse 1982). The pain from this posterior impingement syndrome is most commonly posterolateral, but it should not be confused with peroneal peritendinitis (Burman 1953, 1956, Munk & Davis 1977, Fitzgerald & Coventry 1980, Trevino et al 1981). Lateral radiographs with the foot and ankle in maximal plantar flexion may reveal this abnormality.

Hamilton (1982) also described 'pseudohallux rigidus' and 'functional hallux rigidus'. In the former, the flexor hallucis longus becomes adhesive within its sheath, and movement of the hallux is restricted. In the latter condition, abnormal distal insertions of muscle fibres of the flexor hallucis longus become bound in the fibro-osseous tunnel at the posterior aspect of the talus and restrict dorsiflexion of the hallux when the knee is in full extension and the ankle is maximally dorsiflexed.

Stenosis at the great toe

Gould (1981) described nine patients with stenosis of the flexor hallucis longus as it passes through its sheath between the sesamoid bones of the great toe. This area is subject to repetitive impact loading, especially in runners, and may predispose to fractures or sesamoiditis. Laceration and subsequent scarring of the flexor hallucis longus can also occur in this area (Frenette & Jackson 1977). If the sheath of the flexor hallucis longus is injured in this area, it may heal in a constricted position and result in limited tendon excursion.

Clinical features

Pain in the sesamoid area and inability to flex the interphalangeal joint of the great toe actively when the metatarsophalangeal joint is stabilized in the neutral position are suggestive of stenosis in this area. Radiographs, including sesamoid views, may be helpful in ruling out fractures, cysts, or arthritis.

Treatment

The considerations for treatment of peritendinitis of the flexor hallucis longus are the same as those described for peritendinitis of other tendons. The mainstays of nonoperative treatment are rest, stretching, physical therapy, nonsteroidal anti-inflammatory drugs, and possibly corticosteroids. For stenosis distally, Gould (1981) described trying to break adhesions in the sesamoid area by inflating the tendon sheath with infiltration of 1% lidocaine. If an adequate trial of nonoperative treatment is unsuccessful, tenolysis, as described previously, may be used. Proximal lesions are usually approached from the posteromedial aspect of the ankle with a curvilinear incision.

REFERENCES

Abraham E, Pankovich A M 1975 Neglected rupture of the Achilles tendon: treatment by V-Y tendinous flap. J Bone Joint Surg 57A: 253–255

Abraham E, Stirnaman J E 1979 Neglected rupture of the peroneal tendons causing recurrent sprains of the ankle: case report. J Bone Joint Surg 61A: 1247–1248

Akhtar M, Levine J 1980 Dislocation of extensor digitorum longus tendons after spontaneous rupture of the inferior retinaculum of the ankle: case report. J Bone Joint Surg 62A: 1210–1211

Albert E 1893 Achillodynie. Wiener Medizinische Presse 34: 41–43

Altman D 1966 Managing bursitis in podiatry. J Am Podiatry Assoc 56: 408–410

Anzel S H, Covey K W, Weiner A D, Lipscomb P R 1959 Disruption of muscles and tendons: an analysis of 1,014 cases. Surgery 45: 406–414

Arner O, Lindholm Å 1959 Subcutaneous rupture of the Achilles tendon: a study of 92 cases. Acta Chir Scand (Suppl) 239: 1–51

Arner O, Lindholm Å, Lindvall N 1958–1959a Roentgen changes in subcutaneous rupture of the Achilles tendon. Acta Chir Scand 116: 496–500

Arner O, Lindholm Å, Orell S R 1958–1959b Histologic changes in subcutaneous rupture of the Achilles tendon: a study of 74 cases. Acta Chir Scand 116: 484–490

Arrowsmith S R, Fleming L L, Allman F L 1983 Traumatic dislocations of the peroneal tendons. Am J Sports Med 11: 142–146

Barfred T 1973 Achilles tendon rupture: aetiology and pathogenesis of subcutaneous rupture assessed on the basis of the literature and rupture experiments on rats. Acta Orthop Scand (Suppl) 152: 1–126

Berlin D, Coleman W, Nickamin A 1982 Surgical approaches to Haglund's disease. J Foot Surg 21: 42–44

Bossley C J, Cairney P C 1980 The intermetatarsophalangeal bursa — its significance in Morton's metatarsalgia. J Bone Joint Surg 62B: 184–187

Bosworth D M 1956 Repair of defects in the tendo Achillis. J Bone Joint Surg 38A: 111–114

Brahms M A 1967 Common foot problems. J Bone Joint Surg 49A: 1653–1664

Brody D M 1980 Running injuries. Clin Symp 32(4): 2–36

Brown T D, Fu F H, Hanley E N Jr 1981 Comparative assessment of the early mechanical integrity of repaired tendo Achillis ruptures in the rabbit. J Trauma 21: 951–957

Buck R M, McDonald J R, Ghormley R K 1943 Adventitious bursas. Arch Surg 47: 344–351

Bugg E I Jr, Boyd B M 1968 Repair of neglected rupture or laceration of the Achilles tendon. Clin Orthop 56: 73–75

Burman M 1943 Subcutaneous strain or tear of the dorsiflexor tendons of the foot. Bull Hosp Jt Dis Orthop Inst 4: 44–50

Burman M 1953 Stenosing tendovaginitis of the foot and ankle: studies with special reference to the stenosing tendo-vaginitis of the peroneal tendons at the peroneal tubercle. Arch Surg 67: 686–698

Burman M 1956 Subcutaneous tear of the tendon of the peroneus longus: its relation to the giant peroneal tubercle. Arch Surg 73: 216–219

Burman M S 1934 Subcutaneous rupture of the tendon of the tibialis anticus. Ann Surg 100: 368–372

Burry H C, Pool C J 1973 Central degeneration of the Achilles tendon. Rheumatol Rehabil 12: 177–181

Bywaters E G L 1954 Heel lesions of rheumatoid arthritis. Ann Rheum Dis 13: 42–51

Bywaters E G L 1965 Bursae of the body (editorial). Ann Rheum Dis 24: 215–218

Canoso J J, Wohlgethan J R, Newberg A H, Goldsmith M R 1984 Aspiration of the retrocalcaneal bursa. Ann Rheum Dis 43: 308–312

Cetti R, Christensen S E 1983 Surgical treatment under local anesthesia of Achilles tendon rupture. Clin Orthop 173: 204–208

Cherry J H, Ghormley R K 1941 Bursa and ganglion. Am J Surg 52: 319–330

Clancy W G Jr 1982 Tendinitis and plantar fasciitis in runners. In: D'Ambrosia R, Drez D Jr (eds) Prevention and treatment of running injuries. Charles B Slack, Thorofare, New Jersey, pp 77–87

Clancy W G Jr, Neidhart D, Brand R L 1976 Achilles tendonitis in runners: a report of five cases. Am J Sports Med 4: 46–56

Cohen I, Lane S, Koning W 1983 Peroneal tendon dislocations: a review of the literature. J Foot Surg 22: 15–20

Conwell H E, Alldredge R H 1937 Ruptures and tears of muscles and tendons. Am J Surg 35: 22–33

Cozen L 1965 Posterior tibial tenosynovitis secondary to foot strain. Clin Orthop 42: 101–102

Davidsson L, Salo M 1969 Pathogenesis of subcutaneous tendon ruptures. Acta Chir Scand 135: 209–212

Denstad T F, Roaas A 1979 Surgical treatment of partial Achilles tendon rupture. Am J Sports Med 7: 15–17

De Zwart D F, Davidson J S A 1983 Rupture of the posterior tibial tendon associated with fractures of the ankle: a report of two cases. J Bone Joint Surg 65A: 260–262

Dickinson P H, Coutts M B, Woodward E P, Handler D 1966 Tendo Achillis bursitis: report of twenty-one cases. J Bone Joint Surg 48A: 77–81

Dooley B J, Kudelka P, Menelaus M B 1980 Subcutaneous rupture of the tendon of tibialis anterior. J Bone Joint Surg 62B: 471–472

Eckert W R, Davis E A Jr 1976 Acute rupture of the peroneal retinaculum. J Bone Joint Surg 58A: 670–673

Edna T-H 1980 Non-operative treatment of Achilles tendon ruptures. Acta Orthop Scand 51: 991–993

Edwards M E 1928 The relations of the peroneal tendons to the fibula, calcaneus, and cuboideum. Am J Anat 42: 213–253

Escalas F, Figueras J M, Merino J A 1980 Dislocation of the peroneal tendons: long-term results of surgical treatment. J Bone Joint Surg 62A: 451–453

Evans J D 1966 Subcutaneous rupture of the tendon of peroneus longus: report of a case. J Bone Joint Surg 48B: 507–509

Ferguson A B Jr, Gingrich R M 1957 The normal and the abnormal calcaneal apophysis and tarsal navicular. Clin Orthop 10: 87–95

Fish J B 1982 Ruptured Achilles tendon: a method of repair. Contemp Orthop 5: 21–25

Fisher T R, Woods C G 1970 Partial rupture of the tendo calcaneus with heterotopic calcification: report of a case. J Bone Joint Surg 52B: 334–336

Fitzgerald R H Jr, Coventry M B 1980 Post-traumatic peroneal tendinitis. In: Bateman J E, Trott A W (eds) The foot and ankle: a selection of papers from the American Orthopaedic Foot Society Meetings. Brian C Decker, New York. pp 103–109

Floyd D W, Heckman J D, Rockwood C A Jr 1983 Tendon lacerations in the foot. Foot Ankle 4: 8–14

Fowler A, Philip J F 1945 Abnormality of the calcaneus as a cause of painful heel: its diagnosis and operative treatment. Br J Surg 32: 494–498

Fowler A W 1955 Tibialis posterior syndrome (abstract). J Bone Joint Surg 37B: 520

Fox J M, Blazina M E, Jobe F W, Kerlan R K, Carter V S, Shields C L Jr, Carlson G J 1975 Degeneration and rupture of the Achilles tendon. Clin Orthop 107: 221–224

Fredenburg M, Tilley G, Yagoobian E M 1983 Spontaneous rupture of the posterior tibial tendon secondary to chronic non-specific tenosynovitis. J Foot Surg 22: 198–202

Frenette J P, Jackson D W 1977 Lacerations of the flexor hallucis longus in the young athlete. J Bone Joint Surg 59A: 673–676

Fuglsang F, Torup D 1961 Bursitis retrocalcanearis. Acta Orthop Scand 30: 315–323

Ghormley R K, Spear I M 1953 Anomalies of the posterior tibial tendon: a cause of persistent pain about the ankle. Arch Surg 66: 512–516

Giblin M M 1980 Ruptured tibialis posterior tendon associated with a closed medial malleolar fracture. Aust NZ J Surg 50: 59–60

Gilcreest E L 1933 Ruptures and tears of muscles and tendons of the lower extremity: report of fifteen cases. JAMA 100: 153–160

Gillies H, Chalmers J 1970 The management of fresh ruptures of the tendo Achillis. J Bone Joint Surg 52A: 337–343

Gillström P, Ljungqvist R 1978 Long-term results after operation for subcutaneous partial rupture of the Achilles tendon. Acta Chir Scand (Suppl) 482: 78

Goldman S, Linscheid R L, Bickel W H 1969 Disruptions of the tendo Achillis: analysis of 33 cases. Mayo Clin Proc 44: 28–35

Goldner J L, Irwin C E 1949 Paralytic equinovarus deformities of the foot. South Med J 42: 83–94

Goldner J L, Keats P K, Bassett F H III, Clippinger F W 1974 Progressive talipes equinovalgus due to trauma or degeneration of the posterior tibial tendon and medial plantar ligaments. Orthop Clin North Am 5(1): 39–51

Gould N 1981 Stenosing tenosynovitis of the flexor hallucis longus tendon at the great toe. Foot Ankle 2: 46–48

Gould N 1983 Evaluation of hyperpronation and pes planus in adults. Clin Orthop 181: 37–45

Gould N, Korson R 1980 Stenosing tenosynovitis of the pseudosheath of the tendo Achilles. Foot Ankle 1: 179–186

Griffiths D LL 1952 Tenosynovitis and tenovaginitis. Br Med J 1: 645–647

Griffiths J C 1965 Tendon injuries around the ankle. J Bone Joint Surg 47B: 686–689

Häggmark T, Eriksson E 1979 Hypotrophy of the soleus muscle in man after Achilles tendon rupture: discussion of findings obtained by computed tomography and morphologic studies. Am J Sports Med 7: 121–126

Haglund P 1928 Contribution to the diseased conditions of tendo Achilles (abstract). Acta Chir Scand 63: 292–294

Haldeman K O, Soto-Hall R 1935 Injuries to muscles and tendons. JAMA 104: 2319–2324

Hamilton W G 1982 Stenosing tenosynovitis of the flexor hallucis longus tendon and posterior impingement upon the os trigonum in ballet dancers. Foot Ankle 3: 74–80

Hartmann 1981 The tendon sheaths and synovial bursae of the foot. Foot Ankle 1: 247–269

Håstad K, Larsson L-G, Lindholm Å 1958–1959 Clearance of radiosodium after local deposit in the Achilles tendon. Acta Chir Scand 116: 251–255

Hattrup S J, Johnson K A 1985 A review of ruptures of the Achilles tendon. Foot Ankle 6: 34–38

Hauser E D W 1956 Nonspecific tenosynovitis with effusion at the ankle. Postgrad Med 20: 365–369

Helfand A E, Hirt P R, Madresh A C, DeVincentis A 1971 Triamcinolone acetonide in the treatment of bursitis and other foot disorders. J Am Podiatry Assoc 61: 174–179

Henceroth W D II, Deyerle W M 1982 The acquired unilateral flatfoot in the adult: some causative factors. Foot Ankle 2: 304–308

Heneghan M A, Pavlov H 1984 The Haglund painful heel syndrome: experimental investigation of cause and therapeutic implications. Clin Orthop 187: 228–234

Hertzler A E 1923 Inflammation of the deep calcaneal bursa. JAMA 81: 8–9

Hertzler A E 1926 Bursitides of the plantar surface of the foot (painful heel, gonorrheal exostosis of the os calcis, metatarsal neuralgia). Am J Surg 1: 117–126

Hooker C H 1963 Rupture of the tendo calcaneus. J Bone Joint Surg 45B: 360–363

Howse A J G 1982 Posterior block of the ankle joint in dancers. Foot Ankle 3: 81–84

Inglis A E, Scott W N, Sculco T P, Patterson A H 1976 Ruptures of the tendo Achillis: an objective assessment of surgical and non-surgical treatment. J Bone Joint Surg 58A: 990–993

Ippolito E, Ricciardi-Pollini P T 1984 Invasive retrocalcaneal bursitis: a report of three cases. Foot Ankle 4: 204–208

Isbister J F St C 1974a Calcaneo-fibular abutment following crush fracture of the calcaneus (abstract). J Bone Joint Surg 56B: 567–568

Isbister J F St C 1974b Calcaneo-fibular abutment following crush fracture of the calcaneus. J Bone Joint Surg 56B: 274–278

Jacobs D, Martens M, Van Audekercke R, Mulier J C, Mulier Fr 1978 Comparison of conservative and operative treatment of Achilles tendon rupture. Am J Sports Med 6: 107–111

Jahss M H 1972 Unusual diagnostic problems of the foot. Clin Orthop 85: 42–49

Jahss M H 1974 Pseudotumors of the foot. Orthop Clin North Am 5(1): 67–87

Jahss M H 1982a Spontaneous rupture of the tibialis posterior tendon: clinical findings, tenographic studies, and a new technique of repair. Foot Ankle 3: 158–166

Jahss M H 1982b Disorders of the foot, Vol 1. W B Saunders, Philadelphia. pp 828–868

Jessing P, Hansen E 1975 Surgical treatment of 102 tendo Achillis ruptures — suture or tenontoplasty? Acta Chir Scand 141: 370–377

Johnson K A 1983 Tibialis posterior tendon rupture. Clin Orthop 177: 140–147

Jones D C, James S L 1984 Partial calcaneal ostectomy for retrocalcaneal bursitis. Am Journal Sports Med 12: 72–73

Jones E 1932 Operative treatment of chronic dislocation of the peroneal tendons. J Bone Joint Surg 14: 574–576

Jones H T 1930 Cystic bursal hygromas. J Bone Joint Surg 12: 45–89

Kager H 1939 Cited by Arner et al 1958–1959

Kaplan L, Ferguson L K 1937 Bursitis. Am J Surg 37: 455–465

Keck S W, Kelly P J 1965 Bursitis of the posterior part of the heel: evaluation of surgical treatment of eighteen patients. J Bone Joint Surg 47A: 267–273

Kelly R E 1920 An operation for the chronic dislocation of the peroneal tendons. Br J Surg 7: 502–504

Kettelkamp D B, Alexander H H 1969 Spontaneous rupture of the posterior tibial tendon. J Bone Joint Surg 51A: 759–764

Key J A 1953 Partial rupture of the tendon of the posterior tibial muscle. J Bone Joint Surg 35A: 1006–1008

Kleinman M, Gross A E 1983 Achilles tendon rupture following steroid injection: report of three cases. J Bone Joint Surg 65A: 1345–1347

Krackow K A 1980 Acute, traumatic rupture of a flexor hallucis longus tendon: a case report. Clin Orthop 150: 261–262

Kuhns J G 1943 Adventitious bursas. Arch Surg 46: 687–696

Kulowski J 1936 Tendovaginitis (tenosynovitis): general discussion and report of one case involving posterior tibial tendon. Journal of the Missouri Medical Association 33: 135–137

Kvist H, Kvist M 1980 The operative treatment of chronic calcaneal paratenonitis. J Bone Joint Surg 62B: 353–357

Lagergren C, Lindholm Å 1958–1959 Vascular distribution in the Achilles tendon: an angiographic and microangiographic study. Acta Chir Scand 116: 491–495

Lancet Editorial 1973 Achilles tendon rupture. 1: 189–190

Langenskiöld A 1967 Chronic non-specific tenosynovitis of the tibialis posterior tendon. Acta Orthop Scand 38: 301–305

Lapidus P W 1941 Indirect subcutaneous rupture of the anterior tibial tendon: report of two cases. Bull Hosp Jt Dis Orthop Inst 2: 119–127

Lapidus P W 1953 Stenosing tenovaginitis. Surg Clin North Am October: 1317–1347

Lapidus P W, Seidenstein H 1950 Chronic non-specific tenosynovitis with effusion about the ankle: report of three cases. J Bone Joint Surg 32A: 175–179

Larsen E, Lauridsen F 1984 Dislocation of the tibialis posterior tendon in two athletes. Am J Sports Med 12: 429–430

Lawrence G H, Cave E F, O'Connor H 1955 Injury to the Achilles tendon: experience at the Massachusetts General Hospital, 1900–1954. Am J Surg 89: 795–802

Layfer L F 1980 "Last" bursitis — a cause of ankle pain (letter to the editor). Arthritis Rheum 23: 261

Lea R B 1981 Achilles tendon rupture: results of closed management. In: Moore M (ed) Symposium on trauma to the leg and its sequelae. C V Mosby, St Louis. pp 353–357

Lea R B, Smith L 1968 Rupture of the Achilles tendon nonsurgical treatment. Clin Orthop 60: 115–118

Lea R B, Smith L 1972 Non-surgical treatment of tendo Achillis rupture. J Bone Joint Surg 54A: 1398–1407

Leach R E 1982 Achilles tendon ruptures. In: Mack R P (ed) Symposium on the foot and leg in running sports. C V Mosby, St Louis. pp 99–105

Leach R E, James S, Wasilewski S 1981 Achilles tendinitis. Am J Sports Med 9: 93–98

Lennox D W, Wang G J, McCue F C, Stamp W G 1980 The operative treatment of Achilles tendon injuries. Clin Orthop 148: 152–155

Lindholm Å 1959 A new method of operation in subcutaneous rupture of the Achilles tendon. Acta Chir Scand 117: 261–270

Lipscomb P R November 1942 Non-suppurative tenosynovitis: a clinical and pathologic study. Thesis, Graduate School of the University of Minnesota

Lipscomb P R 1944 Chronic nonspecific tenosynovitis and peritendinitis. Surg Clin North Am August: 780–797

Lipscomb P R 1950 Tendons: Number 1. Nonsuppurative tenosynovitis and paratendinitis. Instr Course Lect 7: 254–261

Lipscomb P R, Kelly P J 1955 Injuries of the extensor tendons in the distal part of the leg and in the ankle. J Bone Joint Surg 37A: 1206–1213
Lipscomb P R, Wakim K G 1961a Regeneration of severed tendons: an experimental study. Proceedings of the Staff Meetings of the Mayo Clinic 36: 271–276
Lipscomb P R, Wakim K G 1961b Further observations in the healing of severed tendons: an experimental study. Proceedings of the Staff Meetings of the Mayo Clinic 36: 277–282
Lipsman S, Frankel J P, Count G W 1980 Spontaneous rupture of the tibialis posterior tendon: a case report and review of the literature. J Am Podiatry Assoc 70: 34–39
Ljungqvist R 1968 Subcutaneous partial rupture of the Achilles tendon. Acta Orthop Scand (Suppl) 113: 1–86
Ljungqvist R, Eriksson E 1982 Partial tears of the patellar tendon and the Achilles tendon. In: Mack R P (ed) Symposium on the foot and leg in running sports. C V Mosby, St Louis. pp 92–98
Lynn T A 1966 Repair of the torn Achilles tendon, using the plantaris tendon as a reinforcing membrane. J Bone Joint Surg 48A: 268–272
Ma G W, Griffith T G 1977 Percutaneous repair of acute closed ruptured Achilles tendon: a new technique. Clin Orthop 128: 247–255
Ma G W C, Griffith T G 1981 Percutaneous repair of acute closed ruptured Achilles tendon: a new technique. In: Moore T M (ed) Symposium on trauma to the leg and its sequelae. C V Mosby, St Louis. pp 358–370
McCarroll J R, Ritter M A, Becker T E 1983 Triggering of the great toe: a case report. Clin Orthop 175: 184–185
McLennan J G 1980 Treatment of acute and chronic luxations of the peroneal tendons. Am J Sports Med 8: 432–436
McMaster P E 1933 Tendon and muscle ruptures: clinical and experimental studies on the causes and location of subcutaneous ruptures. J Bone Joint Surg 15: 705–722
Mann R A 1983 Acquired flatfoot in adults. Clin Orthop 181: 46–51
Mann R A 1985 Biomechanics of the foot. In: American Academy of Orthopaedic Surgeons: Atlas of orthotics, 2nd edn. C V Mosby, St Louis. p 121
Mann R A (ed) 1986 Surgery of the foot 5th edn. C V Mosby, St Louis. pp 293–294
Mann R A, Specht L H 1982 "Posterior tibial tendon ruptures — analysis of eight cases" (abstract). Foot Ankle 2: 350
Mann R A, Thompson F M 1985 Rupture of the posterior tibial tendon causing flat foot: surgical treatment. J Bone Joint Surg 67A: 556–561
Marti R 1977 Dislocation of the peroneal tendons. Am J Sports Med 5: 19–22
Mensor M C, Ordway G L 1953 Traumatic subcutaneous rupture of the tibialis anterior tendon. J Bone Joint Surg 35A: 675–680
Meyerding H W 1938 The treatment of bursitis. Surg Clin North Am 18: 1103–1117
Meyn M A Jr 1975 Closed rupture of the anterior tibial tendon: a case report and review of the literature. Clin Orthop 113: 154–157
Miller B F, Buhr A J 1969 Pump bumps or knobbly heels. Nova Scotia Medical Bulletin 48: 191–192
Miller J W 1967 Dislocation of peroneal tendons — a new operative procedure: a case report. Am J Orthop 9: 136–137
Moberg E 1947 Subcutaneous rupture of the tendon of the tibialis anterior muscle. Acta Chir Scand 95: 455–460
Mortiz J R 1959 Ski injuries. Am J Surg 98: 493–505
Moskowitz E 1971 Rupture of the tibialis anterior tendon simulating peroneal nerve palsy. Arch Phys Med Rehabil 52: 431–433
Mueller T J 1984 Ruptures and lacerations of the tibialis posterior tendon. J Am Podiatry Assoc 74: 109–119
Munk R L, Davis P H 1977 Longitudinal rupture of the peroneus brevis tendon. J Trauma 16: 803–806
Murr S 1961 Dislocation of the peroneal tendons with marginal fracture of the lateral malleolus. J Bone Joint Surg 43B: 563–565
Nicholas J A 1974 Ankle injuries in athletes. Orthop Clin North Am 5(1): 153–175
Nielson A L 1921 Diagnostic and therapeutic point in retrocalcanean bursitis. JAMA 77: 463
Nillius S A, Nilsson B E, Westlin N E 1976 The incidence of Achilles tendon rupture. Acta Orthop Scand 47: 118–121
Nisbet N W 1954 Tendo Achillis bursitis ("winter heel"). Br Med J 2: 1394–1395
Nistor L 1976 Conservative treatment of fresh subcutaneous rupture of the Achilles tendon. Acta Orthop Scand 47: 459–462
Nistor L 1981 Surgical and non-surgical treatment of Achilles tendon rupture: a prospective randomized study. J Bone Joint Surg 63A: 394–399
Norris S H, Mankin H J 1978 Chronic tenosynovitis of the posterior tibial tendon with new bone formation. J Bone Joint Surg 60B: 523–526
O'Brien T 1984 The needle test for complete rupture of the Achilles tendon. J Bone Joint Surg 66A: 1099–1101
Palmer D G 1970 Tendon sheaths and bursae involved by rheumatoid disease of the foot and ankle. Australas Radiol 14: 419–428
Parvin R W, Ford L T 1956 Stenosing tenosynovitis of the common peroneal tendon sheath: report of two cases. J Bone Joint Surg 38A: 1352–1357
Patterson R L Jr, Darrach W 1937 Treatment of acute bursitis by needle irrigation. J Bone Joint Surg 19: 993–1002
Pavlov H, Heneghan M A, Hersh A, Goldman A B, Vigorita V 1982 The Haglund syndrome: initial and differential diagnosis. Radiology 144: 83–88
Percy E C, Conochie L B 1978 The surgical treatment of ruptured tendo Achillis. Am J Sports Med 6: 132–136
Pöll R G, Duijfjes F 1984 The treatment of recurrent dislocation of the peroneal tendons. J Bone Joint Surg 66B: 98–100
Pozo J L, Jackson A M 1984 A rerouting operation for dislocation of peroneal tendons: operative technique and case report. Foot Ankle 5: 42–44
Puddu G, Ippolito E, Postacchini F 1976 A classification of Achilles tendon disease. Am J Sports Med 4: 145–150
Quigley T B, Scheller A D 1980 Surgical repair of the ruptured Achilles tendon: analysis of 40 patients treated by the same surgeon. Am J Sports Med 8: 244–250
Ralston E L, Schmidt E R Jr 1971 Repair of the ruptured Achilles tendon. J Trauma 11: 15–19
Reinherz R P 1984 Management of flexor hallucis longus tendon injuries. J Foot Surg 23: 366–369
Roberts P W 1929a Bursitis of the foot: a neglected cause of disability. Am J Surg 6: 313–317
Roberts P W 1929b Fifty cases of bursitis of the foot. J Bone Joint Surg 11: 338–344
Rubin B D, Wilson H J Jr 1980 Surgical repair of the interrupted Achilles tendon. J Trauma 20: 248–249
Ruch J A 1974 Haglund's disease. J Am Podiatry Assoc 64: 1000–1003

Sammarco G J, Miller E H 1979 Partial rupture of the flexor hallucis longus tendon in classical ballet dancers: two case reports. J Bone Joint Surg 61A: 149–150
Sarma P J 1940 The injection treatment of ganglions and bursae: indications and limitations. Surg Clin North Am 20: 135–140
Sarmiento A, Wolf M 1975 Subluxation of peroneal tendons: case treated by rerouting tendons under calcaneofibular ligament. J Bone Joint Surg 57A: 115–116
Sarrafian S K 1983 Anatomy of the foot and ankle: descriptive, topographic, functional. J B Lippincott, Philadelphia. pp 251–259
Saunders D E, Hochberg J, Wittenborn W 1978 Treatment of total loss of the Achilles tendon by skin flap cover without tendon repair. Plast Reconstr Surg 62: 708–712
Savastano A A 1980 Recurrent dislocation of the peroneal tendons. In: Bateman J E, Trott A W (eds) The foot and ankle: a selection of papers from the American Orthopaedic Foot Society Meetings. Brian C Decker, New York. pp 110–115
Schatzker J, Brånemark P-I 1969 Intravital observation on the microvascular anatomy and microcirculation of the tendon. Acta Orthop Scand (Suppl) 126: 1–23
Schedl R, Fasol P 1979 Achilles tendon repair with the plantaris tendon compared with repair using polyglycol threads. J Trauma 19: 189–194
Scheller A D, Kasser J R, Quigley T B 1980 Tendon injuries about the ankle. Orthop Clin North Am 11(4): 801–811
Scott W N, Inglis A E, Sculco T P 1979 Surgical treatment of reruptures of the tendoachilles following nonsurgical treatment. Clin Orthop 140: 175–177
Scranton P E Jr 1980 Metatarsalgia: diagnosis and treatment. J Bone Joint Surg 62A: 723–732
Sever J W 1912 Apophysitis of the os calcis. New York Medical Journal 95: 1025–1029
Shephard E 1975 Intermetatarso-phalangeal bursitis in the causation of Morton's metatarsalgia. J Bone Joint Surg 57B: 115–116
Shields C L Jr, Kerlan R K, Jobe F W, Carter V S, Lombardo S J 1978 The Cybex II evaluation of surgically repaired Achilles tendon ruptures. Am J Sports Med 6: 369–372
Sim F H, DeWeerd J H Jr 1977 Rupture of the extensor hallucis longus tendon while skiing. Minn Med 60: 789–790
Skeoch D U 1981 Spontaneous partial subcutaneous ruptures of the tendo Achillis: review of the literature and evaluation of 16 involved tendons. Am J Sports Med 9: 20–22
Snook G A 1972 Achilles tendon tenosynovitis in long-distance runners. Med Sci Sports Exerc 4: 155–158
Steffensen J C A, Evensen A 1958 Bursitis retrocalcanea Achilli. Acta Orthop Scand 27: 228–236
Stein S R, Luekens C A 1976a Methods and rationale for closed treatment of Achilles tendon ruptures. Am J Sports Med 4: 162–169
Stein S R, Luekens C A Jr 1976b Closed treatment of Achilles tendon ruptures. Orthop Clin North Am 7(1): 241–246
Stover C N, Bryan D R 1962 Traumatic dislocation of the peroneal tendons. Am J Surg 103: 180–186
Szczukowski M Jr, St Pierre R K, Fleming L L, Somogyi J 1983 Computerized tomography in the evaluation of peroneal tendon dislocation. A report of two cases. Am J Sports Med 11: 444–447
Taylor L W 1981 Achilles tendon repair: results of surgical management. In: Moore M (ed) Symposium on trauma to the leg and its sequelae. C V Mosby, St Louis. pp 371–384
Tehranzadeh J, Stoll D A, Gabriele O M 1984 Open-quiz solution: case report 271. Skeletal Radiol 12: 44–47
Teng M M H, Destouet J M, Gilula L A, Resnick D, Hembree J L, Oloff L M 1984 Ankle tenography: a key to unexplained symptomatology. Part 1: Normal tenographic anatomy. Radiology 151: 575–580
Teuffer A P 1974 Traumatic rupture of the Achilles tendon: reconstruction by transplant and graft using the lateral peroneus brevis. Orthop Clin North Am 5(1): 89–93
Thompson T C 1962 A test for rupture of the tendo Achillis. Acta Orthop Scand 32: 461–465
Thompson T C, Doherty J H 1962 Spontaneous rupture of tendon of Achilles: a new clinical diagnostic test. J Trauma 2: 126–129
Toygar O 1947 Cited by Arner et al 1958–1959
Trevino S, Gould N, Korson R 1981 Surgical treatment of stenosing tenosynovitis at the ankle. Foot Ankle 2: 37–45
Tudisco C, Puddu G 1984 Stenosing tenosynovitis of the flexor hallucis longus tendon in a classical ballet dancer: a case report. Am J Sports Med 12: 403–404
Webster F S 1968 Peroneal tenosynovitis with pseudotumour. J Bone Joint Surg 50A: 153–157
Weston W J 1970 The bursa deep to tendo Achillis. Australas Radiol 14: 327–331
White C S 1913 Retrocalcanean bursitis. New York Medical Journal 98: 263–265
Wicks M H, Harbison J S, Paterson D C 1980 Tendon injuries about the foot and ankle in children. Aust NZ J Surg 50: 158–161
Williams R 1963 Chronic non-specific tendovaginitis of tibialis posterior. J Bone Joint Surg 45B: 542–545
Wrenn R N 1975 Isolated injuries of posterior tibial tendon (abstract). J Bone Joint Surg 57A: 1035
Yancey H A Jr 1977 Lacerations of the plantar aspect of the foot. Clin Orthop 122: 46–52
Zadek I 1939 An operation for the cure of Achillobursitis. Am J Surg 43: 542–546
Zoellner G, Clancy W Jr 1979 Recurrent dislocation of the peroneal tendon. J Bone Joint Surg 61A: 292–294

Tuberculosis

INTRODUCTION

Disease of the ankle and foot accounts for less than 10% of osteoarticular tuberculosis and, in the northern hemisphere, examples are rarely seen. Tuberculosis is now an eminently treatable disease, but the propensity for tuberculous lesions to mimic other pathology and the infrequency of presentation often combine to delay diagnosis and increase morbidity.

In Africa and Asia, particularly on the Indian subcontinent, bone and joint tuberculosis remains common. Population movements in recent decades have increased the incidence of tuberculosis in Britain (Scott & Taor 1982, Sammon 1983, Davies et al 1984) and there is evidence of an increase in the proportion of bony lesions (Scott & Taor 1982). The diagnosis and treatment of tuberculosis of the foot and ankle thus retain their importance in orthopaedic practice. Even in temperate climes such lesions are more common than primary bone tumours (Jacob 1975).

Historical aspects

Bone and joint tuberculosis has been a taxing problem throughout orthopaedic history. Until effective chemotherapy became available surgery was regarded as a desperate measure to effect survival rather than to regain function. Thus Stiles (1912), analysing a series of 29 children with tuberculosis of the ankle, advocated surgery in order to encourage an osseous or firm fibrous ankylosis with eradication of the disease. Three of the 25 children followed up, however, were dead within a year of surgery, six underwent amputation and in only nine was a good long-term result achieved.

The introduction of streptomycin immediately after World War II, and the coincident improvement in living standards in Britain and North America saw a great reduction in the reservoir of infective cases of tuberculosis. The prolonged use of streptomycin rendered 5% of children totally deaf and 20% partially deaf, but it was considered a therapeutic success to gain the healing of a tuberculous joint even if it produced a deaf patient (Bosworth et al 1950).

As other effective antituberculous drugs became available and were used in combination, surgery was used to clear tuberculous granulomata and drain abscesses (Mukopadhaya & Mishra 1957), and the combination of rest, chemotherapy and surgery has remained the standard therapeutic approach.

PATHOLOGY

Incidence

Classically orthopaedic tuberculosis was predominantly a disease of childhood and adolescence, but while this remains true in populations with a large reservoir of untreated tuberculosis, the high-risk groups in temperate regions are now the indigenous elderly and young adults among the Asian immigrants. In England and Wales 4172 cases of tuberculosis were notified in the 6 months from October 1978 to March 1979 (Medical Research Council 1980). Among these notifications, 198 patients suffered from bone and joint tuberculosis; 79 whites, 108 from the ethnic group originating on the Indian subcontinent and 11 of other races. The estimated annual notification rates for orthopaedic tuberculosis were thus 29 per 100 000 for those from the Indian subcontinent ethnic group and 0.34 per 100 000 for whites (Davies et al 1984).

Anatomical distribution

In the rare form of disseminated cystic tuberculous osteitis (multiple pseudocystic tuberculosis of bone) which is a disease of infants and young children (Clinton-Thomas & Young 1955, O'Connor et al 1970) the diaphyses of the bones of the forearms, hands, legs and feet are involved, often symetrically, with multiple expansile lesions. Apart from this variant, osteoarticular tuberculosis is a centripetal disease.

The spine is involved in between 30 and 60% of cases while disease of the hip and knee are the next most common sites (Roaf et al 1959, Jellis 1979a, Sammon 1983, Davies et al 1984). In the series quoted above, tuberculosis of the ankle, tarsus and forefoot was present in between 4% and 12% of patients. In countries where a high proportion of cases present during childhood, there may be an increased proportion of disease of the extremities, possibly because of the peripheral distribution of active reticuloendothelial elements in which the disease may become established (Davies 1946).

Bone and joint infections occur by haematogenous spread from foci in the lungs or gastrointestinal tract, although it is now recognized that such primary foci can exist in many other organs (Crofton & Douglas 1975). Using standard diagnostic methods of investigation, evidence of active or recent tuberculosis elsewhere in the body may be found in between 10 and 20% of patients. In some areas of the world, however, concomitant active pulmonary disease is much more common: 34% in Korea (Medical Research Council 1973); 45% in Hong Kong (Medical Research Council 1974).

Types of lesions

Periarticular granuloma of bone

A granuloma in the metaphysis of the tibia or in the subchondral bone of the talus or other tarsal bones is the usual lesion in the ankle or foot. Infection spreads to the neighbouring joint and in children the epiphyseal cartilage does not act as a barrier. A secondary synovitis occurs with erosion of bone at the synovial attachments and beneath the articular cartilage, but lysis of the articular cartilage is very slow. Eventually cold abscesses and sinuses appear which drain the joint debris. Secondary infection may subsequently complicate the picture. Under favourable conditions, however, the infection may resolve and a fibrous ankylosis develops.

Osteitis of a single bone

Rarely, a central granuloma of the calcaneum may occur (Bosworth 1959, Manzella et al 1979) and occasionally tuberculous osteitis of a metatarsal base or phalanx without spread to the adjacent joints has been seen. In childhood tuberculous dactylitis a phalanx or phalanges may be expanded as if distended by air (Chapman et al 1979) giving the appearance known as spina ventosa.

Synovitis

Primary haematogenous synovitis probably occurs, but in the foot and ankle it is usually possible to demonstrate an adjacent bony lesion from which the infection has spread.

Tenosynovitis

Tenosynovitis and bursitis are usually late sequelae of established infections of the underlying bones.

CLINICAL PRESENTATION

Classically, bone and joint tuberculosis was a disease of childhood but patients may be of any age (Scott & Taor 1982) and of either sex. The onset of disease is insidious, with a history of aching pain in the bone or joint increasing over a period of weeks or months. Swelling of the surrounding tissue is at first soft and decreases overnight but later hardens to a brawny oedema. Hyperpigmentation of the overlying skin occurs in black patients and, in Africa, generations of scarifications from traditional treatment may substantiate the length of history (Fig. 30.1).

Night sweats are a fairly constant feature if specifically enquired for. There is often a history of close tuberculous contact and occasionally of debilitating illness or malnutrition. There is commonly a history of trauma, and although it is difficult to determine any aetiological significance, reports of tuberculosis developing in closed fractures (Stuart 1976) lend some credence to the theory that

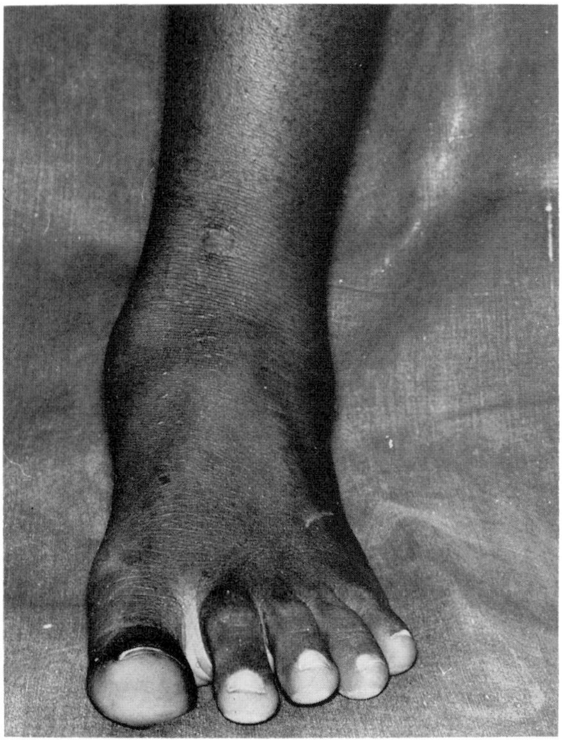

a

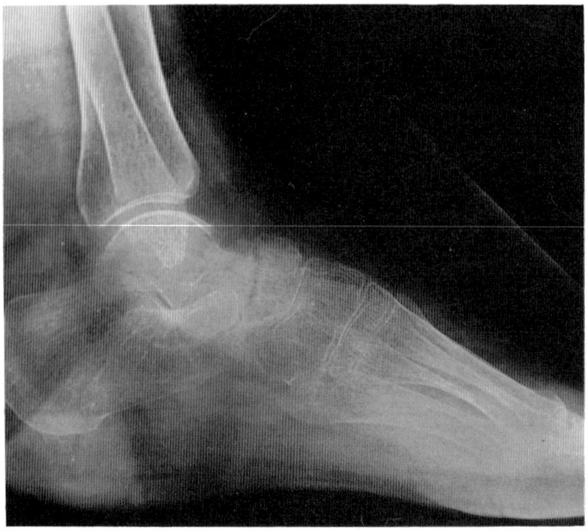

b

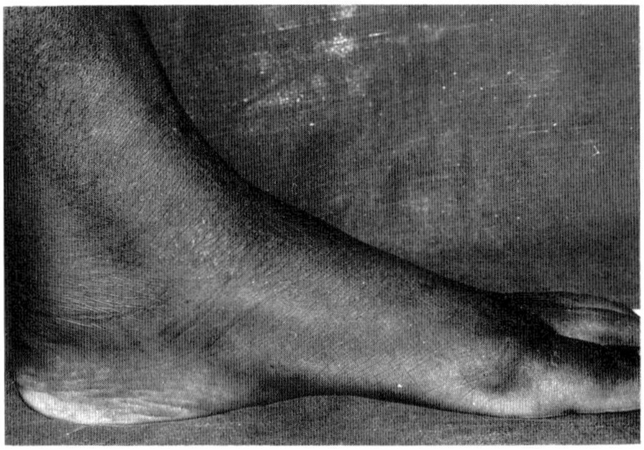

c

Figs. 30.1a,b,c Tuberculosis of the talonavicular joint

Case History
This 20-year-old woman had complained of pain and swelling over the dorsum of the foot for six months. She had received repeated courses of simple analgesics.

There was moderate swelling and tenderness over the talonavicular joint. The overlying skin showed slight hyperpigmentation and the transverse scars of traditional treatment. Dorsiflexion of the foot was limited and weight bearing was painful.

A Heaf test was strongly positive and the ESR 33 mm/h.

Debridement was performed and histology showed typical tuberculous granulation tissue and synovitis.

The patient was treated with streptomycin and Thiazina® and the foot was rested in a walking cast. Painless resolution occurred.

local trauma determines the site of establishment of this haematogenous infection. The stage of the disease at presentation is related to the availability of medical services but, even in Africa, it is now rare to find sinuses at initial presentation (Versfeld & Solomon 1982). The affected joint is usually moderately swollen and stiff with pain at the extremes of passive movement. Involved bones and the joint capsules are diffusely tender.

All such signs are nonspecific and the differential diagnosis on clinical grounds must include any form of subacute, traumatic or chronic arthritis. Acute staphylococcal osteomyelitis and septic arthritis can be excluded clinically unless the signs have been much modified by antibiotic therapy. In the tropics, the warm swollen foot of Kaposi's Sarcoma or the sinuses of Madura Foot may be impossible to distinguish clinically from an advanced tuberculous infection.

Delay in diagnosis is common in temperate regions (Enarson et al 1979) and surgeons should consider the possibility of tuberculosis where any chronic or recurrent lesion is responding poorly to apparently appropriate therapy.

INVESTIGATIONS

Radiology

There is a typical radiological pattern of bone and joint tuberculosis but appearances vary considerably with the age of the patient (Phemister & Hatcher 1933) and between members of the white and coloured races (Chapman et al 1979). Many of the radiographic signs such as soft tissue swelling, periarticular bone atrophy and epiphyseal overgrowth are common to any chronic joint inflammation. In addition, a wide range of uncommon appearances occur, rendering osseous tuberculosis the great mimic of other pathology (Standish et al 1977, Naidoo 1980).

Typically, an area of bone lysis develops in the metaphyseal, subepiphyseal or subchondral bone with surrounding osteoporosis and soft tissue swelling. There is usually little or no periosteal reaction and sclerosis around the lesion is uncommon except in the healing phase.

The margins of the articular bone surfaces are hazy and ill-defined but the joint space is preserved (Fig. 30.2) longer than in pyogenic arthritis because lysis of the sequestrated cartilage is slower.

In predominantly synovial disease, erosion of bone occurs at the synovial attachments. It is often impossible to distinguish, however, whether a bone lesion has spread to an adjacent joint or whether a haematogenous tuberculous synovitis has been responsible for progressive destruction of articular bone. To obtain a histological diagnosis in early cases, it is important to locate the tuberculous granuloma and oblique views (Fig. 30.2c) or tomography may help to locate the target area for biopsy.

Sequestrum formation, usually of the articular cortex, is not uncommon (Phemister & Hatcher 1933, Hunt 1964) but calcification at the margins of tuberculous abscesses or soft tissue granulomata is now rarely seen (La Fond 1958).

Pseudocystic expansile lesions of the phalanges (tuberculous dactylitis, spina ventosa), metatarsals and the os calcis may be seen in disseminated cystic tuberculous osteitis of infants and young children (Clinton-Thomas & Young 1955, O'Connor et al 1970) and tuberculous osteitis of the calcaneum occurs occasionally in older patients (Manzella et al

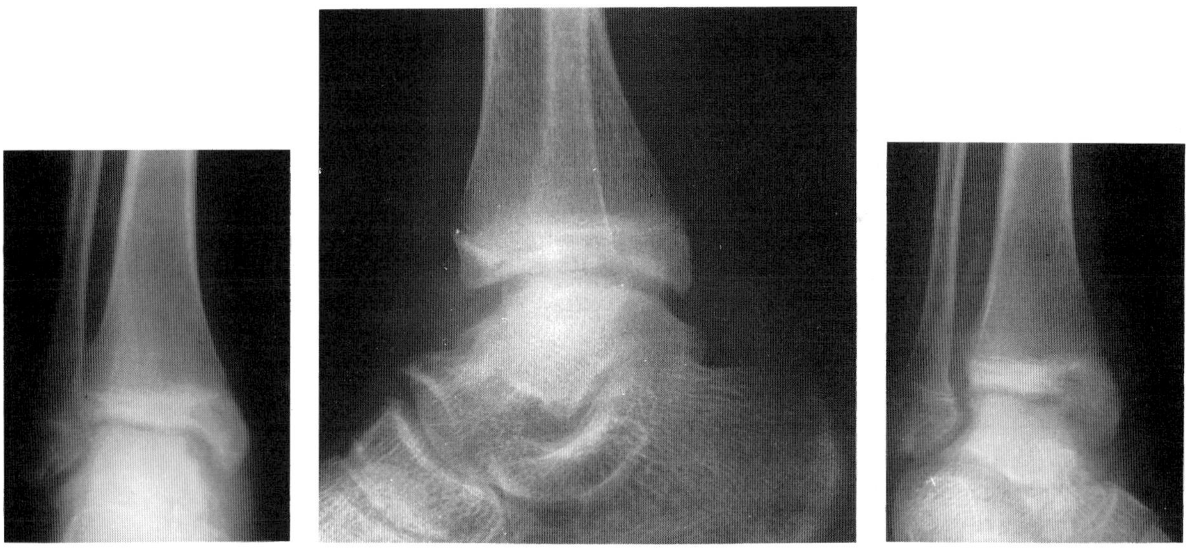

a b c

Figs. 30.2a,b,c Tuberculous arthritis of the ankle

1979). Classical spina ventosa, however, is not pathognomonic of tuberculosis and may occur in other chronic infections (Chapman et al 1979).

The spectrum of radiological appearances produced by bone and joint tuberculosis raises the possibility of a wide range of diagnoses. A metaphyseal lesion in a child, for instance, may mimic that of pyogenic osteomyelitis, a Brodie's abscess or a developmental cyst. Similar osteolytic lesions in adults may be due to tumour deposits, eosinophilic granuloma, osteolytic sarcoma or bone resorption around a radiolucent foreign body. The osteoporosis, periarticular erosions and eventual loss of joint space of tuberculous arthritis may be mistaken for those of rheumatoid arthritis, gout or nonspecific arthropathy unless there are other clues to the diagnosis and the possibility of tuberculosis is constantly borne in mind.

When the presence of osteoarticular tuberculosis is suspected, or indeed, proven, the search for lesions elsewhere in the patient should include radiography of the chest, spine, and renal tract.

In children, bony architecture may undergo remarkable restoration during healing (Papavasiliou & Petrapoulos 1981). During treatment there should be increased bone mineralization and areas of lysis should get smaller while their margins become more easily defined. Sometimes sclerosis of the surrounding bone will be seen.

Other investigations

If tuberculosis is confined to the foot or ankle, anaemia is unlikely to be a feature of the disease. A raised sedimentation rate (ESR), which is usually in the range of 20 mm to 100 mm/60 min (Westergren), and a relative lymphocytosis, are fairly constant features of established disease.

Heaf or Mantoux tests are of limited value. A strongly positive response often accompanies active tuberculosis, but negative testing may indicate freedom from disease or that overwhelming infection or malnutrition have suppressed the patient's immune response.

As evidence of tuberculosis in other systems is sought, bacteriological examination of urine and sputa should be included.

Definitive diagnosis

In over 90% of cases the infective organism is *Mycobacterium tuberculosis*. Infections with *M. bovis* are uncommon and other mycobacteria rarely affect bone.

A definite diagnosis can only be made by isolation of *Mycobacterium tuberculosis* from the lesion but bacteria are comparatively scanty in osteoarticular disease (Débaumont 1966). Positive cultures are usually obtained in 50% of cases from material taken from an infected bone or joint (Davies et al 1984). Positive cultures from other, usually pulmonary, lesions in the patient may raise the total bacteriological proof rate to 70% (Sammon 1983, Davies et al 1984). The use of liquid Lowenstein Jensen culture medium and the injection of material into cortisone-treated guinea pigs may furnish proof of a few more cases (Mathur et al 1980).

Histology

In areas and institutions where the culture of *M. tuberculosis* is not possible or when no growth is obtained, reliance has to be placed on the detection of acid-fast bacilli on smears stained by the Ziehl–Neelsen technique or on the typical histological appearance of a tuberculous granuloma (see Figs. 30.2d and e) with or without demonstration of acid alcohol-fast bacilli in the sections.

The incidence of false negative histological reports is high (Sammon 1983). The tuberculous granuloma may be confined to the primary bone focus and adjacent synovium only (Versfeld & Solomon 1980) whereas the subchondral erosion (Phemister and Hatcher 1933) and general synovitis (Versfeld and Solomon 1980) will show only chronic nonspecific inflammation, probably induced by the dead articular cartilage. The importance of a thorough radiological examination, to guide the biopsy of a representative specimen, cannot be over stressed.

TREATMENT

Treatment of orthopaedic tuberculosis consists of rest, chemotherapy and a variety of surgical interventions, and considerable judgement is needed

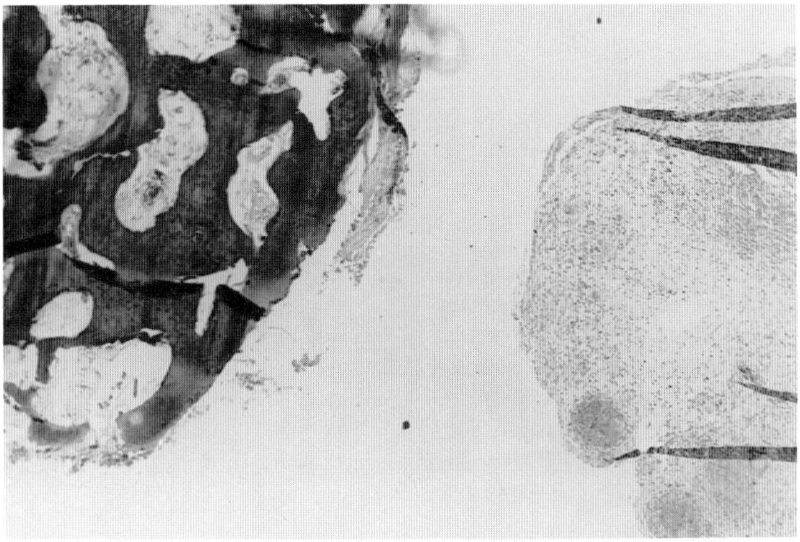

d

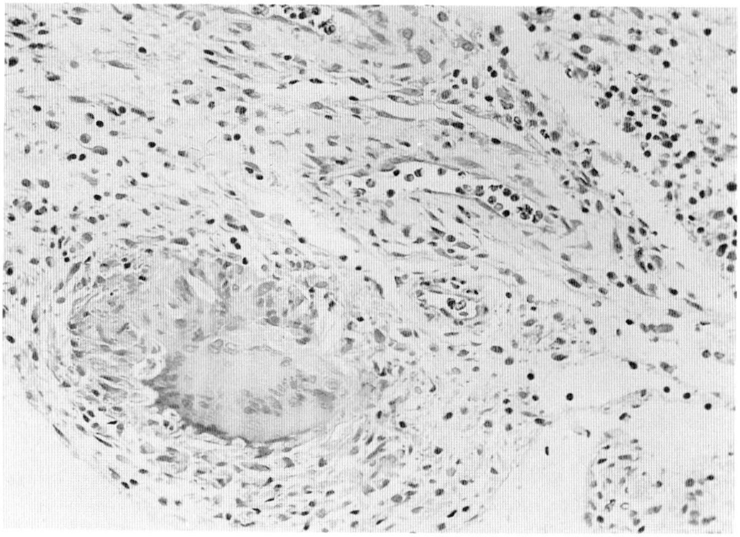

e

Figs. 30.2d,e Low and high power views of the histological appearance from the same patient

Case History

This 14-year-old girl presented with a four month history of gradually increasing pain and swelling of the right ankle. She had experienced night sweats but there was no history of trauma. For several periods of up to three months she had lived with a grandmother who had a chronic cough.

She had wasting of the calf muscles and swelling of the ankle which was most marked behind the lateral malleolus. She was tender over the joint line and the foot was held in moderate plantar flexion. All movements were restricted by pain.

A Heaf test was positive, ESR 64 mm/h and her chest radiograph was normal. The radiographs of the ankle (Figs. 30.2a,b and c) showed typical haziness of the joint outline with preservation of the joint space. The focus of disease in the tibial epiphysis is clearly seen in the oblique view (Fig. 30.2c).

Histological examination showed granulation tissue with giant cells, macrophages and lymphocytes (Figs. 30.2d and e) but no acid-fast bacilli were detected on special staining.

to match therapy with the demands of individual patients.

Surgery

The role of surgery is five-fold:

1. To obtain material for diagnosis
2. To assess the damage to the bone or joint
3. Debridement, which in this context is taken to mean the removal of sequestra, granulomata and any fibrotic barrier to the blood supply of the area
4. Synovectomy if the synovium is excessively thickened
5. Arthrodesis of an irretrievably destroyed joint

In early lesions a single exploration, biopsy and curettage may suffice and healing is achieved by chemotherapy and rest. It may prove impossible, however, to predict whether a damaged joint will heal well enough to bear weight without pain.

When severe destruction has already occurred, especially in the presence of sinuses and secondary infection, initial biopsy and debridement may usefully be followed by several months of chemotherapy before arthrodesis is performed.

As in most bone infections, age has a profound effect on outcome. Remarkably swift recovery may be seen in young children on chemotherapy alone whereas in the elderly, indolent lesions with sequestra formation are the rule. They demand surgical clearance or prolonged chemotherapy.

Chemotherapy

Extensive trials have shown that healing of bony tuberculous lesions is possible with chemotherapy alone (Griffiths 1978) but morbidity may continue for a considerable time and it is often impossible to ensure that patients receive adequate treatment (Jellis 1979b). Surgical clearance and shorter courses of the newer anti-tuberculous agents (rifampicin and ethambutol) with isoniazid have markedly reduced the necessary treatment period and produced an earlier return of the patient to mobility. The chemotherapeutic agents in current use are listed in Table 30.1. Hypersensitivity reactions of the patient or resistance shown by a particular strain of *M. tuberculosis* may necessitate adaptation of the chosen regime and second-line drugs will be needed occasionally (Friedman & Kapur 1973).

Where there is strong clinical and laboratory evidence of a tuberculous lesion, chemotherapy may, with advantage, be started a week or so before surgical intervention. There seems little danger, however, of causing dissemination of untreated disease during surgery. Prolonged preoperative chemotherapy or a 'therapeutic trial' may produce a confusing diagnostic dilemma. Several non-tuberculous infections will respond to anti-tuberculous chemotherapy and prolonged drug treatment may considerably modify the bacteriological and histological pattern of a tuberculous lesion.

The first choice for chemotherapy is a combination of rifampicin, isoniazid and ethambutol (Friedman & Kapur 1973). These drugs have good patient compliance, reach high concentration in bone (Sirot et al 1977) and may considerably shorten the course of treatment needed.

Unfortunately, in the developing countries where tuberculosis is common, cost often precludes the widespread use of rifampicin and ethambutol. Under these circumstances a combination of streptomycin and Thiazina® (see Table 30.1) may be considered standard therapy. Rifampicin and ethambutol are reserved for patients who have had previous antituberculous therapy, or who are known to harbour drug-resistant bacteria. These drugs are also indicated where the patient's resistance to a severe tuberculous infection is thought to be compromised by intercurrent disease or malnutrition.

Operative treatment

Biopsy

If a well localized granuloma (pseudocyst) is present or if a case of diffuse synovitis is being investigated, it may be feasible to employ drill or needle biopsy techniques. However, if tuberculosis is suspected I prefer to combine open biopsy with a thorough assessment of the adjacent joint and probably some degree of debridement.

The approach should be the most direct available, excising any sinuses or passing through abscesses if these exist. A representative specimen of tuberculous granulation tissues should be sought for histological and bacteriological investigation.

Table 30.1 Chemotherapeutic agents in current use

Drug	Dose		Administration	Length of treatment
Streptomycin	Adult	0.75–1.0 g/d		
	Child	15–25 mg/kg/d	Intramuscular	60–90 days
Isoniazid	Adult	300 mg/d		Usually for 18 months but may
	Child	10 mg/kg/d	Oral single dose	be continued for several years if doubt of cure exists
Rifampicin	Adult	600 mg		
	Child	10 mg/kg/d	Oral single dose	90–180 days
Ethambutol	Adult	25 mg/kg/d reducing to 15 mg/kg/d after 60 d	Oral single dose	60 days at full dose then continued at reduced dose for 18 months with isoniazid
Thiacetazone	Adult	150 mg/d		
	Child	5 mg/kg/d	Oral single dose	*18 months with Isoniazid

*Note: Thiacetazone is only used as a first-line drug in direct combination with Isoniazid (Thiazina®, Smith and Nephew Pharmaceuticals); alone it has weak tuberculostatic action.

Debridement should include the removal of sequestra, pus or caseous material, loose or damaged cartilage and any synovium and capsule that is excessively thickened. The bone lesion should be curetted or cut back to normal bone and thick fibrous encapsulation excised.

Assessment

At this stage a decision should be made whether:

1. with rest and chemotherapy the joint may regain an acceptable weight-bearing capacity,
2. it would be in the patient's best interest to perform an immediate arthrodesis, or whether
3. infection, and possibly secondary infection, should be treated before planned arthrodesis is considered.

Special considerations

Age

The higher metabolic activity of childrens' bones renders healing faster and sequestra are less likely to form. Initial surgery should be conservative.

The ankle joint

During exploration the articular cartilage should be thoroughly inspected and loose areas excised. Granulation tissue should be curetted from the talus and tibia. If it is thought that a useful joint may be obtained the wound should be closed and the leg elevated in a split cast for four weeks or until swelling has subsided. A below knee non-weightbearing cast should then be worn for three to six months as judged by the radiological evidence of bony healing.

If the ankle has been extensively damaged, arthrodesis is necessary. It is safe to perform fusion at the time of exploration if the soft tissues are mobile and little bone resection is required. In the presence of sinuses, abscesses or gross bone destruction, however, thorough debridement should be followed by further medical treatment with the ankle elevated in a cast or backslab. Only when swelling has subsided, sinuses have healed and the patient's general condition (as measured by weight gain, falling sedimentation rate and a relative lymphocytosis) has improved, can a formal arthrodesis be planned with assurance of primary healing.

No particular method of arthrodesis has any special advantage over another. The surgeon should choose the method with which he is most familiar and with which he achieves acceptable results. I use a transfibular approach with compression exerted through calcaneal and tibial Denham pins by Charnley clamps. Any incongruities and defects should be packed with cancellous bone from the iliac crest or upper tibial metaphysis.

Tarsus

Disease of the subtalar joint and talus may be treated in a similar manner. Tuberculosis of the talus in a child may result in crushing of the bone necessitating talectomy. In adults, only a minor degree of destruction can be tolerated before peritalar arthrodesis, subtalar fusion or a standard triple arthrodesis will be needed to allow weight bearing free of pain.

Calcaneum

Disease of the calcaneum is rare. If the lesion is centrally situated I prefer to explore the calcaneum through a heel-splitting approach (Gaenslen 1931). This gives wider access than a lateral cortical window and leaves the peroneal tendons undisturbed. The calcaneum is split longitudinally so that tuberculous debris can be curetted from each half of the bone. No cortical bone is removed and the wound is left open. During healing the skin edges invert, so removing pressure from the scar, and there is little change in heel architecture. In a severe infection this is considerably less disabling than excision of the calcaneum, the alternative procedure.

Midtarsal joints

Disease confined to the talonavicular joint, calcaneocuboid joint or between the joints of the cuneiforms and the metatarsal bases, can usually be treated by debridement. After wound healing immobilization in a walking cast for six weeks is usually sufficient for this type of disease. If pain remains a problem, a formal arthrodesis using a block of cancellous bone and compression screw fixation should be performed.

Metatarsals and phalanges

All but minor infections of the second to fifth metatarsals and their phalanges may be speedily eradicated by the subperiosteal resection of the affected bone. After wound healing the support of a firm boot will soon produce a painless foot.

We adopt a more conservative attitude to disease of the great toe and first metatarsal because of their greater role in walking. Debridement and curettage of the lesion should be followed by elevation in a plaster cast until all swelling has subsided and the bone appears strong enough to bear weight.

FUTURE PROSPECTS

It is conceivable that prosthetic replacement of the ankle or the use of Silastic® spacers in the foot, may enable mobility to be retained after eradication of tuberculous infection. However, already there have been reports of recurrence after prosthetic replacement of tuberculous hips (Johnson et al 1979) and there seems little reason to embark on such surgery in the ankle or foot.

In conclusion, I should reiterate that osteo-articular tuberculosis is an eminently treatable disease if recognized at presentation. Unless the possibility of this great mimic is borne in mind, modern chemotherapy and surgery will not be able to restore function to joints destroyed by months or years of undiagnosed tuberculous arthritis (Fig. 30.3).

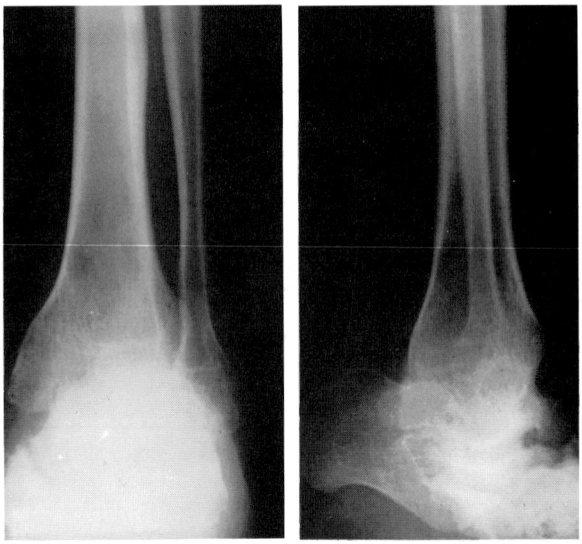

Fig. 30.3 Tuberculosis of the ankle with secondary infection showing loss of the joint space and widespread destruction of the talus

Case History
This 40-year-old man presented with pain and swelling of his left ankle for two days. He also complained of night sweats and loss of weight but no cough. Three years previously he had been treated for 'chronic osteomyelitis' of the ankle by incision and a course of tetracycline. This gave some relief but he had

had recurrent episodes of pain, swelling and discharge of pus since then.

His foot was swollen and held in moderate equinus and there was pain on attempted dorsiflexion. There was a small sinus over the anterior aspect of the ankle.

His white cell count was normal and the ESR 13 mm/h. Culture from the sinus grew gram-positive cocci but a biopsy showed epitheloid granulomata formation and central caseation of the Langhan's giant cells consistent with active tuberculosis.

ACKNOWLEDGEMENTS

I am grateful to Mr W B McGowan FRCS (Edin) Senior Lecturer, Department of Surgery of the University of Zimbabwe, for supplying the clinical details, radiographs and histological slides for Figures 30.2 and 3. I also thank Mr Afzal Ansary AIMBI, Head of the Department of Medical Illustration of the University of Zambia for preparing the illustrations.

REFERENCES

Bosworth D M 1959 Treatment of bone and joint tuberculosis in children. J Bone Joint Surg 41A: 1255–1266
Bosworth D M, Della P A, Fawell R F 1950 Streptomycin in tuberculous bone and joint lesions with mixed infections and sinuses. J Bone Joint Surg 32A: 103–108
Chapman M, Murray R O, Stoker D J 1979 Tuberculosis of the bones and joints. Semin Roentgenol XIV: 266–282
Clinton-Thomas C L, Young W B 1955 Multiple pseudo-cystic tuberculosis of bone. J Bone Joint Surg 37B: 624–631
Crofton J, Douglas A 1975 Respiratory disease, 2nd edn. Blackwell, Oxford. pp 232–233
Davies D U 1946 Synovial membrane and synovial fluid of joints. Lancet ii: 815
Davies P D O, Humphries M J, Byfield S P et al 1984 Bone and joint tuberculosis. A survey of notifications in England and Wales. J Bone Joint Surg 66B: 326–330
Débaumont A 1966 Bactériologie de la tuberculose ostéo-articulaire sous chimothérapie. Adv Tuber Res 15: 125–188
Enarson D A, Fujii M, Nakielna E M, Grzybowski S 1979 Bone and joint tuberculosis a continuing problem. Can Med Assoc J 120: 139–145
Friedman B, Kapur V N 1973 Newer knowledge of chemotherapy in the treatment of tuberculosis of bones and joints. Clin Orthop 97: 5–15
Gaenslen F J 1931 Split-heel approach in osteomyelitis of the os calcis. J Bone Joint Surg 13: 759. Quoted in Crenslaw A H (ed) Campbell's Operative Orthopaedics, 5th edn 1971. C V Mosby Company, St Louis
Griffiths D U 1978 The treatment of tuberculosis of bone and joint. Trans R Soc Trop Med Hyg 72: 559–563
Hunt 1964 Problems in diagnosing osteoarticular tuberculosis. JAMA 190: 95–98
Jacob P 1975 Tuberculosis of bones and joints. In: Sutton D, Granger R G (eds) A textbook of radiology, 2nd edn. Churchill Livingstone, London. p 49
Jellis J E 1979a Symposium: surgical tuberculosis: discussion. Proc Assoc Surg East Afr 2: 54–55
Jellis J E 1979b Tuberculous arthritis and osteitis in Zambia. Proc Assoc Surg East Afr 2: 56–59
Johnson R, Barnes K L, Owen R 1979 Reactivation of tuberculosis after total hip replacement. J Bone Joint Surg 61B: 148
LaFond E M 1958 An analysis of adult skeletal tuberculosis. J Bone Joint Surg 40: 346–364
Manzella J P, Vanvoris L P, Hruska J F 1979 Isolated calcaneal tuberculous osteomyelitis. J Bone Joint Surg 61A: 946–947
Mathur M, Bhatia V N, Agarwal D S, Abbott M G 1980 Detection of acid fast bacilli in material from cases of bone and joint tuberculosis. Indian J Pathol Microbiol 23: 255–260
Medical Research Council 1973 A controlled trial of ambulant out-patient treatment and in-patient rest in bed in the management of tuberculosis of the spine in young Korean patients on standard chemotherapy. A study in Masan, Korea. First report of the working party on tuberculosis of the spine. J Bone Joint Surg 55B: 678–697
Medical Research Council 1974 A controlled trial of anterior spinal fusion and debridement in the surgical management of tuberculosis of the spine in patients on standard chemotherapy: A study in Hong Kong. Fourth report of the MRC working party on tuberculosis of the spine. Br J Surg 61: 853–866
Medical Research Council 1980 National survey of tuberculosis notifications in England and Wales 1978/79: report from the Medical Research Council Tuberculosis and Chest Diseases Unit. Br Med J 281: 895–898
Mukopadhaya B, Mishra N K 1957 Treatment of tuberculous sinuses and abscesses of osteo-articular origin. J Bone Joint Surg 39B: 326–333
Naidoo K S 1980 The great imitator. J Bone Joint Surg 62B: 279
O'Connor B T, Steel W M, Sanders R 1970 Disseminated bone tuberculosis. J Bone Joint Surg 52A: 537
Papavasiliou V A, Petropoulos A V 1981 Bone and joint tuberculosis in children. Acta Orthop Scand 52: 1–4
Phemister D B, Hatcher C H 1933 Correlation of pathological and roentgenological findings in the diagnosis of tuberculous arthritis. Am J Roentgen 29: 736–752
Roaf R, Kirkaldy-Willes W H, Cathro A J M 1959 Surgical treatment of bone and joint tuberculosis. E S Livingstone Ltd, Edinburgh. Ch 2 p 4
Sammon D J 1983 Bone and joint tuberculosis in Glasgow: the present situation. Scott Med J 28: 48–56
Scott J E, Taor W S 1982 The changing pattern of bone and joint tuberculosis. J Bone Joint Surg 64B: 250
Sirot J, Lopitaux R, Cluzel R, Delisle J J, Sauvezie B 1977 Diffusion de la rifampicine dans l'os non infecté chez l'homme. Ann Microbiol (Inst Pasteur) 128B: 299–236
Standish W, Hyndma J, Forsythe M 1977 Skeletal tuberculosis the great imitator. J Bone Joint Surg 59B: 511
Stiles H J 1912 Discussion on the after results of major operations for tuberculous disease of the joints. Br Med J 2: 1356
Stuart D 1976 Local osteo-articular tuberculosis complicating closed fractures. J Bone Joint Surg 58B: 248
Versfeld G A, Solomon A 1980 Tuberculosis of bone and joint. J Bone Joint Surg 62B: 284
Versfeld G A, Solomon A 1982 A diagnostic approach to tuberculosis of bones and joints. J Bone Joint Surg 64B: 446

Pyogenic infections

Text books about lower limb and foot conditions prior to the introduction of antibiotics in the 1940s tended to include a chapter or so on infections. This is given less attention nowadays. Surgical experience with major foot infection mirrors general medical experience over the years. In most developed countries the incidence has lessened with improved standards of living, improved nutrition, hygiene and cleanliness, better shoe wear and protective shoe wear in industry and agriculture. The more effective management of injuries aided by worldwide communication, appropriate preoperative preparation, as well as the availability of adequate chiropody have all played a part in reducing the incidence of foot infection.

Notwithstanding these facts, the introduction of antibiotics has revolutionized the treatment and outcome. Even so, management can still prove difficult.

In the more developed parts of the world a large part of experience is concerned with the increasing age of the population, and patients with diabetes, secondary infection in rheumatoid arthritis, neuropathic disorders and circulatory problems of the lower limbs, both arterial and venous. Added to these are patients with secondary sepsis from ingrowing toe nails and ill-fitting 'fashionable' shoes. Indeed any general or orthopaedic ward will also have its share of patients with secondary sepsis following operative surgery or chiropody.

In the less developed world, experience is probably the same as in the past in, say, Western Europe, with secondary sepsis following trauma by far the most common. Interestingly, with increasing urbanization and industrialization, experience in the large cities of the developing world is faced with ancient problems as well as those presently occurring in the richer countries. So major hospitals in the developing world see a spectrum of cases ranging from those of rural parts of the country (representing the past) to those of the urban areas (representing the present) which includes disorders of the elderly or the more 'well to do' or those secondary to surgery (including advanced prosthetic implantation or arthroplasty).

The importance of major foot infections lies not only with the fact that a great reduction in this incidence is possible, but also, that should infection occur, it is often necessary for these patients to be admitted to hospital or to remain in hospital even if the condition is less life-endangering than hitherto. These factors carry important economic implications for both the individual and the society in which he lives.

AETIOLOGY

Being the distal end of the longest extremity, and having a ready exposure to trauma, the foot has a naturally lessened vitality due to relatively poor circulation compared with elsewhere. There is a reduced potential for healing. As sensation lessens with age, the foot demonstrates the effect of diminished resistance to infection, no matter what the virulence of the organism. Rheumatoid patients, the elderly, those with malnutrition, patients with diabetes and nephritis, alcoholics and the debilitated constitute the 'at risk' patient. These now include immunosuppressed patients, those on steroids and patients with local circulatory problems such as varicose veins and ulcers, arterial insufficiency related to smoking, neuropathies, and gout. Other predisposing local factors include rigid deformity (with corns) and the use of physical agents causing trauma.

Perforating ulcers and bed sores in paraplegic and tetraplegic patients, as well as trophic ulceration from other causes including myelodysplasia, must be included.

Rare causes of infection include ergotism and the injudicious use of tourniquets particularly in the elderly or the diabetic.

Trauma is a factor in localizing the infection, by decreasing the local resistance and with haematoma formation providing a nidus for metastatic infection.

Primary acute infections of the foot

Primary acute haematogenous osteomyelitis of the foot is rare compared to elsewhere. The pathological process is not dissimilar; although acknowledged as part of a bacteraemia, there is probably some degree of septicaemia in every case. The incidence is higher in the poorer communities, but it can attack the fittest and the best fed quite 'out of the blue'. Local trauma usually determines the localization. Acute septic arthritis in neonates is known as Tom Smith's arthritis (1874). In the neonate there is probably an immature defence mechanism. However, persisting reduction in host defences after acute haematogenous osteomyelitis in childhood was not found by Gillespie et al (1983). In adults the condition occurs in patients with lowered resistance and there is reason to believe that in some there is a transient or continued immune deficiency as in Acquired Immune Deficiency Syndrome. Thus any of the 'at risk' patients may suffer the same infection.

Subacute and chronic primary infections of the foot

Such diseases as brucellosis, actinomycosis and other fungal infections are often associated with local trauma as well as a generally poor nutrition and are common in less developed countries in the malnourished. Tuberculosis and fungal infections are dealt with in another chapter.

Chronic primary osteomyelitis seems to affect the calcaneus more frequently than other bones. Osteomyelitis of the metatarsals and other tarsal bones is more frequently secondary to crushing injuries or compound fractures.

Secondary major infections of the foot

Secondary infection is far more widespread. In the less developed parts of the world (as in earlier times elsewhere) the major cause is trauma. The type of case is determined by the environment, whether urban or rural, coastal, forest or desert. For example, within two months one has seen admitted to a District Hospital on the east African coast infections secondary to the following conditions: plantar ulcers with cellulitis (after thorns, sharp objects or sticks have punctured the foot or toes), skin loss following injury by sea urchins or stingray; excessive heat or actual burning applied to relieve the severe pain in these conditions; burns or boiling water; bites of snakes, dogs, crocodiles or other wild animals; old neglected injuries from farming implements (hoes); fungal infections or 'jigger' infestation; abrasions or injuries from coral or rock; hook worm infestation; perforating ulcers from malnutrition; neoplasia (Fig. 31.1), Kaposi's sarcoma and malignant melanoma. Not surprisingly none of these patients wore shoes.

In more developed countries similar examples would include industrial, farming or gardening injuries, lacerations, road traffic accidents, subungual haematoma from great toe crush injuries, blisters, burns, callosities, bunions, bursae, and compound fractures, all of which predispose to secondary infection.

Major infection following compound fractures of the foot from industrial or road traffic accidents and especially from blast or explosive injuries, are a difficult group of cases. They are frequently associated with multiple injuries.

Many have iatrogenic causes such as skeletal pin track infection of the calcaneus, forefoot operations with or without prosthetic implants and poor chiropody. Occasionally after local injections of steroids in plantar fasciitis, in patients of whom some will also have undergone radiotherapy (not an uncommon practice in the past), complication by sepsis is likely to be somewhat resistant to treatment.

Repair of the ruptured tendo Achillis is not infrequently encumbered by low grade infection after wound breakdown (Fig. 31.2) even in the best institutions.

Apart from secondary sepsis following surgery, whether a minor procedure in an office or outpatient casualty department or after major operations,

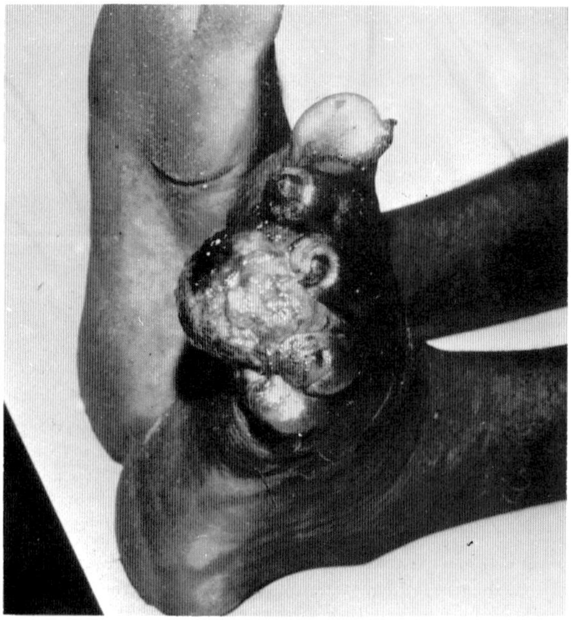

Fig. 31.1a Secondary foot infection in a male patient with malignant melanoma

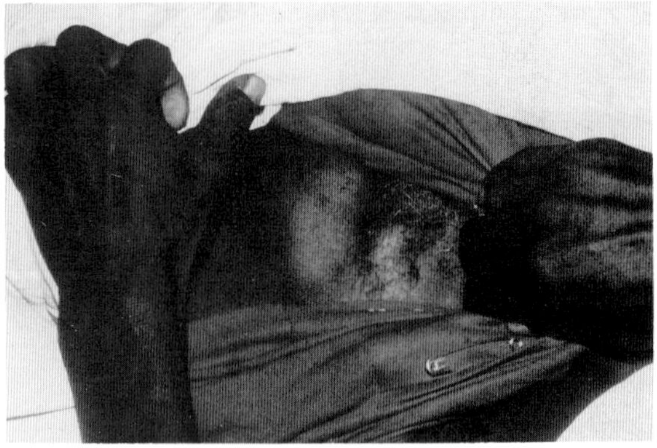

Fig. 31.1b Same patient, enlarged inguinal nodes

Puncture wounds

Secondary infections from puncture wounds form an interesting group. They may be from thorns, needles, pins, 'rusty nails' or splinters of wood. They may result in gram-negative osteomyelitis which is relatively rare, as described by Gordon et al (1974),

secondary infection has to be considered more likely in the 'at risk' patient referred to earlier (Fig. 31.3, 4, 5).

Recent infection of a bunion or ingrowing toenail presents the likelihood of secondary infection if definitive surgery on the same foot is undertaken too early. Moreover the use of local anaesthetic or the use of a tourniquet is unwise in the presence of infection for fear of spread.

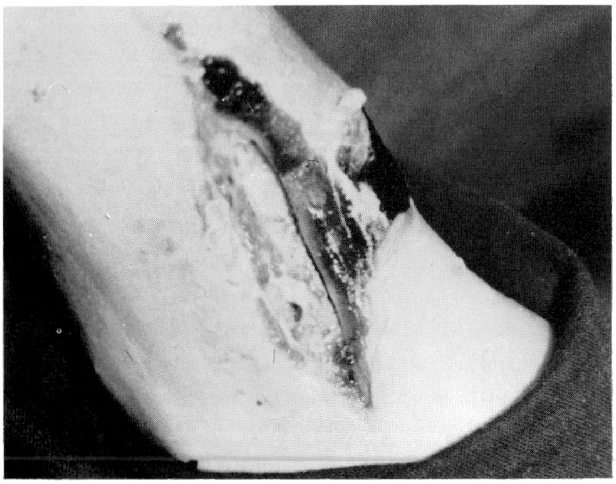

Fig. 31.2a Wound separation with secondary infection after repair of the tendo Achillis

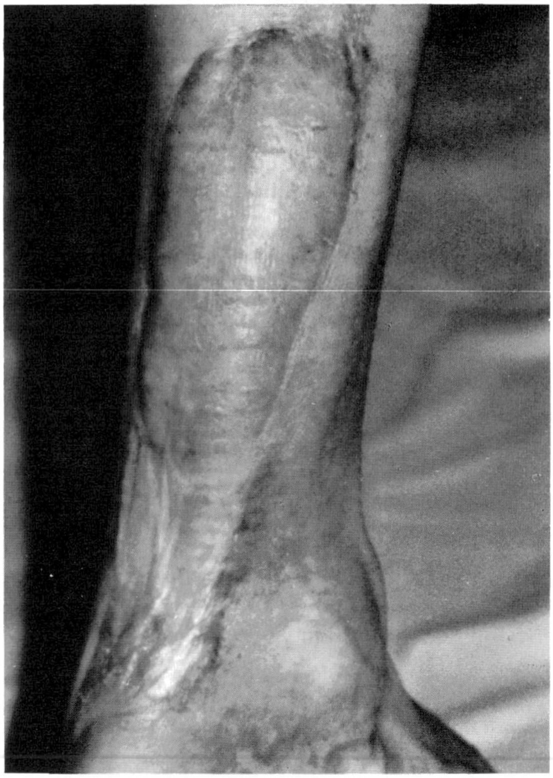

Fig. 31.2b Same case after myocutaneous grafting: standing on the toes

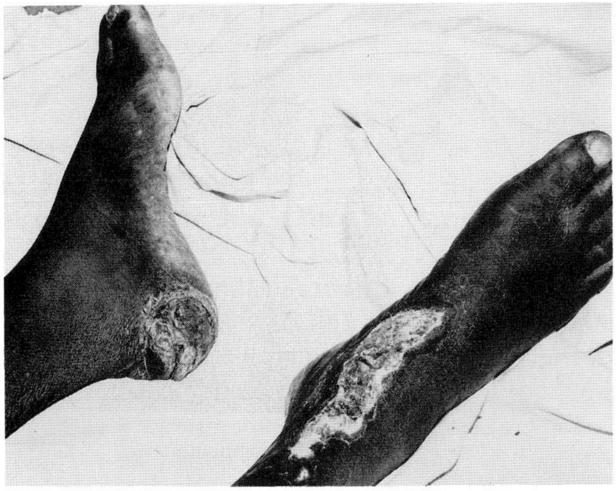

Fig. 31.3 Ulceration of the heel and lower leg in an elderly diabetic who was blind. Secondary infection after trauma with diabetic neuropathy

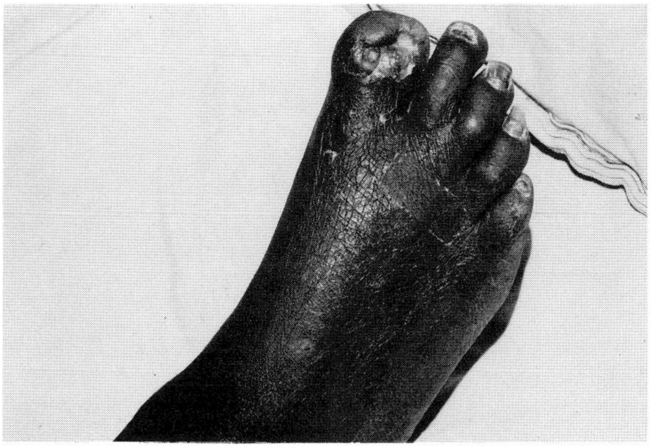

Fig. 31.4 Infection of the great toe, after amputation of the other leg, in a diabetic aged 52 years

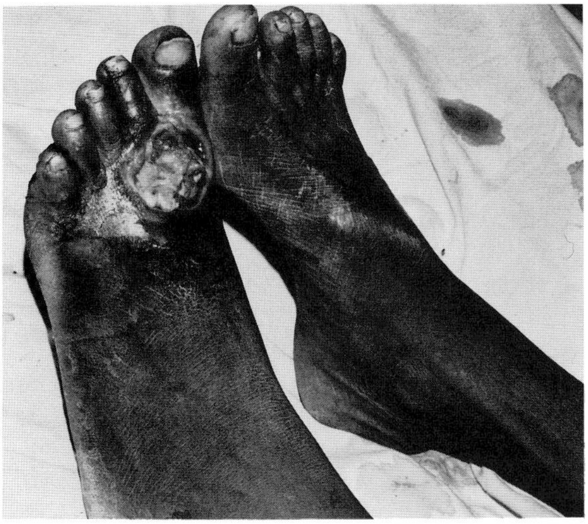

Fig. 31.5a Ulceration of the dorsum of the foot affecting the extensor tendons

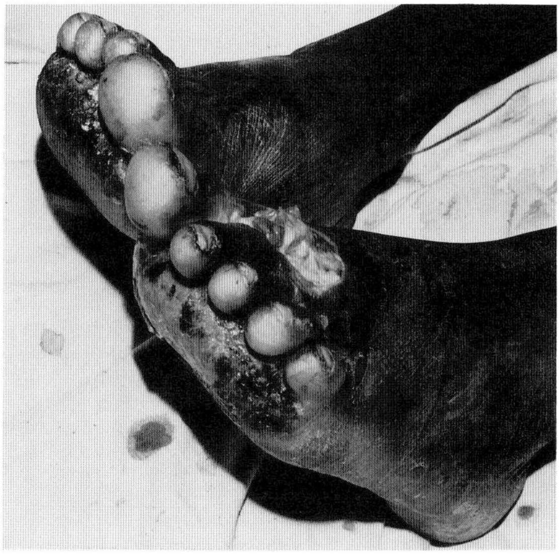

Fig. 31.5b With 'jigger' infestation in the same diabetic patient

Miller & Semian (1975) and Nuber & Anderson (1982). Such puncture wounds can affect all ages. The organism found is not from the usual flora or commensals, but is probably opportunistic from the environment carried in with the foreign body which may be retained.

Pseudomonas aeruginosa osteomyelitis after puncture wounds has been described by MacKinnon (1975). He refers to similar experiences reported by Johanson (1968) describing 11 cases, Minnefor et al (1971), and Hagler (1971). Like Brand & Black (1974), all stress the importance of adequate surgery as well as the use of antibiotics (gentamicin).

Fitzgerald & Cowan (1975) and Lang & Peterson (1976) described osteomyelitis of the foot from puncture wounds in children stating that serious complications ensued if the wound penetrated the physeal plate, joints or articular cartilage, the infection becoming chronic and refractory. Usually there were no systemic problems.

Although infrequent, these injuries are potentially serious and usually aggravated by inadequate treatment of the primary wound. Once established, the infection is best treated by aggressive surgical debridement and the appropriate antibiotics.

PREDISPOSING FACTORS AND PREVENTION

The different aetiological factors described earlier indicate their own preventive measures. Whether it be the fisherman on the east African coast wading out on coral or stung by sea urchins, agricultural or factory workers or barefoot children, protective shoewear is the key. Most especially this applies to patients with loss of sensation such as leprosy patients or diabetics and also to those with poor circulation — the 'at risk' patients. Patients with myelodysplasia and diminished sensation are advised to 'budget their walking' (Hogshead 1966).

In the more sophisticated parts of the world the need for careful chiropody and regular inspection of the feet is well known. Minor foot problems such as ingrowing toe nails, especially in diabetics and those with poor circulation require careful chiropody. This cannot be overemphasized.

Thus prophylaxis takes into consideration the type of footwear, care of the nails and general protection of the feet, care of corns, blisters and abrasions, and even the use of a particular style of scissors. Powerful antiseptics should be avoided to reduce devitalization.

Skin preparation is necessary before phlebotomy or before inoculation in infants to prevent infections or even osteomyelitis as described below. Antisepsis is vital when carrying out any venepuncture or umbilical vein puncture in infants.

Quite simply, sensible shoe wear to protect feet can reduce many hospital admissions and avoids considerable morbidity and even life-threatening problems in the various environments described.

General preparation for surgery

Prior to foot surgery the patient should have a bath or shower preferably with the use of hexachlorophene in an antiseptic detergent. To reduce postoperative infection careful preoperative foot preparation is necessary. Minimally, in the ward, this involves thorough washing with soap and water and other simple local measures such as the use of spirit, but iodine and flavine obscure the colour of the skin and so the state of the circulation. Proflavine is out of favour because of skin toxicity thought to be common in negro races and because of its powerful antigenic character. In the operating theatre preparation with povidone-iodine, followed by the application of tincture of chlorhexidine is probably the best protocol at present available. Any colouring should be washed off with spirit immediately before drying and towelling for the operation.

Regimes differ but all are aimed at reducing secondary operative infection from the skin. Shaving is not usually necessary for feet and is probably contraindicated anyway.

Skin preparation is now less complicated for 'cold' planned operations. The time of admission to hospital before operation should be minimal as the patient soon becomes host to the existing hospital pathogens which are frequently multiantibiotic resistant.

Traditional orthopaedic procedures involved much more and prolonged preparation. However, those who would advocate even less stringent measures than those described here, had best heed the studies described by Cruse (1977) in a prospective study of 30 000 wounds, which showed the significantly lowered incidence of secondary infection from such preoperative skin preparation.

Minor injuries

Casualty departments of hospitals are faced with many injuries which initially appear to be minor, e.g. injuries from glass, thorns, abrasions, minor cuts and burns, but which if not treated carefully could lead to crippling changes due to secondary infection. This entails care of even the seemingly least dangerous injury — 'a mere pin prick'. Apart from thorough cleaning with soap and water and painting the wound with 1% Mercurochrome®, the application of a clean sterile dressing should be considered. Where possible the feet should be exposed to dry. Attention to the subsequent shoe wear and avoiding continued walking in wet and dirty conditions should go a long way in preventing secondary infection.

Major injuries

Compound fractures and more extensive lacerations and wounds require admission to hospital for urgent and perhaps more extensive surgery.

In the operating theatre, after the usual skin preparation, the wounds should be kept moist with saline or Hartmann's solution. Hydrogen peroxide should be used where there is considerable tissue damage and delayed surgery. Dilute chlorhexidine or povidone-iodine aqueous solutions are also recommended. Powerful antiseptics are precluded to avoid further tissue devitalization.

Finally the wounds are washed out with sterile water or saline before proceeding with the necessary debridement (described under Treatment).

CLINICAL PRESENTATION AND DIAGNOSIS

Acute osteomyelitis

Acute haematogenous osteomyelitis may affect any bone of the foot or ankle region but is less common than elsewhere in the limbs; a single bone may be involved or more. Typically it follows relatively minor local recent trauma such as a bruise, although there may be no known incident. There is also frequently a history of infection such as a boil or furunculosis elsewhere and it usually occurs in the ill-nourished, puny child. In the infant the condition may be difficult to diagnose with poor localizing signs initially and hence the presentation as a pseudoparalysis.

The os calcis and talus are the most frequently affected bones in the foot. The patient arrives with local pain, ill with fever and unable to walk on the painful foot. The general toxaemia may seem out of proportion to the local signs in some cases. Later, local swelling, limitation of movement, inflammation, oedema and even blistering of the skin occur. Spreading proximal lymphangitis and then adenitis follow. Rigors may develop, the child becoming rapidly ill and requiring admission to hospital.

Patients with reduced resistance may present late, with severe spreading local changes, but often with relatively little pain and toxaemia. Neonates may be brought in extremis, with the whole limb or foot full of pus.

In acute haematogenous osteomyelitis the brief history is typical. Initially there will be no X-ray changes. In this phase a blood culture is necessary and if positive, the antibiotic sensitivity. Local injection of sterile saline into the area affected followed by aspiration to obtain the organism can be fruitful. The organism may also be obtained from the urine on occasion. A polymorphonuclear leucocytosis in the blood white cell differential count is characteristic, but not the rule in the younger child, the elderly or the debilitated. However, the erythrocyte sedimentation rate (ESR) is almost invariably raised. Above 20 mm/h is significant, even in children and in subacute infections. Changes in the blood counts and sedimentation rates are important in assessing progress and response to treatment.

Recording clinical progress is all important. This not only includes the local signs but also the systemic effects and observations of the temperature; the extent of the pain especially in acute haematogenous osteomyelitis, the spread of the swelling, inflammation, lymphangitis and adenitis, and oedema should be recorded. These observations and records are necessarily made in hospital.

Differential diagnosis

Clinically foot sepsis has to be distinguished from soft tissue trauma, fractures, stress fractures, Still's disease, and perhaps any form of paralysis in children. Additionally, consideration has to be given to gouty conditions, rheumatoid arthritis, arteriovenous malformation, metastatic aneurysm in association with bacterial endocarditis, other forms of polyarthritis including seronegative forms as described by Capen & Scheck (1981), gonococcal infections, benign or malignant lesions (primary or secondary), Sudeck's atrophy or post-traumatic dystrophy and also metabolic bone disease.

Ultimately surgery may be necessary for drainage or biopsy. This carries the advantage of definitive diagnosis by obtaining the actual organism and its antibiotic sensitivity, although this may not be available if antibiotics have already been commenced.

Sickle-cell osteomyelitis

Tests for sickle-cell disease are important particularly where there are multiple sites of osteomyelitis. Both sickle cell trait (AS) and sickle-cell disease (SS or SC) show a tendency for osteomyelitis whether in acute or less acute forms. Sickle-cell disease itself is characterized by osteomyelitis at various sites and is of a recurrent nature associated with crises. The infection may be due to a number of different organisms including *Staphylococcus* as well as *Salmonella* or *Klebsiella* organisms.

Secondary infections of the foot

These are most commonly secondary to trauma such as minor abrasions and puncture wounds, as well as major wounds and compound fractures.

A mild infection is localized, perhaps superficial, with relatively little pain, fever, or illness. It may present as a slight inflammation of the wound, slight swelling, and little discharge or dysfunction; delayed healing may be the worst aspect.

A moderate infection associated with increasing severity is characterized by increased local signs of pain, inflammation, swelling and overlying oedema with a wound showing definite sepsis, the patient becoming febrile.

Severe infection is evident when there are further increased local signs, with further spread and loss of control, lymphangitis and adenitis accompanied by increasing systemic signs: pyrexia, a swinging temperature, tachycardia, malaise and rigors.

Any adjacent cellulitis and a rapid increase in the local and focal signs indicate a severe form of infection with a virulent organism such as β-haemolytic *Streptococcus*, or deep infection due to *Staphylococcus*.

Depending upon the organism, abscess formation ensues. This not only occurs locally in the foot, but may be in the draining lymph nodes.

Even with successful treatment following severe foot infection, there is inevitably delayed healing and frequent permanent disability from stiffness, scarring and deformity.

Complications

These include proximal spread, ultimately causing an inguinal abscess, direct spread and necrosis of adjacent structures in the foot — tarsals, metatarsals and joints. Involved tendons rapidly necrose especially if exposed. Joint destruction and sequestration, with chronic sinus formation are features of chronic infection of the foot.

Increasing skin necrosis occurs with chronic ulceration and secondary infection, aided and abetted by powerful topical applications and careless surgery. Such chronic infection leads to destruction of the tissues causing contractures and deformities of the foot and ankle. This inevitably implies chronic pain, instability and permanent lameness.

With very prolonged chronic osteomyelitis and chronic discharge from a sinus, a Marjolin's ulcer with neoplastic change becomes a possibility (Fig. 31.6).

Sudeck's atrophy — post traumatic dystrophy — is characterized by severe pain and dysfunction often out of proportion to the severity of the injury. It may occur with an uncomplicated injury, but arise with secondary infection. The foot tends to be swollen and shiny with a tendency for cyanosis when dependant. All the tissues atrophy and the joints tend to stiffen.

Ultimately, in severe sepsis with tissue destruction and secondary to severe trauma, gas gangrene may follow. At any stage from the initial acute phase, or even in more chronic forms especially with lowered patient resistance, septicaemia remains a significant possibility, and an important factor to consider in the management of any foot infection.

ANATOMICAL SPREAD OF INFECTIONS

Infection adjacent to the toenail may spread to the dorsal fascial space. Infections of the toe itself,

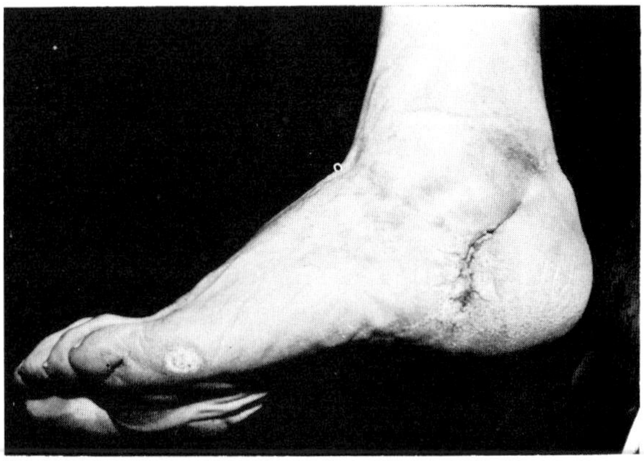

Fig. 31.6 A chronic sinus from the calcaneus with Marjolin's ulcer, 40 years after a war wound

particularly on the plantar surface, may cause a secondary infection of the superficial plantar fascial space. This is the same as the first plantar fascial space of the central compartment (as described in Gray's textbook of anatomy). Interdigital infection, if it spreads to a fascial space, will follow the lumbrical muscles to involve the second and third fascial spaces of the central compartment. An infection of the dorsal subcutaneous space likewise will follow the course of the lumbrical muscles to infect the second and third spaces of the central compartment.

Since the dorsal subcutaneous space and the middle two spaces of the central compartment are connected an infection of the second and third fascial spaces may result in swelling on the dorsum of the foot. In cases of a penetrating wound, the infection may be carried directly to the central compartment.

Cellulitis presenting with swelling, redness and induration, may be associated with a localization of the infection in the deep fascial space and the formation of pus. Deep pus is often present when there is pitting oedema.

Acute suppurative arthritis of any of the joints of the foot due to an infection with pyogenic organisms such as *Staph. aureus, Strep. haemolyticus*, an infection introduced through a puncture wound, secondary to an osteomyelitic abscess penetrating a joint or metastasis through the blood stream, is frequently a problem in children.

CLINICAL BACTERIOLOGY

In osteomyelitis of the feet the range of possible organisms responsible is wide. However, by far the most common is *Staph. aureus*. Whitehouse & Smith (1970) listed other possible organisms affecting the feet: typical and atypical mycobacteria, fungi, Friedländer's bacillus, *Clostridium welchii, Pseudomonas aeruginosa, Neisseria, Strep. pneumoniae* and the salmonellae (usually in sickle cell disease). In addition there are viral infections, variola and rubella affecting the feet as part of a generalized infection in the newborn. They also report the decreasing incidence of congenital syphilis and leprosy, all too common in the less developed parts of the world.

Haemophilus influenzae is not uncommon in the infant in acute joint infection and is of increasing importance according to Nelson & Koontz (1966) and Almquist (1970). *P. aeruginosa* seems to be the common infection in puncture wounds as described above.

According to Antoniou & Conner (1974) coagulase positive organisms tend to cause acute infection and coagulase negative Staphylococci to cause subacute infection. Interestingly they also reported that acute infections affected the calcaneus and subacute ones the talus.

Serratia marcescens acute osteomyelitis of the foot was reported by Thomas et al (1980). One of the patients was elderly and had had an acute sprain of the ankle. The other had cardiac and nephrotic problems. Neither responded to treatment until the appropriate antibiotics (co-trimoxazole and gentamicin) were used. They considered this organism as opportunistic rather than saprophytic.

Acute infection from *Strep. haemolyticus* should be considered in the presence of cellulitis especially in the 'at risk' patient.

Secondary or chronic infection is also usually due to *Staph. aureus* causing abscesses, and is frequently seen with infections from ingrowing toenails, blisters, and following neglect or careless treatment of callosities.

Infections secondary to abrasions, lacerations and other wounds as well as those secondary to surgery (often in diabetics) may be due to mixed infections with *P. aeruginosa, Escherichia coli, Proteus mirabilis* or anaerobic Streptococci. Similar mixed infections and those due to gram-negative organisms are seen in puncture wounds.

Uncommon forms of osteomyelitis due to *Salmonella, Brucella*, coccidioidomycosis, blastomycosis, actinomycosis, Madura foot, lues, leprosy and *Bacteroides* were described by Curtis (1973). Typhoid osteomyelitis of the calcaneus due to direct inoculation was reported by Monsoor (1976), occurring in a six-year-old girl after she had trodden on a nail while playing barefoot in the fields. She was treated successfully by curettage and local and systemic chloramphenicol.

Clostridial myonecrosis (gas gangrene) may follow severe trauma and neglect. It is frequently seen when tissues are devitalized and usually necessitates urgent amputation. Anaerobic streptococcal infection, although it does not usually have such rapid spread, is also likely where there has been severe devitalization.

In no other anatomical region can one see a better illustration of the effect and result of balancing the type of organism and its virulence against the local or general resistance of the host patient in determining the outcome and prognosis. The foot has potentially serious inherent disadvantages compared to other tissues and regions.

X-RAY DIAGNOSIS

X-rays are important not only to demonstrate the late destruction and reactive changes of the bones and joints, but also to localize foreign bodies, e.g. metal and glass. Sinography should be considered in the presence of a chronic sinus; nonopaque foreign bodies as well as sequestra and the presence of bone cavities may be detected in the chronic phase. More sophisticated soft tissue X-rays are useful, including tomography on occasions.

Screening with image intensification may localize foreign bodies during surgery, reducing excessive X-ray exposure and prolonged surgery in these cases. Foreign bodies are notoriously difficult to find in the foot. Gas shadows on X-ray may indicate the presence of anaerobic infection and gas gangrene.

The extent of bone or joint destruction seen helps in planning the treatment and the necessary surgery, including the need for extensive exploration, or in deciding which type of fusion is necessary. Pathological dislocations (Fig. 31.7) will be revealed.

Sudeck's atrophy and disuse atrophy are characterized by gross osteoporosis, but the latter usually has no pain, and may develop from misguided advice for unnecessarily prolonged non-weightbearing.

In subacute and chronic infections, X-ray changes become evident. However, these changes are not necessarily diagnostic. There has been excessive dogma about the radiological differences between pyogenic and tuberculosis infections of the foot, as well as other pathological processes. Smith et al (1971) stated that on X-ray appearance the differential diagnosis also includes metabolic disease and benign and malignant lesions. All these cause osteolysis or reactive periostitis. Indeed, trauma can produce similar changes (e.g. march fracture). These authors illustrated the broad spectrum of subtle X-ray variations which occur with inflammatory lesions of the foot.

Lindenbaum & Alexander (1984) say that the literature contains numerous statements describing

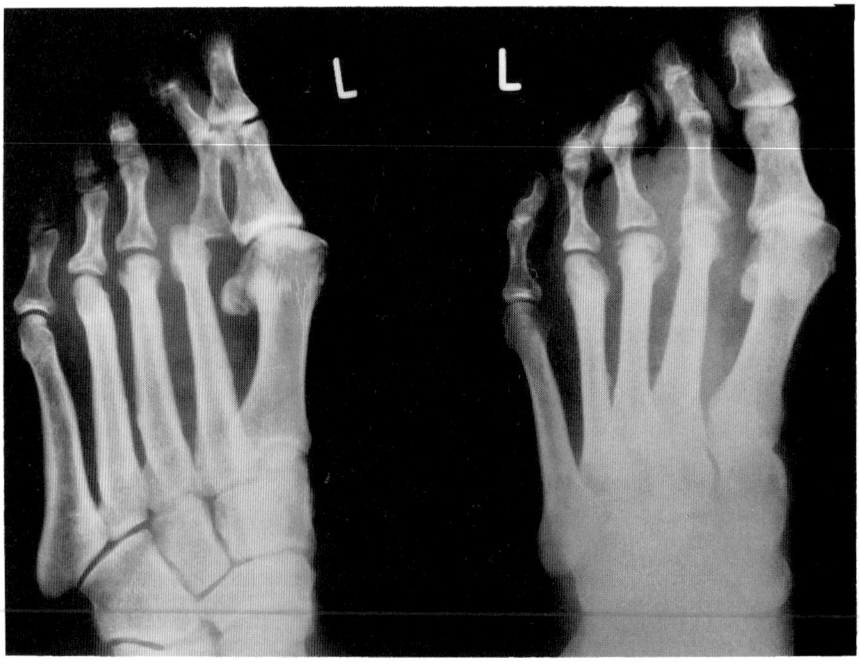

Fig. 31.7 Pathological dislocations with forefoot sepsis in an adult with neuropathy and diabetes

the clinical and radiographic similarities of Ewing's sarcoma and osteomyelitis.

Jaffe & Lichtenstein (1940) had already found that a significant percentage of cases previously reported as osteoid osteoma were in fact cases of osteomyelitis. Kandel & Mankin (1973) found that the most common mistake in diagnosis for osteoid osteoma proved to be osteomyelitis.

Charosky & Marcova (1977) report a case with *S. paratyphi* osteomyelitis at the lower end of the tibia simulating an osteoclostoma.

Again Smith et al (1971) emphasized the late occurrence of X-ray changes in acute osteomyelitis. They drew attention to the frequent failure of the X-rays to reflect the activity of the disease in chronic osteomyelitis and to the fact that X-ray appearances are rarely pathognomonic of a particular disease or diagnosis in the foot.

SPECIAL INVESTIGATIONS

Scintigram radioisotope screening with Technetium 99, methylene disphosphonate can be useful for both acute and chronic cases to localize 'hot spots' due to hyperaemia in osteomyelitis (O'Brien et al 1982, Gilday et al 1975, Hughes 1980, Gelfand & Silberstein 1977). A 'blood pool' can be seen on scanning within 24 hours of the onset in acute osteomyelitis and is a useful procedure in the diagnosis of osteomyelitis in children.

Gallium 67 citrate scanning may demonstrate any leucocytosis locally and is useful in the early diagnosis of infections including secondary infection after surgery (Deysine et al 1975).

Newman et al (1984) have shown that the elevated lactate found in synovial fluid (usually between 3.06 to 20.4 mmol/l^{-1}) is consistent with septic arthritis and that a lower level excludes infection.

Where available anti-Staphylococcal titres should be assessed including teichoic antibodies. The findings of teichonic acid antibodies is considered by Tuazon (1982) of great value in the early diagnosis of acute osteomyelitis caused by *Staph. aureus* and useful in assessing clinical response to treatment; it is not reliable in septic arthritis. These tests can differentiate septic osteomyelitis from tuberculous osteitis in the more chronic case.

Serological investigations may be necessary, for example in *Brucella* infections and *Salmonella* osteomyelitis (typical in sickle cell disease). Such reactions usually have to be repeated to observe changes in the titres before reaching a diagnosis, increasing titres being significant.

More recently sophisticated investigations have been employed in the assessment of the patient's overall resistance and immune studies are worth considering in the unexplained acute infections. Some of these patients have an underlying immune disorder, as in Hodgkin's disease and other related blood and lymphatic disorders.

TREATMENT

Antibiotics

The use of antibiotics is crucial in limb or life-threatening conditions particularly in established acute major infections of the foot. Appropriate antibiotics are chosen from the blood or local culture and tested for antibiotic sensitivity. Where possible antibiotic blood levels should be monitored.

Until the laboratory results are available broad spectrum antibiotics or combinations of these are favoured, especially to cover mixed infections. They should preferably be bactericidal. Depending upon the environment, in acute major infections systemic crystalline penicillin in high doses intravenously still plays a part. In patients who have been in hospital for any length of time, cloxacillin, flucloxacillin, or ampicillin may be necessary. Lincomycin or clindamycin have a place depending upon the organism and sensitivity and the seriousness of the infection. The advantages have to be weighed against possible complications and side effects, in particular the possibility of pseudomembranous colitis from these agents.

Gentamicin, employed against *P. aeruginosa* and other mixed infections, has to be used parenterally. The more recent cephalexin has become necessary for both gram-negative and gram-positive organisms. Co-trimoxazole, together with gentamicin, has also been employed in mixed infections. Carbenicillin and ticarcillin are more recent antibiotics for *Pseudomonas* infections. However, in the absence of systemic effects (a raised temperature and toxity) and without gross local signs of sepsis, the mere finding of *Pseudomonas* can be ignored, especially if the local blood supply is good and the foot infection is resolving. Netilmicin or vancomycin should be used in multiresistant *Staph. aureus* infection.

Intravenous antibiotic therapy is the quickest and best way to provide the necessary blood concentration in serious major foot infections. The regime described by O'Brien et al (1982) is preferred: 100 mg/kg/day of cloxacillin in four divided doses and 30 mg/kg/day of fusidic acid in three divided doses are given in a bolus injection. These achieve serum levels exceeding the usual inhibitory concentrations for staphylococcal strains as reported by Garrod et al (1973). The limb should be splinted and 250 units of sodium heparin per 500 ml of infusion reduces the incidence of superficial thrombophlebitis caused by the fusidic acid. Intravenous therapy is recommended for such cases for three weeks followed by oral therapy for six weeks. The additional use of metronidazole is advisable where anaerobic infection is suspected.

When employed, antibiotics are usually necessary for at least six weeks for major bone or joint infections, but for purely soft tissue infections the period may be less. One is guided by the local and general signs, the level of pain and the blood sedimentation rate during the course of management.

Local instillation of antibiotics into a joint are not necessary in acute infective arthritis, because effective concentrations are present in systemic therapy (Nade 1983). Nevertheless, as a preventative measure, during routine major surgery of the foot in the 'at risk' patient, the use of topical kanamycin or rifampicin should be considered. Bingham et al (1974) had no secondary infections in 700 consecutive cases in three years when using routine topical kanamycin irrigation. The selection of antibiotics for foot infections must take heed of any likely allergies or known patient sensitivities in the usual way.

Especially in the acute infection, the response must be monitored closely and the regime changed if necessary. What would be applicable today may well change in the course of time, especially as hospital pathogenic organisms have a habit of changing their resistance to antibiotics. Combinations of antibiotics may not be the answer indefinitely. The choice of antibiotics must necessarily take into consideration the relative cost, avoiding the habit of using the more costly when there is a genuine choice.

Although antibiotics are still recommended in the debilitated, elderly and those with poor circulation or diabetes, the routine use of antibiotics for lacerations, compound fractures or planned 'cold' operations is unwise, and carries a decided risk of promoting resistant organisms generally in the hospital concerned or in the case itself.

Indeed, antibiotics should be avoided whenever possible. Foot infections are often low grade, subacute, or chronic and not limb or life-threatening. Unnecessary antibiotics invite the culture of resistant or unexpected organisms which themselves *can* be limb or life-threatening. This was dramatically illustrated in the case of chronic foot ulcers and osteomyelitis described by Miscew et al (1979). The patient was treated with oxacillin and although he had no vascular deficiency or diabetes, within 60 hours of the start of parenteral antibiotics, spreading gas gangrene necessitated amputation. This was a rare form of gas gangrene due to *C. sporogenes*.

The leading article by Nade (1983) on acute septic arthritis in childhood, although not confined to the foot, included a comprehensive consideration of the use of antibiotics by himself and other authorities.

Other systemic measures

In addition to appropriate prophylactic antibiotics, to prevent tetanus and gas gangrene antisera should be considered. The use of antiserum in the presence of gas gangrene is generally agreed. It should also be considered prophylactically in severe wounds in which there is delay in treatment and especially those occurring in wartime injuries, in those involved in agricultural work and those with serious devitalizing injuries with much muscle damage and with compound fractures of the foot and lower limb. However, antiserum in tetanus has largely fallen into disuse, certainly as a prophylactic measure, because of the incidence of allergic reactions (including anaphylaxis) to the horse serum from which it is prepared. In the presence of clinical tetanus, special preparations are necessary, including that prepared from human sera.

Antitetanus toxoid immunization is obligatory in soiled wounds, especially in agricultural workers, those with foot injuries in the underdeveloped world and in children running about barefoot. Even minor foot injuries, such as a small puncture wound, in those keen on gardening should be considered for immunization against tetanus.

Other systemic measures include the need for analgesics, sedatives and fluid replacement as well as the treatment of accompanying disorders such as diabetes.

Hyperbaric oxygen therapy has been used in the treatment of chronic osteomyelitis (Morrey et al 1980). Colwill & Maudsley (1968), Maudsley & Colwill (1966) used hyperbaric oxygen in gas gangrene. With reasonably economic means (100% oxygen in 2 atmospheres of pressure undertaken for 2 hours twice daily, in a small one-man chamber) it was possible to reduce the mortality. Hyperbaric oxygen is only an adjunct to surgery and antibiotics, and these two sets of workers related their failures to inadequate surgery.

Local measures

To prevent infection, old injuries, severe injuries with compound fractures and crush injuries should not be closed primarily. This does not mean there should be no surgery. Debridement is necessary, excising severely damaged and devitalized tissues and muscles after the usual wound toilet. Indeed the surgery itself is important, with careful handling of tissues at all times to prevent further devitalization and damage. When left open, the wound is gently packed with gauze and kept moist with saline. The foot should be supported with a well padded plaster of Paris slab in the anatomical position with the ankle at 90° to avoid permanent contractures and deformity. The limb is elevated. After above five days most cases are suitable for secondary suturing to reduce the possibility of gross scarring.

However, some may be left open to granulate and epithelialize. Occasionally split skin grafting is necessary. Some of the more chronic cases or those with considerable skin loss require cross-leg pedicle or myocutaneous grafting as described by Ger (1983) to provide a more supple foot, and the latter also provides a better circulation to combat infection.

It is emphasized that in all severe, contaminated, and crushing injuries, as well as old injuries, primary closure should be avoided. The urge to stitch all lacerations indiscriminately frequently results in secondary infection and necrosis in foot and lower limb injuries.

In established acute infections of the foot undergoing systemic treatment, twice daily inspections are necessary, particularly where conservative measures are being employed. With any lack of response or with signs of spread, more radical measures including open drainage are necessary. Abscess formation necessitates incision and drainage. Aspiration rarely achieves much in the foot at this stage. Dorsal abscesses are drained dorsally, avoiding transverse incisions. In deep plantar sepsis the approach is best carried out on the medial plantar border adjacent to the first metatarsal as described by Henry (1959). The wounds may be left open or packed with saline or boric soaked dressings. Secondary suturing or skin grafting is then necessary. However, if there is a localized abscess and no oedema, tension or cellulitis, primary wound closure is possible.

Plantar incisions, unless there is a pointing abscess, are best avoided as they may leave thickened painful scars and contractures with secondary deformities. Drainage should not be through to the dorsum of the foot.

Gross sepsis with ingrowing toenails requires initial resection or removal of the nail to allow the infection to settle down prior to any definitive surgery regarding the toenail bed. Very severe infection of a toe, especially if bone or joint is involved may necessitate amputation of that toe.

In the foot itself, abscess formation in acute osteomyelitis requires only drainage of the pus found superficially. Radical drilling of the bone is not necessary and indeed potentially harmful, causing unnecessary bone necrosis. Any surgery should be as conservative as possible. Donald's advice (ca.1951) 'do not let the pus out when there isn't any' should be heeded for fear of causing unnecessary further tissue destruction or spread of infection.

Earlier text books on diseases of the foot prior to the introduction of antibiotics, for example that by Hauser (1940), go into considerable detail in describing treatment of infection at each of the anatomical sites and likely complications. Hauser also states that surgical intervention should be avoided unless 'unquestionably indicated'.

An indication for surgery is a localized abscess in the bone, with inadequate drainage, or the presence of a sequestrum. Drainage of the abscess is obtained by opening the cavity with minimum trauma to the surrounding tissue. The local management includes packing of the wound gently with Vaseline® gauze, and supporting the limb in a plaster of Paris cast with a window cut out for sterile dressings. Hauser elevated the limb to about the height of an ordinary pillow to facilitate circulation and to prevent oedema and swelling. The general management has not altered much; he advised rest, fluids (to produce 1500 ml of urine daily), analgesics and sedatives. In those days sulphanilamide was the only antibiotic available and was used for surgical sepsis, especially that due to *Strep. haemolyticus*.

In summary, the principle in the treatment of established severe infection of the foot involves eradication by antibiotics, surgical drainage if necessary, general systemic treatment, local rest and assisting the circulation, usually by elevating the limb. Admission to hospital is generally necessary. With any life-threatening state, amputation should be considered although this is now less often indicated.

Chronic infections and salvage procedures

In the aftermath of acute osteomyelitis, the presence of necrosed cortical bone will be seen at the base of the wound, or on X-ray, or presumed to be there. If still attached to healthy bone there is no urgency to remove it provided there is no gross sepsis. It should be left as long as possible to preserve the architecture of the foot, particularly in children. With sequestrated or loose bone, or bone with gross sepsis and chronic sinuses, surgery is necessary; the infection will not clear until the necrotic material is removed. This includes foreign bodies or implants used in surgery.

Any resulting pain or deformity may necessitate secondary surgery: the excision of bony prominences and the need for limited or extensive arthrodesis where there has been destruction of weight-bearing joints. Radical measures may be necessary to get rid of chronic infection, from partial to total removal of the affected bone. This is possible even after many years of chronic infection with sinuses.

Ultimately, with any spreading infection or with gross destruction which is disabling and deemed to be incurable, some form of amputation may be necessary and indeed beneficial. The likelihood of spread, septicaemia, malignancy, chronic pain and disability can be prevented or overcome.

In some, particularly in diabetics and others with neuropathy and ischaemia the decision to amputate is made by the loss of pain control as described by Catterall (1964). In others selection includes the likelihood of further major foot infection, proximal spread of infection or secondary neoplastic change.

Apart from a window in a plaster cast for dressings (Fig. 31.8), external skeletal fixation has been found useful in gross infection in the tarsal region (see under Talus). This allows the exposure of the wound for dressings and regular inspection without its being obscured by plaster of Paris.

Chronic infection of a weight-bearing joint which has lost its articular cartilage is best treated by means of a formal surgical fusion, especially where the condition remains painful. Spontaneous fusion characteristically may occur, but the foot requires adequate and prolonged support in plaster or in surgical boots while this process is continuing. Properly planned surgery can reduce the morbidity and the length of hospitalization.

The place of continuous passive motion in foot infections has yet to be considered. Although it might be possible to manage infections in this way even with major weight-bearing joint infections such as in the ankle or subtalar joint, most infections of the foot are not confined to the joint and it would therefore be risky to employ continuous passive motion with infection in the tissues, muscles and tendons. These measures are under clinical trial after experimental investigation by Salter et al (1982) in knee infections, where the prospects seem good, although revolutionary.

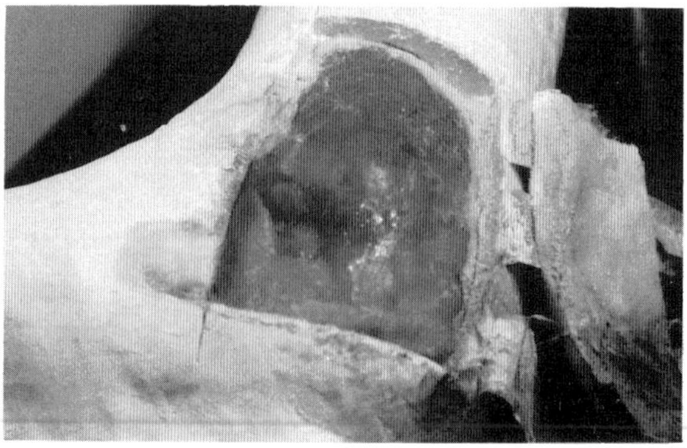

Fig. 31.8 Chronic post-traumatic tarsal sepsis: window in the plaster for dressings

INFECTIONS AT SPECIAL SITES

Tendons

With infection of tendons prevention is better than cure. In trauma where there has been loss of skin, any exposed tendon should be protected by suture or skin grafting as soon as possible. Exposed tendons tend to slough rapidly and once infection is present are usually lost. Deep infection of tendons can be difficult to diagnose, but with the diagnosis of suppuration drainage should be as early as possible.

The loss of tendons (for example the peroneal tendons) can lead to increasing deformity and disability. However, when tendons are lost in the presence of severe injuries and infection, there is often severe bone and joint destruction. Consequently, the related subtalar joint becomes stiff anyway, so that the tendon loss is less important. Moreover, any attempt at secondary tendon transfers or tendon grafts may not be feasible with skin deficiency and scarring from the trauma and infection. Later foot stabilization procedures (e.g. triple arthrodesis) may be preferable.

Radical measures including cross-leg skin grafts or myocutaneous grafts may have to be considered at the earliest stages to preserve exposed vital tendons and indeed the bone and joint structure. Such measures are necessary, for example, after injuries to the Achilles tendon (see Figs. 2a and b).

Sesamoids

Although unusual, infection of the metatarsal sesamoid under the great toe is important in that the diagnosis is frequently late. Infection will not clear until the sesamoid is removed.

Acute osteomyelitis of the metatarsal sesamoid is rare. The responsible organism is usually *Staph. aureus* as reported by Colwill (1969), who described three patients and indicated that five previous cases had been reported. Rome (1963) reported a patient with acute haematogenous osteomyelitis of the sesamoid. Torgerson & Hammon (1969) reported two other cases, one of which was in an adult with diabetes and the other an acute case due to *Staph. aureus* in a 12-year-old.

Acute or chronic infection may be a manifestation of systemic disease and metabolic conditions (such as diabetes or arteriosclerosis), as well as association with rigid deformity, the use of local physical agents and poor shoe wear.

Acute infection of the sesamoid can occur from a neighbouring puncture wound, in which case the organism may be *P. aeruginosa* or *Staph. aureus* according to Nuber & Anderson (1982). The same organism was responsible in the two nondiabetic cases reported by Gordon et al (1974).

Talus

According to Antoniou & Conner (1974) the diagnosis of osteomyelitis of the talus is often made late and the condition is usually subacute. If due to *Staph. aureus* it tends to be the coagulase negative organism. The most common incorrect diagnosis was a ligamentous injury. Most developed an abscess in the bone. Primary haematogenous osteomyelitis was also reported by Skevis (1984) in four children. These had proved difficult to diagnose and again presented late.

Chronic infection of the talus usually responds to local curettage and antibiotics. The antibiotics should be continued for six months. Similarly, plaster fixation may be necessary for six months. Transfixing Steinmann pins or Schantz screws with some form of external skeletal fixation is a useful method, particularly if chronic wounds and sinuses have to be dressed and inspected regularly.

Apart from antibiotics, radical surgery may be necessary in chronic infections of the talus. Such surgery is necessary for adjacent joint infection and destruction if natural ankylosis does not occur. In chronic infections talectomy with tibiocalcaneal fusion can eradicate infection. The calcaneus must be thrust backward to provide a good heel and better leverage for the calf muscles, and a spring in the gait.

Septic necrosis of the talus following trauma was discussed by Mueller (1978). Those with severe devitalization due to high velocity injury were associated with necrosis of the talus and with infection. Further necrosis occurred, setting up a vicious cycle. Recurrence of sepsis in the ankle joint thus indicated that necrosis of the talus was occurring. Following such trauma, necrosis and sepsis yielded a disastrous result. However, excision with a suitable fusion achieved stability in the 12 cases described.

Calcaneus

Local conservative surgery with curettage obtained satisfactory results in 36 cases of chronic osteitis with sinuses from the calcaneus as described by Climescu et al (1967). It was considered that resection of the calcaneus could be avoided. The type of surgery had to be adapted to each case.

Where there are persistent large ulcers of the heel, satisfactory results can be obtained by partial resection of the calcaneus, tailoring the skin incision around the ulcer and carrying out a primary closure as described by Horwitz (1972). This author detailed four cases.

Martini et al (1974) advocated partial or total resection and obtained satisfactory results in 20 cases. A shoe insert for the heel produced a reasonable gait.

The split heel technique of Gaenslen was reported by Broudy et al (1976), describing three children with refractory osteomyelitis and a central sinus. They considered excision unnecessary.

Winkelmann & Schulitz (1977) reported the difficulties experienced in managing 59 cases with chronic infection affecting the calcaneum. Various operations were discussed. Only 10 out of 29 cases followed up had good results. There were frequent deformities, skin trophic changes, scars and ulcers. Amputation was necessary in some. Infection was usually due to *Staph. aureus* but next in frequency were those due to gram-negative organisms. Mueller & Biebrach (1978) discussed their experience with 46 cases over 10 years emphasizing the need for correct early diagnosis and treatment. Only six were eventually symptom-free.

These examples from recent literature illustrate the tendency to chronicity in osteomyelitis of the calcaneus and serve to demonstrate the difficulties in management. The choice of surgery depends upon the site and extent of involvement (tomography and sinography are useful). Although conservative surgery is preferably, subtotal or total resection may be necessary. The results overall may not be satisfactory without proper planning and thorough investigation of the extent of involvement.

Special problems of infants

BCG osteomyelitis at the lower end of the talus in a one-year-old child inoculated three days after birth is reported. This was diagnosed by biopsy, culture, typing and inoculation in the guinea pig. The differential diagnosis lay between osteomyelitis and osteosarcoma. The condition was cleared with surgery and antibiotics (Eng & Aarneland 1966).

Osteitis at the terminal phalanx of the great toe is reported at Pucynski et al (1984) secondary to phlebotomy in an infant.

In infants osteomyelitis has been reported following phlebotomy from the heel. Lilien et al (1976) reported two cases in seven years. These infants required repeated laboratory tests for blood gases during prolonged respiratory assistance. Considering the estimated 6500 cases necessitating phlebotomy at the heel per annum in their Chicago Hospital this complication must be considered exceptionally rare.

Neonatal osteomyelitis reported by Ghibeley (1984) occurred in six cases requiring special care, for example in cardiac and metabolic problems. Incubation, venous cut-downs and umbilical catheterization were necessary. From a septicaemia on the seventh day, the hands and feet were affected with multifocal osteomyelitis due to *Staph. aureus*. The diagnosis was made from local oedema, hypersensitivity of the limb and pseudoparalysis. Tom Smith's arthritis of infants affecting the hip joint can occur from umbilical infection, due to poor hygiene, or poor antisepsis when carrying out venepuncture.

In joint infections in paediatric patients there is a high incidence of *Haemophilus influenzae* in children aged 6 months to 4 years. Thereafter the most common organism is *Staph. aureus*, according to McIntyre et al (1984) in a review of 100 consecutive cases. Nelson & Koontz (1966) and Almquist (1970) reported the increasing importance of *H. influenzae* in the infant. Unusual organisms are likely with penetrating injuries from foreign bodies and with systemic disease altering the immunological status of the child (including treatment with cortisteroids).

AMPUTATIONS

Ultimately, amputation may have to be considered as a life-saving measure in severe, fulminating, spreading infection or gangrene.

Forefoot amputations

Limited amputation may be possible in chronic infections or in the more distal lesions, e.g. a toe, where the structure is lost or unlikely to be saved and there is severe pain.

Hunter (1975) described the results of a minor foot amputation for ischaemia of the lower extremity in both diabetic and nondiabetic patients. He found simple removal of a toe unsuccessful if the vascular supply was poor or could not be improved by vascular reconstruction or sympathectomy or both. He preferred a transmetatarsal amputation.

Transmetatarsal amputation may be feasible and there are numerous references in relation to diabetes and secondary infection in rheumatoid patients favouring this conservative amputation. Rosendahl (1972) described the management of 36 patients with diabetic gangrene. Success depended upon the absence of arteriosclerosis, making a more conservative approach possible. It was emphasized that the diabetes and rehydration should be controlled, and the gangrene well demarcated. There should be careful skin preparation and good bleeding should be seen from the operation field. Schwindt et al (1973) included some cases selected from those without pedal pulses in diabetes. They were reasonably successful even in older patients, but the main complication was intermittent ulceration following operation. Kirsten (1974) achieved success with local amputation in 14 patients with osteomyelitis in the presence of vascular insufficiency. Eight of these had diabetes of adulthood. He advised six weeks of cephalothin.

Partial amputation of the foot for diabetic or arteriosclerotic gangrene constituted 48% of all amputations in an orthopaedic unit in 12 years according to Larsson & Andersson (1978). They achieved success in 60% of 183 amputations in 161 patients, but one-third needed a higher amputation. Subsequently the outcome of the initial operation depended upon the level of amputation, the age of the patient, the interval between the occurrence of the gangrene and the operation, anaemia and pyrexia.

Mid and hindfoot amputations

Maurer et al (1967) reviewed the results of amputation of the hindfoot, Chopart's amputation at midtarsal level. This amputation could be a success if it was possible to prevent the subsequent equinus deformity by a suitable transplant of the extensor tendons to dorsiflex the foot. This is only possible if the sepsis is sufficiently distal to retain part of the cuboid and navicular, or if the ankle is fused.

In Syme's amputation it was found difficult to prevent displacement of the heel pad, which is necessary for good function and appearance. The absence of a palpable tibialis posterior pulsation is in any case a contraindication for a Syme's amputation.

The Syme's amputation in two stages (in which the calcaneus and the talus are removed, but the ankle malleoli trimmed two weeks after the first stage) may be possible in a septic foot if the circulation is satisfactory. This can give a good stump with good function, more satisfactory than a below knee amputation in having a longer lever and being end-bearing. This procedure is recommended in the developing world where prosthetics may not be available.

Hierton (1970) discussed practical aspects in the management of gangrene of the foot. He stressed the need for early medical and surgical treatment in prevention and the provision of special facilities for chronic cases, encouraging active conservative treatment by vascular and orthopaedic surgeons in the working party. Success of the amputation depends on careful surgery.

Below knee amputation

In a below knee amputation there should be a long posterior flap and knee contracture should be prevented. One should aim for a patellar tendon bearing prosthesis so that the patient develops an independent walking ability, with no other walking aid and a painless stump.

The prognosis and outcome with a gangrenous (black) foot was reviewed by Tseng (1975) in a prospective study of 1075 cases between 1958 and 1974. There was a 41.9% mortality rate, increasing in older patients, those with gas gangrene or severe sepsis and with malignancy. The cause of death afterwards was the same as in the general population, except that there was a higher incidence of cardiovascular disease.

REFERENCES

Almquist E E 1970 The changing epidemiology of septic arthritis in children. Clin Orthop 68: 96–99

Antoniou D, Conner A N 1974 Osteomyelitis of the calcaneus and talus. J Bone Joint Surg 56A: 338–345

Bingham R, Fleenor W H, Church S 1974 The local use of antibiotics to prevent wound infection. Clin Orthop 99: 194–200

Brand R A, Black H 1974 Pseudomonas osteomyelitis following puncture wounds in children. J Bone Joint Surg 56A: 1637–1642

Broudy A S, Scott R D, Watts H G 1976 The split heel technique in the management of calcaneal osteomyelitis. Clin Orthop 119: 202–205

Capen D, Scheck M 1981 Seronegative inflammation of the ankle and foot. Clin Orthop 155: 147–155

Catterall R C F 1964 Orthopaedic aspects of diabetic gangrene. J Bone Joint Surg 46B: 785

Charosky C B, Marcova R C 1974 Salmonella paratyphi osteomyelitis. Report of a case simulating a giant cell tumour. Clin Orthop 99: 190–193

Climescu V, Alexandrescu M, Antonesus N 1967 Osteitis of the calcaneus. Rev Med Chir Soc Med Nat Iasi 71/3: 611–617

Colwill M 1969 Osteomyelitis of the metatarsal sesamoids. J Bone Joint Surg 51B: 464–468

Colwill M R, Maudsley R H 1968 The Management of gas gangrene with hyperbaric oxygen therapy. J Bone Joint Surg 50B: 732–742

Cruse P J E 1977 Some factors determining wound infection: a prospective study of 30 000 wounds. In: Polk H C, Stone H H (eds) Hospital Acquired Infections In Surgery. University Park Press, Baltimore Ch 8, p 77

Curtis P H J 1973 Uncommon forms of osteomyelitis. Clin Orthop 96: 84–87

Deysine M, Rafkin H, Teicher I et al 1975 Diagnosis of chronic and postoperative osteomyelitis with gallium 67 citrate scans. Am J Surg 129/6: 632–635

Donald C c.1951 Personal communication

Eng J, Aarneland T 1966 BCG osteitis in a child. Bacteriological investigation. Scand J Resp Dis 47/3: 182–186

Fitzgerald R H J, Cowan J D E 1975 Puncture wounds of the foot. Orthop Clin North Am 6/4: 965–972

Garrod L P, Lambert H P, O'Grady F 1973 Antibiotic and chemotherapy. Churchill Livingstone, Edinburgh

Gelfand M J, Silberstein E B 1977 Radionuclide imaging: use in the diagnosis of osteomyelitis in children. JAMA 237: 245–247

Ger R 1983 Muscle transposition in the management of perforating ulcers of the forefoot. Clin Orthop 175: 186–189

Ghibeley A R 1984 Neonatal osteomyelitis. J Bone Joint Surg 66B: 303

Gilday D L, Paul D J, Paterson J 1975 Diagnosis of osteomyelitis in children by combined blood pool and bone imaging. Radiology 117: 331–335

Gillespie W J, Farmer M H, Fong R, Harding S M 1983 The result of a case study of host defences in haematogenous osteomyelitis of childhood. J Bone Joint Surg 65B: 520

Gordon S L, Evans C, Greer R B 1974 Pseudomonas osteomyelitis of the metatarsal sesamoid of the great toe. Clin Orthop 99: 188–189

Hagler D F 1971 Pseudomonas osteomyelitis: puncture wounds of the feet. Pediatrics 48: 672–673

Hauser E D W 1940 Diseases of the foot. W B Saunders Co, Philadelphia. pp 358–367

Henry A K 1959 Extensile exposure, 2nd edn. E & S Livingstone, Edinburgh. pp 303–308

Hierton T 1970 Practical views on gangrene of the foot. Lakartidningen 67/31: 3461–3500

Hogshead H P 1966 Management of the anaesthetic, paralytic foot in patients with myelodysplasia. J Bone Joint Surg 48A: 1016

Horwitz T 1972 Partial resection of the os calcis and primary closure in the treatment of resistant large ulcers of the heel with and without osteomyelitis of the os calcis. Clin Orthop 84: 149–153

Hughes S 1980 Radionuclides in orthopaedic surgery. J Bone Joint Surg 62B: 141–150

Hunter G A 1975 Results of minor foot amputations for ischaemia of the lower extremity in diabetics and non-diabetics. Can J Surg 18/3: 273–276

Jaffe H L, Lichtenstein L 1940 Osteoid osteoma: further experience with this benign tumour of bone. J Bone Joint Surg 22A: 645

Johanson P H 1968 Pseudomonas infections of the foot following puncture wounds. JAMA 204: 262 264

Kandel S N, Mankin H J 1973 Pyogenic abscess of the long bones in children. Clin Orthop 96: 108–117

Kirsten M D 1974 Osteomyelitis with vascular insufficiency. Curr Ther Res 16/4: 306–310

Lang A G, Peterson H A 1976 Osteomyelitis following puncture wounds in children. J Trauma 16/12: 993–999

Larsson J, Andersson G B J 1978 Partial amputation of the foot for diabetic or arteriosclerotic gangrene. J Bone Joint Surg 60B: 126–130

Lilien L D, Harris V J, Ramamurthy R S, Pildes R S 1976 Neonatal osteomyelitis of calcaneus complication of heel puncture. J Pediatr 88/3: 478–480

Lindenbaum S, Alexander H 1984 Infections stimulating bone tumours. Clin Orthop 184: 193–203

McIntyre W M, Wiley J J, Portner O T 1984 Joint infections in paediatric patients. J Bone Joint Surg 66B: 303

MacKinnon A E 1975 Pseudomonous osteomyelitis following puncture wounds. Postgrad Med J 51/1: 33–34

Martini M, Benkeddache Y, Bekhechi T, Daoud A 1974 Treatment of chronic osteomyelitis of the calcaneus by resection of the calcaneus. J Bone Joint Surg 56A: 542–548

Maudsly R H, Colwil M R 1966 Hyperbaric oxygen in the management of gas gangrene. J Bone Joint Surg 48B: 584

Maurer P, Bombart M, Michant E, Rabeux L, Lefevre B 1967 Amputation of the hind foot. Rev Chir Orthop 53/7: 635–703

Miller E H, Semian D W 1975 Gram negative osteomyelitis following puncture wounds of the feet. J Bone Joint Surg 56A: 535–537

Minnefor A B, Olson M I, Carver D H 1971 Pseudomonas osteomyelitis following puncture wounds of the foot. Pediatrics 47: 598–601

Miskew D B W, Pinzur M S, Pankovich A W 1979 Clostridial myonecrosis in a patient undergoing oxacillin therapy for exacerbation of chronic foot ulcers and osteomyelitis. Clin Orthop 138: 250–253

Monsoor I A 1967 Typhoid osteomyelitis of the calcaneus due to direct inoculation. J Bone Joint Surg 49A: 732–734

Morrey D F, Dunn J M, Heimbach R D, Davis J, Petersen L F A 1980 Hyperbaric oxygen as an adjunct in the treatment of chronic osteomyelitis. J Bone Joint Surg 62B: 132

Mueller K H 1978 Septic necrosis of the talus. Unfallheilkunde 81/8: 532–541
Mueller K H, Biebrach M 1978 Calcaneal osteomyelitis: Biomechanics, clinical features, treatment and results. Unfallheilkunde 81/9: 585–592
Nade S 1983 Acute septic arthritis in infancy and childhood. J Bone Joint Surg 65B: 234–241
Nelson J D, Koontz W C 1966 Septic arthritis in infants and children: a review of 117 cases. Pediatrics 38: 966–971
Newman R J, Curtis G W D, Slach M P E 1984 The value of synovial fluid lactate determination in the rapid exclusion of septic arthritis. J Bone Joint Surg 66B: 290
Nuber D W, Anderson P R 1982 Acute osteomyelitis of the metatarsal sesamoid. Clin Orthop 167: 212–213
O'Brien T, McManus F, MacCauley P H, Ennis J T 1982 Acute haematogenous osteomyelitis. J Bone Joint Surg 64B: 450–453
Pucynski M S, Dvonch V M, Menendex C E, Calwell C C 1984 Osteomyelitis of the great toe secondary to phlebotomy. Clin Orthop 190: 239–240
Rome M 1963 Osteomyelitis of the metatarsal sesamoid. Br Med J 1: 1071
Rosendahl S 1972 Transmetatarsal amputation in diabetic gangrene. Acta Orthop Scand 43/1: 78–83
Salter R B et al 1982 The healing of articular tissues through continuous passive motion: Essence of the first 10 years of experimental investigations. J Bone Joint Surg 64B: 640
Schwindt C D, Lulloff R S, Rogers S C 1973 Transmetatarsal amputations. Orthop Clin North Am 4/1: 31–42
Skevis X A 1984 Primary subacute osteomyelitis of the talus. J Bone Joint Surg 66B: 101–103
Smith T 1874 On acute arthritis of infants: St. Bartholomew Hospital Reports 10: 189
Smith W S, Hensinger R, Whitehouse W 1971 Infections of the foot. J Bone Joint Surg 53A: 1241
Thomas J M, Lowes J A, Tabaqchali S 1980 Serratia marcescens in mixed aerobic infections of bone. J Bone Joint Surg 62B: 389–390
Torgerson W R, Hammond G 1969 Osteomyelitis of the sesamoid bones of the first metatarsophalangeal joint. J Bone Joint Surg 51A: 1420–1422
Tseng W P 1975 Outcome of patients with 'black foot disease'. J Formosan Med Ass 74/1: 37–47
Tuazon C V 1982 Teichoic acid antibodies in osteomyelitis and septic arthritis. J Bone Joint Surg 64A: 762–765
Whitehouse W M, Smith W S 1970 Osteomyelitis of the feet. Semin Roentgenol 5/4: 367–377
Winkelmann W, Schulitz K P 1977 Chronic osteomyelitis in the subtalar tarsus. Orthop Prax 13/11: 848–851

Tropical diseases

INTRODUCTION

Underdeveloped tropical areas have certain factors in common, which render their inhabitants more vulnerable to certains infections and diseases. Many villages are still primitive with crowding, poor community and personal hygiene, use of fields and roadsides for calls of nature, and unsafe water supplies. Transport is frequently inadequate. Many people are of low socioeconomic status, with the added problems of illiteracy and poor communication. There is a lack of faith in such modern medicine as is available and an adherence to traditional medicines and witchcraft. Sweating in the heat is uncomfortable and many remain bare bodied and barefooted, especially in rural areas, increasing the risks of superficial trauma and ulceration and of puncture wounds and infection. Despite the efforts of WHO, government agencies and philanthropic organizations, proper medical facilities, adequate prophylactic methods and sociomedical education are slow to reach the mass of the population. Missionaries are too few and unevenly distributed. Many diseases seen in the developed Western World are also seen in the tropics and are not specially included in this chapter. Similarly, certain topics which are very relevant in underdeveloped tropical countries (e.g. poliomyelitis) are dealt with in other chapters.

LEPROSY

Synonyms: Hansen's infection, Hanseniasis, Hansen's disease, elephantiasis graecorum, leontiasis or satyriasis, korh, maharog or kusth (India)

Leprosy is a chronic granulomatous infection, caused by *Mycobacterium leprae* (discovered by Hansen (1873–74) of Norway), affecting primarily the dermis layer of the skin, peripheral nerves and the muscosa of the upper respiratory tract. Specific cell-mediated immunity, through thymus-sensitized lymphocytes, determines its wide range of clinical manifestations.

Historical background

Egyptian literature describes leprosy in 4600 BC and Indian mythology describes Kings and Queens serving leprosy patients in 3000 BC, whilst Vedas (1400 BC), Charka Samhita (800 BC) and Chinese scripts (600 BC) have all referred to leprosy. The word 'leper' is derived from a Greek word 'lepros' meaning 'scaly'. The Old Testament Hebrew word 'tsara ath' or 'zaraath', denotes the 'scaly condition'. Leviticus considers the disease as an affliction of God upon man for his misdeeds (Lev 13: 1–17; Lev 14: 1–32). Aristotle referred to it as 'leontiasis or satyriasis' and Greek physicians (300 BC) as elephantiasis and later 'elephantiasis graecorum' (Galen 133–202 AD). Slaves and troops from India, Sudan, Egypt, the Middle East and Africa were responsible for the spread of this disease to the western world. Daniezssen & Boeck (1847) recognized the disease.

Sulphone was introduced for treating leprosy in 1941. Since then findings have included those of Shepard (1960) and Rees (1967) who reported possible multiplication of *M. leprae* in the footpad of mice; Kirchheimer et al (1972) who demonstrated abundant multiplication of *M. leprae* when injected into a South American anteater, the immunologically normal nine banded armadillo;

Kwapinski & Kwapinski (1974) who reported bacillary multiplication in newborn snakes; and Waters et al (1978) who successfully infected a primate, the white banded gibbon.

Geographical distribution (Fig. 32.1)

Leprosy remained endemic all over the globe until the end of the Middle Ages. A recent survey indicates a number varying from 11 to 15 million of detected leprosy patients worldwide, the majority of these being in third world countries (Africa, Asia, India, Nepal, Burma, Pakistan, Hongkong, Singapore, China, South America and the Pacific islands) with a lesser incidence in Southern Europe, the Mediterranean islands, Greece, Spain, Portugal, the USA and UK. Denmark, Switzerland and Chile are stated to be free from this disease (Browne 1979).

Aetiology

The causative organism is *Mycobacterium leprae*, mostly curved filamentous, 1 to 10 nm by 0.25 nm, acid and alcohol fast, and the first bacterial pathogen seen to cause disease in humans (Hilson 1965). Usually the organisms are grouped in cigar bundles or clumps in intra- or extracellular masses (globi). The generation time during the logarithmic phase is 12–13 days. The organism has not been cultured in vitro.

Epidemiology

Open lepromatous cases are the only reservoir of the bacilli. Bacilli shed from skin ulcers and nasal secretions gain entry into the host either through cutaneous breaches or the respiratory or gastro-intestinal tracts. *M. leprae* can remain viable for seven days in dried nasal discharges (Daney & Rees 1974). Mosquitoes (Narayana et al 1978) and flies (Geater 1975) may be effective carriers. Factors responsible for spread include:

1. Climate: The hot and humid environment in the tropics has been blamed, but bacilli can thrive almost anywhere in the world though its clinical pattern varies from one country to another. Lepromatous leprosy occurs at a significantly lower incidence in dark-skinned persons (Africans and Indians) than in fair ones (Mongolians and Caucasians). The degree of cutaneous pigmentation may vary inversely with the severity of the disease.

2. Age: Placental transmission is not possible. Infants and children remaining in close and

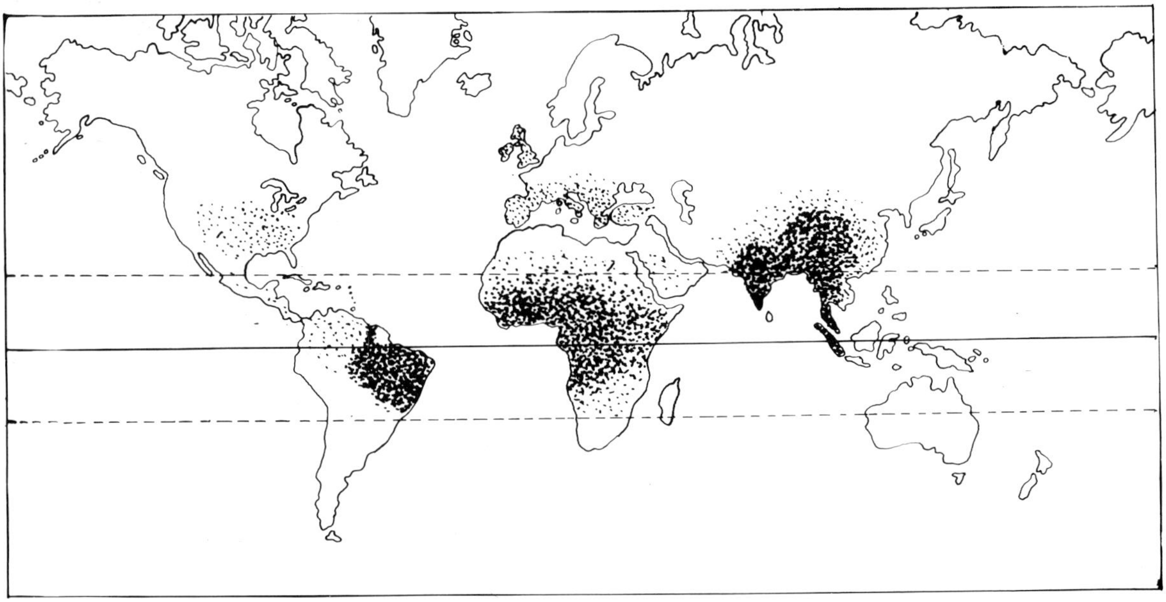

Fig. 32.1 Geographical distribution of leprosy

continued contact with infected parents are more susceptible (60%) (Jopling & Harman 1979).

3. Sex: More chance of exposure and probably a greater susceptibility (WHO 1966) make the male twice as vulnerable.

4. Conjugal leprosy: Though prolonged contact makes it possible, its risk has been exaggerated.

5. Social Status: Low socioeconomic status, illiteracy, poor personal hygiene, sharing of clothing, congested living and under nourishment, encourage the infection.

6. Genetic Factors: Reports of a higher incidence of leprosy in 'O' blood group patients, together with the fact that there is a higher prevalence of lepromatous leprosy in fair-skinned patients, and that identical twins show more concordance in type than non-identical ones, plus the results of a study of cell-mediated immunity, suggest some genetic factors in leprosy.

Immunology

The lepra bacillus is likely to induce an immunological response which may be humoral (which cannot kill the bacilli and hence is useless) or cell-mediated (thymus-sensitized lymphocytes can eliminate the bacilli) as in tuberculosis. BCG if given before clinical manifestations arise, may confer variable immunity.

Immunotherapy with lymphocytes, whole blood or transfer factor has not been successful, as the serum of lepromatous patients contains anti-lymphocytic factors.

Pathogenesis

Entering through the skin, bacilli enter the nerve endings and endoneural fine blood vessels and migrate upwards through the Schwann cells and the axons to localize at the site of predilection in the nerve trunk. There they excite a delayed type of hypersensitivity reaction with aggregation of macrophages, epitheloid and lymphoid cells and with a minimal bacterial population. The lepromatous granuloma leads to intraneural compression, ischaemia and axonal degeneration.

Bacilli entering through respiratory or gastro-intestinal tracts circulate and excite antibody formation to form immune complexes with suppression of cellular immunity. Bacilli multiply unbridled within the macrophages. Well recognized 'globi', foam cells, and macrophage-granulomata, with almost no lymphocytes, dominate the picture. The cortical follicles of the lymph nodes and spleen degenerate and visceral affections set in.

Classification

Leprosy has been classified mainly in relation to host immune response. With the introduction of the infection the bacilli may or may not be completely phagocytosed and quickly destroyed. The defence mechanisms produce a reaction which is usually transient and may produce spontaneous healing in up to 75% of cases. The clinicopathological changes are too immature and unpredictable to be classified other than as 'indeterminate type'. Remission or progress to a 'determinate type' (tuberculoid and lepromatous varieties) depends entirely on the host cell-mediated immune response and bacillary multiplication. In between the two determinate types there is a spectrum of manifestation known as 'borderline' or 'dimorphous' leprosy.

Based upon the immunological spectrum, Ridley & Jopling (1966) have proposed a five-group system of classification of leprosy, which is useful in assessing the disease and its prognosis. The main considerations are the cytological differentiation (epitheloid to macrophages), the degree of lymphocytic infiltration and bacterial population. The five groups, according to severity and infectivity across the spectrum are tuberculoid (TT), borderline tuberculoid (BT), borderline (BB), borderline lepromatous (BL) and lepromatous (LL).

With proper chemotherapy, the borderline type shows an upgrade towards the TT end of the spectrum, and without treatment a downgrade to a subtype of LL, subpolar lepromatous leprosy (known as LLs to differentiate it from polar type, LLp). Group LLp is immunologically stable, LLs is not.

Clinical features

Due to a variable incubation period (2 to 30 years) and bizarre manifestations, one must be vigilant in suspecting and diagnosing leprosy. The clinical features of only the polarized cases are more or less clear.

Indeterminate type

Typically a child with prolonged contact develops one or two hypopigmented weals, papules or pale macules with decreased sweating in an area of normal or slightly depressed sensation. These lesions may persist for months to a year and in 50 to 75% cases there is spontaneous recovery. In others, depending upon cell-mediated immune response and proper treatment, there may be either upgrading towards the tuberculoid pole or downgrading towards the lepromatous pole, or persistence as borderline, unstable leprosy.

Tuberculoid type

The main clinical manifestation in this type of leprosy is the peripheral nerve involvement with or without dermal lesions (Fig. 32.2). The nerves affected are the ulnar, lateral popliteal, greater auricular, median, superficial peroneal, antebrachial cutaneous, posterior tibial, radial and the lateral cutaneous nerve of the thigh. (These are nerves whose mean temperature is 1–2° cooler than those more deeply placed).

Motor loss is mainly manifest in involvement of the ulnar (ulnar clawhand) or ulnar and median (main en griffe), common peroneal (footdrop), and, rarely, radial (wrist drop) nerves. Very rarely there may be trigeminal, olfactory and facial nerve involvement.

Early manifestations consist of sensory disturbances such as paraesthesia, hypoaesthesia or anaesthesia, followed by the gradually increasing effects of the motor loss.

The nerves are thickened and there may be cold abscesses in their course. Anaesthetic skin of the foot and hand can be subjected to repeated, prolonged and greater trauma, leading to trophic ulceration. Anaesthesia, disuse, repeated trauma and trophic ulceration lead to osseous atrophy with shortening and absorption of the digits of the toes and fingers. Chronic corneal ulcers may develop due to sensory loss resulting in corneal opacities.

The dermal lesions (Fig. 32.3) are localized, asymmetric and very few (one to three) in number. A typical tuberculoid dermal lesion is large, anaesthetic, anhydrotic and dry, hairless and more or less saucer-shaped having a sharply raised annular outer edge and a hypopigmented flattened centre. It is usually seen on the extensor surface of a limb, face, back and buttocks. The lesions on the sole and palm are rare and without the raised margin due to the thick and tight skin.

Lepromatous type

The main clinical manifestations in this form are the dermal and mucosal lesions. The neural affections are comparatively late and are an advanced manifestation. Destructive lesions can also be found

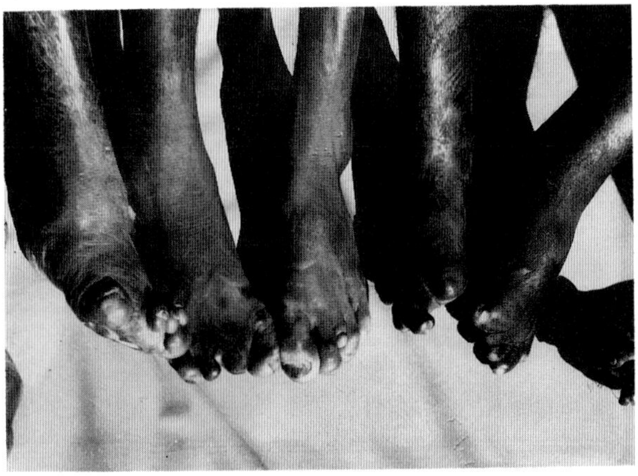

Fig. 32.2 The forefoot is more commonly affected than the hindfoot

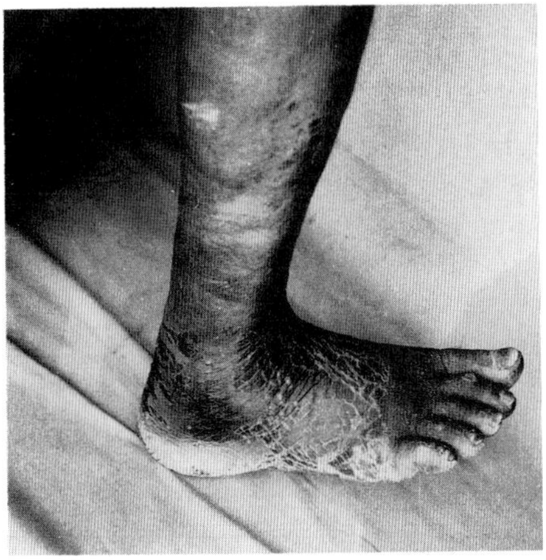

Fig. 32.3 Tuberculoid lesions of the foot — infiltration on the periphery and scaling in the central area, with atrophy

in various other systems and organs of the body, e.g. respiratory, cardiovascular, skeletal, genitourinary, ophthalmic and central nervous systems.

Dermal lesions (macules, papules or nodules) are neither anaesthetic nor anhydrotic and can be found anywhere, but are most commonly seen on the face, extremities and buttocks. In advanced cases the leonine faces may appear.

Mucosal lesions are obvious in the nose and oropharyngeal cavity leading to ulceration, crust formation and bloodstained discharge, perforation of the septum and destruction of bone. Laryngeal lesions produce hoarseness of the voice. Chronic iritis, iridocyclitis and keratitis are common features.

Usually the long short bones of the foot and hand undergo osteoporosis, atrophy and destruction. Trophic changes are mostly seen in the feet. In the phalanges atrophic changes start from the periphery and ultimately the whole diaphysis may look like a stick of bone before dissolution (concentric bone atrophy) (see Figs. 32.18, 19 and 21). In the metatarsals the trophic and absorptive changes usually start in the heads and proceed proximally leading to gradual thinning of the bone which looks like a pencil tip. Ultimately the stumpy end of the toes may remain connected loosely to the foot without any bony continuity.

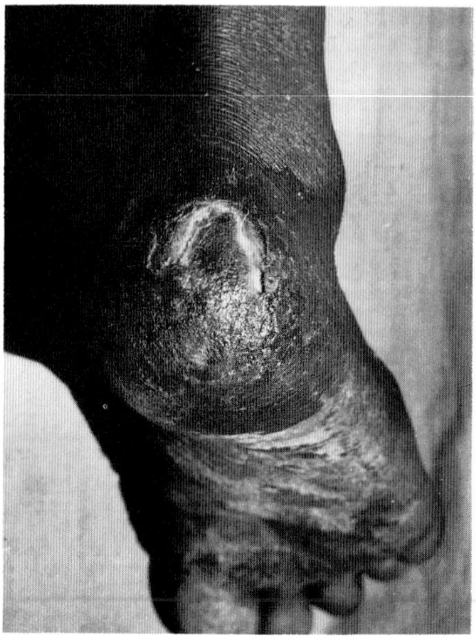

Fig. 32.4 Friction ulcers due to a tight closed boot

The joints of the feet may undergo subluxation, deformity, and ankylosis due to muscular paralysis, disuse, infiltrative lesions in the overlying skin, trophic ulceration and secondary infection through ulcers. Secondary neuropathic joints may also develop due to continued sensory loss which also predisposes to friction lesions (Figs. 32.4, 5 and 6).

Earlier ulcers usually begin as hyperkeratotic (Fig. 32.7) and fissured areas. This may result in a sinus due to infections, which gradually enlarges to a cone-shaped ulcer. Under pressure the ulcer assumes a punched out appearance containing foul smelling necrotic material. Secondary infection may penetrate into the underlying bone leading to pyogenic osteomyelitis.

The lymph glands are enlarged, painless and soft to firm. Persistent lymphoedema of the legs and feet may result in elephantiasis.

Testicular atrophy may lead to sterility and gynaecomastia. Renal failure due to chronic glomerulonephritis, interstitial nephritis or renal

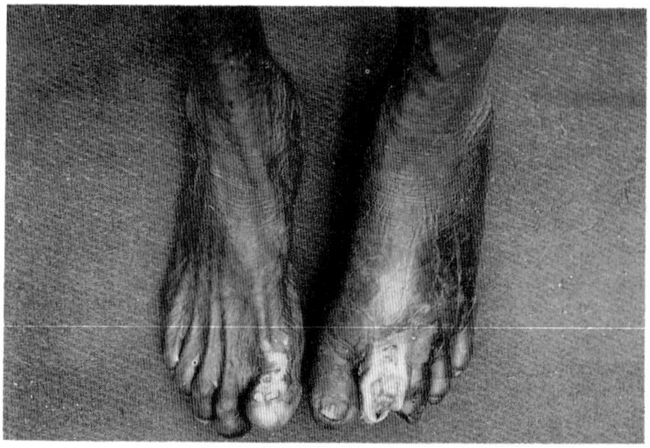

Fig. 32.5 Friction ulcers

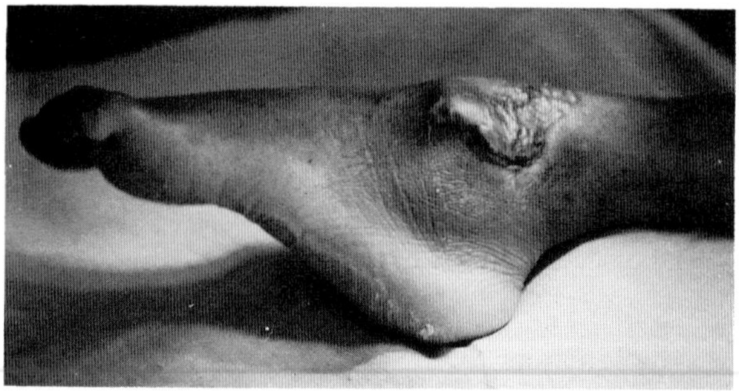

Fig. 32.6 Friction ulcers on the lateral malleolus due to cross-legged sitting habits in Indian culture

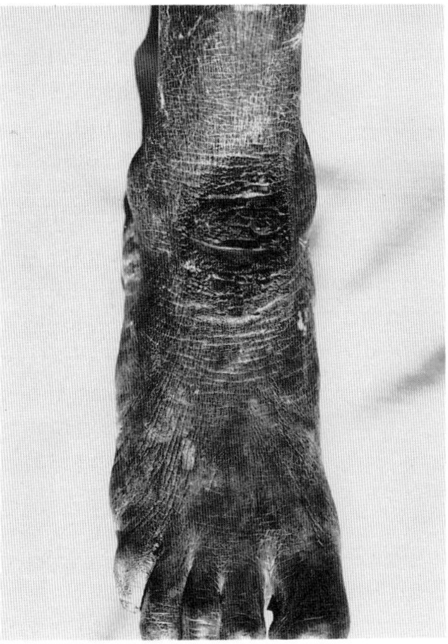

Fig. 32.7 Hyperkeratotic lesion in Lepromatous leprosy

amyloidosis is the common cause of death in the neglected cases.

Borderline or dimorphous type

This type usually occurs in individuals with limited cell-mediated immunity. Here dermal lesions present the mixed picture of tuberculoid and lepromatous types, but there is always marked neural involvement. These cases remain unstable till they polarize to either side depending upon the treatment given and the level of immunity. Usually there is downgrading to a lepromatous type.

Diagnosis

Subjects presenting with hypopigmented or discoloured skin patches, vague sensory complaints like hyperaesthesia, tingling or unnoticed burning of the hands and feet, nonhealing ulcers on the sole, nontraumatic footdrop or persistent blood-tinged nasal discharge must be investigated for leprosy.

Investigations

Leprosy, being a chronic disease, usually has no reactive haematological changes, but more than 50% of patients of treated LL type or BL type and occasionally even untreated ones, suffer from the antigen-induced reactive phenomenon of erythema nodosum leprosum (probably derived from dead lepra bacilli), during which constitutional features appear with polymorphonuclear leucocytosis and raised sedimentation rate. Otherwise, there may be comparative lymphocytosis, a low haemoglobin and little elevation of the sedimentation rate.

Urinalysis

Routine urine examination may not be of any value except with erythema nodosum and in fairly advanced lepromatous cases, when heavy albuminuria may follow the glomerulonephritis and varying kidney damage.

Nasal scrape

Nasal blowings or nasal scrapings taken from the anterior part of the nostril always show enough organisms in the untreated LL type, but are always negative in BB, BT and TT types. In BL types they may or may not be positive.

Skin smear

Skin smears can be taken from active leprosy ulcers or, better, from an active lesion on the ear lobules and dorsum of the fingers. The smear, collected by the 'slit and scrape method' is stained by the Ziehl–Neelson technique. Plenty of AFB are always demonstrable in LL, BL and BB lesions and scanty in BT, but none show in the TT (except during reactions) and intermediate groups.

Bacteriological Index (BI)

The bacteriological index is the measure of the number of bacilli per unit volume of tissue. This should be calculated by examining four to seven smears.

Morphological Index (MI)

This is the assessment of the percentage of the viable bacilli, staining as solid rods as against the dead bacilli which appear fragmented and granular. The

MI is important in assessing the progress of the treatment. Even the LL group should reach zero by six months.

Skin biopsy

This is essential accurately to classify the type of lesion, by properly analysing the histological changes and cell infiltrates. The biopsy material should be taken from the most active part of the lesions (e.g. the edge in tuberculoid (TT) and centre in the lepromatous (LL)) and must include the subcutaneous fat.

Nerve biopsy

This is indicated in pure neural involvements (e.g. TT and BB types) or where the skin biopsy is not informative. A small segment from a thickened peripheral nerve is taken for biopsy.

Sternal marrow puncture

In TT or even in BL leprosy, bacilli can be found in sternal marrow smear examination.

Demonstration of absence of sweating

In doubtful anhydrotic macules (especially in TT) the absence of sweat can be demonstrated by injecting 0.2 ml of 1 in 1000 pilocarpine subcutaneously in the suspected area and a similar amount in adjacent normal skin. Tincture of iodine is painted over the injected areas. After drying the paint, starch powder is sprinkled over them. With normal sweating, the starch will turn blue, but not in an anhydrous area.

Histamine test (Rodriguez & Plantilla 1931)

One drop of a 1 in 1000 solution of histamine diphosphate is placed on a hypopigmented suspicious patch and also on the adjacent normal skin. A shallow puncture is made using a thin needle through the histamine drops. In the normal skin area, a red flare appears within two minutes, but the flare is delayed, faint or absent in TT, BB and indeterminate leprosy. It is particularly useful in diagnosing the indeterminate type of leprosy.

Lepromin test

This intradermal test (injecting the derivative from lepromatous tissue rich in lepra bacilli) was first described by Mitsuda in 1916, but is not diagnostic. It has a definite value in an already diagnosed patient to place him in the spectrum of the disease. It is strongly positive in TT, weak in BT, and negative in BB, BL and LL.

Foot prints (Fig. 32.8)

This simple test is of value in assessing the points of maximum pressure in the anaesthetic sole and progress while treating ulcers.

Radiograph

This demonstrates the pathological changes and amount of destruction in the bone.

Differential diagnosis

The range of manifestations of leprosy is so wide and confusing, that the list of skin, neural and ulcerative conditions to be differentiated is exhaustive.

Foot in leprosy

The affections of the foot are caused both directly by the disease process and secondarily due to nerve involvement, deformity and secondary infection. The true leprosy infection manifests on the dorsum of the foot, mainly in the lepromatous variety and during lepra reactions, as a swollen foot with nodularity and painful joints.

In secondary affections the dominant role is played by nerve damage, mainly of the lateral popliteal, posterior tibial and the calcaneal branch of the posterior tibial nerves.

Mechanism of nerve damage

1. Directly by bacilli

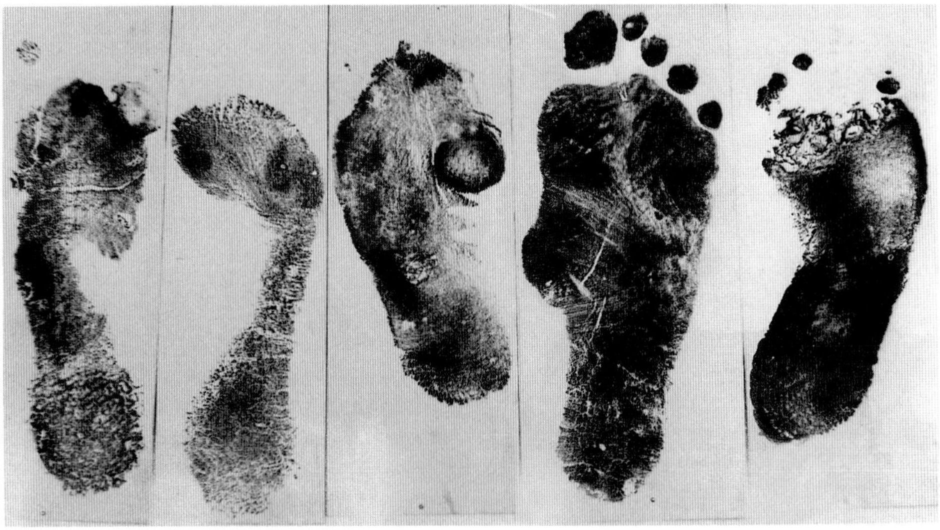

a b c d e

Fig. 32.8 (a) Footprints in leprosy: Absorbed and distorted great toe; fallen 2nd, 3rd and 5th toes; ulcer beneath the anterior end of the tarsal border of the foot
(b) Absorbed and fallen toes; healed ulcer beneath base of fifth toe
(c) Fallen toes; secondary punched-out healing ulcer on the collapsed anterior end of the medial arch; partially healed ulcer on the lateral border of the foot
(d) Collapse of both longitudinal and transverse arches of the foot; partially healed ulcer beneath the base of the great toe and a healed ulcer on the anterior end of the collapsed medial arch
(e) Extensive active deep ulcer beneath the bases of 1st, 2nd, 3rd, 4th and 5th toes with varying absorption of all the toes; secondary varus and adduction deformities of the forefoot

2. By compression
   a. Internal granuloma formation and immuno-complex endarteritis of the vasanervosum leading to inflammatory oedema and compression ischaemia
   b. External pressure over the swollen nerve by the tight surrounding fibro-osseous tunnel leading to venous and lympathic stasis and ischaemia. Movements of the ankle and feet have a milking effect upon the thickened nerve, producing further compression.

Ischaemia of the nerve leads to delayed motor conduction (reversible paralysis). Later, fibrotic constriction strangles the nerve fibrils resulting in irreversible damage. Damage first of autonomic fibres (loss of sweating) is followed by sensory (loss of pain, temperature and touch) and motor fibre loss.

TROPHIC ULCERS

Synonyms: Plantar ulcer, perforating ulcer, neuropathic ulcer, foot pressure ulcer

Plantar ulcer (Price 1959) is a chronic resistant and recurrent ulcer of an anaesthetic foot, where walking is still possible. Of all the complications of leprosy, it is the most unpleasant and annoying. It occurs in about 12% of leprosy patients (Languillon 1964). Males are affected about twice as often as females. Patients with ulcers are almost never below 20 years, and usually have tuberculoid or indeterminate leprosy. Price (1964) has classified these ulcers into:

1. Infected wounds (caused by thorns or sharp nails and burns (Fig. 32.9)
2. Friction ulcers (see Figs. 32.4, 5, 6) usually on the dorsum of the foot, due to sandal straps and unsuitable footwear and on the sole on the projecting part of the deformed foot

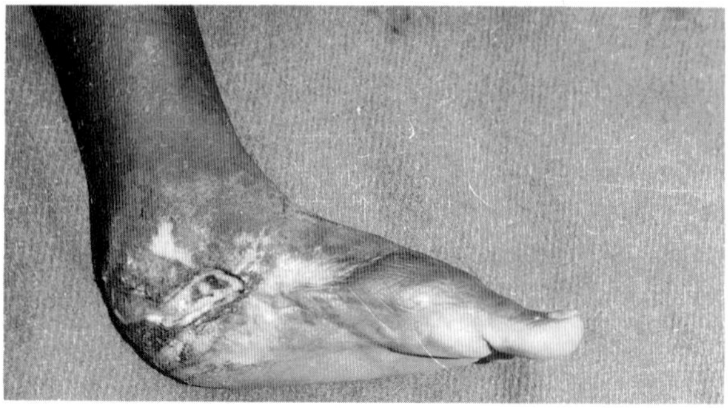

Fig. 32.9 Leprotic foot. Ulcer due to an infected wound. The patient had a burn in childhood: a traumatic abrasion over the scar became infected

3. Plantar ulcers (Figs. 32.10, 11, 12, 13, 14 and 15) occur on any insensitive sole, where the patient still walks. The precipitating factor in producing the ulcer is pressure unbalanced in both amount and time. In leprosy, very fast walking, walking on a hard ground (specially wearing a hard shoe), walking with projecting bony ends in the sole, walking on the edges of a narrow support and walking with footdrop, clawed toes, or a shortened or scarred foot lead to repetitive pressure on a particular hard pressed spot, producing inflammation, necrosis

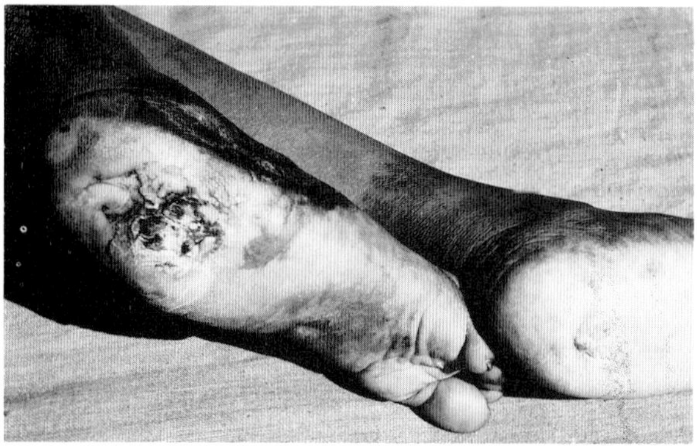

Fig. 32.10 Active heel ulcer

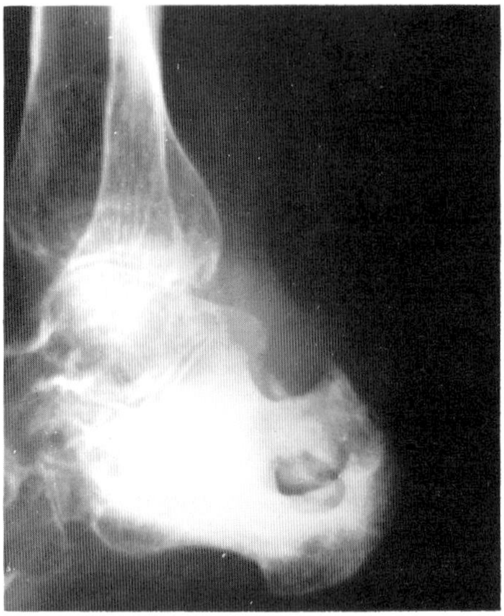

Fig. 32.11 Secondary calcaneal osteomyelitis with sequestrum

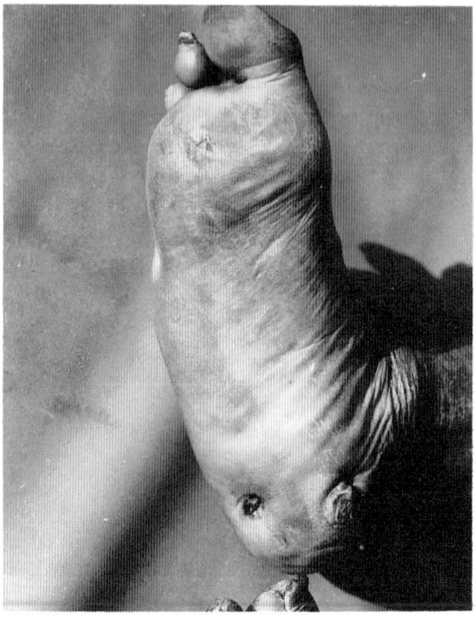

Fig. 32.12 Healed ulcers of the heel, the lateral border of the foot and the base of the second toe

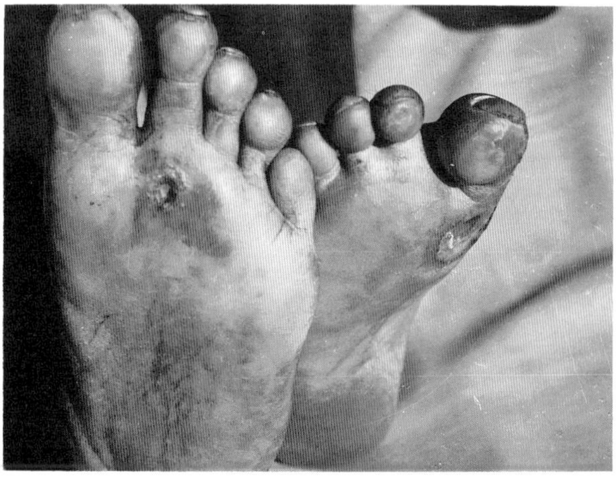

Fig. 32.13 Ulcers at the base of the second left toe and the right big toe

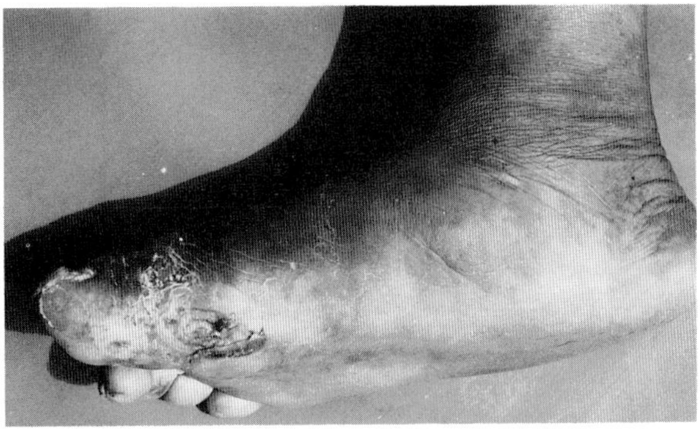

Fig. 32.14 Ulcers at the base and anterior part of the big toe

blisters and ultimately breakdown to trophic ulceration (Brand 1977). These become secondarily infected and, in neglected conditions, deeper destruction of tendons, bones and joints develops, leading to various deformities, falling of digits, and auto-amputations at various levels.

Healing, if it happens at all, occurs as cessation of exudate, epithelial cover and consolidation (Price 1964); the ultimate result is scarring. Further progress involves the evil cycle of scar-ulcer-scar (Anderson 1964). Due to various factors (intrinsic paralysis, ligamentous avulsions and damage and destruction of bones and joints) collapse of the foot (lateral, medial and total) develops. This favours the development of secondary ulcerations. Price (1964) has summarized the natural history of the plantar ulcers in four phases: (a) primary tissue damage, (b) primary plantar ulcer, (c) collapse of the foot and (d) secondary ulceration.

Clawson & Seddon (1960) have concluded that fixed deformities are the most important cause of ulceration. Based on this concept, Lennox (1964) classifies leprosy foot deformities into two main varieties. Primary deformities are due to the disease process, resulting from paralytic muscle imbalance and mostly inevitable (Table 32.1). Secondary

Table 32.1 Primary Deformities (Lennox 1964)

Muscle imbalance	Site of ulcer
Foot drop (with loss of peronei)	Anterolateral border
Foot drop (peronei intact)	Anteromedial border
Claw toes	Dorsum and pulp of toes Metatarsal heads

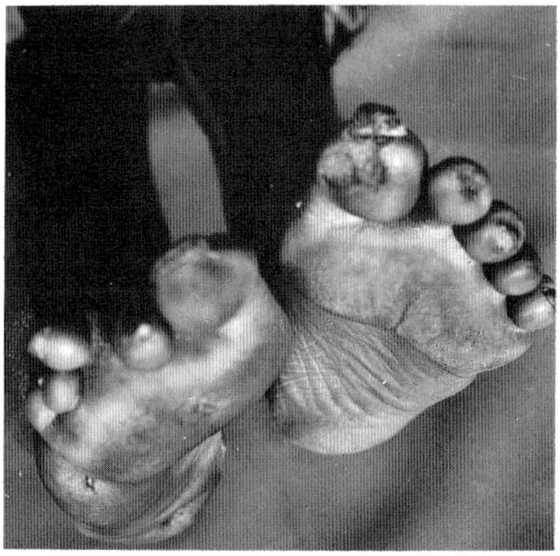

Fig. 32.15 Ulcers of the pads of the toes

deformities usually result from trophic ulceration and secondary infection which should be avoidable (Table 32.2).

Plantar ulcers also may lead to bony destruction. Ulcers on the row of the medial ray lead to damage of the first metatarsal; ulcers on the row of the lateral ray result ultimately in inverted and plantarflexed foot. Forefoot ulceration leads to equinus deformity, and hindfoot ulceration results in calcaneus foot (and vice versa). Osteomyelitis and pathological fracture of calcaneum with avulsion of the weakened posterior tuberosity present an elongated boat deformity of the calcaneum after healing of the ulcer (Figs. 32.16 and 17).

Site of plantar ulcers

The three most common sites are the base of the big toe, the base of the fifth toe and the heel, explained by 'the dynamic pressure triangle of the sole' (Languillon 1964). Other sites include the bases of the 2nd, 3rd and 4th toes, the lateral and medial borders of the foot and the plantar arch.

Bony changes in leprosy foot

These changes, discernible in X-ray, are due to the disease itself and to sensory loss, paralytic deformities and secondary infection. Bones are involved in 'leprous dactylitis', 'concentric bone atrophy' (in phalanges) and tarsal destruction. Leprous dactylitis is manifest as generalized

Table 32.2 Secondary deformities

Muscle imbalance	Site of ulcer
Fixed deformities:	
Shortened equinus foot	Anterior border
Inverted foot (destruction lateral ray)	Lateral border
Shortened foot with destruction of medial ray	Anterior border
Shortened plantigrade foot	Anterior border
Deformity due to joint neuropathy	Centre of sole or instep
Heel deformities	Heel multiple sinuses
Calcaneal deformity	Heel

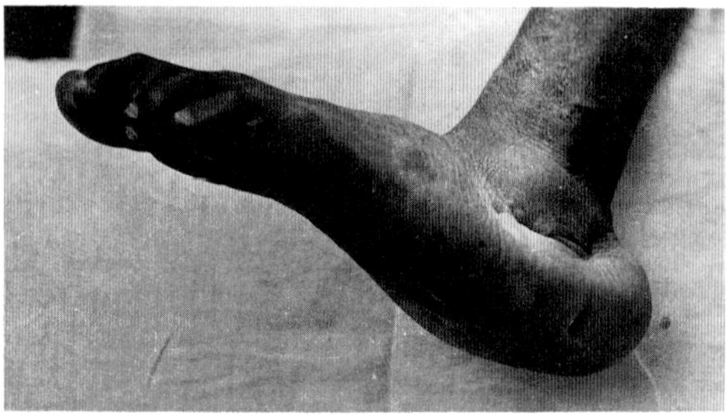

Fig. 32.16 Boat-deformity of the heel, due to pathological crumbling of the calcaneum and upward traction on its posterior rarified end due to tendo Achillis contraction

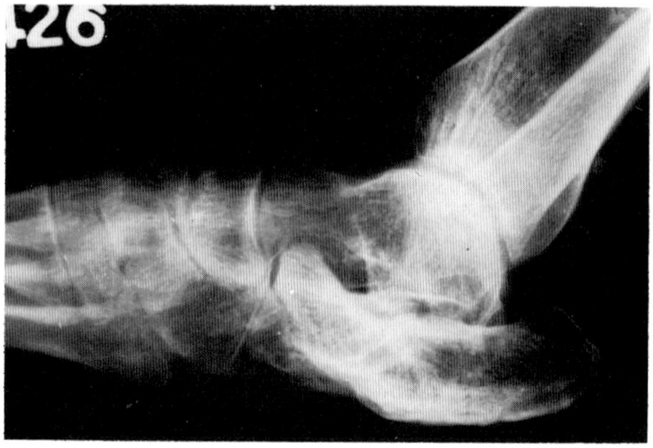

Fig. 32.17 X-ray of same deformity

osteoporosis with a localized area of destruction and periostitis on a subcutaneous prominent bony point.

Anaesthesia and secondary infection lead to osteomyelitis and sequestration, concentric absorption and progressive shortening (Figs. 32.18 and 19), loss of supportive bony structure and deformities.

Pathological fracture, pressure destruction of osteoporosed bone and bony dissolution occurs. These bony changes with deformities should be preventable. By contrast, neurotrophic ulcers in spina bifida (Fig. 32.20) occur without the loss of toe structure seen in leprosy.

Joint changes in leprosy foot

Initial exudative arthritis with or without secondary infections ends in fibrous or even bony ankylosis. With destructive changes dominating, the adjoining bony components of the joint are destroyed leaving a large gap between the two ends. Muscle imbalance (due to paralysis and destruction) leads to various deformities of the joint. Neuropathic changes are also seen in the ankle and foot joints (Figs. 32.21, 22, 23).

Management

General

A good rapport between doctor and patient, proper education about the disease and morale boosting of the patient are essential in order to gain confidence and cooperation of the latter, with which the disease may be finally arrested by therapy without any major deformity or disability of the foot, except for some sensory loss (unavoidable) and motor palsy (which can be compensated).

Segregation. This used to be indicated at the start of treatment, but now except for the initial few weeks in an open LL type, it is unnecessary and avoids

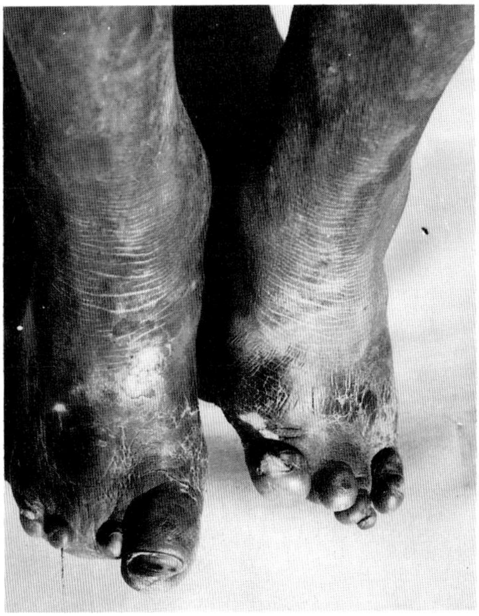

Fig. 32.18 Destruction and variable absorption of the phalanges and the metatarsals, leading to proximal migration of the toe tips

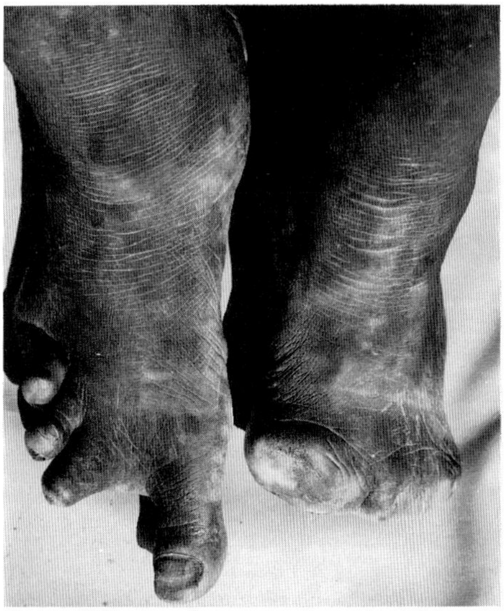

Fig. 32.19 Right foot: variable absorption of 2nd, 3rd, 4th and 5th toe rays, with overriding of fourth toe. Left foot: complete absorption of all the toes

putting stigma upon the patient. For any reaction or during an acute stage, the patient can be managed in any general hospital or even at his home.

General health care. The patient must be properly educated and shown how to take care of his hands, feet and eyes, as a preventive and therapeutic measure.

Specific chemotherapy

Chaulmoogra oil is now historical. Dapsone, diaminodiphenylsulphone (DDS), first reported by Fagen et al in 1943, is the main drug. It is almost nontoxic in the recommended dosage. In TT and BT types 5 to 10 mg daily for the first 6 months, followed by a gradually increased daily dose (to 50–100 mg) should be continued for 5 to 10 years. In LL and BL types 100 mg daily, with or without an accompanying drug (chlorfazimine or rifampicin) should be continued for life to avoid relapse. Primary dapsone resistance has not yet been observed. Injectable dapsone and repository sulphone (acedapsone, DADDS-4, 4′-diacetyl diaminodiphenylsulphone) are used to ensure the administration of therapy and prophylaxis.

Rifampicin, given in single daily dose of 450–600 mg on an empty stomach, is the fastest acting antileprosy drug and is used in LL types with dapsone, in pregnant women (LL type), and in DDS-resistant cases. It is potentially hepatotoxic and nephrotoxic. Besides nausea and abdominal discomfort, yellow or reddish-brown coloration of the urine, sputum, and sweat may occur.

Clofazimine, a riminophenazine dye, is an effective drug acting both as an antibacterial and an anti-inflammatory agent. In resistant cases and in leprosy reactions (erythema nodosum leprosum and lepra), it should be used (100 mg thrice weekly with dapsone or rifampicin). The main complication is a

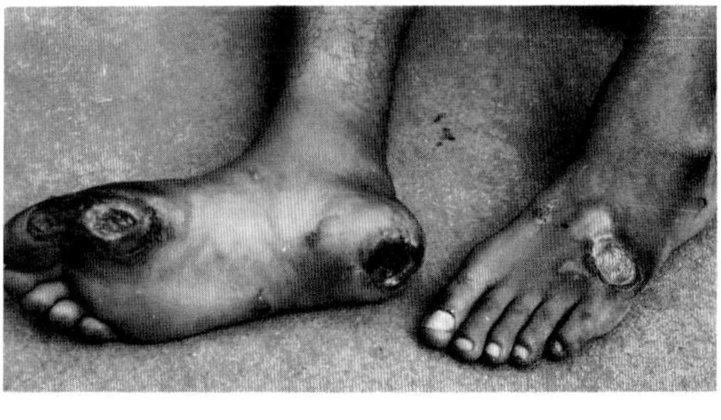

Fig. 32.20 Neurotropic ulcers in a cauda-equina lesion. Toes and other parts of the feet look normal

reddish-brown coloration of the skin, urine and sweat, which gradually clears after stopping the drug.

Second line antileprosy drugs are the thiourea compound thiambutosine (2 mg daily), ethionamide, and prothionamide.

For prophylaxis for child leprosy contacts, dapsone (20–25 mg/week for contacts of 15 years or above) serves the purpose.

BCG vaccination and immunotherapy by 'transfer factor' are controversial. For leprosy reactions (both the lepra reaction and erythema nodosum leprosum) in milder forms, aspirin, paracetamol, indomethacin or oxyphenylbutazone should be added to dapsone or chlorfazimine, but for severe forms steroids must be used with a higher dosage for erythema nodosum.

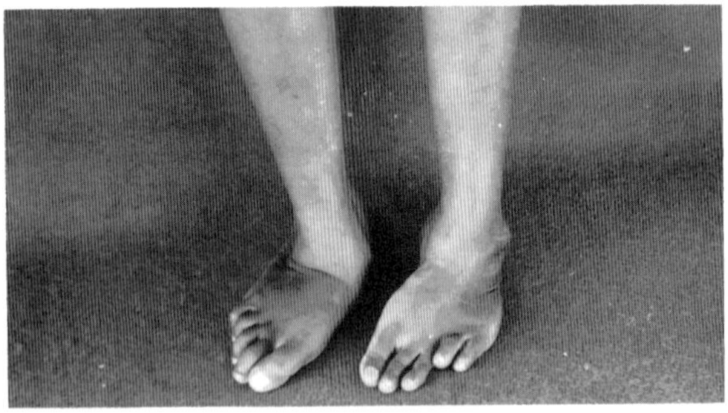

Fig. 32.21 Neuropathic changes in both ankles

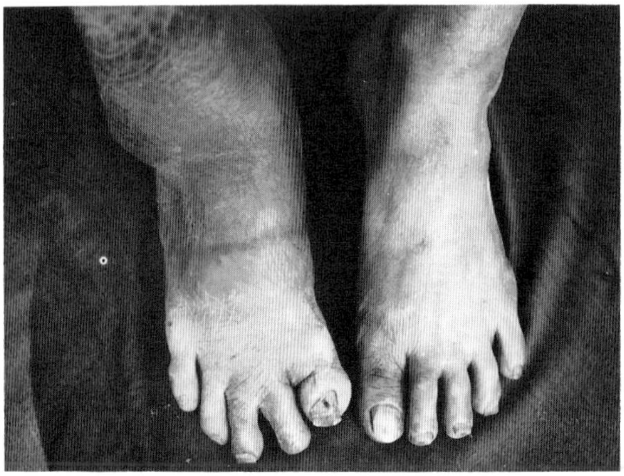

Fig. 32.22 Pathological fracture and neuropathic changes in the right ankle joint

Trophic ulcers

Trophic ulcers can be prevented by proper disease education of the patients and careful foot hygiene. Avoidance of walking barefoot or in nailed footwear and the use of special footwear prepared under supervision of a leprologist are important. The foot should be inspected daily for any thorn or nail prick, and for any black, haemorrhagic or oedematous area and before going to bed it should be soaked in water, mopped dry and gently rubbed with Vaseline®. The nails should be trimmed regularly and callosities and corns carefully shaved off. Walking should be with short steps and sitting on a chair or on the buttocks, avoiding squatting on the feet. If there is footdrop an orthosis should be worn.

A developed ulcer may be acute, subacute or chronic. Acute ulcers may be accompanied by constitutional symptoms, regional lymphadenitis, inflammatory features, and bleb formation, bursting with profuse serosanguinous discharge which becomes foul-smelling with secondary infections. General and local rest with foot elevation, protective dressings and antibiotics help at this stage. Adequate drainage is essential. With the subsidence of acute manifestations, the patient may be allowed up with limited movements in a properly padded plaster with

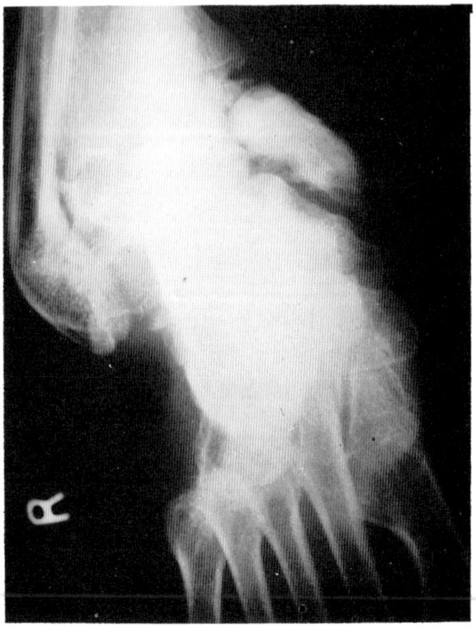

Fig. 32.23 X-ray of same ankle joint

attachments like Bohler's walking iron. Fortunately most trophic ulcers heal in a plaster cast. The freshly healed scar must be protected till it becomes relatively pliable, by using special protective footwear (e.g. the fixed ankle brace walker, FAB walker of Wollstein & Girling 1972) and by walking with slow and short steps.

Resistant ulcers indicate a lack of cooperation by the patient, spreading secondary infection and pyogenic osteomyelitis. Each should be managed on its merits. Thorough debridement, sequestrectomy and an adequate plastic procedure (partial (Fig. 32.24) thickness skin graft, full thickness pedicle flaps or cross-less flaps) may be required for such ulcers.

Polybactrin® and Cicatrin® have been used locally in chronic leprosy ulcers with encouraging results (Susman 1967), but these are costly drugs.

Deformity

Foot deformities should be adequately corrected to prevent the production and recurrence of ulceration.

For footdrop initially a footdrop splint should be tried for at least six months. Thereafter, the deformity can be corrected by tendon transfer (tibialis posterior or peronei to the dorsum of the foot with or without extensor hallucis longus plication) or by a stabilization procedure (Lambrinudi's triple arthrodesis). Fixed deformities like equinovarus will require wedge resection. Persistent ulcers and unstable adherent scars at the metatarsal heads should be resected. Excessive scarring in the forefoot is better managed by forefoot amputation followed by the use of well moulded special footwear.

Equinus deformities usually yield to tendo Achillis lengthening and posterior capsulotomy, but for resistant cases dorsal wedge resection or 'oblique sliding osteotomy' of the foot may be required.

For mobile claw toe (Fig. 32.25) transposition of the flexor digitorum longus to the dorsum of the proximal phalanx can be performed, but in the big toe interphalangeal joint fusion serves better (Ross 1964). Rigid claw toes where the forefoot is relatively intact, should be treated by fusing the interphalangeal joints of the toes. Where there is superficial forefoot scarring, fusion of the interphalangeal joints should be followed by use of resilient-soled footwear, but where there is loss of subcutaneous tissue and metatarsal heads, it is better to amputate the forefoot proximal to the metatarsal heads. Claw toes, with the proximal phalanges grossly hyperextended and a relatively intact forefoot, should be managed by excision of the proximal phalanges of the second to fifth toes through a plantar incision.

Amputation and prosthesis in leprosy

Vexed with repeated ulcers, patients often ask for amputation, but this must be resisted till it is really

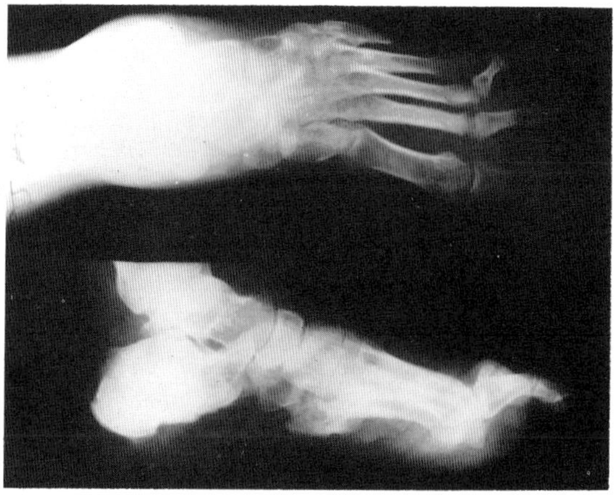

Fig. 32.24 Excision of the fifth metatarsal head was necessary to heal a persistent ulcer

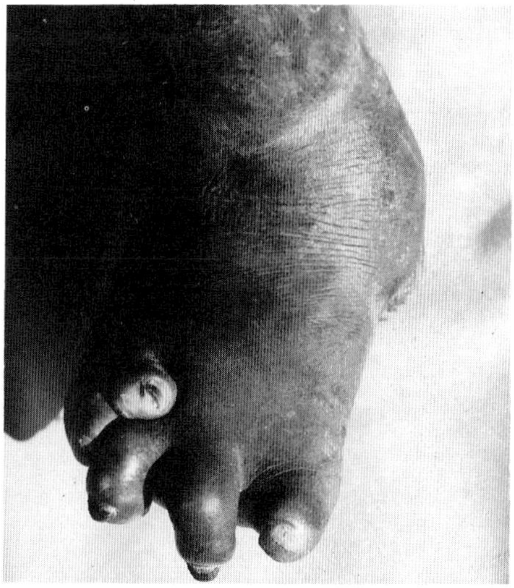

Fig. 32.25 Clawing of toes, 2, 3 and 5; partial absorption of fourth ray with overriding on to the third toe

unavoidable. Resistant trophic ulcers with more or less exposed bone ends and heavily scarred surroundings are the only indication for amputation. A minimum of the foot should be sacrificed.

Amputation has been performed at various levels; the root of the toes, transmetatarsal, transtarsal, Syme's, transankle or even below knee depending upon the areas of gross destruction and the availability of healthy covering flaps.

Prosthetic fittings in such patients require meticulous consideration on account of the insensitive skin (Fig. 32.26). Besides being light and economical attention should be paid to pressure points. Particular attention should be given to the making of a hard socket to prevent breakdown of stump skin (Garst 1971).

Footwear in leprosy foot (Girling 1966, Brand 1977)

The purposes of footwear are: (a) to take care of anaesthetic skin, (b) to prevent undue pressure on the vulnerable sites for trophic ulcers and on scarred areas, (c) to protect from thorns or nails and (d) to substitute for the deficiencies. It is difficult to get an 'all-in-one' design. Usually special footwear is not cosmetically acceptable.

Open slippers have been more beneficial and acceptable, and simple strap microcellular rubber chappals have proved quite useful (Karat 1969). Various materials have been utilized for manufacturing light and useful footwear, such as microcellular rubber, soft to hard leather, vulcanized rubber, automobile tyre walls. Light woods with softly padded tops, plastazote, cork and latex rubber (the latter two being more accepted). The basic facts to be considered when manufacturing such footwear are: (a) no nails should be used, (b) the material should not be too soft (so as to be over compressible) nor too hard to compress, (c) an accurately moulded insole to check instability and to help in distributing plantar pressures of walking and (d) a rigid-soled shoe is needed. In the rural areas wooden clogs, well moulded to sole contour and with some rocking arrangements on the bottom have been tried.

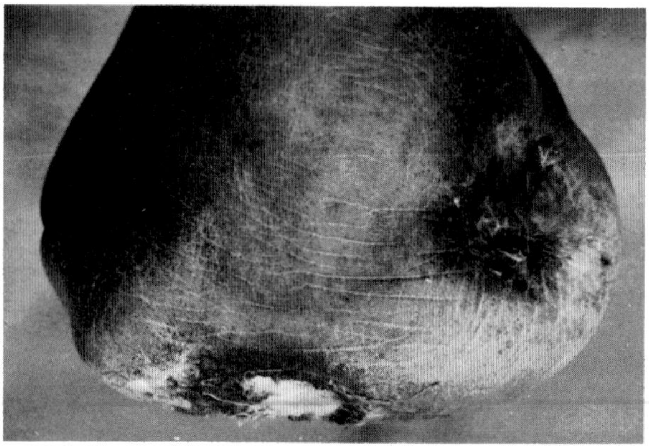

Fig. 32.26 Ulcers on a Syme's amputation stump

Tio et al (1966) have reported more than 75% success with ambulatory treatment of plantar leprosy ulcers in rural areas. The ulcers were plugged with 'zincoil' (75% zinc oxide and 25% cod liver oil) and the patients were instructed to walk in an altered way depending upon the site of ulcer.

Rehabilitation

Properly cared for, no leprosy foot should become a problem in rehabilitating a patient back to his original or a modified occupation. A word of caution: 'patients must not walk on wounded feet' (Ross 1962)

REFERENCES

Brown S G 1979 Mycobacterial diseases — Leprosy. In: Fitzpatrick T B et al Dermatology in General Medicine. 2nd edn. McGraw-Hill Book Company, New York. p 1494

Danielssen, Boeck 1847 Quoted by Browne S C, In: Fitzpatrick T B et al (eds) 1979 Dermatology in General Medicine. 2nd edn. McGraw-Hill, New York. p 1493

Davey T F, Rees R J W 1974 Lepr Rev 45: 121. In: Manson-Bahr P E C, Apted F I C (eds) 1982 Manson's Tropical Diseases. 18th edn. Baillière Tindall, London. p 300

Geater J C 1975 Lepr Rev 46: 279

Hansen G A 1874 In: Rook A, Wilkinson D S, Ebling F J G (eds) 1979 Textbook of Dermatology. 3rd edn. Blackwell Scientific Publications, Oxford. pp 749–765

Hilson G R F 1965 The place of Hansen in the history of microbial disease. Int J Lepr 33: 905

Jopling W H, Harman R R M 1979 Leprosy. In: Rook A, Wilkinson D S, Ebling F J G (eds) Textbook of Dermatology. 3rd edn. Blackwell Scientific Publications, Oxford. pp 749–765

Kwapinski J B G, Kwapinski E H 1974 Pathobiological relationship between *Mycobacterium leprae* and its primitive host. WHO 50: 473

Kircheimer W, Storrs E 1971 Attempts to establish the armadillo (*Dasypus novemcincta linn.*) as a model for the study of leprosy. Int J Lepr 39: 693

Lang-Stevenson A I, Sharrard W J W, Betts R P, Duckworth T 1985 Neuropathic ulcers of the foot. J Bone Joint Surg 67B: 438–442

Mitsuda 1916 In: Park J E, Park K (eds) 1916 Textbook of Preventive and Social Medicine. 10th edn. M/S Banarsidas Bhanot, Jabalpur, India. p 355
Narayanan E, Sreevatsa Raj A D, Kirchimer W F, Bedi B M S 1978 Lepr India 50: 26
Rees R J W 1967 Trans R Soc Trop Med Hyg 61: 581. In: Manson-Bahr P E C, Apted F I C (eds) 1982 Manson's Tropical Diseases. 18th edn. Baillière Tindall. p 299
Rodriguez, Plantill In: Rook A, Wilkinson D S, Ebling F J G (eds) 1979 Textbook of Dermatology. 3rd edn. Blackwell Scientific Publications, Oxford. p 756
Ridley D S, Jopling W H 1966 Classification of leprosy according to immunity. A five group system. Int J Lepr 34(3): 255–275
Shepard C C 1960 The experimental disease that follows the injection of human leprosy bacilli into foot-pads of mice. J Exp Med 112: 445
WHO 1966 Technical Report Series 319

FURTHER READING

Anderson J G 1964 Treatment and prevention of plantar ulcers. A practical approach. Lepr Rev 35, 4A: 251–258
Binford C H, Meyers W M, Walsh G P 1982 Leprosy. JAMA 247: 2283
Brand P W 1965 Leprosy in Tropical Surgery. In: Basu A K (ed) Clinical Surgery No. 8. Butterworths, London. pp 17–50
Brand P W 1977 Leprosy today. Insensitive Feet: A practical handbook on foot problems in leprosy. The Leprosy Mission, London. pp 1–77
Bryceson A, Pfaltzgraff R E 1979 Leprosy. 2nd edn. Churchill Livingstone, Edinburgh. pp 77–80
Garst R J 1971 Prosthesis in leprosy. Lepr Rev 42: 60–68
Girling J, Hameed M A, Selvapanadian A J 1966 Experimental moulded soles and shoe lasts. Lepr Rev 37, 2: 103–107
Goergen T G, Resnick D, Lomonace A, O'Dell C W Jr 1976 Radionuclide bonescan abnormalities in leprosy. Case reports. J Nucl Med 17: 788–790
Hastings R C, Job C K 1978 Reversal reactions in lepromatous leprosy following transfer factor therapy. Am J Trop Med Hyg 27, 25: 995–1004
Jacobson R R, Hastings R C 1976 Lancet ii: 1304. In: Jopling W H 1984 Handbook of Leprosy. 3rd edn. William Heinemann Medical Books Ltd, London. p 84
Jopling W H 1974 Leprosy. Br J Hosp Med, January, 43–50
Jopling W H 1978 Handbook of Leprosy. 2nd edn. Heinemann, London
Jopling W H 1984 Definition Epidemiology and World Distribution. Handbook of Leprosy. 3rd edn. William Heinemann Medical Books Ltd, London. p 1
Karat S 1969 The role of microcellular rubber in the prevention of anaesthetic feet in leprosy. Lepr Rev 40: 165–170
Languillon M C J 1964 Translated by Ross J. Frequency and localization of plantar perforating ulcers of leprosy patients. Lepr Rev 35, 4A: 239–244
Lennox W M 1964 A classification of leprosy foot deformities. Lepr Rev 35, 4A: 245–249
Lennox W M 1965 Plastic surgery of the anaesthetic foot of leprosy. Lepr Rev 36, 3: 109–117
Low J 1947 Lep Rev 18: 54. Quoted by Jopling W H 1984 In: Handbook of Leprosy. 3rd edn. William Heinemann Medical Books Ltd, London. p 4
Pettit J H S, Rees R J W 1964 Lancet ii, 673. Quoted by Jopling W H 1984. In: Handbook of Leprosy. 3rd edn. William Heinemann Medical Books Ltd, London. p 84
Price E W 1964 The etiology and natural history of plantar ulcers. Lepr Rev 35, 4A: 259–266
Price E W 1964 The problem of plantar ulcer. Lepr Rev 35, 4A: 267–272
Rees R J W, Pearson J M H, Water M F R 1970 Experimental and clinical studies on rifampicin in treatment of leprosy. Br Med J 1: 89
Rees R J W, Waters M F R 1972 Recent trends in leprosy research. Br Med Bull 28: 16
Ridley D S 1971 Lepr Rev 29: 45. Quoted by Jopling W H 1984 In: Handbook of Leprosy. 3rd edn. William Heinemann Medical Books Ltd, London. pp 11–12
Rose W F 1962 Etiology and treatment of plantar ulcers. Lepr Rev 33, 1: 25–40
Santoso H, Santoso K 1966 Ambulatory treatment of plantar leprosy ulcers. Lepr Rev 37, 4: 239–244
Sarojini P A, Mshana R N 1983 Lepr Rev 54, 151. Quoted by Jopling W H 1984 In: Handbook of Leprosy. 3rd edn. William Heinemann Medical Books Ltd, London. p 101
Shepard C C et al 1972 Rapid bactericidal effect of rifampicin on *Mycobacterium leprae*. Am J Trop Med Hyg 21: 446
Skinsnes O K 1964 Lepr Rev 35: 106
Skinsnes O K 1980 Int J Lepr 48: 333. Quoted by Jopling W H 1984 In: Handbook of Leprosy. 3rd edn. William Heinemann Medical Books, London. pp 4–6
Trautman J R, Enna C E 1971 Leprosy. In: Tice's Practice of Medicine, Vol 3. Harper & Row, New York. pp 1–38
Walsh G P, Meyers W M et al 1981 Leprosy — a Zoonosis. Lepr Rev 52: (Suppl.1) 77
Warndorff Van Dispen T 1982 Int J Lep 50: 139. Quoted by Jopling W H 1984 In: Handbook of Leprosy. 3rd edn. William Heinemann Medical Books Ltd, London. p 84
WHO Expert Committee on Leprosy 1977 Fifth Report, Geneva. pp 20–26
WHO Expert Committee on Leprosy 1982 Chemotherapy of leprosy for control programmes. WHO Technical Report Series 675, Geneva

TREPONEMATOSIS

Treponematosis includes (a) Yaws (synonyms: framboesia tropica, bouba, buba, patek, pian, parangi) due to *Treponema pertenue*; (b) Pinta (synonyms: carate, mal del pinto) due to *T. carateum* and *T. herrejoni*) and (c) Syphilis: (i) Nonvenereal (Synonyms: njovera, belesh, dichuchwa, skerljero, bejel, nonvenereal childhood syphilis, endemic syphilis) and (ii) Venereal, both due to *T. pallidum*.

Though the epidemiological behaviour and the clinical features of the different treponematoses could be adequately differentiated, the impossibility of cultivating these spirochaetes on artificial media, the common serological reactions and the details of the pathological changes has led to the concept of a unitary theory of the aetiology of these forms of treponematosis.

Regarding the progenitor of this group, Hudsen (1958) believes that ancient Africa was the motherland of the treponemata, where yaws existed first. Gradually, changing environmental factors gave rise to pinta, venereal and nonvenereal syphilis. On the other hand, Hackett (1963) claims 'pinta' to be the original form of treponematosis (15 000 BC), later mutants producing yaws (10 000 BC), nonvenereal syphilis (7 000 BC) and venereal syphilis (3 000 BC). Clinically these treponematoses manifest as primary, secondary and tertiary lesions spread over a prolonged period.

The foot is not affected in the early stages of pinta, but plantar manifestations are seen in even the early stages of yaws and nonvenereal syphilis and infrequently in the secondary stage of venereal syphilis. In tertiary stages, gummatous and destructive lesions can be seen in all these forms, but mostly in yaws.

YAWS

Yaws is a contagious granulomatous disease caused by a nonvenereally transmitted spirochaete, *Treponema pertenue*, mainly involves the skin and bones, and is usually crippling but not fatal.

History (Guthe 1979, Manson-Bahr & Apted 1982)

Yaws primarily existed in Africa almost 10 000 years ago. The earliest record of this disease manifest in bones and joints is from the Mariana Islands in the West Pacific and has been estimated by Stewart & Spoehr (1952) to be from about 854–145 AD. By the eighteenth century, it was found to have spread over Central and South America and Antilles, Oceania and Southeast Asia.

Due to its papillomatous secondary lesions mimicking the raspberry (Fr. framboise), the name framboesia was given to it by the local populace (1778).

Landmarks in its treatment by chemotherapy include the discovery of neoarsphenamine (Ehrlich 1910), bismuth (Lavaditi), arsenicals (Lambert 1923) and penicillin (Guimaraes of Brazil, Findley et al 1943 and WHO 1950)

Geographical distribution (Fig. 32.27)

Yaws is mostly confined to the hot and humid forest regions of the tropics, although it is prevalent in the Far East and China, where it extends into temperate zones.

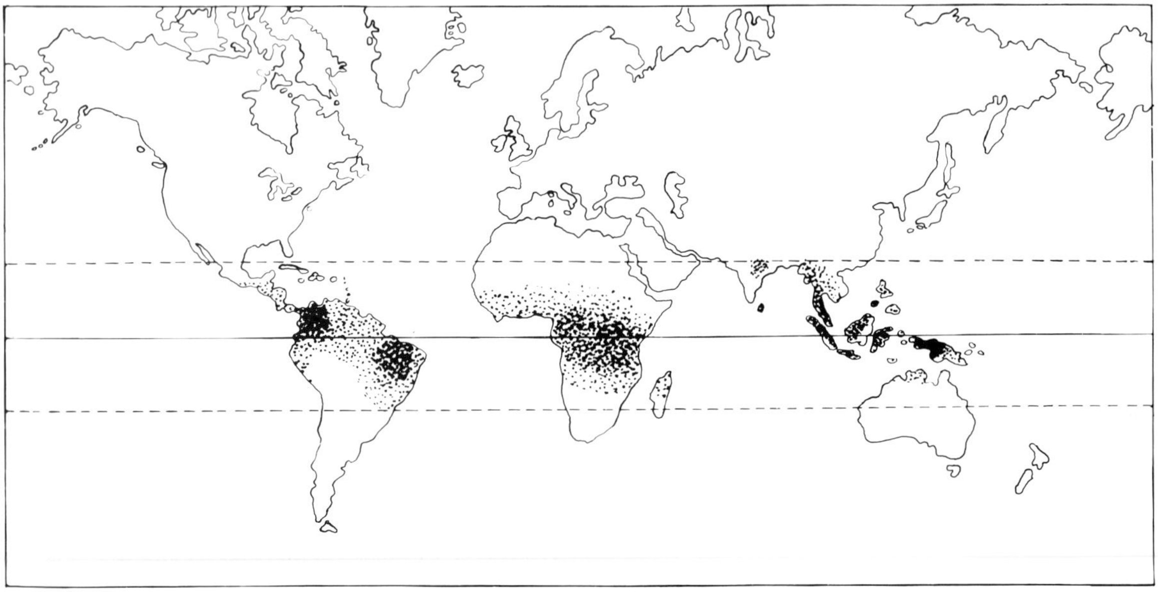

Fig. 32.27 Geographical distribution of yaws

Africa, the motherland of yaws, has still the largest reservoir of this disease (especially on the Ivory Coast and Abidjan). It is endemic in South East Asia (Thailand, Indonesia), in the Pacific Islands, Philippines and Oceania, and in Central and South America (Brazil and Columbia). Scattered pockets of dwindling size exist in India, Burma, Malaysia and Sri Lanka.

With the eradication programme against yaws (WHO) it has ceased to be a public health problem. However, the problem of 'residual yaws' will persist for sometime.

Aetiology

It is a disease of childhood (after 1 year of age) and adolescence. In hyperendemic areas the peak incidence is in the 2–5 years age group, whereas in the low endemic areas the highest seroprevalence is in the older age group. However 70% of infections occur before the age of 15. Males are more frequently affected than females.

The causative organism is *T. pertenue* which very closely resembles *T. pallidum* culturally and morphologically. *T. pertenue* is a tightly coiled, rigid and motile spirochaete (measuring 16 μm × 0.2 μm). It exists in the epidermis of the lesions, the lymph nodes, spleen and bones. No successful culture has been possible in vitro but it can be transmitted to certain animals (monkeys and rabbits). Baboons may act as a reservoir for yaws.

In a hot and humid climate, a rainy season and a low social environment, yaws begins where the highway ends (Vegas 1979). Poor personal hygiene, overcrowding and barefoot walking all predispose to the spread of the disease.

Immunity

There is no natural immunity, but resistance may very slowly be acquired. The incidence of yaws is inversely proportional to that of syphilis, to which there exists strong cross-resistance. However, concurrent infection by both may occur as in the Sudan.

Transmission

The disease is transmitted by direct contact, the organisms from the discharge of the infectious lesion entering through a breach in the epidermis. Transmission from an infected mother to her infant and vice versa is often possible. Spread by fomites is a possibility since the organisms from the discharge of the infectious lesions may survive on the soft, moist, earthen floor. Vectors (*Hippelates*, flies and cockroaches) may spread the infection.

Pathology

With a progressive eradication programme, opportunities for detailed pathological studies of yaws by modern scientific methods are not now possible. However, the records of the past and observations on animal experiments show that immediately after entrance through the breached or intact skin the treponemes are carried to the lymph nodes and also circulate in the body. Lesions are localized either in the skin or the bone, or both, in all three stages of the disease.

Visceral lesions are not a feature of yaws, nor is there endothelial proliferation in the blood vessels, unlike syphilis, though doubts about aortic involvement have been expressed. The CNS is said never to be affected, but Harris's report (1975) of neuro-ophthalmic abnormalities in late yaws confuses the delineation between yaws and syphilis. The basic pathology is the development at the site of cutaneous invasion of a proliferative granuloma containing numerous treponemes in the epidermis. In the primary lesions, acanthosis and multiple papillomatoses form the characteristic features. The oedematous and thickened epidermis shows marked neutrophilic infiltration presenting epidermal microabscesses. A dense lymphocytic, plasma cell and fibroblastic infiltration is seen in the epidermis, which is usually not perivascular.

Clinical features

The incubation period varies between 10 days and 6 months (commonly 3–5 weeks). As in other trepanosomal infections the clinical manifestations of yaws can be divided into three distinguishable stages, primary, secondary and tertiary (Hackett 1957), separated by latent periods.

The early lesions are multiple, nondestructive and contagious whereas the late lesions are destructive and noncontagious.

Primary stage

Synonyms: mamanpion, mother yaws, protopianoma, buba madra

Lesions usually develop at the site of inoculation of infection in an exposed part of the body, three-quarters being on the lower part of the leg and foot (Fig. 32.28). They start with erythematous infiltrated papules, then nodules form which gradually enlarge into a papillomatous, broad-based granuloma exuding whitish-yellow, serous discharge, swarming with treponemes. This later forms a yellow scab. Ultimately typical raspberry lesions are produced which are painless but bleed easily. Constitutional features are mild, occasional and temporary. There may be nonsuppurative, non-specific, painless enlargement of lymph glands persisting for 2–6 months. Mother yaws heal spontaneously without much scarring, although occasionally there may be large atrophic and depressed scars, with a hypopigmented centre. The soles of feet are not a common site for mother yaws, but they may occur at the margins and in the toe clefts.

Secondary stage

The secondary lesions usually appear 8–16 weeks after the onset of the disease, after the primary lesions have healed, but overlap is not infrequent and the period of appearance may also vary widely. The lesions are basically similar to the primary ones, but are multiple and of various sizes. They erupt in successive crops, spread widely, but are very rare on the scalp (Figs. 32.29 and 30). Lesions gradually tend to localize around the body orifices (mouth, nose and urogenital regions), the periaxillary regions and the soles and palms.

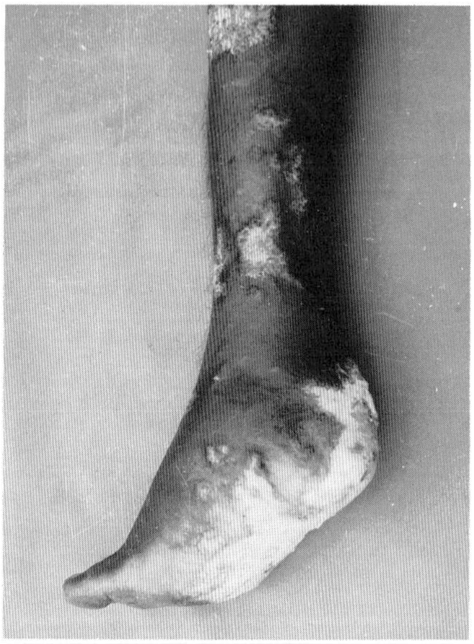

Fig. 32.28 Early framboesiform lesion (the patient had adherent skin at sole and heel following burn in early childhood)

General symptoms such as headache, irregular fever, loss of appetite and weight, pains in the bones and joints and generalized lymphadenopathy may precede the eruptions.

The skin. The exudative (sometimes dry) papillomatous eruptions, usually covered with yellow or brownish crusts, are infectious and except for size and number may resemble mother yaws. These are known as daughter yaws, pianomas, or framboesiomas. Usually they are of two types — the larger ones resembling mother yaws and the smaller ones so-called miniature yaws. However the peripheral extension of the daughter yaws may produce circinate yaws (tineal yaws). Mucosal lesions are very rare, probably appearing as an extension of lesions at the mucocutaneous junction. Usually the cutaneous yaws are painless but they may itch.

Plantar lesions. Those on the sole and palm, where the epithelium is thick and firm, appear late and are painful. The plantar skin becomes dry and peels and is irregularly thickened by hyperkeratotic plaques, cracks and fissures. A cherry-like granuloma appears in the well of the fissured horny layers. The granulomatous tissue is commonly present on the

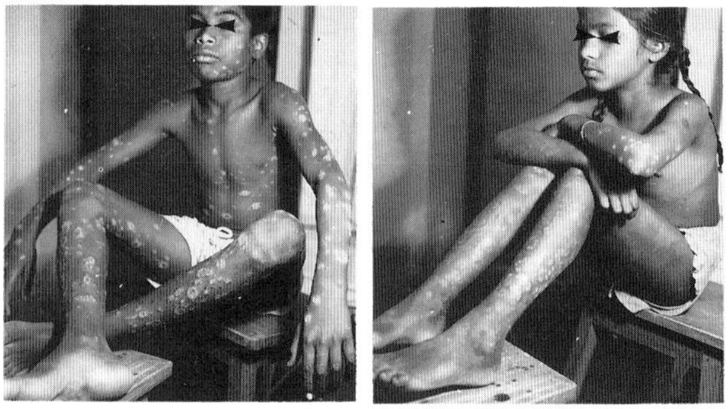

Figs. 32.29 and 30 Secondary eruptions: 'circinate' forms (tineal yaws) can be seen. The two patients are brother and sister (Courtesy of Prof. B. N. Prasad)

outer and inner borders of the sole, and in the clefts of the toes. The yaws on the soles produce painful disability and the patient tries to walk on the margin of the foot, giving rise to the term crab yaws (Fig. 32.31) (Basset et al 1972). The scattered areas of hyperkeratotic plaque on the sole may fall out, leaving behind punched out excavations, known as clavus.

Osseous lesions. The bones are commonly involved in the secondary stage and the order of frequency of involvement is leg, forearm, hand, foot, and skull. They usually produce a deep seated dull ache which is worse at night and in damp conditions. The basic lesions are periostitis and gummatous osteitis. Cortical rarefaction and periosteal bone deposition in the late stages may produce a sabre tibia (in Australia it is called boomerang leg) and bowing of the other long bones of the limbs (Fig. 32.32). Polydactylitis commonly affects children and sometimes may incapacitate them. Usually the secondary bone lesions appear rapidly and resolve spontaneously after a few months or even weeks.

In the hands there may be some thickening, cortical expansion and/or destructive focal rarefaction in the metacarpals and phalanges.

In the foot, the basic osseus lesions are similar to those in the hand and are relatively less common, both in frequency and extent. Tarsal involvement is commoner than that of the metatarsals and phalanges. The destructive changes may reach the surface resulting in ulcers and sinuses.

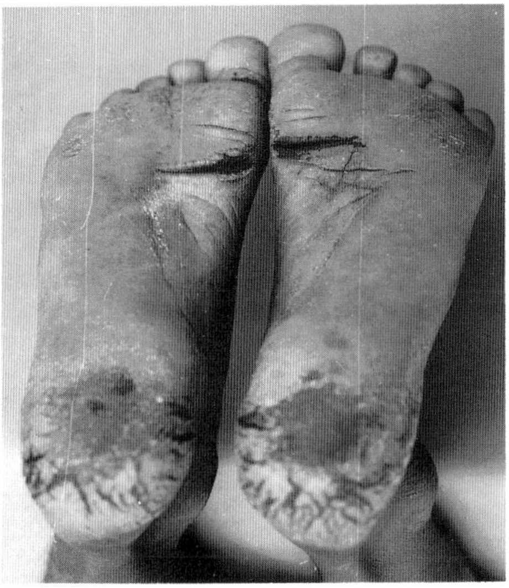

Fig. 32.31 Almost symmetrical 'crab yaws' — late hyperkeratotic lesions with cracks and fissures, partly due to prolonged barefooted walking

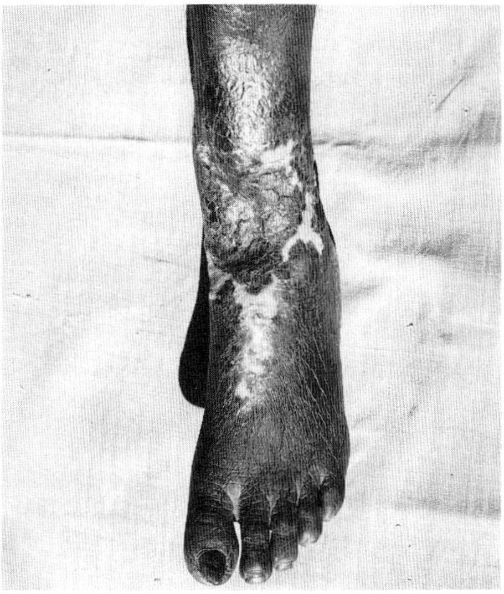

Fig. 32.32 Late yaws with resistant ulcers and tendency to sacre bitia

Late secondary lesions of the skull and facial bones may leave permanent legacies, e.g. gangosa (collapse of the nose with perforation in the palate) and goundou (periosteal deposits across the face on either side of the nasal bridges). A slowly growing, hypertrophic ossification of the nasal bones and frontal processes of the maxilla may rarely lead to blindness.

The joints are not commonly involved, but hydrarthrosis specially in the knee, ankle and elbow may occur. The joint appears as if ensheathed by a gelatinous mass. Rheumatic manifestations may appear in the late stages — rheumatic yaws. Secondary stage lesions may heal spontaneously or with treatment, with or without depigmented scarring. There is usually a latency of about five years after which the tertiary stage lesions develop.

Tertiary stage

In this stage also the main affections are of skin, subcutaneous tissue and bones. The basic reactions are those of active and destructive granulomata, in which the gummatous lesions are at first hard, mobile and painless (Fig. 32.33). Gradually lesions undergo central necrosis with cold abscess

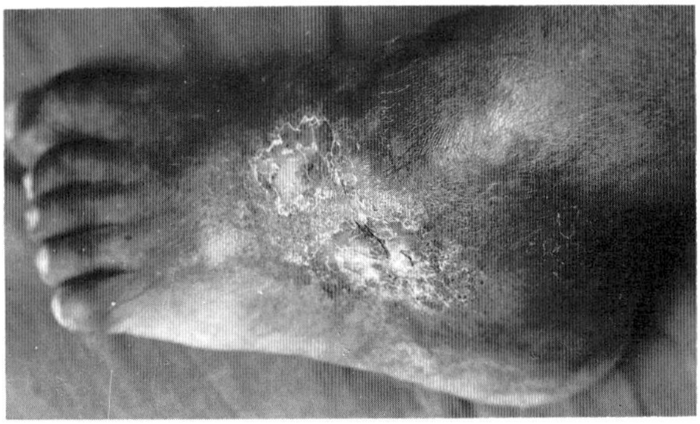

Fig. 32.33 Late yaws — infiltrative lesion mimicking lupus vulgaris

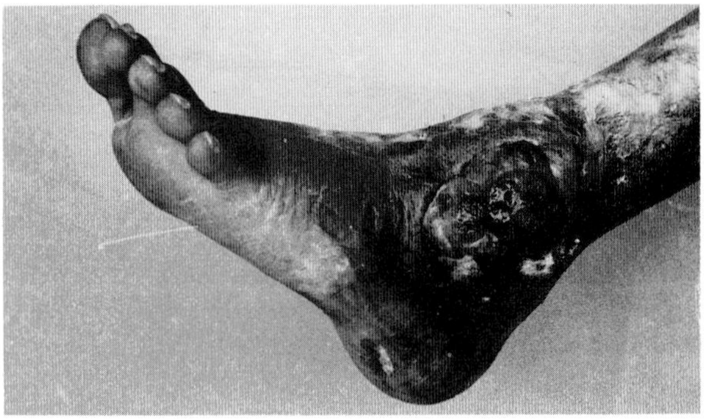

Fig. 32.34 Late yaws — gummatous framboesides

formation. The abscess bursts forming a chronic indolent, slowly progressive ulcer with yellowish slough and deep connections (Fig. 32.34). They ultimately heal with severe scarring, which may lead to disfigurement, and deformity. Keloid formation and secondary elephantiasis may occur. Very rarely the chronic ulcers may end in epithelioma.

The most common legacies are keratoderma and diffuse or localized hyperkeratosis of the sole and palm. Such painful lesions on one side of the sole lead to crab yaws (Lomholt 1979). As in syphilis, hyperkeratotic plaques with fissures oozing serum, or painless minute craters surrounded by hyperkeratotic papules, may develop (see Fig. 32.31) and are known as hormiguillo (Lomholt 1979, Vegas 1979).

Osseous involvement is seen at this stage, and although occurring in only a few bones (tibia (see Fig. 32.32), forearm bones and humerus) is of a serious nature. Where there is osteoperiostitis, thickening of the periosteum, oval cortical rarefaction and necrosis occurs forming a sequestrum. There may be pathological fracture. Skull bone affections, (gangosa and goundou) can be sequelae (Furtado 1955).

Investigations

Isolation of *T. pertenue* from the exudate of the suspected primary and secondary lesions by dark-ground examination or with silver stains is confirmatory.

Inoculations of the treponema have been possible in monkeys, rabbits and hamsters. Serological tests carried out for syphilis (e.g. Wassermann, Kahn etc.) are positive in increasing titre from four weeks after the appearance of the primary lesions. There is evidence of cross immunity with syphilis and vice versa.

Differential diagnosis

Typical early lesions of yaws may not present much difficulty in diagnosis, but framboesiomas may need differentiation from framboesoid leishmaniasis, framboesiform syphilides and paracoccidioidomycosis. Bubides or piamides in yaws should be differentiated from pityriasis versicolor, psoriasis and pityriasis rosea. Early ulcerated leg lesions may be confused with tropical ulcers. Circinate secondary lesions of yaws look like certain fungal infections, e.g. tinea versicolor. The lesions in bejel and pinta mimic yaws lesions and are differentiated on the grounds of areas of prevalence (bejel is seen mostly in the Middle East and among the Bedouin Arabs, pinta in Central and South America and certain Caribbean islands and in Cuba) and by defining the causative organisms.

It is worth remembering that polydactylitis, crab yaws and goundou do not occur in other treponematoses. Yaws does not affect the viscera or the central nervous system and there is no congenital yaws. Hyperkeratotic and allied conditions of the soles resemble keratoma plantare sulcatum, plantar warts, plantar pitting and tropical hyperkeratotic conditions of unknown origin (Hackett & Lowenthal 1960).

In the late stages of yaws, the contractual and destructive lesions should be differentiated from leprosy and tuberculosis.

Treatment

The management of treponemal infections with bismuth preparations and neoarsphenamine have now become more or less historical. Benzathine penicillin G has dramatically revolutionized the treatment and control of yaws (also bejel, pinta and syphilis). The early lesions become dark field negative within 48 hours and disappear within two weeks, even with the single dose treatment. For overt cases the recommended dose schedule (WHO) is as follows:

Adults: total dose 2.4 Mu, as 1.2 Mu given twice at intervals of 4–5 days.

Ages 5–15 years: total dose 1.2 Mu to be given divided at intervals of 4–5 days.

Age below 5 years: single dose of 0.3 Mu.

Latent cases and contacts receive half of the above dosages. Safeguards must be ready for possible Herzheimer reactions to penicillin.

Other antibiotics which may be used with almost comparable efficacy are: tetracycline — 2 g daily for 5 days; chlortetracycline; oxytetracycline — 3 g on first day followed by 2 g on second and third days; chloramphenicol.

Control programme by WHO

WHO has recommended definite policies to control yaws, based upon its endemicity:

1. Total mass treatment: A community having more than 10% prevalence is considered a hyperendemic area and the entire population should be given penicillin in the recommended dosage as for overt cases.

2. Juvenile mass treatment: In areas with an incidence of active cases of between 5–10% (mesoendemic communities), in addition to the actual cases (which are treated with full dosage) all children below 15 years and all contacts should be given the half dose schedule.

3. Selective mass treatment: In hypoendemic communities with prevalence rate less than 5%, only affected cases are treated with full doses and contacts are given half doses.

Eradication programmes have been effective on the mass treatment policies. These are aided by programmes of (a) survey and resurvey — detection — treatment, (b) continued surveillance by basic health services (keen watch — detection — reporting), (c) regular examination of schoolchildren and (d) random survey of villages. Social, economic and environmental improvement, improving domestic and personal hygiene, providing a clean and adequate water supply, the liberal use of soap and better housing conditions are important.

Ulcerated yaws lesions should be adequately dressed and supported. Contractures and deformities may need judicious surgery besides medical treatment. Special footwear is not as important as in leprosy, but plantar lesions should be protected by suitable dressings to avoid secondary infection.

Prognosis

Spectacular results are seen with treatment in the primary and secondary stages, all lesions vanishing in two weeks. Quite late recurrences have been seen. Late tertiary lesions may produce contractures, deformities and incapacitating disabilities. Artificial immunization has not been hitherto possible.

REFERENCES

Basset I, Faye I, Maleville J, Malgras J 1972 Yaws and endemic syphilis In: Marshall J (ed) Tropical Dermatitis. 2nd edn. Excerpta Medica, Amsterdam. p 304

Entlich 1910 In: Beeson P B et al (eds) 1979 Cecil Textbook of Medicine. 15th edn. (Asian Edition). W. B. Saunders Company, Igaku Shoin Ltd, Tokyo. p 506

Findlay et al 1943 In: Woodruff A W 1977 Medicine in the Tropics. Churchill Livingstone, Edinburgh. p 355

Furtado T 1955 Manifestacoes tardias da Framboesia, Brazil, Bele Horizonte. In: Rook A, Wilkinson D S, Ebling F J G (eds) Textbook of Dermatology. 2nd edn. Vol 1. Blackwell Scientific Publications, Oxford. pp 668–674

Guthe T 1979 Non syphilitic treponematoses. In: Beeson P B (ed) Cecil Textbook of Medicine. 15th edn. (Asian Edition). W. B. Saunders Company, Philadelphia. pp 518–522

Hackett C J 1957 An International Nomenclature of Yaws Lesions. WHO Monograph Series No. 36, Geneva

Hackett C J, Lowenthal L J A 1960 Differential Diagnosis of Yaws. WHO Monograph Series 45, Geneva. p 88

Hackett C J 1963 On the Origin of the Human Treponematoses. WHO Bulletin 29: 7, Geneva

Harris J R W 1975 Non venereal treponematoses. In: Morton R S, Harris J R W (eds) Recent Advances in Sexually Transmitted Diseases, Churchill Livingstone, Edinburgh. pp 124–126

Hudson E H 1958 Non-venereal syphilis: A sociological and

medical study of Bejel. In: Manson-Bahr P E C, Apted F I C (eds) 1982 Manson's Tropical Diseases. Baillière Tindall, London. p 416
Lomholt G 1979 Syphilis yaws and pinta. In: Rook A, Wilkinson D S, Ebling F J G (eds) Textbook of Dermatology. 3rd edn. Blackwell Scientific Publications, Oxford. p 740
Manson-Bahr P E C, Apted F I C 1982 Manson's Tropical Diseases. Baillière Tindall, London. p 402
Stewart T D, Spoehr A In: Woodruff A W (ed) 1977 Medicine in the Tropics. Churchill Livingstone, Edinburgh. p 355
Vegas F K 1979 Yaws In: Rook A, Wilkinson D S, Ebling F J G (eds) Textbook of Dermatology. 3rd edn. Blackwell Scientific Publications, Oxford. p 376

FURTHER READING

Fiumara N J 1985 The Treponematoses. In: Moschella S L, Hurley H J (eds) Dermatology, Vol 1. W. B. Saunders Company, Philadelphia. pp 857–865
Woodruff A W 1982 Yaws. In: Scott R B (ed) Price's Textbook of the Practice of Medicine. 12th edn. Oxford University Press. p 110

PINTA

Synonyms: carate (among Carib and Aztec Indians), mal del pinto (Cuba)

Pinta, essentially a disease of childhood and affecting only the skin, is the weakest of the human treponematoses, caused by *T. carateum* which is morphologically indistinguishable from *T. pertenue* and *T. pallidum*. It is geographically isolated in the coloured population of the Americas (e.g. Mexico, Colombia, Peru, Brazil, Venezuela), the West Indies and the South Pacific islands.

History (Guthe 1979, Vegas 1979)

Valdez and Cortez described this disease between 1505 and 1515. Leony Blanco (1939) in Mexico discovered the specific causative organism using dark-field control. Varela (1944) proved the value of penicillin in pinta.

Aetiology

T. carateum gains access mostly through abraded skin. The incubation period is 2 to 3 weeks. There is a weaker cross immunity with syphilis than in yaws and pinta may coexist with syphilis.

Pathology

The essential granuloma slowly develops in the subcutaneous layer along with hypertrophy of the overlying skin, which later undergoes atrophy or depigmentation. Local and regional lymphadenitis may develop.

Clinical features

Progress is through three overlapping stages. In the primary stage, itchy erythematous papules, gradually changing into elevated erythematous patches, develop on the exposed parts of the body (dorsum of the foot and leg, the forearm and dorsum of the hand, elbows, neck, face, buttocks and thigh).

After about a year the secondary stage creeps in, characterized by generalized cutaneous rashes or papules known as pintides; these multiply and may coalesce, and may be hypopigmented, pigmentary or erythematosquamous.

The tertiary stage is manifest 2–5 years later and lesions consist of irregular pigmented spots in different shades of grey, steel, ash or blue (Lawton-Smith 1971).

Eventually depigmented areas appear, especially near bony prominences such as the dorsum of the elbows, malleoli, knees, wrists, on the back of the hands and on the plantar and palmar surfaces.

In the later stages there may be overlap lesions of dyschromia, hypochromia and achromia in the same patient (Figs. 32.35 and 36). Hyperkeratotic scaly lesions with contractures may develop as in yaws, especially in the palms and soles. Ultimately atrophic and depigmented dry lesions manifest especially in the vicinity of the major joints. The skin becomes dry, thinned, and wrinkled with loss of sweat and sebaceous secretion (Marques 1955). Generalized lymphadenopathy without systemic symptoms is seen in the secondary and tertiary stages.

Investigations

Except for the demonstration under dark-field or by

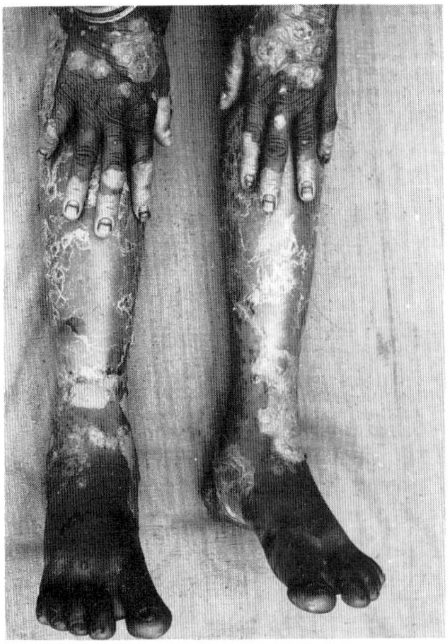

Fig. 32.35 Late pinta with mixed overlap lesions of dyschromia, hypochromia and achromia. Areas with complete loss of melanin mimic vitiligo

phase contrast, of *T. carateum* in serum from scratched lesions or lymph, no other investigation is confirmatory.

Differential diagnosis

Neurodermatitis, tinea, eczema and psoriasis must be differentiated from the early lesions. Late pinta may be confused with erythema dyschromicum perstans, melanosis, various leukodermas and vitiligo, tuberculoid leprosy, dermal tuberculosis, yaws and syphilis.

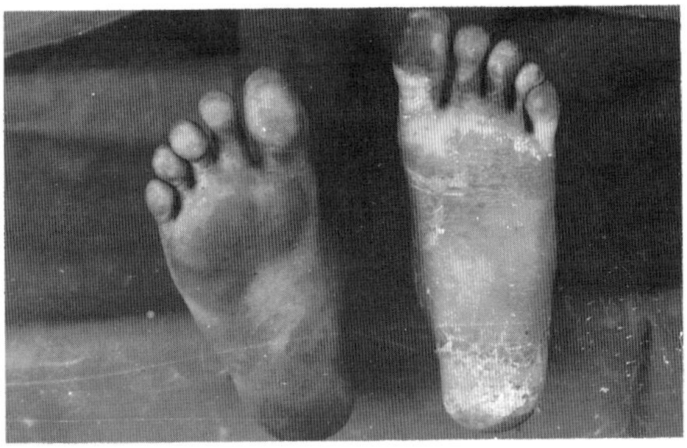

Fig. 32.36 Same as Fig. 32.35 — changes on the sole

Treatment

Repository long acting penicillin (procaine penicillin G in oil with 2% aluminium monostearate) or benzathine penicillin G in total dosage of 2 400 000 units in the drug of choice (Marquez et al 1955). Except for the prolonged depigmented and atrophic lesions of the tertiary stage, other manifestations can be cured with proper treatment.

Prophylaxis

Besides improving social and personal hygiene, a single dose of 1.2 Mu of long acting penicillin is required as a prophylactic measure in mass campaigns in endemic zones.

REFERENCES

Guthe T 1979 Non syphilitic treponematoses — Pinta. In: Beeson P B et al (eds) Cecil Textbook of Medicine. 15th edn. W. B. Saunders Co, Philadelphia. p 524
Leon Blanco 1939 In: Beeson P B et al (ed) 1979 Cecil Textbook of Medicine. 15th edn. (Asian Edition). W. B. Saunders Co, Igaku Shoin Ltd, Tokyo
Lawton-Smith J et al 1971 Neuro ophthalmological study of late yaws and pinta. II The Carcas project. Br J Vener Dis 47: 226
Marquez F et al 1955 WHO Bulletin 13: 229
Varela 1944 In: Beeson P B et al (eds) 1979 Cecil Textbook of Medicine. 15th edn. (Asian Edition). W. B. Saunders Co, Igaku Shoin Ltd, Tokyo. p 524
Vegas F K 1979 Pinta. In: Rook A, Wilkinson D S, Ebling F J C (eds) Textbook of Dermatology. 3rd edn. Blackwell Scientific Publications, Oxford. p 742

FURTHER READING

Fiumara N J 1985 The treponematoses. In: Moschella S L, Hurley H J (eds) Dermatology, Vol 1. W. B. Saunders Co, Philadelphia. p 866
Rhodes A R, Luger A F H 1979 Syphilis and other treponematoses. In: Fitzpatrick T B et al (eds) Dermatology in General Medicine. 2nd edn. McGraw-Hill Book Co, New York. pp 728–729
Willicoe R R 1976 Epidemiology of the spirochaetoses: A worldwide review. In: Johnson R C (ed) Biology of Parasitic Spirochaetoses. New York Academic, New York. pp 133–155

ENDEMIC SYPHILIS

Synonyms: Bejal (Syria), nonveneral childhood syphilis, njovera (Zimbabwe), dichuchwa (Botswana), skerljevo (Bosnia), siti (Gambia), frenjak, sibbens, button scurvy and radesyge

Geographical

Bejel, essentially a childhood chronic treponemal disease, is seen in hot and dry zones (e.g. Syria, Iran, Iraq, Central and South Africa (DuToit 1969), but occurs also in Yugoslavia, Central Asia, Central Australia and Tibet.

Children are the reservoir. Poor hygienic and sanitary conditions and devitalizing mucosal diseases predispose. Causative treponemes are morphologically indistinguishable from *T. pallidum*, *T. pertenue* and *T. carateum*. Cross immunity exists against syphilis.

Clinical manifestations

Endemic syphilis rarely manifests as primary chancres (Merriweather 1959, Schmid & Luger 1962). Secondary lesions, mimicking those of acquired syphilis, are generally distributed over the whole body, but favour warm and moist areas (e.g. lips, tongue, anus, axilla, genitalia, elbows, knees). Cutaneous itchy ulcers may develop. In the tertiary stage erosive ulcers appear in the oropharyngeal and laryngeal areas. Gummatous ulcers, bone changes and condylomata lata may persist for much longer periods. Disabling fissures on thickened skin due to hyperkeratosis of the soles of the feet may be troublesome. Systemic affections are extremely rare.

Diagnosis

The localized epidemiological distribution is perhaps the only real diagnostic criterion.

Treatment

The disease responds quite well to benzathine penicillin G or long acting penicillin (1.2 million units for adults). For late cases, two more such doses at intervals of 3–7 days, and half doses should be given for contacts.

For the foot problems, besides systemic penicillin, care and protection of ulcers and fissures on the sole, the use of dressings and special footwear is essential.

REFERENCES

Dutoit J A 1969 Endemic syphilis in Karoo. S Afr Med J 43(13): 355–358

Merriweather A M 1959 Central Afr J Med 5: 181. In: Rook A, Wilkinson D S, Ebling F J G (eds) Textbook of Dermatology. 3rd edn. 1979. Blackwell Scientific Publications, Oxford. p 727

Schmid E E, Luger A 1962 Serologische untersuchungen bei endemischer syphilis. Dermatologica 124: 53

FURTHER READING

Fiumara N J 1985 The treponematoses. In: Moschella S L, Hurley H J (eds) Dermatology, Vol 1. W. B. Saunders Company, Philadelphia. pp 866–867

Rhodes A R, Luger A F H 1979 Syphilis and other treponematoses. In: Fitzpatrick T B et al (eds) Dermatology in General Medicine. 2nd edn. McGraw-Hill, New York. pp 1726–1727

WHO 1960 Technical Report Series, Geneva. p 190

SYPHILIS

Syphilis, an infectious disease caused by *Treponema pallidum* and mostly transmitted by sexual contact, is not essentially a disease of the tropics, rather more of the civilized world. Its manifestations, through the typical three stages, primary, secondary and tertiary, are bizarre, with a large variety of clinical manifestations.

For the primary chancre, the foot is not a common site. In the secondary stage, papules are more irregularly distributed, and besides the anogenital region, the face, the soles and palms, flexures and folds of skin are especially involved. Localization of papular syphilides to the palms and soles are often missed (Lomholt 1979). Lesions starting as bluish-red erythematous spots, gradually turn into infiltrated and papular ones. In classic cases hyperpigmented papulosquamous lesions involve the palms and soles. The thick epidermal covering gradually peels off leaving scaly collarettes. In late cases epidermal thickening, may develop into small keratotic areas.

In the clefts of toes hypertrophic condylomata lata may appear mimicking tinea pedis. Later psoariatic or keratotic eczematous lesions may appear with flakes and fissures or a warty look.

In the tertiary stage, gummatous ulcers may appear on the leg, ankle and foot mimicking varicose ulcers. Unlike the hand, periosteal reactions and syphilitic osteomyelitis are not common in the phalanges of the foot. Serological tests, both nonspecific (e.g. Wassermann test, VDRL) and specific treponemal tests (e.g. *Treponema pallidum* immobilization (TPI) test; fluorescent treponemal antibody absorption (FTA-ABS) test; Reiter protein complement fixation test (RPCF) and microhemagglutination assay for *T. pallidum* (MHA-TP), and darkfield demonstration of *T. pallidum* confirm the diagnosis. Penicillin, being the most effective, cheapest and safest treponemicide is the drug of choice for all stages of syphilis. The expert ommittee of WHO (1953) has recommended a minimum dose of 2.4 Mu for primary and 4.8 Mu for secondary syphilis. However many clinicians favour a higher dosage even in the primary stage to ensure continuous high penicillin levels.

For the foot problems, along with chemotherapy, local preventive measures by dressing and special footwear are needed.

REFERENCES

Lomholt G 1979 Syphilis, Yaws and Pinta. In: Rook A, Wilkinson D S, Ebling F J G (eds) Textbook of Dermatology. 3rd edn. Blackwell Scientific Publications, Oxford. p 715
WHO 1953 Technical Report Series. p 63

FURTHER READING

Fiumara N J 1985 The Treponematoses. In: Moschella S L, Hurley H J (eds) Dermatology, Vol I. W. B. Saunders Company, Philadelphia. pp 817–857

FILARIASIS

Synonyms: tropical elephantiasis, Malabar legs

Filariasis consists of a group of human diseases caused by seven nematodes of the Filarioidea family and one of the family Dracunculoidea (guinea worm). It is usually transmitted by haemophagous arthropods (mosquitoes), and was the first disease proved to be transmitted by insects.

Historical aspects

The word 'filaria' has been taken from 'filar' which means 'thread-like'. The disease existed in India as early as the 6th century B.C. Clark (1709) in Cochin (Southern India) coined the word 'Malabar legs' for this disease, naming it after the Malabar coast. In Brazil, Woucherer (1866) demonstrated microfilariae in chylous urine. Lewis (1872), in Calcutta, demonstrated microfilariae in peripheral blood. Bancroft (1876) in Brisbane (Australia), discovered the adult female. Cobbold (1877), studied the life cycle of *Filaria bancrofti*. Manson (1878) in China, demonstrated the development of *Wuchereria bancrofti* in mosquitoes (*Culex quinquefasciatus*), and was the first to reveal the phenomenon of periodicity in filarial infections. He also described (1891) the microfilaria of *Dipetatonema perstans*. Bruge (1927), in Indonesia, found the microfilaria of *Brugia malayi*, while Rao and Maplestone (1940) in India, discovered the adult *B. malayi*.

Diethylcarbamazine was discovered to be an effective drug against filariasis in 1946.

Geographical distribution (Fig. 32.37)

Filariasis is distributed worldwide (between 45° North to 25° South latitudes), and is found mainly in Africa, India, the northern parts of South America, Malaysia, Oceania, Tonga and Fiji (WHO 1962). The majority of the sufferers are in Asia. Globally filariasis appears to be on the increase (WHO 1967). Of the various Filarioidea nematodes *W. bancrofti* (Turner 1959) is the most common, followed by *B. malayi* (Ah et al 1974).

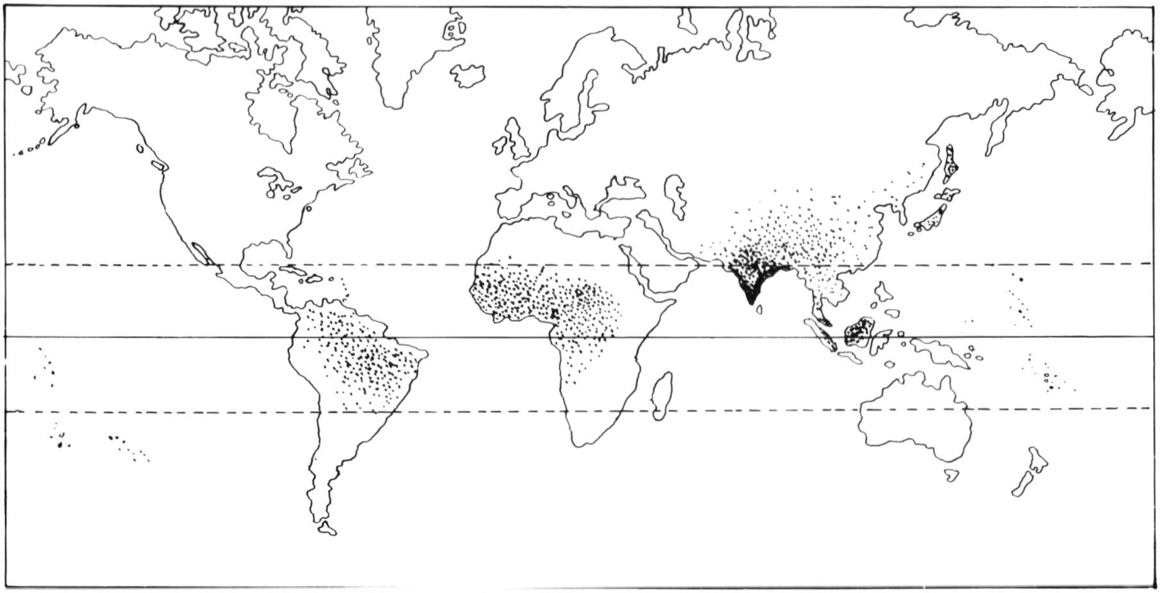

Fig. 32.37 Geographical distribution of filariasis

Of the Filarioidea, the Wuchereria–Brugia complex (producing bancroftian filariasis with lymphatic obstruction and elephantiasis) and onchocerciasis, (responsible for blindness in endemic areas) are important in man. The disease is transmitted through several species of anthropophilic mosquitoes of different genera, *Culex, Aedes, Mansonia* and *Anopheles* (Edeson 1960).

The life cycle of W. Bancrofti (Fig. 32.38)

Man is the only known definitive host. Infective larvae pass from the peripheral blood to the lymphatics, where they mature. Males are usually 40 mm and the females 50–100 mm in length. Mature worms copulate and the viviparous female gives off microfilaria which appear in the peripheral blood one year after infection. Mosquitoes are the intermediate host. When the infected mosquito bites a human being, the larva enters the skin through the puncture wound. In a favourable, hot, moist climate this cycle in the vector lasts for 10–14 days.

Periodicity

The majority of the microfilaria show a biological rhythm for their presence in the peripheral circulation, the controlling mechanism of which is unknown. The majority of *W. bancrofti* and *B. malayi* are nocturnal, but a few may be diurnal in their periodicity.

Host factors favouring infection

A hot, moist climate, bad drainage, pools of stagnant water, and unplanned rapid urbanization and industrialization favour the breeding and thriving of the main vector, i.e. *Culex fatigans* and *Mansonia* mosquitoes. Migration of the infected population is responsible for the dissemination of the disease. Continued reinfection over a prolonged period is necessary for full development of the disease. The microfilaria can pass through the placental barrier. Youths of either sex are the most susceptible, but the infection can occur at any time.

Pathogenesis

The pathogenesis of this disease falls into three stages — inflammatory, obstructive and definitive elephantiasis.

Inflammatory stage

Prolonged repeated infection with the adult worm

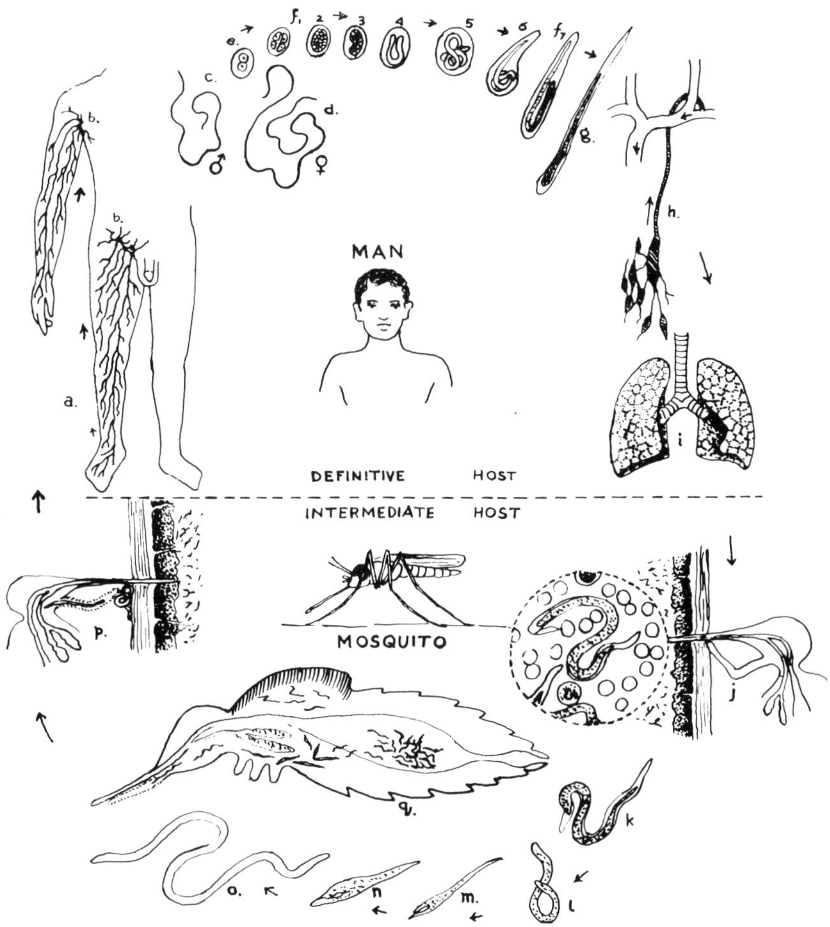

Fig. 32.38 Life cycle of *W. bancrofti*: a, Larva of *W. bancrofti* passing through lymphatics; b, Developed into adult in lymph node; c, Male adult worm; d, Female adult worm; e, Fertilized worm; f, 1–7. Developmental stages of ovum into microfilaria; g, Parturated microfilaria; h, Passing through thoracic duct to venous circulation; i, Staying in pulmonary vessels; j, Sheathed microfilaria sucked by mosquito from cutaneous circulation; k, Sheathed microfilaria; l, Unsheathed microfilaria (within 1 hour); m–n, Sausage form (6–12 hours in thoracic muscles); o, Larva (10 days); p, Larva ejected out through proboscis; q, Development of microfilaria into larva and migration

and later with microfilaria is an essential factor, but the individual's acquired immunosensitivity also plays an important role (Edsom et al 1960, Dondero et al 1975, Schacher & Sahyoun 1967, Denham & Rogers 1975). There is a temporary lymphatic obstruction leading to lymphoedema, which improves with the subsidence of inflammation leaving the lympathic walls weaker. With repeated intermittent rise in lymph pressure, afferent lymphatics become dilated and tortuous, resulting in permanent lymph varices.

Occlusive stages (lymphoedema and elephantiasis)

Maturing worms induce endothelial thickening, obliterative endolymphangitis and fibrin deposition. The death of worms locally produces an epithelioid granuloma and a foreign body giant-cell reaction and even calcification which press upon the lymphatics leading to occlusion. The inflammatory processes gradually lead to permanent fibrotic obliteration of the lymphatic channels, specially those lying in the compact connective tissue of the leg. The regional lymph glands lose their filtering capacity due to fibrosis, which further augments the back pressure producing lymphoedema.

Secondary infection also adds to the lymphatic obstruction. Experimental work by Bosworth & Ewert (1977) in cats has proved the role of β-haemolytic streptococci infection in producing elephantoid tissue. A local abscess may form, which fibroses or ruptures to the surface.

The transudation and spilling of stagnant lymph (rich in protein) due to rupture of the overdilated lymphatics above the obstruction into the surrounding tissues (lymphoedema) leads to cellular proliferation and fibrosis.

Sometimes lymph from the dilated lymphatics ruptures into the hollow space or viscera (chylocele, chylothorax, chyluria, chyloperitoneum).

Gradually those parts of the limb below the obstruction become enlarged with fibrotic infiltration and thickening of the tissues leading to irreversible elephantiasis. Elephantiasis can also be due to obstruction of the venous flow. Skin changes take the form of rough, thickened, warty excrescences due to irregular epithelial hypertrophy, subcutaneous fibrotic thickening and hyperkeratosis. Grooves and transverse folds appear between the heavy, thickened tissue masses. Ulcers may develop in the folds, which heal by fibrosis. Secondary infections are commonly seen in elephantoid tissue resulting in abscesses, which are further responsible for producing scarring. The underlying muscles initially undergo hypertrophy, but ultimately they become atrophic covered by irregular thick layer of fibrofatty tissue.

Histology

The fibro-fatty tissues are oedematous and irregularly infiltrated with mature fibrous tissue, round cells and eosinophils. The lymphatic system in the affected region becomes hypertrophic and dilated with lobulations. Numerous new channels open and the tortuous distended lymphatics may rupture on to the surface. It is very rare to find the filarial worm in the elephantoid tissue. However, a dead or calcified worm (usually detected in X-ray) may rarely be detected in the lymphatic channels and glands.

The development of elephantiasis is not a constant feature of filarial infection. It is difficult to predict which patient will develop the disease and to what extent. Though it is prevalent in all endemic areas, in Samoa and Tahiti the incidence of elephantiasis has been very high, affecting almost every second individual (Manson-Bahr & Apted 1982).

Clinical features

The incubation period is three to 18 months. Though there can be an overlap, the clinical presentation may be considered in relation to the stages of the disease.

Early filariasis or invasion stage

In an endemic area painful lymphadenopathy (inguinal, axillary and epitrochlear), funiculitis, epididymo-orchitis, scrotal or mammary oedema should be taken as a sign of larval infestation and must be investigated. During this stage, there may be a general reaction manifesting with pulmonary symptoms along with an increased eosinophil count, known as tropical pulmonary eosinophilia. After this transitory phase, there may be no manifestations for 2 to 3 years. However, the individual will be a symptomless carrier and the only way to diagnose this dormant phase is the demonstration of microfilaria in the peripheral blood.

Acute inflammatory stage

This state is clinically manifest by (1) filarial fever, and (2) retrograde and centrifugal lymphangitis lasting for a few days. It usually affects the legs in the malleolar region, the testes, spermatic cord and breasts in bancroftial filariasis and the legs or arms in *B. malayi* infection.

Rarely the abdominal lymph varix may rupture and present as an acute 'filarial abdomen' ending even in death.

The affected lymph vessels feel like cords and are acutely tender. The overlying skin is oedematous and itchy and presents congested red streaks running along the course of the affected vessels. Local or regional lymphadenitis and local abscess may develop either overlying the disseminating worms or as a secondary infection. An abscess ultimately bursts producing a sinus.

Chronic obstructive manifestation

Repeated inflammatory reactions end in progressive obstruction of the lymph vessels resulting in various pathologies. There may be no history of an earlier episode, yet chronic filarial manifestations (lymph varices, collections of lymph fluid or chylous fluid in various body cavities, hydrocele, filarial arthropathy, filarial osteomyelitis (Fig. 32.39) (Pandy 1971) and elephantiasis) may be found.

Elephantiasis

Elephantiasis is usually seen in individuals with recurrent infections over prolonged periods who reside in endemic areas for 15–20 years, but in the Pacific area (especially in Samoa and Tahiti) the disease is rampant.

The individual may also present with progressive elephantiasis as a primary complaint. The scrotum, foot, ankle, leg, hands, arm, thigh, mammae, and vulva are the common seats for elephantiasis (in that order). Clinically, the lymphoedema of elephantiasis, can be conveniently divided into four stages (after Chatterjee 1965):

Stage I Static oedema: a feeling of heaviness and a dull ache is accompanied by gravitational, reversible, soft, pitting oedema of the foot and leg and regional lymphadenitis but no skin changes. Features persist or recur over 2–3 years.

Stage II Established lymphoedema with commencing fibrosis: oedema becomes solid and irreversible, lymph glands are firm and the skin becomes thickened and rough.

Stage III Pachydermia: oedema is solid and nonpitting, and the part may be enormous in size with multiple grooves. The skin and subcutaneous tissue becomes hypertrophied, the skin is coarse, rough, scaly, dry and adherent. Progressive fibrosis establishes pachydermia (Fig. 32.40).

Stage IV: Stage III is further complicated by folds, furrows and fissures, nodules and warty projections and indolent wounds and ulcers. The elephantoid tissue is thickest on the dorsum of the foot and leg gradually tapering to merge with normal tissues. Sometimes there is enormous swelling of the foot and ankle without affection of the toes, presenting the 'tortoise foot' (Fig. 32.41). With the development of marked verrucosity the classical 'mossy foot' is produced.

Patients with elephantiasis may suffer episodic febrile attacks (with rigor and sweating, like malaria) known as 'elephantoid fever' (in Fiji it is called 'wanganga', in Barbados 'ague' and in Samoa 'mumu fever').

Investigations

1. A history of the residence in an endemic area.
2. A routine haemogram shows a moderate

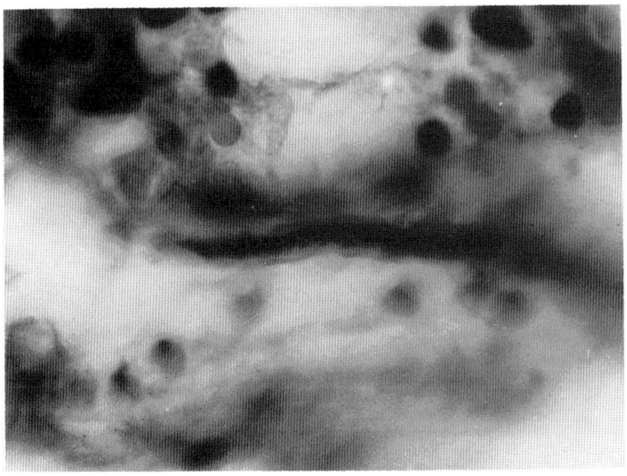

Fig. 32.39 Histological section: Filarial osteomyelitis

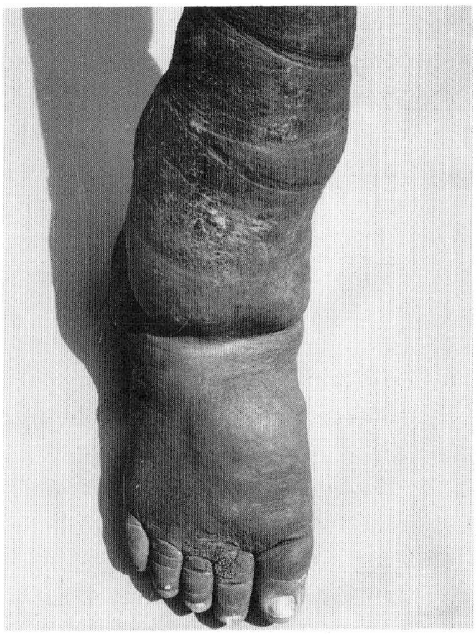

Fig. 32.40 Elephantiasis of the foot and leg with deep transverse grooves, ulcers and pachydermia

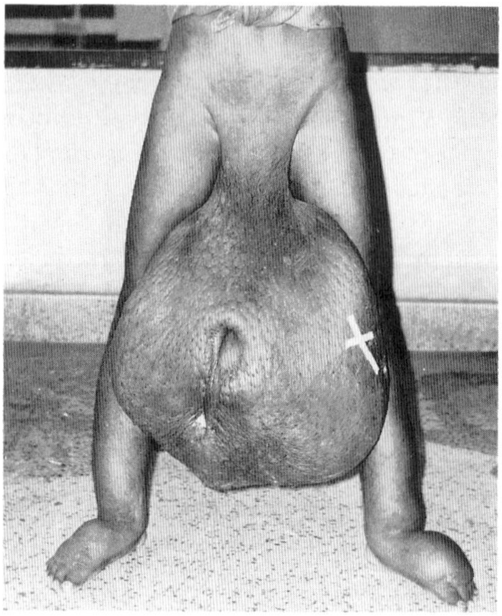

Fig. 32.41 Bilateral elephantiasis of the feet with huge scrotal elephantiasis. 'Tortoise foot' on the left side (Courtesy Dr. S. P. Debuka)

eosinophilia in early and in the recurrent stages of the infection.

3. Urinalysis may show microfilaria or even adult worms during 'chyluria'.

4. Microfilaria in the peripheral blood (taken from the ear lobules or by deep finger-prick) may be demonstrated during the intermediate stages of the disease.

5. Diethylcarbamazine Provocation Test: Even with the nocturnal period forms, microfilaria can be provoked to appear any time in numbers, by administering 100 mg of diethylcarbamazine. Blood should be taken ¾ to 1 hour later. An initial exaggeration of symptoms following the administration of a specific antifilarial drug should be taken as a therapeutic diagnostic test for a suspected filarial infection. Microfilaria or even adult worms may be demonstrated in wet preparations or stained smears of the infected body fluids, e.g. hydrocele or peritoneal fluid.

6. Concentration method (Knott's method): If microfilaria are not found in the peripheral blood, venous blood mixed with formalin (1 ml blood + 9 ml distilled water + 1 ml formalin) is centrifuged and the sediment examined for dead microfilariae.

7. Filtration technique: Heparinized blood is passed through a millipore filter which collects the microfilaria, and these can be examined fresh or stained (Chularek & Desowitz 1970).

8. Centrifuging techniques require the use of an exchange column for diagnosing low-level microfilaraemia and also for estimating numbers.

9. Skin sensitivity test (Fairley 1931) is a quick hypersensitivity reaction. It is performed by injecting intradermally 0.1 ml of antigen prepared from *Dirofilaria*, *Setaria*, or other nonhuman groups or human adult worms. The reactions are observed in the form of weal with pseudopodia occurring in 15–30 minutes.

10. Serological tests: These, though only group-specific, suggest a filarial cause for lymphoedema. The immune response is directed against the microfilaria and is due to humoral (complement fixing, fluorescent and haemagglutinating) and cellular antibodies.

A complement-fixation test is also done with antigen prepared as in the intradermal test and a positive reaction indicates present or past infection. It is positive in only about 25% of *W. bancrofti* infection, whereas there is a very high percentage (85%) in loaiasis.

11. Immunofluorescent antibodies may be antimicrofilarial (co-relating with disease) and antiadult (indicating infection). This is a good method for diagnosing early filariasis.

12. Radiology: Plain X-ray occasionally demonstrates dead and calcified worms. In filarial osteomyelitis, except for local rarefaction, no specific feature is seen.

Lymphangiography (Kinmonth et al 1955) delineates the extent of lymphatic obstruction and may be useful in differentiating several types of lymphoedema. Filarial lymph channels are dilated and limited to below the knee. In Milroy's disease lymph channels are atrophic or absent.

Treatment

During the inflammatory stages treatment consists of rest with the affected part supported, antipyretics, antiallergics and corticoids during reactions, and laxatives or purgatives for constipation.

Specific chemotherapy

Microfilaricidal drugs (antimony, Antrypol® and

arsenicals) kill adult filariae, but are too toxic for general human use. On the other hand microfilaricidal drugs (diethylcarbamazine citrate) are quite effective in controlling the disease. These are not directly lethal but allow the microfilaria to be rapidly phagocytosed by the reticuloendothelial cells, thus clearing them from the circulation. They are more effective against *B. malayi* than *W. bancrofti*.

Due to the rapid and mass destruction of microfilariae and of adult worms, allergic reactions may occur, with pruritus, skin rashes, conjunctival congestion or severe skin lesions. The dosage should be gradually raised over three to four days from 2 mg/kg body weight on the first day, reaching 6 mg/kg, given in three divided doses after meals, and treatment should continue for two to three weeks. Mild side reactions due to the drug itself are common, but never very serious. General reactions like malaise, pyrexia, headache, nausea, vomiting, giddiness, anorexia, drowsiness, and skin rashes may occur by the second to third day and subside within a few days on symptomatic treatment and antihistaminic drugs. Local reactions like acute oedema, aggravation of lymphantitis and lymphadenitis even ending in suppuration may occur.

The liberation of microfilaria usually remains controlled for about five to six months on one course of diethylcarbamazine. It is safe to repeat the course every six months for 24 months to destroy the few surviving adult worms.

Lymphoedema

Measures such as elevation of the limb, prolonged firm sponge-elastic bandaging, spiral elastic stockings, pneumatic stockings, pulsatile air pressure devices, intermittent positive pressure apparatus and the avoidance of prolonged standing or sitting with the leg dependent are effective in the early stages. General measures like weight reduction, fluid and salt restriction, the use of diuretics and prevention of infections should be adopted. Knott's method of bandaging is quite practical and effective in even bigger swellings. The patient lies down with the foot elevated. Using sponge rubber, firm bandage is applied from toes upwards in overlapping fashion. The bandaging is changed daily using more and more pressure. Gradually the fluid is squeezed out and the swelling shrinks to an appreciable extent, which can then be maintained by comfortable elastic stockings. Incipient infection or tinea pedis should be managed by the appropriate antibiotics or antifungal. Prophylactic diethylcarbamazine can be given even in the elephantoid stage to prevent further lymphatic damage.

For chronic elephantiasis only plastic surgical procedures can be beneficial (Gibbon & Tough 1954) but they are required in relatively few patients. The principles of such procedures are the stimulation and establishment of a fresh lymphatic system, or the transfer of normal lymphatics into a lymphoedematous extremity and the removal of massive thickened oedematous fibrofatty masses.

Indications

1. When despite regular conservative treatment, the size of the limb is increasing
2. For recurrent infections in the lymphoedematous limb
3. When the function of the limb is impaired
4. For constant serious skin problems in the elephantoid area
5. For cosmetic considerations, specially when the patient remains emotionally disturbed.

To stimulate the formation of new lymphatic channels, artificial lymphangioplastic procedures like the subcutaneous implantation of thread (Handley 1908) or of fine heterogenous tubes (Chatterjee 1965) have been tried, but none have proved useful. The surgical transfer of normal lymphatic channels from a healthy site to the affected area has been tried with variable success (Gillis & Frazer 1939).

These procedures are aimed at improving function rather than cosmetic appearance. Thompson (1967) suggested burying an intact dermal flap deeper into the oedematous limb to aid lymph drainage. The lymphatics of the flap are supposed to act as a conduit. In the longitudinal plane of the oedematous limb, skin and subcutaneous tissue is excised leaving a 2.5 cm dermal flap, which is tucked into the deeper tissues.

Goldsmith (1967, 1974) has advocated the transposition of intact omentum (rich in lymphatic and vascular vessels) into the affected limb. Along with Alday et al (1972), he has shown the practicability of omental lengthening, sufficient to reach the extremity.

To improve the function and the cosmetic aspect, the wide excision of the large volumes of fibrofatty tissue from the elephantiasis have been practised (Lanz 1911, Charles 1912, Kandoleon 1912, Sistrunk 1927, Ghormley & Overton 1935). Attempts have been made to anastomose the intact superficial lymphatics to the deep lymphatics exposed after excising the diseased tissue. In excisional surgery, the techniques of 'resurfacing the flayed limb' present the main source of controversy. Recommendations range from free skin grafts taken from lymphoedematous skin and other donor sites to variously fashioned and tailored full thickness skin flaps.

McIndoe's modification (1950) of Charles' operation has gained ground. This consists of a wide excision of thickened oedematous tissue after dissecting out the overlying skin as a large full thickness hinged sheet, which is replaced over the raw surface. A pressure bandage maintains even contact. By this technique, the mobility and function of the limb may improve, but usually it remains poor cosmetically and secondary fungal infections, troublesome weeping, eczema and recurrence of papillomatosis on grafted skin mar the good results.

In massive elephantiasis, the patient may insist on amputation. A planned amputation with proper prosthetic fitting is not a bad proposition.

Prevention

This is possible but difficult. It aims at:

1. Elimination of the larval and adult worms from an endemic area
2. Elimination of the larvae of the vector or the control of vector breeding
3. Improvement of rural and urban hygiene.

Methods for eliminating the microfilaria include:

1. Mass drug administration; the WHO expert committee (1967) on filiariasis has recommended diethylcarbamazine in the dose of 6 mg/kg once a month for 12–18 months for the total population at risk
2. Medicated salt; Hawking & Marques (1967) have reported partial control of microfilaraemia after using common salt mixed with diethylcarbamazine. However, it has not been popular
3. Diagnosed cases must be treated properly.

Control of vectors centres around three aspects:

1. Measures to destroy — vector adults or larvae
2. Filaria — preventive engineering techniques
3. Health education, random periodic blood examination in endemic areas and proper surveillance to follow up the known cases and carriers.

Adult mosquitoes are becoming resistant to insecticides like DDT, dieldrin, HCH etc. The spraying of houses and mosquito breeding places with pyrethrum, the aerial low-volume application of malathion and ground generated fogs, have been used to destroy the vector but the processes are associated with other problems and are of limited value.

The WHO technical report (1974) has quoted the successful implementation of a recent 'genetic control of insects programme' by the Filaria Research Unit in Burma for complete elimination of the vector by the mass release of a laboratory strain of *C. fatigans* which were sexually incompatible with the local strain.

To eliminate the larvae, organophosphorus insecticides (e.g. fenthion and dursban) and oils to kill the aquatic stages of the mosquito have been used. Measures to destroy aquatic vegetation, the filling-in of ditches and stagnant water pools, improving of sewage and drainage systems and the proper disposal of industrial and household refuse, have definite roles to play in controlling mosquito breeding.

REFERENCES

Ah H S et al 1974 A simple method for isolation of *Brugia pahangi* and *Brugia malayi* microfilariae. Int J Parasitol 4: 677–679

Bosworth W, Ewart A 1977 Lymphatic patterns of cats infected with *Brugia malayi* and *Streptococcus*. Trans R Soc Trop Med Hyg 71: 21–55

Charles H 1912 In: Latham A M, English T C (eds) A System of Treatment, Vol 3. Churchill Livingstone, London. p 504

Chatterjee P 1965 Filariasis in tropical surgery. In: Basu A K (ed) Clinical Surg No. 8, Butterworth, London. pp 51–103

Chormley R K, Overton L M 1935 Surgical treatment of severe forms of lymphoedema of the leg. Proc Roy Soc 43: 1043

Chularek P, Desowitz R S 1970 A simplified membrane filtration technique for the diagnosis of microfilarae. J Parasitol 56: 623–624

Denham D A, Rodgers R 1975 Structural and functional studies on the lymphatics of cats infected with *Brugia pahangi*. Trans R Soc Trop Med Hyg 69(2): 173–176
Dondero T T, Mullin S W, Balasingham S 1975 In: Manson-Bahr P E C, Apted F I C (eds) 1982 Manson's Tropical Diseases. 18th edn. Baillière Tindall, London. p 179
Edeson D F B, Wilson T, Wharton R H, Laing A B G 1960 Experimental transmission of *Brugia malayi* and *Brugia pahangi* to man. Trans R Soc Trop Med Hyg 54: 229–234
Fairley N H 1931 Serological and intradermal tests in filariasis, preliminary report. Trans R Soc Trop Med Hyg 24: 635–638
Gibbon T, Tough J S 1954 The surgical correction of chronic lymphoedema of the legs. Br J Plast Surg 7: 195
Gillis H, Fraser F R 1935 Treatment of lymphoedema by plastic operation. Br Med J p 96
Goldsmith S H, Delos Santos R, Beattie E J 1967 Relief of chronic lymphoedema by omental transposition. Ann Surg 166: 573
Goldsmith H S 1974 Long term evaluation of omental transposition for chronic lymphoedema. Ann Surg 180: 847
Handley W S 1908 Lymphangioplasty: A new method for the cure of brawny arm of breast cancer and for similar conditions of lymphoedema. Lancet p 784
Hawking F, Marques R J 1967 Control of bancroftian filariasis by cooking salt medicated with di-ethylcarbamazine. WHO Bulletin 37(3): 405–414
Kinmonth J B, Taylor G W, Harper R K 1955 Lymphangiograph: A technique for its use in the lower limb. Br Med J 1: 940
Kondoleon E 1912 Die Operative Be Handlung der Elephonti Astischen Odeme. Zentralbl Chir 39: 1022
Lanz 1911 Quoted by Chatterjee P. In: Basu A K (ed) 1965 Clinical Surgery. Tropical Surgery No. 8, Filariasis. Butterworth, London. p 88
Manson-Bahr P E C, Apted F I C 1982 Manson's Tropical Diseases. 18th edn. Baillière Tindall, London. p 156
McIndoe A H 1950 Discussion on the treatment of chronic oedema of the leg. Proc Roy Soc 43: 1043
Pandey S 1971 Filarial osteomyelitis. Q J Surg Sci 7 (1): 32
St. George J 1975 Ann Trop Med Parasitol 69: 383
Sasa M 1976 Human Filariasis. University Park Press, Baltimore.
Schacher J F, Sahyoun P F 1967 A chronological study of the histopathology of filarial diseases in cats and dogs caused by *Brugia pahangi* (Buckley and Edeson 1956). Trans R Soc Trop Med Hyg 61: 234
Sistrunk W E 1927 Contributions to plastic surgery. Ann Surg 85: 190
Thompson N 1967 The surgical treatment of chronic lymphoedema of the extremities. Surg Clin North Am 47: 445
WHO 1962 Technical Report Series, Geneva No. 233
WHO 1967 Technical Report Series (on Filariasis) No. 359
WHO 1974 Technical Report Series No. 542. WHO Expert Committee on Filariasis, Geneva

FURTHER READING

Alday E S, Goldsmith H S 1972 Surgical technique for omental lengthening based on arterial anatomy. Surg Gynecol Obstet 135 (10): 103
Denham D A, McGreevey P B 1977 Brugian filariasis. Epidemiological and experimental studies. Adv Parasitol 15: 243
Hawking F 1956 The periodicity of microfilariae iv. Stimuli affecting the migration of the microfilariae of *Dirofilaria aethiops, D immitis, D repens, Dipetalonema blanci* and *Litemosoides carinu*. Trans R Soc Trop Med Hyg 50: 397
Lumsden W H R, Evans D A, Kimber C O 1980 Miniature anion exchange centrifugation technique for the diagnosis of microfilaraemia in the field. Trop Med Hyg 74(1): 40–42
Turner L H 1959 Studies in filariasis in Malaya. Trans R Soc Trop Med Hyg 53: 154

DRACUNCULOSIS

Synonyms: dracontiasis, guinea worm, serpent worm, medina worm, dragon worm, naru

Dracunculosis is a chronic human infection caused by the nematode worm *Dracunculus medinensis*, females being solely responsible for clinical manifestations.

Geographical distribution (Fig. 32.42)

Out of an estimated 48 million cases in the world the majority are in Africa and Asia (Harman 1979). The worm is scattered over Africa, the Middle East, India, Pakistan, the Caribbean islands, Brazil, Guyana, southern Russia and certain areas of North and South America. In India, the system of shallow 'step-well' and ponds, in Ghana the rural pools, and in Iran the desert cipterus are the main source of the vector, the *Cyclops*. These are found mainly in dirty, stagnant water and are swallowed by the natives with the water. Gradually the incidence is falling due to preventive measures and the drying-up of the wells, as in the infested areas of Ghana.

In the dry season, when water pools become shallow, the infection rate increases. Children below 5 years are seldom affected, but young adults are the common victims.

The parts mostly involved are the legs and feet (in about 90%), but buttocks, arms, fingers, back (in the water carriers of India), genitalia, abdomen, breasts, head and eyeball are also affected.

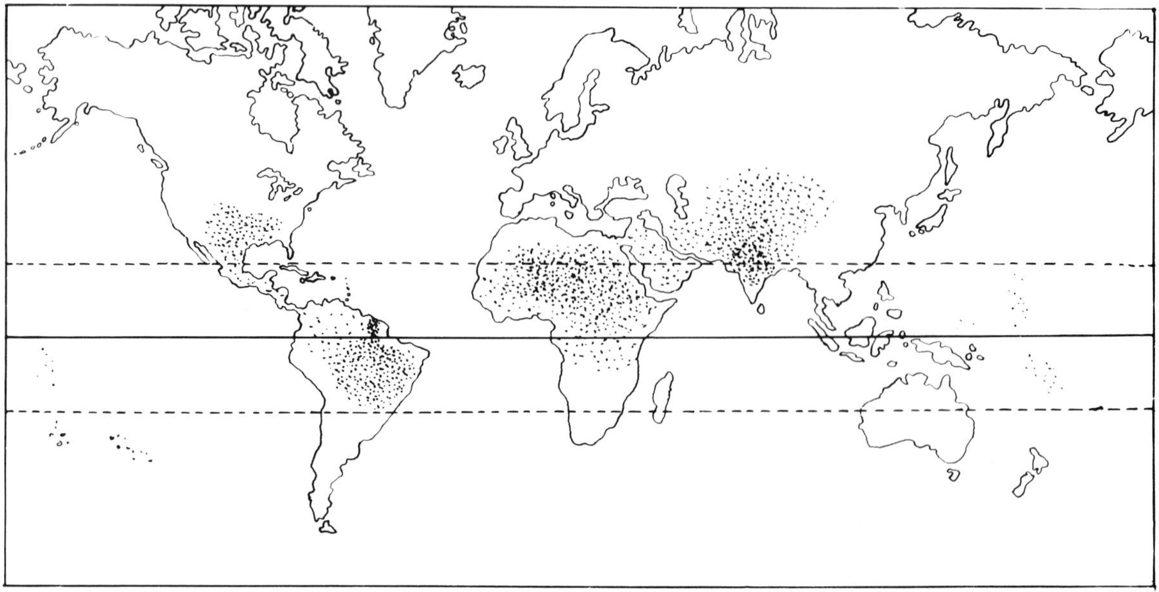

Fig. 32.42 Geographical distribution of guinea worm

Life cycle

D. medinesis (Linn 1758) has two hosts. The definitive host is man, the intermediate host the crustacean *Cyclops*.

The female worm, measuring 60–120 mm by 1.5–2 mm, is solely responsible for the human infestation. Till the gravid stage it remains harmless, lying mostly in the connective tissue. In late gestation, probably exhibiting hydrotropic behaviour, it migrates towards the surface and the periphery where there can be contact with water. Due to the irritating toxic secretion from its head glands, vesicles form in the skin. Upon contact with cold water these vesicles rupture and the packed prolapsed uterus of the worm bursts to eject numerous freely swimming larvae. The female worm dies.

Larvae can remain alive for 3–4 days if the water is clean, but for several weeks in dirty and muddy water, and must find the *Cyclops* to complete their development (Onabamiro 1954). *C. quadricornis* and, in real tropical areas *Tropocyclops multicolor*, and allied species swallow the coiled larvae. These cyclops become infective in man in two weeks. In the stomach of man, the gastric juice dissolves the body wall of *Cyclops* and the larvae are set free. Eventually probably through the lymphatics, these larvae manage to reach the loose retroperitoneal connective tissue and, finally, the subcutaneous tissues by about the forty-third day (Onabamiro 1956). Thereafter the development of both sexes goes on in the connective tissue, reaching maturity by one year. The male dies after copulation and the female shows a tendency to migrate to the subcutaneous region of the lower leg and foot in 82% of cases (Lindberg 1946, 1948). Occasionally the worm may not be able to pierce the cuticle of the host and may die. When this happens there may be local abscesses or the dead worm may undergo calcification to be detected either by palpation as a hard cord, on X-ray or at operation.

Clinical features

Clinical manifestations are due either to toxins liberated from the anterior end of the worm, the presence of a gravid female worm superficially just prior to discharge of the larvae, or to the resultant ulcers due to rupture of the vesicles.

A little before the female worm reaches the surface, the patient may have a slight fever and/or urticaria. By the time the worm is about to pierce through the dermis, general and local reactions develop. The worm may become palpable in the tissues as a firm tortuous cord.

General features may appear as anaphylactic reactions due to the absorption of toxins liberated by the worm, and these are generalized urticaria, pruritus, giddiness, nausea, vomiting, asthma, rigors or diarrhoea.

With the subsidence of the general features local reactions appear, usually at night. The patient feels a sharp pain at the site of worm piercing the cuticle, where a papule develops. For a couple of days, the site remains erythematous, indurated, raised and tender, followed by the appearance of a vesicle in the centre, due to raising of the epidermis over the head of the piercing worm. The patient feels a marked burning sensation and likes to immerse the part in cold water. The vesicle ruptures resulting in a superficial ulcer of about 1.5 cm diameter. The periphery of the ulcer shows spontaneous healing, but at the centre a minute hole is left, through which the head of the worm can be seen protruding.

On contact with water, or after douching the surrounding area with cold water, clear to milky fluid containing numerous motile larvae, is ejected from the uterus of the worm. Occasionally the pellucid tube of the uterus itself may be ejected which may rupture to deliver numerous larvae. This succession of an ejection of larvae can be repeatedly induced till the whole uterus is emptied, which may continue for several weeks. The local lesion gradually heals up in 4–6 weeks provided there is no secondary infection.

With superimposed staphylococcal or streptococcal or other infections, the features may be complicated and become chronic. Hodgson & Barrett (1964) have described chronic dracunculosis consisting of chronic pruritus, chronic suppuration and cyst formation specially in the lower legs and foot. Even tetanus can occur with secondary *Clostridium tetani* invasion.

Rarely, the adult worm may involve a joint (commonly ankles and knee) producing synovitis, arthritis and even ankylosis and contractures (Farah 1979). Serous cavities (peritonitis), extradural space, perineal sac (reported by Lester from Dar-es-Salaam), vagina and retroplacental region have been involved on occasions.

If the worm breaks in the attempted traditional method for its removal (coiled up on a match stick), in several days (Figs. 32.43, 44) secondary infection and abscess formation usually results. The residual worms may remain coiled around a tendon producing a contracture, especially the tendo Achillis and the hamstrings (Figs. 32.45, 46).

Investigations

The differential white cell count shows a high eosionophilia during the appearance of active general and early local symptoms.

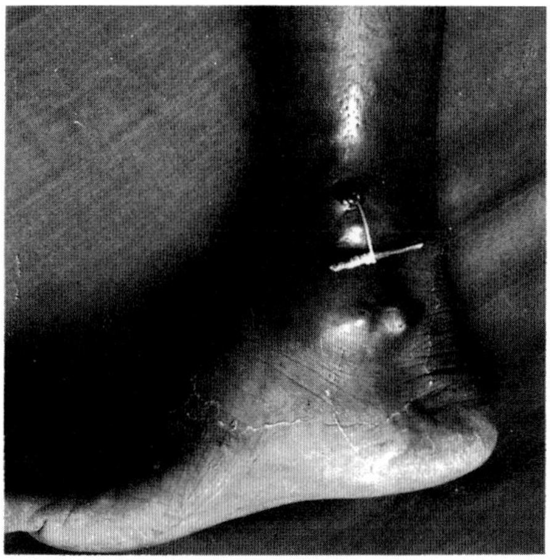

Fig. 32.43 The traditional method of removing the worm by coiling on a match stick. At a distal level two fresh vesicles are appearing

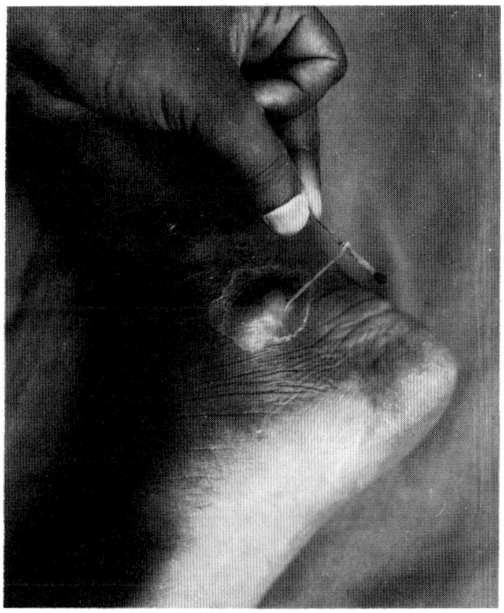

Fig. 32.44 In the same patient, after removing one worm from proximal to the ankle, another worm is being extracted from the distal side two weeks later

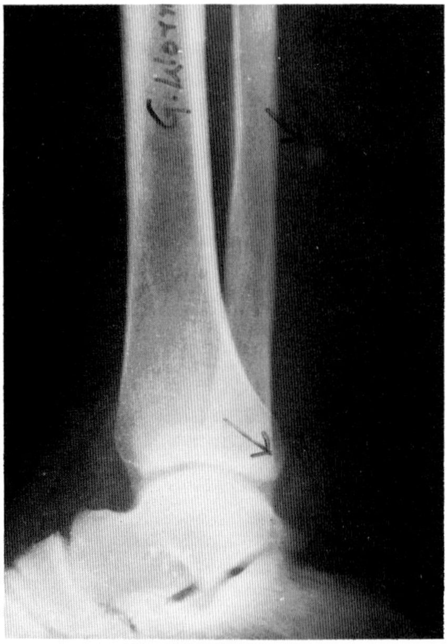

Fig. 32.45 X-ray showing an early calcified remnant of worms at two sites

The milky fluid ejected after cold douching around the vesicular area, if examined under the microscope, shows myriads of coiled up larvae. They are sluggish, but, on coming into contact with a drop of water put under the cover-glass, they show mobility.

Accidentally, the plain X-ray of the part may sometimes show the slender calcified worm lying in the connective tissues (Fig. 32.46). Attempts to inject radio-opaque contrast medium into the worm to render it visible on X-ray have also been made.

Skin sensitivity tests using a 0.25 ml intradermal injection of antigen prepared from ether-free dried powdered guinea-worm, shows a weal of about 2.5 cm in a positive test, though its role has been of dubious value.

Complications

Allergic reactions may be very serious. The victims are usually poor farmers and labourers, who may suffer economically due to the prolonged incapacity. Arthritis and contractures may disable the patient to a variable extent.

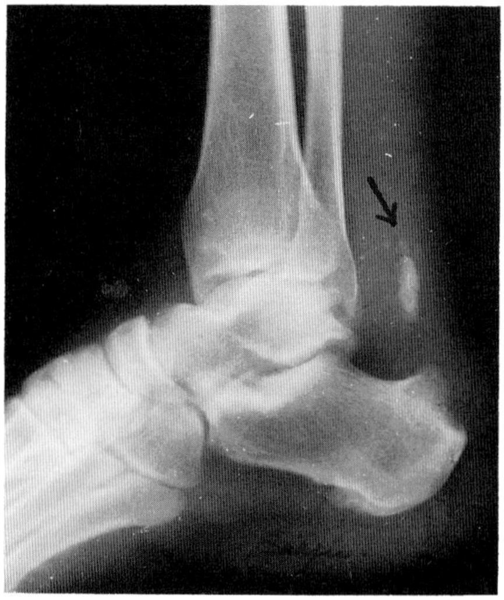

Fig. 32.46 X-ray showing a late calcified worm around the Achilles tendon

Management

Chemotherapy employs several drugs (niridazole, thiabendazole, metronidazole, diethylcarbamazine), which have been found effective in the early stages (Hawking 1956). Sastry et al (1978) have found thiabendazole, in a dose of 50 mg/kg body weight in two divided doses for three days, effective for up to a two-worm infection; for three or more worms they recommend the dose of 75 mg/kg body weight.

Padonu (1973) has claimed complete recovery in 19 days with metronidazole administered in the dose of 400 mg three times daily for five days.

Niridazole, in a dose of 25 mg/kg body weight, in two daily divided doses, has also been claimed to be very effective (Cole 1973, Padonu 1973).

If chemotherapy is effective, manual removal of the worm may not be required. However, usually the worm should be removed, by the traditional method, but with aseptic care. The ruptured vesicle should be cleaned and dressed. Cold compressing and douching of the region for two to three days usually stops the larval discharge. The head of the worm should be identified in the centre of the ulcer, and is caught with forceps and cautiously pulled, while the other hand is used to massage the worm towards the wound to expel it. Gaining a sufficient length, the head end of the worm is tied on a sterile stick and the worm is gradually wound over it (see Figs. 32.43, 44). Each day, 5 to 10 cm or even more of the worm can be extracted and the wound and the stick covered with a sterile dressing. If by chance the worm breaks, it should be left in situ without any surgical attempt at removal. Chemotherapy, antibiotics and antihistaminics should be used. Usually a local abscess and sloughing develops, to be treated on merit.

Joint involvement should be treated with chemotherapy, aspiration and rest.

Prevention

The main prevention is the ensuring of a safe water supply. Measures like improving the source of drinking water, treatment of stagnant water with DDT to kill the *Cyclops*, treating drinking water by boiling or the addition of potash or bleaching powder to the well, help to control the disease.

REFERENCES

Farah F S 1979 Protozoan and helminth infections. In: Fitzpatrick T B et al (eds) Dermatology in General Medicine. 2nd edn. McGraw-Hill Book Company, New York. pp 1652–1653

George J S 1975 Bleeding in pregnancy due to retroplacental situation of guineaworm. Ann Trop Med Parasitol 69: 383

Harman R R M 1979 Parasitic worms and protozes dracunculosis. In: Rook A, Wilkinson D S, Ebling F J G (eds) Textbook of Dermatology. 3rd edn. Blackwell Scientific Publications, Oxford. p 876

Hawking F 1956 Treatment of filariasis. Trop Dis Bull 53: 829

Hodgson C, Barrett D F 1964 Chronic dracunculosis. Br J Dermatol 76: 211–217

Lindberg K 1946 Bull Soc Pathol Exot Filiales 39: 318. Quoted by Rook A, Wilkinson D S, Ebling F J G (eds) 1979 In: Textbook of Dermatology. 3rd edn. Blackwell Scientific Publications, Oxford. pp 876–878

Lindberg K 1948 Seconde enquête epidémiologique sur la dracunculosa dans l'Inde. Bull Soc Pathol Exot Filiales 41: 282

Padonu K O 1973 A controlled trial of metronidazole in the treatment of dracontiasis in Nigeria. Am J Trop Med Hyg 22: 42

Sastry S C, Kumar J K, Lakshmi Narayan V 1978 The treatment of dracontiasis with thiabendazole. J Trop Med Hyg 81(2–3): 32–5

FURTHER READING

Khwaja M S, Dossetor J F B, Lawrie J H 1975 Epidermal guinea-worm abscess. J Neurosurg 43: 627

Onabamiro S D 1954 W Afr Med J 3: 180. Quoted by Manson-Bahr P E C, Apted F I C (eds) 1982 In: Manson's Tropical Diseases. 18th edn. Baillière Tindall, London. p 733

Onabamiro S D 1956 The early stages of the development of *Dracunculus medinensis* (*Linnaeus*) in the mammalian host. Ann Trop Med Parasitol 50: 157

Pardanani D S, Trivado V D, Joshi L G 1977 Metronidazole (Flagyl) in dracunculiasis: a double field study. Ann Trop Med Parasitol 71: 45

Sharma V P, Rathore H S, Sharma M M 1979 Efficacy of metronidazole in dracunculiasis. Am J Trop Med Hyg 28: 658

LARVA MIGRANS

Synonyms: creeping eruption, plumber's itch, sandworm, duckhunter's itch

Larva migrans is a clinical condition characterized by an erythematous, serpentine, tortuous, intracutaneous track, and creeping vesicular eruptions, due to numerous types of moving larvae under the skin.

Geographical distribution

The condition is found in Central and South America, the southern United States of America (along the coast of the Gulf of Mexico and Florida), the Caribbean islands, East and West Africa, the Malay peninsula, parts of the Far East, and Sri Lanka.

Infection is more common during the warm and humid seasons of summer and the early rains. Unprotected skin, exposed on sandy beaches and marshes contaminated with the faeces of cats and dogs, is most at risk.

Common parasites are *Ankylostoma braziliense* and *A. caninum* (dog and cat hookworms). However *Uncinaria stenocephala, A. ceylonicum, Gnathostoma spinigerum, Bunostomum phlebotomum* and *Strongyloides stercoralis* (Larva currens), *Hypoderma* or *Gastrophilus* can also cause similar lesions.

Clinical features

The foot, ankle, leg, hand, buttock, abdomen and

back are affected (Lowe & Augustene 1947, Schwarz 1942).

Larvae penetrate through the bare human skin, but usually not below the layer of the stratum germinativum. A small erythematous papule develops at the point of entry, which becomes raised and vesicles appear. After some time the larvae track through a burrow in the skin lined by stratum corneum at the bottom and stratum granulosum at the roof, at the rate of a few millimeters to a few centimeters a day, usually limited to a small area. The faster migration is referred to as larva currens. There is immense itching and irritation as the migration starts. Initially there is erythema followed by an elevated, indurated, tortuous track (Fig. 32.47) studded with vesicles. The larvae remain ahead of the clinically apparent track. There is local infiltration with eosinophils, lymphocytes and round cells and the lesion is surrounded with an arteriolar flare. Left alone, the track dries up and becomes scaly, but scratching due to the immense pruritus may lead to secondary infection.

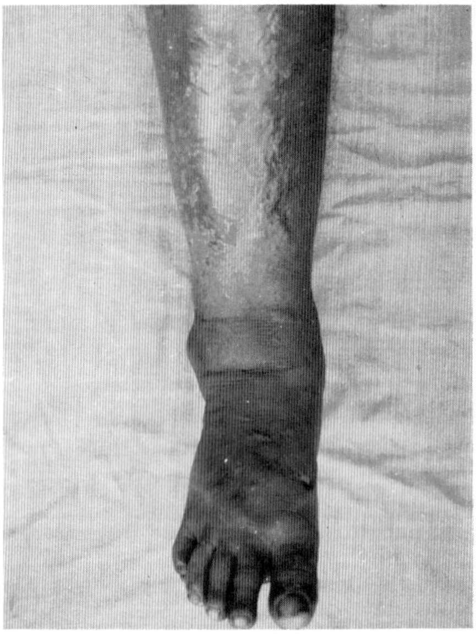

Fig. 32.47 Larva migrans

The typical clinical appearance is the only diagnostic aid. The larvae cannot be extracted from the skin for examination. Usually there is no eosinophilia unless the larvae migrate into the deeper tissues, but 10–35% of eosinophilia and Löffler's syndrome may be associated (Farah 1979). In the human being, the dead-end host, the disease should be self-limiting. It may run a variable course, but 81% of lesions disappear in about 4 weeks (Katz et al 1965). Raised IgE levels have been seen (Harman 1979).

Treatment

The treatment of choice is thiabendazole by mouth, 25 mg/kg body weight daily for two to five days depending upon the magnitude and number of lesions. Katz et al (1965) and London (1965) have suggested single weekly dose therapy by 50 mg/kg body weight till the lesions disappear. Mebendazole in dosage of 100 mg three times a day for six to seven days has been useful.

Freezing of the larvae by cooling with ethyl chloride spray, or carbon dioxide snow exposure has also been used. However, experimentally the larvae have been shown to resist even five minutes of exposure to −23°C. Harland et al (1977) have advocated the topical use of thiabendazole by triturating a 0.5 g tablet with 5 g of petroleum jelly, which is applied daily over the track for five days. Even thiabendazole sprinkled on Elastoplast® can be used over the advancing end of the tunnel.

REFERENCES

Farah F S 1979 Protozoan and helminth infections. In: Fitzpatrick T B et al (eds) Dermatology in General Medicine, 2nd edn. McGraw-Hill Book Company, New York. pp 1650–1651

Harman R R M 1979 Parasitic worms and Protozoa. In: Textbook of Dermatology. 2nd edn. Blackwell Scientific Publications, Oxford. pp 878–880

Katz R, Ziegler, Blank H 1965 The natural course of creeping eruption and treatment with thiabendazole. Arch Dermatol 91: 420

London I D 1965 The treatment of creeping eruption with thiabendazole. Report of 23 cases. Southern Med J 58: 1026

Lowe C V, Augustine D L 1947 Creeping eruption in New England. Report of 2 cases in New England. New Engl J Med 236: 658–661

Schwarz E G 1942 Creeping eruption. Urol Cutan Rev 46: 782

Stone O J, Systemic and topical thiabendazole for creeping eruption. Texas Rep Biol Med 27 (Suppl.2): 658

FURTHER READING

Kahn G, Jonson J A 1971 Serum IgE levels in cutaneous larva migrans. Int J Dermatol 10: 201

TUNGIASIS

Synonyms: jiggers, chigoe, chique

This condition, caused by a small parasite, *Tunga penetrans* (chigoe flea) is mainly seen in South America, the West Indies, tropical Africa, Madagascar and the Indian subcontinent.

The parasites mainly thrive in dry sandy soil. When gravid, the female flea usually tries to enter the sole crevices and fissures, the toewebs or around the toenails. Other parts like buttocks, hands, thighs, genitals or any exposed part may be affected.

The flea immediately starts burrowing through the skin deep into the dermis, and will reach the stratum granulosum in as short a time as ten minutes. Except for the narrow posterior part, the whole of the flea becomes enveloped in the host skin (Fig. 48). A horny mass develops around the burrow which appears as a pit with a black dot in its centre. In one to two weeks, the gravid female distends to the size of a pea as the eggs mature and this causes inflammation and irritation. Itching causes the subject to scratch and the eggs are gradually discharged, and more rarely the whole flea. A localized abscess and later an ulcer may form. Secondary infection may develop with shedding of ulcerated skin. The remnants of the parasite are expelled with the necrotic tissue leaving behind a pitted sole (Figs. 32.48, 49). Regional lymphangitis,

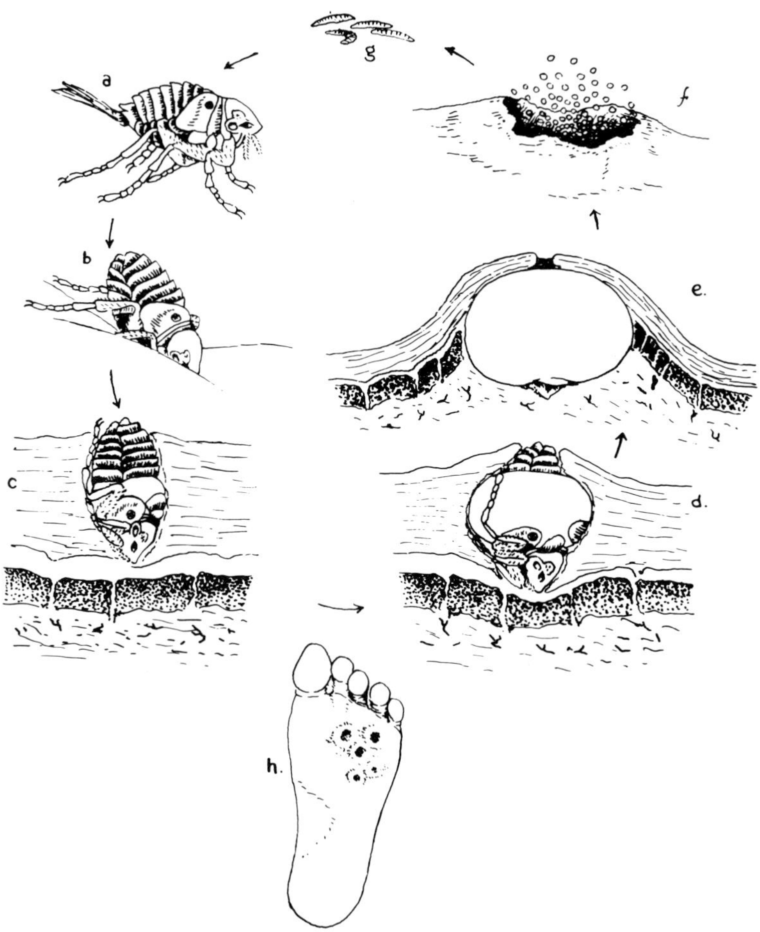

Fig. 32.48 The life cycle of sand flea or jigger: a, Male sand flea; b, Female sand flea penetrating the skin; c–d, Intra cutaneous fertilized female with development of jigger; e, Fully developed jigger; f, Burst jigger, escaping of eggs and formation of ulcer; g, Larval stage (free living); h, Jiggers in the sole of foot (After Manson-Bahr & Apted 1982)

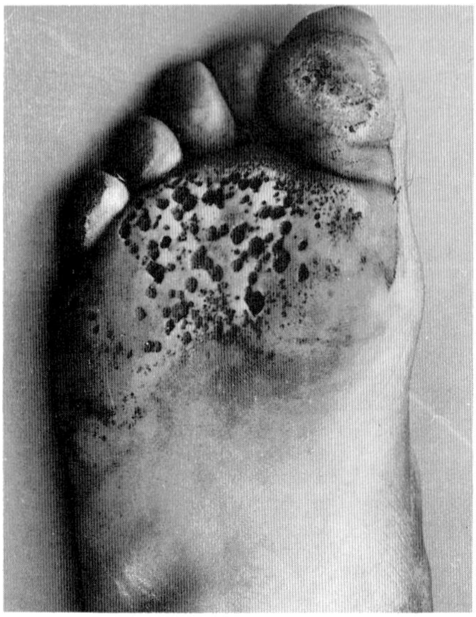

Fig. 32.49 Old unusual jiggers in the sole of the foot

lymphadenitis, or more severe complications may occur such as thrombophlebitis, tetanus or even gangrene (White 1982, Harman 1979).

Usually one or two jiggers are seen at a time, but there may be numerous lesions, producing a honeycomb of solid patches. With lesions beneath the nail, an irregular pocket of pus may form.

Treatment

When detected at an early stage, a thin sterilized needle should be used to enucleate the parasite from the penetrated skin. Care of the ulcer and inflamed area by regular antiseptic dressings should be undertaken. At a later stage it is very difficult to remove the flea, and then they are best killed by turpentine or chloroform or parasiticidal drugs. Usually an ulcer develops after removing the flea, which should be treated with antiseptic dressings till healing occurs.

Since barefoot walking on dirty, sandy soil is the main source of the disease, it can be avoided by using footwear and observing a good standard of hygiene.

REFERENCES

Harman R R M 1979 Tungiasis. In: Rook A, Wilkinson D S, Ebling F J G (eds) Textbook of Dermatology. 3rd edn. Blackwell Scientific Publications, Oxford. p 921

White G B 1982 Fleas. In: Manson-Bahr P E C, Apted F I C (eds) Manson's Tropical Diseases. 18th edn. Baillière Tindall, London. p 820

MYCETOMA

Synonyms: Madura foot, maduramycosis, Vincent's white mycetoma, actinomycosis madurae, pseudo-actinomycosis

Madura foot is a chronic granulomatous systemic fungal disease caused by several species of 'true' fungi, mainly actinomycetes, affecting any part of the body exposed to trauma and resulting in severe damage to skin, subcutaneous tissues and bones. It is typically characterized by a painless, nodular, indurated swelling, suppuration and multiple sinuses discharging coloured granules.

History

Though there is a suggestion that Madura foot was described by Sophocles in the hero of Philoctates, Kaempher first described this condition in 1712 in India. Vandyke Carter (1860) reported the early cases from the Madura area of India.

Mycetoma is caused by two main groups of organism: (a) The true fungi, causing eumycetoma, and (b) The aerobic actinomycetes, causing actinomycetoma. Both groups are characterized by the formation of typical coloured granules ranging from 60 μm to 3 mm in diameter. They occur as saprophytes in soil and on plants or rotting vegetable matter usually during the hot and rainy seasons. The different organisms have been published in the MRC chart in Table 32.3. Poor rural labourers working barefooted in the fields, farms or forests are the main victims, and adult males are affected much more than females. The infection gains entry to the subcutaneous tissues usually through a penetrating injury caused by a thorn or splinter (Abbott 1956).

Geographical distribution (Fig. 32.50)

Mycetoma is known to occur all over the world, but is most common in tropical and subtropical areas (Africa, India, Mexico, Central America, South Vietnam, Senegal, South America and Italy). Abbott (1956) has confirmed its high incidence in the Sudan. Gould (1963) suggested the origin of mycetoma to be due to *Madurella grisea* in northern California.

Immunology

Mycetoma is not a contagious disease. Though it has been seen in the cow, dog and horse, animal to man or human to human cross-infection has not yet been reported. Madura foot patients are deficient in cell-mediated immunity. However type 4 reactions to purified protein antigens and a few cases of actinomycetoma and eumycetoma, with Madura antigens, have been demonstrated.

Precipitating and compliment-fixing antibodies develop in mycetomal infection and their level varies in direct proportion to the activity of infection. If the disease is cured, there may be no demonstrable antibody.

Pathology

The painless swollen foot riddled with numerous nodules and dry or discharging sinuses spreading all over the foot, once seen cannot be mistaken. Nodules develop under the epidermis and rupture into sinuses communicating with abscesses at various depths and having fibrous or epithelial collars around the opening.

With advancing pathology, the Madura foot is easily damaged. On section it is difficult to identify different tissues except for tendons and fascia. Even bony tissue can disappear in the fungal mass. The whole surface presents a pale greyish-yellow, oily and greasy look, an amalgam of the different tissues. The overall look presents a network of cystic spaces containing friable material of different colours, depending upon the variety of mycetoma (see Table 32.3).

Histologically the chronic granulomatous reaction results in dense scar formation. In the cystic spaces, characteristically coloured granules are seen and are discharged in pus through multiple sinuses. Epitheloid, plasma and giant cells in the areas of fibrosis may dominate the picture. Actinomycetoma can be recognized by the positive reaction to gram, hematoxylin and eosin or periodic acid–Schiff

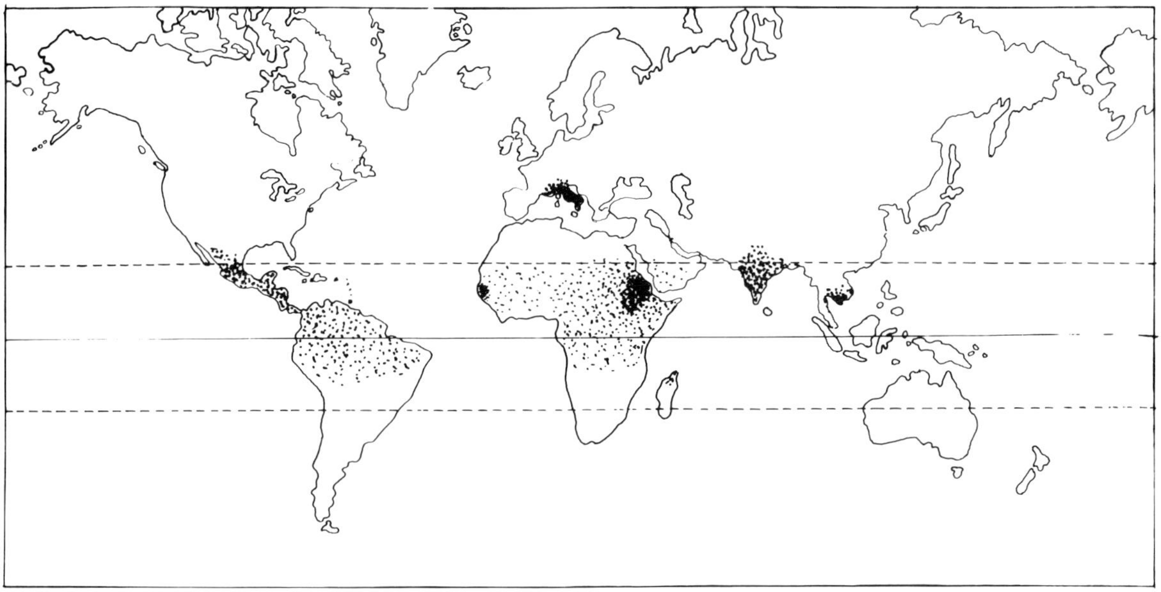

Fig. 32.50 Geographical distribution of mycetoma

Table 32.3 Eumycetes and actinomycetes capable of causing mycetoma

Organism	Colour of grains	Size (mm)	World distribution	Favoured rainfall (cm/year)
Eumycetes				
Madurella	Black	1.0	Africa, South America, India, Madagascar, Indonesia	25–50
M. grisea	Black	1.0	Mainly North and South America	
Leptoshaeria senegalensis	Black	1.0	Senegal and Chad	
Petriellidum (Allescheri) boydii	White or yellow	1.0	Europe, America, Africa	100–200
Acremonium (Cephalosporium) falciforme, A. kilense and A. recifei	White or yellow	1.0	South America, Africa, Europe, India	
Philaophora jeanselmi				
Sopfia rosati				
Fusarium solanae				
Corynespora cassiicola			Sudan	
Actinomycetes				
Nocardia brasiliensis *N. asteroides*	White or yellow	0.5	Cosmopolitan	100–200
Streptomyces	Yellow	0.1	Africa, North and South America, Israel	5–25
Actinomadura (Streptomyces) madurae	Yellow	3.0	Africa, North and South America Vietnam	
A. (S) pelletierii	Red	0.5	Africa, South America	25–100

From MRC (1977); quoted by Manson-Bahr & Apted (1982)

stains, whereas the fungi are identified by their broad ramifying and often irregular mycelium.

The pathology spreads locally but lymphatic spread is rare. Systemic spread may occur in actinomycetoma, but never in eumycetoma.

Clinical features

Irrespective of the causative fungus or actinomycete, the clinical features are essentially the same. The foot is the commonest site (Figs. 32.51 to 58). However,

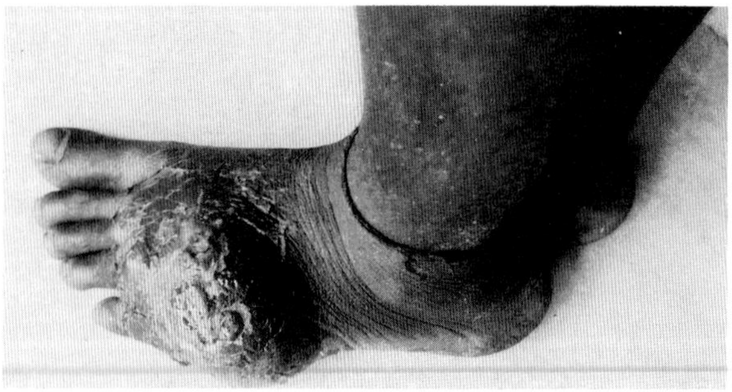

Fig. 32.51 Mycetoma affecting the forefoot, more on the outer side with multiple sinuses

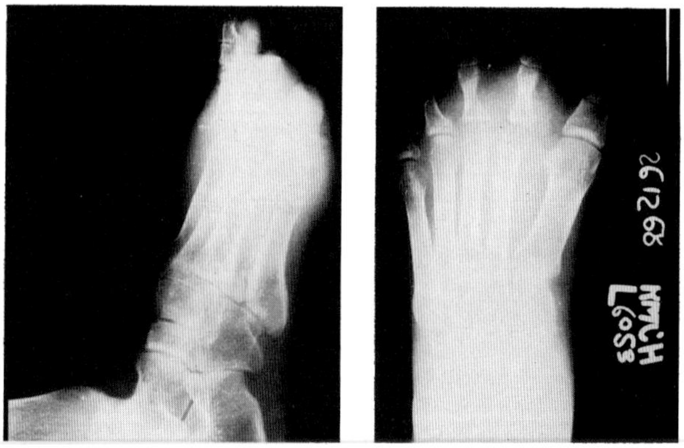

Fig. 32.52 X-ray of the same patient showing mainly soft tissue swelling and an early bony lesion. The patient was happy with a Syme's amputation

hand, face, leg and shoulder may be affected. The course of the disease is prolonged and there may be no history of the initial puncture.

The first manifestation is the appearance of one or more irregular and lumpy, subcutaneous, indurated, pale and painless nodules. Growing slowly, these nodules rupture producing ulcers or sinuses, through which foul-smelling purulent or seropurulent fluid, containing coloured grains of the fungus is discharged. The foot gradually enlarges in size, mostly in its superoinferior dimension (Figs. 32.53 and 54), presenting an ugly look with deformed toes and a plantarflexed ankle (Fig. 32.55). The leg muscles atrophy. Pain and systemic symptoms are conspicuously absent till there is advanced secondary bacterial infection. Usually pyogenic infection does not penetrate the depths till very late, probably because of antibody activity by the fungi. However, secondary infections and long standing disabilities may incapacitate the patient resulting in debility, anaemia and toxaemia. The regional lymph nodes are not affected (less than 1% of those in whom a sinus forms). Other mycetomal infections, such as intraosseous mycetoma, usually affect the upper end of the tibia. Neurological complications and trophic ulceration does not occur in Madura foot.

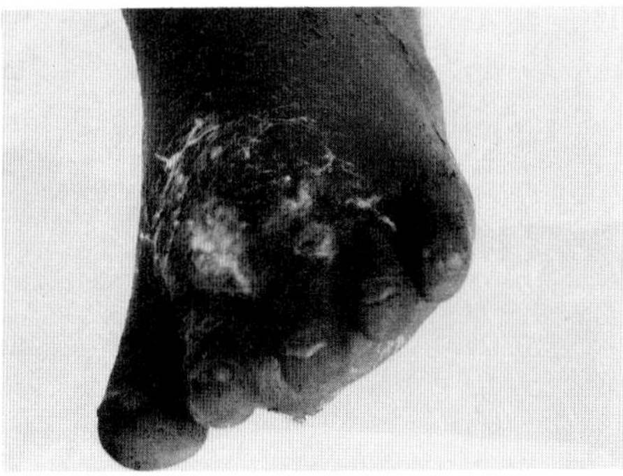

Fig. 32.53 Mycetoma affecting the forefoot with sinuses on the dorsum and sole

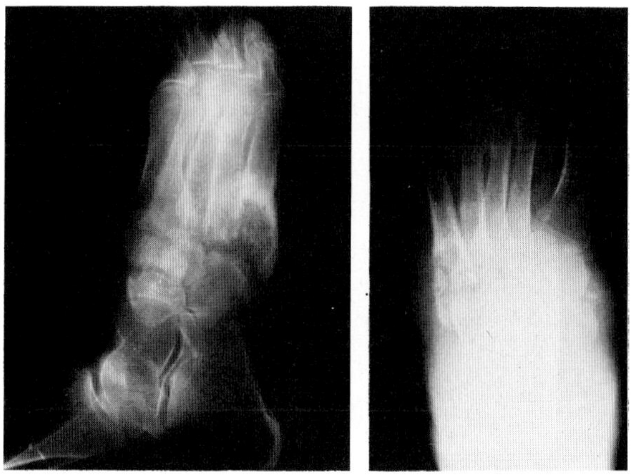

Fig. 32.54 X-ray of Fig. 32.53 showing predominating bony lesions

Investigations

Radiographs reveal soft-tissue swelling with irregular margins and textures, with destructive and proliferative reactions in the underlying bones. Cystic appearances may be seen in the bones.

The demonstration of the characteristic granules is essential to clinch the diagnosis. Direct microscopy of the pus is made by placing the granule in a drop of 10% sodium hydroxide and crushing it under a cover slip to examine for hyphae.

Saline-washed granules must be cultured to demonstrate the responsible fungi.

Serological studies (Gumaa & Mahgoub 1975, Mahgoub 1975) by immunodiffusion and counter-immunoelectrophoresis with the appropriate antigens can be helpful in studying the responsible organism with accuracy. The effectiveness of the chemotherapeutic drug can be well assessed by the serological reactions.

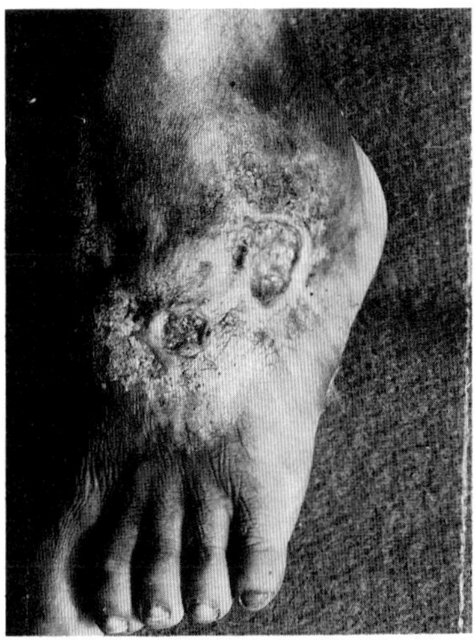

Fig. 32.55 Lesion occupying the dorsum of the hindfoot and ankle

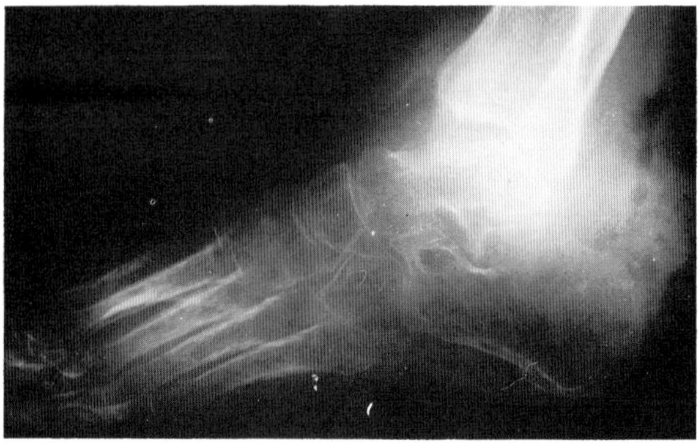

Fig. 32.56 X-ray of Fig. 32.55 — soft tissue swelling; changes within the underlying bones

Management

Medical treatment

Though the clinical manifestations are almost indistinguishable, the differentiation between Eumycetes and actinomycetes is crucial, since the former have resisted the development of any effective chemotherapy while the medical treatment of actinomycetoma is more helpful.

Actinomycetoma. Various drug combinations have been found useful: Dapsone (1.5 mg/kg twice daily) with streptomycin (14 mg/kg daily intramuscularly) or co-trimoxazole with streptomycin or oral rifampicin (4 mg/kg daily) have been used successfully.

Streptomycin, 1 g daily for one month and then on alternate days with either dapsone (100 mg twice daily) or co-trimoxazole is the cheapest regimen (Manson-Bahr 1982). For *Nocardia* infection dapsone alone may be used. However, if mycological assistance is available the drug sensitivity of the isolated organism should be determined. To avoid possible bone marrow depression, regular haematological monitoring should be carried out throughout the treatment (Mahgoub 1976).

The efficiency of the treatment can be checked by assessing the precipitating antibodies which disappear with successful treatment.

Eumycetoma. Though certain fungi have been found relatively sensitive to amphotericin B and griseofulvin in vitro, their clinical efficiency is yet to be proved. However, penicillin and griseofulvin should be used postoperatively to check recurrence.

Surgical treatment

Localized lesions can be best treated by thorough surgical excision. In the case of eumycetoma, due to its resistance to chemotherapy and the inexorability of the disease, complete surgical excision is the only effective management. In most of the advanced cases, planned amputation is the answer (see Figs. 32.51, 52, 57 and 58). In cases where amputation is not desirable or possible, surgical excision followed by local infiltration of 1–2 ml of tincture of iodine into the suspicious areas, every tenth day for two months or more can be tried. Even in severe actinomycetoma, chemotherapy must be tried before surgery. In failed cases surgical procedures are the same as those for eumycetoma.

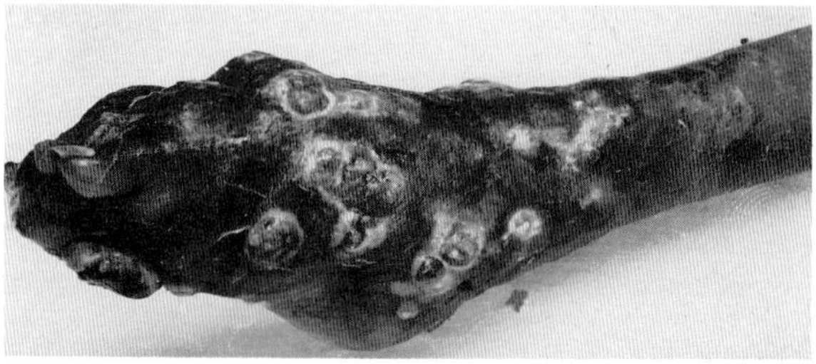

Fig. 32.57 Advanced mycetoma of the foot and lower leg with ulcers and sinuses. Marked equinus deformity

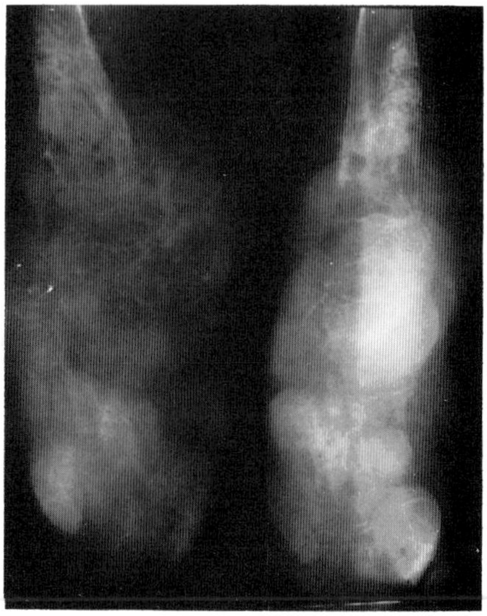

Fig. 32.58 X-ray of Fig. 32.57 showing the bones of the foot and leg grossly affected, rarefied and losing their identity

Prognosis

The disease is very slowly growing and remains localized. Early surgery results in cure without recurrence.

In neglected cases the destruction is progressive and often necessitates amputation.

In the longlasting secondary infection, depression and prolonged disabilities incapacitate the patient and may end in death. It is very seldom self-limiting.

REFERENCES

Abbott P 1956 Mycetoma in Sudan. Trans R Soc Trop Med Hyg 50: 11

Gould W M 1963 Black grain mycetoma originating in Northern California. Report of case caused by *Madurella grisea*. Arch Dermatol 99: 426–428

Gumaa S A, Mahgoub E S 1975 Counter immuno electrophoresis in the diagnosis of mycetoma and its sensitivity as compared to immuno diffusion. Sabouraudia 13(3): 309–315

Mahgoub E S 1975 Pan American Health Organization: 304. Quoted by Manson-Bahr P E C, Apted F I C (eds) 1982 In: Manson's Tropical Diseases. 18th edn. Baillière Tindall, London. pp 473–479

Mahgoub E S 1976 Medical management of mycetoma. WHO Bulletin 54(3): 303–310

Mahgoub E S 1977 Mycosis of Sudan. Trans R Soc Trop Med Hyg 71(3): 184–188

Manson-Bahr P E C, Apted F I C 1982 Mycetoma. In: Manson's Tropical Diseases. 18th edn. Baillière Tindall, London. pp 473–479

Vandyke Carter 1860 Quoted by Utz J P, Shadomy J Deep Fungus Infections. In: Fitzpatrick T B et al (eds) 1979 Dermatology in General Medicine. 2nd edn. McGraw-Hill Book Company, New York. p 1537

TINEA PEDIS

Synonyms: athletes foot, foot ringworm

A chronic infection of the foot with dermatophyte fungi is common in tropical countries specially during the summer and rainy seasons. The causative organisms are either *Trichophyton rubrum, T. interdigitale, T. floccosum* or a mixture. Adolescents and young males are usually affected. Closed, heavy, ill-fitting shoes worn for long periods result in maceration in the interdigital clefts. The exchange of shoes, the use of communal bath tubs, mats and swimming pools favour the spread of infection. In a warm and moist environment, the fungus grows in the stratum corneum of the epidermis. For clinical convenience, the following varieties are recognized:

1. Interdigital: the fourth toe-cleft is usually affected. A sodden, macerated, white layer covering the red, fissured underlying skin is seen. The lesion may spread to the adjoining sole area, the side of the foot, another cleft or even the dorsal surface. A vesiculobullous, pustular or oedematous and erythematous patch or ulcerated lesions may develop. There may be secondary infection (usually staphylococcal), producing features of acute local inflammation, lymphangitis and lymphadenitis.

The patient usually complains of itching, intermittent burning, hyperhydrosis, and malodorous feet.

2. Chronic squamous hyperkeratosis: this is usually caused by *T. rubrum*, affects the sole and the sides of the foot and the palm and is very resistant to treatment. Thickened erythematous areas are covered with powdery, silver-white scales. The toenails may be affected. Except for a feeling of unusual skin roughness, the patient remains symptom-free for a long time.

Differential diagnosis

The typical clinical findings and the demonstration of the causative fungus confirm the diagnosis. Toe-cleft lesions need differentiation from erythrasma, pseudomonas infection (Wood's lamp demonstration of pink fluorescence for the former and greenish blue for the latter), candidiasis, and other bacterial infection. In the hyperkeratotic lesions, yaws, syphilis, psoriasis, keratoderma, and eczema, should be considered.

Treatment

For the acute stage, after applying gentian violet or silver nitrate paint, the foot should be kept at rest till the inflammatory symptoms subside. For the inderdigital variety, Castellani's paint or tincture of merthiolate should be applied. Antifungal powder should be dusted into the toe-clefts and over the sole before putting on the socks, which should be sterilized daily by boiling. It is better to use an open toed shoe. If closed shoes are to be used, they should be sterilized on occasion by formalin vapour.

TINEA UNGUIUM

Synonyms: ringworm of the nails

Chronic infection of the nail plate by the dermatophytes (*Trichophyton* and *Microsporon*), usually in adults, is characterized by discoloured, frayed, deformed, opaque, irregular and brittle nails with the accumulation of hyperkeratotic debris under the anterior end of the nail plate. The lesion spreads from one nail to others and may be bilateral and symmetrical.

There are few symptoms, except intermittent discomfort and visible changes.

The infection has a prolonged chronic course, with a poor prognosis. Behl (1982) quoting Bendek and Sagher, has expressed doubts regarding the primary infection by fungus, believing the tinea unguium is pompholyx due to some septic focus, resulting in dystrophy of the nail and that fungus is a secondary invader of the devitalized nail. Depression in general health and emotional factors are also said to be responsible for the nail changes. Diagnosis is based on the typical appearance and the demonstration of the fungus from the hyperkeratotic debris and nail trimmings.

Treatment

Early proper treatment of tinea pedis will reduce the incidence. Prolonged oral griseofulvin is usually effective. Regular filing of the nail and local applications of antifungal agents such as tincture of iodine or glutaraldehyde also help.

REFERENCES

Behl P N 1982 Practice of Dermatology. 5th edn. Allied Book Agency, Calcutta. p 176

CANDIDIASIS

Synonyms: thrush, moniliasis, monilia, candidosis

Moniliasis is an infection caused by the saprophytic yeast-like fungus *Candida albicans* or allied species. Heat, humidity, moisture, lowered resistance and diabetes favour the organisms. It can affect the skin but mainly attacks the mucous membranes or even the alimentary canal and viscera. In the foot candidia infection produces:

1. Monilial toes: moist, red, macerated and peeling lesions with white, sodden epidermis appear between the toes mimicking tinea pedis.

2. Paronychia: this usually occurs in the fingers, but may also occur in the toes, where chronic inflammatory changes affect the nail folds. The nail fold becomes swollen and red and tends to separate from the nail plate producing a gap filled with cheesy material. The patient complains of dull pain and mild irritation. Gradually the nail becomes distorted and atrophied.

Treatment

Proper cleaning and hygienic care of the foot is essential. Polyene antibiotics (amphotericin, nystatin, natamycin and candicidin) are markedly effective against any form of candidiasis. Topical preparations (spray, powder or lotions) can be safely applied. Gentian violet, tincture of merthiolate, nystatin or imidazole derivatives like clotrimazole, econazole or miconazole lotion or cream may be used locally with good effect.

LOBO'S MYCOSIS

Synonyms: cheloidal blastomycosis, keloidal blastomycosis, George Lobo's disease

This is a rare, chronic, localized, slow-growing, firm, keloid-like lobulated tumorous lesion persisting for up to forty years without affecting the patient's general health. Lobo (1931) described this condition in a patient from the Amazon valley.

South America is the main seat of the disease. It is caused by the fungus *Loboa loboi*, gaining entry through a wound. The exposed parts of the legs, arm and face are affected. Initially the surface lesion appears shining and smooth with or without telangiectatic spots, but later on become verrucous and scaly.

The condition should be differentiated from chromycosis by demonstrating microscopically the causative fungus from biopsy material.

REFERENCES

Lobo J 1931 In: Domonkos A N 1971 Andrew's Diseases of the Skin. 6th edn (Asian edition). W. B. Saunders Company, Philadelphia. p 366

FURTHER READING

Allen H B, Rippon J W 1985 Superficial and deep mycoses. In: Moschella S L, Hurley H J (eds) Dermatology. 2nd edn. Vol 1. W. B. Saunders Co, Philadelphia. pp 785–786
Silva D Quoted in Rook A, Wilkinson D S, Ebling F J G (eds) 1979 Textbook of Dermatology. 3rd edn. Blackwell Scientific Publications, Oxford. pp 856–857

TROPICAL ULCER

Synonyms: tropical sloughing, phagedena, tropical phagedena, tropical phagedenic ulcer, naga ulcer (India)

Tropical ulcer is a clinical syndrome of no definite known aetiology characterized by an initial acute or subacute dermal necrosis followed by a chronic nonspecific persistent ulcer, usually seen in poor patients inhabiting hot and humid areas.

Geographical distribution

Commonly in Africa (commonest in Northern Nigeria), South and Central America and India, but can be seen in other parts of the world.

No definite cause is known (Basset 1969, Canizares 1975, Simons 1952), but minor trauma has been blamed for the initial tissue necrosis. Children and young adults from poor rural areas, labourers and farmers working barefoot and living in crowded, unhygienic surroundings are the usual victims. Anaemia, chronic morbidity and malnutrition (protein and vitamin A deficiencies) (Simons 1952, Thomson 1956) predispose to the condition by devitalizing the tissues. Tropical ulcer may be endemic, e.g. after famine, flood or among refugees and in prison camps.

The role of a specific pathogen is doubted (Roberts & Rook 1979) though the uniform development of the typical ulcer suggests involvement by some specific organism, which becomes active only under certain environmental factors.

In acute lesions, but not closed blebs, *Bacillus fusiformis* and *Borrelia vincentii* are commonly found. However, with the progress of the lesions, several other organisms like Vincent's spirochetes, pseudomonas, proteus, staphylococcus, streptococcus, pneumococcus and diphtheroids may be detected. These are most likely secondary invaders.

Clinical features

Usually there is history of minor trauma, a scratch or an insect or mosquito bite. Soon after the area becomes slightly erythematous and vesicles or bullae containing serous or serosanguinous fluid appear. The surrounding area may be slightly indurated. There may be mild constitutional features with pyrexia. Within 24 to 48 hours the bullae rupture leaving behind a dirty, painful foul-smelling, superficial ulcer. The margin of the ulcer is indurated, and may be undermined or raised. The floor is covered by dirty, purulent, friable slough (Fig. 32.59).

The ulcer spreads rapidly in all directions. The underlying muscles, fascia and tendons die and dissolve and the ulcer encroaches upon bone, where periostitis or osteomyelitis develop. The regional lymph nodes are usually not enlarged, except when there is superimposed infection. The surrounding tissues remain indurated, the skin becomes atrophic, adherent and depigmented. In favourable circumstances the ulcer may start healing within a few weeks with an atrophic scar with hyperpigmented margin.

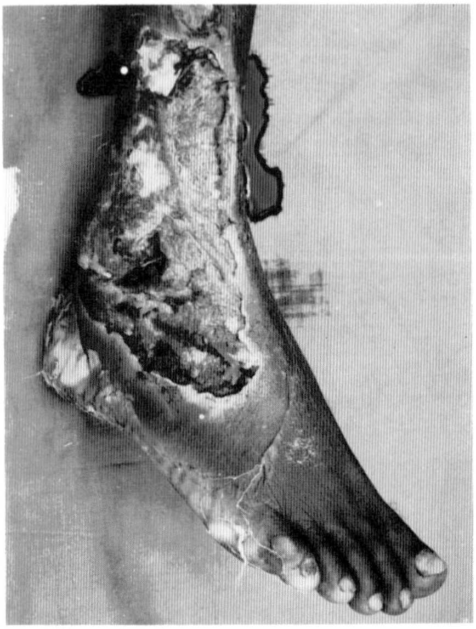

Fig. 32.59 This extensive ulcer developed in 14 days following an insignificant injury caused by the leg of a cot

The margins of longstanding ulcers become hyperplastic and squamous cell epithelioma may develop. Variable contractures, deformities or ankylosis occur and contracting cicatrices may strangulate the circulation necessitating amputation (McLaren 1979). In severe types, the rapid extension of the ulcer debilitates the patient, occasionally resulting in death.

Differential diagnosis

The typical appearance of the ulcer, associated with the demonstration of *B. fusiformis* or Vincents spirochaetes may be taken as diagnostic in the acute stage. Otherwise no specific investigation is helpful. In chronic ulcers only contaminants may be isolated. The chronic tropical ulcer has to be differentiated from the granulomatous ulcers of yaws and syphilis (where serological tests will be helpful) especially as spirochaetes found in tropical ulcers may mimic *Treponema pertenue* (Guthe & Throstein 1980) or *T. pallidum*. Other conditions to be differentiated are tuberculosis, post burn, varicose and Buruli ulcers, veld sores, epithelioma and malignant melanoma.

Management

In the acute stage, rest, nutritious diet and hospital supervision are helpful. The limb should be kept elevated and the wound dressed three times daily with some bland application after irrigating thoroughly with hydrogen peroxide and normal saline. As the ulcer becomes healthy, the number of dressings is reduced to once daily. It is better to carry out a split skin graft on the healthy granulating surface.

If the ulcer is deep, and affecting the underlying bone, excision of the ulcer with curettage or limited excision of the underlying affected bone and skin grafting speeds the recovery.

The patient can be sent home with a plaster cast applied over a dressed wound. The cast should be changed every three to four weeks till the ulcer heals completely. For the very chronic indolent and incapacitating ulcer, the patient may request amputation which should be considered. For secondary epithelioma, a local wide excision along with en bloc lymph gland excision should be attempted if possible; otherwise planned amputation should be done.

Chemotherapy

1 Mu of penicillin in divided dosage should be started. Other antibiotics should be given according to the chemosensitivity of the secondary invaders. Metronidazole (600 mg daily) may assist recovery.

There is no specific preventive measure but improved nutrition and living standards, and the care of injuries will decrease the possibility of developing the tropical ulcer.

REFERENCES

Basset A 1969 In: Simons R D G P, Marshall J (eds) Essays on Tropical Dermatology. Excerpta Medica, Amsterdam. p 25

Brand P 1977 Insensitive Feet: a practical handbook on foot problems in leprosy. The Leprosy Mission, London. pp 16–30

Canizares O 1975 Clinical Tropical Dermatology. Blackwell Scientific Publications, Oxford. p 96

Guthe, Threstein 1980 Non syphilitic treponematosis — yaws. In: Beeson P B et al (eds) Cecil Textbook of Medicine, 15th edn. W. B. Saunders Co, Igaku Shein Ltd, Tokyo. p 521

Languillon M C J 1964 Frequency and localization of plantar perforating ulcers of leprosy patients. Lepr Rev 35, 4A: 239–244
Lennox W M 1964 A classification of leprosy foot deformities. Lepr Rev 35, 4A: 246
McLaren D S 1979 Cutaneous changes in nutrition sciences. In: Fitzpatrick et al (eds) Dermatology in General Medicine. McGraw-Hill Book Co, New York. p 1024
Price E W 1964a The etiology and natural history of plantar ulcer. Lepr Rev 35, 4A: 259–266
Price E W 1964b The problem of plantar ulcer. Lepr Rev 35, 4A: 267–272
Price E W 1959 Studies in plantar ulcers in leprosy. I General. 11 The mechanics of the foot in relation to plantar ulcers. Lepr Rev 30: 98
Roberts S O B, Rook A 1979 Bacterial infections — Tropical ulcers In: Rook A, Wilkinson D S, Ebling F J G (eds) Textbook of Dermatology. 3rd edn. Blackwell, Oxford p 598
Simons R D G P, Anning S T 1952 In: Simons R D G P (ed) Handbook of Tropical Dermatology, Vol 1. Elsevier, Amsterdam. p 413
Thomson I G 1956 Trans R Soc Trop Med Hyg 50: 485. Quoted by Rook A, Roberts S O B 1975 Bacterial infections. In: Rook A et al (eds) Textbook of Dermatology. 2nd edn. Blackwell Scientific Publications, Oxford. p 529

MOSSY FOOT

Synonyms: Various diseases of the foot present as mossy foot – endemic elephantiasis, lymphostatic verrucosis, nonfilarial elephantiasis, mossy foot, lymphoedematous keratoderma or chromblastomycosis

Mossy foot has a clinical presentation in which the dorsum of the foot is swollen and the overlying skin becomes diffusely thickened with a velvety papillomatous surface. However, it may be of 'water bag' type, 'cauliflower'-like or show thickened, fibrotic or irregular warty projections.

True mossy foot results from infection by pigmented fungi and should be differentiated from mycetomal and lymphoedematous elephantiasis.

ENDEMIC ELEPHANTIASIS

Price (1976) has assigned this as 'geo-chemical' disease. Aluminium silicate and silicon have been found to be responsible for producing obstruction of the peripheral lymphatics, thereby producing chronic lymphoedema of the lower limbs — nonfilarial elephantiasis.

Geographical distribution

This disease is more prevalent in areas where the soil is rich in silicon, colloidal iron and aluminium (e.g. red soil resulting from volcanic rocks as in Kenya and Ethiopia (Cohen 1961), Ruanda, Uganda (Loewenthal 1934), West Africa (Manuwa 1935) and Ecuador.

Aetiology and pathogenesis

Poor persons of both sexes in the second decade, working with bare feet, are the main victims. The chemical irritants are absorbed through the sole and produce peripheral lymphatic and lymph node obstruction.

Starting in the skin of the toes, pathological changes slowly proceed proximally up to the knees. In the skin there are lymphatic cuffing of the sweat ducts, small granulomata, birefringent particles and iron staining ferric crystals.

The valves of the peripheral lymphatics of the foot and leg fail to function leading to dilatation of the lumen which contains a reflux of lymphocytes (Manson-Bahr & Apted 1982). Irritation in the lumen initiates hypertrophy and multiplication of the endothelial cells which occlude the lumen. Gradually the lymphatic channel is converted into a thin fibrous band.

The regional lymph nodes also undergo hypertrophy. In the central zone of the gland numerous microphages containing spherical or rod-shaped, tiny, birefringent particles, spread in a disorganized PAS-positive cytoplasm. In early cases granulomata pervade the field.

Clinical features

Swelling starts from the toes and slowly affects the whole foot and leg, limited to just below the knee and usually on only one side, although the contralateral side may be affected. Later, the swollen area may be tender especially in the line of the lymphatics.

In the beginning there may be pitting oedema, 'water-bag' or 'earthworm-bag' feeling to palpation, but in advanced stages extensive fibrosis presents a firm to hard feel. The regional lymph glands are enlarged, tender, and firm in the beginning, but harden slowly.

Usually the subjects are poor and wear sandals, under the strap of which areas of hyperkeratosis and papillomatous warty outgrowths develop. The disease remains painless, developing slowly until elephantiasis or ulcers develop. Thickened skin folds with or without ulcers may develop in front of ankle, but lesions do not affect the sole. Initially the overlying skin becomes diffusely thickened but later it turns velvety, papillomatous and ultimately roughens due to irregular warty projections (Ebling & Rock 1979).

Diagnosis

This is based on the geographical distribution and the insidious progress of the disease, usually occurring in one leg and limited to below the knee.

Investigations

Peripheral blood examination is done to exclude microfilaria; lymphangiography demonstrates either occlusion or varying hypoplasia of the lymphatic vessels below the knee.

Differential diagnosis

Endemic elephantiasis should be differentiated from filarial elephantiasis (where other parts may also be involved, and lymphangiography shows dilated vessels).

Management

In the initial stage, compression therapy by continuous elastic bandages or stockings is useful. Ulcers are chronic and troublesome and should usually be managed conservatively. Prophylaxis is the main aim and proper footwear must be encouraged from early childhood.

REFERENCES

Cohen L B 1961 Idiopathic lymphoedema of Ethiopia and Kenya. East Afr Med J 37: 53

Ebling F J G, Rook A 1979 Disorders of keratinization. In: Rook A, Wilkinson D S, Ebling F J G (eds) Textbook of Dermatology. 3rd edn. Blackwell Scientific Publications, Oxford. p 1307

Loewenthal L J A 1934 On probable inclusion of several diseases in title 'mossy foot'. Ann Trop Med Parasitol. 28: 47

Manson-Bahr P E C, Apted F I C 1982 Endemic elephantiasis. In: Manson-Bahr P E C, Apted F I C (eds) Manson's Tropical Diseases. Baillière Tindall, London. p 21

Price E W 1975 The mechanism of lymphatic obstruction in endemic elephantiasis of the lower legs. Trans R Soc Trop Med Hyg 69(2): 177–80

Price E W 1976 The association of endemic elephantiasis of the lower legs in East Africa with soil derived from volcanic rocks. Trans R Soc Trop Med Hyg 70(4): 333–334

CHROMOMYCOSIS

Synonyms: Chromoblastomycosis, verrucous dermatitis

This is a chronic systemic fungal disease caused by species of *Phialophora*, *Cladosporium* or *Fonsecaea* acquired through the skin by traumatic implantation and characterized by slowly-growing verrucous, ulcerated and crusted or wart-like lesions affecting the skin and subcutaneous tissues.

Historical aspect

Rudolph (1914) first reported a case of chromomycosis from Brazil. Medlar (1915) reported chromomycosis from Boston. Thaxter named *Phialophora verrucosa* as the causative organism, but other fungi have been described.

Geographical distribution

Occurrences have been reported from Cuba, Jamaica, Martinique, Central, South and North

America, South Africa and Madagascar, India, Australia and Northern Europe and a very few from the United States and Britain.

Aetiology

Adult male labourers (especially timber and soil workers) working barefooted in rural areas of the tropics are most susceptible. Numerous fungi have been blamed but the most common are *P. verrucosa, P. pedrosoi, P. compacta, P. dermatitidis, Cladosporium carrioni* and *C. trichoides*. In the tissues these fungi remain single or grouped together and are difficult to distinguish from each other. Each appears as round, thick-walled, 6–12 μ budding cells of the brown colour from which the disease derives its name.

Immunology

The fungi can be seen directly microscopically on potassium hydroxide mounts and also in biopsy sections as deep, pigmented, thick-walled sclerotic cells. They can be cultured and mycelia vary according to genus and species. Precipitation, agglutination and fluorescent antibody tests have been utilized to differentiate the various organisms. Experimentally, infection can be produced in laboratory animals.

Pathology

Histopathologically the infection appears as a foreign body granuloma with isolated micro-abscesses. Six or seven fungal bodies may be seen crowded in a giant cell looking like peas in a pod. Fungal cells are readily discernible with haematoxylin and eosin stains.

Clinical features

Though the lesion in the first reported patient was on the buttock, they are usually seen on exposed sites, especially the feet, legs, hand, forearm, arm, face, neck and shoulders. The general condition is not affected and pathology remains localized in the skin and subcutaneous tissues. The patient may recollect some earlier minor wound.

Primarily a small papule or a nodule or a pustule develops which persists for months. Finally it ulcerates, spreads laterally, becomes dry and crusted and may assume a papular or even wart-like appearance. It may remain flat or grow with a stalk as long as 3 cm and look like a cauliflower. The lesion may heal centrally, but spontaneous cure does not occur. The lesion spreads gradually and may affect the function of the leg or arm in 4–15 years.

The patient complains of considerable itching, but hardly any pain unless ulcers develop. Extensive fibrosis may lead to lymphoedema. The lesion spreads marginally and by lymphatic channels to adjacent areas. There may be satellite lesions due to autoinoculation while scratching. Haematogenous spread producing brain abscesses has also been reported and Desai et al (1966) have reported *C. trichoides* causing cerebral lesions.

Secondary infection may cause lymphoedematous elephantiasis.

Investigations

In examination of the superficial crusts removed from the lesions, dark brown spheroid mycelia-spores 4–8 μ in diameter can be recognized and cultured on media containing chloramphenicol or other antibiotics and incubated at 30°C.

Diagnosis

This is based on a very chronic history, a typical lesion, the demonstration of the spores of the causative organism microscopically from the biopsy specimen and by culture. Early lesions should be differentiated from blastomycosis, tuberculosis, leprosy, leishmaniasis, syphilis and yaws.

Treatment

Medical treatment

There is no certain chemotherapy for these fungi, but oral 5-fluorocytosine 30–50 mg/kg body weight six hourly for several months may be effective. With this therapy blood levels should be monitored, especially in renal-risk cases. In resistant cases amphotericin B may be added, in a dosage of 0.5 mg/kg body weight in 500 ml of 5% glucose intravenously over a six hour period, gradually increasing to a maximum of 1.0 mg/kg body weight.

This should be given on alternate days and a watch should be kept for malaise, nausea, fever, headache and venous thrombosis. Therapy may have to be continued for a month or longer depending upon the response.

Costello et al (1959) have reported successful results following local infiltration of the lesion with 15 mg of amphotericin B dissolved in 3 ml of 2% procaine solution, repeated weekly or at longer intervals for 4 to 8 injections.

Lopes et al (1969) has recommended 5-fluorocytosine by mouth and by local infiltration. Bopp (1974) claimed a cure in two months with no recurrence for six months after giving 500 mg of fluoroytosine six hourly to a total of 400 g combined with 500 mg amphotericin B intravenously on alternate days to a total of 1.5 g.

Heat has also been utilized for treatment based on the concept that the optimum temperature for growth of these fungi lies between 35°C and 39°C. Conti Diaz et al (1966) have claimed cure in cases caused by *P. verrucosa* with infra-red irradiation.

Iodides have also been proposed, but their effectiveness is doubted. Depending on the lesion, electrocoagulation, local infiltration of amphotericin B and copper sulphate iontophoresis have been tried (Behl 1982).

Surgical treatment

For early lesions complete surgical resection is the most effective treatment. When diagnosed, early small localized lesions can also be destroyed by thermal cautery or diathermy.

Local infiltration with amphotericin B and excision with or without skin grafting has been recommended by Whiting & Cloete (1968). However, relapses have been frequent. For stubborn and extensive lesions, amputation may be required to get rid of the disease.

Prognosis

The skin lesions are mostly chronic and compatible with long life. Very rarely distant spread of the disease (e.g. to the brain) may pose serious problems.

REFERENCES

Behl P N 1982 Practice of Dermatology 5th edn. Allied Book Agencies, Calcutta. p 183

Bopp C 1974 Quoted by Manson-Bahr P E C, Apted F I C (eds) 1982 In: Manson's Tropical Diseases. 18th edn. Baillière Tindall, London. p 500

Conti, Diaz I A, Vignale R, Pena De Periera M E 1966 Quoted by Manson-Bahr P E C, Apted F I C 1982 (eds) In: Manson's Tropical Diseases. 18th edn. Baillière Tindall, London. p 501

Costello M J, De Feo C P, Littman M L 1959 Arch Dermatol 79: 184. Quoted by Manson-Bahr P E C, Apted F I C 1982 (eds) In: Manson's Tropical Diseases. 18th edn. Baillière Tindall, London. p 501

Desai C S, Bhatika M L, Mehta R S 1966 Cerebral chromoblastomycosis due to *Cladosporium trichoides* (Bantianum), II Mycopathologic investigations of brain and skin involvement. Neurology 14: 6–18

Lopes et al 1969 Quoted by Manson-Bahr P E C, Apted F I C 1982 (eds) In: Manson's Tropical Diseases. 18th edn. Baillière Tindall, London. p 480

Medlar E M 1915 J Med Res 32: 507. Quoted by Edward D Delamater: Parasitic affections, diseases due to plant parasites. In: Ormsby O S, Montgomery H 1954 Diseases of the skin. 8th edn. Lea & Febiger, Philadelphia. p 1209

Rudolph 1914 Quoted by Utz J P, Shadomy J Deep fungus infections. In: Fitzpatrick T B et al (eds) 1979 Dermatology in General Medicine. 2nd edn. McGraw-Hill Book Company, New York. pp 1556–1561

Whiting D A, Cloete G N 1968 Chemotherapy and conservative surgery in the treatment of Chromoblastomycosis. S Afr Med J 42(34): 885–886

FURTHER READING

A'Doory Y 1972 Chromomychosis. Mountain Press, Montana: Quoted by John P Utz In: Beeson P B et al (eds) 1979 Cecil's Textbook of Medicine. 15th edn. (Asian edition). W. B. Saunders Company, Philadelphia. pp 542–543

Buckley H R, Murray I G 1966 Precipitating antibodies in chromycosis. Sabouraudia 5: 78–80

MacLeod J (ed) 1981 Davidson's Principles and Practice of Medicine: Chromoblastomycosis. 13th edn. (ELBS). Churchill Livingstone, Edinburgh. p 884

De Foe C P, Harber L C 1959 Chromoblastomycosis treated with local infiltration of amphotericin B solution. JAMA 171: 1961

Gordon M A, A'Doory Y 1965 Application of fluorescent antibody procedures to the study of pathogenic dematiacious fungi. II Serological relationship of the genus *Fonsecaea*. J Bacteriol 89: 551

Gugndni H C, Susehan A V, Nwokoloc, Njoku-Obian 1977 Cutaneous cladosporiosis trichoides. J Trop Med Hyg 80(8): 177–178

Howles J K et al 1954 Chromoblastomycosis: Report of 9 cases from a single area in Louisiana. Arch Dermatol 69: 83–90

Klokke A H 1964 Chromoblastomycosis. J Indian Med Assoc 43: 340

Manson-Bahr P E C, Apted F I C (eds) 1982 Chromoblastomycosis. In: Manson's Tropical Diseases. 18th edn. Baillière Tindall, London. pp 479–480
Mead M, Ridley M F 1957 Med J Aust I: 192. Quoted by Beare et al In: Rook A, Wilkinson D S, Ebling F J G (eds) 1965 Textbook of Dermatology. 2nd edn. Blackwell Scientific Publications, Oxford. pp 770–772
Rook A, Wilkinson D S, Ebling F J G (eds) 1979 Textbook of Dermatology. 3rd edn. Blackwell Scientific Publications, Oxford. pp 857–859
Schol-Schwartz M B 1968 Rhinocladiella, its synonym Fonsecaea and its relation to Phialophora. Antonie van Leeuwenhoek J Microbiol 34(2): 119–152
Seeliger H P R, Lacaz C, Das, Ulson C M 1959 International Congress on Tropical Medicine VI. Malar 4: 636. Quoted by Manson-Bahr P E C, Apted F I C (eds) 1982. In: Manson's Tropical Diseases. 18th edn. Baillière Tindall, London. p 502
Sonck C E 1959 Quoted by Beare et al 1975 In: Rook A, Wilkinson D S, Ebling F J G Textbook of Dermatology. 2nd edn. Blackwell Scientific Publications, Oxford. p 772
Woodruff A W 1977 Chromoblastomycosis. In: Woodruff A W (ed) Medicine in the Tropics. Churchill Livingstone, Edinburgh. p 375

LYMPHOEDEMATOUS KERATODERMA

Secondary skin changes developing over a chronic lymphoedematous area are seen in the filarial elephantoid foot, but this may develop in any chronic lymphoedematous area, even in the post-thrombotic oedematous leg and the thickened skin of amputation stumps.

The skin over the affected area first becomes diffusely thickened and then gradually develops a velvety surface with papillomatous and irregular warty projections.

Microscopically, in the epidermal zone, hyperkeratosis, papillomatosis and acanthosis are seen. In the dermis oedematous changes, dilated lymphatics with new vessel formation and patchy sclerosis are found. Chronic inflammatory cells are spread over the area.

ERYTHRASMA

Erythrasma is a common mild, chronic, localized superficial bacterial infection caused by *Corynebacterium* species and characterized by irregular, well-demarcated, brownish-red patches of dry, smooth or creased skin usually occurring in intertriginous areas.

Occurring more in the toe-webs, besides other sites like axillae and groins, morphologically it looks like a fungal infection. A typical 'coral-red' fluorescence is seen under the Wood's lamp and the culture of *Corynebacterium* confirms the diagnosis.

Toe-web infections remain asymptomatic for a long time; slight itching, scaling, fissuring and maceration may occur. Treatment is by proper foot hygiene and 1.0 g daily of oral erythromycin in divided doses for 7 days.

PITTED KERATOLYSIS

Synonyms: dermatolysis plantare sulcatum, keratoderma plantaris, keratoderma palmaris et plantaris

This is a superficial cutaneous infection probably caused by single or mixed infection with *Streptomyces*, *Corynebacterium* and other organisms (Young 1974) and characterized by bilateral circular erosions on the soles and occasionally on the hands.

Numerous discrete, circular or irregular, shallow, superficial lesions with a punched-out appearance appear on the soles and the undersurface of the toes. It is usually associated with hyperhydrosis. There may be fissuring and maceration, accompanied by a foul odour. The condition remains symptomless for a long period, except for mild intermittent itching.

Culture of the organism is difficult.

Histologically filamentous and coccoid micro-organisms may be detected in superficial skin scrapings. The condition has to be differentiated from fungal infections, erythrasma and simple hyperhydrosis.

Treatment

Besides managing the problems of hyperhydrosis, local application of Fucidin® ointment may help.

REFERENCES

Young C N 1974 In: Rook A, Wilkinson D S, Ebling F J G (eds) 1979 Textbook of Dermatology. 3rd edn. Blackwell Scientific Publications, Oxford. p 573

MYCOBACTERIUM ULCERANS INFECTION

Synonyms: Buruli ulcer (in Uganda), Searl's ulcer (in Australia)

Chronic indolent, painless ulcers occurring mostly in the legs in the first and second decades, caused by *Mycobacterium ulcerans (M. buruli)* have been reported widely from the tropics, especially Uganda, Australia, Mexico, Latin America, Africa and Indonesia.

A firm and painless subcutaneous nodule, gradually breaking down to a necrotic rapidly spreading ulcer characterizes the early clinical feature. The ulcer looks shallow, has an undermined edge, and may spread circumferentially. With secondary infection, constitutional changes may appear. In a year the ulcer may heal spontaneously leaving behind marked fibrosis with secondary lymphoedema, contractures and deformities.

The diagnosis can be confirmed by culturing the *M. ulcerans* on a standard medium at 32°C.

Management

In the early stage, the nodule should be excised. When an extensive ulcer develops, thorough debridement of the ulcer and the application of split-thickness skin grafts should be performed. There is no suitable antibiotic.

PASTEURELLA MULTOCIDA INFECTIONS

The lower or ankle region may be the site for a dog, cat, rat, mouse or other animal bite. Local infection with regional adenitis may develop due to infection by *P. multocida* — a small, ovoid, gram-negative bacillus residing as normal flora in the respiratory tract and alimentary canal of these animals.

At the site of the animal bite local inflammatory features develop, followed by cellulitis, abscess formation, local necrosis, sinus formation and ulceration. The discharge may be seropurulent or greyish-yellow and haemorrhagic. If the bite is deeper, osteomyelitis of the underlying bone may occur. Isolation of the organism establishes the diagnosis.

Penicillin and tetracycline can be effective, but the chemosensitivity of the isolated organism should be determined. A local abscess should be surgically drained through a wide incision. The disease is usually arrested with local measures combined with antibiotics.

BOTROMYCOSIS

Synonym: Actinophytosis

Botromycosis is a very rare, chronic, granulomatous reaction to bacterial infection in man, with pus containing pinhead-sized whitish-yellow granules resembling the sulphur granules of actinomycosis. Gram-stained preparations of the crushed granule show clusters of staphylococci (pyogenes). Lesions are mostly on the limbs including the foot (other sites being the perianal region, face, lung, etc.). Some foreign body (like brook straw or a fish bone) is reported as initiating the lesion.

The cutaneous lesion starts with single or multiple abscesses which burst to discharge serous or serosanguinous fluid and end in multiple sinuses with overgranulating masses at their mouths. Healing of the lesions occurs after several months or a year leaving an atrophic scar. Usually the patient's general condition is not affected.

Treatment consists of dressings and suitable antibiotics depending upon the chemosensitivity. Chronic cases may require surgical excision.

PROTOTHECOSIS

Sudman (1974) has indicated the association of *Prototheca zepfii* and *P. wickerhamii* with human disease. Davies et al (1964) has shown and isolated an abundance of *P. zepfii* from the epidermis and dermis of a chronic inflammatory plaque occurring on the dorsum of the foot. The lesion is usually a localized inflammatory plaque or papule in the skin. An abscess may develop in the subcutaneous tissue and very rarely there may be general constitutional changes.

The condition is self-limiting. However amphotericin B may be effective.

REFERENCES

Davies R R et al 1964 A case of human protothecosis. Trans R Soc Trop Med Hyg 58: 448

Sudman M S 1974 Protothecosis: A critical review. Am J Clin Pathol 61(1): 10–19

FURTHER READING

Roberts S O B, Rook A 1979 Protothecosis. In: Rook A, Wilkinson D S, Ebling F J G (eds) Textbook of Dermatology. 3rd edn. Blackwell Scientific Publications, Oxford. p 605

FISH-TANK GRANULOMA

Synonyms: Mycobacterium marinum infection, swimming pool granuloma

This is a chronic, granulomatous, dermal infection mimicking tuberculosis and is caused by an acid-fast bacillus *Mycobacterium marinum*.

In the tropics the source of infection has been traced to fish-tanks, inadequately chlorinated swimming pools, sea-shore and harbour water. Children, adolescents and fishermen are usually affected. The organism invades through breaches in the skin. The elbows are most commonly affected, but the dorsum of the foot, the knee, face and hands are also affected.

The lesion, usually solitary, starts as a verrucous nodule on an inflammatory base. It breaks down to form an ulcer, which may become secondarily infected. Regional lymph nodes are usually not affected, but the infection may spread along superficial lymphatics. Spontaneous healing with scarring may occur in an average of two years.

Histologically the picture closely mimics tuberculosis. Lupus vulgaris, coccidiomycosis, blastomycosis, dermal leishmaniasis, yaws, syphilis, and tularaemia should be considered in the differential diagnosis.

The clinical history, isolating the organism on standard mycobacterial culture and a positive dermal test (reaction to intradermal tuberculin prepared from *M. marinum*) establish the diagnosis.

Treatment

Most of the lesions heal in about two years. After testing the sensitivity, two antituberculosis drugs should be given, rifampicin 600 mg/daily and ethambutol 25 mg/kg body weight (Cortez & Pankey 1973). Minocycline hydrochloride (200 mg daily in divided doses) has been reported to be effective (Loria 1976). Locally electrodesiccation, cryosurgery, heating the part and infiltration with streptomycin have been tried with varying success. Chronic foot lesions can be better treated by excision and closure.

REFERENCES

Cortez L M, Pankey G A 1973 J Bone Joint Surg 55A: 363

Loria P R 1976 *Mycobacterium marinum* infections of the hand. Arch Dermatol 112: 515

PSEUDOMONAS AERUGINOSA INFECTION

Synonym: Tropical immersion foot

Pseudomonas aeruginosa, an aerobic gram-negative bacillus, is an occasional member of normal skin flora, usually occupying the moist cutaneous areas (axilla, groin, anorectal region and external ear). Suppression of the skin gram-positive flora, by local application of antibiotics or after maceration, favours the emergence of these organisms in the toe-webs. This condition, called 'tropical immersion foot', is characterized by well demarcated, macerated, sodden lesions in the web, sometimes with a greenish tinge. The superficial, sodden, crusty plaque may fall off and secondary infection may supervene (Taplin et al 1965). *Bacillus pyocyaneus* may also be isolated from chronic ulcers of the foot or leg, producing typical greenish-yellow or bluish-green pus due to the production of its typical pigments, fluorescein or pyocyanin.

Taplin et al (1966) have reported the development of toe-web lesions by *P. cepacia*, in troops training in swamp conditions.

Organisms can be isolated by bacteriological culture. Green fluorescence in the toe-web lesions can be demonstrated under Wood's light.

The infections are usually resistant to most antibiotics, and chemosensitivity to gentamicin and polymyxin B should be determined. Proper hygiene of the foot and local application of antibiotic spray have proved useful.

REFERENCES

Taplin D et al 1965 Archives of Environmental Health II: 546. In: Rook A, Wilkinson D S, Ebling F J G (eds) 1979 Textbook of Dermatology. 3rd edn. Blackwell Scientific Publications, Oxford. pp 584–585

Taplin D, Zaias N 1966 Tropical immersion foot syndrome. Milit Med 131: 814–815

INFECTION BY OPPORTUNISTIC MYCOBACTERIA

Mycobacterium fortuitum, commonly found in human surroundings, can be pathogenic. Usually it is reported after injection, after vaccination, or after cutaneous abscesses from another source. Regional lymphadenitis is not common, but Azulay et al (1974) have reported the association of severe inguinal lymphadenitis with a granulomatous nodule in one foot of a Brazilian boy, in whom *M. fortuitum* was isolated from both the lesions and the waterpool where the boy had played. The infected lesion required adequate surgical drainage and regular dressings to heal.

REFERENCES

Azulay R D, Neves R G, Estralia R R, Aroradel, Thomas E M 1974 Primary cutaneous lymph nodes complex caused by *Mycobacterium fortuitum*. Rev Ass Med Brazil 20(5): 177–81

FOLLICULAR LESIONS

Folliculitis of different forms has been noticed on the lower legs and ankle region in Indian and African adult males.

Bokhart's follicular impetigo (*Staph. aureus* infection) though common in the scalp is also seen on the lower legs. Desai et al (1964) have reported profuse eruptions of superficial and deep, persistent, follicular pustules on the lower legs and thigh in Indian adults as 'chronic folliculitis of the legs'. Clarke (1952) has described the similar condition occurring in adults of Lagos in West Africa, by the name of 'pustular dermatitis atrophicans of the legs'.

Hitch et al (1968) and Thew et al (1969) have reported recurrent eruptions of follicular, oedematous papules on the legs and trunk in negroes. The lesions are resistant and persist for prolonged periods.

Usually the minor follicular eruptions require no specific treatment. Regular hygienic care of the skin, even by soap and water cleansing, helps in many cases. However the infective eruptions may require specific antibiotic, usually as a topical application.

REFERENCES

Desai S C et al 1964 Indian J Der Vener 30: 89. In: Rook A, Wilkinson D S, Ebling F J G (eds) 1979 Textbook of Dermatology. 3rd edn. Blackwell Scientific Publications, Oxford. pp 556–557

Clarke G H V 1952 A note on dermatitis cruris pustulosa et atrophicans. Trans R Soc Trop Med Hyg 46: 558. In: Rook A, Wilkinson D S, Ebling F J G (eds) 1979 Textbook of Dermatology. 3rd edn. Blackwell Scientific Publications, Oxford. pp 556–557

Hitch J M, Lund H Z 1968 Disseminate and recurrent infundibulo folliculitis. Arch Dermatol 97: 432–435

Thew M A, Wood M G 1969 Disseminate and recurrent infundibulo folliculitis. Arch Dermatol 100: 728. In: Rook A, Wilkinson D S, Ebling F J G (eds) 1979 Textbook of Dermatology. 3rd edn. Blackwell Scientific Publications, Oxford. pp 556–557

CRAB BITE

In the rural tropics, villagers often bathe in ponds and rivers. Sometimes they present with crab bites, usually round the heel. When the pincers pierce the back of the heel, the sudden attempt to withdraw the foot has caused rupture of the Achilles tendon (Fig. 32.60).

Management centres round cleaning and dressing the puncture wounds. Ruptured tendons need repair in early cases and reconstruction if seen late.

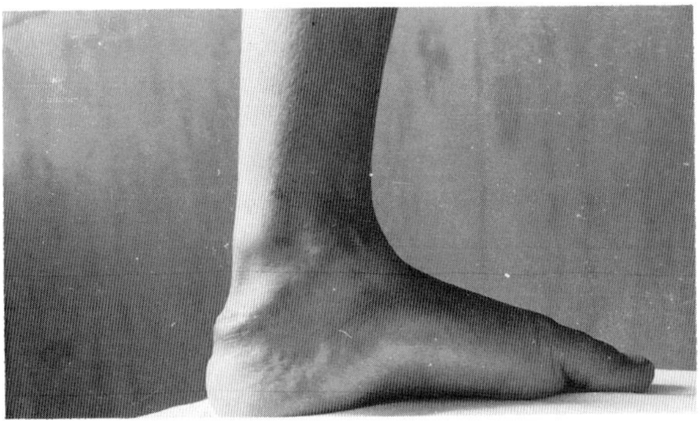

Fig. 32.60 Tendo achillis tear due to crab bite. Healed piercing marks by the prongs visible above and below the site of rupture

RAT BITE

Rodent bite of the foot is often seen in villagers who sleep on the ground in thatched houses or in the fields. However this problem is often encountered in hospital wards, especially in patients with paralysed limbs. The wounds inflicted are usually superficial and heal up with local dressings.

SNAKE BITE

Snake bite is common in the rural tropics, and most of the snake bite deaths occur in tropical Africa and Asia, where venomous snakes are numerous and victims do not avail themselves of whatever inadequate medical care is available. In the tropics most of the bites are on the heel, toes or other parts of the foot and lower leg, as the barefoot victims tread on the snake. There are numerous varieties of poisonous and nonpoisonous snakes, but three families of venomous snakes are usually identified: Elapidae, Hydrophiodae and Viperidae.

The clinical features are a mix of general manifestations (neurotoxic, haematotoxic, nephrotoxic, with fright and emotional reactions) and local lesions (cytotoxic, swelling, ecchymosis pain, necrosis and even gangrene (Fig. 32.61). Proper identification of the type of snake is essential.

Management

General

Rest, reassurance, calming the patient and the management of shock and other vital complications according to the systems involved are the important aspects of general treatment. Polyvalent or specific antivenom and steroids should be given as early as possible.

Local

To delay the absorption of venom, immobilization (preferably in an inflatable splint), rather than the application of a tourniquet, is helpful. Necrotic ulcers need treating on their merits.

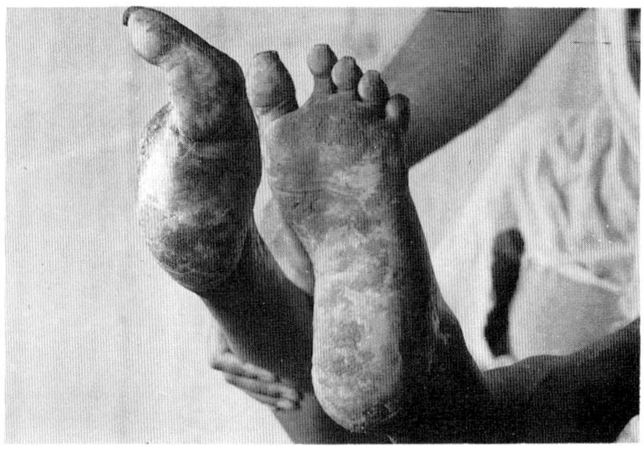

Fig. 32.61 Outer two-thirds of distal foot turned gangrenous and fell off

FURTHER READING

Garfin S R, Mubarak S J, Davidson T M 1979 Rattle snake bites. Curr Concepts Clin Orthop 140: 50
Glass T G Jr 1976 Early debridement in pit viper bites. JAMA 235: 2513
Grace T G, Omer G E 1980 The management of upper extremity pit viper wounds. J Hand Surg 5: 168
Reid H A 1978 Snake bite. In: Scott R B (ed) Price's Textbook of the Practice of Medicine. 12th edn. Oxford University Press. pp 242–244
Strover A E 1964 Some principles of the clinical recognition, assessment and treatment of snake bites. Central Afr J Med 10: 283–288
Swroop S, Grab B 1954 Snake bite mortality in the world. WHO Bulletin 10: 35

SCORPION STING

These arthropods are Arachnids of the Scorpionodae order and are common in the tropics. Their sting produces minor local symptoms and occasionally death. Children and adults with specific sensitivity are the most vulnerable. Dangerous species are *Centruroides* (Mexico and Southern USA), *Androctonus* (Africa), *Buthus* (Asia and Middle East), *Leiurus* (Middle East and Africa) and *Tityus* (South America).

The foot is the most common site affected by the curved sting containing the venom which is located in the tip of the scorpion's tail. Symptoms are local (severe burning pain, swelling, erythema, necrosis, chronic ulcer (Fig. 32.62) and even gangrene) and general, due to neurotoxins which may lead to respiratory failure.

Management

The limb should be immobilized in an inflatable splint. The immediate application of local icepacks gives pain relief. Local infiltration of lignocaine hydrochloride or systemic pethedine may be required. Neurogenic shock and respiratory failure need emergency care. If available, specific scorpion antivenom should be given.

Completely closed shoes afford protection, and houses can be made scorpion-proof.

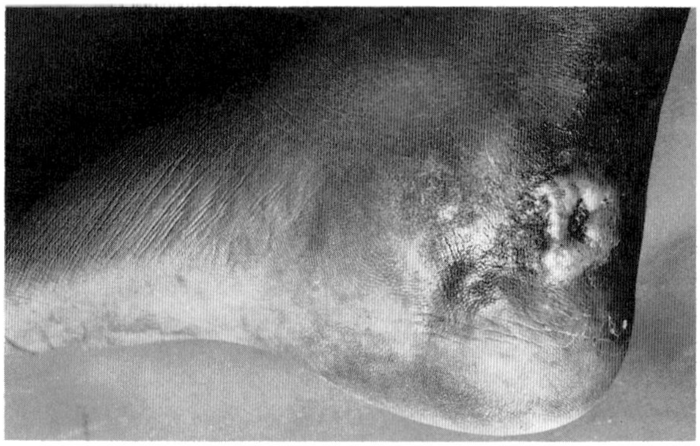

Fig. 32.62 Scorpion sting. The sting became infected resulting in chronic persistent ulcer

FURTHER READING

Chadha J S, Levian A 1979 Honolysis, renal failure and local necrosis following scorpion sting. JAMA 241: 1038
Duggan A 1963 Br Med J II: 181. In: Manson-Bahr P E C, Apted F I C (eds). Mansons Tropical Diseases, 18th edn. Baillière Tindall, London. p 564
Reid H A 1978 Scorpion stings. In: Scott R B (ed) Prices Textbook of the Practice of Medicine. 12th edn. Oxford University Press. p 241
Rimoza M E, Zimmerman D R, Bergeson P S 1980 Scorpion envenomation. Paediatrics 66: 298
Sita Devi P et al 1970 Defibrination syndrome due to scorpion venom poisoning Br Med J 1: 345

MISCELLANEOUS CONDITIONS

Muslim's callus

The Muslim population is large in tropical areas. Their prayer position is typical (Fig. 32.63). On the upper and outer aspect of the left foot, two rounded callosities can always be seen in religious Muslims (Fig. 32.64). These occasionally become infected.

Postural hallux varus

This is occasionally seen in barefoot people (Fig. 32.65).

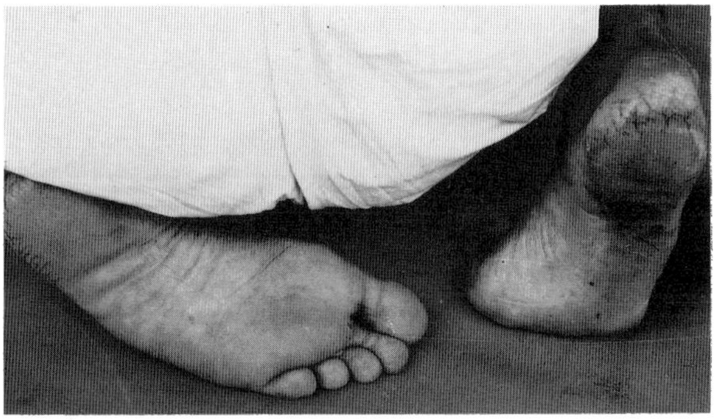

Fig. 32.63 Muslim worship position

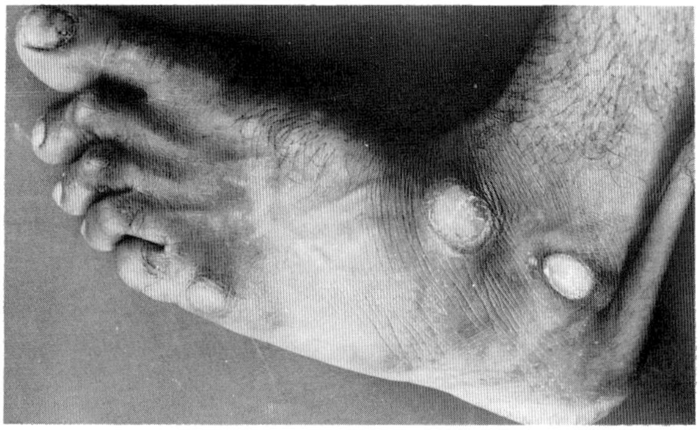

Fig. 32.64 The consequent callosities

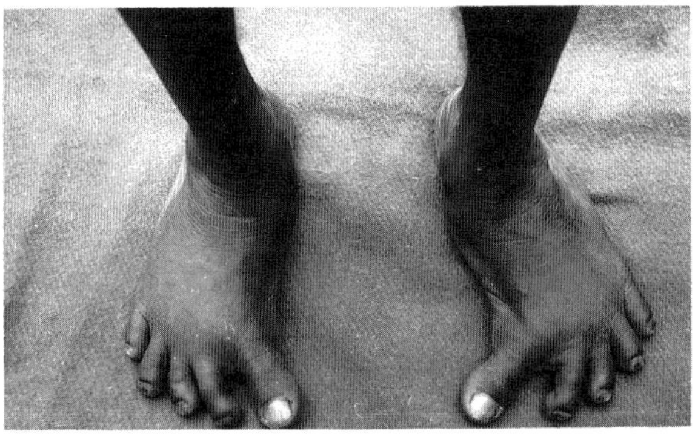

Fig. 32.65 Postural hallux varus in barefoot rural labourers working in hilly and uneven fields

COLD-FIRED FEET

The labourers, farm and field workers, working barefooted develop thick soles and often have an increased threshold for pain. In winter they usually warm their feet over a fire or charcoal burning in earthenware. It is not unusual to see a burn ulcer on the heels on such persons, which may even penetrate to the underlying bone (Fig. 32.66).

Initially they are treated by dressings, avoidance of pressure and suitable antibiotics. In severe cases, surgical excision of the ulcer with infected bone may be required.

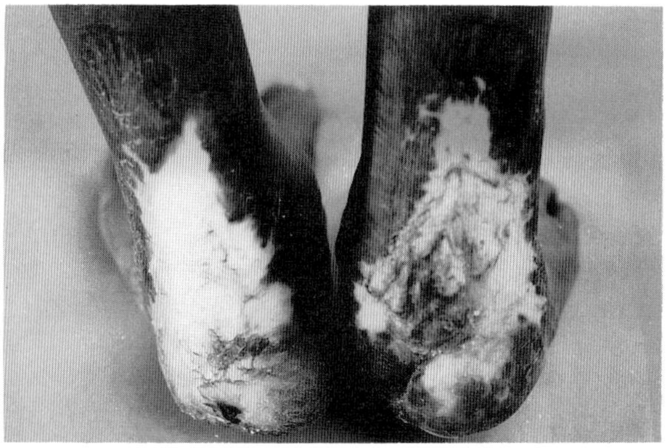

Fig. 32.66 Typical burn on the back of the heel from a rural area where people warm their feet over a fire in winter

XANTHOMATOSIS

This disorder, characterized by the aggregation of xanthoma cells in the skin and internal organs, is often associated with abnormal serum lipids.

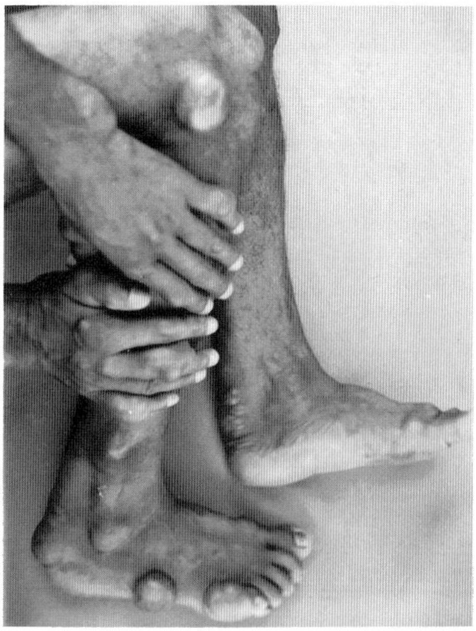

Fig. 32.67 Xanthomatosis in a man aged 43 years

It may be a primary metabolic defect or secondary to hepatic, renal, pancreatic or thyroid disorders or to diabetes with hypercholesterolaemia. Xanthoma tuberosum may affect the feet, which remain asymptomatic except for the cosmetic aspect (Fig. 32.67). The heart, liver and vascular system may be affected with serious complications.

Treatment

General management consists of a low calorie, low cholesterol, low fat diet, care of possible primary causes (e.g. diabetes) and the administration of essential aminoacids. Smaller lesions should be cauterized and bigger ones excised.

SMALL POX

Small pox (variola) has been claimed to be eradicated from the world, but its lesions will continue to be seen for two to three decades. Unlike other parts, the foot is less affected, except for infected pustules which used to be seen on the dorsum and sole. Postvariolar arthritis affecting the ankles may leave its legacies of distorted, ankylosed and painful joints. Management of such joints should be mainly on symptomatic lines and as for any degenerative arthrosis.

ACKNOWLEDGEMENTS

I should like to acknowledge the help of Professor B. N. Prasad (for dermatological diseases), Dr. Pandit (for the diagrams), Dr. S. P. Dubuked, Dr. T. S. Shamshi and Dr. A. K. Pandey (for arranging the text) and Mr. S. C. Agrawal (for the typing). For cutaneous conditions of the foot in the tropics, use has been made of Rook et al 1979 Text Book of Dermatology (Blackwell Scientific Publications, Oxford).

C. G. Iwegbu

Ainhum in Africa

INTRODUCTION

Ainhum is an acquired and progressive constrictive disease affecting mainly the little toe, characterized by a circumferentially spreading and deepening fissure or groove in the plantodigital fold of the toe, which eventually undergoes autoamputation. It is essentially a disease of dark-skinned people. The first description of the disease in the medical literature is credited to Clarke who called it 'dry gangrene of the little toe', (Clarke 1863). Verneuil reported cases of the disease to the Surgical Society of Paris in the same year. Ainhum has since received the attention of many other authors. Isolated case reports have been punctuated by more substantial reports and reviews, including those of da Silva Lima (1867), Weinstein (1912), Spinzig (1939), Browne (1961) and Cole (1965).

Da Silva Lima (1867) was the first to use the word 'ainhum' in the literature and is still being credited with one of the best descriptions of the disease to date. 'Ainhum' is widely believed to have been derived from 'ayun', the Yoruba word for the disease. The condition is particularly common in the Yoruba area of Nigeria. Brazilians of Yoruba origin still live in Brazil today and might have formed the majority of da Silva Lima's patients in 1867.

The terms 'atypical ainhum' and 'pseudo-ainhum' have been freely used in the literature to describe various constrictive diseases, most of which are congenital or of known aetiology. The use of the word 'ainhum' in these conditions should be avoided because the true ainhum is aetiologically and pathogenetically different from them (Browne 1965, Cole 1965).

AETIOLOGY

The aetiology of the disease ainhum (dactylolysis spontanea) has been the subject of much speculation. There were enough hypotheses by the end of the nineteenth century to warrant Wellman's critical analysis of the subject in 1906. The aetiological factors so far incriminated include:

1. Race: Because it is predominantly a disease of Blacks, the increased 'fibrogenetic tendency' of their skin has been incriminated (Browne 1965) but the true condition has been described in a Zulu albino (Follogly 1977) and similar acquired grooves and fissures have been described in the digits of Indians (Aggarwal & Singh 1963), Polynesians (Browne 1961) and white Americans (Shaffer 1947).

2. Age: Most of the patients are aged 30 years or above. Younger patients presenting with the disease should be examined to exclude a predisposing disease, especially chronic tertiary yaws.

3. Sex: The initial claims that males are more frequently affected than women has been disproved. There is no clear sex predilection.

4. Trauma: The observation that the vast majority of the patients walked barefooted most of their lives led to the hypothesis that repeated trauma from stones and other hard objects could be a causative factor. The importance of this factor is however reduced by the fact that the condition also occurs in habitual shoe-wearers (Kean et al 1946). In any case, why should the little toe be selectively involved when all the toes are subjected to the trauma of barefoot walking? Trauma may be important in the facilitation of infection of a previously existing groove.

5. Infection: Various infective organisms have been isolated from ainhum lesions — the chigger,

Sarcopsylla penetrans (Wellman 1908), and *Trichosporon cutaneum* (Kamalam & Thambiah 1981). Pyogenic organisms have also been incriminated (Horwitz 1887). However, the fact remains that no infective agent is found in the overwhelming majority of cases and so, the above organisms are unlikely to be the initiators of the constricting band.

6. Diet: Daynes (1973) suggested that ingestion of plants may account for phocomelia and ainhum, both of which are not uncommon in the Tsolo district of South Africa but his study cannot be considered conclusive.

7. Manifestation of a generalized disease? True ainhum occurs as a distinct and isolated disease. This has been referred to as primary or idiopathic ainhum. However, it appears that the plantar hyperkeratosis of tertiary yaws is a predisposing factor (Browne 1961). Links with syphilis, leprosy, scleroderma and hypothyroidism have been suggested but these remain unconvincing in the case of true ainhum.

PATHOLOGY AND PATHOGENESIS

The little toe is the usual site of the disease. The fourth toe is occasionally affected, but only in association with affection of the little toe (Browne 1965). Affection of the other toes is extremely rare. Bilateral disease is seen in about two-thirds to three-quarters of cases. Characteristically, the lesions are at widely different stages of development (Fig. 33.1). The unaffected toe in unilateral cases commonly

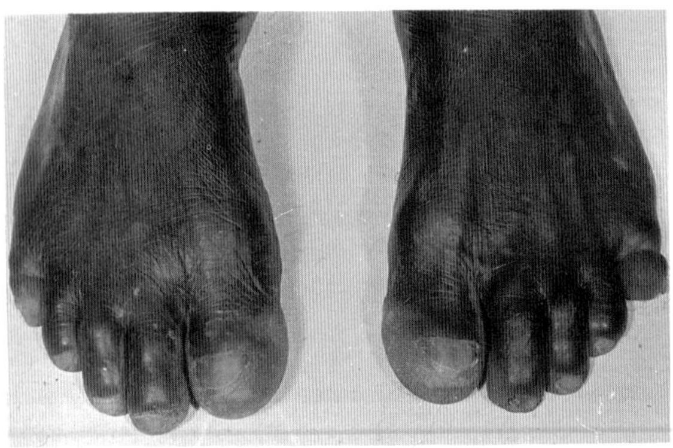

Fig. 33.1 Bilateral ainhum in a 55-year-old man. The lesion is at Stage III on the left and Stage II on the right

becomes affected later. The first evidence of the disease is the appearance of a fissure or groove on the medial aspect of the base of the toe, usually in the plantodigital fold. Sometimes the groove appears distal to the fold (Cole 1965). The fissure spreads circumferentially but fastest in the dorsal direction.

It invariably becomes infected on and off with resulting scarring and accentuation of the constrictive effect. As it deepens, subcutaneous structures such as blood vessels, nerves and tendons become compressed, resulting in the formation of the classical 'bulb' (the oedematous terminal portion of the toe), progressive absorption of the distal part of the proximal phalanx and eventual auto-amputation of the toe at the level of the fissure. The process described can take as long as 20 years to reach completion but the average time in most patients is about 5–10 years. The disease process has been clinically staged as follows (Browne 1961):

Stage I: A sulcus is present at the plantodigital fold

Stage II: The sulcus extends round the base of the toe

Stage III: Complete encirclement of the toe

Stage IV: Autoamputation of the toe.

The essential histological features of the constricting fissure have been described by several authors (Davies & Hewer 1941, Bergner & Winfield 1960, Cole 1965). In the early lesion, the main abnormality is gross thickening of the stratum corneum, with classification of the ducts and of the sweat glands. The dermis is normal. The stratum germinativum is also normal but has thickened papillae and contains no melanin pigment. More advanced lesions show chronic inflammatory reaction with normal vessels and nerves.

The proximal phanlanx around the fissure shows chronic periostitis and a decrease in width due to progressive aseptic bone resorption. The blood vessels remain patent even after the fracture of the phalanx at the level of the fissure (Fig. 33.2). This means that autoamputation of the toe is due to lack of bony support rather than lack of blood supply.

DIAGNOSIS

The disease is easily diagnosed on the basis of the symptoms and physical findings. The most constant

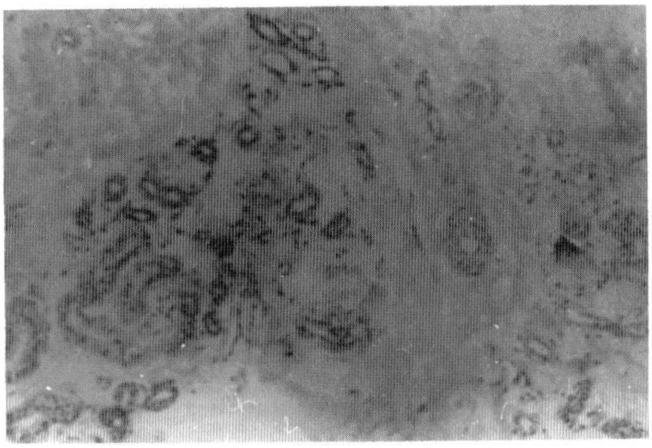

Fig. 33.2 A histological section at the level of the fissure. The blood vessels remain patent even after fracture at the level of the fissure

presenting symptom is pain in the fifth toe which is often associated with ulceration and infection of the fissure. An uninfected fissure rarely causes pain. The intensity of the pain varies from slight in early cases to moderate and severe in the more advanced lesions. It is most severe if the proximal phalanx has fractured ('dangling toe'). Sometimes itching is a major symptom. Oedema of the bulb and sometimes of the dorsum of the foot may be present.

On examination the patient is usually an otherwise healthy rural adult male in the middle age bracket. He walks with a limp. The often mentioned external rotation deformity of the affected toe is not a constant feature as the unaffected toe is usually equally externally rotated.

The size of the fissure depends on the stage of the disease. The classical bulb (Fig. 33.3) is present in the advanced cases. The toe is tender to palpation, especially if the fissure is ulcerated and infected. The toe and the dorsum of the foot may be oedematous in severe cases. Where fracture has occurred, the toe dangles on a narrow cord of tissues ('dangling toe') and is particularly tender to palpation. The anterior and posterior tibial pulses and sensation are usually normal. In unilateral cases, the other fifth toe should always be examined. It is often found to have an early fissure on the medial aspect (see Fig. 33.1).

Predisposing or associated generalized disease

Depending on the environment and other presenting symptoms, evidence for tertiary yaws, syphilis, leprosy, scleroderma or hypothyroidism should be sought, especially in children and young adults.

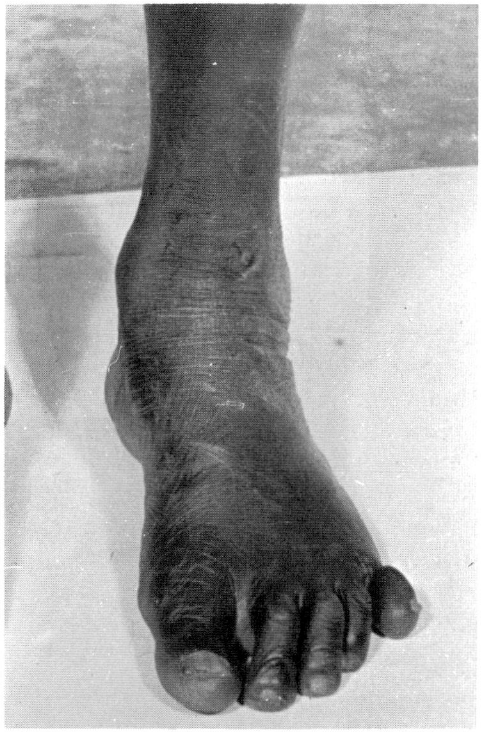

Fig. 33.3 Classical bulb of advanced ainhum

Radiological findings

There is a progressive aseptic absorption of the proximal phalanx, proximal and distalward from the level of the fissure (Fig. 33.4). The absorption, which usually starts from the medial aspect where the fissure is most active, eventually reduces the affected part of the phalanx to a thin bar of cancellous bone which fractures with minimal trauma. After autoamputation, a stump of the proximal phalanx remains (Fig. 33.4) and does not undergo further absorption.

MANAGEMENT

Rational management must be based on what is known of the pathogenesis of the disease. The most important single feature of the disease is the fissure which is produced by a progressively constrictive

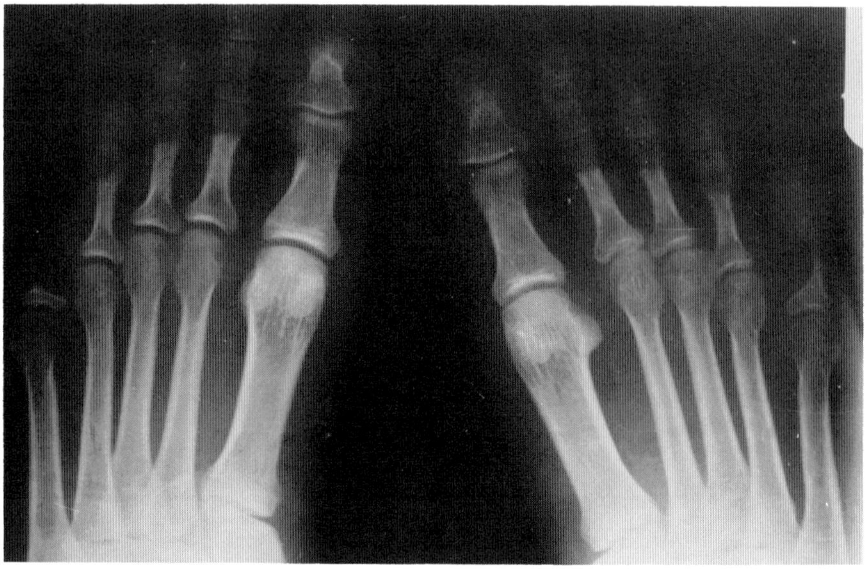

Fig. 33.4 Radiograph of bilateral ainhum. Most of the phalanges of the right fifth toe have undergone resorption. The stump of the proximal phalanx of the left fifth toe after autoamputation is seen

fibrous band. Fissure tear and infection are important but secondary features and bony involvement is a late development. Accordingly, the affected toe can, at least theoretically, be conserved if the fissure is excised in time. Unfortunately, most of the patients present late.

Initial management

The usual presenting symptom is pain, with or without an itch, which almost always results from a tear of the fissure coupled with its infection by pyogenic or fungal organisms. Initial management is therefore directed at the elimination of infection if present by cleaning with a bland antiseptic solution, daily dressing on out-patient basis and systemic broad-spectrum antibiotic. When itching is present, it is usually due to an associated athlete's foot and an antifungal cream usually effects cure.

Definitive treatment

After the infection has been controlled and the fissure tear has healed, the management decision that has to be made is whether to conserve the toe or to amputate it. In general, amputation is the treatment of choice if the fissure has encircled most of the toe, by which time absorption of the distal portion of the proximal phalanx is also advanced (stage III disease). Conservation of the toe may be successful in stages I or II disease.

METHODS OF CONSERVATION OF THE TOE

Nonoperative method

Treatment with drugs

Local injection of steroids into the fibrous band has been reported to give relief from pain, reduce the associated induration and decrease the length of the fissure (Rossiter & Anderson 1976). These authors gave monthly injections of 5 to 7.5 mg of triamcinolone acetonide over a period of 10 months. Long-term results of treatment by this method are not available but it appears that the success claimed is of a temporary nature. Local application of dequalinium chloride has also been reported to be helpful in arresting the constrictive process (Kamalam & Thambiah 1981).

Operative methods

Conservative operative methods that have been used include lumbar sympathectomy (McKnight 1940), longitudinal multiple incisions of the fissure (Cecil & Loebb 1959) and fissure excision followed by Z-plasty (Brown 1959, Allyn & Leider 1963, Kamalan & Thambiah 1981). Lumbar sympathectomy was performed because of the mistaken linkage of ainhum with peripheral vascular disease. Multiple incisions of the fissure did not yield good results.

Fissure excision followed by Z-plasty

This is a rational procedure which removes the fissure, thereby stopping further progression of the constriction and restores an acceptable shape to the toe. It is suitable for the stage I or II disease. The line of the excised fissure serves as the base line from where multiple Z-incisions are made and flaps raised on both sides, rotated accordingly and sewn up in the Z-fashion. The cosmetic result is good (Fig. 33.5).

Amputation of the toe

The natural history of the disease is that the fissure progressively strangulates the toe until auto-amputation occurs. Amputation is therefore a logical method of definitive treatment. Disarticulation at the metatarsophalangeal joint is preferred to amputation at the level of the fissure or just distal to the metatarsophalangeal joint because it does away with the stump of the proximal phalanx which remains after autoamputation and which has been associated with a tendency to injury afterwards, and also because it provides enough soft-tissue flaps for adequate stump closure. Another method of amputation consists of tying off the toe at the level of the fissure.

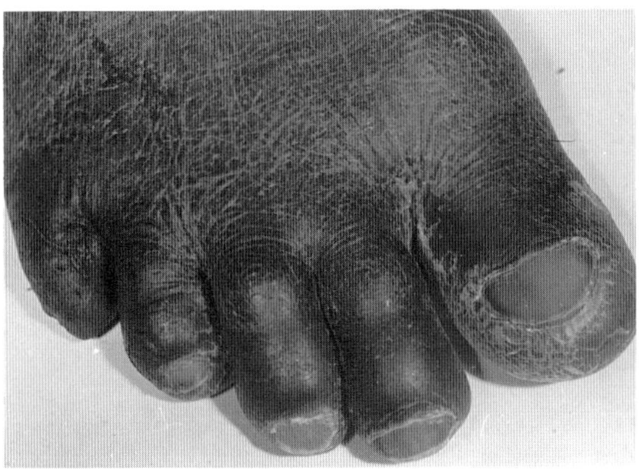

Fig. 33.5 The cosmetic result of Z-plasty is good. This is the same left fifth toe as in Fig. 33.1

Method of disarticulation at the metatarsophalangeal joint

The patient lies supine. The operation is usually performed under local infiltrative anaesthesia using 0.5 or 1% lignocaine without adrenaline but general anaesthesia can also be used with the advantage that a tourniquet can then be applied. The fourth toe is held away from the affected fifth toe which is steadied.

Incision. A transverse incision is made on the dorsum of the toe, at the level of the base of the 4th web space, stretching from the midlateral point laterally to the web space medially. From each end a vertical incision, 2 cm long, is made proximally so that a dorsal and a plantar flap are formed.

Deep dissection. The dorsal flap made up of skin and subcutaneous fat is mobilized to its proximal base. The proximal phalanx is then traced to the metatarsophalangeal joint and mobilized from the metatarsophalangeal distally by cutting the joint capsule and attached tendons. Its mobilization is stopped just distal to the fissure line. The plantar flap is cut transversely at the level of the fissure. Haemostasis is secured throughout the dissection. Any digital nerves seen are cut cleanly across with a sharp knife.

Closure. The flaps are trimmed as necessary before the longer plantar flap is turned over and stitched to the dorsal — dorsally, laterally and medially.

Method of 'tying off' the toe

This is an out-patient procedure used after the proximal phalanx has fractured at the level of the fissure and a 'dangling toe' has resulted. No anaesthesia is used. The toe is cleaned up and a silk tie is applied at the level of the fissure. The toe is then dressed up and the patient instructed to come back to the next weekly clinic. The toe usually drops off within one week. Daily dressing is then applied until healing of the resulting wound is complete.

AINHUM IN ZARIA

Even though the incidence is much higher in humid southern Nigeria where it is often associated with the itchy epidermophytosis, the disease is not uncommon in northern Nigeria. Available records showed that 44 patients were seen with the condition at the Ahmadu Bello University Teaching Hospital, Zaria in the period 1973 to 1984. It is believed that the actual number is greater than this. The notes were complete in only 20 of the 44 patients. Of the 20, 10 were females and 10 were males. Only 2 patients, both females aged 5 and 8 respectively, were below the age of 10. There was bilateral affection in 7 patients so that there were 27 affected toes altogether, all being the fifth toe. Most of the patients presented in stage III or IV and required preliminary treatment of fissure tear and infection before definitive treatment could be given. Amputation was virtually the only procedure used (95%), but the level at which it was carried out was not always clear from the notes.

Because of shortage of beds, most of the patients were operated upon as day cases. Postoperative infection was therefore common in spite of routinely prescribed prophylactic antibiotics. Those hospitalized after operation had a shorter period of morbidity. Some of the patients excluded from the above analysis underwent the procedure of tying off of the toe. It is interesting that they appeared not to have problems with the stump. The treatment of ainhum was carried out mainly by trainee Surgeons.

SUMMARY

Ainhum is an acquired idiopathic progressive constrictive disease chiefly of the fifth toe, characterized by the presence of a fissure or groove. It is therefore to be distinguished from congenital constriction band conditions such as Streeter's syndrome (Streeter 1930, Pillay & Hesketh 1965) and acquired constrictive conditions of known aetiology. The terms 'pseudo-ainhum' and 'atypical ainhum' are best avoided. It is not clear why the fifth toe is selectively affected and or why infection is at the level of the proximal phalanx. A strong genetic link is suggested by prevalence in non-Caucasians and by the presence of a familial history in many of the patients.

It appears that the constrictive process per se is painless and that pain, the usual presenting symptom, arises from tear and infection of the fissure. The histology shows that the blood vessels traversing the fissure to the distal portion of the toe remain patent even after fracture of the proximal phalanx. This shows that autoamputation eventually occurs from lack of bony support rather than from lack of blood supply.

Infection of the torn fissure must be controlled before definitive treatment is embarked upon. The definitive treatment recommended is fissure excision with Z-plasty for stage I or II disease and disarticulation at the metatarsophalangeal joint for the stage III or IV disease. To shorten the period of morbidity, patients should be admitted at least postoperatively for elevation of the legs and for controlled use of prophylactic antibiotics.

ACKNOWLEDGEMENTS

I wish to thank all my Consultant Colleagues in the Department of Surgery for allowing me to study their patients, Mrs Paula Wahlstrom and Mrs Lucy Kangave for their secretarial help and Mrs Peace Uchegbulam for typing the script.

REFERENCES

Aggarwal N D, Singh H 1963 Ainhum: Report of an atypical case. J Bone Jt Surg 45B(2): 376–378

Allyn B, Leider M 1963 Dactylolysis Spontanea (ainhum). Report of a case treated by the surgical procedure known as Z-plasty. JAMA 184 (8): 655–657

Bergner L H, Winfield J M 1960 Ainhum (Dactylolysis Spontanea). Review of the literature and report of a case. Am J Surg 100: 481–485

Brown E C 1959 Bilateral ainhum treated by multiple Z-plasties. Plast Reconstr Surg 23: 550

Browne S G 1961 Ainhum: a clinical and aetiological study of 83 cases. Ann Trop Med Parasitol 55: 314–320

Browne S G 1965 True ainhum: its distinctive and differentiating features in a clinical study based on 100 patients. J Bone Joint Surg 47B: 52–55

Cecil R L, Loebb R F (eds) 1959 A textbook of medicine. 10th edn. W B Saunders Company, Philadelphia. p 424
Clarke 1863 Remarks on topography and diseases of the Gold Coast, West Coast of Africa. Tr Epidemiol Soc Lond 1: 76–105
Cole G J 1965 Ainhum: An account of fifty-four patients with special reference to etiology and treatment. J Bone Jt Surg 47B(1): 43–51
da Silva Lima J F 1867 Estudo Sobre o "Ainhum". Gaz Med Bahia 1: 146
Davies J N P, Hewer T F 1941 Ainhum: Report of a case in England with histological study. Trans Roy Soc Trop Med Hyg XXXV(2): 125–128
Daynes W G 1973 Ainhum: Its possible causation by ingestion of plants. S Afr Med J 47: 320–321
Follogly J G 1977 Classical ainhum in a Zulu albino. Cent Afr J Med 23(11): 253–254
Horwitz O 1887 Case of ainhum occurring in the outdoor surgical department of Jefferson Medical College Hospital. M & S Reporter 56: 649
Kamalam A, Thambiah A S 1981 Ainhum, trichosporosis and Z-plasty. Dermatologica 162: 372–377
Kean B H, Tucker A A, Miller W C 1946 Ainhum: A clinical summary of forty-five cases on the isthmus of Panama. Trans Roy Soc Trop Med Hyg XXXIX(4): 331–334
McKnight R B 1940 A case of ainhum treated by lumbar sympathetic ganglionectomy. NC Med J 1: 76
Pillay V K, Hesketh K T 1965 Intra-uterine amputations and annular limb defects in Singapore. J Bone Jt Surg 47B: 514–519
Rossiter J W, Anderson P C 1976 Ainhum: Treatment with intra-Pesional steroids. Int J Dermat 15: 379–382
Shaffer L J O 1947 Ainhum Report of a case in which the patient was a white woman with diabetes mellitus. Arch Path 43: 170
Spinzig E W 1939 Ainhum Its occurrence in the United States with report of three cases. Am J Roentgenol 42: 246
Streeter G L 1930 Focal deficiencies in foetal tissues and their relation to intra-uterine amputation. Contrib Embryol 22: 1
Verneuil 1863 Affection singulière et non décrite encore des doigts et des mains, par M. le docteur Mirault. Commentaires et discussion pour prouver que cette affection se rattache au rhumatisme, par M. le docteur Verneuil. Gazette Hebdomadaire de Médecine et de Chirurgie 10: 113
Weinstein H 1912 A description of ainhum with report of interesting cases occurring in one family. Proc Canal Zone Med Assoc 4: 110
Wellman F C 1906 Criticism of some theories regarding the etiology of ainhum. JAMA 46: 636–638
Wellman F C 1908 Advanced case of ainhum with some remarks on Sarcopsylla penetrans as the cause of the disease. J Trop Med Hyg 11: 117

Diabetes

INTRODUCTION

Recent advances in the medical treatment of diabetes mellitus have resulted in a dramatic decrease in the life-threatening metabolic disorders. This has not been paralleled by a reduction in the main diabetic complications of retinopathy, nephropathy, vasculopathy and foot disease which are presenting with increasing frequency. This is particularly seen in the lower limb, where the group of symptoms and signs involving neuropathies, angiopathies and infective lesions constitute the 'Diabetic Foot Syndrome'.

The resulting breakdowns with deformity, ulceration, infection and gangrene have become major medical problems today. Reports of a 12% increase in 12 years of hospital admissions for diabetic foot lesions (Kozak & Rowbotham 1984) and a 10% increase in diabetic lower limb amputations (DHSS Amputation Statistics 1974–83) accounting for 21% of all amputations in 1983, confirm this. The increase in diabetic complications is likely to continue, unless a treatable cause is found, for three reasons:

1. Diabetes onset is age related and increases with the general population improved life expectancy. The prevalence of diabetes is approximately 1.5% with 80% presenting over the age of 40.

2. Duration of diabetes is associated with onset of complications, and after 10 years most diabetic feet show some changes of neuropathy or angiopathy.

3. Diabetic complications are progressive with increasing and recurrent susceptibility to foot breakdown.

The cause of diabetes remains unknown, but the previous concept that it was due to a degeneration of the pancreatic beta cells supported by hereditary influences, is no longer acceptable. Opinion suggests that diabetes mellitus can be produced by nearly all the commonly recognized pathological processes such as infections, toxins, immune reactions, inflammatory pancreatitis, specific genetic-protein defects and rarely neoplasia.

PATHOLOGY IN DIABETIC FOOT TISSUES

The classical triopathy of the diabetic foot syndrome is angiopathy, neuropathy and infection with presentation alone or in combination. Neuropathy and infection underlie many diabetic foot problems, but it is the vascular tissue disease which produces the most destructive lesions.

Blood vessels

The increased incidence and severity of complications attributable to macrovascular arteriosclerotic disease such as myocardial infarction and gangrene, especially in the maturity onset diabetic, have been long known. Somewhat later, arteriolar disease was appreciated and, more recently, a microangiopathy involving the capillaries has been recognized. None of the vascular pathologies seen in diabetics is specifically unique to diabetes mellitus; they are qualitatively similar to those occurring in non-diabetics.

Macroangiopathy

Macrovascular disease in the diabetic consists of arteriosclerosis which describes a group of lesions as marked thickening and elasticity loss of the arterial wall. Histopathologically three types are seen involving atherosclerosis, medial calcific sclerosis and diffuse intimal fibrosis.

Atherosclerosis. This may occur in single, multiple or diffuse patterns in any of the lower limb muscular arteries. Development occurs from fatty streaks in the intima progressing to fibrolipid atheromatous plaques which extend into the media causing destruction of the elastic fibres with collagen replacement. Large quantities of extracellular lipid and cholesterol are formed and the plaques may calcify. Segmental stenosis, surface thrombus and plaque emboli or arterial thrombosis progress to produce ischaemia, infarction and gangrene distally. Qualitatively this atherosclerosis is similar in diabetics and nondiabetics, but in the diabetic group, the lesions occur more frequently (Strandness et al 1964) and appear to progress more rapidly (Warren et al 1966). More diffuse involvement of the medium and small arteries in the lower leg and foot occur in diabetics (Haimovici et al 1960, Ferrier 1965, Warren et al 1966). This produces the 'end artery state' of the foot tissues with a limited number of patent supply vessels, loss of collateral circulation and a decreased vascular reserve. Further obstruction or sudden vascular demand can result in ischaemia and gangrene.

Medial calcific sclerosis (Mönckeberg's sclerosis). This involves a progressive calcification of the media of muscular arteries, but, unlike atherosclerosis, does not develop in the large elastic vessels. Calcification occurs around the smooth muscle cells forming plates, rings and finally pipe stems, but the intima is not involved and the lumen not compromised. Medial calcific sclerosis also involves diabetics more severely, at an earlier age and often in association with atherosclerosis, than in the nondiabetic.

Diffuse intimal fibrosis. This affects the larger arteries and as it occurs throughout life, is considered to be an ageing process (Wilens 1951). Normal mechanical haemodynamic forces appear to stimulate fibromuscular proliferation producing the intimal thickening. It is not associated with any specific cell wall damage or lumenal obstruction.

Microangiopathy

Small vessel disease involves the small arteries, arterioles and capillaries presenting as a generalized hyalinization of the wall with intimal proliferation, hypertrophy and fibrosis. The capillary pathology of basement membrane thickening is seen throughout diabetic tissues, but is not pathognomonic as such thickening occurs as an ageing process in nondiabetics. The rate and quantity of this thickening, however, is much greater in diabetic skin and muscle tissues (Kilo et al 1972, Siperstein et al 1968). This thickening has been shown to cause increased permeability in skeletal muscles in diabetics by isotope clearance studies (Trap-Jensen 1971), and may also affect the normal inflammatory response with interference in healing and infections, but this has not been proven.

Pathogenesis of diabetic vascular disease

The concept that the pathogenesis of vascular disease is comparable in the nondiabetic patient but accelerated in the diabetic, is currently accepted. The original 'Response to Injury Hypothesis' has received more recent support suggesting that the primary mechanism is damage and disruption of the arterial endothelium by mechanical, chemical or immune reaction (Ross 1981).

More recent significant research has shown abnormalities in platelet reactions (Cowell et al 1981, Ganda 1980), and in the low density lipoproteins (Reckless et al 1978, Goldstein & Brown 1982, Lopes-Vivella et al 1982) in diabetic patients capable of initiating endothelial injuries. The significance of these changes as primary atherogenic agents is not certain, but their presence at a younger age and the acceleration effect on vascular damage would support their association with the more severe progression of atherosclerosis in the diabetic patient.

Nerves

Diabetic neuropathy is a general term representing a group of disorders of the peripheral nervous system, but the aetiology remains uncertain. Two pathological groups have been suggested with a predominantly metabolic-induced neuropathy in one (Asbury et al 1978) and a vascular cause in the other (Raff et al 1968). These form the basis of a currently accepted classification (Sibley 1982):

1. Metabolic neuropathy
   a) Chronic symmetrical distal polyneuropathy with sensory, motor and autonomic involvement
   b) Acute symptomatic distal neuropathy
2. Vascular neuropathy
   Mononeuritis solitary and multiplex
   (i) Large nerve trunks
   (ii) Radioculopathy
   (iii) Cranial neuropathy
3. Nerve compression syndromes

Chronic symmetrical distal polyneuropathy

This is the commonest diabetic neuropathy with the characteristic symmetry of overlapping nerve terminals most distant from the cell body. The correlation with poor hyperglycaemic control suggests a metabolic cause (Gregersen 1967). The neuropathy is not associated with the severity of the diabetes but more with the degree of control. The mechanism of prolonged hyperglycaemic-induced neuropathy is uncertain. Abnormal endoneural capillary leakage, blood-nerve barrier defects, endoneural toxic oedema, perineural cell basement membrane thickening, and, most recently, abnormal sorbitol and fructose accumulation, have all been reported and critically reviewed (Eliasson 1983).

The main pathological change in this type of neuropathy appears as distal axonal degeneration with loss of the myelin sheath and disappearance of many of the axons (Thomas & Lascelles 1966). With the decrease in motor axons, there is a widespread collateral sprouting of the residual intact ones with reinnervation of denervated muscle fibres. This is incomplete leaving a peripheral motor neuropathy with wasting, weakness and contractures of the small muscles of the foot.

Involvement of the distal sensory nerves by these pathological changes produces a symmetrical neuropathy with loss of touch, pain, proprioception and temperature discrimination sensibility. Demyelination of the proprioceptor and mechano-receptor nerves to the joints and bones leads to secondary intrinsic trophic changes of the Charcot type arthropathies and osteopathies. A similar diffuse degeneration occurs in the autonomic nerves producing the interference in sweating and vasomotor function in the feet.

Acute symptomatic distal neuropathy

This is now rare, having been reported in the past during periods of very poor diabetic control with excessive weight loss and following rapid correction of diabetic acidosis with insulin or tolbutamide. The acute presentation and recovery suggested a metabolic neurapraxia type lesion of motor and sensory nerves.

Mononeuritis — solitary and multiplex neuropathies

These are considered the result of vascular changes in the limb nerves with local ischaemic areas and microinfarcts (Raff & Asbury 1970). Almost any nerve or nerve root may be involved, but the most common mononeuropathies involve the femoral, peroneal, oculomotor, abducens, median or ulnar nerves and the lower lumbar nerve roots. In some cases multiple nerve trunks or nerve roots are involved successively producing the mononeuritis multiplex picture. Despite the severe incapacity, the pathological process appears to be reparative, often with good functional recovery.

Nerve compression syndromes

The nerve trunks of diabetic patients are more susceptible to compression and traction trauma from the latent diffuse neuropathy of metabolic, ischaemic or mixed pathologies (Mulder et al 1961). The posterior tibial nerve in the tarsal tunnel and the peroneal nerve at the fibula neck, the ulna at the elbow and median nerve at the wrist, are at high risk of compressive neuropathies in the diabetic patient.

Infection

There is very little epidemiological evidence to support any higher incidence of primary sepsis in the diabetic patient. However, with the greater frequency of breakdown, especially in the foot, secondary infection is much more common than in the nondiabetic (Pratt 1965, Bessman & Wagner 1975). Studies on humoral immunity between diabetes and infections have shown no immunological incompetence in diabetic patients (Lipcomb et al 1959) or in antibody response in experimental diabetic animals (Dolkart et al 1971). However, many changes in cell-mediated immunity have been recorded and recently reviewed (Axtine 1982). Thus impairment of leucocyte migration and mobilization, decreased granulocyte adherence and diminished leucocyte chemotaxis, phagocytosis and bacteriocidal activity have all been implicated. Also, these abnormalities appear worse in the poorly controlled diabetic and in ketoacidotic states with marked improvement on insulin stabilization.

Basic pathology of much of the diabetic foot infection results from ulceration due to local trauma or high pressure in the presence of insensitive deformed feet and often deficient vascularity. The loss of protective sensibility and delayed healing allows repeated trauma with progressive necrosis of the ulcer through the skin to involve the deeper tissues. Secondary bacterial infection may then follow at any stage giving further tissue destruction with cellulitis, oedema, lymphangitis, abscess, septic arthritis and osteomyelitis possible. Increased tissue pressure and septic thrombosis may obliterate the remaining 'end artery vessels' with resulting gangrene. With slower arterial obstruction, a dry atrophic type of gangrene occurs, but with a more acute blockage, oedema and infection follow giving the wet type gangrene. The third less common 'central gangrene' may occur in the diabetic foot with the midplantar space infection producing obliterative septic thrombosis and extensive tissue necrosis. The skin and peripheral tissues may survive.

Osteomyelitis and septic arthritis are serious lesions of the diabetic foot accounting for over a third of a large series of bone infection patients (Waldvogel et al 1970). Most bone and joint infections in diabetic feet develop from chronic perforating ulcers and, less commonly, from direct penetrating wounds to the neuropathic foot. With deep chronic infection, recurrent ulceration or sinus formation persists with the ever present danger of acute infection flares.

The most common infective organisms in diabetic foot sepsis are streptococci, staphylococci, aerobic gram-negative baccili and anaerobic bacteria (Louie et al 1976). Mixed facultative and obligatory anaerobes have been reported to be mainly responsible for the foul-smelling gas forming infections of the diabetic 'fetid foot' (Fierer et al 1979). Gas formation by nonclostridial organisms in soft tissue infection occurs more frequently in the diabetic patient and must be differentiated from true clostridial infections. (see Fig. 34.17A). These nonclostridial gas-forming infections are much commoner, rarely progress rapidly and usually are systemically nontoxic, being amenable often to local treatment (Bessman & Wagner 1975).

CLINICAL PRESENTATION

The diabetic foot syndrome does not present as isolated vascular, neurological and breakdown complications in the diabetic patient. It forms part of a generalized disorder, most often associated with retinopathy, nephropathy and coronary artery disease (Yamagata & Yamauchi 1969). In the absence of the foot changes, the other complications were much less common as shown previously (Fagerberg 1959). Vascular lesions in the lower diabetic limbs were two to three times more frequent with a neuropathy which itself occurred in most patients with diabetes for over ten years. The presentation of an autonomic neuropathy often precedes the somatic type and may be an indicator of those patients at risk from diabetic foot breakdown (Dearfield et al 1980).

The diabetic patient may present with complications in the lower limbs arising from peripheral vascular disease, neuropathy, deformities and infection, often with combinations of these.

Peripheral vascular disease

Atherosclerosis

Major vessel stenosis or obstruction presents with peripheral ischaemia in diabetics, similar to nondiabetic patients. Intermittent claudication occurs in the calves with increasing severity and decreasing walking tolerance. Night pains from nerve ischaemia progress to rest pain anytime and are often relieved by leg dependency increasing tissue perfusion. A severe sensory neuropathy, however, may result in little pain at all with severe ischaemia. With the atherosclerosis, the main pulses at the foot or knee are often absent, associated with dependency rubor and elevation blanching with delayed venous filling time. Ischaemic skin changes present with shiny, cool, atrophic, hairless skin and with thickened slow-growing nails. With more severe chronic ischaemia, the subcutaneous tissues atrophy and the skin appears tight. With critical ischaemia minor trauma leaves ulcers which become infected with insufficient healing potential and patchy or more diffuse gangrene is then presented.

The diabetic and nondiabetic atherosclerotic vascular disease may present with acute arterial obstruction from emboli or thrombosis. The clinical outcome depends upon the collateral circulation and the duration of the avascular episode before relief. Irreversible changes of the most sensitive tissues, the muscles and nerves occur after 4 to 6 hours. Acute arterial obstruction from a large embolus with little collateral circulation produces the acute severe pain and a pale, waxlike extremity. With arterial thrombosis of an atheromatous plaque, a more cyanotic distal limb occurs. In association with the pain, pallor and pulselessness, the arterial occlusion also produces the paraesthesiae from peripheral nerve ischaemia and paralysis from muscle infarction.

Small vessels

The nonatheromatous peripheral small artery disease common in the diabetic foot produces the 'end artery state'. With little collateral circulation, any single artery obstruction will result in avascular tissue distally. Thus small vessel disease may present with insidious gangrene involving skin patches, toe segments, complete toes or the whole forefoot area. With infected ulcers, septic obliterative arteritis or thrombosis produces spreading gangrenous areas.

Distal artery obstruction from penetrating infection in the toes or web spaces presents with progressive cyanosis, with swelling and then gangrene of the toe. Obliteration of the transverse plantar metatarsal arterial arch may produce gangrene of the middle toes or the whole forefoot. The clinical presentation may often appear confused with good pulsatile arterial vessels at the ankle or even in some toes in the presence of gangrenous areas in the foot unless this nonatheromatous peripheral small artery disease is understood.

Neuropathy

Sensory

The sensory neuropathy in the diabetic foot presents symptomatically in two contrasting forms: one with pain and paraesthesiae and the other with numbness giving loss of pain and temperature appreciation. The latter is much the commoner type and some degree of overlap is seen occasionally.

Clinical differentiation from ischaemic pain is made from the quality of the pain and the state of the peripheral circulation. The hyperalgesic neuropathy produces sharp stabbing or shooting pains occurring at any time and often severe at night, appearing as pseudotabetic in nature. The paraesthesiae is variable with tingling or burning and often hyperaesthetic on contact. Radicular pain, from a mononeuropathy, appears to arise from the spinal roots giving low back pain and variable radiation into the leg, and often associated with dermatomal paraesthesiae, muscle weakness and reflex decrease.

The second and main group of diabetic sensory neuropathies present rarely with symptoms directly as there is decreased sensation to pain, temperature, vibration and proprioception. Feelings described as 'heavy legs' and 'walking on cotton wool' are the main common neuropathic complaints. The loss of superficial and deep pain sensibility produces two main clinical pictures. One is with repeated trauma from mechanical, chemical or thermal injury giving ulceration and ensuing infection. The other is of deformities and disorganisation of the foot from Charcot's type osteoarthropathies which may also produce ulceration over high pressure areas.

These characteristic neuropathic ulcers usually occur on the plantar surfaces, often with round punched-out appearances and variably described as malperforans, plantar, trophic, perforating and pressure ulcers. The loss of deep sensibility also presents with painless deep infections involving soft tissue spaces, bone and joints spreading insidiously from the penetrating ulcer in the unwary patient. Insensitive toes commonly produce breakdown lesions from extrinsic footwear pressure, foot heating devices and minor mechanical trauma. Intrinsic pressure from nail in-growths, underlying prominent bone and toe deformities with breakdown are often the first presenting sign of a sensory neuropathy.

Motor

Motor neuropathy presents with weakness and atrophy and later fibrous contracture of the intrinsic foot muscles producing various forefoot deformities. This results in alteration of the normal foot compliance on weight bearing with increased local pressures. Associated with the sensory neuropathy, results of these motor nerve changes are a further liability to ulceration and infection. The diabetic amyotrophy may present with wasting and weakness of the calf with dynamic equinovalgus foot deformities with an abnormal gait and weight bearing.

Autonomic

Autonomic nervous system involvement in diabetic neuropathy presents with loss of sudomotor function giving a dry, flaky skin. Cracks and fissures may be present with secondary infection. Loss of the skin thermoregulation with vasomotor instability may produce both vasodilation and vasoconstriction with decreased or increased foot temperatures variably. Loss of the small arterial and arterovenous shunting control may present local ischaemic areas in the skin and deeper tissues with inability to divert the circulatory requirements to damaged new sites.

Deformities

Contractures

The foot deformities presenting in diabetic patients are similar to those in nondiabetics but appear to occur more frequently and to progress more severely. These deformities present in the early phases with dynamic contractures from muscle weakness and atrophy, but later become fixed joint contractures.

The forefoot deformities are the most common and are frequently associated with breakdown problems. Hammer, claw and angular deformities commonly occur in the lesser toes and the 'cock-up' claw toe and valgus deformities most frequently in the hallux.

Further pressure from the contractures occurs over the medial side of the first metatarsal head with a bunion bursitis reaction and under the head on the sesamoid bones. The hallux may underride the second toe giving further clawing with plantar and dorsal pressure sites. Any adjacent toe contracture may produce nail pressure or a soft corn element. Plantar callosities may develop under any of the metatarsal heads with dynamic or fixed depression secondary to the intrinsic muscle contractures.

Midfoot deformities occur with a forefoot plantaris associated with contracture of the plantar intrinsic and calf flexor extrinsic muscles. The resulting pes cavus gives the forefoot claw toes and the hindfoot high pressure loads. Occasionally a pes planovalgus deformity may develop from invertor weakness and a dropped foot from dorsiflexion loss.

The hindfoot deformities may present with prominence of the calcaneum on either the plantar surface with atrophy of the heel pad or posteriorly at the tendo Achillis insertion, often being associated with a pes cavus contracture. Reactive hyperkeratosis of the heel with secondary fissuring and breakdown from the increased pressure loads also occurs.

Nail deformities

Deformities of the toenails are common in the general population, but appear to involve almost all patients with diabetes. These deformities are associated with atrophy, infection, both fungal and bacterial, local trauma, footwear pressure and poor nail hygiene.

The common deformities producing local pressure and infection are from curved edges giving the ingrowing toenail (onychocryptosis), the thickened horny nail (onychogryphosis), horny nailbed epithelial growth (onychophosis) and the thickened discoloured nail from fungal infection (onychomycosis). As the sensory neuropathy usually starts in the toes, these nail deformities are under considerable risk from local breakdown and infection.

Osteoarthropathies

Deformities of the diabetic foot are also produced by structural changes resulting from Charcot's neuropathic joint (Charcot 1868), or bone changes, often in combination (Jordan 1936, Heiple & Cammarn 1966). These changes are usually associated with a full sensory neuropathy and often follow foot trauma (Boehm 1962).

This osteoarthropathy may develop in the acute form with a warm, swollen foot followed by rapid disruption of the bones and joints giving the deformed Charcot foot. In the chronic type, slower progressive degenerative-type changes occur, often followed by subluxation, dislocation and fractures. In both forms, osteopathy with osteolysis, sclerosis, fragmentation and ectopic bone formation may occur producing the diabetic neuropathic deformed foot. Differentiation from a low-grade infection is necessary.

The osteoarthropathy most commonly occurs in the forefoot with deformities of the metatarsal and phalangeal bones and joints (Fig. 34.1a), often associated with ulceration (Kelly & Coventry 1958). The second, less common site is in the midfoot region involving the metatarsal-tarsal and midtarsal joints and bones (Fig. 34.1b). Collapse of the longitudinal arch with midtarsal joint subluxation may produce the 'rocker bottom foot' (Fig. 34.1c). The third and least common neuropathic osteoarthropathy deformity presents in the hindfoot, with spontaneous fracture of the calcaneum or talus and often disruption of the subtalar joint and rarely the ankle joint. A severe planus, valgus or adduction deformity is produced.

Infection

Infection of the diabetic foot often presents as the first sign of a peripheral neuropathy or angiopathy. Three basic anatomical forms of the most major foot infections involve the malperforans, nonsuppurative cellulitis of the foot dorsum and abscess in the deep tissues (Meade & Mueller 1968, Bose 1979). The infected abscesses may involve the deep spaces of the

a

c

b

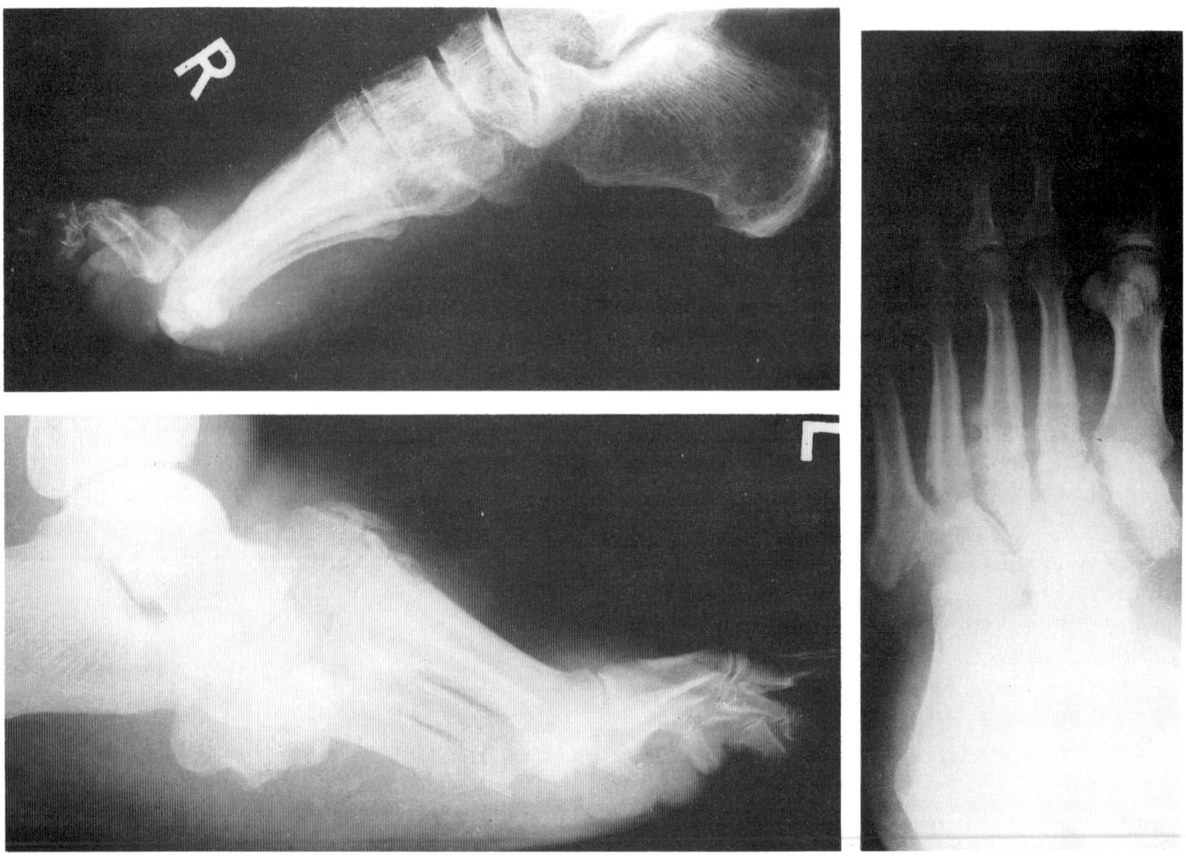

Fig. 34.1 Diabetic neuropathic osteoarthropathies: a, Forefoot metatarsophalangeal joints dislocation; b Forefoot metatarsotarsal joints subluxation; c, Midtarsal joints dislocations (rocker foot — see Fig. 34.9)

foot, the bones and joints. Many of these lesions are progressive, starting with a superficial ulcer, proceeding to a deeper one, then developing abscess formation in the tissues, and if the circulation is compromised, ending with gangrenous lesions, as shown from a study of the natural history (Meggitt 1973, 1976).

Ulceration

This presents most commonly with areas of high pressure or friction over bony prominences. The commonest site is under the metatarsal heads (Fig. 34.2a) with toe deformities and over the pulp and nail of the next toe ends. Ulceration over the first metatarsal bunion, fifth metatarsal bunionette and base of the fifth metatarsal are also common sites from shoe friction pressure.

These ulcerative lesions appear as two types: with a corn or callus hyperkeratosis reaction, often with incomplete sensibility loss; or as a 'punched out' perforating ulcer with little reaction and usually in a fully insensitive area. The individual ulcers may present as a relatively clean lesion with a necrotic sloughing base or with an infected pus discharging centre with or without surrounding cellulitis.

Other ulcers may occur in the neuropathic foot from direct mechanical, thermal or chemical trauma. Ischaemic ulcers also present spontaneously or with trauma, mainly on the toes or dorsum of the foot, and progress to healing or further breakdown dependent upon the adequacy of the circulation.

Dorsal cellulitis

A spreading inflammatory lesion presenting as cellulitis and swelling on the dorsum of the foot is usually secondary to surface infection in the nails, toes or web space (Fig. 34.2b). A systemic reaction with pyrexia is often present and a deeper abscess may occasionally develop.

Abscess

The common sites for abscess formation are in the toes, web spaces, flexor sheaths, the central, medial and lateral plantar spaces and in the heel. Presentation of the abscess occurs with little or no pain and the patient often remains walking so 'pumping' the infection widely. Loculated pus usually presents with deep extension of a pyogenic infection from either an open surface ulceration or a closed previous lesion or penetrating injury. Two forms are seen clinically: involving the closed abscess formation with extensive foot swelling and systemic reaction, or with open draining ulcer or sinus without loculation.

The toe abscess may involve paronychia, pulp, volar spaces and flexor tendon sheaths. The web space abscess presents with swelling and cellulitis extending to the adjacent toes and dorsum of the forefoot. The abscess of the central plantar space occurs with severe swelling of the sole spreading shortly to the dorsum of the foot, together with loss of the longitudinal arch and skin creases. Further proximal spread along the flexor tendons and sheaths gives induration around the ankle and occasionally a calf abscess. Abscesses of the medial and lateral plantar spaces produce local swelling and dorsal oedema, usually being associated with infected ulceration over the first or fifth metatarsal head.

Osteitis

Diabetic osteomyelitis is often associated with vascular deficiency and local abscess formation. Most cases follow chronic ulceration and sinuses with infective discharge. Variable pain, swelling and erythema are the local signs. The commonest sites of osteomyelitis are associated with those of the ulcerations, mainly the toes, metatarsals (Fig. 34.2c) and calcaneum in the heel. Septic necrosis, fragmentation and sequestrum formation may occur. A small sinus may communicate with a large abscess cavity with infected bone and constitute the 'volcano lesion' which may erupt into a full spreading abscess at any time.

Septic arthritis

This commonly presents with swelling, stiffness and variable pain in the interphalangeal or metatarso-phalangeal joints underlying a penetrating ulcer. Contracture, subluxation or dislocation may occur with recurrent episodes of swelling, redness and often a discharging sinus. Associated infection spread to adjacent bones or tissue spaces may give

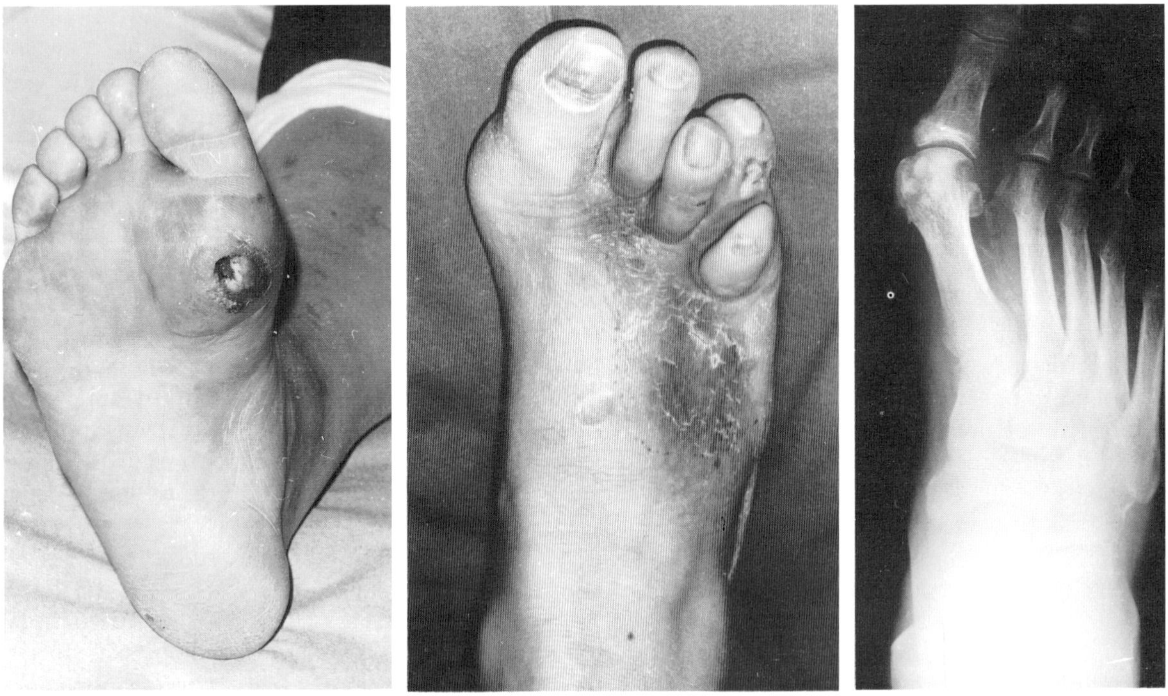

Fig. 34.2 Diabetic foot infections: a, Deep plantar ulceration, 1st metatarsal head; b, Dorsal cellulitis from 4th toe abrasion; c, Osteitis abscess, 1st metatarsal head

further abscess formation. These chronic septic arthritis lesions carry a poor prognosis for healing and danger of spreading (Margo 1967, Singer & Rossi 1968).

RADIOLOGICAL CHANGES IN THE DIABETIC FOOT SYNDROME

Plain film X-ray examination of the foot is essential for diagnostic and progress monitoring of the often asymptomatic diabetic limb with neuropathic and infective abnormalities. The radiological features of neuropathic and infective lesions in the foot have been reported from large series (Schwartz et al 1969, Cofield et al 1983), but the differentiation between the two is often very difficult (Hodgson et al 1948, Whitehouse 1978).

Major disorganisation of the skeletal structures in the neuropathic diabetic foot is not uncommon and may involve spontaneous fractures (Johnson 1967) and spontaneous dislocations (Newman 1979).

Skeletal changes

Osteomyelitis

This is usually associated with soft tissue swelling, ulceration or abscess occurring mainly in the forefoot, occasionally in the heel and rarely in the midfoot bones. The X-ray changes invariably appear as cortical erosions, local diffuse osteoporosis, periosteal reactions, cortical and medullary bone destruction and bone collapse with fragmentation and fracture.

Septic arthritis

Diffuse local osteoporosis, subchondral bone resorption, collapse of the articular surface and deformities with subluxation and dislocation are the main radiological features. With more advanced infection, the bone adjacent to the joint may actually disappear with osteomyelitis changes in the shaft and subperiosteal reaction.

Neuro-osteopathy

Radiological appearances of diabetic neuropathic osteopathy show demineralization, osteolysis and fractures. Osteolysis appears as localized bone resorption defects, most often involving the ends of the phalanges and distal metatarsals. Thinning of the shafts may produce the 'hour glass' deformity whereas resorption of the head region produces the 'pencil-shaped' appearance which, if it is flattened, gives the 'pestle and mortar' deformity. These bone changes may remain static, undergo slow progression or develop a massive acute osteolysis with extensive destruction.

Spontaneous fractures may occur painlessly in the calcaneum, metatarsals and phalanges, but these are far less common than the other bone changes. They are often associated with neuropathic joints and can proceed to callus healing.

Neuroarthropathy

The specific radiological changes in the neuropathic joint present as a wide spectrum from joint swelling and osteoporosis, osteophytosis and periostitis, through cartilage loss, joint collapse and fragmentation to subluxation and dislocation. Often multiple changes are present in various joints constituting the Charcot osteoarthropathy picture. Three patterns are commonly seen (see Figs. 34.1a–c):

Forefoot changes involving the metatarsophalangeal and interphalangeal joints, often associated with toe deformities and plantar ulceration.

Midfoot involvement with disorganisation of three joint groups. Most commonly, the metatarsotarsal joints (Lisfranc) with often spontaneous displacement dorsolaterally. Secondly, the talonavicular-cuneiform medial column as part of the anterior pillar may collapse the longitudinal arch. Thirdly, the lateral column with destruction of the calcaneocuboid joint results in plantar lateral deformity. Disorganisation of the foot at the intertarsal joint level may occur producing not only the severe planus foot but also reversal of the longitudinal arch to produce the 'rocker bottom' deformity.

Hindfoot neuropathic changes can occur involving the subtalar and ankle joint with severe valgus deformity.

Soft tissue changes

These are shown radiologically as increased density with oedema, irregularity of the skin surface with ulceration and subcutaneous cystic areas from gas formation (see Fig. 34.17a). Bone or calcified debris is seen adjacent to neuropathic joints, osteolysis or osteomyelitic lesions. Vascular calcification in the foot arteries is commonly due to arteriosclerotic changes and may extend to the distal metatarsal and digital vessels (see Fig. 34.2c). Superficial cutaneous or skin calcification may be due to local ischaemia or calcified venous thrombosis. Occasionally foreign bodies are seen embedded in the foot such as needles, tacks or glass fragments confirming the insensitive neuropathic foot.

'AT RISK' DIABETIC FOOT CONCEPT

The concept of the 'at risk' diabetic foot (Fig. 34.3) is derived from a combination of the loss of protective sensibility, the lowered resistance to infection with delayed healing and the development of deformities with high pressure areas. Early assessment of the severity of these complications with instigation of appropriate treatment is essential if the 'at risk' diabetic foot is not to be lost. Long term prophylactic treatment is then essential for both feet.

ASSESSMENT OF THE DIABETIC FOOT

As diabetes mellitus is a progressive multisystem disease, it is essential to have a full general body assessment under the diabetic physician's care before undertaking a local evaluation of the diabetic foot condition. Also, the patient's mental, physical and mobility status is recorded.

The local assessment of the diabetic foot severity is shown in Fig. 34.4.

Vascularity assessment

Clinical

Clinical parameters indicating a reduced arterial

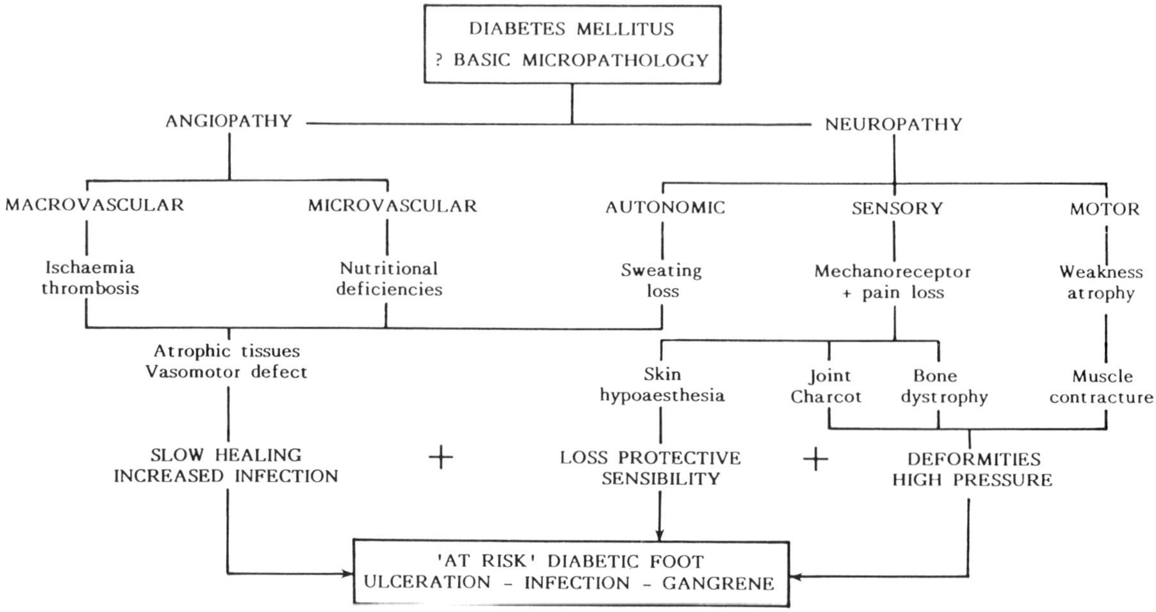

Fig. 34.3 Pathogenesis of diabetic foot breakdown: 'at risk' concept

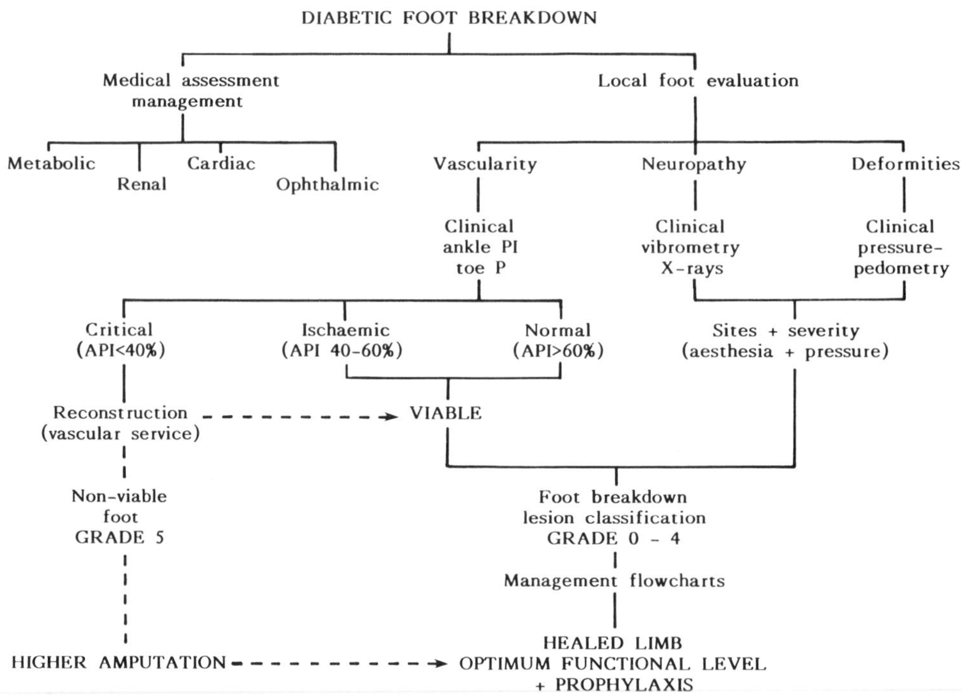

Fig. 34.4 Diabetic foot breakdown: general management flow chart. API = ankle pressure index

flow and poor tissue nutrition provide more of a qualitative diagnosis than a quantitative evaluation. In the early major vessel disease, there are often few clinical signs. In the more severe macrovascular disease, intermittent claudication and walking tolerance distance is a rough guide to the severity of the vascular disease.

Pressure index

Blood flow varies directly with the systolic blood pressure and this pressure at a given level may be used as an index of tissue perfusion to the local area supplied.

The noninvasive pressure index test is used as a crude, but practical, evaluation of the vascular status in the lower limb (Yao 1970, Carter 1973). The segmental systolic pressure is accurately recorded using 12 cm cuffs placed on the thigh, calf and ankle and listening over the artery below with a Doppler ultrasound (10 MHz) probe (Figs. 34.5a,b). The brachial artery pressure is also recorded and a 'Pressure Index' is calculated using the leg as a percentage of the arm pressure (Fig. 34.5c).

The 'Ankle Pressure Index' (API) is used as a guide to the circulation in the foot and prognosis for healing (Wagner & Buggs 1978). Recent evaluation of this API test has shown its coefficient of variation to be $< 10\%$ (Quin et al 1977) and changes of $> 15\%$ are considered significant (Baker & Dix 1981).

As there may be distal vessel obstruction beyond the ankle, then, more recently, toe pressure (TP) measurements have also been included using a photoplethysmograph. (Holstein et al 1978, Barnes et al 1981). These assessments of the foot vascularity are recorded and the patients divided into three groups with a prognosis for healing:

a 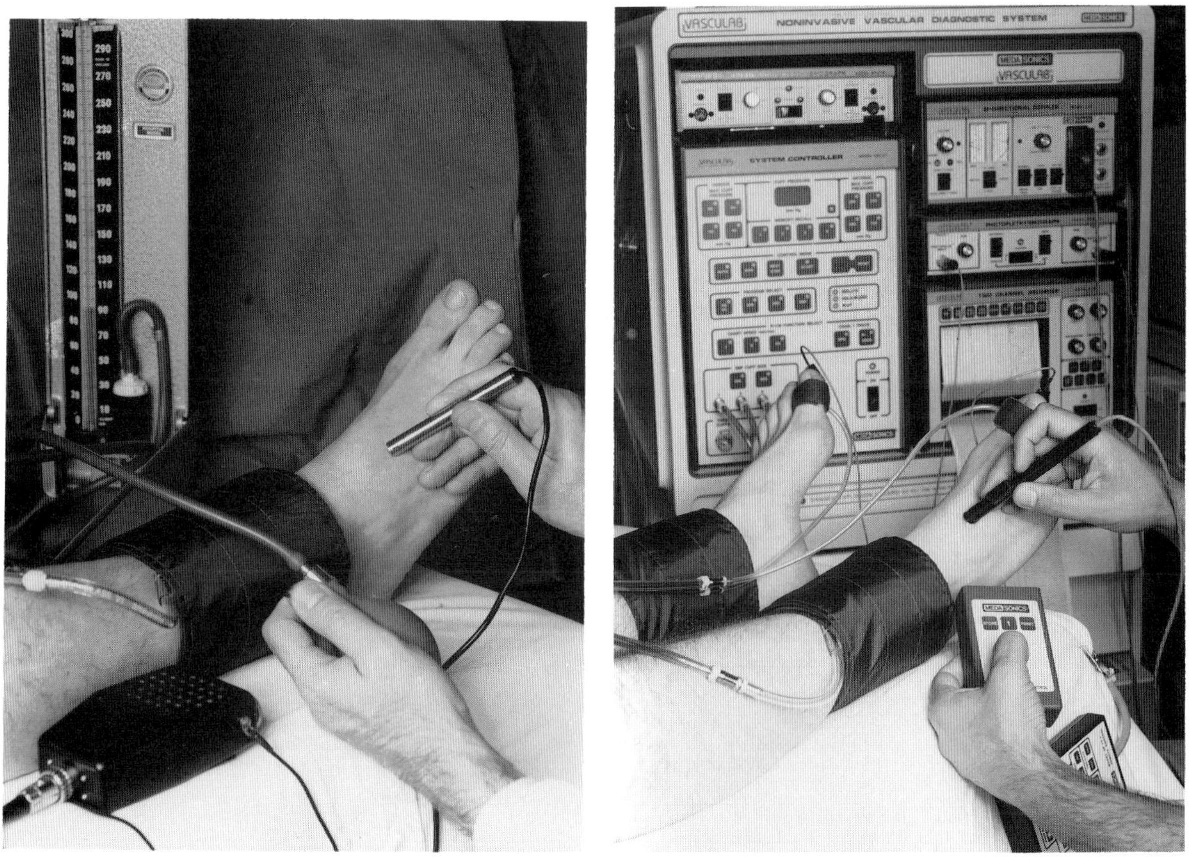 b

Fig. 34.5 Foot vascularity pressures assessment: a, Simpler Doppler probe, audio unit and sphygmomanometer; b, Vasculab Doppler and toe photoplethysmograph

'VASCULAB' DOPPLER

Addenbrookes Hospital
Hill's Road, Cambridge
CB2 2QQ

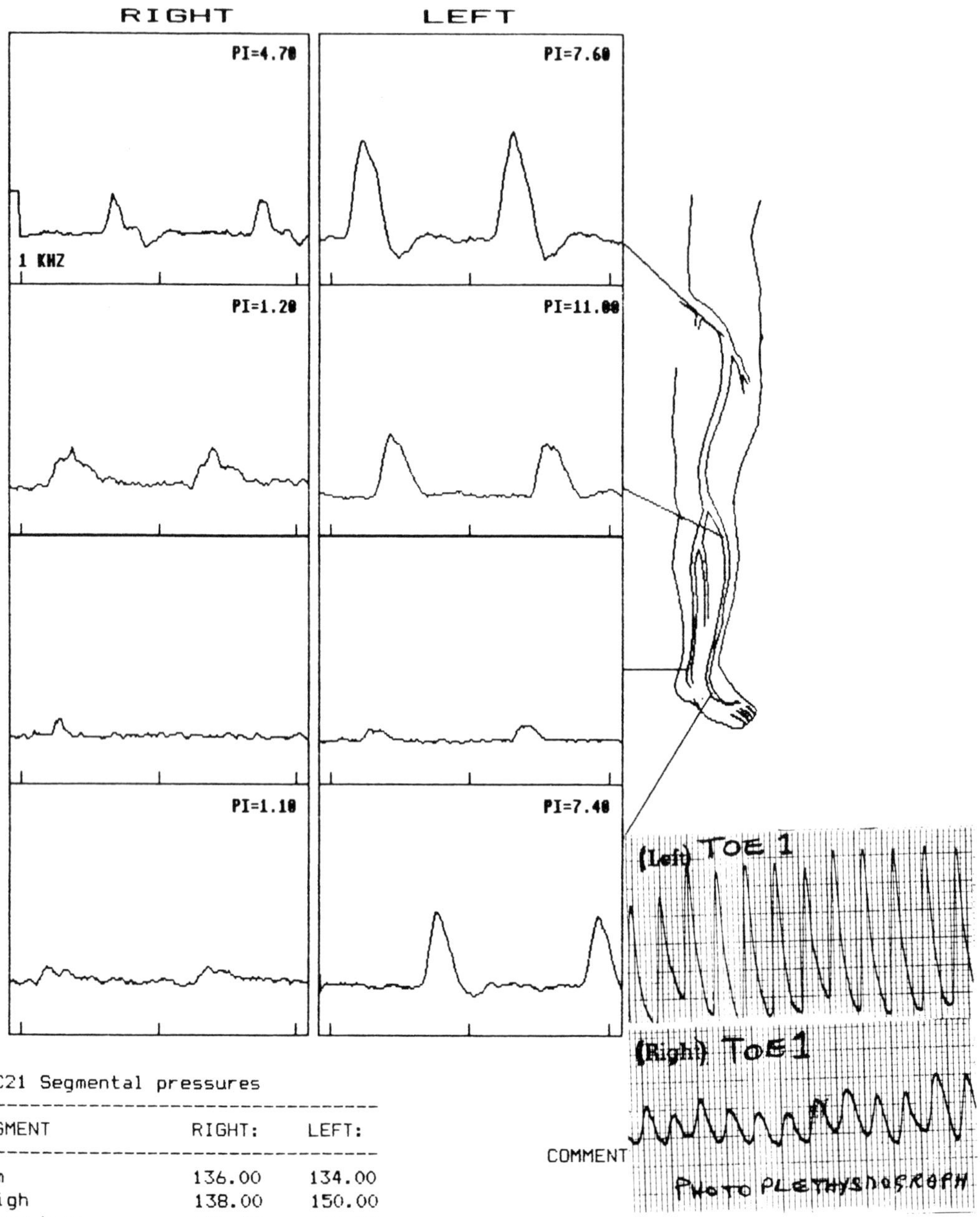

VSC21 Segmental pressures

SEGMENT	RIGHT:	LEFT:
Arm	136.00	134.00
Thigh	138.00	150.00
Above knee	100.00	145.00
Below knee	80.00	140.00
Ankle	65.00	126.00
Toe	34.00	80.00
Ankle:arm Index	0.48	0.93
Toe:arm Index	0.25	0.59

COMMENT

SIGNATURE

Fig. 34.5c Vasculab Doppler computer printout: pressures, wave forms and pulsatility indices with diffuse right arteriopathy

1. Critical ischaemia API $< 40\%$ TP < 30 mmHg
2. Viable ischaemia API 40–60% TP 30–60
3. Normal range API $> 60\%$ TP > 60

More direct techniques of measuring the tissue blood flow have been developed using isotope (XE^{133}, Tc^{99}, I^{125}) clearance following subdermal injections and monitoring transcutaneous oxygen tension, but these require a laboratory set-up and complex instrumentation.

Contrast arteriography

This provides assessment of the site, extent and degree of patency of the larger peripheral vessels. The investigation is not without risk and is indicated when vascular reconstructive surgery is necessary for arterial disease. The segmental blood pressure recordings provide a more accurate screening test now with a drop of 40 mm or more suggesting a stenotic segment or occlusion between the segments. This, together with distal pressure levels within the critical range, requires arteriographic evaluation.

For lesions above the femoral artery, transbrachial or translumbar arteriograms are performed and below, a transfemoral technique is used. The radio-opaque dye with serial radiographs can demonstrate occlusions, stenoses, aneurysmal dilations and atheromatous areas in all the major arteries from the pelvis to the foot.

The recent introduction of digital subtraction angiography (DSA) with computerized image subtraction and dynamic range enhancement is proving to be a valuable tool. Visualization of all the foot and toe vessels is obtained with intra-arterial DSA.

Neuropathy evaluation

Clinical

Standard clinical sensory examination of the diabetic foot provides a general assessment of the degree of impairment and distribution of touch (cotton wool, brush or bristle) and pain (pin prick). These are recorded as normal, reduced or absent and the extent of involvement as none, patchy or diffuse. Vibration (tuning fork) and position sensibility (toe movements) can be recorded as present or absent. Temperature appreciation at various levels is difficult but heat and cold extremes of 45°C and 0°C with warm water and ice respectively in test tubes provide a positive or negative response.

Vibrometry

For more accurate and repeated comparable testings, vibration threshold sensibility is measured using a mains driven vibrometer (Bio Thesiometer) (Hockaday et al 1982, Bloom et al 1984). Sensory nerve impairment by conduction testing and autonomic neuropathy testing with galvanic skin stimulation, provide qualitative results only with little clinical value. Similarly, motor neuropathy assessment with conduction tests are of diagnostic use only.

Pressure distribution assessment

Corns, calluses and ulcerations with bony prominences are clinical indications of high pressure areas in many diabetic neuropathic feet. Modern pedobarometers are used to evaluate the high plantar pressures in the 'at risk' neuropathic feet (Stokes et al 1975, Betts et al 1980) and also for testing the efficiency of surgery and orthotic footwear in reducing these dangerous pressures. Newer pressure pedometers with static and dynamic foot recordings suitable for clinical use are under evaluation at present.

NATURAL HISTORY AND CLASSIFICATION OF DIABETIC FOOT LESIONS

A classification of diabetic foot complications based essentially on the underlying pathology as septic, neuropathic, ischaemic and mixed groups, has improved the understanding of the aetiology of the lesions (Oakley 1954). A clinical classification developed from a study of the natural history of the progressive foot breakdown (Fig. 34.6) has been presented (Meggitt 1972, 1973, 1976). This involved six grades of severity from the early 'at risk' potential lesions to progressive ulceration, abscess, osteomyelitis and finally to gangrene. Occasionally closed deep lesions occurred secondary to penetrating

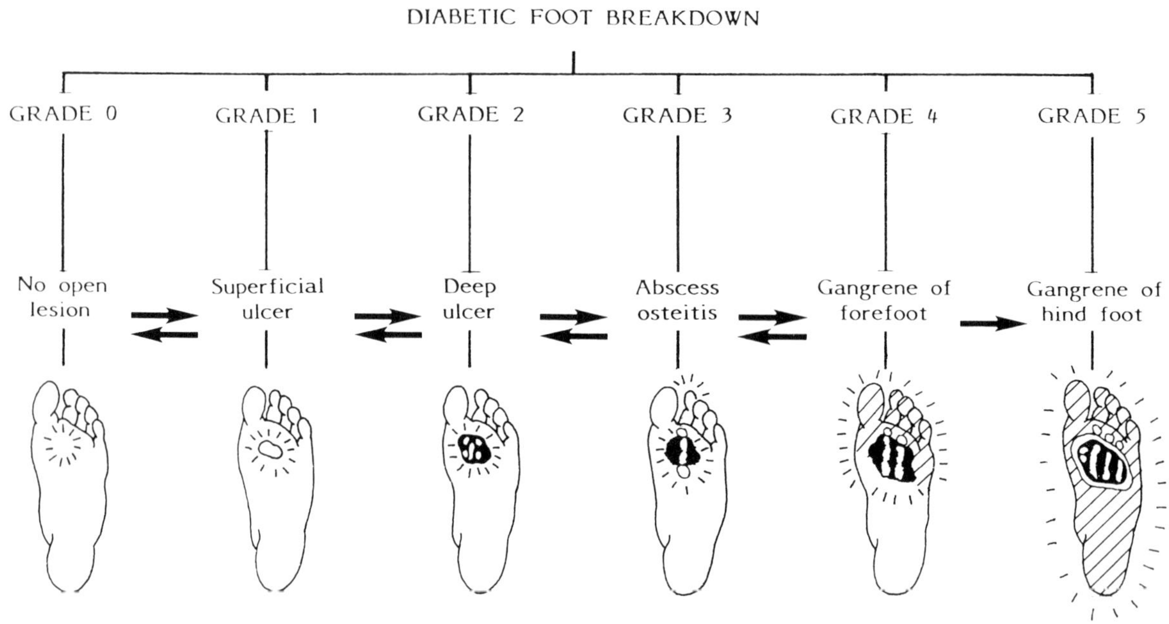

Fig. 34.6 Clinical classification of diabetic foot lesions

injuries, infections with small skin defects and previously healed lesions. This grading system is as follows:

- Grade 0: There is no open lesion but potential breakdown with high pressure deformities and sensory neuropathy
- Grade 1: The lesion is superficial through the skin only with or without underlying bony prominences
- Grade 2: The ulcer is deep penetrating to tendon, joint or bone
- Grade 3: There is deep abscess formation with plantar space and tendon sheath infection, osteomyelitis or septic arthritis
- Grade 4: Gangrene is present locally in the toes or more diffuse over the forefoot
- Grade 5: Gangrene has spread and involves the hindfoot requiring a higher amputation

TREATMENT PROGRAMMES

A working hypothesis that diabetic foot breakdown is due to local pressure or trauma in the presence of tissue nutritional deficiencies with microvascular disease, impaired sensibility, foot deformities and lowered resistance to infection provides a rationale for treatment. The clinical classification (Fig. 34.6) has been used as the basis for a comprehensive management framework with the development of treatment flow sheets and applied to a prospective study of diabetic foot lesions (Meggitt 1972, 1973, 1976). These flow sheets formed a sequence of treatment steps for each lesion grade obtained by matching the requirements for healing against the optimum available materials and techniques. Use of this clinical classification and further development of the flow sheets with application to other dysvascular feet has been reported (Wagner 1979, 1981).

A patient being referred with a diabetic foot problem first undergoes full general assessment and optimal treatment under the care of the diabetic medical unit. Foot evaluation of the vascularity level, neuropathic severity and the deformity-pressure sites is undertaken and recorded before the lesion itself is considered. With the vascularity at the critical or severe ischaemic level (Doppler ankle index $<40\%$ or toe pressure <30 mmHg), with clinically reduced arterial flow and ischaemia, then urgent vascular reconstructive service referral is undertaken. With higher pressure indices, grading of the lesion and its appropriate treatment then follows.

Grade 0

This is essentially the 'at risk' diabetic foot (Fig. 34.7) showing degrees of neuropathy and deformities but with no open lesion. Treatment is essentially preventative with full patient education and relief of pressure over danger areas.

Education

Advice on daily feet inspection with a bathroom mirror, washing with soap and water only and application of lanolin cream to prevent drying is given. Direct external heat to the insensitive feet should be avoided, especially from hot water bottles, electric pads and blankets, fires and car heaters.

Orthotic footwear

The principle of 'cushioning the foot' on a total contact moulded resilient insole has provided maximal plantar pressure distribution during weight bearing. A clearance of at least 1 cm depth of insole from the lowest point of the foot is necessary to prevent 'bottoming out' (Fig. 34.8a). This insole is then fitted into a custom-made extra depth shoe or boot with a firm sole. A rocker sole is added for foot stiffness and an ankle ortholene or metal bar brace fitted for any ankle weakness.

For emergency prescription or for house use in the elderly, the direct thermomouldable extra depth plastazote insole and shoe is fitted with the use of an infrared oven in a few minutes from stock (Fig. 34.8b). In the overweight patient with neuropathic feet and deformities, often Charcot type in which the

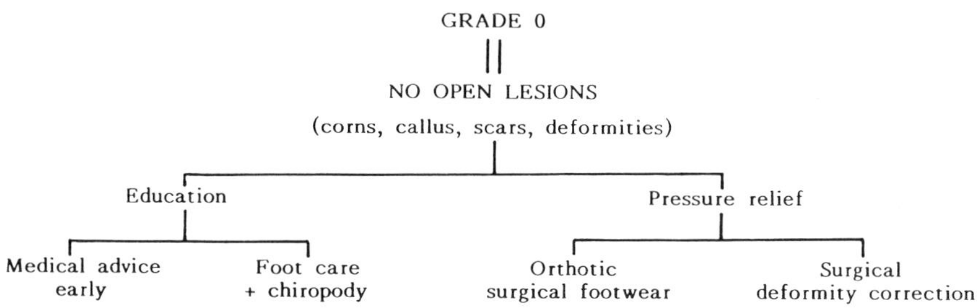

Fig. 34.7 Grade 0: 'at risk' foot treatment flow sheet

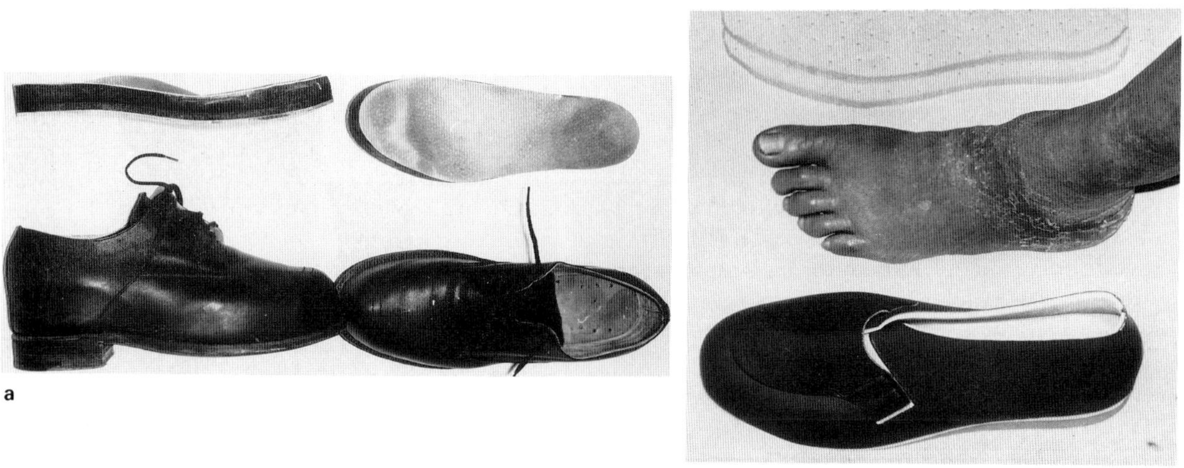

a

b

Fig. 34.8 Orthotic extra-depth footwear: a, Definitive shoe with composite high-medium density plastazote moulded insole leather covered; b, Temporary thermomouldable plastazote shoe and insole

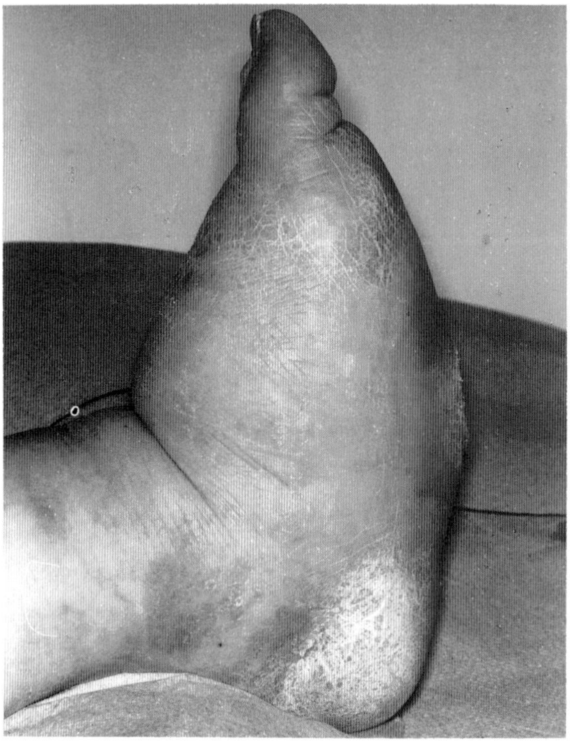

a

Fig. 34.9a Charcot left foot — rocker bottom (see Fig. 34.1c)

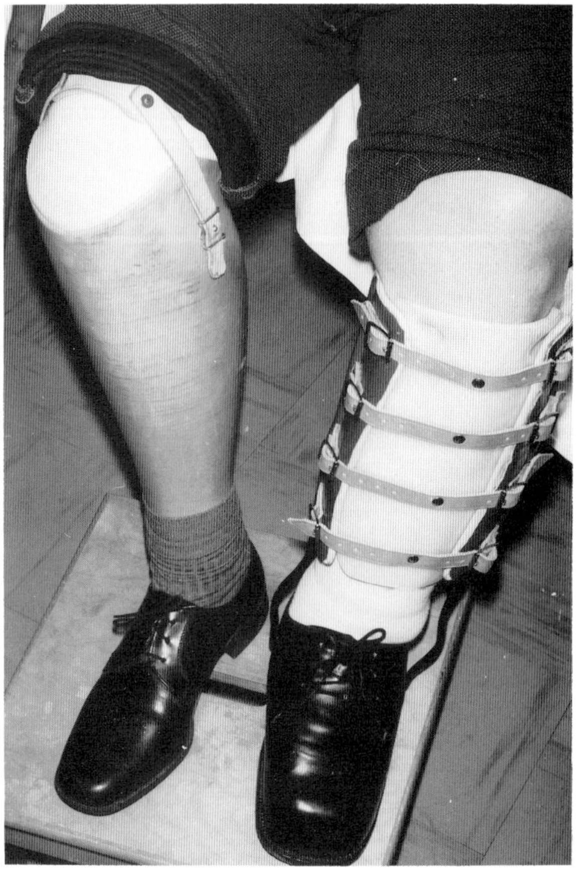

b

Fig. 34.9b Orthotic footwear with higher loading tibia brace

plantar surface is too small to obtain insole pressure relief, the load is transferred higher with a patella tendon-tibial condylar bearing brace (Figs. 34.9a,b).

With the acute Charcot osteoarthropathy, the foot is rested elevated and then mobilized in a well moulded plastic cast.

Prophylactic surgery

If conservative treatment with orthotic footwear is not sufficient, then surgical relief of intrinsic pressure by correcting the deformities is undertaken. With adequate assessment and selection, successful treatment of ingrowing toe nails with wedge resections or matrix ablations, hallux valgus with metatarsal osteotomy or Keller's arthroplasty, claw toes with tendon transfers or arthrodeses, and metatarsal head protrusion with osteotomies or Fowler's procedure, have all been undertaken (Fig. 34.10).

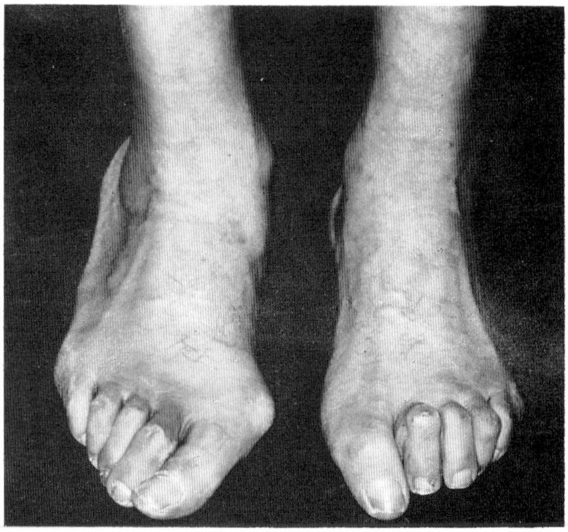

Fig. 34.10 Neuropathic forefeet deformities with recurrent ulceration: prophylactic surgery indicated (API = 76%, TP = 43 mmHg)

Grade 1

If the Grade 1 (Fig. 34.11) superficial ulcer has a necrotic base, this is debrided to provide a clean viable one. With ulcers on the foot dorsum, smaller ones will epithelialize but larger ulcers (> 1 inch diameter) will require a skin graft. An elastic tubular bandage and a moulded plastazote boot are used.

On the plantar surface similar treatment is used for small ulcers, but if not seen to be healing or with larger ones, a well moulded below-knee walking synthetic or plaster cast is applied with a rocker soled overboot (Fig. 34.12). This provides even load distribution on the sole and allows the patient to remain safely walking. The cast can be changed two to four weekly but healing rapidly occurs in the viable foot. Once healed the further management is as in Grade 0.

Grade 2

Ulcer penetration to the deeper tissues forms the Grade 2 lesion (Fig. 34.13) and usually requires a surgical debridement of all necrotic tissue, often without anaesthetic in the insensitive foot. Chemical desloughing agents (Malatex®, Aserbine®, Flamazine®) and antiseptic packing (eusol, povidone-iodine, chlorhexidine, proflavine) are usually necessary to cleanse the cavity. With dorsal foot lesions the plastazote boot is used. On the plantar surface or sides, a below-knee walking cast is used with a walking heel or stirrup and a cut-out window over the lesion allowing daily dressing access. (Figs. 34.14a,b).

Where there are large bony prominences with slow healing or recurred ulceration, then relief of the intrinsic pressure is undertaken surgically. Thus Keller's bunionectomy arthroplasty, metatarsal head excision or elevation osteotomies, claw toe straightening and exostectomies of any prominent bone may be required. With these usually small wounds, primary closure is undertaken using a Silastic® Yates' type drain and intravenous antibiotic cover. With smaller, less clean wounds, standard antiseptic ribbon gauze pack is used. Following rest and elevation, once the cavity is granulating satisfactorily, treatment continues as for the Grade 1 lesion. If healing does not occur, further surgical debridement is necessary with partial or complete ray resections, partial foot amputations or even a Syme's amputation as described as Grades 3 and 4.

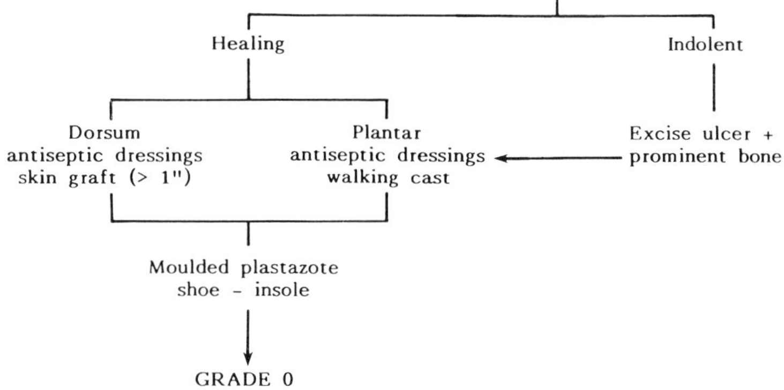

Fig. 34.11 Grade 1: superficial ulcer treatment flow sheet

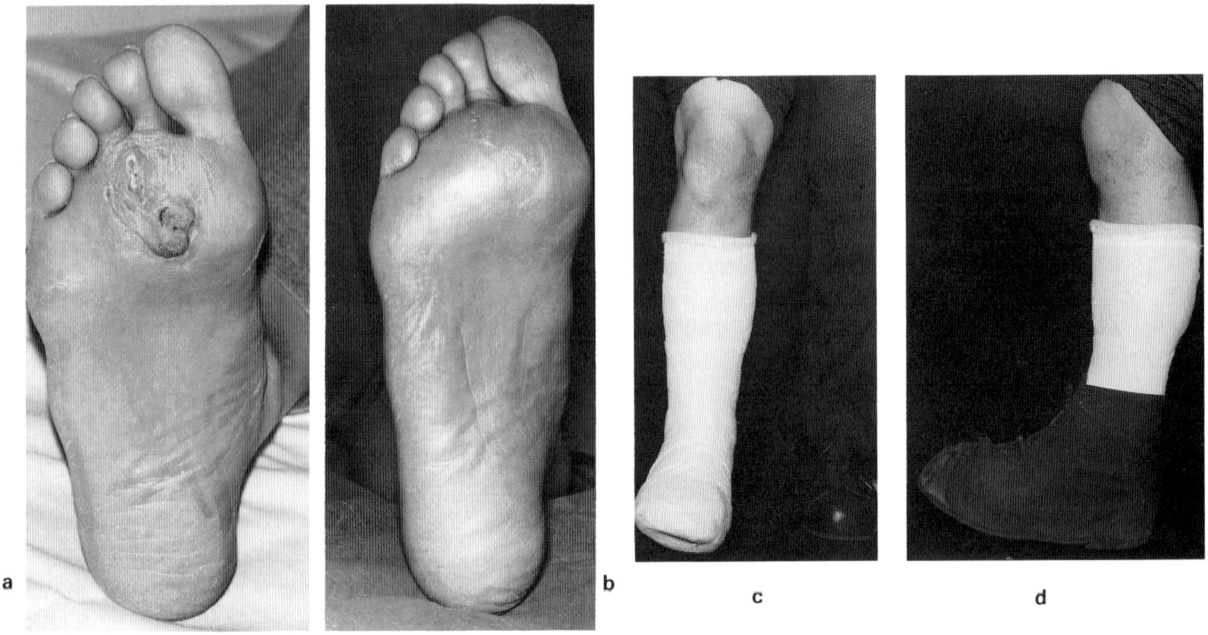

Fig. 34.12 Walking cast treatment of plantar ulcers a, Grade 1 plantar ulcer in anaesthetic forefoot; b, Lesion healed with 8 weeks in cast; c, Walking cast used with even moulding over all foot; d, rocker cast boot fitted

Grade 3

This lesion (Fig. 34.15) involves a deep abscess, often with osteomyelitis and joint involvement, presenting either as an acute infection or a chronic flare with intermittent discharging sinuses. Urgent treatment with limb rest and elevation, intravenous antibiotics and diabetic control is necessary. An acute fluctuant abscess (Fig. 34.16) is treated primarily with incision, drainage and curettage on a

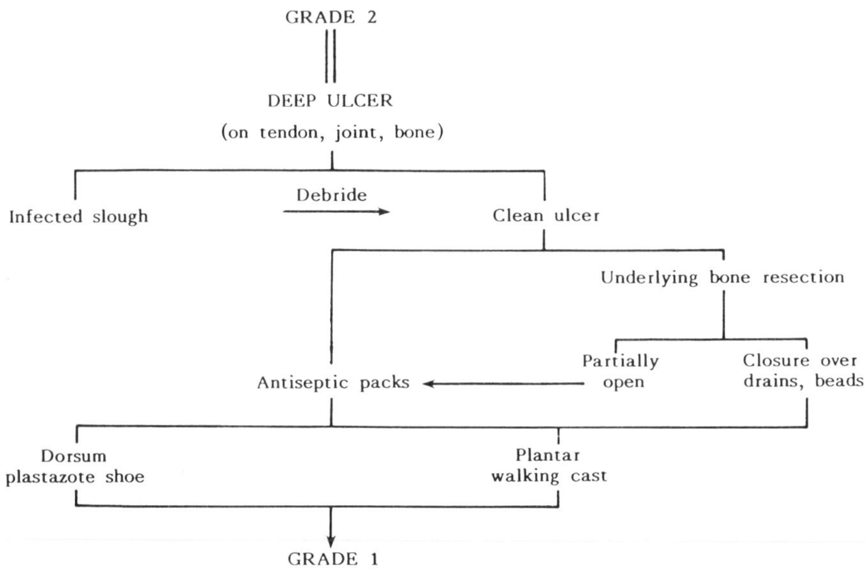

Fig. 34.13 Grade 2: deep ulceration treatment flow sheet

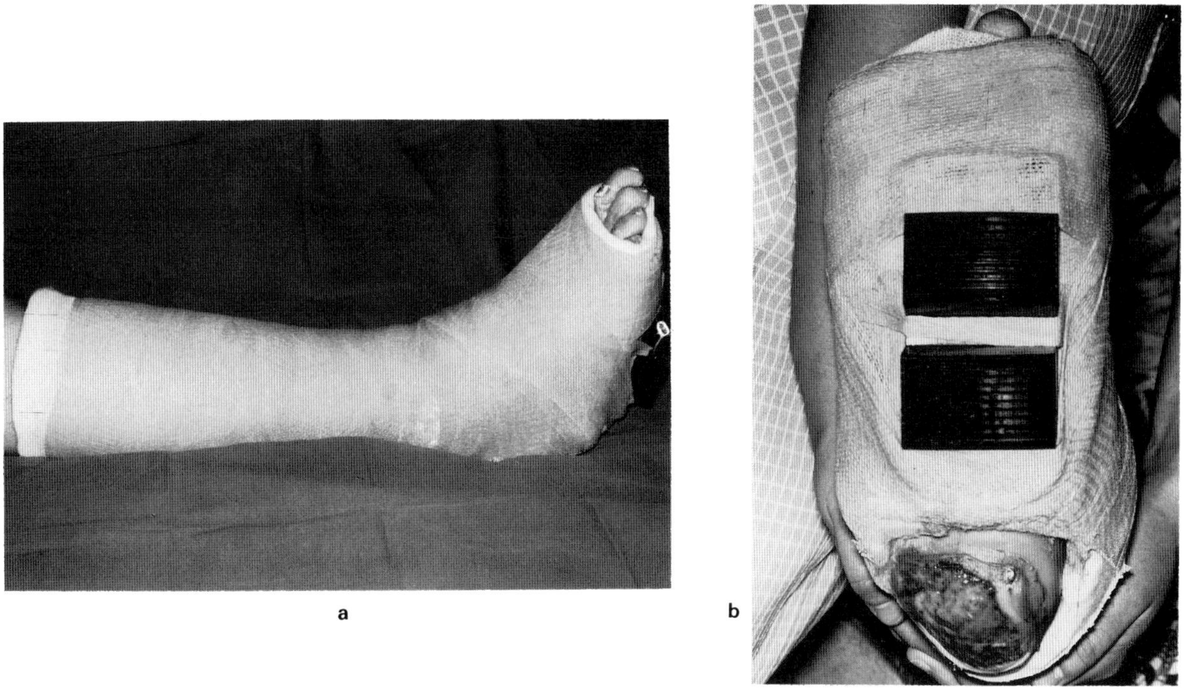

Figs. 34.14a,b Grade 2 ulcer over heel: walking synthetic cast with rocker, weight relief and replaceable window for dressings

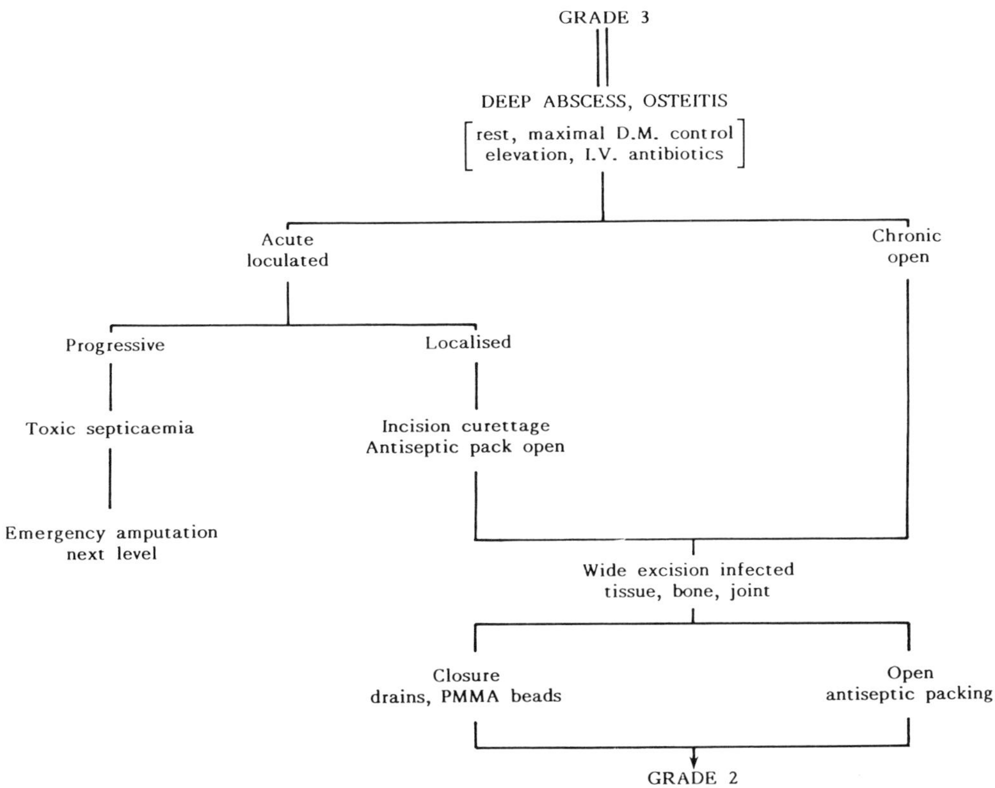

Fig. 34.15 Grade 3: deep abscess — osteitis treatment flow sheet. PMMA = Polymethylmethacrylate

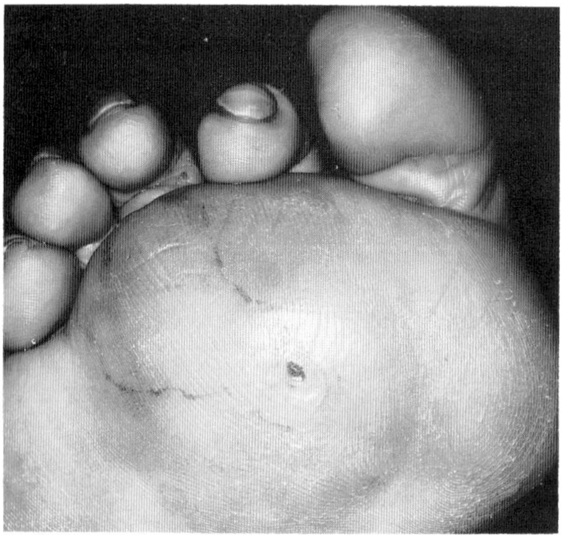

Fig. 34.16 Grade 3 lesion with acute midplantar abscess from previous ulcer with fluctuation area marked

semiurgent basis with open antiseptic packing. Once the acute lesion is localized, treatment is the same as with the chronic lesion involving a wide excision of all necrotic tissue under continuing appropriate antibiotic cover. In the diabetic, these chronic infections are often deceptive with a small surface sinus and a deep 'volcano lesion' involving bone, joint and tendon. Surgical debridement procedures often require partial, multiple or complete ray resections, transmetatarsal, tarsometatarsal or Syme's amputations.

The residual cavity is treated by closure and kept sterile by an antibiotic irrigation-drainage system or by the more recent method of local depot high level antibiotics using the polymethylmethacrylate bead chains (e.g. with gentamicin). One bead is left through a separate stab incision and the chain can be extracted within two to three weeks (Figs. 34.17a,b). The slow, high level, antibiotic release is far in excess of the mean inhibitory concentrations for all bacteria, providing a rapid local control of infected cavities after adequate surgical debridement (Wahlig et al 1978). Very encouraging results of the system in Cambridge in a series of infections have been obtained in a continuing study. The reliability and simplicity of this implant technique has considerable advantages over the more complex nursing intensive irrigation-drainage systems.

With smaller cavities left partially open, antiseptic gauze packing is undertaken. Once the lesions have healed and progressed to a granulating ulcer, further management continues as under Grade 2.

Grade 4

With Grade 4 lesions of gangrene (Fig. 34.18) involving the toes or forefoot, a partial foot amputation is mandatory if the vascular assessment at the ankle is satisfactory (Figs. 34.19a,b). General treatment involves leg elevation and rest, optimum metabolic control and systemic antibiotics. Locally the gangrene is treated with regular antiseptic soaks

a

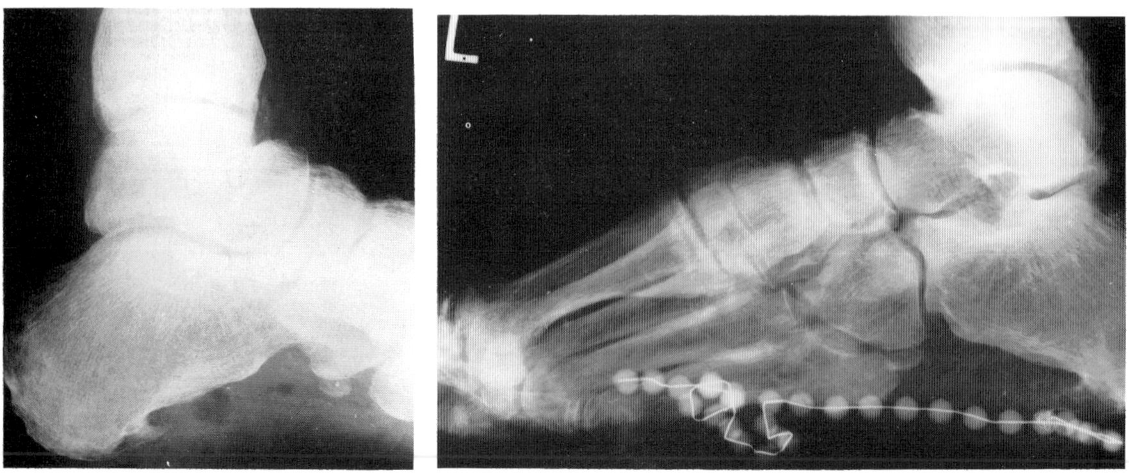

b

Fig. 34.17 Acute on chronic abscess from heel ulcer: a, Nonclostridial gas formation; b, Gentamicin bead chain in large debrided abscess cavity

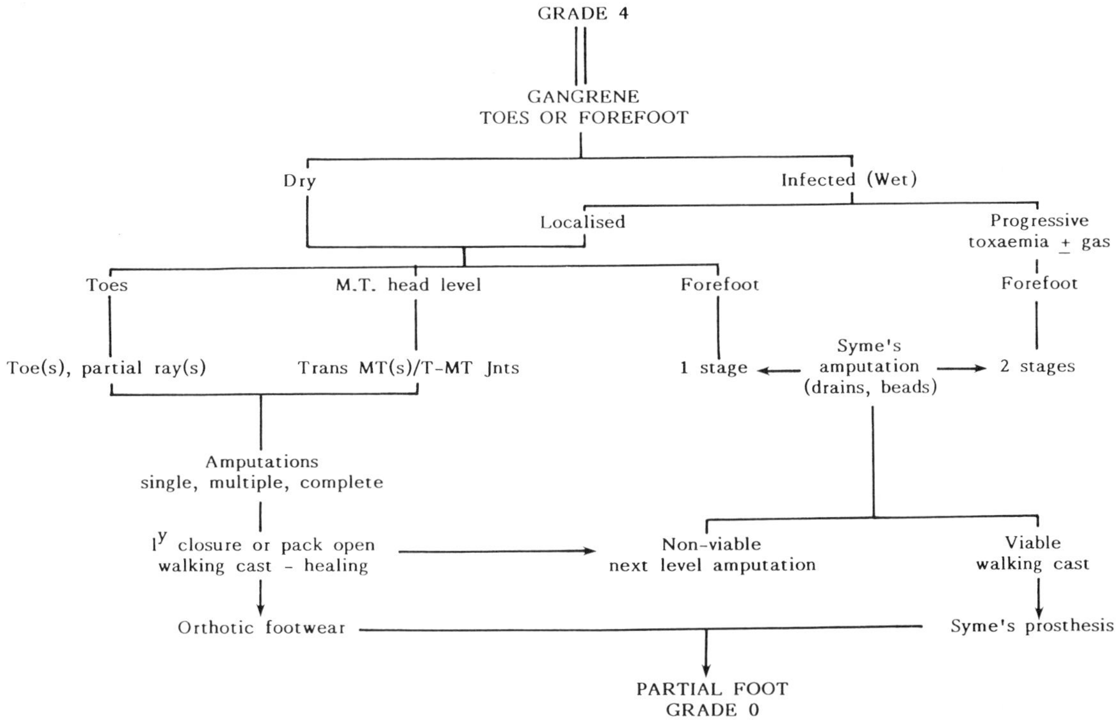

Fig. 34.18 Grade 4: forefoot gangrene treatment flow sheet

(e.g. povidone-iodine solution). Almost any combination of resections of the foot may be undertaken (Fig. 34.20) to provide viable flap closure involving toes, rays and metatarsal disarticulation as partial, complete, single or multiple procedures.

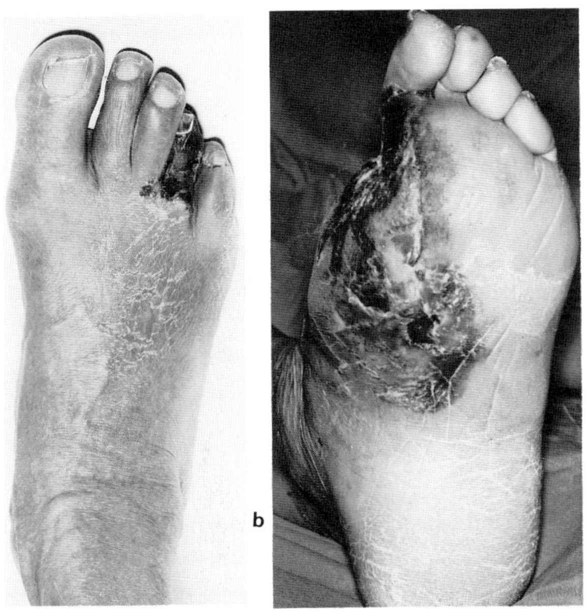

a b

Fig. 34.19 Grade 4 lesions: a, Localized 4th toe gangrene: for partial ray resection (API = 72%); b, Extended gangrene after hallux resection: for Syme's amputation (API = 55%)

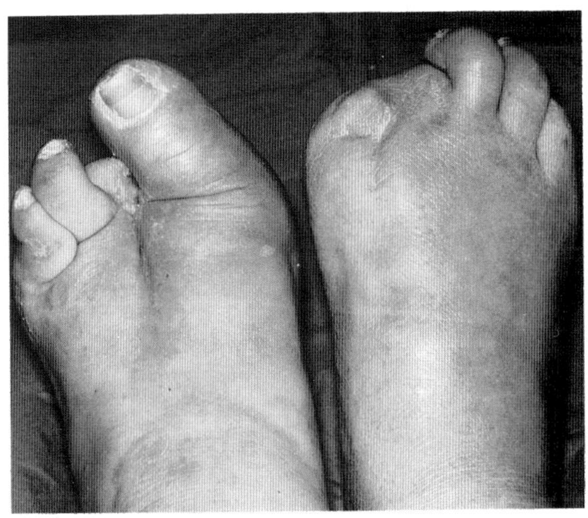

c

Fig. 34.20 Multiple toectomies and partial ray resections for localized infection and gangrene: five procedures over 12 years with still functionable feet

With the now rare infected wet type of gangrene with progressive severe toxaemia and often septicaemia, amputation of the life-threatening limb is an emergency and should be undertaken at the next safe and viable level.

Toe amputation

This is indicated for localized gangrene of the toes as well as for chronic lesions with ulceration, phalangeal osteitis and septic arthritis. The amputation is undertaken through healthy skin with adequate racket, fishmouth or eccentric flaps. With amputations of the hallux, the base of the proximal phalanx is preserved if possible to maintain the weight-bearing tissue. With this, or, if necessary, with disarticulation through the first metatarso-phalangeal joint, the extensor hallucis longus tendon is sutured to the dorsal capsule under a little tension so preserving its dorsiflexion and inversion function in the forefoot. Similarly, the lesser long toe extensors are reattached to the dorsal capsules with basal amputation when possible.

Ray resection

When gangrene extends to the base of the toes or chronic infection involves the metatarsals, then partial or complete ray resection is necessary. All necrotic tissue is excised with ideally a racket incision bring the long 'handle' proximally over the dorsum of the foot to avoid plantar surface scarring. When there is associated metatarsal ulcer, this can be included in a plantar skin wedge excision. The metatarsal bone is excised cleanly with a small airsaw, or, if necessary, disarticulated at the metatarsotarsal joint. Closure is partial with gauze packing or completely over a low vacuum drain or gentamicin beads. Once the wound is healing satisfactorily, the patient is mobilized in a walking cast as in Grade 3 management. If reinfection or breakdown occurs with adequate tissue vascularity, then either a further local resection is undertaken, or, if necessary, a more proximal amputation at the transmetatarsal, tarsometatarsal or Syme ankle level (Fig. 34.21).

Transmetatarsal amputation

Transverse amputation through the metatarsals is indicated when the gangrene or chronic infection extends to the base of multiple toes and into the distal forefoot, or with healing failure of toectomies or partial ray resections. This transmetatarsal amputation for diabetic gangrene and infection has been reported in large series to provide a functional and durable foot (McKittrick et al 1949, Wheelock 1961, Baddeley & Fulford 1965).

The transmetatarsal amputation technique (see Fig. 34.21) involves a curved incision across the dorsum of the foot through all tissues at the level of the bone divisions. At the sides, the incision is taken vertically and then distally to approximately half an inch from the web space to give a long plantar flap, slightly longer on the medial side to allow for the greater foot depth.

The metatarsal shafts are divided from the dorsum with an oblique plantar undercut, and with retraction, dissection is carried forward along the metatarsal plantar surfaces to complete the amputation. With some recent longer term pressure studies, a plantarvalgus deformity occurs from tendon imbalance giving high medial stump loading. The extensor hallucis longus is sutured to the periotsteum or via a drill hole through the dorsum of the first metatarsal section end. The lesser extensor tendons may be sutured similarly. Closure in two layers over drains or antibiotic beads without tension follows.

Further support with a semipermeable adhesive dressing (e.g. OpSite) can be provided to the suture line followed by a well padded posterior cast splint. Once the incision is healed, a walking cast is applied until mature. An extra depth moulded plastazote shoe with insole and end filler is fitted followed by similar permanent protective orthotic footwear.

Lisfranc amputation

Disarticulation amputation through the tarso-metatarsal joints (Lisfranc joints) is indicated when the gangrene or chronic infection extends proximally to the metatarsal head level with insufficient skin for a transmetatarsal amputation.

A previous problem with the Lisfranc amputation was the development of an equinovarus deformity

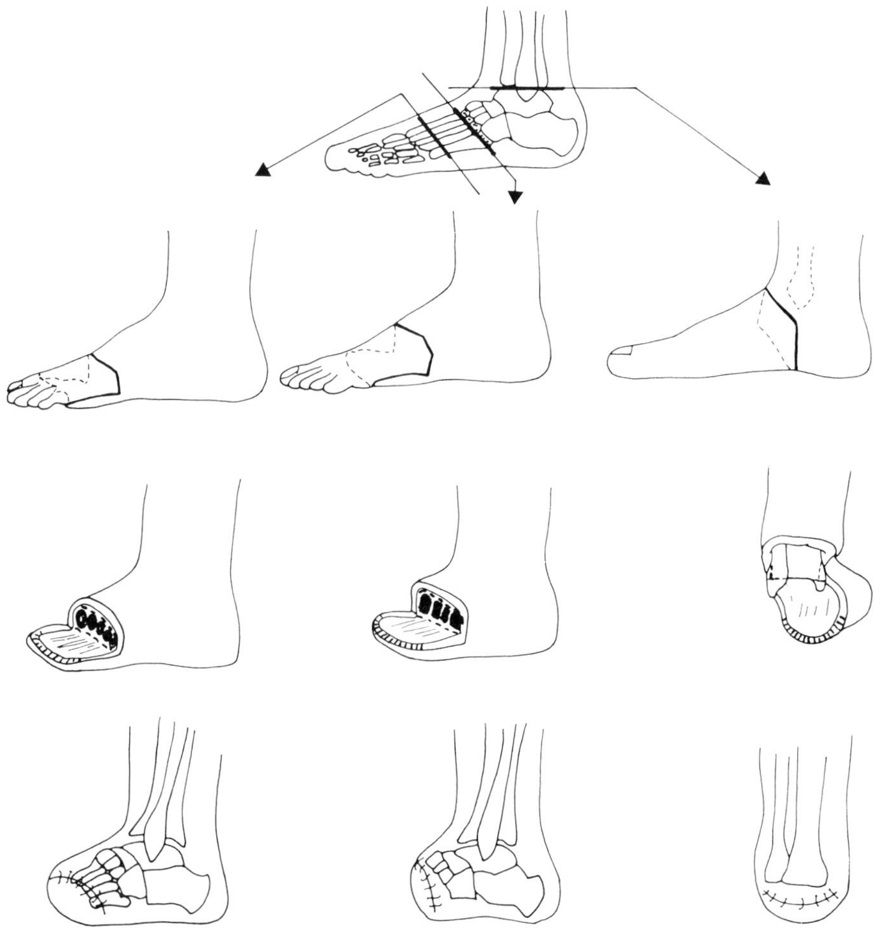

Fig. 34.21 Principles of major foot amputations

from imbalance loss of the long toe extensors and peroneus brevis. This can be overcome with rebalance of the foot by suturing the toe extensors and peroneus brevis laterally. A series of Lisfranc amputations undertaken in Cambridge over the last 10 years are so far very encouraging, and without significant deformity (Fig. 34.22a). A tendo Achillis lengthening was held in reserve but has not been required as yet. The patient is able to wear a normal boot or shoe using a soft calf leather lightweight zip closure bootee with a moulded polypropylene sole plate and toe filler. (Fig. 34.22b).

The alternative is a Syme's amputation with full prosthetic requirement long term. The technique of the Lisfranc amputation (see Fig. 34.21) is similar to that of the transmetatarsal with a transverse dorsal incision over the tarsometatarsal joint level and providing a long plantar flap. The peroneus brevis tendon is sutured to the remaining lateral capsule of the fifth metatarsaltarsal joint. The long toe extensors are sutured to the remaining dorsal capsules of the cuboidmetatarsal joints, beginning with the extensor hallucis longus in the middle and the lesser tendons laterally under moderate tension by providing a little eversion and dorsiflexion of the foot to achieve the dorsiflexion-valgus balance. Postoperative management is similar with the walking cast followed by the 'Lisfranc zip appliance' from the prosthetic service.

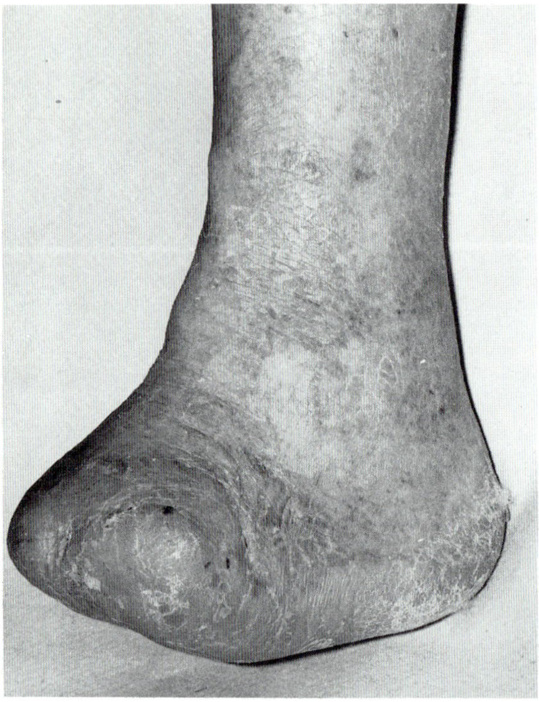

a

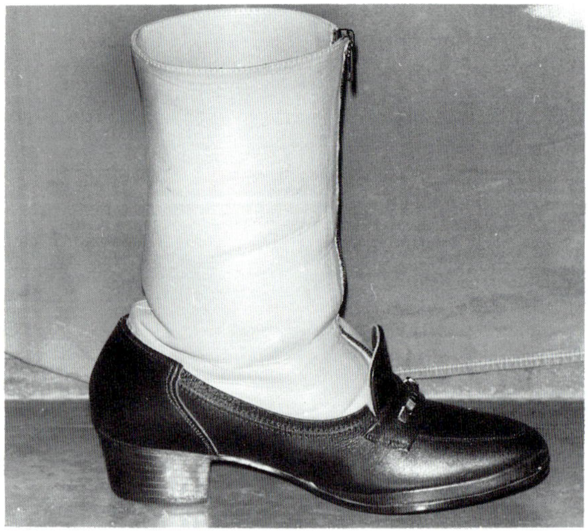

b

Fig. 34.22 Lisfranc amputation with tendon rebalance. a, Healed stump with eversion and dorsiflexion control; b, 'Zip-in' partial foot (ZIP) appliance in normal shoe

Syme's amputation

The indications for a Syme's amputation are if the gangrene or deep infection extends proximally in the forefoot where partial foot amputations are not possible or have failed to heal. Contraindications are if the necrosis extends to the heel flap level, if the foot has chronic oedema or if the heel itself has ulceration or infection. Adequate vascularity of the hindfoot is essential (API > 40%). The presence of a sensory neuropathy in the heel is not a contraindication (Harris 1956, Baker & Stableforth 1969).

Although the ankle disarticulation amputation was described over 100 years ago (Syme 1843), it did not become widely accepted until the last 40 years (Alldredge & Thompson 1946, Harris 1961). Reports have also indicated the successful use of the Syme's amputation in peripheral vascular disease (Warren et al 1955, Dale 1961, Mazet 1968). A modified Syme's amputation has been developed as a two-stage procedure involving primary disarticulation and then later, when healed, a secondary stump formation for salvage of failed forefoot reconstructive surgery (Hulnick et al 1949) and after infected war wounds (Spittler et al 1954). The procedure has been successfully applied to the diabetic foot with gangrene with the same rationale (Wagner 1979).

Before the introduction of the vascularity pressure index for diabetic foot healing (Carter 1973), clinical selection of the two-stage Syme's amputation in diabetic foot breakdown showed a 55% successful salvage rate from an otherwise higher amputation (Meggitt 1973, 1976). However, use of the Doppler ankle pressure index improved the selection of this two-stage Syme procedure in the diabetic with a reported over 90% success rate (Wagner et al 1980).

The original reasoning for the two-stage procedure was difficulty in controlling the infection and often doubtful vascularity. This is much less valid today with wide spectrum antibiotics, improved surgical techniques and better tissue vascularity evaluation. As this modified Syme's amputation requires two operations, prolonged hospitalization and difficulty in mobilizing between the procedures, the single stage Syme's amputation is being revived.

This is being confirmed in a Cambridge series where over the last 7 years, the one-stage Syme amputation for diabetic midfoot gangrene or chronic infection has been used with adequate vascularity (API > 40%), with no failure from secondary infection. In comparison with the previous two-stage series, however, the disability period, hospitalization and time to provisional limb fitting was more than halved. A Syme's amputation in one stage is now considered indicated for most unsalvagable foot breakdown lesions extending to the midfoot level and the two-stage procedure reserved only for the severe acutely infected forefoot.

The Syme's amputation stump is very functional with end bearing (Figs. 34.23a,b) and allows an easily donned and doffed prosthesis. The energy requirements are much less in a Syme's amputation walker than in higher levels, this being significant with many diabetics having cardiovascular complications (Waters et al 1976).

The operative technique (see Fig. 34.21) involves an incision from the tip of the lateral malleolus extending transversely across the ankle just below the distal tibia to a point opposite, usually 1 cm below the tip of the medial malleolus. The incision continues vertically down the sides to the sole and transversely across at right angles to the foot. The tendons are divided under tension to retract and vessels ligated. The ankle joint capsule is opened anteriorly with dissection down the sides of the talus to divide the collateral ligaments from the inside. With the aid of a bone hook in the talus first and then the calcaneum, dissection is carried out posteriorly, taking care to protect the neurovascular bundle posteromedially.

a

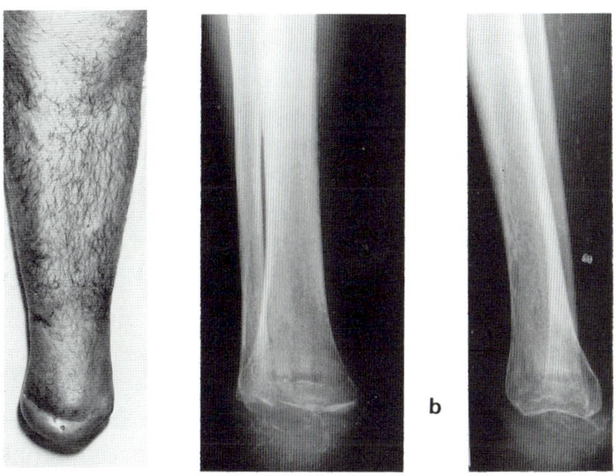

b

Fig. 34.23 Syme's amputation: a, Stable end bearing stump; b, X-Ray showing ankle disarticulation level and malleoli bevelling

The tendo Achillis and posterior attachment of the long plantar ligaments are divided by sharp dissection, but the rest of the os calcis is delivered subperiosteally working from side to side to preserve the pressure tolerant fibrofatty heel pad intact. On reaching the plantar incision level, the amputation is completed cleanly with the Syme's knife. After plantar vessel ligation and nerve division away from the suture line, the malleoli are dissected and excised level with the abraded tibial articular surface. The remaining sharp corners are rounded off with vertical bone resection by approximately 1 cm. Closure in two layers of the periosteum to deep plantar fascia and of the skin with absorbable sutures follows over either an irrigation-drainage tube or antibiotic beads with a non-vacuum overflow drain laterally.

With the two-stage procedure, the wound is closed after the disarticulation, and when healed, 6 to 8 weeks later, the malleoli are resected through lateral incisions. With removal of the drains (5 days) or beads (10 to 14 days), a well moulded synthetic walking below-knee cast is applied and the patient mobilized. Once mature, the Syme prosthesis is fitted.

Grade 5

Once gangrene or severe infection has extended to the hindfoot, then a higher amputation is mandatory. Reassessment of the segmental vascularity pressure index will determine whether the next best level at the below-knee site is possible, or whether a higher through-knee or above-knee amputation is necessary.

RESULTS AND PROGNOSIS

The clinical classification and treatment flow charts were first applied to a group of 151 diabetic foot lesions in 1971–2 (Meggitt 1973, 1976) showing 78% local healing, 16% Syme's amputation salvage and 6% higher amputation in Grades 1, 2 and 3. In Grade 4, 33% were healed locally, 35% with a Syme's and 32% with a higher amputation. With the introduction of the Doppler ankle pressure index selection, a further report from the same centre (Rancho Los Amigos Hospital, USC) showed 93%

successful healing in infected and gangrenous foot lesions (Wagner 1981).

When the Doppler was first used in Cambridge in 1978, its value was uncertain. A study of clinically selected foot lesions for treatment was correlated later with the initial Doppler ankle pressure index. The results (Table 34.1) showed that 75% of foot lesions with API < 40% failed initially; two patients in the critical ischaemia range did heal their Syme's but with cold poor quality stumps with one breakdown at 11 months and the other patient dying of a cardiopathy at 6 months. Only 3% with API > 40% required a higher amputation. Thus the Doppler API was shown to be a reliable guide to selection for foot healing.

The results of a further investigation from 1983 are shown (Table 34.2) using API > 40% for the hind and midfoot and toe pressures > 30 mmHg for the forefoot as treatment selection guides. Thus 70% were healed locally, 23% with a partial foot amputation and only 2% required a higher amputation in Grades 1, 2 and 3. In Grade 4, healing occurred locally in 46%, with a partial foot amputation in 46% and with a higher amputation in 8%.

Thus the Clinical Grading Classification, the Doppler vascular assessment and the treatment flow charts are shown to provide a functional framework for management of the diabetic foot breakdown lesions.

Table 34.1 Diabetic foot treatment results: clinical vs retrospective API

Lesion grade No. Feet (failures)	1-2-3 58	4 17	Total 75	Healed %
API > 60%	37(1)	8(0)	45(1)	98
API 40–60%	17(0)	3(1)	20(1)	95
API < 40%	4(4)	6(4)**	10(8)**	20

**2 Syme's API 38% and 35% healed with one failed later

The diabetic vasculopathy is a progressive disease and the problem of further breakdown must be considered. Longer term follow-up reports, however, indicate that once healed, only between 4 and 10% required a revision amputation within 1 to 10 years with an average of 4½ years with partial foot amputations (Larsson & Anderssen 1978). The contralateral limb remains at risk and must be fully assessed and treated at the same time as the presenting foot breakdown. The earlier prognosis for the contralateral limb amputation in a large series of unilateral amputees has been recorded as between 20 to 30% after 3 years (Baddeley & Fulford 1965, Mazet 1967), but does represent the more severe groups.

The longevity prognosis in this group of diabetic patients with partial foot amputations, has received little reports in the literature. Higher amputations, however, perhaps indicating more generalized vascular disease, with 'in hospital' and '3 month' mortalities following surgery in a large recent series has ranged from 9% to 16% (Ebskov & Josephsen 1980). In the same report, the mortality after 4 years was recorded as 22%. This does not agree with the previous suggestions that diabetic patients have more risk for their life than for their other limb.

The future of the diabetic life and limbs, however, must depend upon the elucidation of the basic pathology of the metabolic derangement and complications. Until then, treatment of the diabetic foot syndrome remains essentially empirical. It depends upon an efficient health care system to provide early detection and prophylaxis, improved assessment and treatment of the breakdown lesions and effective rehabilitation to return the patient to the optimum functional level.

Table 34.2 Results of diabetic foot treatment with API > 40%

Lesion grade	Total feet (No.)	Healed locally (%)	Trans MT Lisfranc (%)	Syme's %	Higher amputation (%)
1-2-3	47	75	11	12	2
4	20	46	21	25	8

REFERENCES

Alldredge R H, Thompson T C 1946 The technique of the Syme amputation. J Bone Joint Surg 28: 415–436
Asbury A K, Johnson P C, Bennington J L (eds) 1978 Diabetic neuropathies. In: Pathology of peripheral nerves Vol 9: Major problems in pathology. W B Saunders Co, Philadelphia
Axtine S G 1982 Infection and diabetes mellitus. In: Bressler R, Johnson D J (eds) Management of diabetes mellitus. Wright, Bristol. Ch 9, p 175
Baddeley R M, Fulford J C 1965 A trial of conservative amputations for lesions of the feet in diabetes mellitus. Br J Surg 52: 38
Baker G C W, Stableforth P G 1969 Syme's amputation. A review of sixty seven cases. J Bone Joint Surg 518: 482–487
Baker J D, Dix D 1981 Variability of Doppler ankle pressures with occlusive disease: An evaluation of ankle index and brachial-ankle pressure gradient. Surgery 89: 134
Barnes R W, Thornhill B, Nix L, Rittgers S E, Turley G 1981 Prediction of amputation wound healing. Roles of Doppler ultrasound and digit photoplethysmography. Arch Surg 116: 80
Bessman A N, Wagner F W 1975 Non-clostridial gas gangrene: report of 48 cases and review of the literature. JAMA 23: 958
Betts R P, Franks C I, Duckworth T, Burke J 1980 Static and dynamic foot pressure measurement in clinical orthopaedics. Med Biol Eng Comput 18 (5): 674
Bloom S, Till S, Sönksen P, Smith S 1984 Use of biothesiometer to measure individual vibration thresholds and their variation in 519 non-diabetic subjects. Br Med J 288: 1793
Boehm J J 1962 Diabetic Charcot's joint. N Engl J Med 267: 185
Bose K 1979 A surgical approach for the infected diabetic foot. Int Orthop 3: 177
Carter S A 1973 The relationship of distal systolic pressures to healing of skin lesions in limbs with arterial occlusive disease with special reference to diabetes mellitus. Scand J Chir Lab Invest 31 Suppl 128: 239
Charcot J M 1868 Sur quelques arthropathies qui paraissent d'une lesion du cerveau ou de la moelle épinière. Archives de Physiologie Normale et Pathologique 1: 161
Cofield R H, Morrison M J, Beabout J W 1983 Diabetic neuropathy in the foot: patient characteristics and patterns of radiographic change. Foot Ankle 4: 15
Cowell J A, Lopes-Vivella M, Halushka P V 1981 Pathogenesis of atherosclerosis in diabetes mellitus. Diabetes Care 4: 121
Dale G M 1961 Syme's amputation for gangrene for peripheral vascular disease. Artif Limbs 6: 44
Dearfield J E, Daggett P R, Harrison M J G 1980 The role of autonomic neuropathy in diabetic foot ulceration. J Neurol Sci 47: 203
DHSS Amputation Statistics for England, Wales and N Ireland 1974–1984
DHSS Amputation Statistics for England, Wales and N Ireland 1983
Dolkart R E, Halpern B, Perlman J 1971 Comparison of antibody responses in normal and alloxan diabetic mice. Diabetes 20: 162
Ebskov B, Josephsen P 1980 Incidence of reamputation and death after gangrene of the lower extremity. Prosthet Orthot Int 4: 77
Eliasson S G 1983 Neuropathy and the diabetic foot. In: Levin M A, O'Neal L W (eds) The Diabetic Foot, 3rd edn. Mosby, St. Louis, Ch 2, p 76
Fagerberg S E 1959 Diabetic neuropathy, a clinical and histological study on the significance of vascular affectations. Acta Med Scand 164: Supp 345
Ferrier T M 1965 Vascular lesions in diabetes. Br Med J 2: 819
Fierer J, Daniel D, Davis C 1979 The fetid foot: lower extremity infections in patients with diabetes mellitus. Rev Infect Dis 1: 210
Ganda O P 1980 Pathogenesis of neurovascular disease in the human diabetic. Diabetes 29: 931
Goldstein J L, Brown M S 1982 Lipoprotein receptors: genetic defence against atherosclerosis. Clin Res 30: 417
Gregersen G 1967 Diabetic neuropathy: influence of age, sex, metabolic control and duration of diabetes on motor conduction velocity. Neurology 17: 972
Haimovici H, Shapiro J H, Jacobson H G 1960 Serial femoral arteriography in occlusive disease. Am J Roentgenol Radium Ther Nucl Med 83: 1042
Harris R I 1956 Syme's amputation. The technical details essential for success. J Bone Joint Surg 38B: 614–632
Harris R I 1961 The history and development of Syme's amputation. Artif Limbs 6: 4
Heiple K G, Cammarn M R 1966 Diabetic neuropathy with spontaneous peritalar fracture dislocation. J Bone Joint Surg 48A: 1177–1181
Hockaday T D R, Hilson R M, Smith B 1982 Correlates of deterioration in pedal vibration sensory threshold over 5 years from diagnosis of maturity onset diabetic patients. Diabetologica 23: 174
Hodgson J R, Pugh D G, Young H H 1948 Roentgenologic aspects of certain lesions of bone: neuropathic or infections? Radiology 50: 65
Holstein P, Naer I, Tonnesen K H, Sager P 1978 Distal blood pressure in severe arterial insufficiency. In: Bergan J J, Yao J S T (eds) Gangrene and severe ischaemia of the lower extremities. Grune & Stratton, New York, Ch 5
Hulnick A, Highsmith C, Boutin F J 1949 Amputations for failure in reconstructive surgery. J Bone Joint Surg 31A: 639
Johnson J T H 1967 Neuropathic fractures and joint injuries: pathogenesis and rationale of prevention and treatment. J Bone Joint Surg 49A: 1
Jordan W R 1936 Neuritic manifestations in diabetes mellitus. Arch Intern Med 57: 307–66
Kelly P J, Coventry M B 1958 Neurotrophic ulcers of the feet: review of 47 cases. JAMA 168: 388
Kilo C, Vogler N J, Williamson J R 1972 Muscle capillary basement membrane changes related to ageing and to diabetes mellitus. Diabetes 21: 881
Kozak G P, Rowbotham J L 1984 Diabetic foot disease: a major problem. In: Kozak G P et al (eds) Management of diabetic foot problems. W B Saunders Co, Philadelphia. Ch 1, p 3
Larsson U, Andesson G 1978 Partial amputation of the foot for diabetic or arteriosclerotic gangrene. J Bont Joint Surg 60B: 125
Lipcomb H, Dobson H L, Greene J A 1959 Infection in the diabetic. South Med J 52: 16–23
Lopes-Vivella M F, Sherer G K, Lees A M et al 1982 Surface binding, internalisation and degradation by cultured human fibroblasts of low density lipoprotein isolated from type 1 (insulin dependent) diabetic patients: changes with metabolic control. Diabetologica 22: 430
Louie T J, Bartlet J G, Tally F P, Gorbach S L 1976 Aerobic and anaerobic bacteria in diabetic foot ulcers. Ann Intern Med 85: 461

Margo M K 1967 Surgical treatment of conditions of the forepart of the foot. J Bone Joint Surg 49A: 1665
Mazet R 1967 The geriatric amputee. Artif Limbs 11: 33
Mazet R 1968 Syme's amputation. J Bone Joint Surg 50A: 1549
McKittrick L S, McKittrick J B, Risley J S 1949 Transmetatarsal amputation for infection or gangrene in patients with diabetes mellitus. Ann Surg 130: 826–842
Meade J W, Mueller C B 1968 Major infections of the foot. Med Times 96: 154
Meggitt B F 1972 Orthopaedic management of diabetic foot breakdown: classification and local treatment framework for preventative leg amputations, Orthop Seminars — Los Angeles County University, S California 5: 311
Meggitt B F 1973 Orthopaedic management of foot breakdown in the diabetic patient. J Bone Joint Surg 55B: 882
Meggitt B F 1976 Surgical management of the diabetic foot. Brit J Hosp Med 16: 227
Mulder D W, Lambert E H, Bastron J A 1961 The neuropathies associated with diabetes mellitus. A clinical and electromyographic study of 103 unselected diabetic patients. Neurology 11: 275
Newman J H 1979 Spontaneous dislocation in diabetic neuropathy. J Bone Joint Surg 61B: 484
Oakley W 1954 Diabetes in surgery. Ann Royal Coll Surgeons 15: 108
Pratt T C 1965 Gangrene and infection in the diabetic. Med Clin N Amer 49: 987
Quin R O, Evans D H, Fyfe T 1977 Evaluation of indirect blood pressure measurement as a method of assessment of peripheral vascular disease. J Cardiovasc Surg 18: 109
Raff M C, Asbury A K 1970 Ischaemic mononeuropathy and mononeuropathy multiplex in diabetic mellitus. N Engl J Med 279: 17
Raff M C, Sangalong V, Asbury A K 1968 Ischaemic mononeuropathy multiplex associated with diabetes mellitus. Arch Neurol 18: 487
Reckless J P, Betteridge D J, Wu P 1978 High density and low density lipoproteins and prevalence of vascular disease in diabetes mellitus. Br Med J I: 883
Ross R 1981 Atherosclerosis: a problem of the biology of the arterial wall cells and their interaction with blood components. Atherosclerosis 1: 293
Schwartz G S, Berenyi M R, Siegel M W 1969 Atrophic arthropathy and diabetic neuritis. Am J Roentgenol 106: 523–529
Sibley W A 1982 The neuropathies of diabetes mellitus. In: Bressler R, Johnson D G (eds) Management of diabetes mellitus. Wright, Bristol. Ch 12, p 251
Singer A, Rossi G 1968 Radical local surgery in diabetic gangrene. J Mt Sinai Hosp NY 35: 390
Siperstein M D, Unger R H, Madison L L 1968 Studies of muscle capillary basement membranes in normal subjects, diabetic and prediabetic patients. J Clin Invest 47: 1973
Spittler A W, Brennan J J, Payne J W 1954 Syme amputation performed in two stages. J Bone Joint Surg 36A: 37
Stokes I A F, Faris I B, Hutton W C 1975 The neuropathic ulcer and loads on the foot in diabetic patients. Acta Orthop Scand 46: 839
Strandness D E, Priest R E, Gibbons G E 1964 Combined clinical and pathologic study of diabetic and non diabetic peripheral arterial disease. Diabetes 13: 366
Syme J 1843 Amputation at the ankle joint. Lond Edinb Monthly J Med Sci 3: 93
Thomas P K, Lascelles R C 1966 The pathology of diabetic neuropathy. Q J Med 35: 489
Trap-Jensen J 1971 Permeability of small vessels in diabetes. In: Lundback K, Keen H (eds) Blood vessel disease in diabetes. The Publishing House 'Il Ponte', Milano. Acta Diabetol Cat 8 Suppl I: 192
Wagner F W 1979 A classification and treatment program for diabetic, neuropathic and dysvascular foot problems. In: The American Academy of Orthopaedic Surgeons Instructional Course Lectures 28, C V Mosby Co, St Louis. p. 143
Wagner F W 1981 The dysvascular foot: a system for diagnosis and treatment. Foot Ankle 2: 64
Wagner F W, Buggs H 1978 Use of Doppler ultrasound in determining healing levels in diabetic dysvascular lower extremity problems. In: Bergan J J, Yao J S T (eds) Gangrene and severe ischaemia of the lower extremities. Grune and Stratton, New York p. 131
Wagner F W, Russ J, Webb J, Buggs H 1980 Syme's amputation of the diabetic foot: results utilising preoperative Doppler evaluation. In: Bateman J E, Trott A W (eds) The Foot and Ankle. Brian C Decker, New York. Ch 15, p. 127–130
Wahlig H, Dingelden E, Bergmann R, Reuss K 1978 The release of gentamicin from polymethylmethacrylate beads. J Bone Joint Surg 60B: 270
Waldvogel F A, Medoff G, Swartz M N 1970 Osteomyelitis: a review of clinical features, therapeutic considerations and unusual aspects. N Engl J Med 282: 198
Warren R, Thayer T R, Achenbach H, Kendall L G 1955 The Syme amputation in peripheral vascular arterial disease. Surgery 37: 156
Warren S, Le Compte P M, Legg M A (eds) 1966 The pathology of diabetes mellitus, 4th edn. Lea and Febiger, Philadelphia. Ch 4
Waters R L, Perry J, Antonelli D, Hislop H 1976 Energy cost of walking of amputees. The influence of level of amputation. J Bone Joint Surg 58A: 42
Wheelock F C 1961 Transmetatarsal amputations and arterial surgery on diabetic patients. N Engl J Med 264: 316–320
Whitehouse F W 1978 On diabetic osteopathy: a radiographic study of 21 patients. Diabetes care I (5): 303
Wilens S L 1951 The nature of diffuse intimal thickening of arteries. Am J Pathol 27: 825
Yamagata S, Yamauchi Y 1969 Diabetic neuropathy and triopathy. Diabetes: Proceeding of the Sixth Congress of the International Diabetes Federation, Stockholm, Amsterdam. Excerpta Medica Foundation
Yao J S T 1970 Haemodynamic studies in peripheral vascular disease. Br J Surg 57: 761

P. A. Revell and B. C. Sommerlad

Tumours

In this chapter, tumours and tumour-like conditions have been divided into those that appear to arise from the skin or immediately subcutaneous tissue, those that arise from soft tissue (excluding synovium), those which may arise from synovial tissue or at least show synovial characteristics, and those which arise from bone. The divisions may not be clear-cut as the tissue of origin of some tumours is uncertain and as tumours may spread to involve adjacent tissue.

SKIN

The skin of the foot is prone to most of the tumours and tumour-like conditions occurring elsewhere in the body. However, the skin of the sole is histologically different from that of the dorsum, having profuse eccrine glands, no sebaceous glands, very thick stratum corneum and no hair. This gives a guide as to the sort of tumours which occur at each site. Disorders of the skin of the foot may be part of a generalized disease.

Many of these conditions will be dealt with later (Chapter 38). Only the common and important tumours will be discussed here (Table 35.1).

Diagnosis

Diagnosis first depends on an adequate history. The duration of the lesion is all-important and change in a previously quiescent lesion should be viewed with suspicion. A history of previous trauma may be important but may be a 'red herring'. A search should always be made for similar swellings elsewhere, with particular care being taken to examine the other foot.

Examination, by demonstrating mobility on deep tissues, should confirm that the tumour arises from the skin. Variation of colour in a pigmented lesion may be important. Ulceration of a skin tumour may indicate malignancy, especially if the margins are raised and indurated. Examination of popliteal and groin lymph nodes should be routine.

If doubt about the diagnosis remains, excision biopsy (if the lesion is small) or incision biopsy (if large) is indicated.

Table 35.1 Tumours and tumour-like conditions of skin

Congenital	Haemangioma
	Lymphangioma
	Neurofibromatosis
	Hamartoma
Traumatic	Keratoses—callosities and corns
	Inclusion dermoid cysts
Infective	Pyogenic granuloma
	Warts
	Specific infections (tuberculosis, mycoses, leprosy and yaws)
'Degenerative' and miscellaneous	
	Sarcoidosis
	Epidermal cysts
	Granuloma annulare
Neoplastic	Benign fibrous histiocytoma
	Acquired digital fibrokeratoma
	Sweat gland tumours
	Basal cell carcinoma
	Squamous cell carcinoma
	Malignant melanoma
	Kaposi's sarcoma
	Dermatofibrosarcoma protruberans
	Deep tumours which may present in the skin

General principles of management

Because of the tendency of the sole of the foot to produce hyperkeratotic, fissured scars, and of the dorsum of the foot to produce scars which rub on footwear, unnecessary operations must be avoided. Especially on the weight-bearing sole, a benign lesion, which will respond to nonsurgical measures such as cryotherapy, should not be surgically excised.

Where surgical excision is necessary on the weight-bearing sole, the aims should be to produce as little scar as possible on and adjacent to the weight-bearing area, to preserve as much subcutaneous fat as possible, to leave fibrous attachments to bone as undisturbed as possible and to preserve sensation.

Unfortunately, there is little spare skin on the dorsum of the foot and still less on the sole. Removal of a tumour therefore frequently necessitates skin replacement. Split skin grafts may be satisfactory on the dorsum and on non-weightbearing areas of the sole. Grafts on weight-bearing sole tend to be protected by the patient by alteration of gait, if possible (Sommerlad & McGrouther 1978), this being more easily achieved on the heel than on the forefoot (Fig. 35.1). Random local skin flaps and muscle flaps (Ger 1975) are useful in certain situations. Distant flaps, lacking the specialized skin and subcutaneous tissue of the sole, are best avoided if possible. Neurovascular island flaps from toes which are to be amputated or from web spaces, may be useful for small defects. The instep flap, based on the medial plantar nerves and vessels (Shanahan & Gingrass 1979, Harrison & Morgan 1981) may be used either as an ipsilateral island pedicled flap, a contralateral pedicled flap (requiring subsequent division) or as a free microvascular flap. This may be the most suitable form of reconstruction for a significant area of weight-bearing sole.

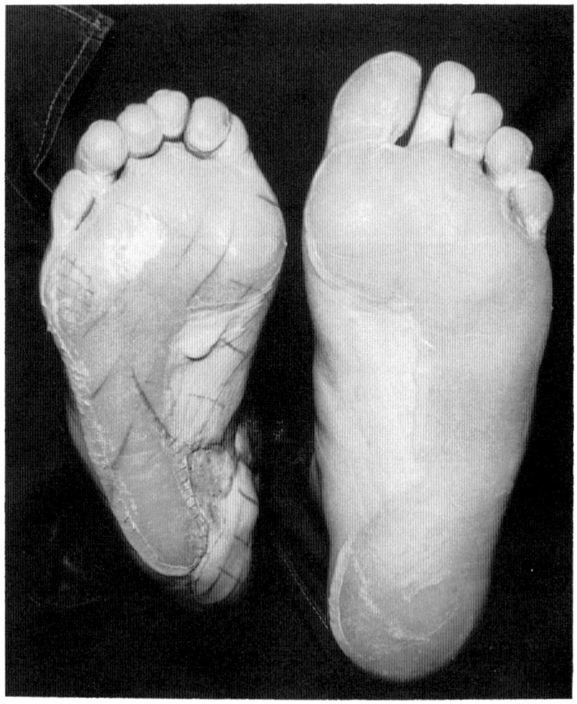

Fig. 35.1 Demonstration of weight-bearing patterns (by asking the patient to walk on coloured paint) show that a skin graft used for heel cover does not actually take weight and is avoided by the patient

Common tumours and tumour-like conditions of skin

Traumatic

Keratoses, callosities and corns. The skin of the sole of the foot responds to abnormality within or abnormal pressure without, by excessive production of keratin (Jahss 1982) (Fig. 35.2). In callus, the parakeratin is relatively diffuse; in corns, there is a localized central core of keratin. Pressure of callus may produce underlying necrosis or adjacent fissuring (especially in vulnerable patients such as diabetics). Treatment consists of shaving and paring and subsequent avoidance of pressure by modification of footwear.

Inclusion dermoid cysts. The absence of a relevant history does not exclude penetration by a foreign

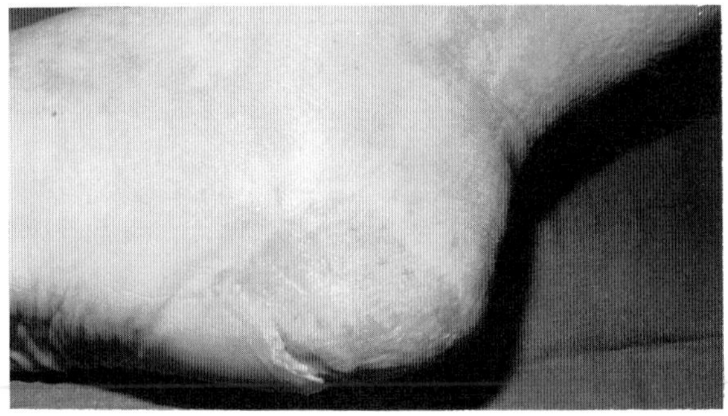

Fig. 35.2 Hyperkeratosis of the sole adjacent to a split skin graft over the heel (with fissuring)

body and the diagnosis should always be considered when there is an intradermal or subcutaneous swelling (Rowley et al 1978). Soft tissue penetration X-rays may show the offending foreign body. Treatment consists of excision of the entire cyst with its foreign body (if present).

Infective

Pyogenic granuloma. The pyogenic granuloma may follow recognized injury. It is usually red, partly compressible, may or may not be ulcerated or crusted and tends to bleed with minor trauma (Berlin et al 1972). Histologically, the lesion looks like chronic granulation tissue containing many capillaries, simulating a capillary haemangioma. Curettage and diathermy is usually the first line of treatment, although recurrence is not uncommon.

Warts. Warts are discussed in Chapter 38. The surgeon may see them when excessive keratin formation may suggest a neoplasm or underlying foreign body. He must resist all requests to excise them, because the disease is self-limiting, better treated by less radical means and the scar resulting from excision is likely to be a permanent source of trouble from hyperkeratosis and fissuring (Fig. 35.3).

Specific infection. Infections such as tuberculosis, mycoses, leprosy, sarcoidosis and yaws, are discussed elsewhere, but may be mistaken for tumours.

'Degenerative' and miscellaneous

Epidermoid cysts. Epidermoid cysts can occur on the dorsum of the foot, where they are not common but may occasionally be large.

Granuloma annulare. This condition may be mistaken for a basal cell carcinoma. It occurs commonly on the dorsum where it usually presents as a raised, reddish lesion, often in the form of a doughnut and sometimes composed of discrete papules. No treatment is necessary if the diagnosis is made, as the lesion will almost certainly regress spontaneously.

Neoplastic

Benign fibrous histiocytoma (dermatofibroma or sclerosing haemangioma). The fibrous histiocytoma or dermatofibroma is a benign tumour, presenting usually as a small, firm reddish brown and sometimes almost green, painless nodule in the skin. It may be single or multiple and the extremities of adults are most commonly affected. Fibrous histiocytoma is rare on the soles of the feet (Bedi et al 1976) but does occur (Fig. 35.4).

Occasionally these lesions are darker coloured or black, due to heavy deposition of haemosiderin, and under these conditions there may be clinical confusion with malignant melanoma. A firm consistency and the presence of a central dimple on lateral compression is a useful clinical sign in making the distinction from melanoma (Fitzpatrick & Gilchrest 1977). The fibrous histiocytoma may occasionally be more deeply situated in the soft tissue of the extremities, again usually in young adults. They are yellow or white, well circumscribed masses on naked eye examination.

Histological examination shows that the fibrous histiocytoma is made up of fibroblasts, histiocytes, capillaries and young or mature collagen in varying proportion. The exact name used by the pathologist may vary according to the appearance and sclerosing haemangioma is considered to be the same type of lesion as fibrous histiocytoma (Gross & Wolbach 1943). Many now prefer to use the term fibrous histiocytoma regardless of the particular features present in a given lesion (Enzinger & Weiss 1983).

The collagen fibres in these tumours are typically arranged in an intertwined mat-like or 'storiform' pattern, or radiate from a central point in a whorled arrangement. Hyperplasia of the overlying epidermis occurs in over 80% of fibrous histiocytomas (Schoenfeld 1964).

In most cases, a definite clinical diagnosis can be made and no treatment is required unless the lesion is large or causing discomfort. On occasions, a benign fibrous histiocytoma may extend to several centimetres in diameter, arousing suspicion of malignancy which is not confirmed by histological examination.

Acquired digital fibrokeratoma. Acquired digital fibrokeratoma is a benign tumour, occurring at any age, but predominantly in middle-aged men. It is a typically solitary sessile or pedunculated lesion, found usually on a toe, though occasionally on the sole of the foot (Verallo 1968) and may be present for

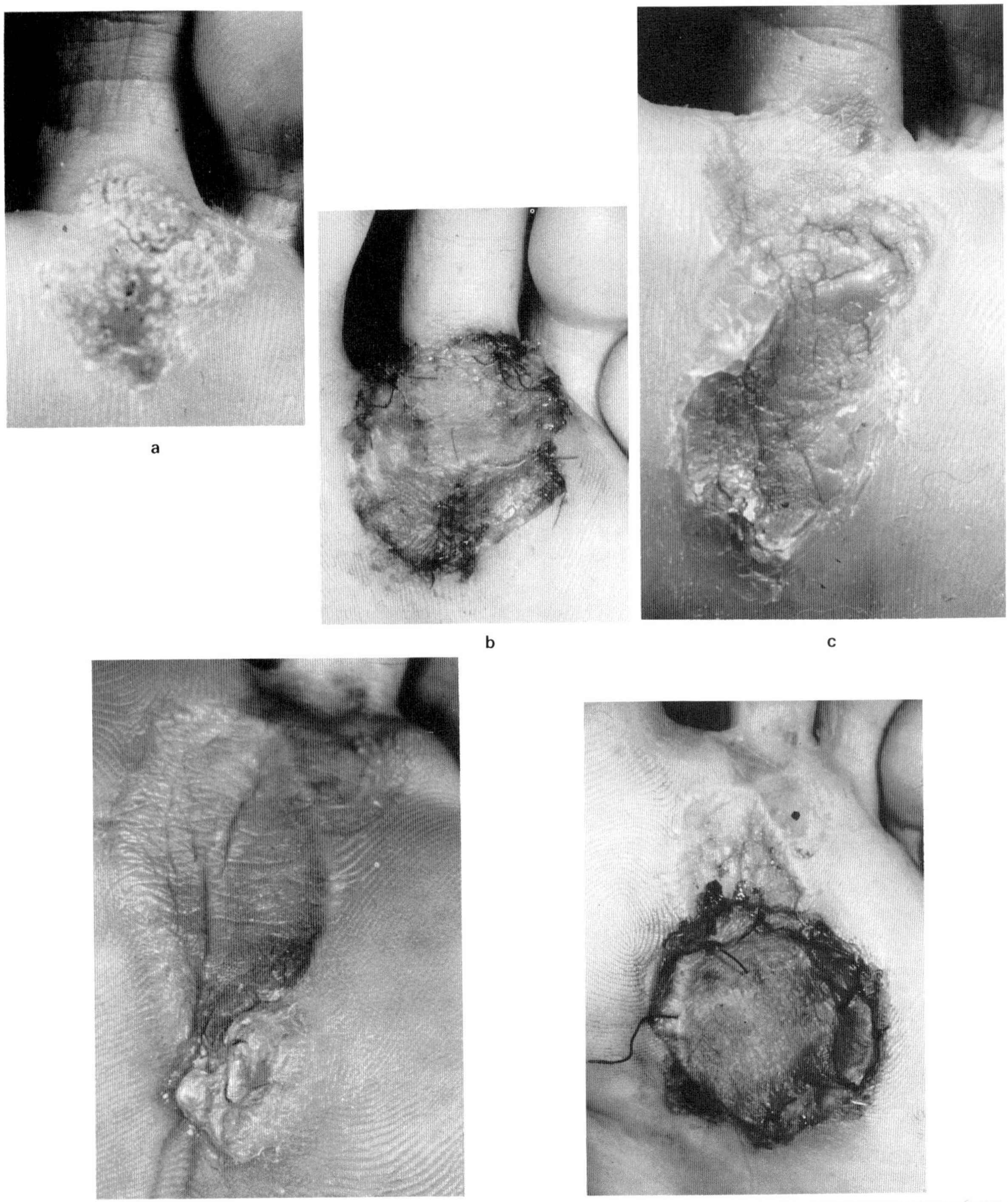

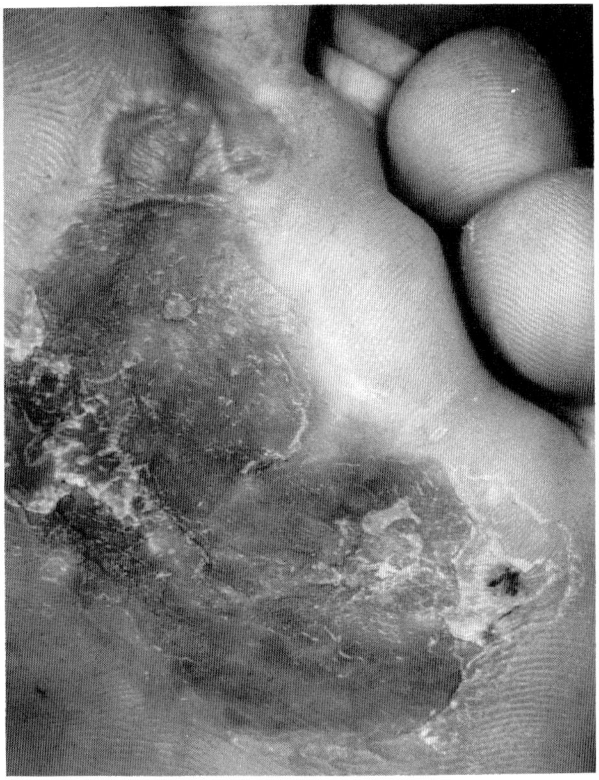

f

Fig. 35.3 (a) Resistant plantar warts; (b) Treated by excision and graft; (c) Fissuring at the margin of the graft; (d) Increasing hyperakeratosis at the margin of the graft; (e) Wider excision and graft; (f) The most recent appearance following still further excision. This demonstrates that excision of the skin of the sole of the foot must be a last resort. Split skin grafts on weight-bearing sole (particularly the forefoot) are totally unsatisfactory

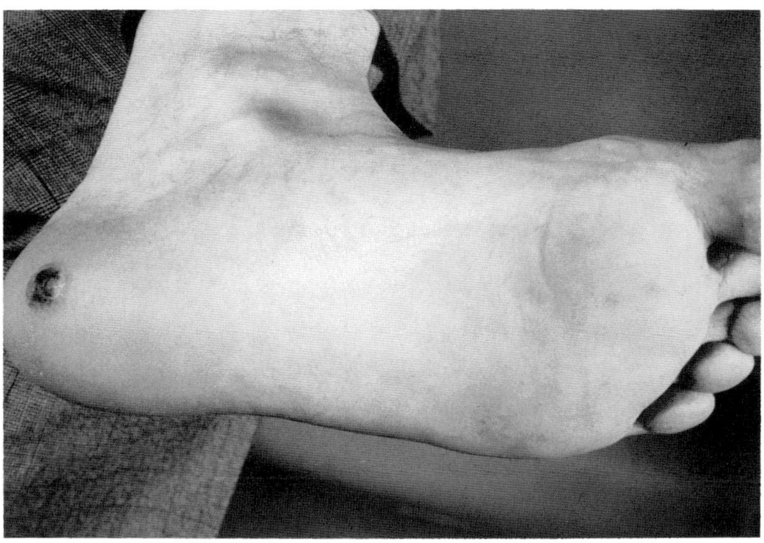

a

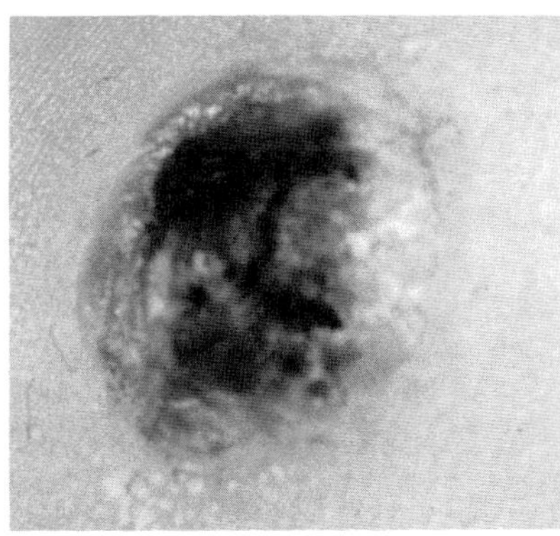

b

Fig. 35.4 A histiocytoma (dermatofibroma) of the sole of the foot: (a) Postion; (b) Close-up — a rare condition months or years before the patient seeks medical advice.

Histology reveals hyperkeratosis and acanthosis of the epidermis with thickened branching rete ridges, which cover a vertically arranged core of thick interwoven collagen bundles in which there are variable numbers of elastic fibres (Lever & Schaumberg-Lever 1983, Bart et al 1968, Hare & Smith 1969). The lesion may resemble a rudimentary supernumerary digit clinically, but is readily distinguished on pathological examination. More detailed accounts are available elsewhere (Verallo 1968, Bart et al 1968, Hare & Smith 1969, Hemric & Allen 1979). Treatment is by curettage and cautery or local excision.

Sweat gland tumours. Because of the high density of eccrine glands on the sole of the foot, one might expect a relatively high incidence of sweat gland tumours, but few have been reported (Forman & Streigold 1982). The eccrine poroma is the most common. It presents as a red swelling on the sole. Histopathological examination shows ducts traversing solid masses of basophilic tumour cells extending into the dermis. Treatment is by local excision.

Malignant sweat gland tumours are extremely rare in the foot.

Basal cell carcinoma. The ubiquitous basal cell carcinoma in fact occurs very rarely on the foot (Kurzer & Patel 1979). It occasionally occurs on the dorsum of the foot or ankle, either as a typical raised, pearly 'cystic' lesion or, more commonly, as a crusted and somewhat indurated lesion which may well be disregarded by the patient for some time. Basal cell carcinoma of the sole is rare but not unknown (Robinson 1979). Treatment involves excision, usually with split skin grafting.

Squamous cell carcinoma. The typical, low-grade, actinic squamous cell carcinoma may occur on the dorsum of the foot where treatment consists of excision and grafting. The sole of the foot is one of the more common sites of the verrucous carcinoma or epithelioma cuniculatum (Seehafer et al 1979, Schwartz & Burgess 1980). These are proliferative lesions, sometimes looking rather warty or friable. They are often foul-smelling. Not all squamous cell carcinomata of the sole of the foot are of this histological type (Fig. 35.5). Wide local excision is indicated (Demuth & Snider 1980) and reconstruction may be difficult, requiring specialized flaps. Lymph node metastases are not uncommon.

Subungual squamous cell carcinoma occurs occasionally on the toes and is often diagnosed late. Distal amputation is indicated.

Malignant melanoma. The foot is a relatively common site for this potentially lethal tumour (Sondergaard & Olsen 1980), the incidence on the sole and dorsum being approximately equal. Malignant melanoma of the foot has been well reviewed recently (Fuselier et al 1985).

Lentigo maligna may occur on the dorsum of the foot, presents as a flat brown to black lesion with irregular margins, and may progress from a superficial noninvasive lesion to invasive nodular melanoma. Histopathological examination reveals intraepidermal pleomorphic melanocytes, these cells varying from near normality to extreme abnormality.

Superficial spreading malignant melanoma presents as a flat or slightly raised pigmented lesion which may vary in colour from black or brown to tan, red, white or even bluish (Fig. 35.6). Histopathological examination shows atypical melanocytes arranged singly or in nests within the dermis. There may be lateral extension in the epidermis and dermal invasion in irregular cords and nests. The superficial spreading malignant melanoma may enter an invasive nodular phase (Fig. 35.7). The level of dermal invasion can be classified according to Clark's level (Clark 1969) and the depth measured in millimetres from the granular cell layer of the epidermis to the depth of the tumour (Breslow 1970).

True nodular melanoma occurs as a nodule, usually uniform dark brown or black in colour. Histologically, it is characterized by direct invasion into the dermis wherever intraepidermal tumour exists.

The acral lentiginous melanoma occurs in the foot as a plantar or subungual tumour (occurring also on the hand or on mucosal surfaces). Initially, it presents as a flat, irregular, brown or black lesion. Later it may become more raised and palpable (Fig. 35.8).

Histopathological examination demonstrates large pleomorphic melanocytes in the basal layer. In early lesions, the cells have large nuclei and prominent long dendrites. In later invasive tumours, the cells may be spindle-shaped and nonpigmented.

Subungual melanoma most commonly affects the

a
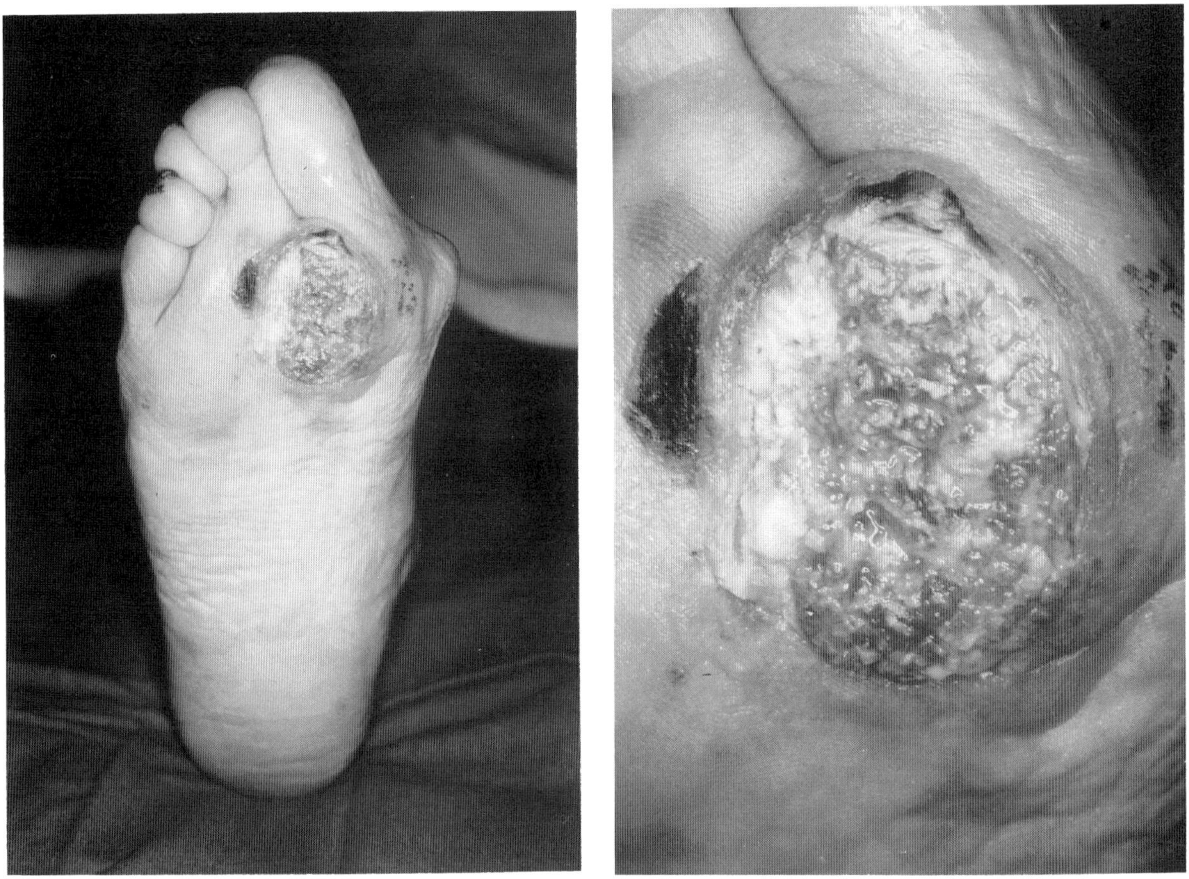
b

Fig. 35.5 A well-differentiated squamous cell carcinoma of the sole of the foot: (a) Position; (b) Close-up

big toe. Initially, it presents as a flat brown or black pigmentation of the matrix, nail bed and perhaps eponychium and paronychium. Later, there may be alteration of the nail bed which may separate.

Surgery remains the mainstay of primary treatment of malignant melanoma. Superficial spreading lesions (less than 0.7 mm in thickness) may be adequately treated by local excision with margins of approximately 1 cm. The greater the nodularity and invasiveness, the wider should be the ideal resection. In the sole of the foot, excision should leave as much weight-bearing subcutaneous tissue and skin as is compatible with adequate clearance. Split skin graft is the usual method of reconstruction (Petersen 1968) but primary flap reconstruction, particularly of the weight-bearing forefoot, may be indicated to maintain a mobile patient. Amputation of the toe, at least at the interphalangeal joint, is indicated for proven subungual melanoma. Radical groin lymph node dissection is accepted as the treatment for clinically involved glands. Prophylactic gland dissection is more controversial. The prognosis of acral lentiginous melanoma of the sole and subungual region appears to be poor (Arrington et al 1977, Feibelman et al 1980, Coleman et al 1981).

Although lower extremity lesions in general carry a good prognosis, malignant melanoma of the foot seems generally to be an exception (Petersen 1968, Keyhani 1977, Day et al 1981).

Kaposi's sarcoma. Kaposi's sarcoma or multiple idiopathic haemorrhagic sarcoma is a condition which has an insidious onset, affects males more often than females and is more common in particular parts of the world such as Eastern Europe and Africa south of the Sahara. There is an association with lymphoma and leukaemia, long-term immunosuppressive treatment and in homosexuals with acquired immunodeficiency syndrome (AIDS) (Cox & Helwig 1959, Reynolds et al 1965, O'Brien & Brasfield 1966, Strachley et al 1975, Harwood et al 1979, Gottlieb et al 1981, Friedman-Kien 1981, Siegal et al 1981).

Lesions most commonly occur first on the legs and feet, commencing on one side, but tending to become bilateral and symmetrical. Kaposi's sarcoma is characterized by the presence of bluish-red or dark brown plaques or nodules particularly on the distal parts of the lower limbs and on the arches and soles of the feet where they may become hyperkeratotic. These plaques may undergo ulceration at a later stage, and there is then often lymphoedema of the lower extremity. The clinical course may be indolent, the local disease alone may be progressive or dissemination may occur. Visceral lesions occur in about 10% of cases (Tedeschi 1958) and involve lymph nodes, gastrointestinal tract, liver, lungs and heart. There is a higher incidence of fatal systemic involvement in sub-Saharan Africans and young

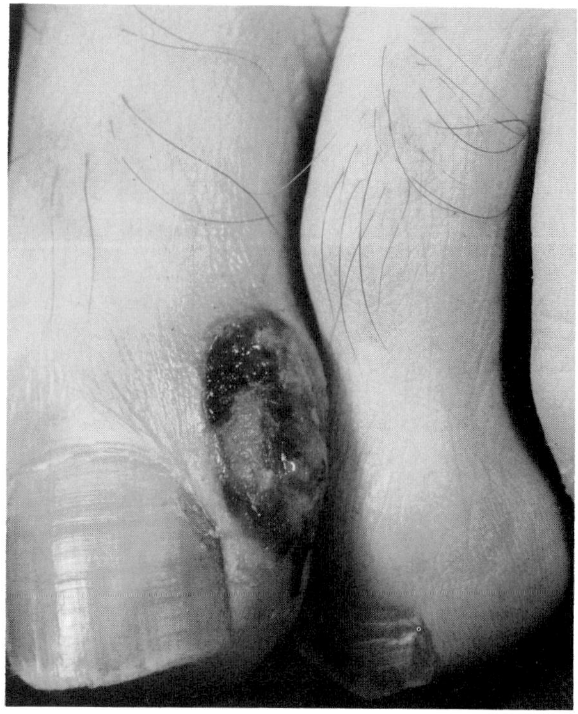

Fig. 35.6 A histologically proven superficial spreading malignant melanoma of the left great toe in a 40-year-old man. Despite a Breslow thickness of 0.9 mm, this patient developed inguinal groin gland metastases and subsequently cerebral metastases. This tends to support the view that malignant melanoma of the foot carries a rather poorer prognosis than elsewhere

a

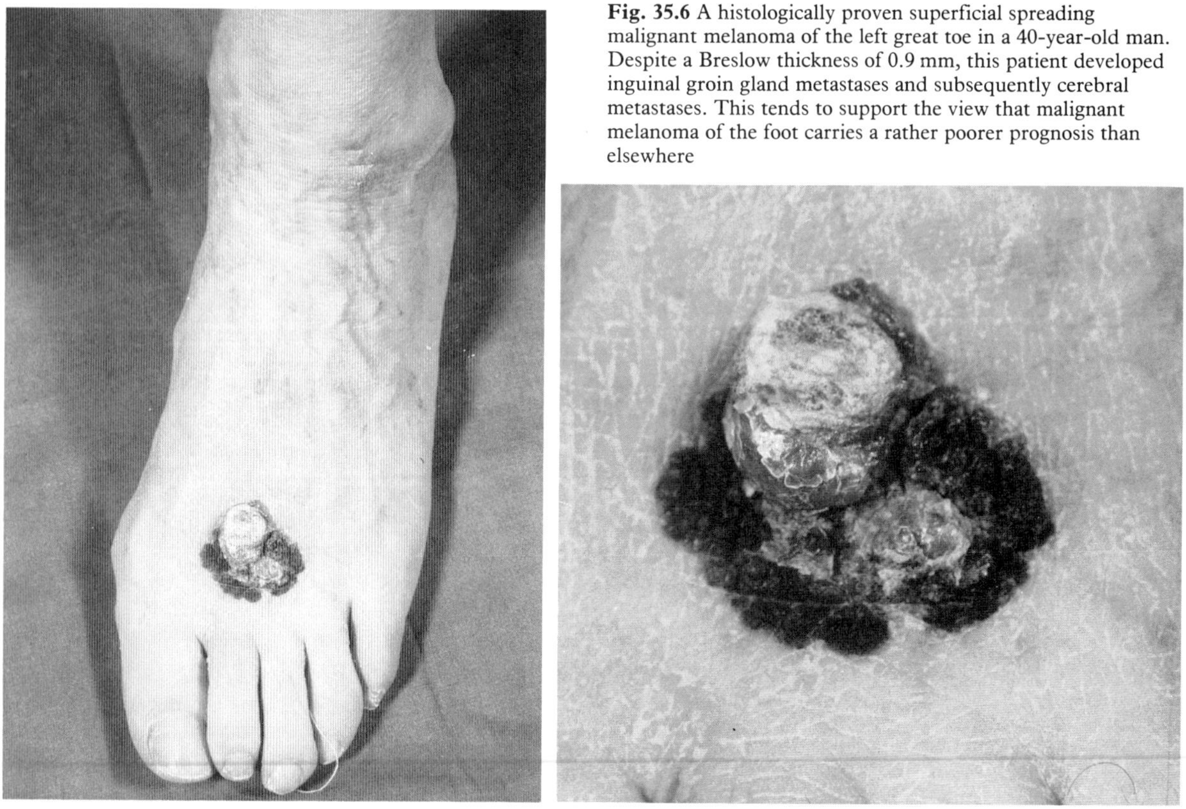

b

Fig. 35.7 A superficial spreading malignant melanoma of the dorsum of the foot with nodule: (a) Position; (b) Close-up

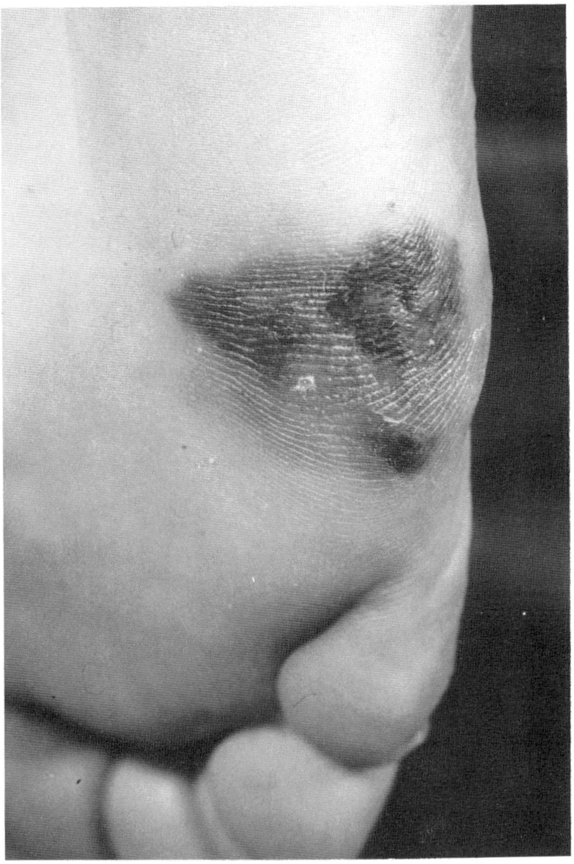

Fig. 35.8 An acral lentiginous melanoma of the sole of the foot

homosexual men in the United States of America (Gottlieb et al 1981, Friedman-Kien 1981).

The clinical differential diagnosis of lesions on the foot comprises a long list of conditions, including pyogenic granuloma, neurofibroma, pemphigus vulgaris, verrucae, lichen planus, psoriatic eruption, hyperkeratotic tinea pedis, glomus tumour, haemangioma, angiosarcoma, foreign body reaction, melanoma, sarcomas of various types and infective conditions such as leprosy, filariasis and maduromycosis (Cargialosi & Schmoll 1976).

Histology shows two types of change; vascular formations with prominent endothelial cells, and spindle cell areas containing vascular slits. The presence of inflammatory cells in early lesions gives an appearance resembling granulation tissue (Lever & Schaumberg-Lever 1983).

Treatment is largely by medical means using radiotherapy and systemic cytotoxic drug therapy. Surgical excision may be useful for small isolated lesions or as a palliative procedure in fungating lesions not responding to other methods of treatment.

Dermatofibrosarcoma protruberans. This tumour may occur in the foot (Sheital et al 1978) where it appears as a raised, firm, irregular, usually dull red swelling within the skin. It may appear to be multinodular and inspection and palpation frequently suggests subcutaneous extension.

Histology shows whorled fibrous tissue with a degree of pleomorphism. Treatment consists of wide local surgical excision, usually with split skin graft. Local recurrence is frequent but distant metastases are rare.

Deep tumours which may present on the skin. Haemangioma, the fibromatoses, glomus tumour, malignant fibrous histiocytoma, epithelioid sarcoma and fibrosarcoma, may all present within the skin. These will be discussed in the next section.

TUMOURS AND TUMOUR-LIKE CONDITIONS OF SOFT TISSUE (EXCLUDING SYNOVIUM)

Some tumours of the foot arise within subcutaneous fat, from plantar aponeurosis, or from blood vessels, tendons and nerves situated more deeply. (Table 35.2). The origin of some tumours is obscure.

Diagnosis

Once again, the duration of the lesion is of major importance. Examination should reveal the depth of the tumour. In this group of conditions, the skin is mobile over the tumour unless it becomes secondarily involved. X-rays confirm lack of skeletal involvement (unless bone, too, is secondarily involved or eroded) and may show an unsuspected deep foreign body. Exploration and biopsy may be the only way to make a final diagnosis.

General principles of management

Management obviously depends on whether the lesion is benign or malignant.

Nonneoplastic swellings (such as haemangiomata and plantar fibromatoses) require surgery only if the diagnosis is uncertain or the condition is causing troublesome symptoms.

Table 35.2 Tumour and tumour-like conditions of soft tissue (excluding synovium)

Congenital	Haemangioma
	Arteriovenous malformation
	Neurofibromatosis
	Hamartoma
Traumatic	Traumatic neuroma
	Traumatic aneurysm
	Deep retained foreign bodies
'Degenerative' and miscellaneous	
	Digital mucous cyst
	Recurrent infantile digital fibroma
	Fibromatoses:
	Cicatrical fibromatosis
	Keloid
	Nodular fasciitis
	Plantar fibromatosis
	Aggressive fibromatosis
	Congenital generalized fibromatosis
Neoplastic	Tumours of fat:
	Lipoma
	Liposarcoma
	Tumours of nerve:
	Neurofibroma
	Neurilemmoma
	Malignant schwannoma
	Tumours of blood vessels
	Capillary haemangioma
	Cavernous haemangioma
	Haemangiopericytoma (benign)
	Glomus tumour
	Angiosarcoma (malignant)
	Haemangiopericytoma (malignant)
	Tumours of fibrous tissue:
	Fibroma
	Fibrosarcoma
	Dermatofibrosarcoma protuberans
	Tumours of doubtful origin:
	Granular cell myoblastoma
	Malignant fibrous histiocytoma
	Epithelioid sarcoma
	Tumour of muscle:
	Leiomyoma
	Leiomyosarcoma
	Rhabdomyosarcoma
	Miscellaneous tumours
	Extraskeletal chondroma or chondrosarcoma
	Clear cell sarcoma of tendons and aponeuroses

Benign neoplasms are generally treated by surgical excision. Wherever possible, incision should avoid weight-bearing areas and weight-bearing plantar subcutaneous fat should be preserved.

Malignant soft tissue tumours, unless radiosensitive, require radical surgery which may mean partial or complete amputation of the foot. The various types of incomplete salvage amputations in the foot will be described in Chapter 61.

Common conditions

Congenital

Haemangioma. Haemangiomas are vascular tumours produced by the proliferation of vessels and considered by many to be hamartomatous malformations rather than true neoplasms. They may be subdivided into various types, including capillary, cavernous, hypertrophic and cirsoid/racemose (Pack & Miller 1950, Stout 1953).

Haemangiomas are the most common tumours of infancy and childhood. They are relatively rare in the foot, where they may occur in skin, subcutaneous tissues, muscle and other soft tissues or bone. However, 142 cases of lower extremity haemangioma involved the foot in the early study of Weaver (Someren & Merritt 1978). A capillary haemangioma is seen as a red, slightly raised skin lesion. A cavernous haemangioma in subcutaneous tissue presents as a palpable mass with poorly defined borders, and there may be oedema and pain (Margileth & Museles 1965). The latter may be due to nerve compression. The soft spongy mass has been described as resembling a 'bag of worms' or like 'spaghetti' by an Italian author (Carnevali 1938). If the lesion is close to the epidermis, there may be local red, brown, blue or purple discolouration of the skin. Such discolouration is not seen with all haemangiomas, particularly those occurring more deeply, and the diagnosis should be borne in mind in cases where there is a localized tumour-like swelling. Pulsation of the lesion is not a frequent feature and is indicative of a high arterial input.

The differential diagnosis includes ganglion and other cystic lesions, lipoma, fibroma, neuroma, haematoma, arteriovenous fistula, pigmented villonodula synovitis and malignant soft tissue tumour (Borden & Shea 1976, Cox 1976, Midenberg & Kirschenbaum 1983).

Pathological examination usually shows a capillary haemangioma to be situated in the dermis but extending into subcutaneous fat and underlying muscles. Histology shows a network of capillary-like vascular channels of variable calibre which may contain blood. The extent of local involvement by haemangioma can be assessed preoperatively by skin temperature studies, plethysmography, venography and arteriography (Watson & McCarthy 1940).

The typical capillary or cavernous haemangioma is noticed some time after birth, increases in size for months (or occasionally years) and then begins to resolve spontaneously. No treatment is indicated unless growth is rapid. If resolution is slow, and preventing the wearing of footwear, the injection of sclerosant, perhaps combined with compression, may be indicated. This must be performed with care, as considerable necrosis can result. Very rarely, surgical excision may be necessary. Vessel ligation or embolization usually produce only temporary improvement, but may be very useful in reducing flow prior to surgery. Surgical excision should be performed under tourniquet with careful bipolar coagulation of divided vessels. Blood loss may still be considerable when the tourniquet is released. Haemangioma may involve muscles, neurovascular bundles and even bone, and complete removal will probably be impossible. However, persistence of a haemangioma beyond the first two to three years suggests a degree of arteriovenous shunting and if arteriovenous shunts can be embolized and excised, the remaining haemangioma may regress.

The management of persisting high-flow haemangiomata may be a difficult problem. The management of haemangioma of the foot is, generally, complicated by the need for a child to begin walking early (Borden & Shea 1976, Cox 1976, Midenberg & Kirschenbaum 1983, Politz 1976, Bernhard et al 1983).

A relatively uncommon related lesion is the angiokeratoma circumscriptum which may occur on the foot (Fig. 35.9) and which frequently occurs following wide excision and skin grafting. The Argon laser may be useful in this condition.

Arteriovenous malformations. Although many haemangiomata have a degree of arteriovenous shunting, when such shunts are multiple they may cause gigantism of the limb and even high output cardiac failure. There may be capillary haemangiomatous involvement of the skin, dilated veins, obvious temperature increase and possibly thrills or bruits at the site of large shunts. Embolization offers the best chance of control.

Neurofibromatosis (von Recklinghausen's disease). Neurofibromatosis is inherited as an autosomally dominant trait with an incidence of around 1:3000 live births. Clinically, it is divisible into peripheral and central forms, overlap between which is minimal in any individual kinship. It is the peripheral form of the disease which is important in considerations of foot involvement.

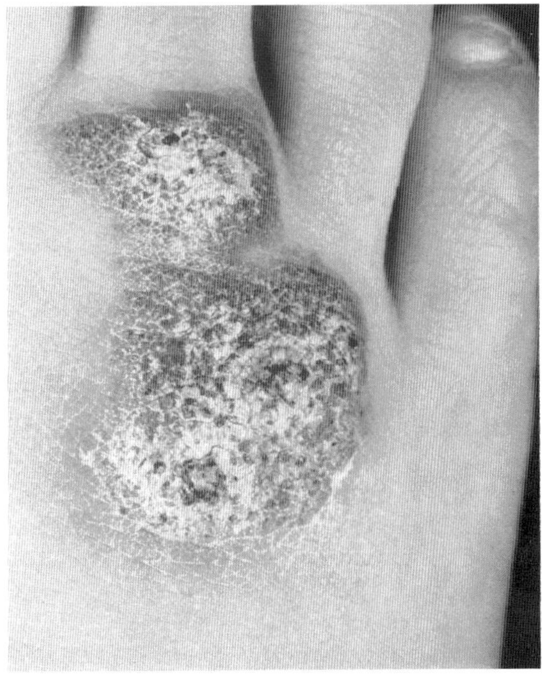

Fig. 35.9 Angiokeratoma circumscriptum of the dorsum of the foot

The clinical manifestations include the presence of macular pigmented lesions resembling freckles, called 'cafe au lait' spots which are present early in life and become more numerous with increasing age.

Neurofibromas usually begin to appear in childhood or adolescence and are slowly growing tumours. Pathologically, they may be localized, plexiform or diffuse neurofibromas, the last of these being the rarest (Enzinger & Weiss 1983). Plexiform neurofibroma involves a major nerve which becomes distorted and converted to a 'bag of worms'. The multiple neurofibromas of von Recklinghausen's disease give rise to significant morbidity and mortality and are usually so numerous as to make surgical excision of all tumours impossible. It is not possible to predict which lesions, if any, will undergo malignant transformation, although it is likely that those who have had the disease for many years have the greatest risk of such a development (Guccion & Enzinger 1979).

In the absence of a strong suspicion of malignancy, surgery has to be selective and it has been suggested that it be reserved for lesions which are large, painful or strategically placed so that they impair function significantly (Enzinger & Weiss 1983). The development of a sarcoma typically presents as rapid enlargement or pain in a pre-existing neurofibroma, and either symptom should lead to biopsy followed, on confirmation of malignancy, by radical local excision or amputation.

In the foot, the neurofibroma may present as a deep swelling, tending to be more mobile transversely than longitudinally and associated with a nerve. Unfortunately, in neurofibromatosis, there may be more extensive involvement of skin and subcutaneous tissue in a plexiform neurofibroma (Fig. 35.10). Finally, there may be gross skeletal deformity with gigantism or dysplasia.

Treatment, if indicated, consists of surgical excision. The isolated small neurofibroma can be excised as it rarely involves a major nerve. The plexiform neurofibroma can be reduced in size if not completely excised, as the tumours tend to be particularly lax, although vascular.

Hamartoma. Hamartoma, involving tissues of many origins and producing gross deformity of the foot, may occur. Histology of tissue removed shows no evidence of neurofibromatosis (Fig. 35.11).

Traumatic

Traumatic neuroma. A traumatic neuroma may present, in the sole of the foot, as a nodule which may be occasionally painful or tender.

It is due to excessive proliferation of the nerve fibre at a site of injury or surgery, occurring, presumably, where regenerative nerve fibres are unable to grow in an orderly fashion into the distal severed end of the nerve sheath.

Macroscopically, it is a well circumscribed,

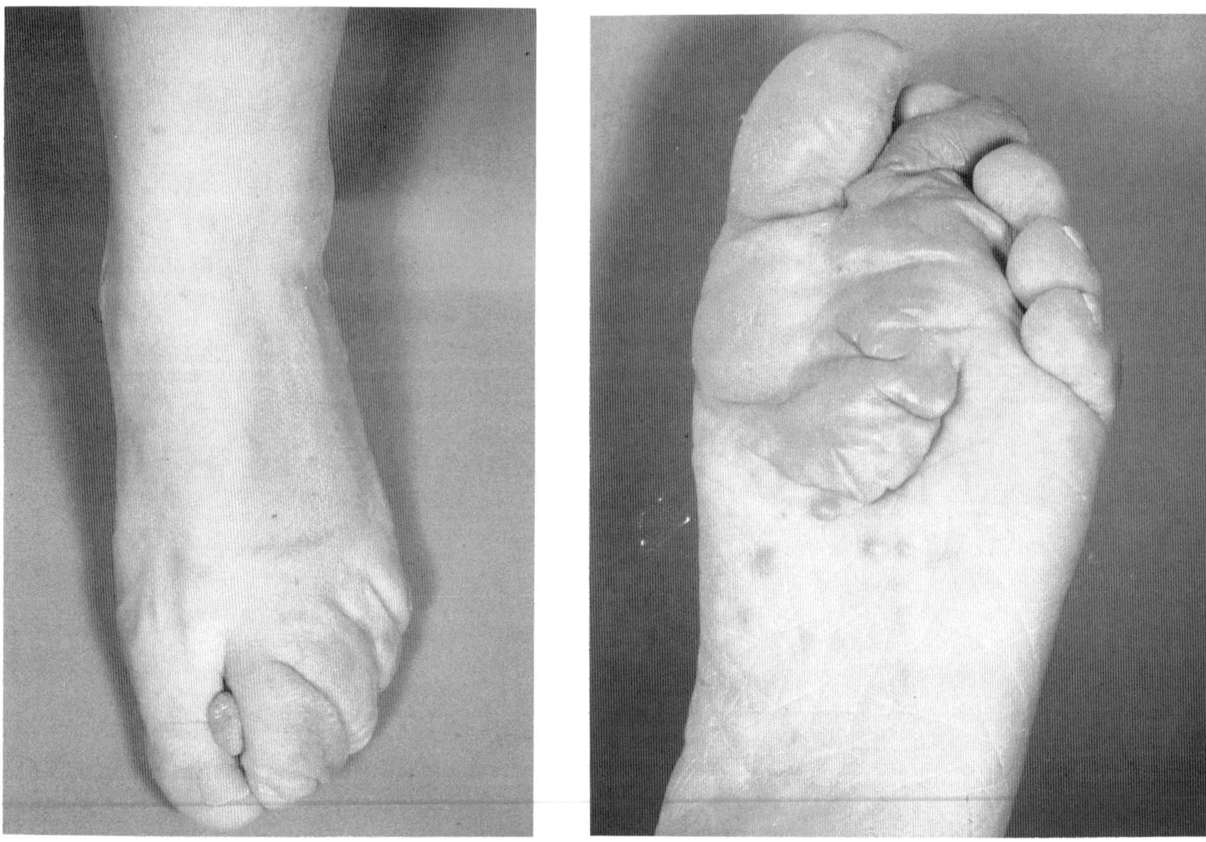

Fig. 35.10 Diffuse plexiform neurofibromatosis of the foot (in a patient with von Recklinghausen's disease)

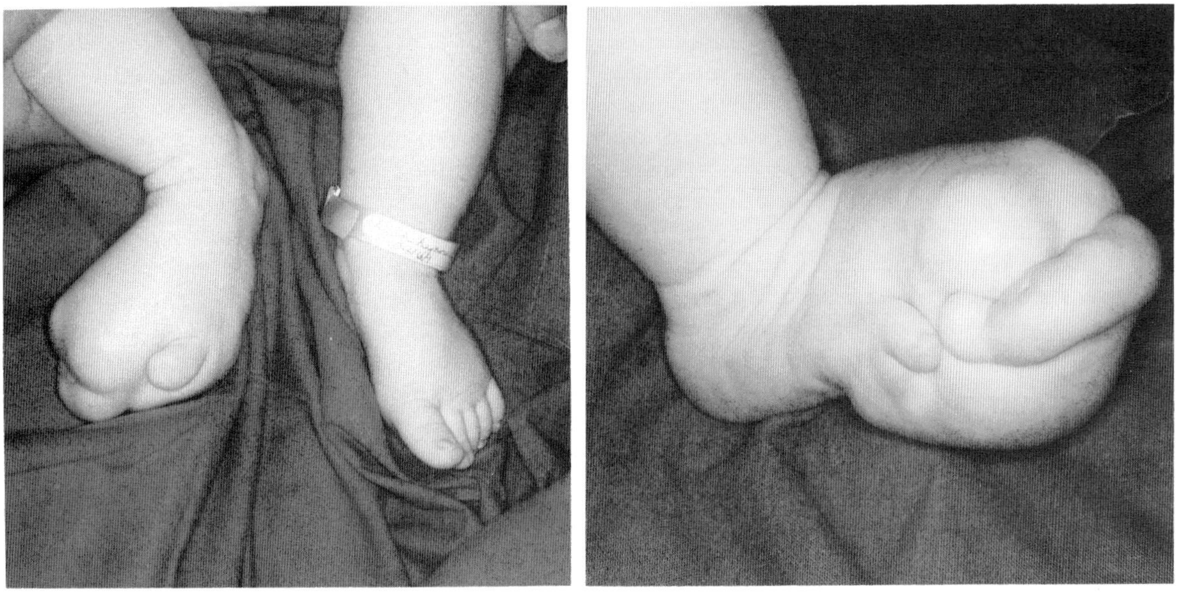

a b

Fig. 35.11 Congenital hamartoma of the foot: (a) Comparison with left foot; (b) Lateral view

whitish-grey nodule in continuity with the affected nerve, and microscopy shows a random overgrowth of nerve fibres, Schwann cells and fibroblasts forming fibrous tissues.

Surgical excision is indicated if the diagnosis is in doubt or if the lesion has become symptomatic. Surgery may involve repair of the nerve, dissection of the neuroma if part of the nerve remains in continuity, or excision and burying of the nerve end if pain has been a problem.

Neuroma of the heel affects the medial calcaneal nerve and may be related to direct trauma, the overloading effects of obesity, or calcaneal eversion associated with pronation (Altman & Hinkes 1982).

Morton's neuroma (Morton's metatarsalgia) is described in Chapter 22.

'Degenerative' and miscellaneous

Digital mucous cyst. Digital mucous cysts are benign lesions that occur in the subcutaneous tissues of the toes, particularly on the dorsum near the distal interphalangeal joint and close to the nail bed. They occur at any age and in either sex. Presentation is with a translucent-looking cystic swelling of variable size with little or no tenderness. Occasionally, patients may describe spontaneous rupture with discharge of gelatinous fluid, but the lesion may recur. On other occasions, the lesion spontaneously disappears. Differential diagnosis includes ganglion, lipoma, fibroma, epidermal cyst, nodular pigmented villonodular tenosynovitis and sarcomas of various types.

Pathologically, there is a central myxoid cystic area surrounded by fibrous tissue. Some authorities regard the lesions as ganglia of the distal interphalangeal joint.

Treatment should be directed at complete local excision. This may involve full-thickness skin grafting or local flap cover (if joint or nail bed is exposed) if the overlying skin cannot be peeled off and closed primarily. References to this lesion, sometimes referred to as a myxoma, are available elsewhere (Lever & Schaumberg-Lever 1983, Grosse 1937, Stout 1948, Sugar 1981, Enzinger & Weiss 1983).

Recurrent infantile digital fibroma. Single or multiple nodules are present on the toes (and fingers) in recurrent infantile digital fibroma. A little over 50 cases have been reported in the literature, including those occurring in the hand (Coskey et al 1979, Santa Cruz & Reiner 1978, Shapiro 1969). They are usually either present at birth or appear in the first year of life, though development later in childhood sometimes occurs. Recurrent digital fibromas are characteristically circumscribed, reddish-pink nodules which undergo spontaneous involution.

Histopathological examination shows interlacing bundles of collagen fibres with numerous fibroblasts in the dermis and sometimes extension of this process into subcutaneous fat. Characteristic eosinophilic inclusion bodies, 3–10 μm diameter, are present in many of the fibroblasts, and the ultrastructure and significance of these inclusions are discussed elsewhere (Lever & Schaumberg-Lever 1983).

Treatment of recurrent digital fibroma should be conservative, with surgical excision reserved for those occasions where there is significant impairment of function because of the lesion. Surgery may well produce even further deformity.

Fibromatoses. Plantar fibromatosis (Fig. 35.12) may be confused clinically with soft tissue tumours. Its management is discussed in Chapter 36. Nodular fasçiitis may occur in the foot and may be difficult to differentiate histologically from fibrosarcoma.

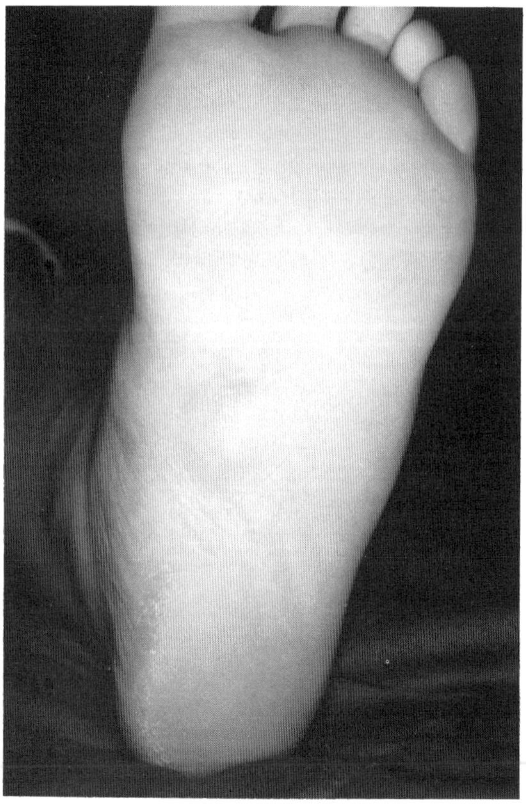

Fig. 35.12 Plantar fibromatosis in a young female

Neoplastic

(a) Tumours of fat

Lipoma. The lipoma is a benign neoplasm of fat which may contain variable amounts of fibrous and vascular stroma. It presents as a soft swelling which is usually asymptomatic and not tender, although just occasionally it may produce discomfort.

Lipomas in the foot are usually situated just beneath the skin (Lisch et al 1982). They may occur within tendon sheaths in the foot or ankle, where they may present with mild discomfort and swelling of the involved tendon sheath (especially peroneal, tibialis anterior and tibialis posterior). Lipomas are the commonest benign soft tissue tumours anywhere in the body, and comprise 50% of such lesions in the lower extremity, although occurrence in the foot is relatively infrequent (Booher 1965).

Lipomas may occur at any age and in either sex, but are more common in middle-aged females and rarely affect children. Radiological examination reveals a tumour with a characteristic radiolucency (Cavanagh 1973), while the macroscopic and microscopic appearances are similar to those of normal adipose tissue. Differentiation from low-grade liposarcoma by the histopathologist is on the basis of the presence of pleomorphic lipoblasts. Development of a liposarcoma in a lipoma is uncommon. Liposarcoma of the foot is excessively rare, though single cases have been reported (Booher 1965, Kauffman & Stout 1959, Sugar & Murphy 1955).

Treatment of lipoma is by complete surgical excision after which local recurrence is very unusual (Booher 1965).

(b) Tumours of nerves

True nerve tumours of the foot are rare. They include neurilemmoma, neurofibroma, neuroblastoma and primary malignant nerve sheath tumours (Berlin et al 1975).

Neurofibroma. The neurofibroma may occur singly or as part of neurofibromatosis (von Recklinghausen's disease). A search should always be made for 'cafe au lait' spots or other signs of the generalized disease. Solitary neurofibromas are evenly distributed over the body surface and affect the dermoid subcutaneous tissues. They are slowly-growing, painless lesions, mostly seen in young adults. Solitary neurofibromas are the commonest nerve tumours in the foot (Berlin et al 1975).

Macroscopic examination shows a whitish-grey tumour which may form a fusiform expansion on a larger nerve. Histologically, the appearances are variable but there are interlacing spindle cells, collagen fibres and mucin present and some may be frankly myxoid.

Treatment, if indicated, consists of surgical excision.

Neurilemmoma. The neurilemmoma, (or schwannoma) is an encapsulated nerve sheath tumour which may occur at any age but is more common between the ages of 20 and 50 years (Geschickter 1935). They are relatively rare occurrences on the foot (Luke 1976). Neurilemmoma is a slowly growing lesion, usually causing little in the way of pain or neurological problems, and situated in relation to a nerve. One series included four cases in the foot and there were symptoms of pain, tenderness and paraesthesia (White 1967).

On sectioning, the cut surface has a pink, white or yellow appearance, while histological examination reveals characteristic appearances known as Antoni A and B patterns in a tumour made up of spindle cells with variable amounts of collagen fibre deposition (Enzinger & Weiss 1983).

The tumour is encapsulated, being surrounded by the epineurium, so that complete removal should be possible without damage to the related nerve. Temporary loss of nerve function may occur but should return (Geschickter 1935). Incomplete excision is needed for cases where attempts at complete removal would give rise to permanent damage to the related nerve (if important).

Malignant schwannoma. This tumour is rare, commonly metastasizes and should be treated by amputation if there is no evidence of distant spread.

(c) Tumours of blood vessels

Haemangiomata. Haemangiomata tend to involve multiple tissues and may be situated primarily subcutaneously. They have been discussed previously.

Glomus tumour. Glomus bodies are arteriovenous anastomoses surrounded by a nerve plexus. The glomus tumour is a benign tumour considered to be a hamartoma of the glomus body (Carroll & Berman 1972). They are found particularly in the distal part of the upper and lower extremities and the face. In the foot, the glomus tumour occurs in the papillary dermis of the sole or under the toenails. There may be red or blue discolouration of the skin or nail bed (LaPorta et al 1976, Quigley 1979). The lesion can often be accurately localized by the patient by direct pressure at a specific point. Both cold and pressure produce severe local pain. Glomus tumours may be present at any age, but subungual lesions have been described under the age of 25 years (Vineyard 1975). They are spherical, compressible lesions of small size (often less than 0.5 cm in diameter). Rarely, X-rays show erosion of distal phalanx.

Macroscopically, the lesion is blue, red or violaceous and may resemble a small haemorrhage when located subungually. Histological examination shows blood vessels lined by normal endothelial cells and surrounded by a solid proliferation of round or cuboidal epithelioid cells. The differential diagnosis includes haemangioma, neuroma, skin appendage tumour, haemangiopericytoma and Kaposi's sarcoma.

Treatment is by surgical excision, which produces immediate relief of symptoms. Subungual glomus tumours require prior removal of the nail, longitudinal incision of the nail bed, and removal of the tumour, which can often be readily ennucleated, and the bed curetted. The nail bed should then be repaired under magnification, by fine sutures to minimize subsequent distortion.

Recurrence is unusual and metastases are extremely rare (Lumley & Stansfeld 1972, Symmers 1973).

(d) Tumours of fibrous tissues

Fibrosarcoma. Fibrosarcoma is rare in the foot. It presents as a firm nodule and may be confused with the benign fibromatoses.

Histological differentiation may be difficult. The fibrosarcoma is composed of reticulin and collagen, with predominantly spindle-shaped cells. In a well differentiated tumour, the cells may be polarized and mitoses rare. Biopsy confirms the diagnosis and differentiation. If well differentiated, wide local resection may be resorted to but recurrences may occur. The poorly differentiated, advanced or recurrent tumour should be treated by amputation. Metastases are not uncommon (Campbell 1982).

(e) Tumours of doubtful origin

Granular cell tumour (granular cell myoblastoma). The granular cell tumour is rarely diagnosed clinically, usually discovered as an incidental finding on physical examination, and is an unusual tumour in the foot, occurring more frequently in the head and neck and upper limb (Strong et al 1970, Vance & Hudson 1969). It may occur at any age but is more frequent over the age of 40 years.

The granular cell tumour is a poorly circumscribed lesion and histological examination shows the presence of large uniform cells with eosinophilic cytoplasm and monotonously similar nuclei distributed in bands or nests. Electron microscopical examination shows these cells to have a characteristic appearance and a relationship to Schwann cells is favoured by most pathologists. Treatment is by local excision and recurrence is rare, although metastases occur very occasionally.

Malignant fibrous histiocytoma. This tumour, increasingly recognized elsewhere in the body, is rare in the foot (Smith et al 1976). It may appear as a poorly demarcated nodule or as diffuse thickening beneath and involving the skin. Growth tends to be rapid. It may arise deeply or within subcutaneous tissue. Histologically, it is classically composed of spindle-shaped cells arranged in a 'storiform' pattern and accompanied by pleomorphic giant cells and inflammatory cells. Treatment consists of wide local excision and this may involve amputation in the foot.

Epithelioid sarcoma. Epithelioid sarcoma was first clearly described by Enzinger (1970). It is a slowly growing neoplasm, occurring mainly in the extremities including the feet, which were the site of involvement in 9% of cases in one series (Enzinger & Weiss 1983). This tumour occurs mostly in adolescents and young adults (age 15–35 years) though no age group is completely exempt, and men are affected about twice as often as women.

The tumour may occur subcutaneously, within plantar aponeuroses or with tendon sheaths. If situated subcutaneously, the tumour may appear as an apparently trivial nodule, sometimes described as 'woody, hard' or it may cause ulceration of the overlying skin. It may be mistaken for a foreign body granuloma. If arising from aponeurosis, it may appear as a poorly defined swelling and may be mistaken for plantar fibromatosis (Fig. 35.13).

Naked eye examination shows a glistening grey-white or grey-tan mottled surface, with focal areas of necrosis or haemorrhage, while light microscopy shows a distinctive nodular arrangement of tumour cells which may undergo central necrosis. This nodular aggregate of tumour cells may be multiple. Detailed descriptions of the histopathology are available elsewhere (Lever & Schaumberg-Lever 1983, Enzinger & Weiss 1983). Vascular and perineural invasion are seen in surgical excision specimens (Pratt et al 1978, Moore et al 1975) and local recurrence is seen in about 85% of cases where there has apparently been initial complete excision because of this diffuse spreading of the lesion (Enzinger & Weiss 1983). The tumour tends to spread locally along nerves, fascial planes and tendons, and these areas should be particularly examined by the histopathologist. Metastases to the lymph nodes and later to the lungs may occur (Pratt et al 1978).

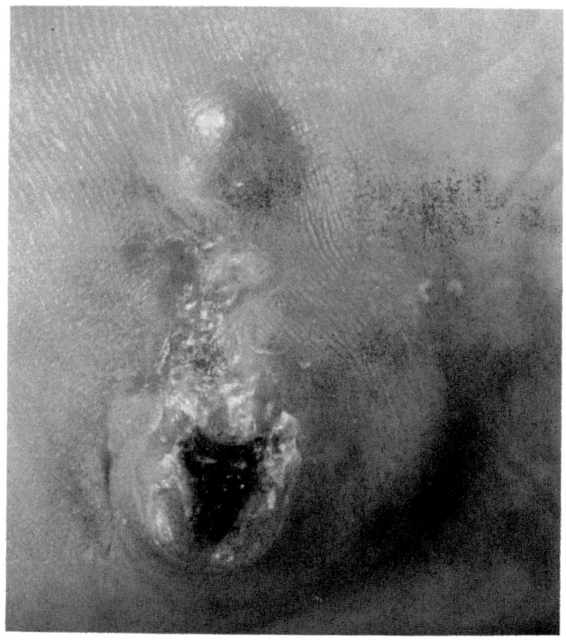

Fig. 35.13 Epithelioid sarcoma of the sole of the foot, which was initially thought to be due to plantar fibromatosis. Following local excision (which confirmed the diagnosis), there was early recurrence and the patient had a below-knee amputation. He remains well seven years later

The differential diagnosis includes a number of benign conditions in which there are superficial small nodules, such as infective granulomatous lesions, rheumatoid nodules, nodular fasciitis, fibrous histiocytoma, and squamous carcinoma in the case of superficial ulcerated lesions. Larger, deeply situated lesions require differentiation from the fibromatoses, other sarcomas such as synovial sarcoma, fibrosarcoma and angiosarcoma.

Because of the marked tendency for this lesion to recur, adequate treatment requires radical local excision, with amputation if there is involvement of a toe. Amputation should be considered in other sites if there is recurrence. Lymph node metastasis is fairly common and some would argue that lymph node resection should be included in the primary management. Radiotherapy and long-term chemotherapy may be helpful but have not been conclusively shown to improve prognosis.

(f) Tumours of muscle

Rhabdomyosarcoma. Rhabdomyosarcoma, although a rare tumour, is one of the more common soft tissue malignancies of childhood. There are various histological varieties of rhabdomyosarcoma, namely embryonal, botryoid, alveolar and pleomorphic types, and overlapping between these may occur in individual cases (Horn & Enterline 1958). Rhabdomyosarcoma usually occurs in infants and young children, less frequently in older children and adolescents, and rarely, if ever, in adults over the age of 45 years (Enzinger & Weiss 1983). Just over 7% of 588 cases occurred in the lower limb in one series and these affected mainly the foot.

Clinical presentation is with an enlarging deep-seated mass which may be closely associated with striated muscle. Pain and neurological defect may occur because of direct nerve invasion and, while erosion of bone is rare with rhabdomyosarcoma, it is in the hands and feet that this feature is sometimes seen. Distal tumours in one series were mostly interosseus in location, although one involved the arch of the foot (Ransom et al 1977).

Macroscopic examination reveals an ill-defined firm or rubbery-grey to pinkish-tan coloured tumour, invading into surrounding soft tissues and sometimes showing areas of haemorrhage and necrosis. The histological type of tumour in the foot is variable, although mixed and alveolar types were present in one series (Patcher & Alpert 1964). The histological differentiation from poorly differentiated round and spindle-cell sarcomas like neuroblastoma, Ewing's sarcoma, angiosarcoma, synovial sarcoma, malignant melanoma and malignant lymphoma may be difficult.

Treatment should be by surgical excision. Except in low-grade, well encapsulated tumours, this will mean amputation. Surgery may be combined with radiotherapy and adjuvant chemotherapy. The presence of disseminated tumour and the location of the primary tumour on the extremity are significant prognostic features (Ransom et al 1977).

Inadequately treated rhabdomyosarcomas recur and metastases are mainly to the lungs, lymph nodes and bone marrow, followed by other viscera, namely heart, brain, meninges, pancreas, liver and kidney.

Miscellaneous tumours

Extraskeletal chondroma. Chondromas sometimes occur in extraskeletal connective tissue and, when they do so, they are found mainly in the soft tissues of the hands and feet, chiefly the former. There is no connection to underlying bone, though association with tendon, tendon sheath or joint capsule may be present (Murphy & Wilson 1958, Someren & Merritt 1978) and the lesion is usually solitary. Multiple chondroid nodules suggest the possibility of synovial chondromatosis (q.v.).

Clinical presentation is as a slowly growing mass, which is rarely painful or tender, and adults between the ages of 30 and 60 years are mainly affected. X-ray may show calcification.

Pathological examination shows a well dermarcated, firm, round or oval lesion which histologically has the features of a benign cartilaginous tumour. There may be fibrosis, ossification or myxoid change.

Fibrochondroma, osteochondroma, myxochondroma, and focal calcification may be present towards the centre of the lesion, potentially giving problems with differentiation from tumoural calcinosis in a heavily calcified lesion. Differential diagnosis includes chondroma arising from the outside of the bone (periosteal or juxtacortical chondroma), low-grade chondrosarcoma and synovial chondromatosis, though the latter tends to occur in relation to larger joints like the knee, hip and elbow.

Treatment is by local excision. Further detailed information is available in the literature (Dahlin & Salvador 1974, Chung & Enzinger 1978, Lichtenstein & Goldman 1964).

Clear cell sarcoma of tendons and aponeuroses. Clear cell sarcoma is a deeply located soft tissue tumour which may be related to malignant melanoma in that there are histological resemblances to the latter, including the presence of melanin (Bearman et al 1975, Boudreaux & Waisman 1978, Toe & Saw 1978).

A common feature is involvement of tendons and aponeuroses. Clinical presentation is with a slowly growing mass which is tender and painful in about 50% of cases, and the duration of symptoms ranges from a few weeks to several years. Young adults (age 20 to 40 years) are mainly affected, but occasionally cases in younger and older patients have been described. Most clear cell sarcomas are situated in the lower limb (Enzinger 1965) and 38% occurred in the foot, heel or ankle in one series (Enzinger & Weiss 1983).

Naked eye examination reveals a lobulated or multinodular mass with a grey-white cut surface, frequently attached to a tendon or aponeurosis and with no connection to the overlying skin. Histopathological examination shows nests of clear, round or fusiform cells with vesicular nuclei and prominent nucleoli. Intracellular melanin is detected with special stains and by electron microscopy (Kauffman & Stout 1959). The differential diagnosis is from other sarcomas, particularly synovial sarcoma, fibrosarcoma and nerve sheath tumours.

Clear cell sarcoma is a highly malignant tumour which metastasizes to the lung, regional lymph nodes and bone. Radical excision is required, with amputation if necessary, together with chemotherapy and radiotherapy. Removal of regional lymph nodes should be considered and performed, particularly if there is lymphadenopathy. Local experience suggests a particularly good response to radiotherapy and chemotherapy with vincristine and bleomycin (Sugar & Murphy 1955, Radstone et al 1979). Late metastases are not uncommon.

TUMOURS AND TUMOUR-LIKE CONDITIONS OF SYNOVIUM

Several tumours and tumour-like conditions either arise from the synovium of the joints and tendon sheaths of the foot and ankle, or have appearances suggesting a synovial origin (Table 35.3).

Table 35.3 Tumours and tumour-like conditions of synovium

'Degenerative' and miscellaneous	
	Ganglion
	Local pigmented villonodular synovitis (giant cell tumour of tendon)
	Diffuse pigmented villonodular synovitis (giant cell tumour of tendon)
	Synovial chondromatosis
Neoplastic	Synovial sarcoma

Diagnosis

A tumour of synovial origin may be suspected because of the apparent site of the swelling within or adjacent to synovial structures. The appearances of the malignant synovial sarcoma may be deceptively benign.

General principles of management

The benign conditions of synovium have a marked tendency to recurrence following excision. This may be related to their situation within the fibrous flexor sheath where longitudinal spread and seeding is presumably unobstructed.

Perhaps for the same reason, the malignant synovial sarcoma tends to spread readily within the fibrous flexor sheath and the sort of spread suggestive of malignancy may occur late.

Common conditions

'Degenerative' and miscellaneous

Ganglion. The most common site for a ganglion in the foot is the dorsum over the tarsals (Slavitt et al 1980). (Fig. 35.14). The swelling may be hard and indistinguishable from an exostosis. An X-ray will confirm the soft tissue nature of the swelling. Microscopic examination shows cellular areas with mucinous degeneration, often in the form of multilocular cysts.

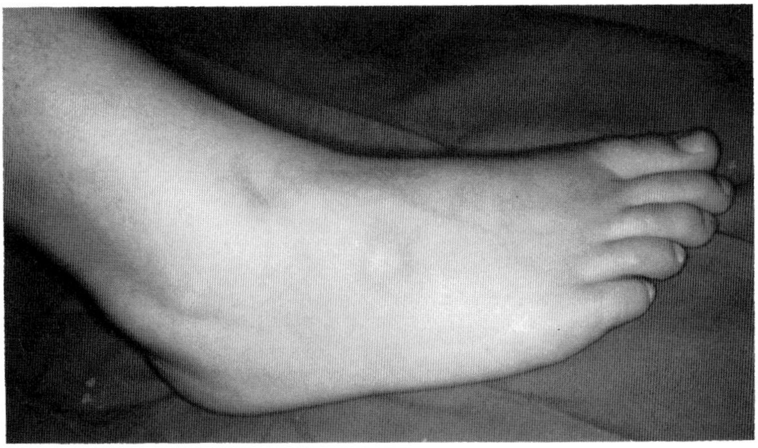

Fig. 35.14 Ganglion of the dorsum of the foot

Up to 50% of ganglia spontaneously disappear. If treatment is indicated, some authorities advocate aspiration and instillation of hydrocortisone. However, generally, if treatment is indicated, adequate surgical excision gives the best chance of cure but recurrence is not uncommon.

Local pigmented villonodular synovitis (giant cell tumour of tendon sheath). Localized (nodular) villonodular tenosynovitis (or giant cell tumour of tendon sheath) can occur at any age, but more commonly occurs between the ages of 30 and 50 years, and in women a little more often than in men. It occurs predominantly in the hand but may also affect the foot and ankle. The tumour is a slowly growing lesion, occurring in joints or tendon sheaths. Radiological examination shows a soft-tissue mass and, in a small number of cases, there may be erosion of bone.

The macroscopic appearance is of a localized nodule, usually mottled yellow or brown, ranging in size between 0.5 cm and 3 cm in diameter, although those occurring in the foot may be larger and more irregularly shaped. Sectioning reveals a pinkish-grey cut surface, which may be flecked with yellow or brown due to lipid or haemosiderin.

Histologically there is a discrete nodular proliferation of macrophages and fibroblast cells, forming collagen, with giant cells, foam cells and pigment-laden macrophages also present — features shared with the diffuse form. This raises the possibility that the lesion may be due to a reactive hyperplastic inflammatory reaction (Jaffe et al 1941). The exact appearances vary from lesion to lesion, depending on the proportion of macrophages, giant cells, foam cells and collagenization.

Although giant cell tumours are benign, they have a tendency to recur after surgical removal. Recurrence has been quoted as between 10 and 30% (Enzinger & Weiss 1983, Byers et al 1968). Excision involves pursuing the often tortuous route of the tumour to achieve complete removal.

Diffuse pigmented villonodular tenosynovitis (giant cell tumour of tendon sheath). Diffuse pigmented villonodular tenosynovitis mainly affects the large joints such as the knee, though involvement of the ankle and foot occurs in a significant proportion of cases (Enzinger & Weiss 1983). The toe is an uncommon site. Typical symptoms are limitation of movement, pain, tenderness and joint effusion, the latter often due to haemarthrosis. Radiography shows a soft tissue mass and there may be erosion of related bone. At surgery, the synovial membrane is diffusely thickened and brownish-yellow in colour. Microscopy reveals a macrophage and fibroblast proliferation with giant cells, collagen deposition and the presence of pigment-laden macrophages and foam cells.

Treatment is by synovectomy, with curettage of any bony component, but experience shows that there is a high recurrence rate, probably between 40 and 50% (Enzinger & Weiss 1983, Byers et al 1968). The aim should be complete removal of the lesion at first operation, if this is possible without causing severe disability to the patient.

Synovial chondromatosis. Synovial chondromatosis is a term used to describe two quite different conditions, sometimes referred to as primary and secondary chondromatosis. Primary chondromatosis is a condition in which nodules of metaplastic chondroid tissue develop within the synovial soft tissue. Patients may be of any age, and the larger joints are usually those affected, although involvement of toes and the ankle has been described (Jeffreys 1967, Villacin et al 1979, Murphy et al 1962). Primary chondromatosis is typically a monarticular disease, presenting with pain, swelling and limitation of movement. Physical examination shows tenderness, and there may be a mass or effusion. Radiological examination may reveal a soft tissue swelling and there is sometimes erosion of related bone, suggesting the possibility of a malignant tumour.

Pathological study shows chondroid nodules, which may be so numerous as to form an almost continuous mass, and some may break away to become loose bodies in the joint space. By light microscopy there are lobulated collections of chondrocytes, characteristically arranged in small clusters within related matrix. Cellular pleomorphism and the presence of binucleate cartilage cells may at times be alarming, but chondrosarcomatous change is exceedingly rare, if it occurs at all (Murphy et al 1962, Goldman & Lichtenstein 1964, Dunn et al 1974, King et al 1967).

One of the chief problems is that the locally erosive character and the histological appearances may lead to the erroneous diagnosis of malignancy. The behaviour of these cartilaginous lesions in the foot is benign (Dahlin 1978). The differential diagnosis is from other loose bodies as formed in secondary chondromatosis, which is perhaps better named synovial osteochondromatosis.

Treatment is by local excision of the affected synovial membrane and the removal of loose bodies. Recurrence of the problem after surgery is well known and is not an indication of malignancy.

Secondary synovial chondromatosis is more common than the primary form already described (Villacin et al 1979, Milgram 1977a,b, Milgram & Addison 1976, McIvor & King 1962) and better termed synovial osteochondromatosis since the loose bodies present in the joint space and incorporated in the synovial membrane comprise both articular cartilage and underlying bone. Large joints are usually those affected, but loose osteochondromatous bodies are sometimes found in the foot and ankle (Villacin et al 1979). In general, they form as a result of such processes as osteochondritis dissecans, osteochondral fractures and traumatic damage and joint disintegration in degenerative, and possibly inflammatory, disease (Villacin et al 1979, Milgram 1977a).

Neoplastic

Synovial sarcoma — malignant. Synovial sarcoma comprises about 8% of soft tissue malignancies. It occurs most frequently in the lower extremities and, in approximately 20% of cases, occurs in the foot or ankle (MacKenzie 1966, Wright et al 1982). It is said to be the commonest sarcoma of the hands and feet. The tumour arises from periarticular structures but not, apparently, directly from synovium (Ryan et al 1982). In fact, many tumours appear to arise when no synovial structures are present (MacKenzie 1966). The tumour presents at any age, but most commonly in young adults, and usually as a painful lump.

Microscopically, the tumour consists of two neoplastic cellular elements, the fibrosarcomatous spindle cell and the pseudoepithelial or glandular cell. Fissures, spaces or clefts, suggestive of synovial cavities, are usually found.

Treatment consists of wide resection. The surgeon should not be misled by apparent encapsulation. The general view is that, at least, ray amputation (if involving a digit) or more proximal amputation (if involving major joints) is the correct treatment. Lymph glands are relatively uncommonly involved (Chimenti et al 1982).

TUMOUR AND TUMOUR-LIKE CONDITIONS OF BONE AND CARTILAGE

Diagnosis

Tumours, or tumour-like conditions of bone and cartilage (Table 35.4), present usually as swellings or because of pain. The age of incidence and the rapidity of growth may suggest the diagnosis. X-ray may be definitive but biopsy may be necessary to confirm the diagnosis.

Table 35.4 Tumours and tumour-like lesions of bone and cartilage

Congenital	Abnormal metatarsals or phalanges Abnormal tarsals—e.g. accessory navicular Neurofibromatosis (with skeletal deformity)
Traumatic	Bony spurs Exuberant callus
Miscellaneous	Solitary bone cyst Aneurysmal bone cyst Fibrous dysplasia Eosinophilic granuloma
Neoplastic	Vascular tumours: Haemangioma Lymphangioma Haemangioendothelioma Haemangiopericytoma Angiosarcoma (malignant) Chondroid-forming tumours: Chondroma Osteochondroma Chondromyxoid fibroma Chondroblastoma Chondrosarcoma (malignant) Osteoid-forming tumours: Osteoid osteoma Subungual exostoses Osteoblastoma Osteosarcoma (malignant) Giant cell tumour Marrow tumours: Ewing's sarcoma Lymphoma Myeloma Metastatic

Principles of management

The borderline between benign and malignant tumours is blurred and some bony tumours (for example, giant cell tumour of bone) rarely metastasize. It is therefore essential that an accurate diagnosis is made before definitive treatment is performed. Although the diagnosis may be made on history, X-ray and macroscopic appearance, if there is any doubt biopsy should be taken for paraffin section diagnosis. In general the benign noninvasive tumours are treated by curettage, with or without cancellous bone grafting, while the more aggressive tumours are treated by resection.

Common conditions

Congenital

Bony prominences at the site of previous accessory toes, skeletal anomalies such as accessory navicular bones, or skeletal deformity due to hamartoma or neurofibromatosis are unlikely to pose diagnostic problems.

Traumatic

Bony spurs secondary to repeated trauma, and exuberant callosity at a fracture site, may be confused with bony tumours.

Miscellaneous

Solitary bone cyst. The solitary bone cyst usually appears during childhood or adolescence, most commonly in the os calcis (Campbell 1982). X-ray shows a well demarcated cyst with a sclerotic margin.

If seen in the os calcis, it may be safe to carry out no specific treatment. If the cyst is in another bone, if the diagnosis is in doubt, or if pathological fracture occurs, surgery is indicated. The cyst contains clear fluid and is lined by a thin membrane. At operation, it is curetted and the cavity packed with cancellous bone chips.

Aneurysmal bone cysts. This tumour-like condition is a cystic lesion surrounded by a thin shell of bone. In the past, it was often confused with what is now called giant cell tumour of bone. Aneurysmal bone cysts occur most commonly in the second and third decades and may be painful. X-ray is suggestive but exploration may be necessary. When entered, blood-filled cavities are seen, interspersed by strands of reddish-brown soft tissue. Bleeding may be profuse but it is reduced by removal of the abnormal tissue. Histology shows spaces lined by fibrous tissue (with multinucleated giant cells) and occasionally strands of bone.

Curettage and bone grafting is the usual treatment and recurrence is rare.

Fibrous dysplasia. This may be monostotic or polyostotic (especially in Albright's syndrome). In the foot, there may be palpable swelling or deformity. X-ray shows lysis which is well demarcated. Treatment, if necessary, consists of biopsy, curettage and packing with bone chips.

Eosinophilic granuloma. This condition affects children and adolescents and presents as pain or swelling. X-rays show lysis. On exploration, a granulomatous lesion is found. If proven histologically, the treatment is curettage and packing with bone chips.

Histology shows granulations with histiocytes, leucocytes and especially eosinophils.

Neoplastic

(a) Vascular tumours

Haemangioma, lymphangioma, haemangioendothelioma, haemangiopericytoma and angiosarcoma may all rarely involve bone.

(b) Chondroid-forming tumours

Chondroma. The enchondroma is a benign tumour of mature cartilage, usually occurring centrally in the short tubular bones of the hands and feet. Such lesions, arising centrally in the bone, are referred to as enchondromas. They may occur singly or they may be multiple in enchondromatosis (Ollier's disease). In Maffucci's syndrome, there are multiple enchondromas associated with haemangiomas.

They are likely to be asymptomatic, although pathological fracture may occur and cause pain. They are frequently a chance finding on radiological examination, which shows a centrally placed area of radiolucency, most often situated in the diaphyseal region (Fig. 35.15). Macroscopically, the tumour is a lobular bluish-grey mass resembling cartilage, and light microscopy reveals a benign tumour composed of chondrocytes and cartilage matrix.

Treatment is by curettage and insertion of cancellous bone chips. It is usually unnecessary to treat the multiple lesions of Ollier's disease.

Osteochondroma and related lesions. Osteochondroma, or cartilage-capped exostosis, is the commonest benign bone tumour but rarely is it found in the distal extremities (Dahlin 1978, Fuselier et al 1984). An even rarer lesion has been described and given the name 'bizarre parosteal osteochondromatous proliferation of the hands and feet' (Nona et al 1983). These lesions, too, may occur singly or they may be multiple. They occur at almost any age and in the foot present on the proximal

a

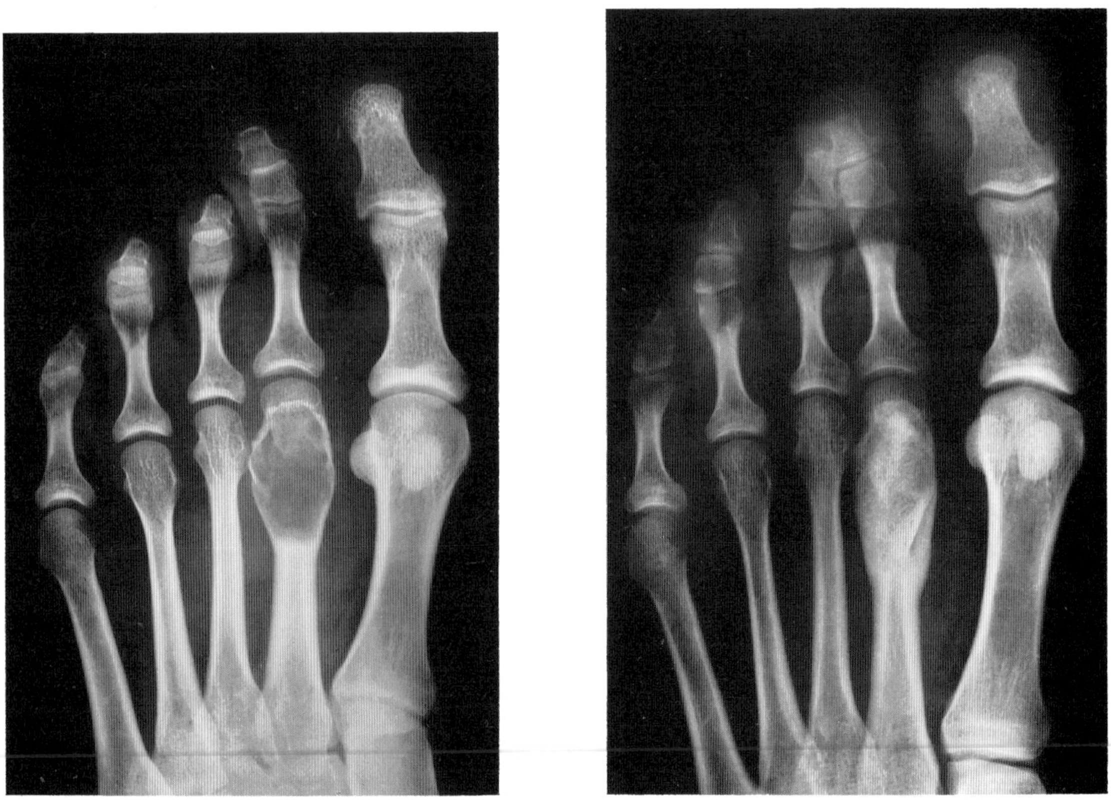

b

Fig. 35.15 (a) A chondroma of the second metatarsal; (b) Following curettage and cancellous bone-grafting phalanges or metatarsals (of which few examples have been described). They are painless, unless involved in pathological fracture or pressure against an adjacent nerve.

The cartilage cap contains bizarre binucleate chondrocytes and these appearances mimic chondrosarcoma.

X-ray shows the cortex continuous with the cortex at the base of the exostosis and there may be patchy calcification at the margin of the cancellous bone under the cartilage.

The lesions can be treated by excision but recurrence may occur in over 50% of cases (Nona et al 1983).

Chondromyxoid fibroma. Chondromyxoid fibroma is a rare localized tumour affecting males more often than females, presenting at any age in adults, though usually in the second and third decades, and involving the long bones, particularly of the lower limb (Spjut et al 1971, Dahlin 1978). It is not uncommon in the foot (Campbell 1982).

Local pain, which may be of some duration, is a common presenting symptom and there may be local tenderness. Radiological examination shows a well circumscribed area of rarefaction and there may be expansion of the outline of the bone.

Macroscopically, chondromyxoid fibroma is a grey-white mass with variable amounts of myxoid, cystic or haemorrhagic change. Histology shows myxomatous, fibrous and chondroid areas and oval, round or spindle-shaped cells, resembling the chondroblasts seen in chondroblastoma.

Treatment is by local excision. Recurrence may occur after curettage and insertion of bone chips and should be treated by local resection if feasible. Sarcomatous change, if it occurs, is an extreme pathological rarity (Dahlin 1978).

Chondroblastoma. Chondroblastoma is a rare tumour occurring in the epiphyseal part of a long bone, usually the femur, tibia or humerus. Occasional cases of involvement at other sites have been described, including the small bones of the hand (Neviaser & Wilson 1972) and foot (Ross & Dawson 1975, Campbell 1982). The majority of patients present in adolescence or adult life. Localized pain is a common clinical feature, although this was absent in a case of chondroblastoma occurring in a toe (Ross & Dawson 1975). There may be considerable swelling. Radiological examination shows a radiolucent area surrounded by a narrow zone of sclerosis, and there may be spotty calcification within the tumour (McLeod & Beabout 1973).

Naked eye examination shows a grey or grey-brown tumour with a gritty surface and sometimes cystic or spindle-shaped chondroblasts with chondroid matrix and multinucleated giant cells, showing a lace-like focal calcification (Spjut et al 1971).

Treatment should aim at complete local removal by curettage and packing with bone chips, or excision. In the case of a toe, amputation may well be the most suitable choice (Ross & Dawson 1975).

Chondrosarcoma. Chondrosarcoma, a malignant cartilage-forming tumour of bone, occurs most frequently in the age range 30 to 60 years. Involvement of the small bones of the hand and foot is exceptional and only a small number of cases has been described in the latter, involving either the tubular bones or the tarsus (Dahlin 1978, Jakobson & Spjut 1960, Miki et al 1978, Lewis et al 1975, Patcher & Alpert 1964).

Local pain and swelling are the usual presenting complaints. Radiological examination shows an expansile destructive mass, often containing mottled radiodensities representing calcification or ossification within the tumour.

The naked eye appearance is that of a bluish-grey lobular mass, while histology shows a tumour in which cartilage matrix is being formed by malignant chondrocytes showing nuclear and cytoplasmic pleomorphism. Multinucleate tumour cells and mitoses may be present. The question of the chondrosarcoma in the hands or feet taking origin from a pre-existing benign enchondroma is not yet resolved, although this would seem unlikely on the basis that enchondromas have a high frequency while chondrosarcomas in this site are rare (Patcher & Alpert 1964).

Treatment should aim at complete and wide local excision, with the possibility of prosthetic joint replacement. The involved bone and the soft tissue surrounding it should be excised. In more high-grade chondrosarcomas, amputation is the treatment of choice. Radiotherapy is not indicated, chondrosarcoma being a radio-resistant tumour.

(c) Osteoid-forming tumours

Subungual exostosis. A subungual exostosis is a benign bone tumour, found adjacent to or beneath the nail on the distal phalanx of a digit. It is a relatively uncommon tumour, which is comprised of trabecular bone with a fibrocartilaginous cap (Dahlin 1978, Evison & Price 1966, Landon et al 1979). These lesions are not related to osteochondromas (exostoses) seen elsewhere in the skeleton and they are not found in patients with multiple hereditary exostoses (Landon et al 1979).

Presentation is with a mass in the distal part of the digit, with elevation of the nail bed and often local pain. The vast majority of cases occurring in the foot in one study were present on the great toe (Landon et al 1979). A lateral radiograph shows a dorsal bony outgrowth on the distal part of the phalanx.

Surgery involves first removal of the nail. As much of the nail bed as possible should be preserved. Through a longitudinal incision, the exostosis is excised with osteotomy at the base and complete removal of the fibrocartilaginous cap. The nail bed should then be repaired.

Osteoid osteoma. Osteoid osteoma is a benign bone-forming tumour, usually affecting the diaphysis or metaphysis of a long bone in the lower limb, particularly the femur and tibia. The great majority of affected patients are aged between 5 and 25 years (Dahlin 1978, Byers 1968). In the foot, the osteoid osteoma is probably the most common osteoid-forming tumour (Dahlin 1978, Jaffe & Lichtenstein 1940, Kahn et al 1983, Peridue & Olin 1980, Campbell 1982). Osteoid osteoma and osteoblastoma are histologically similar lesions, there being no criteria for their separation apart from size, in that osteoid osteomas are less than 1 cm in diameter and typically surrounded by sclerotic bone (Byers 1968, McLeod et al 1976). An osteoid osteoma causes progressively more severe pain and relief from this is obtained with salicylates. Night pain is almost always present and is commonly severe enough to disturb sleep (Dahlin 1978).

Radiological examination typically shows a small area of radiolucency, with a surrounding area of sclerotic bone (Fig. 35.16) (Swee et al 1979); tomography and scintigraphy may be valuable in localizing the lesion where typical radiological features are absent yet the diagnosis is suspected (Winter et al 1977). If situated subperiosteally, there may be some new bone formation adjacent to the tumour (Fig. 35.17).

Macroscopic examination may reveal a friable red-grey 'nidus' of tumour in the centre of sclerotic bone, though finding this nidus may prove difficult and radiology of excised bone should be considered as an aid to its detection.

Histologically, the nidus is composed of cellular, highly vascular tissue with benign osteoblasts lining the surface of osteoid trabeculae, which themselves show a totally random arrangement, while the surrounding bone shows sclerosis (Dahlin 1978). The differential diagnosis includes chronic abscess, other benign or malignant tumours, fibrous dysplasia, bone cysts and healing fractures, particularly stress fractures (Freiberger et al 1959).

Treatment is by complete excision en bloc and the nidus can be identified on an X-ray of the biopsy specimen. In the phalanges and metatarsals, curettage is carried out and the nidus looked for histologically. The prognosis is excellent. Unfortunately, cases occur in which there is return of pain and local recurrence, most likely due to inadequacy of primary excision.

Osteoblastoma. Osteoblastoma is a benign bone-forming tumour with histological similarity to osteoid osteoma, but differentiated from the latter on the basis of size. Osteoblastomas are more than 1.5 cm in diameter (McLeod et al 1976). Although there is a marked tendency for osteoblastomas to occur in the vertebrae, other sites include the ilium, ribs and long bones. The short tubular bones of the hand and foot are sometimes affected (Spjut et al 1971, Dahlin 1978), and the talus and os calcis (Giannestras & Diamond 1958, Khermosh & Schujman 1977). Pain may be present but is not a marked feature, in contrast to osteoid osteoma. Radiological appearances are nonspecific, the lesion sometimes being radiolucent, sometimes more dense, with a variable amount of sclerosis demarcating the margin. These appearances may be mistaken for osteosarcoma, chondrosarcoma, aneurysmal bone cyst, or even osteoid osteoma (Khermosh & Schujman 1977).

The diagnosis is confirmed by biopsy. Naked eye appearance is of a vascular and haemorrhagic dark purple lesion, with a gritty cut surface, lacking a dense reactive margin but often with a surrounding

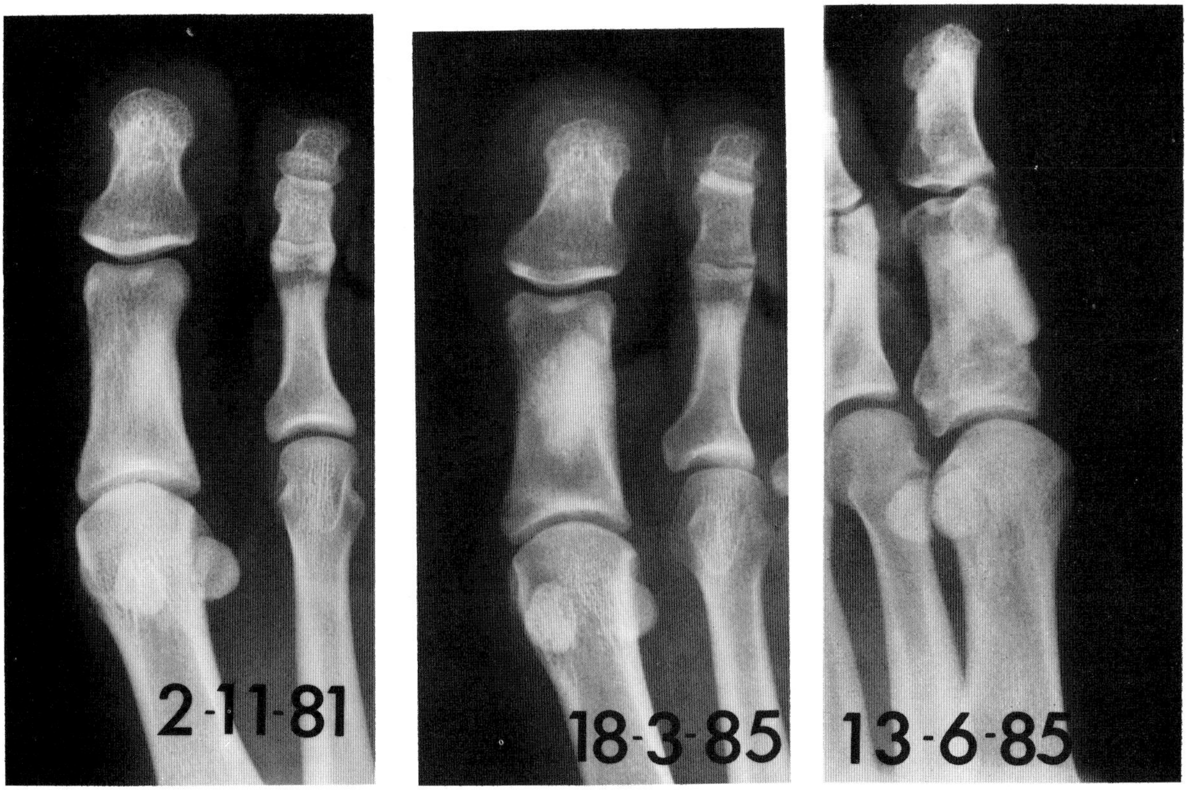

a b c

Fig. 35.16 (a) An X-ray to show an early osteoid osteoma of the proximal phalanx of the great toe; (b) A follow-up X-ray three and a half years later to show considerable enlargement; (c) Following excision and bone grafting

thin shell of new bone. Histology shows a connective tissue stroma containing osteoid and bone trabeculae formed by benign osteoblasts.

Treatment should be local removal of the lesion by conservative surgery, either by excision or by curettage and packing with bone graft if necessary, to fill any defects. Local recurrence does occur.

Osteosarcoma. Osteosarcomas are, by definition, malignant tumours showing evidence of osteoid or bone formation by the malignant tumour cells. Most cases occur between the ages of 10 and 20 years and boys are affected more often than girls. Osteosarcoma may occur in any bone, although the lower femur, upper tibia, upper femur and upper humerus are most frequently involved. The sites of involvement have been summarized elsewhere for five series of cases (Revell 1981). This shows that between 1 and 2% of osteosarcomas occur in the ankle or foot and this is confirmed by other sources (Dahlin 1978, Dahlin & Unni 1977).

Pain and local swelling are the most common modes of presentation and a long history is unusual. The radiological appearances are variable, but there is usually evidence of bone destruction and the tumour mass, which often shows evidence of ossification or calcification in the radiograph, may extend into the surrounding soft tissue. Skeletal surveys, computerized tomography and radio isotope scanning may all be valuable in assessing the clinical extent of the disease.

Naked eye appearances vary according to the composition of the tumour, which may be osteoblastic, chondroblastic, fibroblastic or telangiectatic. Histological features are similarly extremely variable. Classicially, a malignant proliferation of spindle-shaped or oval cells, with variable numbers of mitoses, shows evidence of bone or osteoid formation (Fig. 35.18). Haematogenous metastasis to the lungs and other bones is the usual form of spread. Differential diagnosis is between osteosarcoma

a
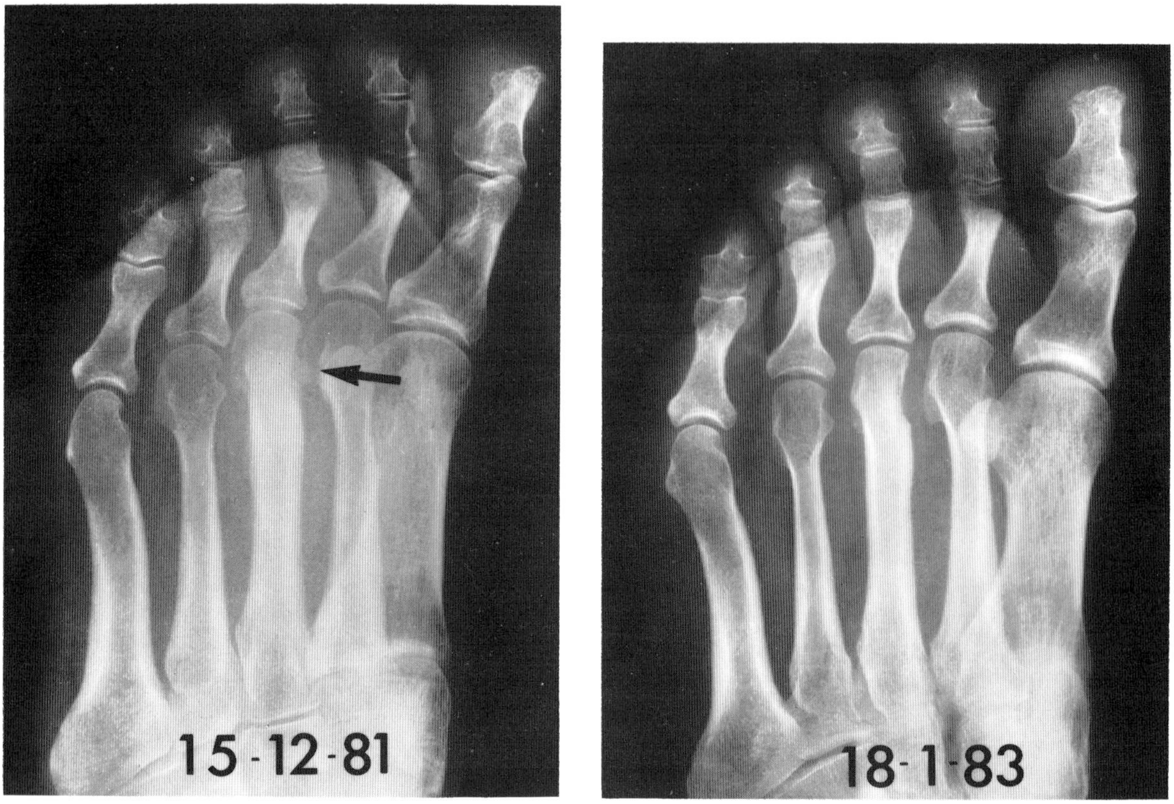

b

Fig. 35.17 (a) An X-ray to show a small subperiosteoid osteoma of the head of the middle metatarsal. The patient presented with obscure forefoot pain; (b) A postoperative X-ray to show the small bony defect following excision

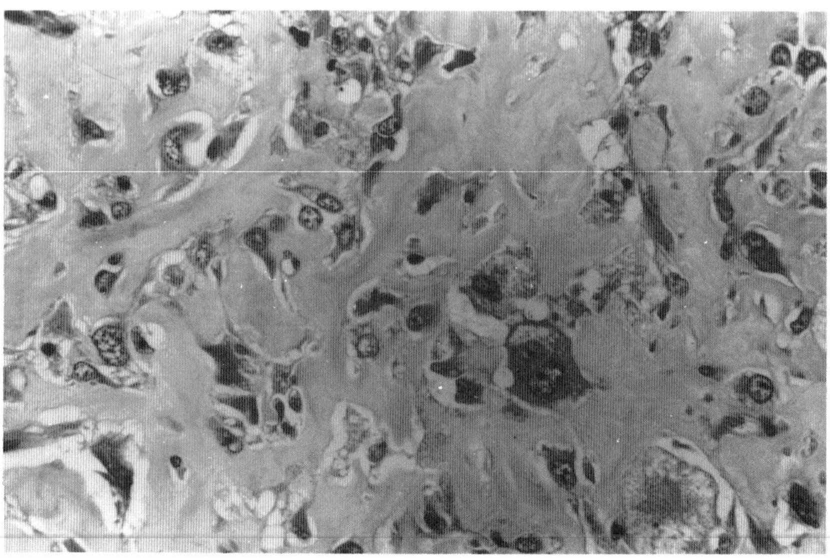

Fig. 35.18 The histological appearance of an osteosarcoma showing numerous malignant osteoblasts with nuclear and cytoplasmic pleomorphism. The cells are producing osteoid matrix. Haematoxylin-eosin × 700

and other destructive malignant tumours, and it is essential that an adequate biopsy is available in order that an accurate diagnosis can be made in view of the close similarities there might be to other sarcomas, for example, chondrosarcoma or fibrosarcoma in large parts of any individual lesion.

Surgical treatment should be directed at complete removal with a wide margin of normal tissue. In the foot, this is likely to involve amputation although limb preservation is being used with prosthetic replacement for osteosarcoma at other sites. Radiotherapy and chemotherapy are important adjuvant features in the modern management of osteosarcoma.

(d) Giant cell tumour (osteoclastoma)

Giant cell tumours (osteoclastomas) occur mostly in the age range 20 to 55 years and affect women more often than men (Dahlin 1978, Schajowicz 1961, Hutter et al 1962, Goldenberg et al 1970). Giant cells are often present in other bone lesions in considerable numbers, particularly nonosteogenic fibroma, chondroblastoma, chondromyxoid fibroma, aneurysmal bone cyst and the so-called 'brown' tumour of hyperparathyroidism, and these are a potential source of confusion in biopsy interpretation, together with nodular villonodular tenosynovitis.

Giant cell tumours are more often in the epiphyseal region of long bones, frequently around the knee, but may be present almost anywhere, including the hands and feet where they are most commonly located in the tarsal or metatarsal bones. A giant cell lesion affecting the small bones of the foot is more likely to be due to hyperparathyroidism or bone involvement with localized nodular tenosynovitis (Murphy & Ackerman 1956).

The clinical presentation of a giant cell tumour of bone is with pain and swelling, and a mass palpable on physical examination may crepitate. Particularly if there is extensive soft tissue involvement, the overlying skin may be red. There are no specific radiological features, the observed eccentric position of a lytic lesion as being an osteoclastoma (Jaffe et al 1940) is considered to be nonspecific (Spjut et al 1971, Dahlin 1978).

Macroscopic examination shows an heterogeneous cut surface showing solid, pale yellow fibrous areas alternating with cysts, grey-red vascular tissue, necrosis and haemorrhage. The bone is expanded and the overlying cortex thinned. Light microscopy shows multinucleate giant cells, intermixed with numerous oval or spindle-shaped cells (Fig. 35.19). Systems of grading have been devised in the past (Hutter et al 1962, Jaffe et al 1940) but have unfortunately proved of no value in predicting the

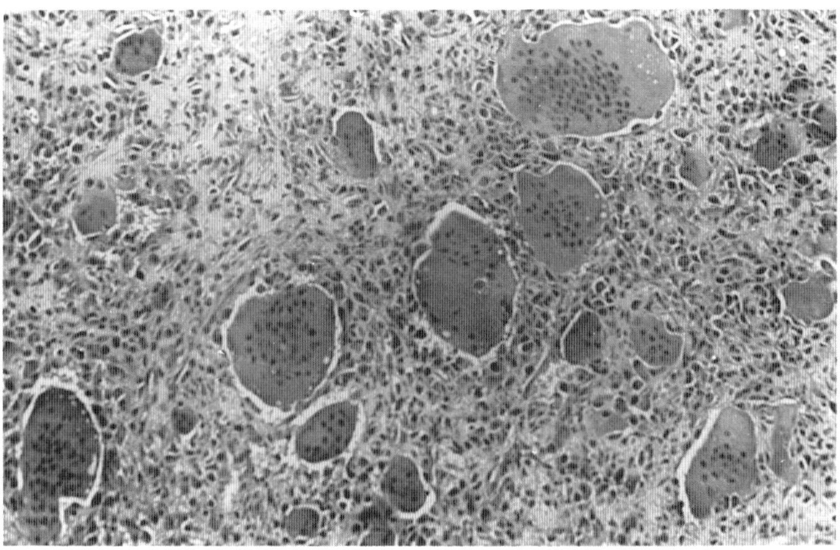

Fig. 35.19 Histological appearance of giant cell tumour of bone showing spindle-shaped cells and giant cells containing numerous nuclei. Haematoxylin-eosin × 350

way in which an individual lesion will behave (Spjut et al 1971, Dahlin 1978), since some tumours' apparently benign histological appearance may unexpectedly assume a malignant course.

Although treatment by curettage has been practised in the past, it is increasingly realised that total excision of the tumour and its surrounding shell of bone (and, if involved, soft tissue) is the treatment of choice, especially in a small bone. This may be difficult in some sites in the foot. Following curettage, the recurrence rate is approximately 50%, and of these, 10% metastasize (Goldenberg et al 1970). More radical excision and amputation should be reserved for cases of multiple recurrent tumour.

Radiotherapy should not normally be used because of the possible risk of inducing malignant change, and because giant cell tumours are anyway relatively radio-resistant.

(e) Marrow tumours

Ewing's sarcoma. Ewing's sarcoma is an uncommon malignant tumour arising in bone, the usual sites being the femur, tibia, humerus, ilium and ribs, and occurring mostly before the age of 20 years. Small numbers of cases in the ankle, tarsals, metatarsals and phalanges have been described (Dahlin 1978, Marcove & Charosky 1972, Dunn et al 1976, Bhansali & Desai 1963, Campbell 1982).

The most common symptoms are swelling and pain; the latter may be intermittent initially. Physical examination shows a palpable tender mass, and the bony temperature and erythrocyte sedimentation rate may both be raised, sometimes together with a leucocytosis (Dahlin 1978, Bhansali & Desai 1963). These features may lead to an erroneous diagnosis of osteomyelitis, and this was certainly the case in one specific report relating to Ewing's sarcoma in a great toe (Dunn et al 1976). It is frequently stated that Ewing's sarcoma can be distinguished by its radiological appearances alone, the lytic tumour mass being surrounded by multiple layers of subperiosteal reactive new bone to give an 'onionskin' appearance. Ewing's sarcoma may, however, be equally difficult to distinguish from osteosarcoma, eosinophilic granuloma, malignant lymphoma, metastatic disease or osteomyelitis.

Macroscopically, it is a soft, grey-white lesion and light microscopy shows a small round cell tumour arranged in cords, nests or sheets, sometimes with a rosette pattern. The demonstration of glycogen granules at light and electron microscopical level aids in the differentiation of the small round cell tumours of bone (Dahlin 1978, Revell 1986).

Opinions differ as to the best mode of treatment for Ewing's sarcoma, some favouring radiotherapy, others surgical excision. In the foot, the radiotherapy required may produce significant disability to necessitate subsequent amputation. One large study (Bhansali & Desai 1963) concluded that surgery was the superior treatment when feasible, and amputation should be strongly considered in lesions of the foot. Where there is evidence of metastases, radiotherapy and/or chemotherapy is indicated.

(f) Metastatic

Much the most common malignancy affecting bone is metastatic carcinoma, with the likeliest primary sites being lung, breast, prostate, thyroid and kidney. Metastatic carcinoma usually involves the more centrally placed bone marrow containing parts of the skeleton, namely the spine, ribs, pelvis, proximal femur and skull. Spread to the distal parts of the limbs is decidedly uncommon, there being a little over 50 documented cases of such an occurrence in the foot and ankle (Sundberg et al 1982, Gall et al 1976, Zindrick et al 1982). Lung, colon and urogenital carcinomas were the most frequent source of metastases to the foot and ankle, followed by breast, cervix, uterus, ovary, prostate and submandibular gland (Sundberg et al 1982, Gall et al 1976, Kumar & Kovi 1978, Gelberman et al 1975, Harkonen & Olin 1980). The metastatic lesions have no particular predilection for a specific part of the foot, involving multiple sites, the os calcis, the talus, a phalanx, metatarsal or other tarsal bone. The differential diagnosis includes osteomyelitis, gout, and the peripheral arthropathy of Reiter's syndrome or rheumatoid arthritis. Radiology, tomography and radio isotope scanning methods are all useful in making the diagnosis and technetium scanning is a particularly effective way of detecting metastatic disease (Revell 1986).

Treatment should be aimed at maintaining maximum function and mobility, with short hospitalization in these patients who are likely to be terminally ill. Radiotherapy and external splinting may prove sufficient to control pain and limit local growth, although amputation may sometimes be required if these less invasive procedures are ineffective.

REFERENCES

Altman M I, Hinkes M P 1982 Heel neuroma. A case history. J Amer Podiatry Assoc 72: 517-519

Arrington J H III, Reed R J, Ichinose H, Krementz E T 1979 Plantar lentiginous melanoma: a distinctive variant of human cutaneous melanoma. Am J Surg Pathol 1: 131

Bart R S, Andrade R, Kopf A W et al 1968 Acquired digital fibrokeratomas. Arch Dermatol 97: 120-129

Bearman R, Noe J, Kempson R 1975 Clear cell sarcoma with melanin pigment. Cancer 36: 977-984

Bedi T R, Pandhi R K, Bhutania L K 1976 Multiple palmoplantar histiocytomas. Arch Dermatol 112: 1001-1003

Berlin S J, Block L D, Donick I I 1972 Pyogenic granuloma of the foot. A review of the English literature and report of four cases. J Am Podiatry Assoc 62: 94-99

Berlin S J, Donick I I, Block L D, Costa A J 1975 Nerve tumours of the foot: diagnosis and treatment. J Am Podiatry Assoc 65: 157-166

Bernhard L M, Brant R G, Bakst M J, Coleman W B, Nickamin A 1983 Hypertrophic haemangioma vs haemangiopericytoma. J Foot Surg 22: 308-313

Bhansali S K, Desai P B 1963 Ewing's sarcoma. Observations of 107 cases. J Bone Joint Surg (Am) 45: 541-553

Booher R J 1965 Lipoblastic tumours of the hands and feet: review of literature and report of 33 cases. J Bone Joint Surg (Am) 47: 727-740

Borden J I, Shea T P 1976 Cavernous haemangioma of the foot. A case report and review. J Am Podiatry Assoc 66: 484-490

Boudreaux D, Waisman J 1978 Clear cell sarcoma with melanogenesis. Cancer 41: 1387-1394

Breslow A 1970 Thickness, cross-sectional areas and depth of invasion in the prognosis of cutaneous melanoma. J Am Surg 172: 902-915

Byers P D 1968 Solitary benign osteoblastic lesions of bone: osteoid osteoma and benign osteoblastoma. Cancer 22: 43-47

Byers P D et al 1968 The diagnosis and treatment of pigmented villonodular synovitis. J Bone Joint Surg (Br) 50: 290-305

Campbell C J 1982 Tumours of the foot In: Jahss M H (ed) Disorders of the foot, 1st edn. W B Saunders, Philadelphia. Ch 34 pp 986-988

Cargialosi C P, Schmoll S J 1976 Kaposi's sarcoma of the foot. J Am Podiatry Assoc 66: 525-527

Carnevali S L 1938 Sugli angioma dei muscoli striati. Arch Orthop 54: 476-507

Cavanagh R C 1973 Tumours of the soft tissues of the extremities. Semin Roentgenol 8: 73-89

Carroll R E, Berman A T 1972 Glomus tumours of the hand. Review of the literature on twenty-eight cases. J Bone Joint Surg (Am) 54: 691-703

Chimenti S, Calvieri S, Ribuffo M 1982 Synovial sarcoma of the foot. J Dermatol Surg Oncol 8: 882-886

Chung E B, Enzinger F M 1978 Benign chondromas of soft parts. Cancer 41: 1414-1424

Clark W H Jnr In: From L, Bernardina E A, Mihm M C 1969 The histogenesis and biologic behaviour of primary human malignant melanomas of the skin. Cancer 29: 705-727

Coleman W P, Loria P R, Reed R J, Krementz E T 1981 Acral lentiginous melanoma. Ach Dermatol 116: 773

Coskey R J, Nabbai H, Rahbari 1979 Recurring digital fibrous tumour of childhood. Cutis 23: 359-362

Cox F H, Helwig E B 1959 Kaposi's sarcoma. Cancer 12: 289-298

Cox K L 1976 Subcutaneous haemangioma of the foot — a case report. J Am Podiatry Assoc 66: 519-521

Dahlin D C 1978 Bone tumours. General aspects and data on 6221 cases. 3rd edn. Thomas, Springfield. p 111

Dahlin D C, Salvador H 1974 Cartilaginous tumours of the soft tissues of the hands and feet. Mayo Clin Proc 49: 721-726

Dahlin D C, Unni K K 1977 Osteosarcoma of bone and its important recognizable varieties. Am J Surg Pathol 1: 61-72

Day C L, Sober A J, Kopf A W 1981 A prognostic model for clinical stage I melanoma of the lower extremity. Am Surg 193: 599

Demuth R J, Snider B L 1980 Primary squamous cell carcinoma of the plantar surface of the foot. Am Plast Surg 4: 310-314

Dunn E J, McGavran M H, Nelson P, Greer R B 1974 Synovial chondrosarcoma. J Bone Joint Surg (Am) 56: 811-813

Dunn E J, Yuska K H, Judge D M, Garner F L, Varano L A 1976 Ewing's sarcoma of the great toe. Clin Orthop 83: 224-231

Enzinger F M 1965 Clear cell sarcoma of tendons and aponeuroses. An analysis of 21 cases. Cancer 18: 1163-1674

Enzinger F M 1970 Epithelioid sarcoma. A sarcoma simulating a granuloma or a carcinoma. Cancer 26: 1029-1040

Enzinger F M, Weiss S W 1983 Soft tissue tumours. C V Mosby, St Louis

Evison G, Price C H G 1966 Subungual exostosis. Br J Radiol 39: 451-455

Feibelman C E, Stoll H, Maize J C 1980 Melanomas of the palm, sole and nailbed: a clinicopathological study. Cancer 46: 2492-2504

Fitzpatrick T B, Gilchrest B A 1977 Dimple sign to differentiate benign from malignant pigmented cutaneous lesions. New England J Med 296: 1518

Forman W R, Streigold H 1982 Eccrine poroma: review of literature and case reports. J Foot Surg 21: 330-334

Freiburger R H, Loitman B S, Helpern M, Thompson T C 1959 Osteoid osteoma: a report of 80 cases. Am J Roentgenol 82: 194-199

Friedman-Kien A E 1981 Disseminated Kaposi's sarcoma syndrome in young homosexual men. J Am Acad Dermatol 5: 468-471

Fuselier C O, Binning T, Kushner D et al 1984 Solitary osteochondroma of the foot: an in-depth study with case reports. J Foot Surg 23: 3-24

Fuselier C O, Cachia V V, Wong C et al 1985 Selected soft tissue malignancies of the foot: an in-depth study with case reports. J Foot Surg 24: 162-204

Gall R J, Sim F H, Pritchard D J 1976 Metastatic tumours to the bones of the foot. Cancer 37: 1492-1495

Gelberman R H, Salamon P B, Huffer J M 1975 Bone metastasis from carcinoma of the uterus. Clin Orthop 106: 148-150

Ger R 1975 The surgical management of ulcers of the heel. Surg Gynecol Obstet 140: 909-911

Geschickter C F 1935 Tumours of the peripheral nerves. Am J Cancer 25: 377-410

Giannestras N J, Diamond J R 1958 Benign osteoblastoma of the talus. J Bone Joint Surg (Am) 40: 469–478
Goldenberg R R, Campbell C J, Bonfiglio M 1970 Giant cell tumour of bone. An analysis of two hundred and eighteen cases. J Bone Joint Surg (Am) 52: 619–664
Goldman R L, Lichtenstein L 1964 Synovial chondrosarcoma. Cancer 17: 1233–1240
Gottlieb G J et al 1981 A preliminary communication on extensively disseminated Kaposi's sarcoma in young homosexual men. Am J Dermatopathol 3: 111–114
Grosse R E 1937 Recurring myxomatous, cutaneous cysts of the fingers and toes. Surg Gynecol Obstet 65: 289–302
Gross R E, Wolbach S D 1943 Sclerosing haemangiomas: Their relationship to dermatofibroma, histiocytoma, xanthoma and to certain pigmented lesions of the skin. Am J Pathol 19: 533–551
Guccion J G, Enzinger F M 1979 Malignant schwannoma associated with von Recklinghausen's neurofibromatosis. Virch Arch (Pathol Anat) 383: 43–57
Hare P J, Smith P A 1969 Acquired (digital) fibrokeratomas. Br J Dermatol 81: 667–670
Harkohen M, Olin P E 1980 Rectal carcinoma metastasizing to a toe. Acta Med Scand 207: 235–236
Harrison D H, Morgan B D G 1981 The instep island flap to resurface plantar defects. 34: 315–318
Harwood A R et al 1979 Kaposi's sarcoma in recipients of renal transplants. Am J Med 67: 759–765
Hemric J R, Allen H B 1979 Acquired digital fibrokeratoma. Cutis 23: 304–306
Horn R C, Enteline H T 1958 Rhabdomyosarcoma: A clinicopathological study and classification of 39 cases. Cancer 11: 181–199
Hutter R V P, Worces J N, Francis K C, Forte F W, Stewart F W 1962 Benign and malignant giant cell tumours of bone. A clinicopathological analysis of the natural history of the disease. Cancer 25: 1377–1383
Jaffe H L, Lichtenstein L 1940 Osteoid osteoma: further experience with this benign tumour of bone. J Bone Joint Surg 22: 645–682
Jaffe H L, Lichtenstein L, Portis R B 1940 Giant cell tumour of bone. Its pathologic appearance, grading, supposed variants and treatment. Arch Pathol 30: 993–1031
Jaffe H L, Lichtenstein L, Sutro C J 1941 Pigmented villonodular synovitis. Arch Pathol 31: 731–765
Jahss M H 1982 Examination. In: Jahss M H (ed) Disorders of the foot, 1st edn. W B Saunders Company, Philadelphia
Jakobson E, Spjut H J 1960 Chondrosarcoma of the bones of the hand. Report of three cases. Acta Radiol 54: 426–432
Jeffreys T E 1967 Synovial chondromatosis. J Bone Joint Surg (Br) 49: 530–534
Kahn M D, Tiano F J, Little R C 1983 Osteoid osteoma of the great toe. J Foot Surg 22: 325–348
Kauffman S L, Stout A P 1959 Lipoblastic tumours of children. Cancer 12: 912–925
Keyhani A 1977 Comparison of clinical behaviour of melanoma of the hands and feet: a study of 283 patients. Cancer 40: 3168–3173
Khermosh D, Schujman E 1977 Benign osteoblastoma of the calcaneus. Clin Orthop 127: 197–199
King J W, Spjut H J, Fechner R E, Vanderpool D W 1967 Synovial chondrosarcoma of the knee joint. J Bone Joint Surg (Am) 49: 1389–1396
Kumar P P, Kovi J 1978 Metastases to bones of the hands and feet. J Natl Med Assoc 70: 837–840
Kurzer A, Patel M 1979 Basal cell carcinoma of the foot. Br J Plast Surg 32: 300–301
Landon G C, Johnson K A, Dahlin D C 1979 Subungual exostoses. J Bone Joint Surg (Am) 61: 256–259
LaPorta G A, Davis W S, Scarlet J 1976 Glomus tumour of the foot. Discussion and case report. J Am Podiatry Assoc 66: 528–533
Lever W F, Schaumberg-Lever G 1983 Histopathology of the skin. 6th edn. Lippincott, Philadelphia
Lewis M M, Marcove R C, Bullough P G 1975 Chondrosarcoma of the foot. A case report and review of the literature. Cancer 36: 586–589
Lichtenstein L, Goldman R L 1964 Cartilage tumours in soft tissues, particularly in the hand and foot. Cancer 17: 1203–1209
Lisch M, Mittleman M, Albin R 1982 Digital lipoma of the foot: an extraordinary case. J Foot Surg 21: 330–334
Luke R D 1976 Neurilemmomas of the foot. J Am Podiatry Assoc 66: 547–549
Lumley J S P, Stansfeld A G 1972 Infiltrating glomus tumour of lower limb. Br Med J 1: 484–485
McIvor R R, King D 1962 Osteochondromatosis of the hip joint. J Bone Joint Surg (Am) 44: 87–97
MacKenzie D H 1966 Synovial sarcoma: a review of 58 cases. Cancer 19: 169–180
McLeod R A, Beabout J W 1973 The roentgenographic features of chondroblastoma. Am J Roentgenol Radium Ther Nucl Med 118: 464–471
McLeod R A, Dahlin D C, Beabout J W 1976 The spectrum of osteoblastoma. Am J Roentgenol Radium Ther Nucl Med 126: 321–335
Marcove R L, Charosky C B 1972 Phalangeal sarcomas simulating infection of the digits. Clin Orthop 83: 224–231
Margileth A M, Museles M 1965 Current concepts in diagnosis and management of congenital haemangiomas. Paediatrics 36: 410–416
Midenberg M, Kirschenbaum S E 1983 Benign cavernous haemangioma of the ankle. J Foot Surg 22: 294–297
Miki T, Yamamuro T, Oka M, Urushidani H, Itokazu M 1978 Chondrosarcoma developed in the distal phalangeal bone of the third toe. Clin Orthop 136: 241–243
Milgram J W 1977a The classification of loose bodies in human joints. Clin Orthop 124: 282–291
Milgram J W 1977b The development of loose bodies in human joints. Clin Orthop 124: 292–303
Milgram J W, Addison R G 1976 Synovial osteochondromatosis of the knee. J Bone Joint Surg (Am) 58: 264–266
Moore S W, Wheeler J E, Hefter L G 1975 Epithelioid sarcoma masquerading as Peyronie's disease. Cancer 35: 1706–1710
Murphy W R, Ackerman L V 1956 Benign and malignant giant cell tumours of bone. A clinical evaluation of thirty one cases. Cancer 9: 317–339
Murphy A F, Wilson J N 1958 Tenosynovial osteochondroma in the hand. J Bone Joint Surg (Am) 40: 1236–1240
Murphy F P, Dahlin D C, Sullivan C R 1962 Articular synovial chondromatosis. J Bone Joint Surg (Am) 44: 77–86
Neviaser R J, Wilson J N 1972 Benign chondroblastoma in the finger. J Bone Joint Surg (Am) 54: 389–392
Nona F E, Dahlin D C, Beabout J W 1983 Bizarre parosteal osteochondromatous proliferations of the hands and feet. Amer J Surg Pathol 7: 245–250
O'Brien P H, Brasfield R D 1966 Kaposi's sarcoma. Cancer 19: 1497–1502

Pack G J, Miller T R 1950 Haemangiomas: Classification and treatment. Angiology 1: 405-426
Patcher M R, Alpert M 1964 Chondrosarcoma of the foot skeleton. J Bone Joint Surg (Am) 46: 601-607
Peridue R L, Olin F H 1980 Osteoid osteoma of the talus, a case study. J Am Podiatry Assoc 70: 353-355
Petersen N C 1968 Malignant melanoma of the foot. Scan J Plast Reconst Surg 2: 144-153
Politz M J 1976 Haemangioma of the digits. Two cases. J Am Podiatry Assoc 66: 515-518
Pratt J, Woodruff J M, Marcove R C 1978 Epithelioid sarcoma. Cancer 41: 1472-1487
Quigley J T 1979 A glomus tumor of the heel pad. J Bone Joint Surg (Am) 61: 443-44
Radstone D J, Revell P A, Mantell B S 1979 Clear cell sarcoma of tendons and aponeuroses treated with bleomycin and vincristine. Br J Radiol 52: 238-241
Ransom J L, Pratt C B, Shanks E 1977 Childhood rhabdomyosarcoma of the extremity. Results of combined modality therapy. Cancer 40: 280-281
Revell P A 1981 Diseases of bones and joints. In: Berry C L (ed) Paediatric pathology. Springer, Berlin. pp 451-485
Revell P A 1986 The Pathology of bone. Springer, Berlin
Reynolds W A, Winkelmann R K, Soule E H 1965 Kaposi's sarcoma. Medicine (Baltimore) 44: 419-443
Robinson J K 1979 A gigantic basal cell carcinoma on the plantar arch of a foot: report of a case. J Dermatol, Surg, Oncol 5: 958-960
Ross J A, Dawson E K 1975 Benign chondroblastoma of bone. J Bone Joint Surg (Br) 57: 78-81
Rowley L C, Winston L, Hovermale T, Ruskin J 1978 Epithelioid inclusion cyst of the foot: a literature review and case report. J Am Podiatry Assoc 68: 829-833
Ryan J R, Baker L H, Benjamin R S 1982 The natural history of metatarsal synovial sarcoma: experience of the Southwest Oncology Group. Clin Orthop 164: 257-260
Santa Cruz D J, Reiner C B 1978 Recurrent digital fibroma of childhood. J Cutan Pathol 6: 339-346
Schajowicz F 1961 Giant cell tumours of bone (osteoclastoma): a pathological and histochemical study. J Bone Joint Surg (Am) 43: 1-29
Schoenfeld R J 1964 Epidermal proliferations overlying histiocytomas. Arch Dermatol 90: 266-270
Schwartz R A, Burgess G H 1980 Verrucous carcinoma of the foot. J Surg Oncol 14: 333-339
Seehafer J R, Rahman D, Soderstrom C W 1979 Epithelioma cuniculatum: verrucous carcinoma of the foot. Cutis 23: 287-290
Shanahan R E, Gingrass R P 1979 Medial plantar sensory flap for coverage of heel defects. Plast Reconstr Surg 64: 295-298
Shapiro L 1969 Infantile digital fibromatosis and aponeurotic fibroma. Arch Dermatol 99: 37-42
Sheitel P L, Scheffer N M, Hawthorne F A 1978 Dermatofibrosarcoma protruberans. J Foot Surg 17: 174-176
Siegal F P et al 1981 Severe acquired immunodeficiency in male homosexuals, manifested by chronic perianal ulcerative herpes simplex lesions. N Engl J Med 305: 1439-1444
Slavitt J A, Behesht F, Lenet M, Sherman M 1980 Ganglions of the foot: a six year retrospective study and a review of the literature. J Am Podiatry Assoc 70: 459-465
Smith L S, Lenet M, Sherman M 1976 Malignant fibrous histiocytoma. A rare soft tissue tumour of the foot. J Am Podiatry Assoc 66: 459-464
Someren A, Merritt W H 1978 Tenosynovial chondroma of the hand: A case report with a brief review of the literature. Human Pathol 9: 476-479
Sommerlad B C, McGrouther D A 1978 Resurfacing the sole. Br J Plast Surg 31: 107-116
Sondergaard K, Olsen G 1980 Malignant melanoma of the foot. A clinicopathological study of 125 primary cutaneous malignant melanomas. Acta Pathol Microbiol Scand 88: 275-283
Spjut H J, Dorfman H D, Flechner R E, Ackerman L V 1971 Tumours of bone and cartilage. In: Atlas of tumour pathology (fascicle 5). Armed Forces Institute of Pathology, Washington DC
Stout A P 1948 Myxoma, the tumour of primitive mesenchyme. J Surg 127: 706-719
Stout A P 1953 Tumours of the soft tissues. In: Armed Forces Institute of Pathology Atlas of Tumour Pathology, Section II, Fascicle 5. Washington DC
Strachley C J et al 1975 Kaposi's sarcoma in a renal transplant recipient. Arch Pathol 99: 611-613
Strong E W, McDivitt R W, Brasfield R D 1970 Granular cell myoblastoma. Cancer 25: 415-422
Sugar M H 1981 Benign myxomas of the digits: a surgically resistant neoplasm. J Foot Surg 20: 67-69
Sugar S, Murphy B M 1955 Liposarcoma of the foot. Case Report. J Michigan State Med Soc 54: 468-469
Sundberg S B, Carlson W O, Johnson K A 1982 Metastatic lesions of the foot and ankle. Foot Ankle 3: 167-169
Swee R G, McLeod R A, Beabout J W 1979 Osteoid osteoma. Radiology 130: 117-123
Symmers W St C 1973 Glomus Tumours. Br Med J 2: 50-51
Tedeschi C G 1958 Some considerations concerning the nature of the so-called sarcoma of Kaposi. Arch Pathol 66: 656-684
Toe T K, Saw D 1978 Clear cell sarcoma with melanin. Report of two cases. Cancer 41: 235-238
Vance S, Hudson R 1969 Granular cell myoblastoma. Am J Clin Pathol 52: 208-211
Verallo V V 1968 Acquired digital fibrokeratomas. Br J Dermatol 80: 730-736
Villacin A B, Brigham L N, Bullough P G 1979 Primary and secondary synovial chondrometaplasia. Histopathologic and clinicoradiologic differences. Human Pathology 10: 439-451
Vineyard W 1975 Glomus tumour. Clin Dermatol 2: 1-10
Watson W L, McCarthy W D 1940 Blood and lymph vessel tumours. Surg Gynecol Obstet 71: 569-588
White N 1967 Neurilemmomas of the extremities. J Bone Joint Surg (Am) 49: 1605-1610
Winter P F et al 1977 Scintigraphic detection of osteoid osteoma. Radiology 122: 177-178
Wright P H, Sim F H, Soule E H, Taylor W F 1982 Synovial sarcoma. J Bone Joint Surg 64A: 112-122
Zindrick M R, Young M P, Daley R J, Light T R 1982 Metastatic tumours of the foot: case report and literature review. Clin Orthop 170: 219-225

Plantar fibromatosis

Plantar fibromatosis is a benign disease of the plantar fascia (Pedersen & Day 1954). It has been known for a long time, probably first being described by Sir Astly Cooper, but was best characterized by Dupuytren in 1832 when he mentioned foot lesions in two of his cases of classic contractures of the hand which bear his name (Meyerding & Shellito 1948). The disease consists of fibrous nodules which develop within the plantar fascia. They are usually found on the medial side of the fascia near the highest point of the longitudinal arch, but may of course occur anywhere. Classically the nodules extend out toward the skin but larger nodules also protrude toward the inner portion of the sole of the foot. In contrast to contractures of the fingers, seen in Dupuytren's of the hand, toe contractures are not seen (Stoyle 1964).

ANATOMY

A review of the anatomy of the plantar aponeurosis shows that it arises from a strong thick attachment on the medial tubercle of the calcaneus. The more pronounced medial band traverses the longitudinal arch attaching to the undersurface of the first metatarsal band and also to the first cuneiform. At about midfoot the aponeurosis divides into digitations which proceed toward the toes. Deeper fibres form transverse fasciculi between the longitudinally running bands (Hollishead 1964). Distal to the transverse fasciculi, the digital nerves and vessels lie within the connective tissue, and continue forward to the toes. Across the metatarsal head area the digitations are united by a thin band of transverse fibres, the superficial transverse metatarsal ligament. Distally the fascial digitations split to pass around the flexor tendons strengthening the sheaths. Lateral slips of the aponeurosis end in thin and somewhat insignificant digital extensions. For this reason contractures of the toes almost never occur, and nodules are seldom seen on lateral bands (Curtin 1962). It is important to remember that the plantar aponeurosis sends septa from its deep surface to attach to the first and fifth metatarsals, dividing the foot into three compartments.

The medial and lateral plantar nerves and blood vessels enter the foot together. They pass under the flexor retinaculum and traverse under the abductor hallucis where they separate. The lateral neurovascular bundle courses obliquely under the plantar structures penetrating the lateral intermuscular septum lateral to the flexor digitorum brevis. The medial bundle continues forward under the abductor hallucis, coursing more superficially and appearing between the abductor and the medial border of the flexor digitorum brevis just underneath the plantar aponeurosis. At this point, at about the base of the metatarsals or at the midfoot, it divides into its digital branches. Cutaneous branches pierce the plantar fascia and supply the skin of the medial side of the foot. The common digital nerves lie immediately deep to the plantar aponeurosis. The lateral plantar nerve also gives off plantar cutaneous branches which pierce the deep fascia and supply the lateral side of the sole. It is somewhat analogous to the ulnar nerve in the hand as, although it gives rise to fewer digital branches, it does supply most of the intrinsic muscles of the foot.

PHYSICAL FINDINGS

Clinically the overlying skin may be unaltered, dimpled, fissured or fixed as a result of the underlying nodules. The best method of palpating and measuring the nodule is to dorsiflex the foot and the toes. This tenses the plantar fascia and one can easily and accurately measure the length and width of a nodule.

Patients usually present with nodules that are at least 1 cm in diameter. However smaller nodules can be palpated by a physician if one suspects their presence, such as when evaluating a patient with palmar fibromatosis. The nodules, even the larger ones, are usually nontender, and moveable within the confines of the plantar fascia.

PATHOLOGY

On gross examination the nodule is firm, solid and of a yellowish/orange colour when cut (Curtin 1962). Microscopically the nodule consists of islands of proliferating fibroblasts on a relatively acellular collagenase background. On low power there is a nodular multicentric growth pattern. In Allen's (1955) series inflammatory cells were seen in every case. Lymphocytes were seen in perivascular locations. The fibroblast nuclei are elongated fusiform, oval and contain scant chromatin material and one to two pale nucleoli.

It is well known that without supplying the relevant clinical data a pathologist simply reviewing the slide may entertain an erroneous diagnosis of fibrosarcoma. Both tumours lack encapsulation and diffusely spread (Curtin 1962). However fibrosarcoma of the foot is an extremely rare tumour and malignant degeneration of a clinical plantar fibroma is not thought to occur.

Meyerding (1948) attempted to stage the disease. He divided it into active disease and resting disease. The active stage is early with the gross detection of nodules that might be tender or somewhat painful. During this stage there is increased fibroblastic activity and cellular proliferation with perivascular round cell infiltration. The resting stage is later in the disease with hard nontender nodules.

OCCURRENCE

The actual incidence of this condition is hard to estimate. Meyerding's comprehensive twenty year review was based on patients with Dupuytren's contractures of the hands or with plantar fibromatosis. He found only 24 patients with foot involvement and 12 patients (1.5%) with foot and hand involvement. It was noted that there may be many more cases of foot nodules, but in general the feet have not always been evaluated particularly when the patients were being examined for contractures of the hand. Plantar fibromatosis is not common.

Allen (1955) reviewed a 50 year experience at the Mayo Clinic with soft tissue tumours of the foot. 69 had plantar fibromatosis and nine had malignant neoplasms. Jahss (1982) showed a slight male preponderance of 62% in his series with 39% of cases being bilateral. There was an association with epilepsy in 7% of cases and the occurrence of Dupuytren's contractures of the hands in 37%.

There is a definite increase in Dupuytren's contractures of the hands and plantar fibromatosis in patients with epilepsy (Lund 1941). When 361 epileptics were studied 50% of the males had Dupuytren's disease of the hand as did 32% of the females. Plantar fibromatosis was seen in 25 patients. This was compared to 1021 control brewery workers of whom only one had plantar fibromatosis (Allen et al 1955).

The disease seems to increase with advancing age although most patients are in the fourth or fifth decade. There seems to be no positive factors with regard to the patient's history particularly with regard to their occupation, level of activity, possible trauma or family history for this condition.

Radiographically there may not be any changes although at times a very large nodule can be seen in the soft tissue especially in a tangential projection. The differential diagnosis probably should include (1) old scars, (2) callosities, (3) chondroma, (4) exostosis and (5) possible fibrosarcoma. Other conditions also present with distinct nodules in the palms and soles. Juvenile aponeurotic fibroma is such a condition seen in children and adolescents (Keller & Baez-Giangreco 1975). The tumours are small, painless, and lesions on the trunk have also been described. Microscopically a spotty calcification is seen in these tumours, which along with the low number of mitoses seen, leads to a correct diagnosis and differentiation from fibrosarcoma.

TREATMENT

There is probably no indication to treat a patient with plantar fibromatosis unless the nodules are large enough to cause discomfort or disability. Initially it is probably best to observe the nodules on two or three separate occasions over a period of several months. It is possible accurately to measure the length and width of the nodules and this should be recorded so that the course of the disease can be evaluated. Frequently the nodules do not grow. However, if the patient is seen at an earlier stage, the nodules can increase in size and others, perhaps previously not appreciated, may be palpated.

Historically radiation has been described as a treatment, but apparently has had no effect on the lesions. Other nonoperative treatments such as local infiltration of hydrocortisone or local anaesthetic or ultrasound treatments are of no value. There is really no reason to attempt to aspirate a nodule on the sole of the foot. The most obvious diagnosis should be a solid plantar fibromatosis and the pathologic anatomy of this area does not lead to the development of a cystic fluid-filled lesion such as a ganglion or a bursa. Early treatment should consist of modifying the patient's shoes to accommodate the nodules should they be tender. This can be done by excavating a portion of the inner sole and perhaps filling in with a softer lining material (Cracchiolo 1982).

The decision to remove these nodules surgically should be based on the patient's discomfort. Obviously large nodules which cause significant discomfort should be excised. It is not necessary to biopsy these nodules, but a complete excision is indicated.

A recurrence rate of these nodules has been reported. Allen's study (1955) indicates that 15 of 28 (54%) recurred after a single excision. In seven cases two excisions were performed and in four of these there was recurrence. In three patients, three or more excisions were performed. Probably the explanation for recurrence is an incomplete removal of the nodule. Conservative excision such as resecting only the palpable nodule is not adequate as other areas of involvement may exist.

At times patients present with a single small palpable nodule which may be symptomatic. Although it may be tempting to excise the small nodule, it can usually be treated conservatively. It is better to observe such a patient as other nodules may become palpable and justify, both to the patient and the surgeon, the need to perform an adequate excision of the plantar aponeurosis.

One must appreciate the extensive involvement of this disease and the anatomy of the plantar fascia which may extend deep within the sole of the foot toward the metatarsal shafts. Also it is now appreciated that complete excision of the plantar fascia, particularly the medial band, is essential to prevent a recurrence (Curtin 1962). In addition, experience with the palmar aponeurosis has shown that removal of the entire fascia yields the best results (Curtin 1962). Reoperation on the foot, like the hand, also leads to poorer results due to additional postoperative fibrosis.

OPERATIVE TREATMENT

Adequate exposure of the plantar fascia particularly the medial band is essential. The skin incision is critical and the plantar approach as devised by Curtin (1962, 1965) provides the optimal exposure for this condition.

In the past, incisions on the plantar aspect of the foot were condemned. The common approach to the sole of the foot was through the medial incision of Henry (1963) who stated that 'incisions to the sole are best avoided'. He advocated approaching from the medial side of the arch, dividing the skin and superficial fascia on the inner side of the foot from the hallux metatarsal head to the heel. This would require extensive subcutaneous dissection of the lateral flap. Unfortunately skin incisions placed high on the medial side of the longitudinal arch are precarious. The undermining necessary to expose even the medial band of the plantar fascia disrupts the arterial supply to the lateral plantar skin flap and also encourages venous congestion which leads to skin necrosis (Curtin 1965).

It is preferable to place the patient in the prone position and to perform the operation under tourniquet control (Fig. 36.1). The skin incision begins on the plantar surface of the foot just medial and anterior to the medial aspect of the calcaneus. It proceeds distally in a lazy curve turning more sharply lateral, but posterior to the head of the first

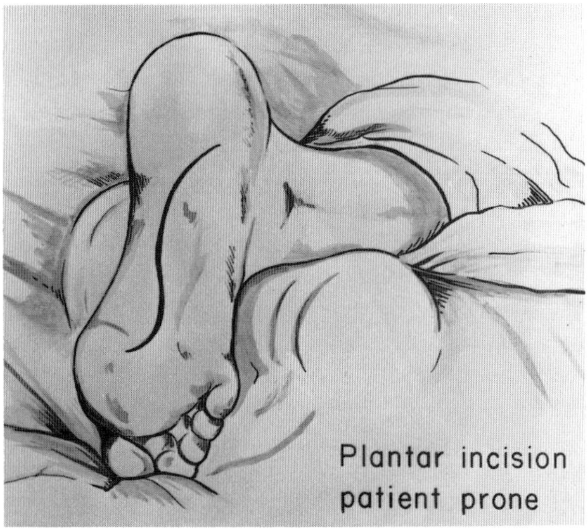

Fig. 36.1 A schematic drawing of the patient placed in the prone position. This gives the most comfortable view of the plantar aspect of the foot and outlines the incision. The distal leg should be supported on a sterile towel roll to prevent pressure on the toes. In this position the surgeon has good control of the extremity and can perform the operation with minimal assistance

metatarsal. It is possible to avoid any potential weight-bearing surface that is under a bony prominence. The plantar fascia is exposed proximally and transected from its attachments to the calcaneus (Fig. 36.2).

Distal dissection proceeds with care to avoid injury to the medial or lateral plantar nerve. Since the medial and lateral plantar nerves pass under the abductor hallucis proximally in the foot, care must be taken to avoid deep pressure or dissection in that area (Fig. 36.3). Once the plantar fascia has been transected from the calcaneus it can be held away from the underlying muscle belly of the flexor digitorum brevis. At about the midfoot these nerves may first be seen as they course on either side of the flexor brevis. More distal dissection brings the common digital branches into view; these lie just beneath the fascia, and care must be taken to avoid their injury. For all these reasons, it is easier and safer to begin the dissection proximally and proceed with care distally.

Unfortunately, most nodules are in the mid portion of the medial plantar fascia which is also in the area of the medial plantar nerve. At times, loop magnification is most helpful in performing a safe dissection. Dissection should be carried out to the

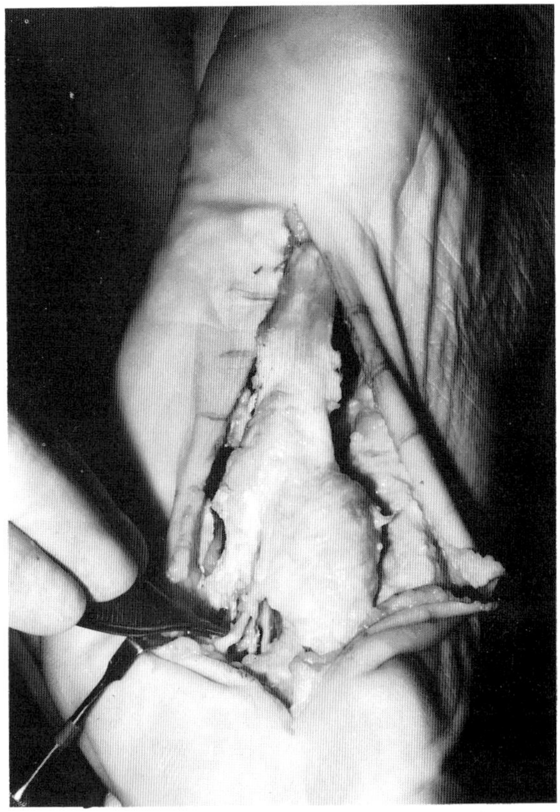

Fig. 36.2 The plantar fascia exposed from the calcaneus distally with a very large fibroma along the medial half of the fascia. Under tourniquet control good visualization of the structures including tendons and vessels is possible

metatarsal heads but should not proceed distally because of the lack of involvement of the fascial bands in the area of the toes. Excessive lateral excision of the fascia is usually unnecessary since most of the nodules have always been found within the medial portion of the fascia. Nodules should be dissected within the mass of the plantar fascia and should be traced if they proceed toward the more distal portions of the foot (Fig. 36.4). This is frequently seen in larger nodules especially involving the deeper fascial extensions to the first metatarsal.

Meticulous haemostasis is necessary because skin flaps are usually present. If tourniquet control has been utilized, the tourniquet should be deflated and haemostasis secured. Suction drainage is essential particularly where large nodules or multiple nodules have been removed creating a dead space. A compression dressing should be placed and kept on

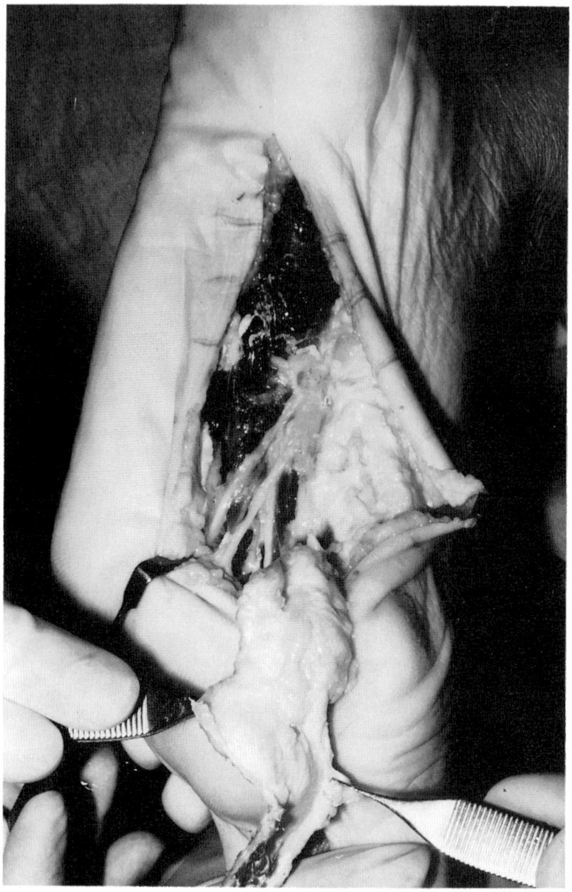

Fig. 36.3 The plantar fascia released from the calcaneus and reflected distally. Under the fascia one can see the fleshy muscle of the flexor digitorum brevis, tendons and nerves

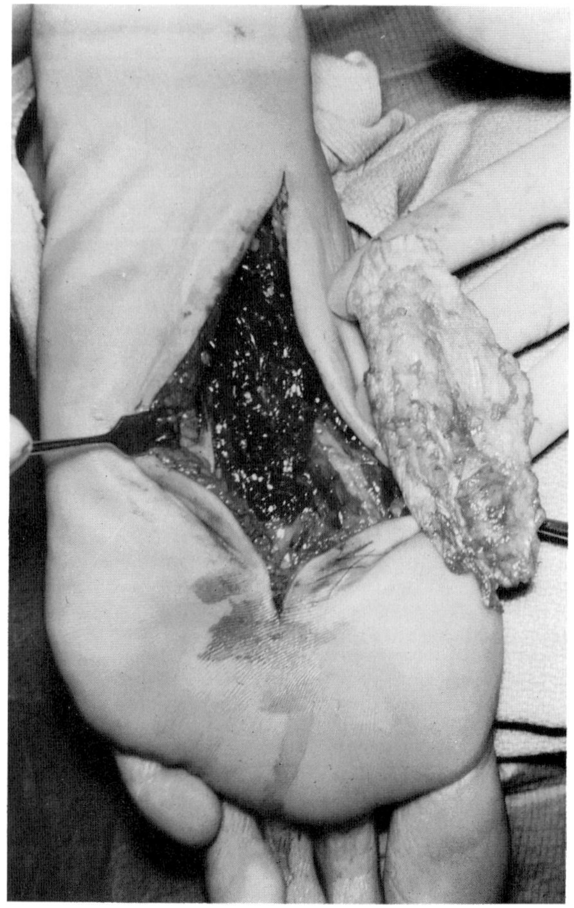

Fig. 36.4 The transected specimen with the underlying flexor digitorum brevis. Note that the majority of the fascia removed contains the medial one-half to two-thirds of the plantar fascia with the complete nodule

the patient for seven to ten days. The patient should be kept at bed rest, being up only indoors and using bilateral support such as crutches or a walker. Every precaution should be taken to ensure good wound healing. The wound should be inspected prior to discharge from hospital and at approximately 7 to 10 days later, and the interrupted sutures should probably be removed no earlier than 14 to 21 days postoperatively.

SUMMARY

Plantar fibromatosis is a benign condition of the plantar fascia where either a large single nodule or multiple nodules form. Involvement of the palmar fascia is more common and the condition seems at least to be more common in patients with Dupuytren's contractures of the hands as well as in epileptic patients.

Treatment is frequently unnecessary. However when significant pain and discomfort are caused by the nodule, complete excision of the plantar fascia, particularly the medial band, is indicated. A careful clinical history is necessary so that a proper diagnosis can be made following microscopic examination of the specimen. This benign lesion should not be confused with fibrosarcoma.

Proper surgical excision is through a plantar incision which will adequately expose the plantar fascia. Recurrences will only occur if the fascia has been incompletely excised. Meticulous dissection and haemostasis as well as proper drainage and skin closure are necessary if wound healing is to be optimal. A proper compression dressing as well as avoiding dependency and weight bearing aid in the healing process.

REFERENCES

Allen R A, Wollner L B, Ghormley R K 1955 Soft tissue tumors of the sole with special reference to plantar fibromatosis. J Bone Joint Surg 37A: 14–26

Cracchiolo A 1982 Office Practice: footwear and orthotic therapy. Foot Ankle 2 (4): 242–248

Curtin J W 1962 Surgical therapy for Dupuytren's disease of the foot. Plast Reconstr Surg 30: 568–576

Curtin J W 1965 Fibromatosis of the plantar fascia: surgical technique and design of skin incision. J Bone Joint Surg 47A: 1605

Henry A K 1963 Extensile Exposure. The Williams and Wilkins Co. Baltimore

Hollishead W A 1964 Anatomy for Surgeons. Volume 3. Harper and Row, New York

Jahss M H 1982 Disorders of the Foot. W.B. Saunders Co., London pp 841–842

Keller R B, Baez-Giangreco A 1975 Juvenile aponeurotic fibroma. Clin Orthop 106: 198–205

Lund M 1941 Dupuytren's contracture and epilepsy. The clinical connection between Dupuytren's contracture, fibroma plantae, periarthrosis humeri, helodermia, induratio penis plastica and epilepsy, with an attempt at a pathogenic evaluation. Acta Psychiat Neurol 16: 465–492

Meyerding H W, Shellito J G Dupuytren's contracture of the foot. J International Coll Surg 11: 595

Pedersen H E, Day A J 1954 Dupuytren's disease of the foot. JAMA 154: 33

Stoyle T F 1964 Dupuytren's contracture in the foot. J Bone Joint Surg 46B: 218

C. Barnes

Systemic disease

INFLAMMATORY ARTHROPATHIES

The inflammatory arthropathies, using rheumatoid arthritis as the model of this group of diseases, affect the joints of the feet and ankles in the vast majority of patients. These diseases may be classified in a simplified form as follows:

1. Rheumatoid arthritis
2. Seronegative spondarthritis
   a. ankylosing spondylitis
   b. psoriatic arthritis
   c. reactive arthritis
      i. sexually acquired (SARA), 'Reiter's syndrome'
      ii. post-dysenteric
   d. colitic (enteropathic)
3. Associated with systemic connective tissue diseases, especially systemic lupus erythematosus
4. Viral infections, e.g. rubella
5. Miscellaneous
   a. associated with erythema nodosum
   b. Behçet's syndrome
   c. anaphylactoid (Henoch–Schönlein) purpura
   d. Clutton's joints
   e. acne arthritis

Rheumatoid arthritis

Rheumatoid arthritis is considered in Chapter 25. However, it must be noted that the symmetrical small joint polyarthritis of rheumatoid disease involves the metatarsophalangeal joints, but not the interphalangeal joints of the toes (Table 37.1).

Table 37.1 Patterns of joint involvement

		OA	RA[a] SLE	Seronegative[b] Spondarthritis	Gout
Hands:	Metacarpophalangeal		+	+	(+)
	Proximal interphalangeal		+	+	(+)
	Terminal interphalangeal	+		+	
	1st carpometacarpal	+			
Wrists			+	+	(+)
Sacroiliitis				+	
Ankles	Subtalar		+	+	+
Feet:	Midtarsal	+	+	+	+
	1st metatarsophalangeal	++		(+)	++
	2nd–4th metatarsophalangeal		+	+	(+)
	Interphalangeal			+	
Plantar fasciitis / Achilles tendinitis				+	

[a] = usually symmetrical involvement; [b] = often asymmetrical involvement

Metatarsal pain frequently is the presenting symptom of the disease.

Radiologically erosions are often seen in the metatarsophalangeal joints before appearing in the small joints of the hands or wrists even if symptoms in the feet are mild or absent. Thus diagnostic radiographic investigation of a case of possible rheumatoid arthritis, or the progressive assessment of an established case, requires posteroanterior films of both hands and feet as a minimum. Progression of disease shown by increasing erosive changes in the metatarsophalangeal joints is seen in Fig. 37.1.

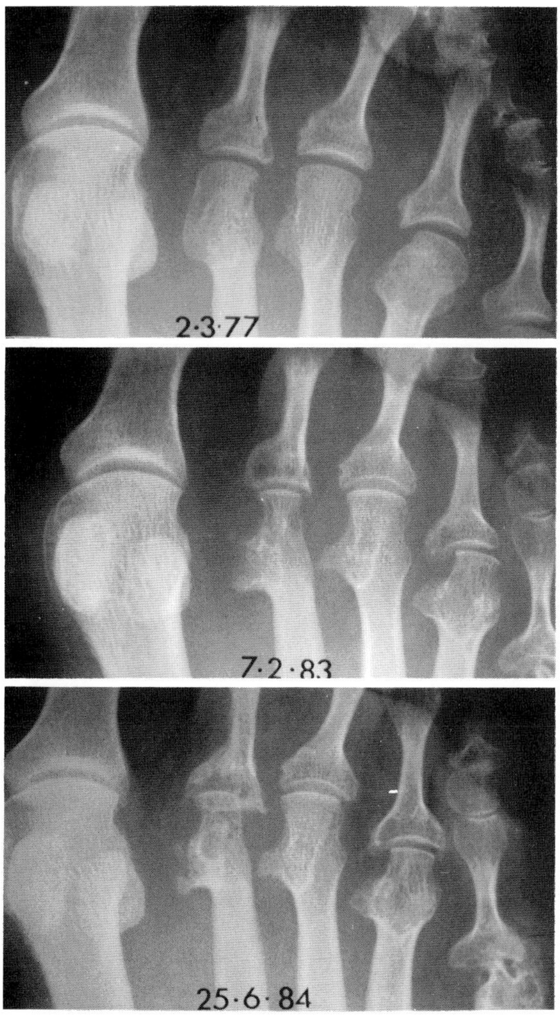

Fig. 37.1 Rheumatoid arthritis: progressive radiological erosions of the metatarsophalangeal joints

Seronegative spondarthritis

The definition of inflammatory arthritis with negative tests for rheumatoid factor (seronegative), in contrast to rheumatoid arthritis in which 75% of patients are seropositive, does not depend solely on laboratory tests for rheumatoid factor. As shown in Tables 37.1 and 2 the pattern of joint involvement, the spectrum of extra-articular manifestations and the association with the histocompatibility antigen HLA-B27 distinguishes this group from rheumatoid arthritis.

The term 'seronegative spondarthritis' has been adopted by some in preference to seronegative arthritis to emphasize the frequent involvement of the sacroiliac joints and spine (spondylitis) in this group of diseases (Moll et al 1974). It has been shown that sacroiliitis and spondylitis are present more often than expected in patients with ulcerative colitis (Wright & Watkinson 1965, Macrae & Wright 1973), Crohn's disease (Haslock & Wright 1973–4), psoriatic arthritis but not in psoriasis alone (Jajic 1968, Moll & Wright 1973) and sexually acquired reactive arthritis (Reiter's syndrome) (Wright 1963, Lawrence 1974, Olhagen 1983).

Similarly an increased prevalence of inflammatory bowel disease (Jayson et al 1970, Brewerton & James 1973) prostatitis and urethritis (Mason et al 1958) in patients with ankylosing spondylitis has been shown, as well as an increased incidence of all these features in first degree relatives of patients.

This has led to the formulation of diagnostic criteria to distinguish these spondarthritides from other forms of inflammatory arthritis as follows (Moll et al 1978, Wright et al 1983):

1. Absence of serum rheumatoid and antinuclear factors
2. Absence of subcutaneous 'rheumatoid' nodules
3. Inflammatory peripheral arthritis
4. Radiological sacroiliitis with or without ankylosing spondylitis
5. Clinical 'overlap' between members of the group
6. Tendency to familial aggregation
7. Significant association with HLA-B27 antigen (Ebringer & Shipley 1983).

Pattern of joint involvement

The pattern of peripheral joint involvement in the

Table 37.2 Seronegative spondarthritis

	Genitourinary	Gastrointestinal	Eyes	Skin mucosal	Nails	HLA-B27†
Ankylosing spondylitis	Prostatitis		Uveitis			90+%[1]
Psoriatic arthritis			Uveitis Conjunctivitis Keratoconjunctivitis sicca	Psoriasis	Pitting Hyperkeratosis and dystrophy	S: 50–100%[2] P: 9 –28%
Reactive arthritis						
SARA	Urethritis Cervicitis		Uveitis Conjunctivitis	Psoriasis/ skin rash Keratoderma Circinate balanitis Mouth ulcers (painless)	Hyperkeratosis and dystrophy	60–80%[3]
Post-dysenteric		Infective dysentry				
Colitic (enteropathic)		Ulcerative colitis Crohn's	Uveitis	Erythema nodosum Pyoderma gangrenosum Mouth ulcers (painless)	Clubbing	UC: 19%[4] Cr: 4% S: 33–91%[5] P: 5–29%

(In the SARA and Post-dysenteric rows, braces join the Eyes, Skin mucosal and Nails entries so that they apply to both rows.)

†Normal ≤ 8% Caucasians
S = Sacroiliitis/spondylitis
P = Peripheral arthritis only
UC = Ulcerative colitis only
Cr = Crohn's disease only
[1]Brewerton et al (1973), Schlosslein et al (1973), Arnett (1979), Keat et al (1979)
[2]Brewerton et al (1974a, b), Masi (1979), Kammer et al (1979)
[3]Morris et al (1974), Harris et al (1975), Olhagen (1983), Aho (1983), Sheldon & Pell (1983), Masi (1979), Arnett (1979), Keat et al (1979)
[4]Dekker-Saeys et al (1978)
[5]Brewerton et al (1974a, b), Brewerton & James (1975), Masi (1979)

seronegative spondarthritides differs from rheumatoid arthritis, osteoarthritis and gout (see Table 37.1), and possible involvement of the sacroiliac joints as well as those of the hands and feet must be taken into account. The major differences in the pattern of joint involvement, therefore, are that in the seronegative group (a) the terminal interphalangeal joints of the fingers and interphalangeal joints of the toes are often affected (Fig. 37.2), (b) sacroiliitis is common (see above), (c) asymmetrical involvement is usual, and (d) plantar fasciitis and Achilles tendonitis are common.

Nevertheless, the histological appearance of the synovium may be indistinguishable from rheumatoid arthritis although rheumatoid factor is not present in the synovial plasma cells.

Ankylosing spondylitis

Sacroiliitis and spinal involvement are characteristic of ankylosing spondylitis but peripheral joints may be affected in up to 50% (Sharp 1957), and may be the presenting feature in 15% (Sharp 1965) of such patients. The peripheral joints most commonly affected are the hips and knees presenting as monarticular synovitis, but the interphalangeal joints of the toes, ankles and subtalar joints may similarly be involved.

Inflammation at the site of attachment of ligament/tendon to bone is characteristic and is known as an enthesopathy (Ball 1971, 1983). This leads to cortical erosion, new bone formation and ossification into the ligament and is typically seen in the development of spinal bony ankylosis, radiologically being the 'bamboo spine' of advanced severe cases. Many other sites may be affected by this process and in the foot at the attachment of the Achilles tendon and plantar fascia to the calcaneum, leading to pain and tenderness at these sites. Radiological erosion and new bone (spur) formation are seen. The latter has the fluffy appearance associated with inflammatory periostitis in contrast to well corticated 'hard' calcaneal spurs which are not of clinical significance (Fig. 37.3).

Psoriatic arthritis

The prevalence of skin psoriasis is approximately 2% of the population and the overall incidence of arthritis in these patients is approximately 5% (males 1.5–5.8%; females 4.1–7.9%) (Wright 1978, Kammer et al 1979).

Moll & Wright (1973) defined five clinical forms of psoriatic arthritis.

1. Polyarthritis with predominant involvement of terminal interphalageal joints (and one can add not

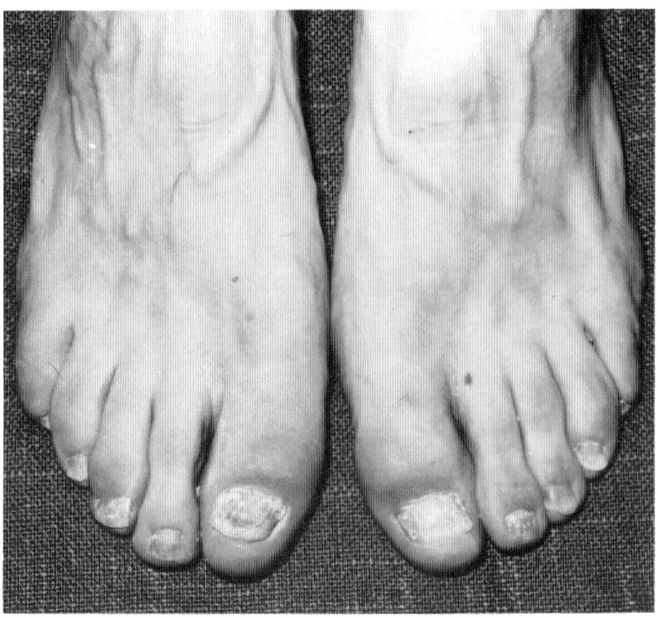

Fig. 37.2 Involvement of the interphangeal joints of the toes

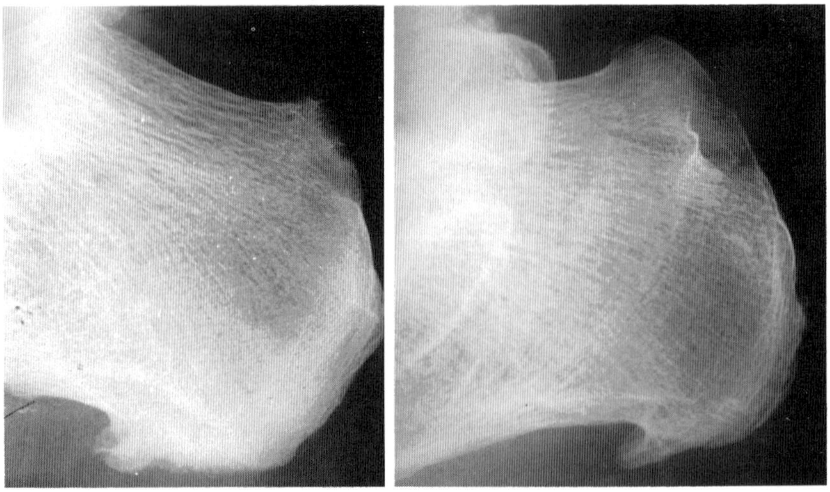

Fig. 37.3 Calcaneal spurs — right an innocent 'hard' well corticated spur: left a 'fluffy' spur due to periostitis in Reiter's syndrome

infrequently involvement of the interphalangeal joints of the toes)

2. Severe deforming, destructive arthritis with ankylosis, and rarely 'arthritis mutilans' affecting hands and feet (Fig. 37.4)
3. Symmetrical polyarthritis resembling rheumatoid arthritis
4. Asymmetrical oligoarthritis
5. Ankylosing spondylitis (approximately 5% of all psoriatic arthritis).

The psoriasis may be detected as nail pitting alone, or be asymptomatic but present in the scalp, umbilicus or natal cleft. There is no direct relationship between exacerbations or the severity of skin and joint disease. Nail dystrophy (hyperkeratosis, pitting and ridging) are more common in patients with terminal interphalangeal joint involvement (Fig. 37.5). Radiographic changes of peripheral joints include periarticular osteoporosis, loss of cartilage joint space and erosive destruction of joints. The latter is frequently asymmetrical, as is the arthritis clinically so that some joints are severely destroyed while others nearby remain normal (Fig. 37.6).

Reactive arthritis

The eponymous term Reiter's syndrome or disease, defined as the association of arthritis, conjunctivitis and urethritis, is being replaced by the term reactive arthritis. This may be defined as inflammatory arthritis following, or as a reaction to, infection, which may be dysenteric or genital, the latter then acquiring the title of 'Sexually Acquired Reactive Arthritis' (SARA) (Keat et al 1979). In fact Reiter himself described the postdysenteric rather than the sexually acquired form.

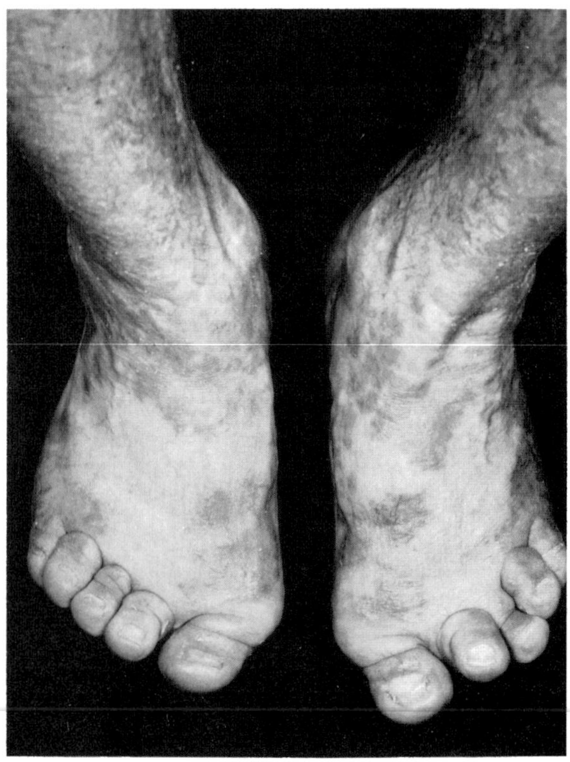

Fig. 37.4 Severe psoriatic arthritis

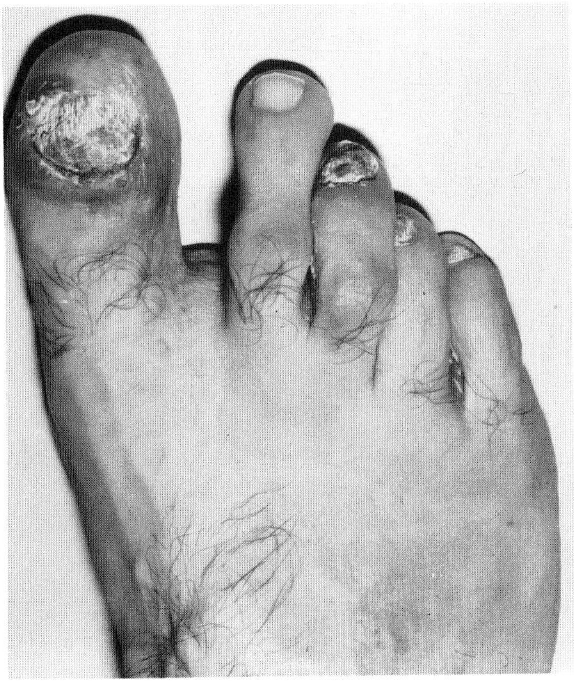

Fig. 37.5 Nail dystrophy in psoriasis

Infections associated with arthritis, therefore, are nongonococcal urethritis (Catterall 1983), with an association in a substantial proportion of cases with chlamydial infection and infective enterocolitis (dysentery) due to *Shigella* species, *Salmonella* species, *Klebsiella* species and *Yersinia enterocolitica* (Amor et al 1983, Good 1983, Aho et al 1983, Ford 1983a, b). Masi (1979) recorded an incidence of 1.7% of Reiter's syndrome in association with nongonococcal urethritis, 9% postdysenteric arthritis after *Salmonella* infection and 33% after *Yersinia* infection.

Thus the features of reactive arthritis are:

1. Developing two to four weeks after an episode of infective enterocolitis *or* coincident with or preceded by urethritis and/or conjunctivitis
2. An infective organism cannot be isolated from the blood. In postdysenteric forms the organism cannot be isolated from joint fluid although chlamydia has been isolated from the joint fluid of patients with SARA
3. The arthritis frequently resolves within six months although recurrent and chronic destructive forms occur.

Lower limb joint involvement is characteristic of this group leading to pain, swelling and stiffness of the interphalangeal joints of the toes, metatarsophalangeal, midtarsal and subtalar joints and of the ankles. Progressive joint destruction tends to lead to rigidity of the foot (Fig. 37.7). Thus the flat, immobile foot and toes, with severe limitation of the ankle and subtalar joints and valgus heel, occurs in severe, chronic and advanced cases. Achilles tendonitis and plantar fasciitis are common, as in ankylosing spondylitis.

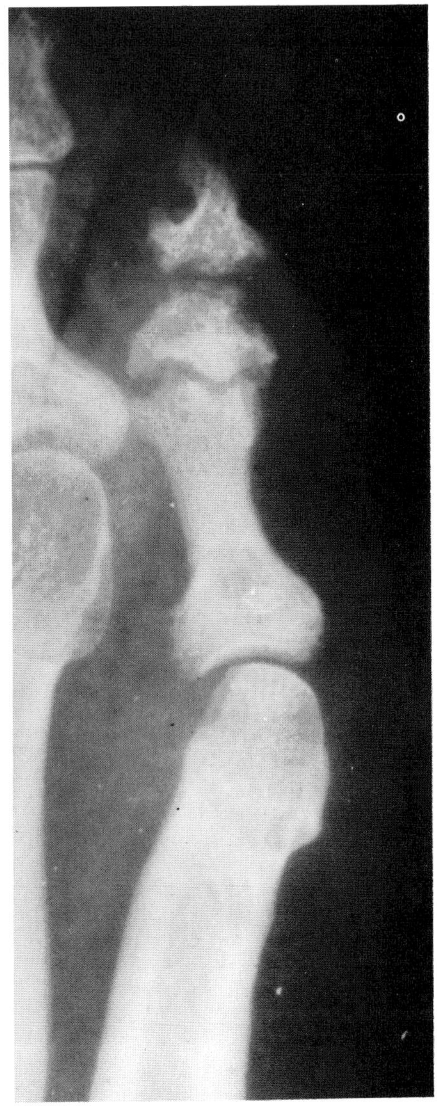

Fig. 37.6 Psoriatic arthritis — radiograph showing erosive damage in the fifth toe interphalangeal joint

While keratodermia (Fig. 37.8) and nail dystrophy

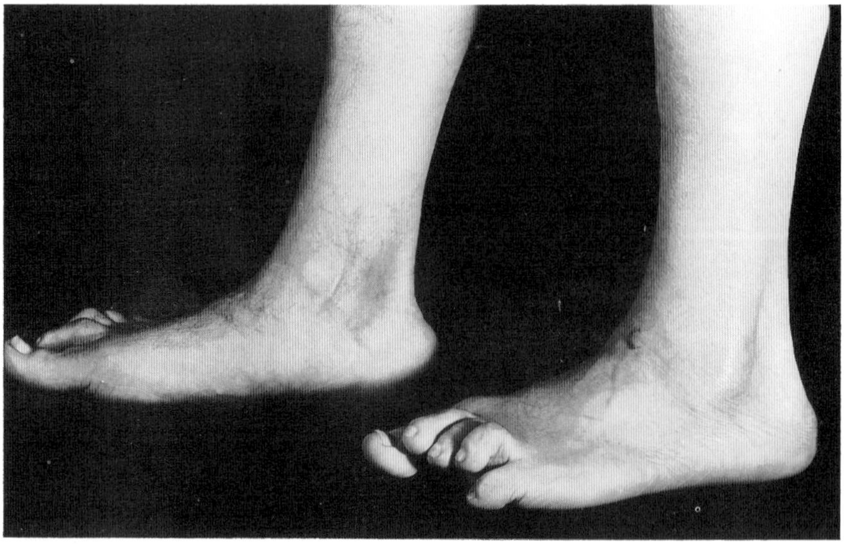

Fig. 37.7 The rigid flat foot of Reiter's syndrome (from Barnes C G 1980 *The Practitioner*, 224, 45–57, with permission of the editor)

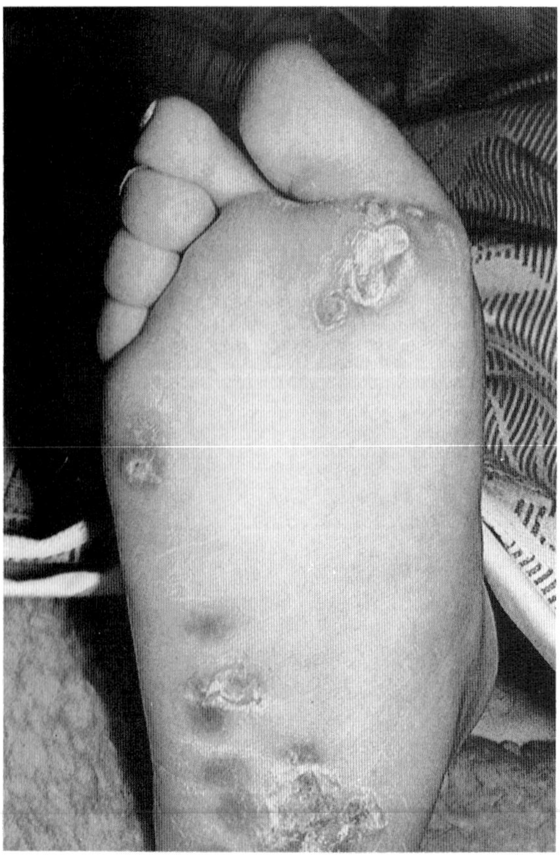

Fig. 37.8 Keratoderma in Reiter's syndrome

are typical of the sexually acquired reactive arthritis (Reiter's syndrome) they may also occur in the postdysenteric type.

Colitis (enteropathic) arthritis

Dekker-Saeys et al (1978) confirmed the three patterns of joint involvement in patients with inflammatory bowel disease in whom they found 13% to have a peripheral arthritis, 10% asymptomatic sacroiliitis and 3.7% classical ankylosing spondylitis. Peripheral arthritis has also been shown to occur in 12% of patients with ulcerative colitis and 22% of those with Crohn's disease (Haslock 1978). Although episodes of acute, nondestructive inflammation of large joints, usually the knees, are characteristic, very occasionally peripheral small joints are involved as in ankylosing spondylitis.

Pyoderma gangrenosum

Pyoderma gangrenosum (Fig. 37.9) is a condition of unknown cause with necrosis and ulceration of skin, usually affecting the lower legs and less frequently the thighs and rarely the arms. It may accompany inflammatory bowel disease, especially ulcerative colitis (Perry & Brunsting 1957), and thus may be associated with colitic arthropathy. It has also been

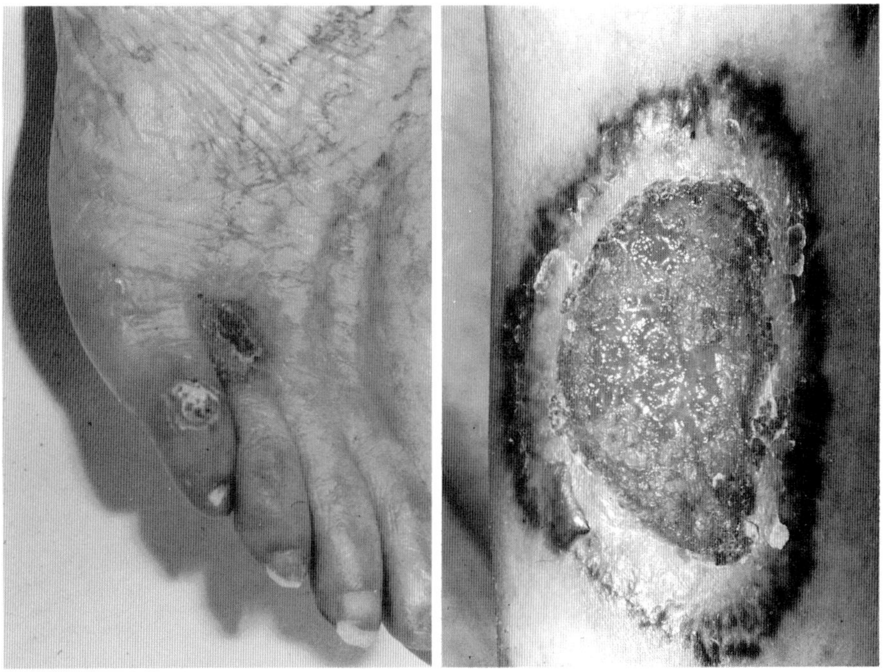

Fig. 37.9 Pyoderma gangrenosum

recorded as occurring with typical rheumatoid arthritis and to be associated with a progressive, erosive seronegative arthritis affecting mainly upper limb and sacroiliac joints (Holt et al 1980).

Systemic connective tissue diseases

A symmetrical inflammatory polyarthritis, resembling rheumatoid arthritis, may be the presentation of any of the systemic connective tissue diseases especially Systemic Lupus Erythematosus (SLE).

Arthralgia often exceeds objective signs of synovitis. The arthritis is mild and usually nondeforming and nondestructive. As in all cases of inflammatory arthritis close enquiry and examination is required for evidence of associated systemic features (Table 37.3). Thus arthritis and vasculitis may both present in the feet (Fig. 37.10).

Rheumatoid factor tests are positive in approximately one-third of patients, antinuclear antibody tests in almost 100% of SLE and 30% of other conditions. DNA binding assays are positive in SLE in which leucopenia may be present also.

A positive fluorescent antinuclear antibody test with a speckled pattern is the immunological marker of the so-called 'Mixed Connective Tissue Disease'. In these cases DNA binding assays are usually normal and extractable nuclear antibody (ENA) assays are positive with specificity for RNA. Whereas this was originally thought to represent a separate disease entity (Sharp et al 1972) it is now apparent that these patients follow the disease pattern of SLE, systemic sclerosis or occasionally rheumatoid arthritis.

Raynaud's phenomenon

Raynaud's phenomenon, while often benign and idiopathic in young females, is a prominent feature of the systemic connective tissue disorders with which they may present. Although this commonly affects the hands, involvement of the feet is not unusual, and in the most severe cases leads to ischaemic lesions of the tips of the fingers and toes.

The development of Raynaud's phenomenon in middle age must always be regarded as a possible onset of a connective tissue disorder, especially systemic lupus erythematosus or systemic sclerosis. The skin changes of systemic sclerosis (scleroderma) affect the feet (Fig. 37.11) less often than the hands.

Table 37.3 Major clinical features of the systemic connective tissue diseases

Systemic lupus erythematosus
polyarthritis
alopaecia
skin rash (for example, 'butterfly')
renal involvement
leucopenia
rheumatoid factor tests positive in approximately 30%
positive antinuclear antibody and DNA binding tests
absence of radiological erosions
neuropsychiatric lesions
Polyarteritis nodosa
arteritis
mononeuritis multiplex (see p. 795)
pulmonary involvement
'asthma'
pulmonary opacities
leucocytosis
eosinophilia (with pulmonary involvement)
abdominal pain
hypertension
haematuria
Systemic sclerosis
skin involvement (scleroderma)
telangiectasia
polyarthritis
subcutaneous calcinosis
dysphagia
hypertension
fibrosing alveolitis
renal involvement
polymyositis
Dermatomyositis
characteristic skin rash
heliotrope periorbital rash
facial oedema
scaling erythema of face, trunk, arms and thighs which is irritating and burning
'collodion' patches over the dorsum of finger joints
telangiectasia around nail beds
inflammatory proximal myopathy

Viral infections

Metatarsophalangeal joints and ankles, together with the small joints of the hands, wrists and knees, may be involved in a symmetrical inflammatory synovitis in association with viral infections. The synovitis is usually mild and nondestructive but with marked arthralgia. This may precede, be coincident with, or follow a few days after the development of other features of the infection. The arthritis resolves completely without residual joint damage in a variable time from a few days to a few weeks during which time it may be migratory or persistent and

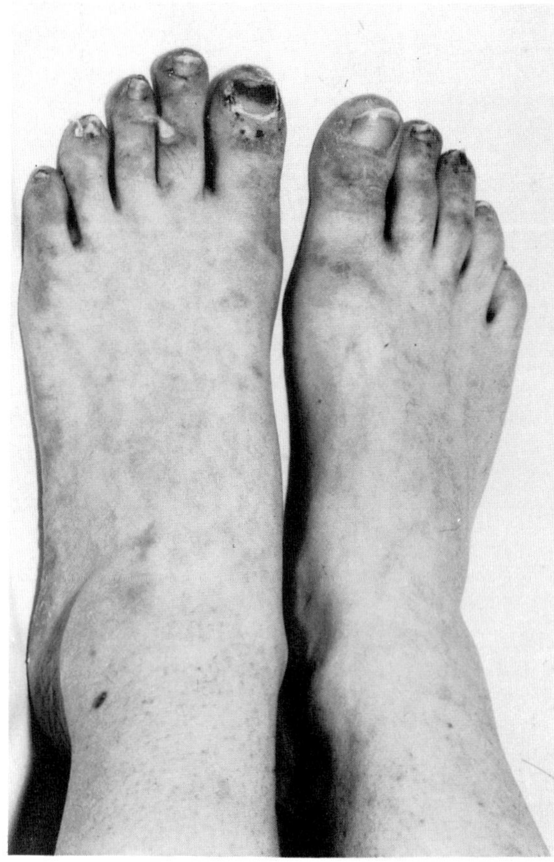

Fig. 37.10 Vasculitis and arthritis in systemic lupus erythematosus

accompanied by myalgia, tenosynovitis and carpal tunnel syndrome.

This has been described most commonly in association with rubella (Chambers & Bywaters 1963), and after rubella immunization (Spruance & Smith 1971), in young females. Rubella virus has been isolated from infected joints. Other infections associated with similar joint manifestations include infectious mononucleosis, mumps (Lass & Shepherd 1961, Ghosh & Reddy 1973), viral hepatitis (Schumacher & Gall 1974), influenza, chicken pox (Friedman & Naveh 1971) and smallpox (Ansell 1978).

Erythema nodosum

Arthralgia and a benign self-limiting symmetrical polyarthritis may accompany up to 75% of patients with erythema nodosum of any cause, which may

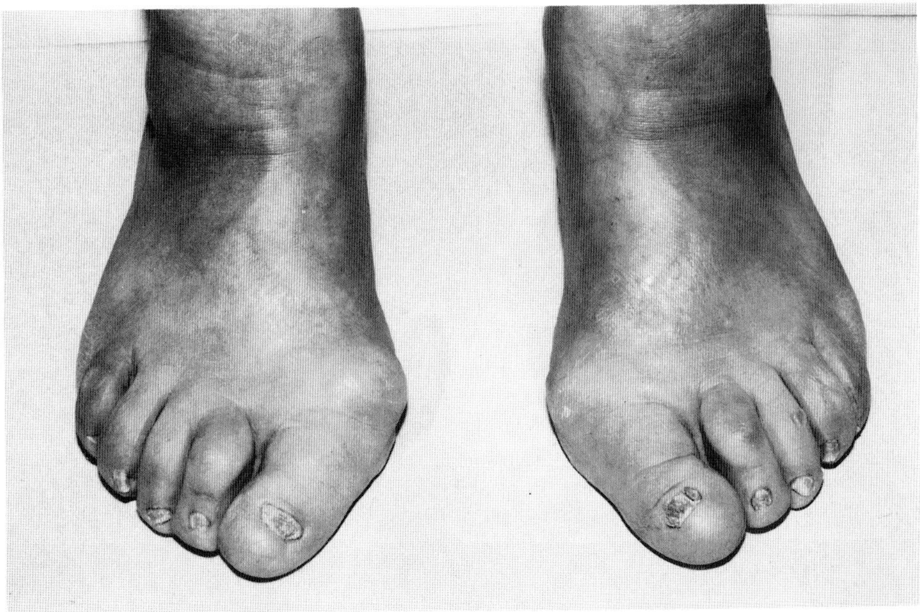

Fig. 37.11 Systemic sclerosis

include streptococcal infections, sarcoidosis (Lofgren's syndrome), tuberculosis, Behçet's syndrome, ulcerative colitis, leprosy, meningococcal infections, fungal infections and sulphonamides (Blomgren 1974).

Severe, often confluent, erythema nodosum around the distal part of the lower leg and ankle, with warmth, redness, tenderness, pain on movement and hence stiffness may mimic a synovitis of the ankle (Fig. 37.12).

Involvement of the ankles

A number of unrelated conditions may present as, or include, an inflammatory arthritis of the ankles but rarely if ever involve smaller joints of the feet.

Palindromic rheumatism

Palindromic, or episodic, rheumatism presents attacks of acute joint inflammation lasting for up to seven days. These occur irregularly, affecting one or two joints at a time, commonly the ankles (Fig. 37.13), knees, hands, wrists and elbows. The involved area is swollen, red, hot, stiff, painful and tender, the swelling and redness often being

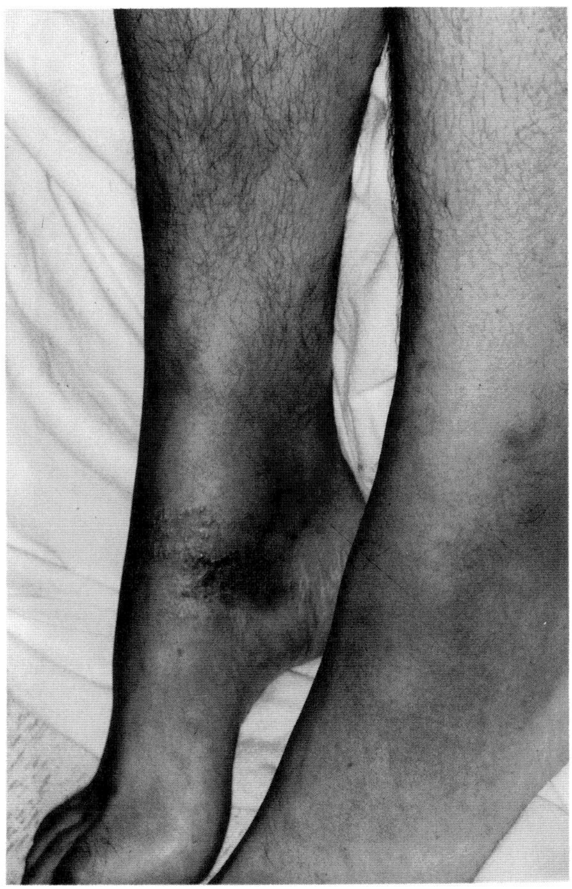

Fig. 37.12 Erythema nodosum

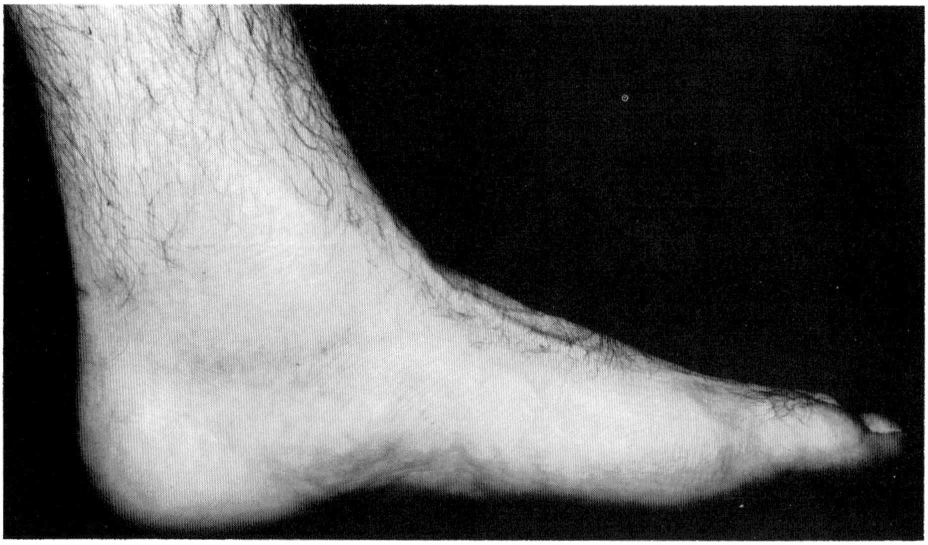

Fig. 37.13 Palindromic rheumatism — acute episode involving the ankle

periarticular. There is nevertheless a true synovitis present (Wajed et al 1977).

In approximately half of these patients the disease progresses to a more typical continuous polyarticular pattern of rheumatoid arthritis, positive tests for rheumatoid factor often developing during the palindromic phase.

Treatment of the acute attack requires full doses of anti-inflammatory analgesics, and if the attacks are frequent regular use of these drugs will prevent or alleviate such attacks. In those with very severe and acute attacks of palindromic rheumatism, in whom rheumatoid factor tests are positive, treatment with gold injections or penicillamine is indicated as in rheumatoid arthritis.

Anaphylactoid (Henoch-Schönlein) purpura

Anaphylactoid purpura arises from vasculitis of arterioles and capillaries which histologically may include a necrotizing arteriolitis (Gairdner 1948). The cause remains unknown, but an allergic response to streptococci (Bywaters et al 1957), various foods, insect bites and drugs, especially penicillin (Casser 1956), has been incriminated. Levinsky & Barratt (1979) detected both circulating and skin bound immune complexes which include IgA.

Papular nonthrombocytopaenic purpura develops on the buttocks and legs, and typically on the soles of the feet, and occasionally on the upper half of the body. Widespread ecchymoses and skin necrosis may develop.

Henoch originally described the gastrointestinal lesions of haemorrhage and oedema of the intestinal wall, with colicky abdominal pain, intestinal haemorrhage or intussusception (Allen et al 1960).

Medium and large sized joints are the site of inflammatory synovitis usually affecting the ankles, knees and hips in the lower limbs, and less commonly involving the wrists and elbows.

Additional features may include acute proliferative or focal glomerulonephritis which may become chronic and hypertension and renal failure, and also intracranial and ocular haemorrhage (Derham & Rogerson 1956, Lewis & Philpott 1956, Bywaters et al 1957, Vernier et al 1961).

Clutton's joints

A nonspecific inflammatory synovitis, developing in children and young adults with congenital syphilis, characteristically affects the knees symmetrically and much less frequently the ankles and elbows (Gray & Philp 1963). The synovitis is nondestructive and self-limiting.

Acne arthritis

Oligoarticular arthralgia and inflammatory arthritis affecting predominantly lower limb joints (knees and ankles) have been described as a rare association of severe acne (acne fulminans; acne conglobata) in male patients (Burns & Coleville 1959, Davis et al 1981, Clement et al 1982). Joint fluid and blood cultures remain sterile, and reduced delayed hypersensitivity (Rajka 1977, Palatski 1977), reduced serum complement levels (Lane et al 1976) and circulating immune complexes (Davis et al 1981, Clement et al 1982) have been detected. It has been suggested, therefore, that this may represent a form of 'reactive arthritis' (q.v.) related to skin infection.

Table 37.4 Clinical features of vasculitis

Subcutaneous nodules	— along affected vessels
Skin	— necrotic lesions seen (Fig. 37.14) — livedo reticularis — nonthrombocytopenic purpura
Cardiovascular system	— hypertension
Gastrointestinal	— abdominal pain — intestinal infarction — mucosal ulceration
Renal	— hypertension — renal failure
Pulmonary	— asthma — radiological opacities and cavitation
Central nervous system	— cerebral infarction — epilepsy
Peripheral nervous system	— mononeuritis multiplex

VASCULAR DISEASE

Vasculitis

Vasculitis, classically polyarteritis nodosa, may be part of any of the systemic connective tissue diseases, but also occurs in rheumatoid arthritis (q.v.) and anaphylactoid (Henoch–Schönlein) purpura (q.v.). Thus, these occur in conjunction with arthralgia and arthritis, myalgia and polymyositis, all producing clinical features resulting from the vasculitis itself. These features depend entirely on the effects of vascular occlusion resulting from the inflammatory involvement of the vessel wall, intimal proliferation and healing with fibrosis, each of which may result in thrombosis. The clinical features of the vasculitis are shown in Table 37.4. In the foot this may present as skin necrosis (Fig. 37.14), arthritis or arthralgia, and the effects of a mononeuritis multiplex (q.v.).

Atheromatous peripheral vascular disease

The classical clinical symptoms of intermittent claudication may be accompanied by severe ischaemic lesions in the feet. Thus cold, painful cyanotic feet, with absent peripheral pulses are typical of this situation. Hypertension, obesity, cigarette smoking and diabetes mellitus are predisposing causes to atheroma.

Thromboangiitis obliterans (Buerger's disease)

Acute inflammation with thrombosis of peripheral arteries and veins characterizes Buerger's disease. Men are affected almost exclusively, between the ages of 20 and 40 years. The cause remains unknown but cigarette smoking is closely related to the clinical manifestations of intermittent claudication, Raynaud's phenomenon and peripheral gangrene affecting the feet more than the hands.

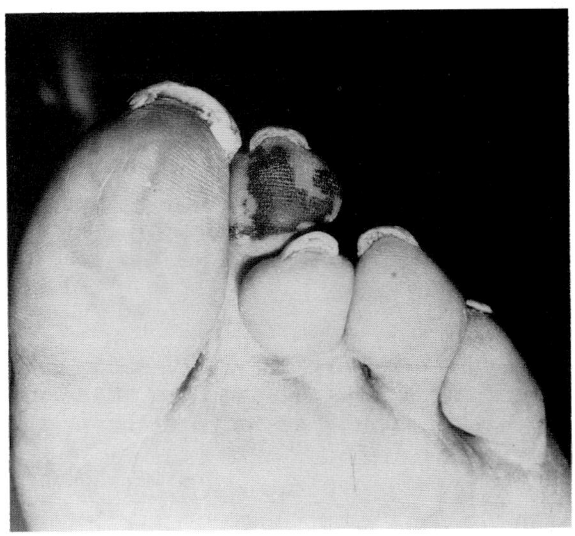

Fig. 37.14 Skin necrosis in polyarteritis nodosa (by permission of the publishers and editor of *Clinical Rheumatology* Currey H L F (ed) 1980)

CRYSTAL ARTHROPATHIES

Introduction

The crystal arthropathies (crystal deposition disease) include the two major diseases of gout due to urate crystals, and pyrophosphate arthropathy or pseudo-gout. However there is now an increasing awareness of many other crystals which may be identified in articular and periarticular tissue and of the possible pathogenetic role of these crystals. Thus hydroxy-apatite, carbonate apatite, calcium triphosphate, carbonate and oxalate, and cholesterol are only some of the crystals identified (Dieppe et al 1983). Remarkably, crystals were first identified by van Leuwenhoek in 1679 using his most primitive microscope.

Crystallization of urate is responsible for the clinical manifestations of gout, hence the terminology crystal arthropathy, crystal-induced disease, crystal synovitis or crystal deposition disease. The fact that urate crystals themselves were responsible for inflammation was proposed by Garrod (1859, 1876) and demonstrated by Freudweiler (1901). McCarty & Hollander (1961) then detected urate crystals by polarized light microscopy, these being strongly negatively birefringent needle-shaped crystals.

The mechanism by which crystals induce inflammation has been extensively investigated. A simple mechanism was originally postulated, the sequence being solute excess → crystal formation → phagocytosis by polymorphonuclear leucocytes → release of chemical mediators of inflammation. This was partially confirmed by the finding of intracellular crystals in phagocytes and high levels of acid phosphatases (etc.) in joint fluid, but it is now apparent that the mechanism is more complex. Crystallization of urate in a hyperuricaemic individual is itself dependant on a number of factors including solute excess, hydration, pH, temperature, local tissue damage, trauma, exercise, etc., and there are similarly a number of inhibitors. Having crystallized, the urate is not only phagocytosed by polymorphonuclear leucocytes, but also by platelets with the release of ADP, ATP and serotonin, the crystals are bound to proteins, mainly albumin, complement and Hageman factor activation occurs and there is an interaction with acute phase proteins (Platt & Dick 1983, Scott 1983, Fiddis et al 1983).

Hyperuricaemia is not synonymous with gout. Population studies have revealed biochemical hyperuricaemia to be present in up to 14% of men (Popert & Hewitt 1962). The prevalence of gout is probably correlated to the height of the serum uric acid level (Mikkelson et al 1965, Hall et al 1967) although Fessel (1972) reported that only three of 66 men with high uric acid levels developed gout in the following four years. Urate levels in the population follow a normal distribution curve (Sturge et al 1977).

Crystals of calcium pyrophosphate dihydrate were detected in joint fluid in 1962 (Kohn et al), being weakly positively birefringent rhomboid-shaped crystals, and shown to be responsible for the features of pyrophosphate arthropathy.

Radiology

Radiological changes are a late feature of gout, consisting of the formation of radiolucent bony tophi appearing as large erosions which may calcify, narrowing of joint space, secondary degnerative changes and occasionally bony ankylosis (Fig. 37.15) (Hughes et al 1968). Thus radiographs do not contribute to the diagnosis of acute gout. Conversely the presence of radiological chondrocalcinosis articularis is a major diagnostic feature of pyrophosphate arthropathy.

Pyrophosphate arthropathy

The acute form of pyrophosphate arthropathy, being an acute crystal synovitis, resembles gout and hence is often known as 'pseudo gout'. Although this occurs more commonly in the knee, the ankles and first metatarsophalangeal joints may be the site of the acute synovitis. In contrast to urate gout, shoulders and hips may similarly be involved.

Chronic pyrophosphate arthropathy is indistinguishable from osteoarthrosis, with or without episodes of acute crystal synovitis (Mitrovic 1983). Rarely polyarticular synovitis occurs mimicking rheumatoid arthritis.

Diagnosis depends on the presence of radiological chondrocalcinosis, most frequently seen in the hyaline and fibrocartilage of the knee (Fig. 37.16), and the detection of calcium pyrophosphate dihydrate (CPPD) crystals, which may be within polymorphonuclear leucocytes, by examination of joint fluid by polarized light microscopy.

Fig. 37.15 Bony ankylosis in severe chronic gout: a, radiograph of 1st toe interphalangeal joint; b, histology of midtarsal joints (from Hughes et al 1968: by permission of the editor of the *Annals of the Rheumatic Diseases*)

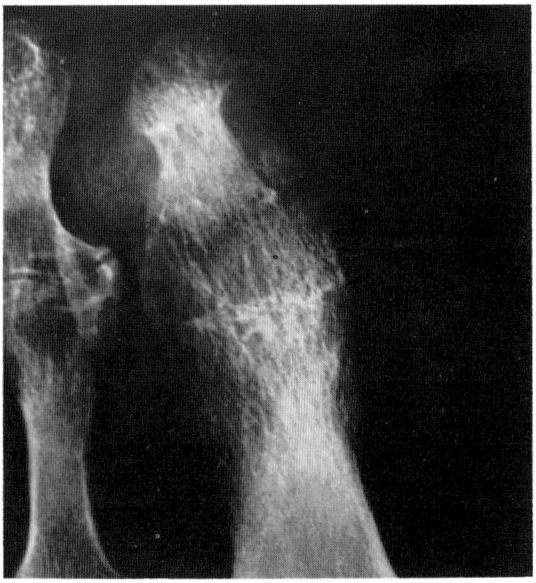

a

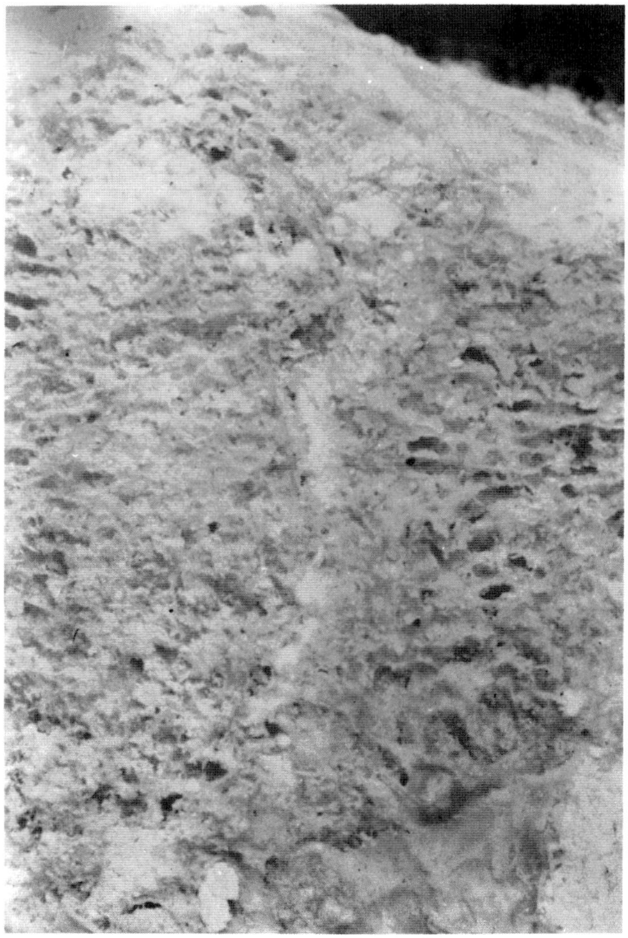

b

The metabolic basis for the deposition of CPPD crystals is still incompletely understood.

The original series reported from Czechoslovakia was of the inherited form of the disease (Zitnan & Sit'aj 1963), since when further descriptions have come from Chile, the Netherlands, Sweden, France and the USA, raising the question of a possible abnormality of inorganic phosphate metabolism. Pyrophosphate deposition is also associated with hyperparathyroidism, haemochromatosis, hypothyroidism and hypophosphatasia (Caswell et al 1983).

Radiological chondrocalcinosis and pyrophosphate arthropathy increases with age, especially in those over 60 years old. Men are affected at a younger age than women and have recurrent acute attacks and less destructive disease. Women tend to have more chronic and polyarticular disease with destructive changes especially in knees and shoulders (Dieppe et al 1982, Doherty 1983).

INFECTIVE ARTHROPATHIES

Monarticular inflammation of a joint must be considered as being due possibly to infection until proved otherwise.

Acute infective arthritis due to pathogenic organisms may complicate direct trauma. However, haematogenous spread from a distant source of infection occurs in patients with underlying predisposing disease such as diabetes mellitus, rheumatoid arthritis, leukaemias, corticosteroid treatment for any reason, and general debility.

The affected joint is red, hot and extremely painful. Diagnosis is made by microbiological

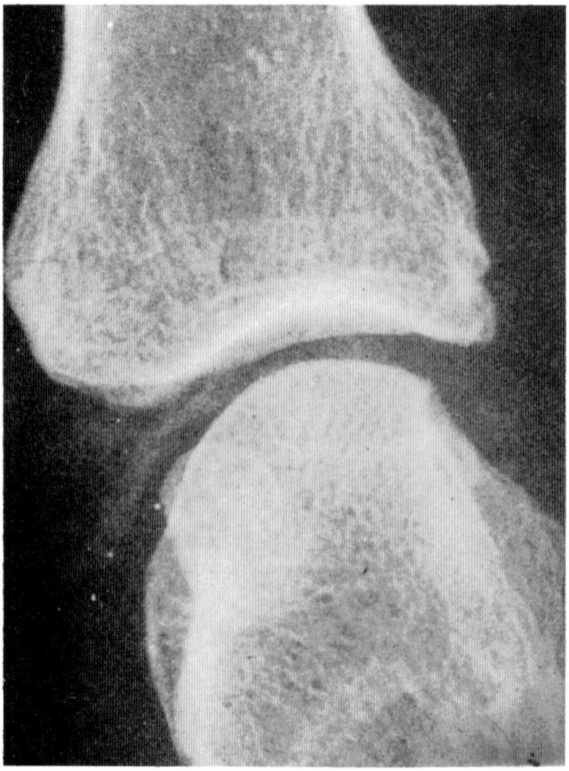

Fig. 37.16 Chondrocalcinous articularis

examination of joint fluid or synovium and treatment is with the appropriate antibiotic.

Gonococcal arthritis

Gonococcal arthritis is usually monarticular, but may occasionally appear to be migratory or polyarticular. Ankles, midtarsal and metatarsophalangeal joints may be affected as may be the knees and wrists (Gelfand et al 1975). It occurs within three weeks of genital infection, which should be sought, and may be accompanied by a typical pustular, erythematous or macular skin eruption on the palms and soles (Ackerman et al 1965) which probably reflects the septicaemic phase of the disease.

Tuberculosis

Involvement of the ankle and tarsal joints, or of the metatarsal bones, may occur in tuberculosis, bone and joint tuberculosis still being prevalent in the United Kingdom (Newton et al 1982, Halsey et al 1982, Davies et al 1984). It must be suspected especially in immigrant patients from the Indian subcontinent and in British patients with a history of previous tuberculosis.

Tuberculosis infection other than that of the involved bone or joint, for example pulmonary, is detectable in only a minority of patients.

Diagnosis depends on the rapid development of radiological osteoporosis and destructive lesions, on a strongly positive (1/10 000) Mantoux test, but most importantly on the histology and bacteriological culture of biopsy material.

HYPERTROPHIC OSTEOARTHROPATHY

Clubbing of the nails (Fig. 37.17), swelling of joints with local pain and tenderness most commonly involving the ankles and wrists, and radiological periostitis (Fig. 37.18) are the characteristic features of hypertrophic osteoarthropathy. The overlying skin is red, warm and oedematous and tenderness extends to the distal part of the long bones of the

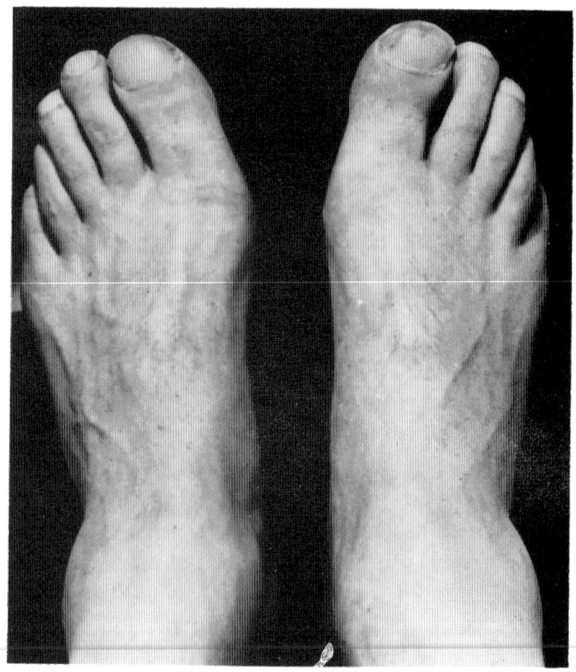

Fig. 37.17 Hypertrophic osteoarthropathy — clubbing of the toe nails

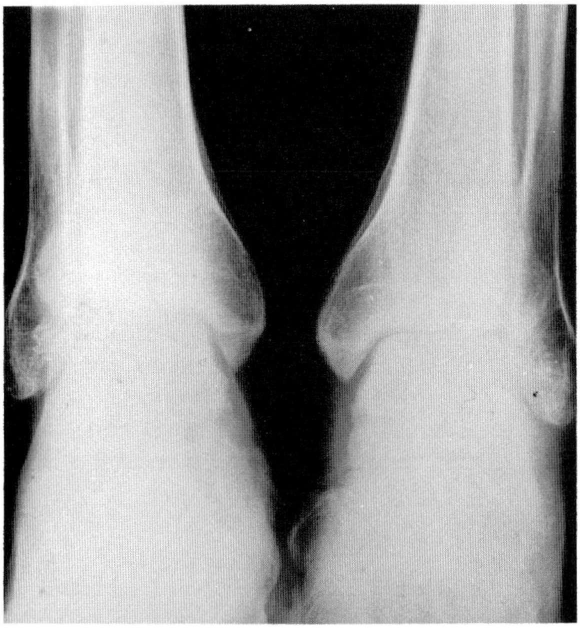

Fig. 37.18 Hypertrophic osteoarthropathy — periostitis of the tibia

Table 37.5 Causes of hypertrophic osteoarthropathy

Pulmonary-neoplastic[1]	Bronchial carcinoma All primary lung neoplasties (except cylindromic adenoma) Metastases from other sites Pleural fibrosarcomata
Non-neoplastic[2]	Bronchiectasis Empyema Tuberculosis Aspergillosis
Congenital cyanotic heart disease[3]	
Gastrointestinal	Biliary atresia[4] Biliary cirrhosis[5] Portal cirrhosis[6] Intestinal lymphoma[7] Ulcerative colitis[8] Crohn's disease[9] Gastrointestinal neoplasms[10] Pseudomembranous enterocolitis[11]
Hodgkin's disease[12]	
Cystic fibrosis[13]	

[1]Flavell 1956, Stenseth et al 1967, Yacoub et al 1967, le Roux 1968
[2]Yacoub & Simon 1966
[3]McLaughlin et al 1967
[4]Cavanaugh & Holman 1965
[5]Mendlowitz 1942
[6]Buchan & Mitchell 1967, Han & Colins 1968, Epstein et al 1979
[7]Bakhshandeh et al 1971
[8]Honska et al 1957, Farman et al 1976
[9]Neale et al 1968, Fielding & Cooke 1971
[10]Hollis 1967
[11]Ueno et al 1981
[12]Mullins & Lenhard 1971
[13]Wasser et al 1982

forearm and lower leg. A mild synovitis of the knees may also be present, although the synovial fluid does not contain the high cell count characteristic of an inflammatory condition.

A narrow band of periosteal new bone is present radiologically, especially at the distal ends of the radius and ulna, tibia and fibula (Fig. 37.18), but this may also be seen affecting the bones of the hands and feet, vertebrae and clavicles (Yacoub & Simon 1966, Greenfield et al 1967).

Formerly the condition was known as hypertrophic pulmonary osteoarthropathy since it is most commonly secondary to pulmonary pathology, bronchial carcinoma being the most frequent. However many causes which are not primarily pulmonary have been identified leading to the omission of the word pulmonary from the name of the disease. Causes identified are listed in Table 37.5. From this it will be seen that the majority of primary pathologies are pulmonary or gastro-intestinal, and the report of hypertrophic osteo-arthropathy in cystic fibrosis (Wasser et al 1982) interestingly links these two systems. A coincidence of both hypertrophic osteoarthropathy and metastatic synovial and bony deposits from a bronchial neoplasm has been reported (Fam & Cross 1979). Nevertheless, the pathogenesis is unknown. It has been suggested that periostitis is responsible for the clinical manifestations and that that may be dependent on vagal stimulation (Dixon 1963). It has been demonstrated that the rheumatological manifestations may regress after vagotomy (Flavell 1956, Yacoub 1965, le Roux 1968) or after parasympathetic blocade (Lopez-Enriques et al 1980, Schwartz 1981) without removal of a primary bronchial neoplasm. Removal of the primary cause, where possible, will lead to a resolution of hypertrophic osteoarthropathy and this has also been achieved by chemotherapeutic treatment of neoplastic disease (Evans 1980).

Pachydermoperiostosis (Touraine-Solente-Gole syndrome)

This is a rare primary form of hypertrophic osteoarthropathy. It has been shown to be inherited by a Mendelian dominant or sex-linked trait affecting males (Fischer et al 1964, Rimoin 1965). Clubbing, periostitis, skin and scalp thickening (pachydermia) and painful swelling around the knees, wrists and ankles are characteristic. The latter is due to the periostitis without synovitis (Calabro et al 1966). Bone marrow failure has been reported (Metz & Dowell 1965).

The disease usually presents at about the time of puberty and progresses for up to five years thereafter (Calabro et al 1966, Salfeld & Spalckhaver 1966).

Thyroid acropachy

Long standing severe hyperthyroidism, often with pretibial myxoedema and exophthalmos, may rarely be associated with clubbing and periostitis. The latter leads to swelling of the hands and feet, with thickened, coarse and fissured skin possibly due to lymphatic obstruction (Scanlon & Clemett 1964, Williams 1967, Ford 1970, Bland et al 1979, Rothschild & Yoon 1982).

METABOLIC AND ENDOCRINE DISORDERS

Hyperlipoproteinaemias

Five groups of hyperlipoproteinaemias have been identified (Fredrickson et al 1967, Rifkind 1970) (Table 37.6). Tendon xanthomata may occur in Types II and III, frequently in the Achilles tendon (Glueck et al 1968) and a polyarthritis may occur in Types II and IV. Large joints tend to be affected in Type II, the symptoms being migratory, lasting for up to one month in an individual joint. The ankles may be involved and it is debated whether the swelling, redness and tenderness is due to a true synovitis (Glueck et al 1968) or a periarthritis (Rooney et al 1978).

A histologically proven synovitis may cause a large and small joint polyarthritis in Type IV hyperlipoproteinaemia (Buckingham et al 1975).

Hyperuricaemia occurs in association with Types III, IV and V hyperlipoproteinaemia (hypertriglyceridaemias) with an increased incidence of gout, obesity and diabetes (Berkowitz 1964, 1966).

Hyperparathyroidism

Hyperparathyroidism may lead to five forms of rheumatic manifestations (Holt 1978):

1. Bone pain resulting from fracture or trabecular collapse which may involve metatarsal bones, from periosteal new bone formation or from osteomalacia. In the latter case local bone tenderness is present, pain may arise from tendon insertions and neuropathy and myopathy may also be present (Patten et al 1974).

2. An erosive small and medium sized joint polyarthritis. Bywaters et al (1963) attributed the erosions to collapse of subchondral bone although Resnick (1974) reported articular without subperiosteal erosions. Subchondral bone collapse may occur, usually at the tibial plateau at the knee, with an associated synovitis, all of which may be traumatic.

3. Chondrocalcinosis articularis and pyrophosphate arthropathy (q.v.).

Table 37.6 Hyperlipoproteinaemias

Type	Cholesterol	Triglycerides	Tendon	Joints	Plasma uric acid
I	N/+	++++			
II	+++	N/+	Xanthomata	Polyarthritis	
III	++	++	Xanthomata		↑
IV	N/+	++		Arthralgia Arthritis	↑
V	++	+++			↑

N = normal

4. Secondary (renal) hyperuricaemia and gout.

5. Fusion of sacroiliac joints (Bunch & Hunder 1973) and tenderness at points of tendon attachment to bone likened to ankylosing spondylitis and the associated enthesopathy (Ball 1971, 1983).

Thus in the foot hyperparathyroidism may present as a small joint polyarthritis, as a 'March' fracture or as (secondary) gout. Symptoms of the associated hypercalcaemia (polyuria, fatigue, weight loss, vomiting, depression) are likely to be more prominent than the rheumatological symptoms.

Acromegaly

Acromegaly may be associated with low back ache (Bluestone et al 1971), carpal tunnel syndrome, coarse crepitus with variable noninflammatory effusions of large joints without pain, entrapment neuropathies especially carpal tunnel syndrome, and fatigue sometimes with a mild proximal myopathy.

Thus in the foot, the principal feature is a diffuse enlargement as also seen in the hand. Radiologically, early widening of the cartilage joint space and late degenerative changes are seen. Prominent tufting of the terminal phalanx also develops, best seen in the fingers, but which may also be present in the toes (Bluestone et al 1971). Thickening of the soft tissue of the heel pad seen radiologically is a supporting diagnostic feature.

Hypothyroidism

Muscle cramps (q.v.), entrapment neuropathies (carpal tunnel or tarsal tunnel syndromes (Frymoyer & Bland 1973)) and tenosynovitis of the dorsum of the foot (Dorwart & Schumacher 1975) may all produce symptoms referable to the foot in hypothyroidism. Examination of the foot includes eliciting the ankle jerk which, with other reflexes, is characteristically slow in relaxation in hypothyroidism.

Hyperthyroidism

Thyroid acropachy is considered on page 792. In severe hyperthyroidism proximal myopathy with weakness and cramp, spreading distally in the most severely affected cases, may develop.

Diabetes mellitus

Five principal complications, or manifestations, of diabetes affect, and therefore may present in, the foot. These are neuropathic (Charcot's) joint disease, peripheral neuropathy, peripheral vascular disease and possibly Dupuytren's diathysis (Gray & Gottlieb 1976), each of which are considered separately within this chapter. The fifth is gout, but there are doubts whether this is a true association. There is an association between obesity and hypertriglyceridaemia with both hyperuricaemia and diabetes (Berkowitz 1966). Two large population studies (Hall et al 1967, Mikkelson et al 1965) failed to demonstrate a statistical clinical relationship between the two diseases.

HAEMATOLOGICAL DISORDERS

Haemophilia

90% of haemorrhages in patients with haemophilia (haemophilia A: factor VIII deficiency) or Christmas disease (haemophilia B: factor IX deficiency) occur in joints or muscles. Severe joint damage develops in these patients with less than 2 iu/dl (2% of normal) factor VIII or IX levels respectively resulting from frequent and apparently often spontaneous bleeding (Ahlberg 1967).

The chronic joint damage appears to result from several mechanisms including synovitis, synovial fibrosis and cartilage destruction, the latter arising from mechanical, chemical and enzymatic processes (Stein & Duthie 1981). Knees, elbows and ankle/subtalar joints are most commonly affected, followed by hips and shoulders, small joints of the hands and feet rarely being involved. The proportion of bleeds into joints decreases in lower limb and increases in upper limb joints during adolescence, but the overall number of haemarthroses usually falls rapidly in adult life (Aronstam et al 1979, Barnes & Colvin 1983). Chronic synovitis may also result from repeated haemarthroses.

Damaged joints are vulnerable to repeated haemarthroses, severe local muscle wasting usually develops, thus the final outcome is joint limitation and deformity. Radiologically the changes are those of severe degenerative joint disease with prolific new bone formation and often large bone cysts (Fig. 37.19).

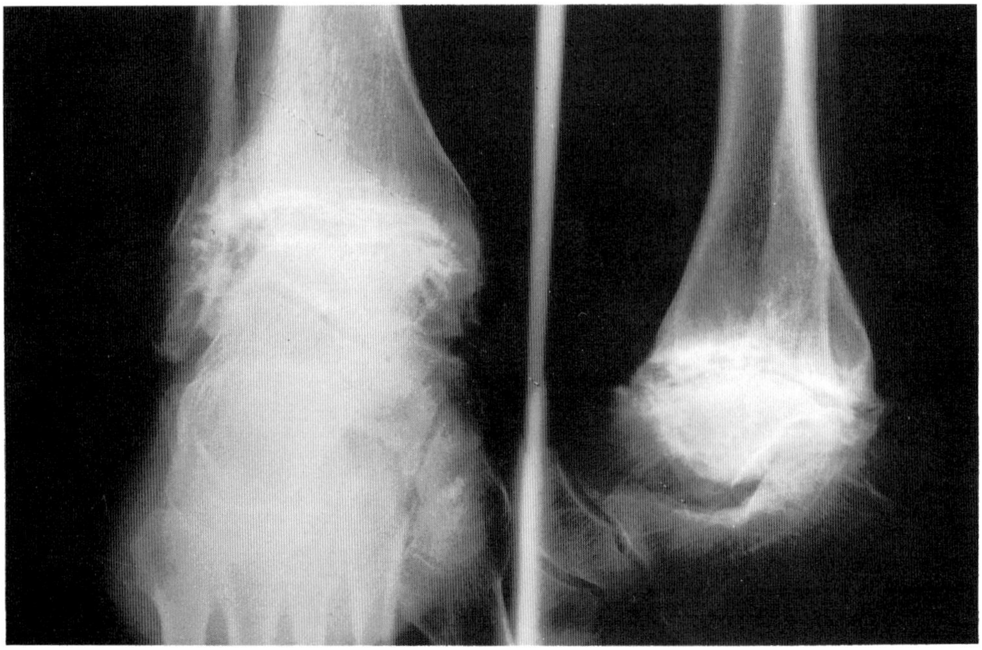

Fig. 37.19 Haemophilia — chronic arthritis of the ankle

It is essential that intravenous replacement of the missing factor is given immediately on the development of a haemarthrosis. With modern treatment using concentrated preparations of factor VIII and IX and home treatment programmes, aspiration of affected joints is very rarely required.

Long-term management of chronic joint damage requires a home programme of physiotherapy to maintain associated muscle power and prevention, or correction, of deformity. Lightweight plastic splints for the ankle/subtalar joints will relieve stress on a limited joint and improve comfort. Surgical arthrodesis of the ankle/subtalar joints is appropriate for the most severely affected cases with gross joint damage, where the knees especially are not themselves a limiting factor.

Leukaemia

Acute leukaemia in childhood may present with bone and joint pain and migratory synovitis, resembling juvenile arthritis. Since the latter may include fever, weight loss, lymphadenopathy, splenomegaly, anaemia and leucocytosis, the differential diagnosis may be difficult (Barnes 1978).

Haemoglobinopathies

Bone and joint changes in sickle cell disease (Hb_{S-S}) and its variants (Hb_{A-S}, Hb_{S-Thal}) include:

1. Pathological fractures due to cortical thinning, itself due to erythroid hyperplasia.
2. Bone infarction due to sickle cell crises. These crises are usually due to hypoxia which leads to the formation of sickle cells in vivo due to a physicochemical alteration of Hb_S. The sickle cells then form thromboses presenting as fever, abdominal pain, and joint or bone pain, the latter due to infarction. Joint pain may be associated with effusion or haemarthrosis, or haemorrhage into subchondral bone.
3. Dactylitis causing painful swelling of the hands and feet. Periostitis of metacarpals and metatarsals is present radiologically.
4. Septic arthritis and osteomyelitis with a high incidence of *Salmonella* infection of bone (Barrett-Connor 1971, Engh et al 1971).

NEUROLOGICAL DISORDERS

Peripheral neuropathies

The causes of peripheral neuropathies have been outlined in Chapter 10 where the electrodiagnostic abnormalities have also been described, and are listed in Table 37.7. The majority of patients have 'cryptogenic' neuropathy thus implying an unknown cause.

Patients present with burning dysaesthesiae, numbness or parasthesiae in the feet and toes, extending up into the lower legs in the more severe case. In such cases peripheral weakness, for example foot drop, is also present.

The signs are those of a glove and stocking loss, or diminution, of sensation, peripheral weakness and absent peripheral tendon reflexes. Clinically and by investigation features of the possible causes need to be sought, and the diagnosis confirmed by nerve conduction studies.

Neuropathic arthropathy (Charcot's joints)

Loss of pain sensation has been regarded as the cause of joint destruction known as Charcot's joints. It is unlikely, however, that this is the true cause as some patients with this condition do experience pain. However there is a combination of impairment of pain sensation and positional sense in most patients which, together with trauma, may lead to the joint destruction.

Table 37.7 Causes of peripheral neuropathy

Cryptogenic:	Cause unknown
Metabolic:	Diabetes mellitus (15%) Diabetic amyotrophy Porphyria Amyloidosis Uraemia
Toxic:	Arsenic Lead Mercury Thallium
Vitamin deficiencies:	Vitamin B (including thiamine and B_{12}) Alcoholic Pyroxamine Pantothenic acid
In rheumatic diseases:	Rheumatoid arthritis
Drug induced:	Gold salts Isoniazid Metronidazole Nitrofurantoin Phenytoin Vincristine
Neoplastic:	Bronchial Lymphoreticular Gastric
Genetic:	Charcot–Marie–Tooth

The classical description by Charcot was of joint destruction in syphilitic tabes dorsalis. Other causes now identified include diabetes mellitus, syringomyelia, leprosy, congenital indifference to pain, Charcot–Marie–Tooth disease, paraplegia, meningomyelocele, subacute combined degeneration of the cord, and familial amyloid polyneuropathy.

Lower limb joints, including those of the foot, are involved especially in tabes dorsalis, diabetes mellitus with painful involvement of the tarsus (Sinha et al 1972), paraplegia and Charcot–Marie–Tooth disease (Bruckner & Kendall 1969).

Joint destruction with hypertrophic bone formation is usual although an atrophic resorptive radiological picture has been described in diabetes, in that case affecting upper more than lower limb joints (Schwartz et al 1969).

Mononeuritis multiplex

A mononeuropathy implies a lesion of an individual nerve. Thus the symptoms and signs are those of motor and sensory deficit in the distribution of the affected nerve distal to the lesion. An isolated foot drop may thus develop. This may arise from mechanical injury or nerve entrapment. Multiple lesions due to vasculitis (q.v.) of the vasa nervorum thus affect a number of individual nerves, and summation of such lesions would lead to a symmetrical picture resembling a glove and stocking neuropathy. Such summation of nerve lesions is usually evident in a careful assessment of the patient's history. This occurs classically in polyarteritis nodosa but also in systemic lupus erythematosus and rheumatoid arthritis, and also in diabetes mellitus although then the cranial nerves are usually affected.

Acquired neurological disorders

Motor neurone disease and hereditary neuropathy (Charcot–Marie–Tooth disease) need to be considered in cases of acquired pes cavus, and in the development of foot drop and perhipheral muscle wasting and weakness. Although upper limb abnormalities develop earlier than the lower limb the signs are those of combined upper and lower motor neurone lesions in motor neurone disease.

Multiple sclerosis may present in a number of apparently unrelated forms arising from the dispersion of neurological lesions in time and space. Thus presentation in the feet may be with isolated sensory symptoms, isolated peripheral nerve palsies, or the development of upper motor neurone lesions leading to lower limb spasticity.

CRAMPS

Muscle cramp is a usually painful, involuntary contraction of muscle lasting for a few seconds to several minutes. Electromyographically high frequency motor unit discharges are present with a repetition rate of 200–300 per second (Kimura 1983). It is extremely common, tends to increase in incidence and also in fequency in the individual patient with age, and often occurs at night.

Muscles of the lower leg and foot are most frequently involved causing a 'spasm', for example with extreme extension and abduction of the hallux. Frequent and severe cramps may lead to a more persistent aching after the acute episode.

The majority of cases of cramp occur in otherwise healthy subjects, or follow periods of unaccustomed exercise. Rarely they result from peripheral ischaemia, hyponatraemia, hypokalaemia due to acute diarrhoea or the excessive use of diuretics, hypocalcaemia or hypothyroidism (Joekes 1979). Cramps may also occur in patients with peripheral neuropathy of any cause or in early cases of motor neurone disease.

DUPUYTREN'S DIATHESIS

Dupuytren's syndrome presents in the hand as a flexion deformity of the fingers resulting from thickening and contraction of the palmar fascia. This occurs in 1–3% of the population, men being affected more frequently than women, is most common in Northern Europe and is rare in coloured peoples (Hueston 1962, Viljanto 1973). There is a strong inherited predisposition, expressed as a dominant inheritance in men (Early 1962).

Rarely this is part of a wider spectrum of manifestations which is then known as Dupuytren's diathesis or disease (Lynch & Jayson 1979), which includes nodules in the palmar and plantar fasciae, epilepsy, gum hypertrophy, stiff shoulders, Peyronie's disease and Garrod's pads (Lettin 1964, Hueston 1975). A high incidence of Dupytren's syndrome has been reported in patients with diabetes mellitus (Lynch & Jason 1979, Noble et al 1984).

Fibrous nodules associated with proliferation and thickening of the plantar fascia (Gabbiani & Manjo 1972, Viljanto 1973) may thus produce severe discomfort on weight bearing and be the presenting, or most prominent symptom of the syndrome.

PAGET'S DISEASE OF BONE

Paget's disease of bone is usually asymptomatic and monostotic. Its cause remains unknown and it is characterized by excessive resorption and deposition of bone. This leads to the production of abnormal bone with characteristic radiological changes of loss of normal trabecular pattern, marked thickening of the cortex and expansion of the bone, and the presence of a coarse trabecular pattern. Abnormal bone is often sharply demarcated from normal bone at which site fractures may occur (Brailsford 1954, Grainger & Laws 1957, Barry 1961).

Long bones, pelvis, vertebrae and the skull are most commonly affected and involvement of the small bones of the hands and feet is very rare with the exception of the occasional monostotic involvement of the calcaneum (Barry 1969). Thus significant involvement of the bones of the feet is extremely rare, is usually a radiological incidental finding and does not require any treatment.

PIGMENTED VILLONODULAR SYNOVITIS

Pigmented villonodular synovitis presents as a swelling, which is often painless, of a joint or tendon sheath. Both sexes at any age may be affected although Rao & Vigorita (1984) have reported a female:male ratio of 2:1 and a younger mean age in those with lower limb involvement compared with those with involvement of the hands.

Joints most commonly involved are those of the fingers and the knees (Granowitz & Mankin 1967, Rao & Vigorita 1984) but involvement of the hips, shoulders, elbows, wrists, ankles and toes is not unusual. Rao & Vigorita (1984) reported a 9% incidence in the toes, and 2.5% in the ankles in a series of 81 patients, compared with 58% in the wrists and hands and 28% in the knees. In that series pain was mild or absent when the ankles, toes or hands were involved compared with mild to severe pain in the majority of involved knee joints. Tenderness is uncommon except in the knees.

Villous, nodular or villonodular lesions may be present in both joints and tendon sheaths, localized nodular proliferation producing the clinical feature of a mechanical derangement. Aspiration of the affected joint reveals a heavily blood-stained fluid.

Radiologically the early feature is the presence of soft tissue swelling while the adjacent bone and joint remains normal. Marginal erosion of juxta articular bone, cystic changes, narrowing of the joint space representing cartilage erosion and localized osteoporosis develop as late radiological features (Breimer & Freiberger 1958, Smith & Push 1962, Schajowicz & Blumenfeld 1968, Pantazopoulos et al 1975, Rao & Vigorita 1984).

The differential diagnosis includes any cause of haemarthrosis, including coagulation disorders, trauma, malignant tumours and synovial haemangiomata, and also synovial sarcoma and fibrous xanthomata, the latter especially when there is tendon sheath involvement (Jones et al 1969).

Histologically the villi are covered by synovial lining cells; sheets of compact round and polyhedral cells, many of which are multinucleate, are present in the stroma of the synovium. Excessive amounts of haemosiderin are present in both the synovial lining cells and stroma. Foamy histiocytes, plasma cells and lymphocytes are present in the stroma and synovial lined clefts are often present. Excessive numbers of mitoses may be present. The lesion may be encapsulated by fibrous tissue (Clark 1958, Nilsonne & Moberger 1969, Schumacher et al 1982, Rao & Vigorita 1984).

Complete excision of the lesion by synovectomy is the treatment of choice although recurrences may occur for which radiotherapy has been advocated (Granowitz et al 1976, Rao & Vigorita 1984).

The classification and aetiology of pigmented villonodular synovitis remains uncertain. The name was introduced by Jaffe et al (1941) as a description of the chronic proliferative synovium which is dark brown due to the presence of haemosiderin. It has been classified as a benign haemangioma, a low grade malignant tumour and an inflammatory granulomatous condition, and it may follow local trauma (Byers et al 1968, Bobechko & Kostvik 1968, Granowitz et al 1976, Molnar et al 1971, Vilppula et al 1982). Despite the possible confusion with malignant neoplasia (single joint involvement, blood stained fluid, radiological bone destruction and increased number of mitoses) it is probably more accurate to classify the diffuse form as a chronic inflammatory granulomatous condition of unknown cause, although the nodular form probably represents a benign neoplastic proliferation of synovium. Metastasis does not occur.

REFLEX SYMPATHETIC DYSTROPHY
(Sudeck's atrophy)

Reflex sympathetic dystrophy or Sudeck's atrophy was first described following trauma in 1864 by Mitchell et al (Kozin et al 1976a). This has been described as usually occurring in the upper limb, for example the 'shoulder-hand syndrome'. Clinically it is recognized that the same syndrome may affect the lower limb, albeit less commonly (Kim et al 1979).

The periphery, and occasionally the knee (Kim et al 1979) becomes diffusely painful and swollen with red, shiny, moist and tender skin. Movement is limited and painful. Radiologically, patchy osteoporosis is typical and radioisotope bone scans show increased uptake, in the lower limb this being around the knee, ankle (Kim et al 1979) and foot, and usually affecting the hand in the upper limb (Kozin et al 1976b). This is usually considered to represent hypervascularity.

Although the syndrome is usually strictly unilateral following trauma, or accompanying a painful limited proximal joint (shoulder-hand syndrome) Kozin et al (1976a, b) demonstrated both a nonspecific synovitis of the small joints of the affected hand and also involvement of the contralateral extremity.

Treatment is by intensive active mobilizing physiotherapy of the proximal and distal limb joints, with appropriate analgesics, and in very severely affected cases treatment with corticosteroids (Kozin et al 1976a) or by sympathetic blockade with intravenous guanethedine or reserpine (Benzon et al 1980).

REFERENCES

Ackerman A B, Miller R C, Shapiro L 1965 Gonococcemia and its cutaneous manifestations. Arch Dermatol 91: 227–232

Ahlberg S 1967 Treatment and prophylaxis of arthropathy in severe haemophilia. Clin Orthop 53: 135–146

Aho K 1983 Yersinia reactive arthritis. Brit J Rheumatol 22 (Suppl 2): 41–45

Aho K, Ahvonen P, Juvakoski T, Kousa M, Leirisalo M, Laitinen O 1983 Immune responses in Yersinia-associated reactive arthritis. Ann Rheum Dis 38 (Suppl): 123–126

Allen D M, Diamond L H, Howell D A 1960 Anaphylactoid purpura in children (Henoch–Schonlein syndrome). Amer J Dis Child 99: 833–854

Amor B, Kahan A, Orfila J, Thomas D 1983 Immunological evidence of chlamydial infection in Reiter's syndrome. Ann Rheum Dis 38 (Suppl): 116–118

Ansell B M 1978 Infective arthritis. In: Scott J T (ed) Copeman's textbook of the rheumatic diseases, 5th edn. Churchill Livingstone, Edinburgh. Ch 31, p 808

Arnett F C 1979 Incomplete Reiter's syndrome: clinical comparisons with classical triad. Ann Rheum Dis 38 (Suppl): 73–78

Aronstam A, Rainsford S G, Painter M J 1979 Patterns of bleeding in adolescents with severe haemophilia A. Brit Med J 1: 469–470

Bakhshandeh K, Nasr K, Haghighi P, Haghshenas M 1971 Clubbing and osteoarthropathy associated with primary upper small intestinal lymphoma. J Trop Med Hyg 74: 117–119

Ball J 1971 Enthesopathy of rheumatoid and ankylosing spondylitis. Ann Rheum Dis 30: 213–223

Ball J 1983 The Enthesopathy of ankylosing spondylitis. Brit J Rheumatol 22 (Suppl 2): 25–28

Barnes C G 1978 Miscellaneous and uncommon rheumatic conditions. In: Scott J T (ed) Copeman's textbook of the rheumatic diseases, 5th edn. Churchill Livingstone, Edinburgh. Ch 33, p 844

Barnes C G 1980 Less common forms of arthritis. The Practitioner 224: 45–60

Barnes C G, Colvin B T 1983 Haemophilia. Reports on Rheumatic Diseases 85

Barrett-Connor E 1971 Bacterial infection and sickle cell anaemia. Medicine (Baltimore) 50: 97–112

Barry H C 1961 Sarcoma in Paget's disease of bone in Australia. J Bone Joint Surg 43A: 1122–1134

Barry H C 1969 Paget's disease of bone. E & S Livingstone Ltd, Edinburgh

Benzon H T, Chomka C M, Brunner E A 1980 Treatment of reflex sympathetic dystrophy with regional intravenous reserpine. Anaes Analgesia 59: 500–502

Berkowitz D 1964 Blood lipid and uric acid inter-relationships. JAMA 190: 856–858

Berkowitz D 1966 Gout, hyperlipaemia and diabetes. JAMA 197: 77–80

Bland J H, Frymoyer J W, Newberg A H, Revers R, Normal R J 1979 Rheumatic syndromes in endocrine disease. Semin Arthritis Rheum 9: 23–64

Blomgren S E 1974 Erythema nodosum. Semin Arthritis Rheum 4: 1–24

Bluestone R, Bywaters E G L, Hartog M, Holt P J L, Hyde S 1971 Acromegalic arthropathy. Ann Rheum Dis 30: 243–258

Bobechko W P, Kostvik J P 1968 Childhood villonodular synovitis. Can J Surg 11: 480–486

Brailsford J F 1954 Pagets disease of bone. Br J Radiol 27: 435–442

Breimer C W, Freiberger R H 1958 Bone lesions associated with villonodular synovitis. Am J Roentgen 79: 618–629

Brewerton D A, Caffrey M F P, Hart F D, James D C O, Nicholls A, Sturrock R D 1973 Ankylosing spondylitis and HL-A27. Lancet 1: 904–907

Brewerton D A, Caffrey M, James D C O 1974a The histocompatibility antigen (HL-A27) and its relation to disease. J Rheumatol 1: 249–253

Brewerton D A, Nicholls A, Caffrey M, Walters D, James D C O 1974b HL-A27 and arthropathies associated with ulcerative colitis and psoriasis. Lancet 1: 956–957

Brewerton D A, James D C O 1975 The histocompatibility antigen (HL-A27) and disease. Semin Arthritis Rheum 4: 191–207

Bruchner F E, Kendall B E 1969 Neuroarthropathy in Charcot–Marie–Tooth disease. Ann Rheum Dis 28: 577–583

Buchan D J, Mitchell D M 1967 Hypertrophic osteoarthropathy in portal cirrhosis. Ann Intern Med 66: 130–135

Buckingham R B, Bole G G, Bassett D R 1975 Polyarthritis associated with Type IV hyperlipoproteinaemia. Arch Int Med 135: 286–290

Bunch T W, Hunder G C 1973 Ankylosing spondylitis and primary hyperparathyroidism. JAMA 225: 1108–1109

Burns R E, Coleville J M 1959 Acne conglobata with septicemia. Arch Dermatol 79: 361–362

Byers P D, Cotton R E, Deacon O W, Lowy M, Newman P H, Sissons H A, Thompson A D 1968 The diagnosis and treatment of pigmented villonodular synovitis. J Bone Joint Surg 50B: 290–309

Bywaters E G L, Isdale I, Kempton J J 1957 Schonlein-Henoch purpura. Q J Med 50 (NS26): 161–175

Bywaters E G L, Dixon A St J, Scott J T 1963 Joint lesions of hyperparathyroidism. Ann Rheum Dis 22: 171–187

Calabro J J, Marchesano J M, Abruzzo J L 1966 Idiopathic hypertrophic osteoarthropathy (pachydermoperiostosis): onset before puberty. Arthritis Rheum 9: 496

Casser L 1956 Anaphylactoid purpura following penicillin therapy. J Med Soc NJ 53: 133–134

Caswell A, Guilland-Cumming D F, Hearn P R, McGuire M K B, Russell R G G, 1983 Pathogenesis of chondrocalcinosis and pseudogout. Metabolism of inorganic pyrophosphate and production of calcium pyrophosphate dihydrate crystals. Ann Rheum Dis 42 (Suppl): 27–37

Catterall R D 1983 Clinical aspects of Reiter's Disease. Brit J Rheumatol 22 (Suppl 2): 151–155

Cavanaugh J J A, Holman G H 1965 Hypertrophic osteoarthropathy in childhood. J Paediatr 66: 27–40

Chambers R J, Bywaters E G L 1963 Rubella synovitis. Ann Rheum Dis 22: 263–268

Clark W S 1958 Pigmented villonodular synovitis. Bull Rheum Dis 8: 161–162

Clement G B, Vasey F B, Fenske N A, Bridgeford P, Germain B F, Espinoza L R 1982 Acne arthritis: clinical manifestations, human leukocyte antigens and circulating immune complexes. Arthritis Rheum 25 (Suppl): 51, Abstract 58
Currey H L F 1980 Mason & Currey's Clinical Rheumatology, 3rd edn. Pitman Medical, London p 124
Davies P D O, Humphries M J, Byfield S P et al 1984 Bone and joint tuberculosis. J Bone Joint Surg 66B: 326–330
Davis D L E, Viozzi F J, Miller F, Blodgett R 1981 The musculoskeletal manifestations of acne fulminans. J Rheumatol 8: 317–320
Dekker-Saeys B J, Meuwissen S G M, Berg-Loonen E M Van der, DeHaas W H D, Meijers K A F, Tytgat G N J 1978 Ankylosing spondylitis and inflammatory bowel disease. Ann Rheum Dis 37: 30–41
Derham R J, Rogerson M M 1956 The Schonlein-Henoch syndrome with particular reference to renal sequelae. Arch Dis Child 31: 364–368
Dieppe P A, Alexander G M, Jones H et al 1982 Pyrophosphate arthropathy: a clinical and radiological study of 105 cases. Ann Rheum Dis 41: 371–376
Dieppe P, Doherty M, MacFarlane D 1983 Crystal-related arthropathies. Ann Rheum Dis 42 (Suppl): 1–3
Dixon A St J 1963 Unusual effects of bronchial carcinoma and other lung tumours. Thorax 18: 197
Doherty M 1983 Pyrophosphate arthropathy — recent clinical advances. Ann Rheum Dis 42 (Suppl): 38–44
Dorwart B B, Schumacher H R 1975 Joint effusions, chondrocalcinosis and other rheumatic manifestations in hypothyroidism. Am J Med 59: 780–790
Early P F 1962 Population studies in Dupuytren's contracture. J Bone Joint Surg 44B: 602–613
Ebringer A, Shipley M (eds) 1983 Pathogenesis of HLA-B27 associated diseases. Br J Rheumatol 22 (Suppl 2)
Engh C A, Hughes J L, Abrams R C, Bowerman J W 1971 Osteomyelitis in the patient with sickle-cell disease. J Bone Joint Surg 53A: 1–15
Epstein O, Ajdukiewicz A B, Dick R, Sherlock S 1979 Hypertrophic hepatic osteoarthropathy. Clinical, roentgenologic, biochemical, hormonal and cardiorespiratory studies, and review of the literature. Am J Med 67: 88–97
Evans W K 1980 Reversal of hypertrophic osteoarthropathy after chemotherapy for bronchogenic carcinoma. J Rheumatol 7: 93–97
Fam A G, Gross E G 1979 Hypertrophic osteoarthropathy, phalangeal and synovial metastases associated with bronchogenic carcinoma. J Rheumatol 6: 680–686
Farman J, Twersky J, Fierst S 1976 Ulcerative colitis associated with hypertrophic osteoarthropathy. Dig Dis 21: 130–135
Fessel W J 1972 Hyperuricaemia in health and disease. Semin Arthritis Rheum 1: 275–299
Fiddis R W, Vlachos N, Calvert P D 1983 Studies of urate crystallisation in relation to gout. Ann Rheum Dis 42 (Suppl): 12–15
Fielding J F, Cooke W T 1971 Finger clubbing and regional enteritis. Gut 12: 442–444
Fischer D S, Singer D H, Feldman S M 1964 Clubbing: a review, with emphasis on hereditary acropachy. Medicine (Baltimore) 43: 459–479
Flavell G 1956 Reversal of pulmonary hypertrophic osteoarthropathy by vagotomy. Lancet 1: 260–262
Ford D K 1983a Yersinia-induced arthritis and Reiter's syndrome. Ann Rheum Dis 38 (Suppl): 127–128
Ford D K 1983b Cell-mediated immunity to U. urealyticum (Mycoplasma) in patients with Reiter's syndrome. Ann Rheum Dis 38 (Suppl): 129–130
Ford P M 1970 Thyroid acropachy. Proc R Soc 63: 284–285
Fredrickson D S, Levy R I, Lees R I 1967 Fat Transport in lipoproteins — an integrated approach to mechanisms and disorders. N Eng J Med 276: 34–44, 94–103, 148–156, 215–225, 273–281
Freudweiler M 1901 Experiment elle untersuchungen uber die Enistehung der Gichtknoten. Dtsch Arch Klin Med 69: 155 (English translation Arthritis Rheum 1965: 8, 267–288)
Friedman A, Naveh Y 1971 Polyarthritis associated with chicken pox. Am J Dis Child 122: 179–180
Frymoyer J W, Bland J 1973 Carpal tunnel syndrome in patients with myxedematous arthropathy. J Bone Joint Surg 55A: 78–82
Gabbiani G, Manjo G 1972 Dupuytren's contracture: fibroblast contraction? An ultrastructural study. Am J Pathol 66: 131–147
Gairdner D 1948 The Schonlein-Henoch syndrome (anaphylactoid purpura). Q J Med NS 17: 95–122
Garrod A B 1859 The nature and treatment of gout and rheumatic gout. Walton and Maberley, London
Garrod A B 1876 A treatise on gout and rheumatic gout (rheumatoid arthritis). 3rd edn. Longman, London
Gelfand S G, Alfonse T M, Gareia-Kutzbach A 1975 Spectrum of gonococcal arthritis. Evidence for sequential stages and clinical subgroups. J Rheumatol 2: 83–90
Ghosh S K, Reddy T A 1973 Arthralgia and myalgia in mumps. Rheumatol Rehabil 12: 97–99
Glueck C J, Levy R I, Fredrickson D S 1968 Acute tendinitis and arthritis. JAMA 206: 2895–2897
Good A E 1983 Shigellae and Reiter's syndrome. Ann Rheum Dis 38 (Suppl): 119–122
Grainger R G, Laws J W 1957 Paget's disease — active or quiescent? Br J Radiol 30: 120–124
Granowitz S P, Mankin H J 1967 Localised pigmented villonodular synovitis of the knee. J Bone Joint Surg 49A: 122–128
Granowitz S P, D'Antonio J, Mankin H L 1976 The pathogenesis and long term end results of pigmented villonodular synovitis. Clin Orthop 114: 335–351
Gray M S, Philp T 1963 Syphilitic arthritis. Ann Rheum Dis 22: 19–25
Gray R G, Gottlieb N L 1976 Rheumatic disorders associated with diabetes mellitus. Semin Arthritis Rheum 6: 19–34
Greenfield G B, Schorasch H A, Shkolnik A 1967 The various roentgen appearances of pulmonary hypertrophic osteoarthropathy. Am J Roentgenol 101: 927–931
Hall A P, Barry P E, Dowber T R et al 1967 Epidemiology of gout and hyperuricaemia: a long-term population study. Am J Med 42: 27–37
Halsey J P, Reeback J, Barnes C G 1982 A decade of skeletal tuberculosis. Ann Rheum Dis 41: 7–10
Han S Y, Colins L C 1968 Hypertrophic osteoarthropathy in cirrhosis of the liver. Radiology 91: 795–796
Harris J R W, Gelsthorpe K, Doughty R W, Lee D, Morgan R S 1975 HL-A27 and W10 in Reiter's syndrome and non-specific urethritis. Acta Derm Venereol (Stockholm) 55: 127–130
Haslock I, Wright V 1973–4 The arthritis associated with intestinal disease. Bull Rheum Dis 24: 750–754
Haslock I 1978 Enteropathic arthritis. In: Scott J T (ed) Copeman's textbook of the rheumatic diseases, 5th edn. Churchill Livingstone, Edinburgh. Ch 23, p 567
Hollis W C 1967 Hypertrophic osteoarthropathy secondary to

upper gastrointestinal tract neoplasm. Ann Intern Med 66: 125–130
Holt P J A, Davies M G, Saunders K C, Nuki G 1980 Pyoderma gangrenosum. Clinical and laboratory findings in 15 patients with special reference to polyarthritis. Medicine (Baltimore) 59: 114–133
Holt P J L 1978 Endocrine disorders and metabolic bone disease. In: Scott J T (ed) Copeman's textbook of the rheumatic diseases, 5th edn. Churchill Livingstone, Edinburgh. Ch 28, p 707
Honska W L, Strenge J, Hammarsten J F 1957 Hypertrophic osteoarthropathy and chronic ulcerative colitis. Gastroenterology 33: 489–492
Hueston J T 1962 Digital Wolfe grafts in recurrent Dupuytren's contracture. Plast Reconstr Surg 29: 342–344
Hueston J T 1968 Dupuytren's contracture and specific injury. Med J Aust 1: 1084–1085
Hueston J T 1975 Dupuytren's contracture selection for surgery. Br J Hosp Med 13: 361–370
Hughes G R, Barnes C G, Mason R M 1968 Bony ankylosis in gout. Ann Rheum Dis 27: 67–70
Jaffe H L, Lichtenstein L, Sutro C J 1941 Pigmented villonodular synovitis, bursitis and tenosynovitis. Arch Pathol 31: 731–765
Jajic I 1968 Radiological changes in the sacro-iliac joints and spine of patients with psoriatic arthritis and psoriasis. Ann Rheum Dis 27: 1–6
Jayson M I V, Salmon P R, Harrison W J 1970 Inflammatory bowel disease in ankylosing spondylitis. Gut 11: 506–511
Joekes A M 1979 Cramp. Clin Rheum Dis 5: 873–881
Jones F E, Soule E H, Coventry M B 1969 Fibrous xanthoma of synovium (giant-cell tumour of tendon sheath, pigmented synovitis). A study of one hundred and eighteen cases. J Bone Joint Surg 51A: 76–86
Kammer G M, Soter N A, Gibson D J, Schur P H 1979 Psoriatic arthritis: a clinical, immunological and HLA study of 100 patients. Semin Arthritis Rheum 9: 75–97
Keat A C, Scott J T, Ridgway G, Maini R N, Pergrum G D 1979 Sexually acquired reactive arthritis. Ann Rheum Dis 38 (Suppl): 52–54
Kim H J, Kozin F, Johnson R P, Hines R 1979 Reflex sympathetic dystrophy syndrome of the knee following meniscectomy: report of three cases. Arthritis Rheum 22: 177–181
Kimura J 1983 Neuromuscular diseases characterised by abnormal muscle activity. In: Electrodiagnosis in diseases of nerve and muscle: principles and practice. F A Davis, Philadelphia. Ch 26, p 549
Kohn N N, Hughes R E, McCarty D J, Faires J S 1962 The significance of calcium phosphate crystals in the synovial fluid of arthritic patients: the 'pseudogout syndrome'. II Identification of crystals. Ann Intern Med 56: 738–745
Kozin F, McCarty D J, Sims J, Genant H 1976a The reflex sympathetic dystrophy syndrome. I. Clinical and histologic studies: evidence for bilaterality, response to corticosteroids and articular involvement. Am J Med 60: 321–331
Kozin F, Genant H K, Beckerman C, McCarty D J 1976b The reflex sympathetic dystrophy syndrome. II. Roentgenographic and scintigraphic evidence of bilaterally and of periarticular accentuation. Am J Med 60: 332–338
Lane A M, Leyden J I, Spiegel R J 1976 Acne Arthralgia. J Bone Joint Surg 58A: 673–675
Lass R, Shepherd E 1961 Mumps arthritis. Br Med J 2: 1613–1614
Lawrence J S 1974 Family survey of Reiter's disease. Br J Vener Dis 50: 140–145
Le Roux B T 1968 Bronchial carcinoma with hypertrophic pulmonary osteoarthropathy. S Afr Med J 42: 1074–1075
Lettin A W F 1964 Dupuytren's diathesis: a case report. J Bone Joint Surg 46B: 220–225
Levinsky R J, Barratt T M 1979 IgA immune complexes in Henoch–Schonlein purpura. Lancet 2: 1100–1103
Lewis I C, Philpott M G 1956 Neurological complications of the Schonlein–Henoch syndrome. Arch Dis Child 31: 369–371
Lopez-Enriquez E, Morales A R, Robert F 1980 Effect of atropine sulfate in pulmonary hypertrophic osteoarthropathy. Arthritis Rheum 23: 822–824
Lynch M, Jayson M I V 1979 Dupuytren's disease and contracture. In: Dixon A St J (ed) Soft tissue rheumatism. Clin Rheum Dis 5: 837–840
Macrae I, Wright V 1973 A family study of ulcerative colitis, with particular reference to ankylosing spondylitis and sacroiliitis. Ann Rheum Dis 32: 16–20
Masi A T 1979 Epidemiology of B27-associated diseases. Ann Rheum Dis 38 (Suppl): 131–134
Mason R M, Murray R S, Oates J K, Young A C 1958 Prostatitis and ankylosing spondylitis. Br Med J 1: 748–751
McCarty D J, Hollander J L 1961 Identification of urate crystals in gouty synovial fluid. Ann Intern Med 54: 452–460
McLaughlin G E, McCarty D J Jr, Downing D F 1967 Hypertrophic osteoarthropathy associated with cyanotic congenital heart disease. Ann Intern Med 67: 579–587
Mendlowitz M 1942 Clubbing and hypertrophic osteoarthropathy. Medicine (Baltimore) 21: 296–306
Metz E N, Dowell A 1965 Bone marrow failure in hypertrophic osteoarthropathy. Arch Intern Med 116: 759–764
Mikkelson W M, Dodge H J, Valkenburg B 1965 The distribution of serum uric acid values in a population unselected as to gout of hyperuricaemia. Tecumseh, Michigan 1959–1960. Am J Med 39: 242–251
Mitrovic D R 1983 Pathology of articular deposition of calcium salts and their relationship to osteoarthrosis. Ann Rheum Dis 42 (Suppl): 19–26
Moll J M H, Wright V 1973 Psoriatic arthritis. Semin Arthritis Rheum 3: 55–78
Moll J M H, Wright V 1973 Family occurrence of psoriatic arthritis. Ann Rheum Dis 32: 181–201
Moll J M H, Haslock I, Macrae I F, Wright V 1974 Associations between ankylosing spondylitis, psoriatic arthritis, Reiter's disease, the intestinal arthropathies and Behçet's syndrome. Medicine (Baltimore) 53: 343–364
Moll J M H, Haslock I, Wright V 1978 Seronegative spondarthritides. In: Scott J T (ed), Copeman's textbook of the rheumatic diseases, 5th edn. Churchill Livingstone, Edinburgh. Ch 24, p 578
Molnar Z, Stein W H, Stoltzner G H 1971 Cytoplasmic tubular structures in pigmented villonodular synovitis. Arthritis Rheum 14: 784–787
Morris R I, Metzger A L, Bluestone R T, Terasaki P I 1974 A useful discriminator in the arthropathies of inflammatory bowel disease. N Engl J Med 290: 1117–1119
Mullins G M, Lenhard R E 1971 Digital clubbing in Hodgkin's disease. Johns Hopkins Med J 128: 153–157
Neale G, Kelsall A R, Doyle F H 1968 Crohn's disease and diffuse symmetrical periostitis. Gut 9: 383–387
Newton P, Sharp J, Barnes K L 1982 Bone and joint tuberculosis in Greater Manchester. Ann Rheum Dis 41: 1–6
Nilsonne U, Moberger G 1969 Pigmented villonodular

synovitis of joints. Histological and clinical problems in diagnosis. Acta Orthop Scand 40: 448–460
Noble J, Heathcote J G, Cohen H 1984 Diabetes mellitus in the aetiology of Dupuytren's disease. J Bone Joint Surg 66B:322–325
Olhagen B 1983 Urogenital syndromes and spondarthritis. Br J Rheumatol 22 (Suppl 2): 33–40
Palatski R 1977 Delayed hypersensitivity and febrile acne conglobata. Acta Dermat (Stockholm) 57: 51–53
Pantazopoulos Th, Stavrou S, Stamos C, Kehayas G, Hartofilaleidis-Gerofalidis G 1975 Bone lesions in pigmented villonodular synovitis. Acta Orthop Scand 46: 579–592
Patten B M, Bileyikian J P, Mallette L E, Prince A, Engel W K, Aurback G D 1974 Neuromuscular disease in primary hypoparathyroidism. Ann Intern Med 80: 182–193
Perry H O, Brunsting L A 1957 Pyoderma gangrenosum: a clinical study of 19 cases. Arch Dermatol 75: 380–386
Platt P, Dick W C 1983 Crystals and inflammation. Ann Rheum Dis 42 (Suppl): 4–7
Popert A J, Hewitt J V 1962 Gout and hyperuricaemia in rural and urban populations. Ann Rheum Dis 21: 154–163
Rajka G 1977 Cell mediated immunity and acne conglobata. Acta Dermatol (Stockholm) 57: 141–143
Rao A S, Vigorita V J 1984 Pigmented villonodular synovitis (giant cell tumour of the tendon sheath and synovial membrane). J Bone Joint Surg 66A: 76–94
Resnick D L 1974 Erosive arthritis of the hand and wrist in hyperparathyroidism. Radiology 110: 263–269
Rifkind B M 1970 The hyperlipoproteinaemias. Br J Hosp Med 4: 683–692
Rimoin D L 1965 Pachydermoperiostosis (idiopathic clubbing and periostosis). Genetic and physiological considerations. N Eng J Med 272: 923–931
Rooney P J, Thind J, Madkour M M, Spender D, Dick W C 1978 Transient polyarthritis associated with familial hyperbetalipoproteinaemia. Q J Med 187 (NS47): 249–259
Rothschild B M, Yoon B H 1982 Thyroid acropathy complicated by lymphatic obstruction. Arthritis Rheum 25: 588–590
Salfeld K, Spalckhaver I 1966 Zur Kenntnis der Pachydermoperiostosis. Derm Woch 152: 497–511
Scanlon G T, Clemett A R 1964 Thyroid acropachy. Radiology 83: 1039–1042
Schajowicz F, Blumenfeld I 1968 Pigmented villonodular synovitis of the wrist with penetration into bone. J Bone Joint Surg 50B: 312–317
Schlosslein L, Tevasaki P I, Bluestone R T, Pearson C M 1973 High association of an HL-A antigen, W27, with ankylosing spondylitis. N Engl J Med 288: 704–706
Schumacher H R, Gall E P 1974 Arthritis in acute hepatitis and chronic active hepatitis. Am J Med 57: 655–664
Schumacher H R, Lotke P, Akthreya B, Rothfuss S 1982 Pigmented villonodular synovitis: light and electron studies. Semin Arthritis Rheum 12: 32–43
Schwartz G S, Berenyi M R, Siegel N W 1969 Atrophic arthritis and diabetic neuritis. Am J Roentgen 106: 523–529
Schwartz J A 1981 Pro-banthine for hypertrophic osteoarthropathy. Arthritis Rheum 24: 1588 (letter)
Scott J T 1983 Gout. Ann Rheum Dis 42 (Suppl 1): 16–18
Sharp G C, Irwin W S, Tan E M, Gould R G, Holman H R 1972 Mixed connective tissue disease. An apparently distinct rheumatic disease syndrome associated with a specific antibody to an extractable nuclear antigen (ENA). Am J Med 52: 148–159
Sharp J 1957 The differential diagnosis of ankylosing spondylitis. Br Med J 1: 975–978
Sharp J 1965 Ankylosing spondylitis: a review. In: Dixon A St J (ed), Progress in clinical rheumatology. Churchill, London p. 180
Sheldon P J, Pell P 1983 Yersinia arthritis in the Midlands: clinical and immunological features in ten cases during 1980–1983. Br J Rheumatol 22 (Suppl 2): 46–49
Sinha S, Munichoodappa C S, Kozak G P 1972 Neuro-arthropathy (Charcot joints) in diabetes mellitus. Medicine (Baltimore) 51: 191–210
Smith J H, Pugh D J 1962 Roentgenographic aspects of articular pigmented villonodular synovitis. Am J Roentgen 87: 1146–1156
Spurnance S L, Smith C B 1971 Joint complications associated with derivatives of HPV-77 rubella virus vaccine. Am J Dis Child 122: 105–111
Stein H, Duthie R B 1981 The pathogenesis of Chronic haemophiliac arthropathy. J Bone Joint Surg 63B: 601–609
Stenseth J H, Clagett O T, Woolner L B 1967 Hypertrophic pulmonary osteoarthropathy. Dis Chest 52: 62–68
Sturge R A, Scott J T, Kennedy A C, Hart D P, Buchanan W W 1977 Serum uric acid in England and Scotland. Ann Rheum Dis 36: 420–427
Ueno Y, Cassell S, Barnett E V 1981 Hypertrophic osteoarthropathy and pseudomembranous enterocolitis. J Rheumatol 8: 825–828
Van Leuwenhoek A 1679 See McCarty D J Pathogenesis and treatment of crystal produced inflammation In: McCarty D J (ed) Arthritis and allied conditions, 9th edn Lea and Febiger, New York 1979: p 1245
Vernier R L, Worthen H G, Patersen R D, Colle E, Good R A 1961 Anaphylactoid purpura. Pediatrics 27: 181–193
Viljanto J A 1973 Dupuytren's contracture: a review. Semin Arthritis Rheum 3: 155–176
Vilppula A H, Yli-Kerttula U I, Aine R A T, Ojala A T 1982 Pigmented villonodular synovitis. Scand J Rheumatol 11: 145–149
Wajed M A, Brown D L, Currey H L F 1977 Palindromic rheumatism. Clinical and serum complement study. Ann Rheum Dis 36: 56–61
Wasser K B et al 1982 Pulmonary hypertrophic osteoarthropathy in cycstic fibrosis: a survey of 375 patients. Arthritis Rheum 25 (Suppl): 5154, Abstract E94
Williams B L 1967 Acropachy in a case of thyrotoxicosis. Proc R Soc Med 60: 899–900
Wright V 1963 Arthritis associated with venereal disease. Ann Rheum Dis 22: 77–89
Wright V, Waktinson G 1965 Sacroiliitis and ulcerative colitis. Br Med J ii: 675–680
Wright V 1978 Psoriatic arthritis. In: Scott J T (ed) Copeman's textbook of the rheumatic diseases, 5th edn. Churchill Livingstone, Edinburgh. Ch. 21, p 537
Wright V, Neumann R, Shinebaum R, Cooke E M, 1983 Pathogenesis of seronegative arthritis. Br J Rheumatol 22 (Suppl 2): 29–32
Yacoub M H 1965 Cervical vagotomy for pulmonary osteoarthropathy. Brit J Dis Chest 59: 28–31
Yacoub M H, Simon G 1966 Hypertrophic osteoarthropathy and intrathoracic inflammatory conditions. Brit J Dis Chest 60: 81–86
Yacoub M H, Simon G, Ohnsorge J 1967 Hypertrophic pulmonary osteoarthropathy in association with pulmonary metastases from extrathoracic tumours. Thorax 22: 226–231
Zitnan D, Sitʼaj S 1963 Chondrocalcinosis articularis. Ann Rheum Dis 22: 142–170

Skin disorders

DERMATITIS

The terms dermatitis and eczema tend to be used synonymously by most British dermatologists. Dermatitis/eczema may be divided into two main categories, exogenous, where an external factor can be incriminated, or endogenous, where there is no obvious aetiological factor (Table 38.1).

Incidence. The incidence of dermatitis varies considerably and usually accounts for 20% of patients seen in dermatological clinics in the U.K.

CONTACT DERMATITIS (Cronin 1980)

This is a dermatitis induced by external factors and is divided into irritant contact dermatitis and allergic contact dermatitis. The distinction is not always easy to make on clinical grounds and even histology does not always help.

A primary irritant reaction occurs when a substance which is always capable of causing skin damage is applied in a sufficiently strong concentration. Allergic contact dermatitis is due to delayed type hypersensitivity (type IV allergy) and there is a characteristic delay between induction of the sensitivity and development of the dermatitic reaction on subsequent exposure to the antigen.

Table 38.1 Categories of dermatitis

Exogenous dermatitis	Contact dermatitis irritant allergic Infective dermatitis Asteotic dermatitis Stasis dermatitis
Endogenous dermatitis	Atopic dermatitis Nummular or discoid dermatitis Seborrhoetic dermatitis

Clinical features (Fig. 38.1). Irrespective of the cause, the clinical features of the dermatitic reaction are similar. The main symptom is itch which may be severe.

In acute dermatitis, erythema with papules and vesicles is the initial change seen which progresses to

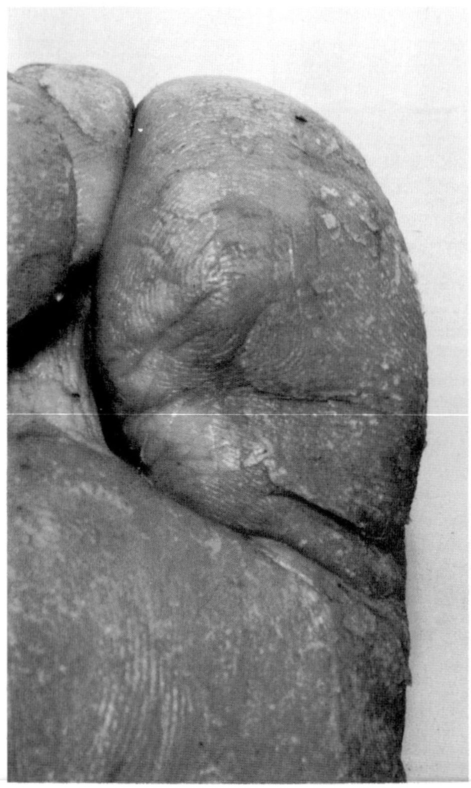

Fig. 38.1 Shoe dermatitis: chronic dermatitis on the plantar surface of the great toe. The sensitizer was rubber adhesive on the insole of the shoe

exudation and crusting. In the chronic phase, dry scaling lichenified fissured plaques are seen. Secondary hyperpigmentation occurs due to chronic scratching and following inflammation.

On the palms and soles where the stratum corneum is thick and resistant the vesicles tend to coalesce to produce large bullae (up to 2 cm in diameter) which may eventually rupture. The vesicles often look like deep seated sago grains with minimal erythema. This appearance is called cheiropompholyx. Pain and not itch may be the predominant feature in this situation.

Irritant contact dermatitis

Primary irritant reactions on the feet are not common but do occur in those engaged in wet work with inadequate protective footwear. It is a major problem in the military who may spend hours in wet footwear while on manoeuvres.

Allergic contact dermatitis

There are many factors which influence the development of allergic contact dermatitis of the foot. There is increased percutaneous absorption due to occlusion caused by shoes and socks. Sweating may further irritate the skin and has the effect of leaching out chemicals like dichromate salts from leather. Friction plays a part in the development of allergic contact dermatitis by damaging the stratum corneum and increases the ease of penetration of the antigen.

There are three major groups of agents which commonly cause allergic contact dermatitis on the foot: (1) footwear — components of shoes and stockings; (2) medicaments and cosmetics; (3) foot appliances.

Shoe dermatitis (Jordan 1972). Shoe induced contact dermatitis is a common problem and is frequently misdiagnosed. The pattern of the dermatitis is often helpful in that shoe dermatitis usually begins on the dorsum of the big toe and spreads to involve the dorsal aspects of the other toes (Fig. 38.2). The dermatitis may take on the shape of the shoe. Characteristically, the interdigital webs are clear. The skin on the dorsum of the foot is thinner and has numerous hair follicles through which antigen may be introduced. Involvement of the sole is the other common site involved and in some series it may be the only affected site.

Secondary infection readily occurs and inappropriate use of medicaments, especially antifungals, may result in generalized dermatitis severe enough to require hospitalization.

Causes of shoe dermatitis. The structure of shoes tends to be the same irrespective of style. They are made in four parts: the sole which usually consists of a leather insole, a fabric or rubber mid sole and an outer sole of leather, rubber or plastic; the upper portion consists of outside leather, rubber or plastic; the box toe and the lining. Adhesive is used throughout.

Rubber box toes are the commonest sensitizers. Celastic and thermoplastic material rarely sensitize and are useful alternatives for patients sensitive to rubber.

Rubber occurs even in so-called all-leather shoes either as rubber adhesive or in the box toe. The rubber accelerators, mercaptobenzothiazole and tetramethylthiuram monosulphide as well as the antioxidant monobenzyl ether of hydroquinone are the commonest rubber sensitizers. Monobenzyl ether of hydroquinone may cause leukoderma and the condition may be misdiagnosed as vitiligo.

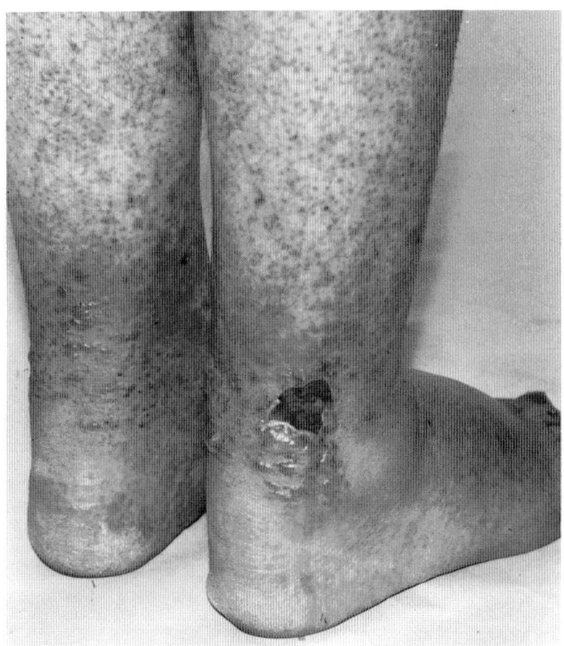

Fig. 38.2 Acute allergic dermatitis with blister formation and oedema due to rubber in stockings

Leather. Dichromate sensitivity occurs frequently in patients with shoe dermatitis. Sweating is a factor in the development of the shoe dermatitis as not all patients who are dichromate sensitive have foot dermatitis. Sweat is known to leach out chromates from chrome tanned leather. The hexavalent chromium salt is considered the most likely sensitizer. Leather may also be tanned by vegetable tannins and these are now a very important cause of shoe dermatitis. Dermatitis from tree tannins has not been reported. Formaldehyde is used as a tanning agent in white kid leather shoes. It is usually so well bound in the leather that it is a rare cause of shoe dermatitis.

Dyes in leather. The azoaniline dyes are the principal group of dyes used in leather. They are a rare cause of dermatitis. They may give rise to trouble if the shoes are redyed or if dye is leached from fabric or plastic shoes. Paraphenylenediamine is the usual allergen in these cases. The dermatitis due to dyes takes the shape of the shoe uppers.

Other causes of shoe dermatitis. In nickel sensitive patients, nickel plated arch supports and eyelets may cause a foot dermatitis. Fungicides used as antimildews in shoes are a rare cause of shoe dermatitis.

Diagnosis. Accurate history taking, the presence and localization of the eruption, help to make the diagnosis. A high index of suspicion is important. Patch testing is necessary to help identify the putative antigen. It is important that not only is patch testing carried out to the various constituents of footwear but also to all the patient's footwear, especially slippers.

Stocking dermatitis (Cronin 1966). Dermatitis from stockings, socks or tights is uncommon in women and rare in men. The reported sensitizers are disperse dyes in nylon and rubber in support stockings.

Clinical features. The characteristic pattern affects where the stocking has closest contact with the skin. This is on the dorsum of the foot, around the heel and occasionally on the sole, the popliteal fossae and the band around the waist if tights are worn. The whole leg may be involved or occasionally only the foot, which may mimic a shoe dermatitis.

A lichenoid dermatitis has been reported in southern Italy amongst women wearing black stockings while in mourning. This was due to paraphenylenediamine (PPD) (Meneghini 1971). Elastic bands round the feet may give rise to a localized band of eczema in rubber-sensitive patients. Nylon itself has not been shown to be a sensitizer in stockings as in all cases dyes or rubber chemicals have been incriminated.

Medicament dermatitis of feet. The present preoccupation with soft, sweet smelling feet has led to an amazing variety of readily available medicaments to achieve this aim. All of these have the ability to sensitize some patients. The incidence will increase if they are applied to already inflamed skin. Patch testing to constituents and preservatives of these medicaments is required to make the diagnosis. Occasionally photosensitizing fungicides used for the treatment of athlete's foot may give rise to an allergic photo-contact dermatitis. Over a period of time the dermatitis becomes lichenified and hyperpigmented and the diagnosis may be difficult.

Occupational dermatitis. Rubber boots worn by fishermen or in other industries are well recognized as causing foot dermatitis (Ross 1969).

Treatment. The most important first step is the removal of the offending sensitizer as cure will not be achieved if exposure persists. Bed rest with elevation of the feet is necessary if severe. The feet should be soaked in a 1:8000 solution of potassium permanganate twice a day for 15–20 minutes. Soaks or compresses of 0.5% silver nitrate or 1:80 solution of sodium hypochlorite renewed at 6–8 hourly intervals will speed the resolution of the exudative phase. Strong topical corticosteroids with or without occlusion may be used. As soon as possible, weaker or diluted corticosteroids should be used. Occasionally oral corticosteroids may be indicated in severe cases or where there is widespread dissemination not responding to topical therapy. A reducing dose regimen will help prevent a rebound phenomenon. Systemic antibiotics are indicated only if secondary bacterial infection is a problem.

On recovering, open toed shoes or sandals are recommended until the skin hardens and complete resolution takes place. Control of hyperhidrosis has meant that some patients are able to wear shoes to which they are sensitive. Patients should be advised on wearing cotton or natural fibre rather than synthetic socks and avoiding occlusive shoes.

It may be a major problem trying to free shoes of sensitizers. Shoes with thermoplastic or celastic box toes or plastic and canvas shoes free of rubber or rubber adhesives may be obtained; and vegetable tanned leather shoes for those sensitive to chromate. Most shoe manufacturers are helpful in providing lists of their shoes free of certain sensitizers.

ASTEOTIC ECZEMA (Fig. 38.3)

Asteotic eczema tends to occur in the elderly, especially those in long-stay, high dependency units where frequent bathing is carried out. While the whole skin may be involved the lower legs and dorsum of the feet are the sites of predilection.

The skin has a characteristic dry, wrinkled, crazy-pavement appearance. As the condition worsens cracking, erythema and oozing may occur. This is aggravated by continued scratching and thickened fissured lesions may eventually develop.

Treatment

Rehydration of the skin by the substitution of aqueous cream or a bath oil for soap and a reduction in bathing is essential. Liberal amounts of white soft paraffin or emulsifying ointments will help to keep the skin hydrated and to achieve normal suppleness. Topical corticosteroid ointments are only indicated if marked inflammatory changes are present.

ATOPIC DERMATITIS

Definition

Atopic dermatitis is a chronic recurrent disease starting in infancy and may be associated with other atopic disorders of asthma and hayfever. The prevalence of this disorder is estimated at between 1.1 and 4.3% of the general paediatric population.

Aetiology

In most cases there is a family history of atopy but the transmission is not that of a simple dominant trait. Several immunological abnormalities have been recognized in atopic patients. The most frequent is the high incidence of positive prick tests to common allergens like house dust mite, pollens, animal danders and some foods which correlate well with an elevated serum IgE. Serum IgE levels fluctuate, often being elevated during exacerbations. Despite increasing knowledge of the physiological and immunological abnormalities the basic process giving rise to the dermatitis is unknown.

Clinical features

The disease occurs from 2 months onwards and is not present at birth. It may settle at the age of 2–3 years only to recur later on in childhood, adolescence

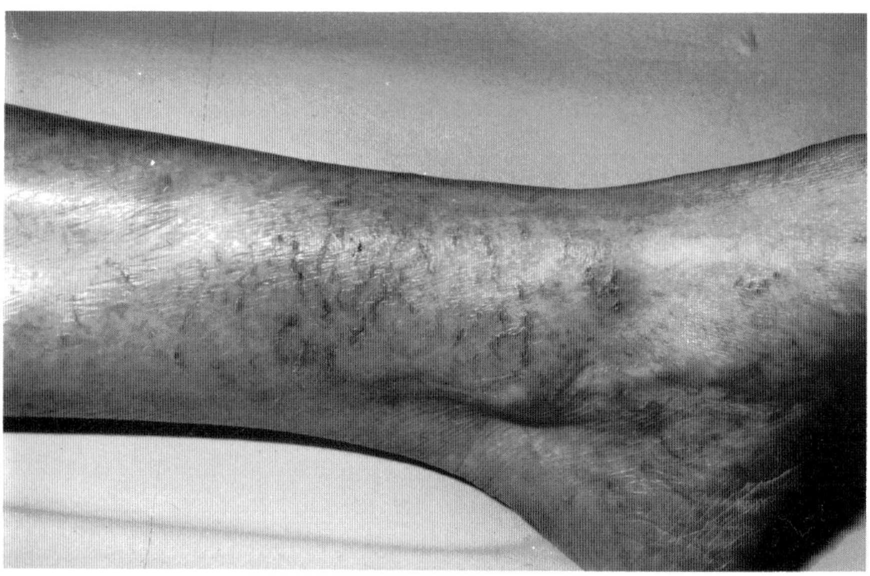

Fig. 38.3 Asteotic dermatitis. The lower leg is a common site

or adulthood. At different ages varying patterns of dermatitis occur.

In infancy the face and scalp are the areas primarily involved. The dermatitis is red, oozy and scaling. As the child gets a little older a characteristic flexural pattern develops involving the antecubital and popliteal fossae, around the ankles and in front of the wrists. In some children a reverse pattern of the dermatitis may occur, i.e. fronts of knees, ankles and extensor forearms which carries a poorer prognosis for complete clearance. In the childhood phase the dermatitis is more chronic with dry lichenified plaques. Lichenification is thickening of the skin with exaggerated skin markings. Papules and excoriations are frequent. Hypo or hyper-pigmentation frequently occurs due to scratching especially over joints. Intense itch is a feature.

In children atopic dermatitis may be localized to the feet, particularly on the dorsum and tips of the toes, especially the great toe. The soles of the feet are not usually involved with atopic dermatitis unless infected or irritated by footwear.

Associated features

Ichthyosis. Dominant ichthyosis is common and usually manifests as mild perifollicular hyperkeratosis on outer upper arms and thighs. The more severe the ichthyosis the poorer the prognosis for recovery.

Infection. Broken skin is easily infected and infection, especially staphylococcus, may exacerbate the eczema. The atopic skin handles herpes simplex poorly at times and widespread dissemination may occur giving rise to Kaposi's varicelliform eruption or eczema herpeticum.

Asthma and hayfever. There is no correlation between the severity of dermatitis and of the asthma or hayfever. The association of urticaria and angio-oedema with food allergy is well recognized.

Miscellaneous factors. Atopic skin is sensitive to environmental changes — excessive atmospheric dryness, rough wool fabrics and sweating may irritate the skin and start the itch/scratch cycle with resultant deterioration in the patient's dermatitis.

Diagnosis

The diagnosis is based on history and clinical features. Prick tests to house dust mite, pollens and danders and serum IgE levels do not improve the diagnostic accuracy, nor do they significantly influence management.

Treatment

Management of atopic dermatitis is never easy. The parents must be involved and the treatment with long-term objectives discussed. The fact that the diathesis is inherited and treatment is not going to cure this tendency must be emphasized at the outset.

Treatment is aimed at treating the itch/scratch cycle. This can be achieved by rehydrating the skin by careful avoidance of strong detergents on the skin. The use of oil, reducing the number of baths and the liberal use of nonperfumed emollients are very important. The avoidance of friction from shoes or excess occlusion and the wearing of soft cotton next to the skin will considerably improve the patient's comfort.

Topical corticosteroids in an appropriate strength are extremely useful. Prolonged use of strong corticosteroids, especially with occlusive dressings, may result in systemic absorption as well as local skin atrophy, erythema and telangiectasia. Routine systemic corticosteroids should be avoided but are occasionally necessary. Topical antibiotics, because of their ability to sensitize, should be restricted. Appropriate systemic antibiotics may be required if secondary infection is a problem.

Occlusive paste bandaging containing hydrocortisone, ichthamol or tars are especially useful for chronic lichenified and persistently excoriated plaques of dermatitis.

Itch is usually worse at night but responds reasonably to the sedative antihistamines like promethazine and trimeprazine in adequate doses. The daytime use of these antihistamines is not logical as these drugs act centrally producing sedation, rather than as a peripheral histamine blocker.

JUVENILE PLANTAR DERMATITIS

(Synonym: forefoot eczema) (Fig. 38.4; Ashton et al 1985)

Definition

This is a scaling, fissuring disorder mainly involving the forefoot of prepubertal children.

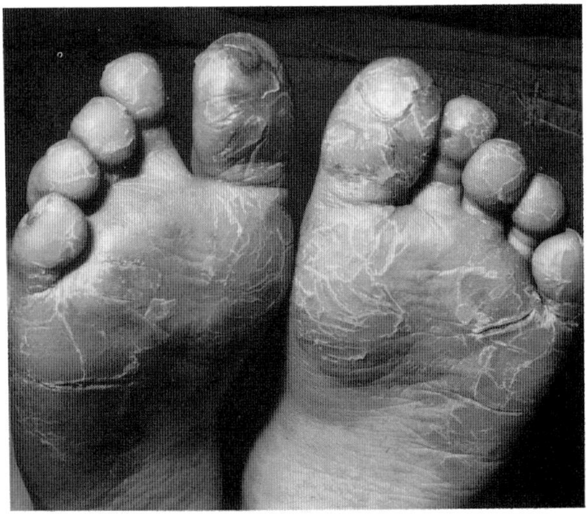

Fig. 38.4 Juvenile plantar dermatosis, with glazed fissured appearance of the skin of the forefoot

Aetiology

The aetiology is obscure and the condition has only been widely recognized in the past decade. Its appearance coincided with the increase in synthetic footwear and socks for children. This type of footwear is occlusive and interferes with sweating. There is marked reduction in sweating in the involved skin as shown by using staining techniques which demonstrate active sweat glands.

Extensive allergy testing to various components of shoes and socks have failed to demonstrate that allergic contact dermatitis plays a role in its aetiology. Reports on the incidence of atopy varies widely and there is no clear evidence that this condition is commoner in atopic than nonatopic children.

Clinical features

The skin changes involve primarily the anterior foot and toes. The skin texture is altered and the glazed sheen of the skin is characteristic. Scaling and fissuring is seen especially on the dorsum of the great toes and the pads of the other toes. There is sparing of the interdigital spaces and parts of the toes not in close apposition with the footwear. Pain due to the deep fissuring is the main symptom and can make walking difficult. The fissuring follows the skin creases and a deep fissure can occur at the base of the great toe.

Histology

There is mild acanthosis with focal spongiosis around the sweat duct as it goes through the horny layer. Some of the distal coils are narrow and some are blocked.

Differential diagnosis

This condition is often misdiagnosed as fungal but the sparing of the webs and the age of the patient helps to rule it out. Fungal infections are uncommon in prepubertal children. Allergic contact dermatitis can usually be ruled out on clinical grounds or by patch testing.

Treatment

Treatment is unrewarding. Prolonged bed rest and total avoidance of footwear and socks is sometimes useful but this advice is impractical. Changing to all-leather shoes helps a small minority of children. Pure cotton or wool socks should be encouraged. Some dermatologists recommend the wearing of two pairs of socks or insoles made of cork or felt to increase the absorption of sweat.

Topical steroids should be avoided as they may cause atrophy of the skin and more importantly, they do not work. Simple emollients like aqueous cream BP, yellow soft paraffin or emulsifying ointment applied twice a day are more helpful.

Prognosis

There is apparent spontaneous resolution at puberty.

NUMMULAR DERMATITIS (Fig. 38.5)

This is a dermatitis of unknown aetiology characterized by nummular or coin-shaped lesions scattered over the limbs and trunk. It tends to occur in middle-aged men and is associated with dry skin.

Clinical features

Coin-shaped lesions are moderately well demarcated with a papulovesicular periphery and a centre which tends to heal. Oozing and crusting are common

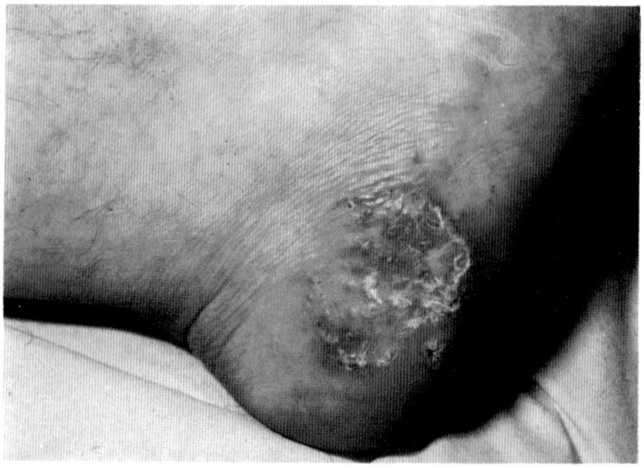

Fig. 38.5 Nummular dermatitis. Chronic plaque on heel with vesicle formation and scaling. Histology confirmed and dermatitic changes

features as the vesicles are thin walled and easily ruptured. Dry scaling fissured or lichenified plaques may occur. Itch and scratching are a major feature. It may also present as a solid plaque over the ankle when it is known as lichen simplex chronicus.

Treatment

This type of dermatitis tends to recur especially in the winter and is easily aggravated by excess washing.

Topical corticosteroids or coal tar preparations are useful in reducing symptoms and clearing the rash but do not appear to influence recurrence. Paste occlusive bandaging is also useful as it forms a barrier, albeit temporary, against the roving scratching finger nails or heels.

STASIS DERMATITIS

Stasis dermatitis is a manifestation of prolonged venous hypertension which gives rise to poor tissue perfusion and nutrition. It occurs more commonly in middle-aged obese women than men. About one-third of patients give a past history of deep venous thrombophlebitis, major trauma or prolonged periods of immobility. It is more common in people who stand for prolonged periods.

Clinical features

Stasis dermatitis has a predilection for the area just above the medial malleolus of the ankle overlying the most inferior perforating vein. It is characterized by pigmentation, oedema and varicosities. As the disease progresses induration and inflammation giving rise to fibrosis and scarring occur. The clinical pattern is called lipodermatosclerosis. Ulceration may occur with further scarring. Pigmentation occurs early and is due to the deposition of haemosiderin following rupture of small venules. It starts as small light brown macules which enlarge and darken and may cover large areas of the lower leg and foot.

Erythema and oedema is usually accompanied by pruritus. Scratching results in lichenification and an exudative vesicular dermatitis. The injudicious use of topical preparations may worsen the situation by giving rise to a primary irritant and/or allergic contact dermatitis. Local spread may be associated with a more widespread patchy dermatitis known as an 'id' (autosensitization) reaction. Secondary infection gives rise to considerable pain and increased oozing and crusting.

Prolonged oedema leads to progressive deterioration and eventually results in fibrosis which clinically is manifested by induration of the tissues. Recurrent thrombophlebitis, cellulitis and trauma aggravate the fibrosis. Small white atrophic scarring occurs within the hyperpigmented area and is known as atrophe blanche.

Ulceration occurs, usually following minor trauma. Ulcers may heal with scarring or progress in some patients to involve large areas of the lower leg. The edge is soft and irregular with a necrotic base which may penetrate deeply to reveal underlying tendon and bones. Secondary bacterial infection usually gives rise to rapid expansion of the ulcer and considerable pain. Recalcitrant ulcers are seen where there is significant fibrosis.

Management

General advice in an effort to reduce venous pressure is paramount. Weight reduction, avoidance of standing still (walking improves the muscle pump) and good surgical support stockings should be emphasized. Elevation of the legs to or above the level of the heart when the patient is sitting down and raising the end of the bed 8–10 in at night should be recommended. The patient must understand that the normal sitting position with the feet on the floor or on a low ottoman is useless.

Treatment of dermatitis

If exudative, use potassium permanganate 1:8000 solution baths for 15 minutes twice daily. When the dermatitis is dry topical corticosteroids of appropriate potency for the degree of inflammation are useful. Ointments are more emollient and contain fewer preservatives. A zinc oxide (Unna) boot may be useful by providing a soothing dressing under which a topical steroid may be applied. It should be changed every 2 to 7 days but it is cumbersome and makes bathing and the wearing of shoes difficult.

Treatment of ulceration

A myriad of treatments exist for the management of stasis ulcers. For mild ulceration, elevation, soaks with saline, silver nitrate 0.25% solution or aluminium acetate 1:20 or 1:40 solution, and most importantly, time, are indicated.

Grafting with 'pinch' grafts to the ulcer base or excision and split thickness grafting may be considered.

Severe chronic ulcers may respond to repeat applications of an Unna boot. Macromolecular dextran beads and a variety of other expensive synthetic dressings are available but their superiority in healing ulcers has not been shown conclusively.

Topical antibiotics should be avoided if possible and systemic antibiotics are only required for deeper infections.

PSORIASIS (Cram 1981)

Definition

Psoriasis vulgaris is a chronic inflammatory dermatosis characterized by reddish papules and plaques associated with fine silvery scaling. It has a predilection for extensor surfaces. There is epidermal hyperplasia and a two-fold increase in epidermal turnover rate in the active lesion.

Incidence

Psoriasis affects 2% of the population. It affects both sexes equally and may occur at any age. It is inherited as a simple autosomal dominant trait with incomplete penetrance.

Aetiology

The basic defect in psoriasis is unknown.

Trauma to the skin either physical or chemical, may elicit psoriasis in a susceptible subject. This is called the Koebner or isomorphic phenomenon. Puberty and the menopause are associated with an increased incidence of psoriasis.

Histology

There is epidermal thickening (acanthosis) with elongation of rete ridges. The granular level is absent and hyperkeratosis and parakeratosis are present. There is an increase in mitotic activity in the basal and suprabasal cells. Small intraepidermal accumulations of leucocytes form the classical microabscesses of Munro.

Clinical features

The clinical lesion has three main features:

1. The lesion is thickened and clearly demarcated from normal skin.

2. The dull pink-red colour often described as salmon-pink is especially helpful in diagnosing plantar lesions. The colour reflects the increased vasculature and dermal blood flow. Auspitz's sign is characteristic of psoriasis and is produced by blunt scraping off of the scale revealing puntate bleeding points.

3. The amount of scaling is variable and is a fine loosely adherent silvery scale.

Psoriatic lesions are modified by site. The most common forms of psoriasis on the foot are (1) plaque type psoriasis; (2) psoriatic keratoderma of the sole; (3) interdigital psoriasis; (4) psoriasis of nails; (5) exfoliative and erythrodermic psoriasis; (6) arthropathic psoriasis and (7) pustular psoriasis of palms and soles.

Plaque type psoriasis (Fig. 38.6). Stable plaque type psoriasis occurs on the feet and lower limbs as part of widespread psoriasis. Lesions tend to be symmetrical with well demarcated scaling and erythematous plaques. Waxy yellow hyperkeratotic rupioid lesions

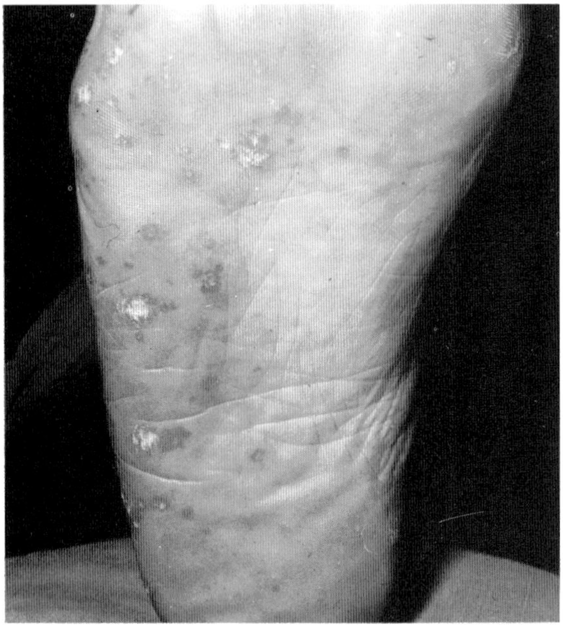

Fig. 38.6 Psoriatic plaques on plantar surface

occur alone or in association with pustules especially on the sole. Similar but smaller lesions occur in Reiter's disease.

Psoriatic keratoderma (Fig. 38.7). This presents as sharply marginated hyperkeratotic scaly plaques which are symmetrical and bilateral. They usually occur on the heels and beneath the instep. Deep painful fissures may occur associated with the thickened yellow keratoderma. Palmar hyperkeratosis of varying degrees usually accompanies it. The absence of vesiculation is helpful in distinguishing this form of psoriasis from hyperkeratotic dermatitis.

Interdigital psoriasis (Waisman 1961). Psoriasis localized to the interdigital spaces has been referred to as 'white psoriasis'. It may occasionally occur in the absence of psoriasis elsewhere but is usually accompanied by psoriatic changes in the toe nails and psoriasis elsewhere.

The lesions are characterized by thick white hyperkeratosis with ulceration and fissuring between the toes or at their bases. Secondary bacterial infection with occasional cellulitis is not uncommon.

The type must be differentiated from erythrasma and interdigital dermatophyte infection.

Psoriasis of nails. Nail changes are present at some stage of the disease in almost all patients.

Discrete punctate pits which occur in lines are characteristic but not specific to psoriasis. They may occur in alopecia areata and chronic dermatitis.

Separation of the nail from the bed is called onycholysis and usually starts at one side of the nail. Subungual hyperkeratosis is due to subungual hyperplasia and accumulation of entrapped stratum corneum. Periungual changes, swelling, diffuse erythema and desquamation are frequent. Nail growth is increased both in the affected and clinically normal nails.

Exfoliative and erythrodermic psoriasis. Spread of psoriasis to become generalized may occur spontaneously or may follow systemic infection or some external factor. Pitting oedema associated with exfoliative erythroderma of the lower limbs is frequently seen and congestive cardiac failure may occur due to increased demands on cardiac output.

Psoriatic arthropathy is of two forms: (1) a rheumatoid like erosive peripheral arthropathy with a predilection for the distal interphalangeal joints which is seronegative for rheumatoid factor, and (2) ankylosing spondylitis which is associated with a high incidence of HLA-B27 especially in those patients with sacroiliitis.

Pustular psoriasis (Fig. 38.8). A localized form involving the palms and soles occurs in middle-aged patients but its relationship to psoriasis is in some dispute. It is immunogenetically distinct and the positive associations of HLA-B27 and BW17 seen in psoriasis vulgaris is lacking.

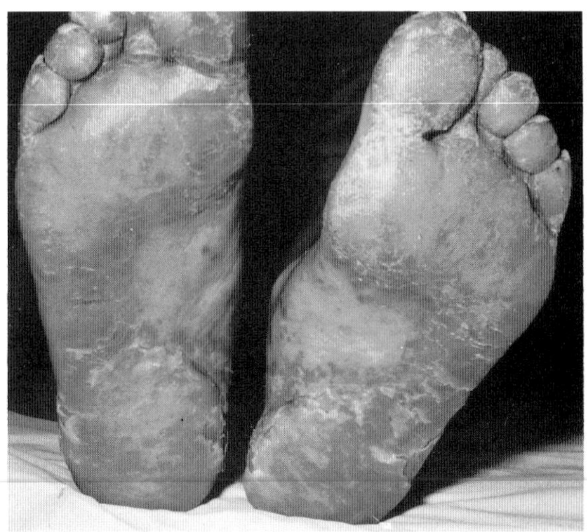

Fig. 38.7 Psoriatic keratoderma on the plantar surface

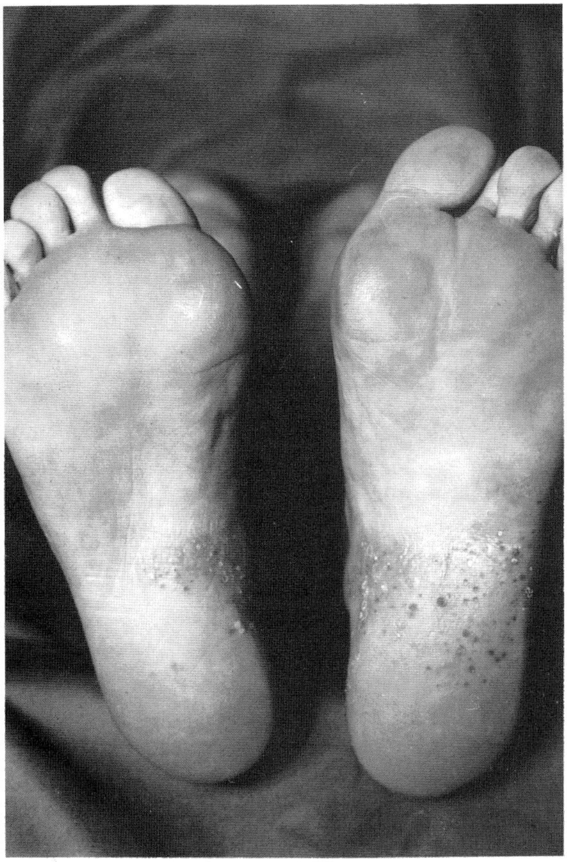

Fig. 38.8 Pustular psoriasis with the characteristic sterile pustules at different stages of evolution

Clinical features

The rash is usually bilateral and remarkably symmetrical. It starts on the instep of the plantar arch as showers of sterile pustules on erythematous plaques. This is often associated with a burning sensation or itch. The pustules dry out and form brown crusts which gradually exfoliate leaving an erythematous base. Recurrent crops of pustules occur so early pustules and exfoliating brown crusts are present in the same plaque.

Marked pain and disability occurs when the lesions extend on to weight-bearing areas. Nail changes with puntate stippling and onycholysis is very common.

Differential diagnosis

In the absence of psoriasis elsewhere the disorder must be distinguished from chronic hyperkeratotic lichenified eczema, Reiter's disease, Bowen's disease, lichen planus and drug eruption.

Treatment

Topical preparations containing salicylic acid, dithranol or tar, form the first line of treatment. This may be combined with ultraviolet light. Topical corticosteroids may be used but the side effect of atrophy limits their use.

Systemic treatment is used for more severe psoriasis. Photochemotherapy is successful in inducing clearance of psoriasis and also appears to be useful in maintenance of remission. A photosensitizing drug, usually 8-methoxypsoralen, is prescribed before exposure to ultraviolet light at 360 nm (UVA).

Immunosuppressive and cytostatic agents tend to be reserved for older patients with resistant psoriasis. Methotrexate, hydroxyurea and azathioprine are the main second line drugs and their use is limited by their side effects, both short and long term.

Etretinate, a synthetic aromatic retinoid, has recently been introduced but its role in the management of psoriasis has yet to be fully assessed. Side effects include teratogenicity and the long half-life limits its usefulness.

Course

Psoriasis is unpredictable and undergoes spontaneous remissions and relapses. Guttate psoriasis following a sore throat tends to clear in several months. Generalized pustular and erythrodermic psoriasis are associated with appreciable morbidity and mortality.

REITER'S SYNDROME (Callen 1979)

The classical triad in Reiter's syndrome is a seronegative arthritis, nonspecific urethritis and conjunctivitis. The components of the triad may not all occur at the same time and incomplete forms occur.

An infectious aetiology has been suggested as Reiter's Syndrome has been seen in susceptible patients after dysenteric illness and venereal disease.

Clinical features

The soles of the feet are almost always involved but the dorsal aspects of the feet and hands, finger nails and scalp are common. The initial lesion is a dull macule which rapidly becomes papular and pseudo-vesicular. The colour changes from yellow to orange-red as the lesion rapidly thickens to form a conical hyperkeratotic plaque which is limpet-like. A scaly collarette is sometimes present. New lesions may coalesce forming an irregular heaped-up dull yellow mass.

Some lesions are frankly pustular from the outset and are indistinguishable from pustular psoriasis of palms and soles. Flaccid bullae filled with cheesy yellowish-brown contents may cover the foot. This type of skin change is referred to as keratoderma blennorrhagicum and occurs in 8% of venereal cases but only in 1% of postdysenteric ones. Keratoderma is usually self-limiting and resolves within months. Evolution into widespread erythroderma infrequently occurs but may be potentially fatal.

Nail changes are common with pustules occurring under the nails which may be friable and shed. Painless red swelling at the nail base may evolve into parakeratotic scaling giving rise to nail thickening and ridging.

Treatment

Topical corticosteroid is the treatment of choice for keratoderma but psoriatic lesions elsewhere should be treated as for psoriasis.

LICHEN PLANUS (Altman & Perry 1961)

Lichen planus is an uncommon dermatosis which may run a protracted course and is of unknown aetiology. Similar eruptions may be precipitated by drugs including practolol and gold. A lichenoid rash indistinguishable from lichen planus may occur in patients with graft versus host disease.

Clinical features

The rash develops rapidly and is usually extremely itchy. The lesions may appear on the skin and mucus membranes. The characteristic lesion is a small polygonal violaceous flat-topped papule. Its surface shows a delicate white network (Whickham's striae). The lesions are often linear and related to trauma demonstrating a Koebner phenomenon. The papules may coalesce to form large plaques. They heal leaving marked postinflammatory hyperpigmentation.

It has a predilection for the flexor surfaces of upper limbs, extensor surface of the lower limbs, the penis and buccal mucosa. Vesicles and bullae are uncommon but are occasionally the prominent feature.

The appearance of lichen planus varies according to its position. It tends to be chronic and hypertrophic on the shins and ankles. The lesions may become warty and thickened with fine adherent scale. Excoriation and ulceration is frequently seen as these lesions are particularly itchy. As the plaques involute hypopigmentation and atrophy may occur.

Lichen planus of the soles is usually papular or nodular and the lesions are situated along the margin rather than the centre of the sole. Their colour is more likely to be yellow or pink than violaceous. When the lesions coalesce and thicken they may resemble calluses.

A rare form of lichen planus occurs on the foot which is associated with cicatrical alopecia. It is characterized by bullae and deep painful slow-healing ulcers on the soles. Gradual but permanent loss of the toe nails occurs. The toes show bleeding and granulating ulcers surrounded by atrophic pigmented skin.

Histology

The diagnostic features of lichen planus are seen irrespective of the clinical picture. There is hyperkeratosis, a thick granular layer, irregular acanthosis and liquifaction degeneration of the basal layer with individual cell death (colloid bodies). In the dermis there is a dense cellular infiltrate hugging the epidermis which gives rise to the characteristic 'saw-tooth' appearance of the dermoepidermal junction.

Course

Most cases of lichen planus clear in one to two years. The development of squamous carcinoma is very uncommon in hypertrophic lichen planus. This is not the case in ulcerative lichen planus of the feet where there is a tendency for squamous carcinoma to develop unless the area is grafted.

Treatment

Therapy does not greatly influence the course of lichen planus. The relief of itch is paramount but may be difficult. Antihistamines do not help unless sedation is achieved.

Topical corticosteroids, occlusive bandaging with corticosteroid or tar helps to reduce the irritation. Systemic corticosteroids should only be used for extensive disease, where progressive nail destruction is occurring or when ulceration has occurred.

Intralesional triamcinolone is very useful in hypertrophic lichen planus.

Nail changes in lichen planus. The nails are involved in 10% of cases of lichen planus. This usually is a minor feature of the disease. Thinning of the nail plate as it emerges from the cuticle gives rise to longitudinal ridges and linear depressions. Pterygium, which is an overgrowth of the cuticle and adhesion between the dorsal nail fold and the nail plate, is frequently seen. The great toes are most often affected. There are usually changes of lichen planus at the nail fold. The more severe changes are usually permanent but the nails are rarely shed. These nail changes are similar to the changes due to impaired peripheral circulation or trauma.

The overlap syndrome lichen planus/lupus erythematosus exists which shows features of both diseases, the lesions being reddish-blue chronic atrophic patches which occur on the extremities.

PITYRIASIS RUBRA PILARIS (PRP)
(Griffiths 1976)

Definition

This is a group of rare, chronic, inflammatory dermatoses characterized by the presence of fine horny follicular papules.

Aetiology

The cause is unknown but in the juvenile type a positive family history is often found. There are two peaks in the age of onset, the largest incidence between the ages of 40 to 60 and a much smaller peak in the first decade. That the two types are identical diseases, is in considerable doubt. When PRP occurs in the adult it may be difficult to differentiate from psoriasis.

Clinical features

The onset of PRP is often abrupt. Erythroderma which starts on the upper half of the body gradually becomes generalized. The slowly developing follicular keratosis is characteristic of the disease and involves not only the extremities but the trunk and face. The papules are firm red pinhead lesions topped with a horny cap. 'White islands' of apparently normal skin may be seen within the erythroderma. The black horny follicular plugs in the hair follicles on the dorsa of the digits are a diagnostic sign of the disease. Diffuse yellow thickening of the palms and soles gives rise to the 'keratodermic sandal of PRP'.

Circumscribed juvenile PRP occurs on bony prominences like knees and elbows where follicular keratosis and spotty parakeratosis are seen. There is keratodermic sandal may not be well developed.

Atypical PRP is probably a variant of ichthyosiform erythroderma.

Course

Classical PRP in the adult tends to clear without relapse in 1–3 years but the course may be prolonged in children.

Histology

Large follicular horny plugs are seen in areas of follicular hyperkeratosis. Elsewhere diffuse hyperkeratosis and spotty parakeratosis are seen. There is mild irregular acanthosis and liquifaction degeneration of the basal cell layers. A mild, chronic inflammatory cell infiltrate is seen in the upper dermis.

Treatment

The efficacy of any mode of therapy in this condition must be considered in the light of its tendency (in the adult) to undergo spontaneous remission. In the erythrodermic, exfoliative phase systemic corticosteroids may shorten this stage. Azathioprine, methotrexate and PUVA all appear to be helpful. Etretinate, an oral retinoid, has been shown to be very successful in improving not only the keratoderma but also the follicular hyperkeratosis in these patients.

INFECTION

The skin has a normal resident population of micro-organisms which probably do not invade into the intact stratum corneum but remain in the loose surface layer. The normal skin flora includes *Staphylococcus*, *Corynebacterium*, *Acinetobacter* and *Streptococcus*. There is 'normal' carriage of dermatophytes in patients who do not develop clinical disease. Up to 9% of normal webs in one series had fungi isolated (Leyden & Kligman 1978).

The degree of hydration of the stratum corneum has a very important influence on the skin flora. Increasing the quantity of water at the skin surface greatly increases the number of micro-organisms. This is of particular importance in the case of the feet where occlusive footwear and sweating can so alter the flora that extensive dermatophytosis and bacterial infection may occur. Drying of the skin results in a reduction of micro-organisms.

DERMATOPHYTE INFECTIONS (Leyden & Kligman 1978)

Athlete's foot is a term which is applied to the white macerated itchy disorder of interdigital spaces. It is important to realize that all interdigital infection is not fungal and isolation of fungus from overt clinical ringworm is reported in less than 25% of cases.

Clinical features

The spectrum of tinea pedis in the interdigital webs ranges from minimal dry scaling to a highly inflammatory reaction.

The change from mild disease to severe infection occurs with prolonged occlusion and sweating with superhydration of the stratum corneum. This allows bacterial invasion and the fungus appears to be driven deeper into the stratum corneum. The main dermatophytes that cause interdigital ringworm are *Trichophyton rubrum*, *Trichophyton interdigitale* and *Epidermophyton floccosum*. These are anthropophilic species and humans are the primary host.

The main clinical variety is an itchy peeling inflamed, moist and fissured toe space, the fourth and fifth spaces being the most commonly involved. Extension to involve the other spaces, the dorsum and plantar surfaces gradually occurs. *T. rubrum* produces a chronic fine scaling on the soles and the nails are frequently involved. A more inflammatory reaction with the development of pompholyx blistering is seen with *T. interdigitale*. This may closely resemble eczema.

A widespread papular rash called a dermatophytide may be associated with highly inflammatory tinea pedis.

Diagnosis

This is made by identifying the causative organism. Skin scrapings from dry scaling interdigital webs are usually positive. The recovery rate of fungus is dramatically reduced in severe infection and increases when the secondary bacterial infection is treated.

Treatment

Topical antifungal agents, e.g. miconazole or clotrimazole are useful for uncomplicated tinea pedis. Magenta paint is cheap and useful for inflammatory tinea pedis but is messy. Whitfield's ointment is cheap but not always effective and can be irritant to inflamed skin. Antibiotics, either local or systemic, will be necessary where bacterial infection complicates tinea pedis.

Physical separation of the toes with cotton wool pledgets and the wearing of open shoes will reduce maceration.

The regular use of tolnaftate is recommended to those who frequent swimming pools or communal changing rooms.

Differential diagnosis

Erythrasma and occasionally *Candida albicans* may cause a clinical picture indistinguishable from tinea pedis. A macerated interdigital wart, soft corns or condylomata lata may present like athlete's foot.

Eczema rarely affects the interdigital spaces and involves the medial rather than the lateral toe spaces.

CANDIDIASIS (Fig. 38.9; Ray & Wuepper 1978)

Candidiasis or moniliasis is caused by a yeast-like fungus. Healthy intact skin is fairly resistant to infection. It is an opportunistic pathogen and causes disease only in the presence of an underlying host defect, such as poorly controlled diabetes mellitus and prolonged antibiotic therapy. On the foot candidiasis may present as interdigital infections, paronychia and onycholysis and rarely as candida granuloma.

Interdigital candidiasis gives rise to eroded, macerated tissue with fissuring and is also known as erosio interdigitalis blastomycetica. The fourth web space is commonly affected. Sweating, closely opposed toes, the wearing of tight occlusive socks which prevent evaporation of sweat all predispose to interdigital candidiasis.

Paronychia and onycholysis produced by *Candida* infections of the toe nails is much less common than in fingernails. The skin surrounding the nail fold becomes red, swollen and tender. The posterior nail fold is raised from the underlying nail. Moisture and sweat in the posterior nail sulcus leads to persisting infection. The nail becomes opaque and dystrophic and may progress to separation of the nail plate from the underlying nail bed (onycholysis). Several or all nails are usually affected.

CANDIDA GRANULOMA

Candida granuloma is regarded as a variant of chronic mucocutaneous candidiasis. Lesions on the feet, face and scalp are common. The nodules are multiple and break down to form fungating crusted surface due to oozing. There may be evidence of serious bacterial infection in these patients. Defects in delayed hypersensitivity are present in some but not all patients.

BACTERIAL DISEASES

Erythrasma (Noble 1981)

Erythrasma is a disease of sweaty, macerated skin. It occurs principally in the axillae, groins and toe webs but may occur where any two skin surfaces are opposed.

It is characterized by erythema, scaling and maceration, and may resemble a fungal infection. The classical feature of this disease is its coral red fluorescence under Wood's light. This fluorescence is due to the production of porphyrins by *Corynebacterium minutissimum*. About 20% of normal young adults carry the bacterium with no evidence of clinical disease.

Treatment. Topical antibacterial or germicidal soaps may be useful in reducing scaling and bacterial counts. Erythromycin orally for two weeks may be necessary if severe infection occurs. Recurrence is not uncommon.

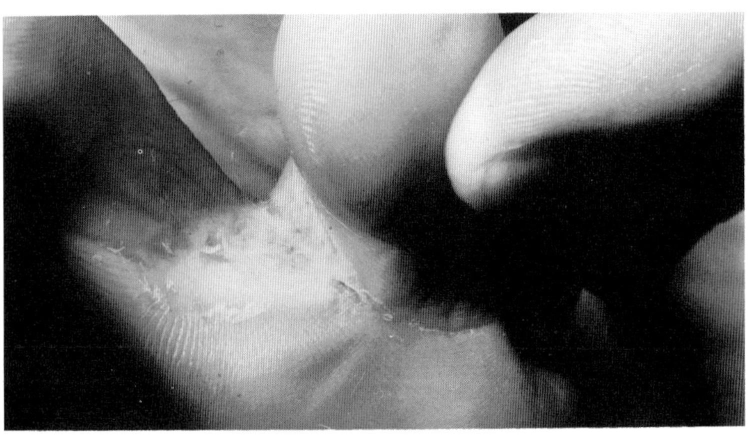

Fig. 38.9 Interdigital candida with pseudomonas overgrowth

Erysipelas

Erysipelas is a superficial form of cellulitis due to streptococci. It was initially described on the face but in two-thirds of patients it occurs on the legs. The usual site of entry of the infection is broken skin in the toe webs.

The infection results in a sharply demarcated, erythematous, swollen, hot plaque. Vesicles may be present on the periphery, usually at the advancing edge.

The lymphoedematous limb is more prone to recurrent streptococcal infection which may result in the development of elephantiasis nostras verrucosa.

Treatment. Oral penicillin is the treatment of choice. There is a case for long-term low dose penicillin in patients with lymphoedema to prevent recurrent attacks.

Pitted keratolysis (Tilgren 1979)

Pitted keratolysis is a common superficial infection of the plantar surface associated with hyperhidrosis. Crateriform pits are seen in the stratum corneum which vary in size from small discrete lesions to large areas of superficial erosion. *Corynebacterium* species have been isolated from the keratolytic areas. The lesions respond to oral erythromycin and treatment of the hyperhidrosis.

Impetigo

Impetigo is a superficial bacterial skin infection caused by staphylococci and to a lesser extent by streptococci. It tends to occur in school children. The golden yellow 'stuck on' crusts occur mainly on the face but may occur anywhere on the body except the palms and soles.

Bullous impetigo is a variant of impetigo and occurs in newborn and younger children. The blisters are flaccid and are less easily broken than in impetigo. On the soles the blisters are tense with minimal surrounding erythema.

Extensive impetigo may be associated with lymphadenopathy and pyrexia. Impetigo due to streptococcus occurs in about one-third of cases in the U.K.

Treatment. Scrupulous attention to hygiene is essential to prevent spread of the disease.

Topical antibiotics, e.g. neomycin or tetracycline, may be adequate for mild infection. Systemic antibiotics, penicillin or flucloxacillin, are the drugs of choice for more severe infection.

WARTS (Massing & Epstein 1963, Bunny 1982)

Warts are caused by the papovavirus and are the commonest virus infection in man. Fifteen types of human papillomavirus (HPV) have been identified so far. Two clinical patterns are found on the foot:

> Type I: deep solitary painful warts, associated with HPV-1 and HPV-4
> Type II: mosaic plantar warts, associated with HPV-2

In neither of these two types is oncogenicity suspected.

Incidence. The incidence of warts is increasing. Plantar warts are contagious and spread in areas like swimming pools and communal showers is common.

Clinical manifestation. The plantar wart (verruca plantaris, myrmercia) is a well circumscribed, round, usually solitary lesion with a rough keratotic surface surrounded by a smooth collar of thickened horn. The normal skin creases are obliterated. If the cap is pared down small bleeding points from the oozing capillary loops are evident. Most warts occur at pressure points either under metatarsal heads, the heels or under the toes. Considerable pain on walking and a cluster of tiny satellite warts may occur around a larger wart.

Mosaic warts

Mosaic warts are also known as superficial spreading warts and are associated with HPV-2 virus. The term describes the closely grouped warts which may coalesce to form a plaque. The angular outline of the individual warts may be seen when the surface is pared. They tend to be painless but deep fissuring of the plaques may be extremely disabling. They tend to persist.

Differential diagnosis. The main differential diagnosis of the solitary verruca is a callus. The obliteration of skin lines and the absence of punctate bleeding points on paring should help to distinguish them.

Treatment. Treatments for warts abound and each culture and age has its own folk cures. Spontaneous remission occurs and 67% will clear within two years. Spontaneous remission is often heralded by increasing pain and haemorrhage into the wart before it involutes. Itching sometimes precedes resolution.

The response of warts to treatment is inversely proportional to their duration, the age of the patient, the number of warts and type. Mosaic warts tend to persist while single deep warts respond readily. Treatment must be tried for at least 12 weeks before it is deemed to have failed. Keratolytic agents like salicylic acid in strengths varying from 10–60% are useful in the management of warts. 3% formalin causes desiccation of the wart and may cause fissuring even when restricted to plantar warts. Formalin is capable of sensitization and for this reason is best avoided. Glutaraldehyde is an antimicrobial agent and acts like formalin. Podophyllin (15–25%) has a potent antimitotic effect and should be applied weekly. This drug is highly irritant and the normal skin should be protected. It should not be used in pregnancy. It is one of the more effective treatments of mosaic warts.

Cryotherapy is the most popular mode of treatment at present. Carbon dioxide and liquid nitrogen are the two freezing agents available, the latter being more efficient. It is widely available and may be applied using cotton buds or special delivery systems. It is not necessary to provoke blister formation. Excessive blistering may be rewarded by new warts being formed at the periphery. Warts need to be treated at three week intervals or less. Longer intervals reduce the cure rate by half. Care must be taken to make sure that treatment does not end with scarring. Warts will eventually clear but a painful scar may be a permanent reminder.

EPIDERMODYSPLASIA VERRUCIFORMIS (EV) (Lawandowsky & Lutz 1922)

Definition. EV is a rare inherited cutaneous disease characterized by nodular or verrucous lesions which may occur anywhere on the body. They tend to be most numerous on the face, neck and backs of hands and feet. Its viral origin has been confirmed by inoculation experiments and electron microscope demonstration of the virus.

The clinical course is of persistence with spontaneous resolution being rare.

Two variants of EV occur:

1. HPV-3 induced — benign

The clinical picture resembles an extensive flat wart but occurrence is usually in childhood and there may be a familial incidence. In some cases confluent pigmented plaques, particularly on the legs, may occur. Malignant degeneration does not occur.

2. HPV-5

This occurs in childhood and is probably inherited as an autosomal recessive trait. Clinically, the lesions are scaly red macules or hypo or hyperpigmented macules resembling pityriasis versicolor. They are extensive and long lasting.

Malignant changes occur within 2–20 years, especially in lesions on light exposed areas. The malignant changes are usually Bowen's disease (in situ squamous carcinoma) and occasionally invasive squamous cell carcinoma. Malignant change only occurs with HPV-5 so that the oncogenic potential appears to be related to the virus type rather than the extent of the T-cell defect.

Treatment. This is unsatisfactory, and all the usual modalities for treatment of warts may be attempted. Oral retinoids may be beneficial as may α-Interferon, when injected into the benign and premalignant lesion of patients with EV.

MOLLUSCUM CONTAGIOSUM (Postlethwaite 1981)

Molluscum contagiosum is a viral infection of the skin caused by a pox virus. The virus is found worldwide and may occur at any age. The incubation varies from 14–50 days. Spread is probably by direct contact and outbreaks have centred on swimming pools. Molluscum lesions are discrete, shiny, pearly white dome-shaped papules with a central punctum through which a white cheesy material of molluscum bodies may be expressed. They occur mainly on the trunk with plantar and palmar lesions being uncommon.

Diagnosis

Microscopy examination of the expressed contents of a molluscum shows the characteristic viral particles.

HAND-FOOT-AND-MOUTH DISEASE
(Tindall & Miller 1972)

Definition

Hand-foot-and-mouth disease is a disease usually of childhood caused by the coxsackieviruses. It may occur as an epidemic disease where it is associated with coxsackie A16 or as sporadic cases associated with A5 and A9. A similar clinical picture occurs in infection with enterovirus 71.

Clinical features

It is characterized by the presence of small, painful, oral ulcers, usually lasting about 5–10 days. The vesicular stage is transient and the typical oral lesion is a shallow grey ulcer surrounded by an erythematous halo. The skin lesions, varying in number, appear either simultaneously with or shortly after the oral lesions. Involvement of the palms and soles is common. Each blister, which arises from an erythematous base, is greyish in colour and tends to be oval or linear running in or parallel to the skin creases. They may be painful, especially when on the soles of the feet and resolve within 7–10 days.

Diagnosis

Coxsackie A virus is isolated from stool specimens and innoculated in suckling mice. There are no specific serological tests for the disease.

Treatment

There is no specific treatment but symptomatic relief may be obtained from analgesics or topical local anaesthetic in the mouth.

HERPES VIRUS

Herpes simplex infection

Herpes virus hominis is unique to humans and is spread by close contact. After the initial infection the virus lies dormant in the posterior root ganglion and episodically migrates to the skin or mucus membrane, where it will be shed. There are two types of herpes virus which can be distinguished by their cultural characteristics and biochemical enzymatic studies: Type I tends to involve the lips, face and nongenital sites; Type II is usually isolated from anogenital lesions but is not a rigid pattern.

Clinical manifestations. Primary herpetic lesions are uncommon on the foot but zosteriform herpes simplex infection does occur. The primary infection is characterized by painful vesiculation and erosion of the involved skin, local lymphadenopathy and systemic upset. Primary infection lasts about 2–6 weeks before subsiding spontaneously.

Recurrent lesions are usually not accompanied by systemic upset and are less painful and shorter lived. Recurrences are unpredictable and may be precipitated by sunburn, fever or trauma.

Complications. Kaposi's varicelliform eruption is a widespread cutaneous infection by herpes simplex (type I) in patients with atopic dermatitis, Darier's disease and epidermolytic hyperkeratosis. The onset is sudden with fever and a widespread vesiculopustular eruption. Secondary bacterial infection is frequent.

In some patients recurrent herpetic infection is followed 7–10 days later by erythema multiforme. This hypersensitivity reaction is a nonspecific response to the herpes simplex virus. Erythema multiforme may be bullous and is often debilitating.

Treatment. Topical 5% idoxuridine applied early in the course of the disease reduces virus shedding time and speeds healing. Avoidance of triggering factors may be possible in some cases. Topical, oral or parenteral acyclovir has been shown to be useful in primary herpetic infections where it shortens viral shedding time, eases pain and speeds healing. Treatment does not influence recurrent episodes.

SPIROCHAETAL INFECTIONS

Syphilis (synonym: lues)

Syphilis is an infection caused by the spirochaete *Treponema pallidum*. It has four clinical stages, primary, secondary, latent and tertiary. The primary, secondary and early latent phases comprise early infectious syphilis whereas the other phases are regarded as late, noninfectious syphilis.

Primary syphilis. The chancre, occurring typically 18–21 days after infection, is usually the first cutaneous marker of syphilis and occurs at the site of inoculation of the skin by the spirochaete. It tends to be located on the genitalia but extragenital chancres are not uncommon. Chancre on the big toe has been reported. The typical lesion is a painless red papule or encrusted erosion which over a period of weeks becomes round and indurated giving the characterized rubbery consistency. The chancre heals in 4–6 weeks without treatment. Regional lymphadenopathy is frequent with discrete rubbery nontender enlarged lymph nodes.

The diagnosis is made by examining the serous exudate from the chancre with darkfield illumination, provided no topical or oral antibiotics have been used. The serological tests for syphilis do not become positive for 1–3 weeks after the development of the chancre.

Secondary syphilis. The lesions of secondary syphilis develop 6 weeks to 6 months after the initial infection and about 6 weeks after the development of the chancre. The early lesions are symmetrical, macular and transient. The macular lesions are characteristically a light pink colour which become brownish red. Later they become maculopapular, papular or papulosquamous and less frequently scaly pigmented and pustular. The papular lesions have a coppery colour and occur on the palms and soles. Vesicles and bullae are not found.

Condylomata lata starts as a papular lesion of moist areas of the anogenital region and occasionally in the toe webs. They may form a soft red mushrooming mass with a smooth weeping surface.

Generalized painless lymphadenopathy, hepatosplenomegaly and alopecia may be present. Systemic upset with fever, malaise and a sore throat is common. Serological tests are positive in high titres. As with primary syphilis, secondary syphilis undergoes spontaneous resolution. Therapy is indicated to prevent progression of the disease.

Latent syphilis. When the lesions of secondary syphilis resolve, a latent period occurs which lasts a few months or for the patient's lifetime. No lesions either systemic or cutaneous are present in this stage but the specific treponemal tests, fluorescent treponemal antibody absorption test (FTA-ABs) and microphaemagglutination Treponema Pallidum (MHA-TP) test are positive.

Tertiary syphilis. Lesions of tertiary syphilis may occur as soon as 6 months after infection but are more common after 2–3 years. They are not infectious but tend to be destructive and heal with scarring. Gummata occur as single or disseminated lesions in a serpiginous pattern on the lower leg. They may be restricted to the skin but can involve viscera, subcutaneous tissue or bone. They start as a small nodule which enlarges and develops central necrosis which is extensive and leads to punched-out deep indolent, deeply infiltrated ulcers. The lower leg is the most frequent site and may simulate ulcers due to venous hypertensive disease.

Biopsy shows an obliterative end arteritis and/or mixed granulomatous infiltrate of plasma cells, lymphocytes, epitheloid cells and fibroblasts extending from the epidermis to the subcutis. Occasionally tuberculosis will be simulated but well organized granuloma are uncommon.

In neurosyphilis trophic ulcers occur due to anaesthesia of the feet.

Congenital syphilis. Congenital syphilis occurs in children born to syphilitic mothers and infection is transmitted across the placenta at about the fifth month. It is unlikely to occur in mothers who have syphilis for more than four years. Congenital syphilis may be manifest in the neonatal period or may not appear until later in childhood.

The early skin lesions are usually maculopapular bright red which fade to a coppery colour. Secondary pustule formation occurs in lesions that occur a year or more after birth. The eruption has a marked predilection for the lower legs and face, with truncal sparing. A purely papular lesion may occur which becomes infiltrated with coalescence. These are seen on the soles and palms which are diffusely thickened and then desquamate leaving a bright red shiny surface and heal leaving radiating scars. Gummata may occur in children who have stigmata of congenital syphilis at birth.

Syphilitic pemphigus. This is a rare manifestation of congenital syphilis. The bullous eruption occurs on the palms and soles. The bullae are large and rapidly become purulent and rupture leaving large eroded areas. The localization to the feet and the large size of the bullae help to differentiate it from bullous impetigo or pemphigus neonatorum.

Treatment

Penicillin is the drug of choice for all stages of syphilis. Penicillin-allergic patients may be treated with tetracycline or erythromycin. These alternate drugs have been less extensively evaluated than penicillin in the treatment of syphilis and every effort should be made to treat the patient with penicillin.

MYCOBACTERIAL INFECTION (Cott et al 1967)

The mycobacteria are acid-fast bacilli which characteristically produce chronic granulomatous lesions which may ulcerate and disseminate. In man the most important are *Mycobacterium tuberculosis* and *Mycobacterium leprae*.

The other major group of mycobacteria to cause human disease are the opportunistic or atypical mycobacterium. They are found in soil, water and excreta. They differ from mycotuberculosis by being nonvirulent in guinea pigs, able to grow at room temperature, resistant to pretherapy with isoniazid and unable to form nicotinic acid. Runyon has divided them into four groups as outlined in Table 38.2.

Mycobacterium marinum infection.

Synonyms: 'Fish tank granuloma', 'Swimming pool granuloma' (Linell & Norden 1954)

Definition. A chronic granulomatous skin lesion produced by direct inoculation by *M. marinum*. The organism's natural habitat is water and it is found in the crevices and grooves in the cement walls of swimming pools which have been identified as the focus of outbreaks of the disease.

Clinical features. The lesions develop on traumatized skin and commonly on the dorsal aspects of the feet, the fronts of the knees and sometimes the elbows. It usually occurs in adolescents who forsake the steps or ladders of the pool and prefer to climb out on to the deck.

A small reddish papule develops at the site of inoculation after a 3–4 week incubation period. The lesion enlarges to form a hard reddish-brown nodule which sometimes ulcerates and may be covered with a greyish exudate or even becomes verrucous. Lymphangitis or regional adenopathy does not occur. In some instances satellite nodules may develop along the line of the lymphatics resembling a sporotrichoid infection.

Spontaneous healing occurs with scarring within a year but persistence for up to 45 years has been recorded. The response to therapy with antituberculosis agents is variable and is only indicated for resistant or severe disease. Minocycline, tetracycline and cotrimazole have all been reported as successful but only in very small groups of patients. Skin testing with purified protein derivative (PPD) is positive.

Infection with other atypical mycobacteria

Cutaneous infection with atypical mycobacteria other than *M. marinum* is rare. They produce lesions similar to those of *M. marinum* but infection is not transmitted by water.

M. kansasii may produce lesions in a linear path or on the draining lymphatics resembling a sporotrichoid.

Mycobacterium ulcerans (Buruli) infection

Synonyms: Seal's ulcer (Australia); Buruli ulcer (Africa)

This is a common infection endemic to many tropical

Table 38.2 Classification of mycobacteria (Runyon 1959)

Group		Growth at room temperature		Species
I	Photochromogens	2–3 weeks	Yellow colour on exposure to light	*M. marinum* *M. kansasii*
II	Scotochromogen	2–3 weeks	Yellow pigment when grown in dark	*M. scrofulaceum*
III	Nonchromagen	2–3 weeks		*M. intracellulare*
IV	Rapid grower	3–5 days		*M. fortuitum*

areas. Children between 5 and 14 years are most commonly affected in cases reported from Africa. The lesions tend to occur on the lower legs and feet following trauma, the ulcer rapidly developing from the painless subcutaneous nodules. The ulcer may be 10–25 cm in diameter with deeply undermined edges and is usually single and shallow with a whitish-yellow necrotic base. Satellite lesions may occur. Lymphadenopathy is not a feature and the patient experiences no systemic upset despite the large ulcer size. Spontaneous healing usually occurs within 9–12 months but may occasionally persist. The subsequent scarring over the ankle may lead to contracture and disability.

BULLOUS DISORDERS

FRICTION BLISTERS

Friction blisters occur commonly on the feet where the epidermis is both thick and firmly attached to the underlying tissue.

Friction is reduced if the skin is dry, greasy or very wet but not if moist, so powder and silicone may help prevent friction blisters. Two pairs of socks, with a thin sock next to the skin, means that movement is between shoe and thick outer sock rather than skin/shoe. Sterile aspiration of a friction blister within 12 hours of its formation, followed by a pressure dressing results in readhesion of the roof. The roof of a blister should not be removed unless secondary infection occurs.

EPIDERMOLYSIS BULLOSA (Gedde-Dahl 1971)

Epidermolysis bullosa (EB) is a term applied to a large group of genetically determined disorders which are characterized by blistering of the skin and of mucosal membranes. The blisters may result from minor trauma and arise spontaneously. At least seven different forms have been identified which are genetically distinct diseases mediated by different mechanisms.

Epidermolysis bullosa simplex (Weber–Cockayne type) (Cockayne 1938)

The commonest type is epidermolysis bullosa simplex which is transmitted by an autosomal dominant gene. Bullae usually develop in the first year when the child begins to walk or crawl. Clear, tense bullae occur at sites of trauma, usually hands and feet. They heal without scarring or milia formation, milia being small subepidermal keratin cysts 1–2 mm in size. When they occur in the course of the blistering disorders they represent retention cysts. Heat increases the tendency to blister particularly in patients with palmar-plantar hyperhidrosis. The condition may improve at puberty but tends to persist.

Recessive dystrophic epidermolysis bullosa (Fig. 38.10)

More severe and widespread blistering occurs in the other forms especially recessive dystrophic epidermolysis bullosa. Bullae appear at birth or in early infancy. They are large and flaccid, sometimes haemorrhagic and may occur spontaneously. The bullae heal with milia formation and atrophic scarring. Pseudo webbing due to scar tissue covers the fingers and toes producing gross deformities. Nails are shed early on and sclerosis of the finger tips develops. Rarely large eroded nonhealing areas occur on the extensor surface of the limbs.

The mucus membranes are usually involved with oral bullae, erosions and ulcers complicating early feeding. Oesophageal casts may be shed and strictures occur in early childhood. These strictures interfere with adequate nutrition and chronic anaemia results. Aspiration pneumonia may occur and in those who survive long enough, carcinoma of the cardia.

Surviving children are usually physically retarded but mentally normal. Squamous carcinoma, sometimes multiple, have developed in the scarred atrophic skin especially on the legs. Leukoplakia followed by carcinoma has also been reported in the mouth.

Treatment. This is unsatisfactory. In the milder forms, protection from trauma and the use of topical or systemic antibiotics if infection occurs is all that can be offered to these patients. Reduction in sweating improves blistering on the soles. Skilled

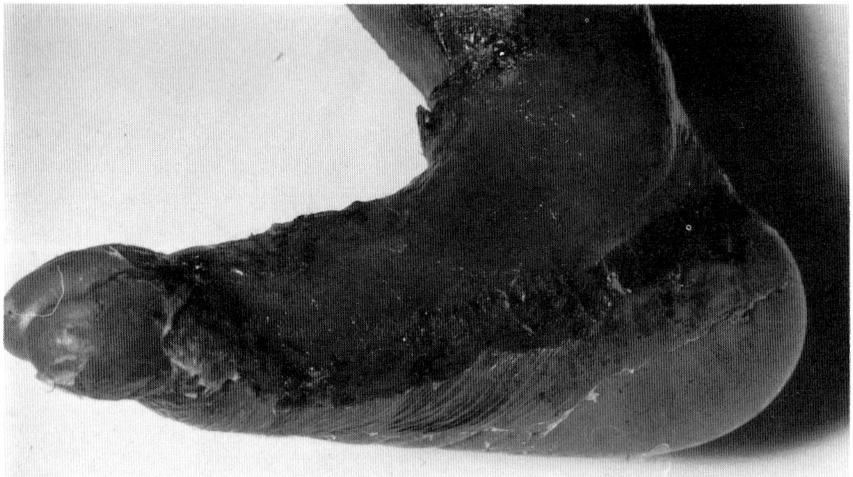

Fig. 38.10 Epidermolysis bullosa. Blistering, erosions and pseudo webbing in a child with epidermolysis bullosa recessive type

nursing and suitable antibiotic control of infection improves survival in children with the recessive dystrophic types of EB. High doses of corticosteroids are no longer recommended. Plastic surgery is required repeatedly in order to maintain function of fingers and hands. Phenytoin with its effect on collagenase activity does not significantly alter the disease.

PEMPHIGOID

This is an uncommon autoimmune disease of the elderly with an IgG antibody directed against the basement membrane.

Clinical features

The typical lesion is a large tense unilocular blister on an area of urticated erythema. The eruption is symmetrical and involves the trunk and limbs. Prodromal itch occurs occasionally. Pemphigoid tends to run a chronic benign course and is likely to go into spontaneous remission within a few years of onset.

PEMPHIGUS VULGARIS

This is an uncommon disease of unknown aetiology characterized by the presence of an IgG antibody to the intercellular cement. The attack causes intra-epidermal blisters which are thin roofed and easily rupture.

Pemphigus is most commonly seen in the 40–60 years age group and if untreated is eventually fatal. The blisters rupture easily leaving large, raw, tender erosions. Mucus membranes are frequently involved.

Treatment of pemphigus

High dose prednisolone is required to suppress blister formation and life long maintenance therapy is usually necessary. Azathioprine may be used for its steroid spring effect.

NAILS (Dawber & Baran 1986)

Abnormalities of the nails may be divided into congenital or acquired.

CONGENITAL ABNORMALITIES

These are extremely uncommon. They present either alone or in association with other ectodermal defects.

Pachyonychia congenita

Marked hypertrophy of the nail bed and the nail with thickening and hyperkeratosis is the main feature of this rare condition. The nail is often normal at birth but shortly afterwards becomes discoloured. Keratoderma may be associated with it. Surgical ablation of the nail bed has been used in the management of this condition.

Nail patella syndrome

In this dominantly transmitted disorder the nails are absent or rudimentary. The thumb nails are always involved but not necessarily other nails. Skeletal abnormalities are frequent and a small or absent patella is the most common finding.

ACQUIRED NAIL DISORDERS

Subungual haematoma

Subungual haematomas are very common in the great toe nails and are usually due to crush injury. The shear force causes separation of the nail from its bed which is in itself painful but it is the accumulation of blood under the nail that causes the severe pain.

Treatment. Treatment by complete removal, under local or general anaesthesia, of the toe nail may be carried out. The main disadvantage to that line of treatment is that the nail bed is exposed and this can be temporarily disabling. Decompression of the nail has the advantage of immediate relief of pain and also the nail is left in situ to protect the nail bed until it is pushed off by the growing nail.

Drilling the nail with a heated paper clip or the blunt end of a sailmaker's needle will allow blood to burst through the hole. No pressure must be used and as the needle cools rapidly it needs to be reheated frequently. If care is taken the procedure is painless as the needle should not touch the nail bed.

Onycholysis

In this condition there is painless separation of the nail from its bed. Drugs that give rise to photosensitive reactions can cause onycholysis. This occurs even in toe nails which have not been exposed to light, as with benoxyprofen (Opren). The mechanism is unknown. Accumulation of dirt under the nail and vigorous attempts to clean it out sometimes leads to secondary infection and pain. The nail bed may be colonized with *Candida albicans* and *Pseudomonas pyocyanea* but while this may result in discolouration of the nail, the infection is usually silent.

Onycholysis may occur secondarily to a variety of skin and general medical conditions. It is a feature of nail involvement in psoriasis, pityriasis rubra pilaris, dermatitis and fungal infection.

Onychogryphosis

This progressive abnormal thickening of the toe nails, commonly the great toe nail, tends to occur in the elderly. It is due to prolonged pressure on the nail bed and once started is difficult to control. This used to be called Ostler's nail as it was a frequent sequelae to injury caused by horses standing on the ostler's foot. It may progress to a horn which causes further pressure and may curve back into the toe causing ulceration.

Twenty nail dystrophy

This is a dystrophy seen mainly in children where all the nails are involved. The nails are thin, ridged and roughened and often split.

There is some controversy as to its relationship with lichen planus. Histological data are available only in 3 cases — one showing features of lichen planus while the others showed a spongiotic parakeratotic picture.

Yellow nail syndrome

This syndrome of slow growing yellow thickened nails usually follows the development of lymphoedema. The nails are excessively curved in the long axis and onycholysis may be present. The cuticles are usually lost.

It is infrequently seen in patients with congenitally abnormal lymphatics. The lymphoedema usually involves the legs but other areas may be affected. The degree of abnormality seen in these lymphatics ranges from apparently normal vessels through its atresia or varicosity. All nails of hands and feet may be involved.

Tinea unguium

In this condition there is invasion of the nail plate with dermatophytes. The dermatophytes which are commonly involved in toe nails are usually associated with tinea on the palms and soles. These dermatophytes are *Trichophyton rubrum*, *T. interdigitale* and *Epidermophyton floccosum*. *T. rubrum* and *T. interdigitale* easily invade the nail plate and are more commonly found than *E. floccosum*.

It tends to be a condition of adults but the elderly, easily traumatized toe nails are particularly susceptible to infection.

Clinical features. Irrespective of the causative organism the clinical features are the same. The earliest sign is patchy discolouration along the free nail edge. The colour may be white or yellow. As it spreads the discolouration spreads towards the nail base and the colour darkens to brown or black. The nail becomes progressively thickened with heaped up subungual hyperkeratosis. The changes may progress to complete destruction of the nail.

While infection usually starts with one nail others may become infected but the degree of invasion varies and changes may be minimal. Infection is usually painless but where gross destruction of the nails has occurred patients often complain of pain and discomfort when wearing shoes.

Diagnosis. Nail clippings should be taken for mycological examination, as should scrapings from the interdigital web and sole of the foot.

Treatment. While tinea pedis responds well to griseofulvin its use in the management of tinea unguium is dubious. In young patients with normal nail growth griseofulvin will usually eradicate tinea unguium. However, many authors consider treatment of tinea in the toe nails to be completely ineffective. Even the advent of the imidazole drugs has added little to the therapeutic battery. If treatment is to be undertaken then it must be for prolonged periods (1–2 years). Avulsion of a single infected toe nail may be a useful adjuvant to griseofulvin therapy.

Differential diagnosis: The clinical features may suggest psoriasis but pitting is not a feature of fungal infection. Lichen planus and eczema may also cause a dystrophy indistinguishable from fungal infection.

Scopulariopsis

S. brevis is a saprophytic mould which may invade the great toe nails, other nails occasionally being involved. There is marked thickening of the nail with a cinnamon discolouration often limited to the lateral border of the nail.

Treatment. Avulsion of the toe nail if infection is limited to one nail is usually effective. Miconazole under polythene occlusion may be useful.

Hendersonula toruloidea infection

This plant pathogenic fungus may cause tinea pedis and unguium in tropical areas or in immigrants from Africa or Asia. Two types, A and B, have been identified according to different growth patterns. Type A is usually found in West Indians and type B in those from the Indian subcontinent. The clinical features are similar to dermatophyte infection with interdigital and nail involvement. It is often accompanied by a paronychia which is not normally a feature of dermatophytosis. It may coexist with ringworm.

Scytalidium hyalinum

This is another plant fungus recently described as infecting the hands and feet in West Indians. It is indistinguishable from dermatophytosis.

Ingrowing toe nail

The soft tissue of the lateral nail fold is penetrated by a pointed spicule of nail which results in pain, secondary infection and often the formation of granulation tissue. The great toe nails are most commonly affected. Improper nail trimming and illfitting footwear contribute to the development of ingrowing toe nails.

Treatment: consists of removing the nail spicule and treating the infection with soaks, painting with antiseptic paints such as silver nitrate and occasionally oral antibiotics if cellulitis occurs. Proper chiropody and well fitting shoes will help prevent recurrence.

Surgery is only indicated if conservative means have failed.

Tumours

A variety of benign and malignant tumours may occur involving either the nail matrix, nail fold or nail bed. The paronychial areas surrounding the matrix and nail bed are the areas most commonly involved with tumour.

Warts

Periungual and subungual warts occur quite commonly in the finger nails but are less frequent in the toe nails. Treatment is notoriously difficult at times. There is a definite risk of nail deformity due to matrix damage from certain modalities of therapy, e.g. curettage and electrodesiccation.

Subungual exostosis

In this condition a bony lump appears below the nail. It is not a true exostosis as the tumour consists of normal mature bone. It occurs mainly in children and adolescents and is most commonly found in the great toes.

The lesion presents as a hard lump under the skin of the distal nail bed. The overlying portion of nails is often rubbed away by shoe pressure. Although it often resembles subungual warts or an ingrowing toe nail ulceration does not occur.

Confirmation of the diagnosis is by X-ray which clearly demonstrates the bony lesion lying lateral to the distal phalanx.

Pyogenic granuloma (Granuloma telangecticum) (Fig. 38.11).

This lesion usually occurs after trauma. It involves the hyponychium and enlarges to involve the nail bed. Removal of the nail and either surgical excision or electrodesiccation usually cures the lesion.

Fibromas (Fig. 38.12)

These occur in 50% of patients with tuberous sclerosis. They are usually periungual but may occur subungually. Grooving of the nail is a common manifestation. They occur after puberty and usually stigmata of the disease are well established. Surgical excision will cure the lesion.

Junctional naevi

Linear pigmented bands are frequently seen in the nails of coloured races. Naevus cells in the matrix produces the pigmented bands which may vary in colour from light brown to black.

It is important in the differential diagnosis of subungual melanoma and any alteration from the original naevus should be biopsied to rule out a malignant change.

Glomus tumours

Glomus tumours are vascular tumours arising in the dermis of the nail bed. They are intensely painful when even the lightest pressure is applied. Removal of the nail plate and excision of the lesion results in a complete cure.

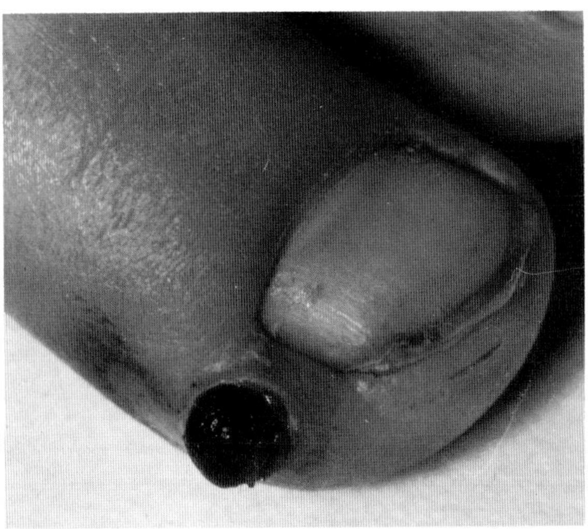

Fig. 38.11 Pyogenic granuloma on the second toe of a child

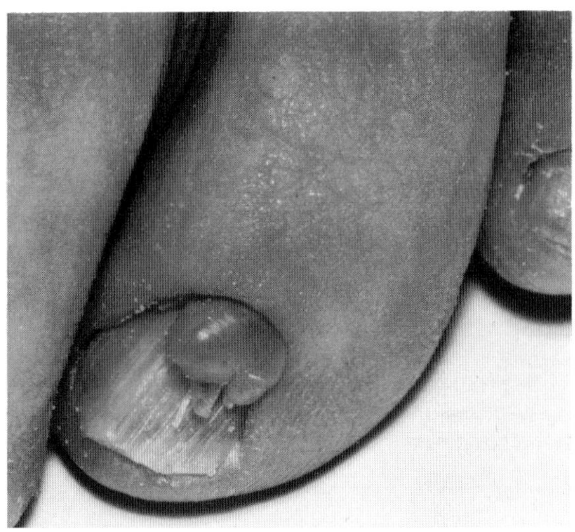

Fig. 38.12 Periungual fibroma in a patient with eploia

Myxoid cysts

Myxoid cysts are more commonly seen on the dorsal aspect of the distal digits, usually abutting the nail. Pressure of the tumour on the nail may result in longitudinal ridging and thinning of the nail. They contain clear viscous mucoid material which may be discharged intermittently. They are regarded as degenerative cysts and are frequently associated with osteoarthritic distal interphalangeal joints.

Malignant tumours

Malignant tumours of the nail are fortunately very rare. They include basal and squamous cell carcinoma and malignant melanoma. Subungual kerato-acanthoma may also occur.

TUMOURS

ECCRINE POROMA (Hyman & Brownstein 1969)

Definition

This is a benign growth of the distal eccrine sweat duct.

Clinical features

The lesion occurs on the nonhair-bearing areas of the foot and occasionally the palm. It presents as a nontender smooth reddish tumour which may protrude from a shallow cup-shaped depression which forms the base. It bleeds readily and may vary in size from 2–12 mm in diameter. Pigmented lesions have been reported. While the lesions tend to be singular, multiple lesions do occur.

Incidence

This is an uncommon tumour and affects both sexes equally. It tends to be a disease of middle-age.

Histology

The histological features are characteristic with solid masses of small uniform basophilic epithelial cells with intercellular bridging. Splits or cleft-like lumina may be found with attempts at forming a cuticle. The adjacent epidermis becomes thickened and hyperkeratotic. Vascular dilation with hyper-plastic capillaries may be present.

Treatment

Local excision is curative. Curettage with electro-desiccation of the base may be adequate.

Differential diagnosis

This lesion may simulate Kaposi's sarcoma, malignant melanoma, basal cell carcinoma or a pyogenic granuloma.

MALIGNANT ECCRINE POROMA OR POROCARCINOMA

Malignant change may occur in an eccrine poroma of long duration or may arise de novo. It may present localized and indistinguishable from an eccrine poroma or as an ulceration nodule. Cutaneous and visceral metastases have been recorded as causing death.

ARSENICAL KERATOSES (Yeh 1973)

Definition

Inorganic arsenicals were widely used in the past for the treatment of psoriasis, dermatitis and anaemias. They are well recognized carcinogens which cause both skin and visceral malignancies.

Clinical features

The characteristic arsenical keratosis is a discrete, hard, wart-like keratotic lesion of 2–4 mm. The lesions are multiple and occur predominantly on the palms and soles but may occur on any part of the skin. These lesions occur a decade or more after exposure to arsenic. They resemble actinic keratoses and are premalignant. Their malignant potential is low.

The other stigmata of chronic arsenical ingestion

may be present, i.e. hyperpigmentation, intra-epidermal carcinoma (Bowen's disease) and multiple basal cell carcinoma.

Histology

Hyperkeratosis and acanthosis is present with a downward proliferation of the rete ridges.

Treatment

Treatment of multiple keratoses of the soles of the feet is difficult. Freezing with liquid nitrogen, cautery and diathermy have all been used but care is needed to prevent the development of painful scars. Topical 5-fluorouracil or podophyllin may also be used to good effect.

The oral retinoid etretinate has been used in other hyperkeratotic conditions to good effect. Its use in this condition has not been evaluated in extensive trials although early results are promising.

KAPOSI'S SARCOMA (Multiple idiopathic haemorrhagic sarcoma) (Reynolds et al 1965)

Definition

This is a malignant tumour of vascular tissue.

Aetiology

Kaposi's sarcoma is a common tumour amongst elderly male Africans and middle-aged Europeans where it runs a relatively benign course. It has been well recognized in association with lymphoma, leukaemia and immunosuppression, i.e. post renal transplant, and may occur in 6–12% of these patients. A rapidly progressive disseminated form is seen in patients with the Acquired Immune Deficiency Syndrome (AIDS) (Friedman–Kien 1981). It has been associated with a pathogenic retrovirus (HTLV-III/LAV).

Clinical features

The initial lesions usually occur on the soles of the feet as bluish-red or black macules which spread and coalesce to form a large plaque. Rubbery angiomatous nodules with oedema may then develop. The nodules ulcerate and have a foul smelling discharge. The disease slowly advances with more nodules developing and increasing lymphoedema.

In the early stages of the disease spontaneous resolution of some or all the nodules may occur leaving atrophic hyperpigmented scars. Later on, macules, patches and nodules appear on the faces, ears, soft palate and the trunk. The disease becomes slowly progressive. Gangrene of the feet may occur.

Involvement of bone and the small bowel is common and is indicative of disseminated disease. Bone changes are characteristic and show cyst formation, rarefaction and erosion of the cortex. In the elderly, it runs a relatively benign course if confined to the skin. Once visceral involvement occurs death is rapid.

Diagnosis

The histological picture is variable. The early lesions resemble granulation tissue while in the late phase prominent endothelial cells are seen lining the vessels with spindle-shaped cells lying peripherally.

Treatment

In elderly men, conservative radiotherapy has been used with marked resolution of the tumours. Combined chemotherapeutic regimes have not to date resulted in the salvage of any patient with Kaposi's sarcoma in AIDS sufferers.

VERRUCOUS SQUAMOUS CELL EPITHELIOMA (Epithelioma cuniculatum plantare) (Reingold et al 1978)

Definition

This rare tumour of the plantar surface of the foot is a variant of squamous cell carcinoma.

Clinical features

The exophytic tumour has a cauliflower-like or verrucoid ulcerating surface which is often associated with a foul discharge. At first the lesion closely resembles a recalcitrant plantar wart. It is capable of great local destruction with deep punctation of the underlying fascia and may destroy the metatarsal bones and go on to invade the skin on the dorsum of the foot as the tumour penetrates deeply. While capable of great local destruction it has little tendency to metastasize. The development of regional lymph node metastases has been documented.

Histology

A large deep biopsy is essential for the diagnosis of verrucous carcinoma. In the upper portion the tumour shows hyperkeratosis and acanthosis and resembles a verruca. The rest of the tumour is composed of large downward projections of well differentiated epithelia or squamous carcinoma, which compress the collagen bundles and push them aside.

Treatment

Local wide excision is important. Amputation may be necessary if bone is involved. Radiation should not be used as it has led in some instances to the development of metastatic squamous carcinoma.

Differential diagnosis

The diagnosis is often difficult and it must be distinguished from an intractable plantar wart, giant keratoacanthoma, deep fungal infection and pseudo-epitheliomatous hyperplasia.

MALIGNANT MELANOMA

Definition. An uncommon malignant tumour which arises from epidermal melanocytes. Cutaneous malignant melanoma (MM) are usually divided into four types:

1. Lentigo maligna melanoma (LMM)
2. Superficial spreading (SMM)
3. Acral lentiginous melanoma (ALM)
4. Nodular melanoma (NM).

In the first three types an early horizontal growth phase exists — melanoma in situ, where the tumour is confined to the epidermis. After a varying length of time an invasive or vertical growth phase occurs. Invasive melanoma arising from melanoma in situ tends to have a better prognosis than nodular melanoma arising de novo.

Acral lentiginous melanoma in situ

ALM in situ has only recently been recognized as a separate entity. Characteristically, it occurs on the hairless skin of the palms and soles and also in the subungual and periungual areas. Clinically uneven pigmentation with an irregular ill-defined edge is seen. If it occurs in the nail bed, matrix or nail, it presents as a pigmented longitudinal band.

Diagnosis of ALM in situ is difficult and may not be recognized clinically or even histologically. Wide excision at this stage offers excellent prognosis.

Acral lentiginous melanoma

ALM is the invasive form of ALM in situ. The earliest lesions are irregular macular lesions with uneven pigmentation. They may be present for a considerable time — up to 7 years, and are usually ignored by the patient.

Itch is sometimes present even before any discernible change in pigment occurs. Pigmentary changes are common and may either increase or decrease in colour with an irregular border. The skin surface markings are lost in association with the early pigmentary changes. Blue-black or pink nodules are often found within the tumour. Bleeding is a sinister sign and is often associated with ulceration and necrosis in the tumour.

No one sign is a specific indicator of malignancy as all may occur simultaneously. However any previously uniformly pigmented lesion on the sole of the foot which shows alteration in the pigment either centrally or peripherally, or develops elevated nodules with an inflammatory edge, should be regarded with a high index of suspicion.

Histology. In contrast to its aggressive biological behaviour the histological features are sometimes rather benign with large melanocytes many of which show dendritic spindle shapes which tends to indicate a benign course but not in ALM.

Incidence. There is a slight female predominance in most series of 3:2. It has a peak incidence in the sixth decade for women and a decade later for men.

There is considerable epidemiological evidence implicating the role of sunlight in the formation of malignant melanomas. It is obvious that sunlight is not the only factor in inducing melanoma on the foot and the role of repeated trauma is difficult to assess.

Prognosis. Prognosis is poor for ALM as tumefaction, ulceration and metastases often occur after a short time. Prognosis is directly related to tumour thickness. Volar melanomas less than 1 cm deep and those in the horizontal growth phase have a better prognosis and usually only require local wide excision. The overall five year survival rate varies from 11–15%.

VASCULAR DISORDERS

LUPUS ERYTHEMATOSUS

This autoimmune disorder presents in two forms — chronic discoid lupus erythematosus which is confined to the skin and systemic lupus erythematosus where internal organs are involved.

Chronic discoid lupus erythematosus (Fig. 38.13)

This condition affects both sexes equally and occurs commonly on the light exposed areas of the face. Lesions occur elsewhere and involvement of the plantar foot is not uncommon. It is an asymmetrical rash and is aggravated by sunlight.

Clinical features. It is characterized by well defined slightly scaly, erythematous plaques with some degree of atrophy and follicular plugging. When the scale is removed the classical 'carpet-tack' appearance is seen. As the disease progresses atrophy, scarring and depigmentation occur. Involvement of hairy areas gives rise to scarring alopecia.

Histology. Liquefaction degeneration of the basal layer, dermal oedema and a patchy lymphocytic infiltrate is seen. Hyperkeratosis and follicular plugging is readily identified.

Treatment. Therapy includes the use of potent topical steroids, avoidance of ultraviolet light, antimalarial drugs such as hydroxychloroquine and very occasionally, systemic corticosteroids. Retinal damage due to antimalarial drugs is a well recognized complication.

Systemic lupus erythematosus

This is a multisystem disease which usually occurs in females of 20–50 years. It is characterized by the presence of antibodies to nuclear antigens and especially to purified double stranded DNA. Immunofluorescence studies show deposition of immunoglobulins at the basement membrane.

Clinical features. Nailfold capillary dilatation and chilblain-like plaques are seen on the digits, more easily on the fingers, but are clearly visible on the toes. Splinter haemorrhages and small periungual infarcts due to vasculitis are also clearly seen. Raynaud's phenomenon may be present but is usually mild.

Treatment. Treatment includes systemic steroids, azothioprines, antimalarials, and occasionally plasmaphoretics has been advocated.

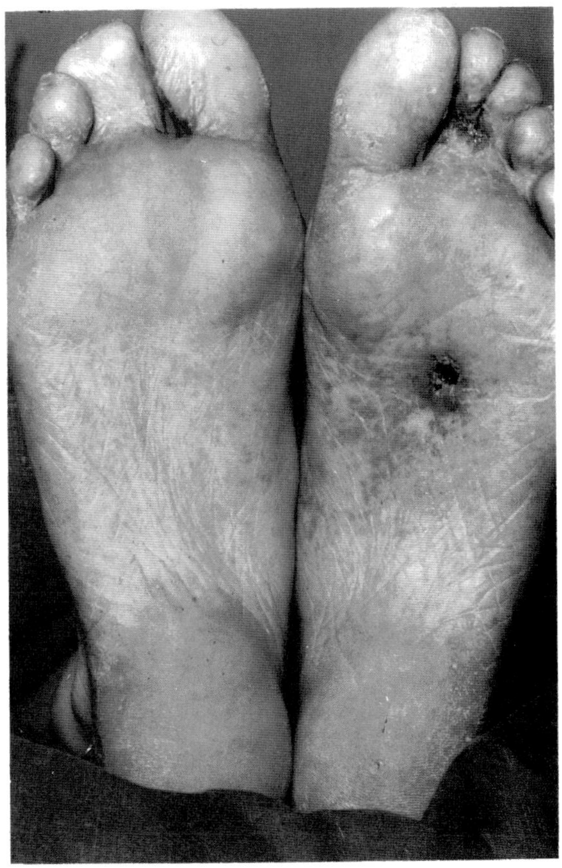

Fig. 38.13 Discoid lupus erythematosus on the plantar foot with active area centrally and extensive scarring. Incidental webbing of second and third toes is present

The prognosis in SLE is variable but it tends to run a chronic course with intermittent exacerbations. Severe vasculitis, renal and central nervous system involvement carries a significantly poor prognosis.

SCLERODERMA

Scleroderma occurs in two forms — a localized cutaneous form called morphoea and a systemic form. Both forms are uncommon.

Morphoea (Fig. 38.14)

In this idiopathic disorder there is localized sclerosis of the skin. Morphoea consists of a hardened plaque with a violaceous colour around the edge of the lesion. The centre becomes more indurated and white in colour surrounded by a hyperpigmented rim. There is loss of hair and reduction of sweat production in the smooth shiny plaques. Atrophy of the underlying muscles and bones occurs giving rise to considerable disability. Lesions tend to resolve and soften over many years (5–10 yr). Treatment is rarely necessary.

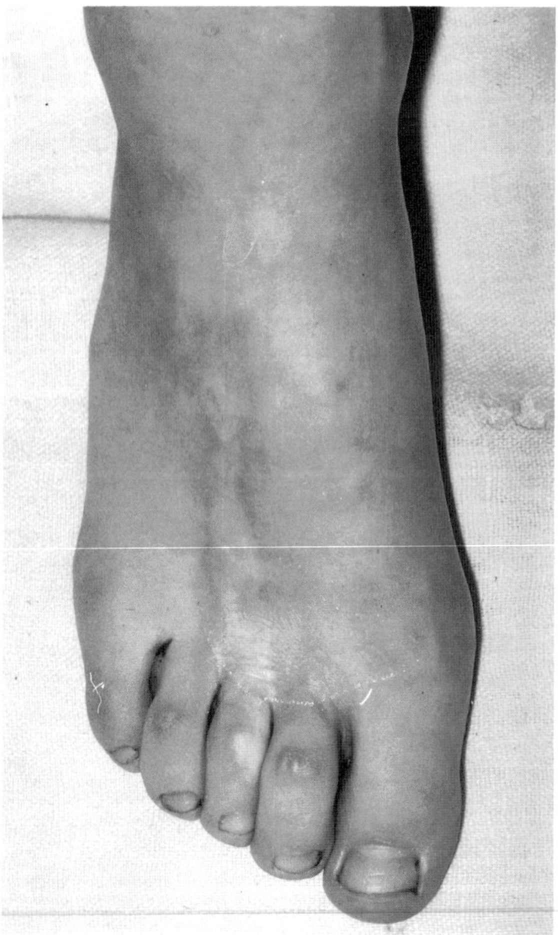

Fig. 38.14 Linear morphoea (scleroderma). Localized area of scleroderma on dorsum of foot

Systemic sclerosis

This rare disorder is characterized by increased collagen deposition in all systems. Arterial constriction and occlusion occurs in many internal organs.

Raynaud's phenomenon is the usual presenting symptom and may be present for many years before more obvious signs of the disease occur. Severe digital ischaemia with ulceration gives rise to loss of digital pulp. Progressive induration of the skin leads to restriction and deformity of the digits. Cutaneous calcinosis is commoner on the fingertips than on the feet and causes tender nodules which often ulcerate.

The facies are characteristic with lack of facial expression, beaked nose, perioral furrows, reduction in mouth size and telangectasia on the cheeks.

Treatment. This is unsatisfactory and vasodilators like nifedipine may help peripheral perfusion. Steroids, immunosuppressive drugs and penicillamine have little useful effect on the systemic changes. Avoidance of cold, an absolute ban on smoking, and physiotherapy to preserve function are more important than drug therapy.

Prognosis: depends on the presence and the degree of renal, cardiac and pulmonary involvement.

MISCELLANEOUS

CORNS (or clavi)

Corns are painful, clearly demarcated hyperkeratotic lesions and occur mainly on the dorsolateral aspects of the fifth toes or the dorsal prominence of the hammer toe. They are acquired lesions and are induced by pressure exerted by footwear on bony prominences. They can be differentiated from calluses by the presence of a translucent central hyperkeratotic core which projects downwards. This core interrupts the normal skin papillary lines. They may be extremely painful and disabling, especially in the elderly.

SOFT CORNS (Fig. 38.15)

Corns occur in the interdigital web of the fourth and fifth toes. They are soft and may be extremely macerated so resembling a dermatophyte infection. They are often exquisitely painful and recurrent infection giving rise to cellulitis on the dorsum of the foot is not uncommon. They result from friction of the condyle of the phalanges of the fifth toe and the condyle of the metatarsal head of the fourth. Occasionally opposing soft or 'kissing' corns may occur.

CALLUS

Callus may be found at any point on the forefoot where excess friction or abnormal pressure occurs, due to improperly fitting shoes. It is most commonly found on the sole of the foot under the first and fifth metatarsal heads. When found under the second metatarsal head it may represent a congenitally short first metatarsal which throws excess weight on the second metatarsal. Paring of the calluses reveals no bleeding points as in a wart nor the translucent core of a corn. The papillary lines are preserved.

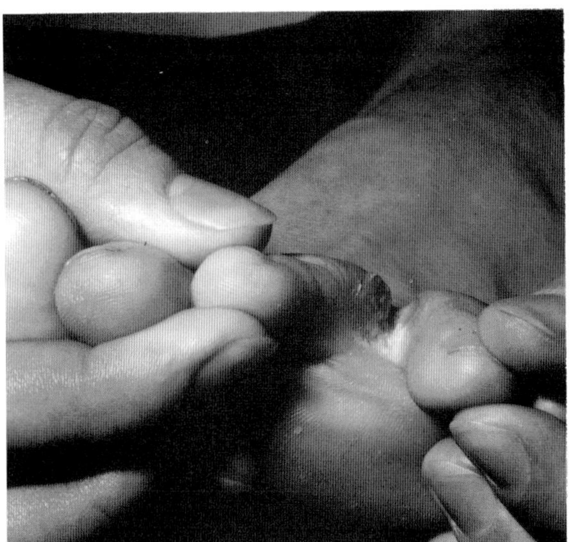

Fig. 38.15 Interdigital corn with maceration of web space simulating interdigital fungal infection

PRAYER NODULES

Hyperkeratosis of the lateral and anterior aspects of the ankles is common. It may be induced by certain sitting or squatting habits as in children or certain religious groups. The nodules also occur in certain sports like surfboard riding where there is an associated hyperkeratosis of the knees and tibial tubercles. Tailors who adopt the crossed leg position develop callus on the outer border of the fifth metatarsal.

The position adopted to induce these lesions is acute inversion of the foot so that the rim of the lateral talar condyle is being continually rubbed against the skin.

PIEZOGENIC PEDAL PAPULES (Schlappner et al 1972)

These are flesh coloured papules which appear on the medial aspects of the heels. They are usually asymptomatic and are visible on weight bearing. They are often overlooked as most patients are examined recumbent.

The papules are true herniations of subcutaneous fat through defects in connective tissue into the dermis. This extrusion of fat with its blood vessels and nerves could account for the pain on standing in some patients.

Treatment

Cushioning of the shoe or supportive orthopaedic devices may help to relieve pressure on the heel.

FOREIGN BODY REACTIONS

Foreign bodies in the skin are a common problem. Granulomatous reactions may occur at the site of entry in the skin.

EPIDERMOID INCLUSION CYSTS

These are nontender tumours that occur on the palms and soles. They result from traumatic implantation of chemically inert material and are most often seen in middle-aged men.

Treatment

They are easily curetted off or excised.

SILICA GRANULOMAS (Epstein 1955)

Silica in the form of glass, quartz, sand or flint may give rise to silica granuloma which develop months or even years after the initial injury has healed. It is the conversion of silica to silica colloid in the tissues that is thought to account for the granuloma formation. The silicates in the spines of sea urchins may also produce a sarcoidal granuloma and even local osteitis. They present as red-brown or violaceous maculopapules. Ulceration is rare. The lesions may spontaneously remit but can be treated surgically or by local injection of corticosteroid.

Foreign bodies i.e. splinters or other objects may introduce micro-organisms into the skin. Staphylococcal and streptococcal infections may give rise to cellulitis. Sporotrichosis may be transmitted by infected thorns.

HAIR

Hair acting as a foreign body results in a number of reactions. This usually depends on the site and depth of penetration. Mild erythema, abscess and sinus formation as well as chronic granuloma may all be associated with hair reactions.

HAIR SINUSES OF THE FEET (Price & Popkin 1976)

A very characteristic syndrome occurs when a hair penetrates the skin of an interdigital web, usually the fourth. This is often unsuspected and the patient may present with a long history of recurrent episodes of pain, swelling or cellulitis. Examination reveals oedema of the adjacent dorsal foot, with a pinhole sinus present in the base of the web. This is often hidden beneath an accumulation of macerated skin. Surgical excision of the sinus tract is curative.

Hair penetrating the foot is an occupational hazard of hairdressers and dog groomers. Hyperkeratotic tender nodules on the heels and toes and abscess formation on the toes have all been reported in hairdressers.

CALCANEAL PETECHIAL 'BLACK HEEL' (Fig. 38.16)

In this condition a speckled black lesion appears on the back or side of the heel just above the junction of the hyperkeratotic skin of the sole of the foot and the thinner skin above. It occurs as the result of rupture of small papillary capilla due to a shearing force and is commonly seen in adolescents involved in football, basketball and squash.

Clinical features

It is usually a painless condition with the sudden development of a black lesion which on closer examination is made up of closely grouped black dots.

Diagnosis and treatment

Gentle paring of the skin reveals that the black pigment comes away in the horny layer. Treatment is not indicated but a softer heel piece in the shoe or a felt pad may help.

The main importance of this condition is that it must be differentiated from malignant melanoma or a tattoo.

GRANULOMA ANNULARE

This granulomatous condition of children and young adults may be an indicator of latent diabetes.

Aetiology

The aetiology is unknown. The histological features

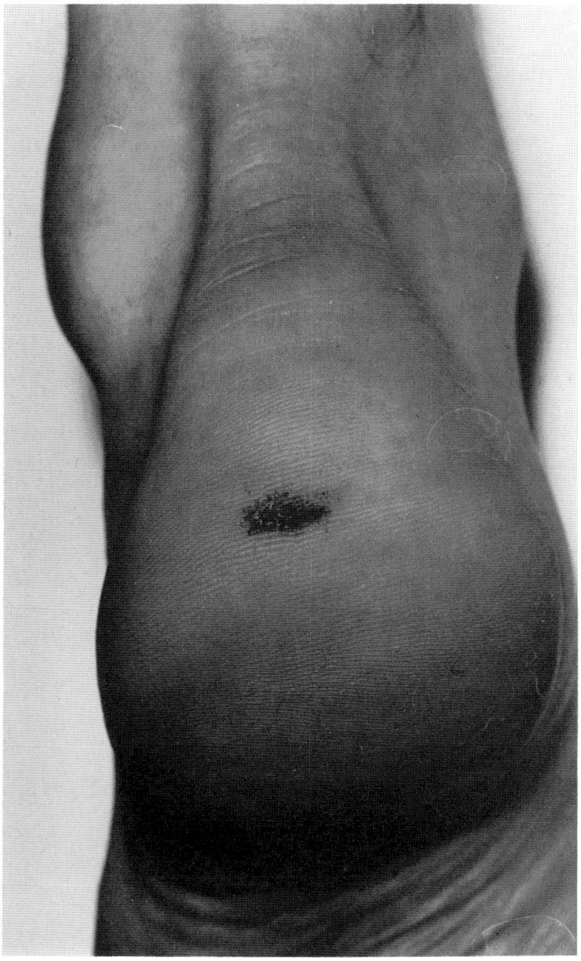

Fig. 38.16 Black heel. The characteristic punctate haemorrhage can be readily seen

may merge into those of necrobiosis lipoidica. It is commoner in females than in males.

Clinical features

The lesions are commonly found on the extensor aspects of the hands, feet, arms and legs. The lesions are pink or flesh coloured papules or nodules which form rings. There is a characteristic beading and blanching of the ring of white dermal papules.

Treatment

No treatment is necessary as the lesions resolve spontaneously but its course may be influenced by local or intralesional corticosteroids.

AINHUM AND PSEUDOAINHUM (Cole 1965)

Ainhum (dactolysis spontanea)

Definition. Ainhum is a condition characterized by the development of constricting bands around digits resulting in autoamputation. Other types of constricting bands may mimic it and are called pseudoainhum.

Incidence and epidemiology. Ainhum is traditionally regarded as a disease of middle-aged barefoot Africans involving exclusively the fifth toe and is of unknown aetiology. However, it is known to occur all over the tropics in both sexes, all ages and races. An incidence of 2% is reported from Nigeria.

Classification. This condition can be divided into the following categories:

1. True ainhum
2. Pseudoainhum:
   a) Congenital amniotic bands
   b) Related to specific disease — hereditary; nonhereditary; miscellaneous
   c)Traumatic — thermal or chemical burns; frostbite; mechanical injuries; elastic bands; etc.

Clinical features. Ainhum usually affects the fifth toe and tends to be bilateral. The fissure or groove is the characteristic feature of this condition. In the beginning it appears on the medial side of the base of the toe at the plantardigital fold. The groove encircles the toe gradually getting deeper until eventually the toe undergoes autoamputation. Oedema and resorption of underlying bone develops with the increasing constriction and secondary infection and crusting of the skin is common. The condition is frequently very painful. The rate of constriction varies but usually takes many years. Other digits may be involved.

Congenital constricting bands (amniotic band syndrome) (Raque et al 1972)

The constricting bands in pseudoainhum are always circumferential and may involve a limb or the trunk. The defect may be deep enough to cause amputation of a limb in utero, and a terminal scar is visible at the end of the stump.

The distal parts of the extremities are more

commonly involved, usually the digits or the leg and forearm. In cases where the defect is proximal, the distal limb is usually abnormal and syndactyly, microdactyly and club foot may be present. Gross oedema and chronic elephantiasis of the foot and ankle has also been reported. The incidence is unknown and figures vary from 1 in 1200 live births to 1 in 15000 live births.

Acquired bands

Constriction of the digits by artefacts is sometimes seen in young children and occasionally in adults. Hair, rubber bands, thread or fibre may cause constriction and gross oedema of the digit so that the ligating band is not readily recognized.

Acquired bands are seen secondary to a variety of conditions. Severe dermatophyte infection in children may result in the development of pseudoainhum which should resolve completely with appropriate chemotherapy. Pseudoainhum may occur in conditions where there is vascular insufficiency or decreased sensation. Constricting scar formation may follow trauma, frostbite or burns.

Pseudoainhum with subsequent loss of digits is seen in a number of hyperkeratotic conditions. It is a common consequence of the verrucous hyperkeratotic plantar lesions of yaws. In Vohwinkel's syndrome (keratoma hereditarium mutilans), a rare hereditary form of hyperkeratosis, the constricting bands develop at puberty. Constricting bands around the digits may occur in Mal de Meleda proximal to the nailfolds.

Pathology. The histology in ainhum and pseudoainhum is similar. The constricting bands which are essentially scars extend deep through the dermis into the subcutaneous layers and may impinge on underlying bone. The epidermis may be hyperkeratotic and slightly acanthotic.

Treatment. Surgery is the treatment of choice. Z-plasty has been recommended for early ainhum and congenital constricting bands. Early amputation for the more advanced cases will reduce pain and secondary infection.

FROSTBITE (Killian 1981)

This is discussed elsewhere in more detail (Chapter 52). Frostbite is rare in civilian populations but common in soldiers in winter military campaigns. It accounted for 9% of all British casualties in the Falkland Islands war in 1982.

Minor frostbite occurs with brief exposure to extreme cold and usually results from inadequate protection from the cold. Severe frostbite tends to occur in the elderly, vagrant, alcoholic or immobile patient.

Pathophysiology

Cold induced venous constriction causes raised venous pressure with decreased capillary flow and capillary sludging. Antisludging agents like low molecular weight dextrans have been advocated in the past but no beneficial effect has been shown in man.

Management

Population education on the dangers of extreme cold may help reduce the number of cases of minor frostbite.

Surgical intervention after a clear line of demarcation between living and dead tissue has been established as the treatment of choice. Aspiration of blisters, elevation and exposure of the frostbitten limb helps to relieve pain. Tetanus toxoid and prophylactic antibiotics should be given in the first week. Thereafter antibiotics are only required if the demarcation area becomes infected. Sympathectomy helps reduce pain and resolution of oedema and hastens demarcation.

ERYTHEMA MULTIFORME

Erythema multiforme is a form of vasculitis and probably represents an immunological reaction to a wide variety of factors. Infections such as herpes simplex and mycoplasma and drugs (especially sulphonamides) are recognized precipitating factors but in over 50% of cases no provocative factor can be identified.

Clinical features

There are three main clinical variations but the

hallmark lesion of the disease is the iris or target lesion. This has a central discoloured area surrounded by one or more rings of erythema. The papular form is the commonest type and involves the palms, soles and forearms. The lesions are purple and vary in size from pinhead papules to 2–3 cm plaques.

In the vesiculobullous form vesicles and blisters occur in the centre of the rings. Mucosal involvement is common.

Severe forms of the disease occur and may be fatal as in the Stevens-Johnson syndrome where severe systemic upset, stomatitis, conjunctivitis, pneumonitis and renal failure may occur.

Treatment

The disease is usually self-limiting in 2–3 weeks and treatment is reserved for the most severe cases. Prednisolone in high doses is used but there is no evidence to show that it is effective. Identification and treatment of a precipitating factor, i.e. herpes simplex, may prevent relapse.

URTICARIA

Urticaria is a common skin disorder which affects about 20% of the population during their lifetime. It is caused by a transient increase in capillary permeability giving rise to local dermal oedema. In over 70% of patients it will be of the idiopathic variety with the remainder being physical, cholinergic or allergic urticaria.

Clinical features. Urticaria is an itchy condition characterized by the development of erythematous swellings in the skin. These are transient and usually last about 30 minutes but in the case of urticarial vasculitis may last 2–3 days. The size of the lesions vary from a few millimetres to several centimetres in diameter.

On the soles of the feet, because of the structure of the skin, weals are not readily seen. Diffuse erythema and oedema may be seen and a burning sensation, which may be severe, is more common than itch.

The physical urticarias are urticarias induced by pressure, heat, cold and sunlight.

Pressure urticaria

This is probably a variant of dermographism and tends to occur on the buttocks and feet, 4–6 hours after pressure. The swellings are painful and appear to be indurated as the lesions spread subcutaneously. The mechanism in this condition is obscure and the cause of the delay is unknown.

Treatment. H1 antihistamines are usually effective but the sedative side effects limit their usefulness. Some of the newer antihistamines, e.g. terfenadine, which are relatively free of sedation, should be tried first.

REFERENCES

Altman J, Perry H O 1961 The variation and course of lichen planus. Arch Dermatol 84: 733

Ashton R E, Russell-Jones R, Griffiths A 1985 Juvenile plantar dermatosis. A clinicopathologic study. Arch Dermatol 121: 225

Bunney M H 1982 Viral Warts: their Biology and Treatment. Oxford University Press, Oxford

Callen J P 1979 The spectrum of Reiter's disease. J Am Acad Dermatol 1: 75

Cockayne E A 1938 Recurrent bullous eruption of feet. Br J Dermatol 50: 358

Cole C J 1965 Ainhum, an account of fifty-four patients with special reference to etiology and treatment. J Bone Joint Surg 47: 43

Cott R E, Carter D M, Sall T 1967 Cutaneous disease caused by atypical mycobacterium: review of two chromagen infections and review of the subject. Arch Dermatol 95: 259

Cram D L 1981 Psoriasis: current advances in etiology and treatment. J Am Acad Dermatol 4: 1

Cronin E 1966 Shoe dermatitis. Br J Dermatol 79: 617

Cronin E 1980 Contact Dermatitis. Churchill Livingstone, Edinburgh. Ch 3 p 36

Dawber R P R, Baran R 1986 The Nails. In: Rook A, Wilkinson D S, Ebling F J G, Champion R H, Burton J L (eds) Textbook of Dermatology, 4th edn. Blackwell Scientific Publications, Oxford. Ch 54, p 2039

Epstein E 1955 Silica granuloma of the skin. Arch Dermatol 71: 24

Friedman-Kien A E 1981 Disseminated Kaposi's sarcoma syndrome in young homosexual men. J Am Acad Dermatol 5: 468

Gedde-Dahl T Jr, 1971 Epidermolysis Bullosa: A Clinical, Genetic and Epidemiological study. Johns Hopkins Press, Baltimore

Griffiths W A D 1980 Pityriasis rubra pilaris. Clin Exp Dermatol 5: 105

Heyman A B, Brownstein M G 1969 Eccrine poroma. Dermatologica 138: 28

Jordan W P 1972 Clothing and shoe dermatitis. Postgrad Med J 52: 143

Killian H 1981 Cold and Frost Injuries. Springer, Berlin

Lewandowsky F, Lutz W 1922 Eis Fall einer bisher nicht beschrieben Hauterkrankung (Epidermodysplasia verruciformis). Arch Dermatol Syphilol (Berlin) 141: 193

Leyden J J, Kligman A M 1978 Interdigital athlete's foot. The interaction of dermatophytes and resident bacteria. Arch Dermatol 114: 1466

Linell F, Norden A 1954 Macrobacterium balnei. A new acid fast bacillus occurring in swimming pools and capable of producing skin lesions in humans. Acta Tuberc Scand (suppl) 31: 1

Massing A M, Epstein W L 1963 Natural history of warts. A two year study. Arch Dermatol 87: 306

Meneghini C 1971 Lichenoid contact dermatitis. Contact Dermatitis Newsletter 9: 194

Noble W C 1981 In: Microbiology of Human Skin. Lloyd-Luke, London p 79

Postlethwaite R 1981 Molluscum Contagiosum. In: Braude Al (ed) Medical Microbiology and Infectious Diseases. Saunders, Philadelphia p 1700

Price S M, Popkin G L 1976 Barber's interdigital hair sinus. A case report in a dog groomer. Arch Dermatol 112: 523

Raque C J 1972 Pseudoainhum constricting bands of the extremities. Arch Dermatol 105: 434

Ray T L, Wuepper K D 1976 Experimental cutaneous candidiasis in rodents. J Invest Dermatol 66: 29

Reingold I M, Smith B R, Graham J H 1978 Epithelioma cuniculatum pedis, variant of squamous cell carcinoma. Am J Clin Pathol 67: 561

Reynolds W A, Winklemann R K, Soule E H 1965 Kaposi's Sarcoma. (Review) Medicine (Baltimore) 44: 419

Ross J B 1969 Rubber boot dermatitis in Newfoundland. A survey of 30 patients. Canad Med Ass J 100: 13

Runyon E H 1959 Anonymous mycobacteria in pulmonary disease. Med Clin N Am 43: 273

Schlappner O L A, Wood M G, Gerstein W, Gross P R 1972 Painful and non-painful piezogenic pedal papules. Arch Dermatol 106: 729

Tilgren W 1979 Pitted keratolysis (keratolysis plantare sulcatum) Ultrastructural study. J Cutan Pathol 6: 18

Tindal J P, Miller G D 1972 Hand, foot and mouth disease. Cutis 9: 457

Waisman M 1961 Interdigital psoriasis ("white psoriasis") Arch Dermatol 84: 733

Yeh S 1973 Skin cancer in chronic arsenicism. Hum Pathol 4: 469

H. L. F. Currey

Crystal arthropathies

INTRODUCTION

This chapter covers a group of joint disorders which result from the deposition in articular tissues of a variety of metabolic products ('metabolic deposition diseases'). The clinical manifestations of these disorders depend, not so much on the chemical composition of the substance deposited, as on the physical presence of the crystalline material within the joint tissues. The crystal arthropathies (Table 39.1) include two common diseases: gout and pyrophosphate arthropathy. Ochronosis (alkaptonuria) is an excessively rare inborn error of metabolism, mentioned here only to complete the classification. Finally, crystals of hydroxyapatite (the mineral component of bone) have been identified in synovial fluids in a number of circumstances. However, their possible role in the pathogenesis of joint disease and in the production of symptoms remains a matter for speculation at present. Each of these four conditions is discussed below.

In addition to these naturally occurring diseases, a wide range of crystalline materials produces inflammation when injected into the joints of experimental animals. Also, the occasional acute flare which follows a therapeutic injection of (crystalline) corticosteroid into a joint probably represents a similar reaction.

GOUT

Gout is a disorder in which an excess of uric acid in the plasma — hyperuricaemia — leads to precipitation of urate in the tissues. In the joints this causes recurrent episodes of acute inflammatory arthritis. Untreated, this may later progress to local accumulations of urate as 'tophi' and chronic destructive joint changes. Fortunately, for most patients the drug allopurinol provides effective control of both the underlying metabolic defect and the clinical features.

Table 39.1 Metabolic and crystal-induced arthropathies

Disorder	Material deposited	Distribution of arthritis	Clinical features
Gout	Urate	Peripheral small joints	Initially acute and episodic; later chronic deforming arthritis
Pyrophosphate arthropathy (Pseudogout)	Calcium pyrophosphate dihydrate	Larger limb joints	Acute episodic and/or chronic 'degenerative' arthritis
Apatite associated arthritis	Hydroxy-apatite	?	Inflammatory episodes in OA? Chronic destructive arthritis?
Alkaptonuria (Ochronosis)	Homogentisic acid metabolites	Central joints (mainly spine)	Chronic 'degenerative' arthritis

The disease is known to be of great antiquity. It remains a common disorder, and affects predominantly adult males, often with familial clustering. As described below, plasma levels of uric acid depend on the interplay between many influences. However, gout is described as 'primary' when the hyperuricaemia is due mainly to an inborn metabolic fault, and 'secondary' when it results mainly from an environmental factor or acquired disease state.

The clinician dealing with disorders of the foot needs to be familiar with gout. Apart from the characteristic acute podagra of the first metatarsophalangeal joint, other joints in the foot and the ankle joint are commonly affected. Diagnosis can be difficult; gout may closely mimic a local infective lesion, and vice versa. Further, while modern drug therapy should be highly effective in the management of gout, there continues to be widespread misunderstanding of how these newer drugs should be deployed.

Clinical features

Primary gout is predominantly a disease of men, and the first attack usually occurs between the ages of 20 and 50. A tendency to gout — like frontal baldness — appears to be inherited as an autosomal dominant trait, with male sex hormone status exerting a 'permissive' effect on its expression (Hippocrates noted that eunuchs were spared both conditions). Complications include urate stone formation in the urinary tract (urate urolithiasis) and a metabolic nephropathy ('gouty kidney').

The acute attack

The initial attack characteristically involves one or other first metatarsophalangeal joint ('podagra'). The patient may be awoken with a dull ache in this joint which, over the next few hours builds up to an almost intolerably acute pain. The joint becomes swollen and red. Walking may become impossible, and even the weight of the bedclothes may be unbearable. Untreated the joint reverts to complete normality over the following week to ten days. There follows a symptom-free ('intercritical') period, lasting weeks, months or even years, before the next attack occurs. This then follows a similar pattern, returning perhaps to the same or the opposite first metatarsophalangeal joint, or some other peripheral joint. Proximal limb joints (shoulder and hip) are seldom involved. Acute attacks may be triggered by trauma, surgical operations, or a sudden lowering of the plasma urate level (as occurs for example when allopurinol therapy is introduced). The mechanism of this is not understood.

Chronic tophaceous gout

Untreated, this sequence of acute episodic attacks may continue for years. However, there is usually a gradual change in the pattern, with the individual attacks becoming less acute, lasting longer, and the joints failing to return completely to normal between attacks. With the passage of time this can evolve into a picture of widespread peripheral polyarthritis and gross, crippling joint deformities with occasional superadded subacute flares in individual joints.

The deformities are due to solid deposits of monosodium urate or 'tophi'. These usually originate in the cartilage of joints and enlarge to produce irregular lumps related to peripheral joints (Fig. 39.1). Similar masses arising from the cartilage of the pinna of the ear appear as cream-coloured nodules on the helix (Fig. 39.2), a site where they should always be sought as an important diagnostic lead. Tophi also penetrate into subchondral bone to produce large radiological 'erosions' (Fig. 39.3). These are a late feature, therefore (unlike the early erosions of rheumatoid arthritis) not useful in diagnosis.

Many cases of gout do not progress to a chronic tophaceous stage. Pointers to a severe outcome are a first attack at a young age, e.g. below 25 years, and a short interval between the first attack and the appearance of tophi, e.g. within four years. Fortunately modern methods of management have made it possible in most cases to prevent or even reverse chronic tophaceous lesions.

Urinary tract complications

Gout may be complicated by urinary tract stone formation or by an interstitial metabolic nephropathy. The liability to stone formation is due to the fact that many gouty patients excrete an abnormally high daily load of uric acid in the urine. Uric acid is relatively insoluble, particularly in an acid

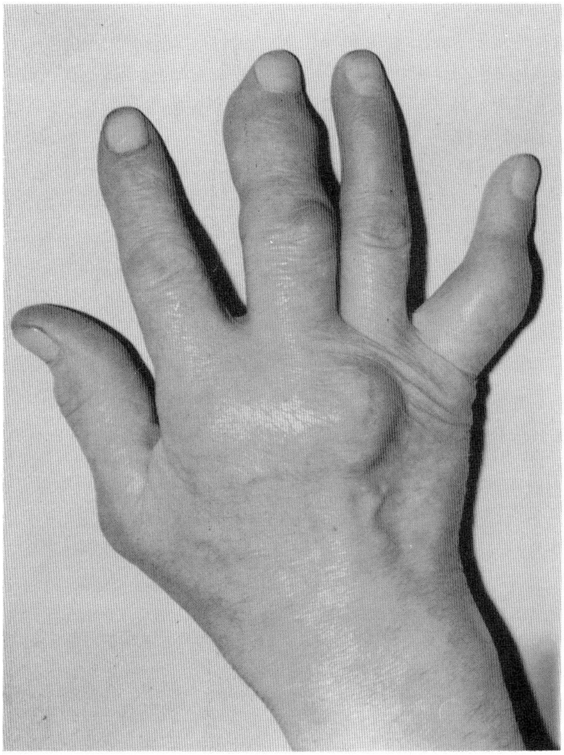

Fig. 39.1 Gouty tophi in the hand

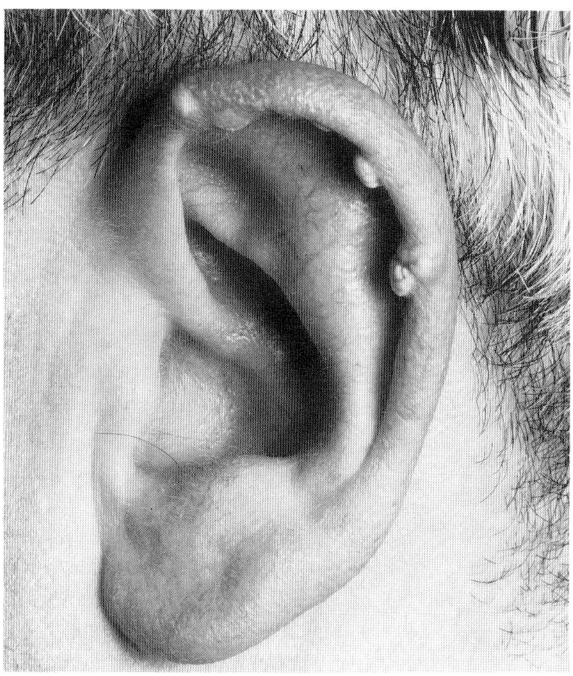

Fig. 39.2 Gouty tophi on the helix of the ear (reproduced by permission from Currey 1970)

environment. Hence the two renal processes of concentration and acidification both predispose to crystallization of uric acid out of solution to form stones (urate urolithiasis) or 'gravel'. A hot, dry environment predisposes to stone formation, and ill-understood, genetically determined aspects of renal tubular function are probably also involved. The link between uric acid stone formation and clinical (articular) gout is less close than might be expected. Most gouty patients do not develop stones, and most patients with uric acid stones do not have gout.

The clinical features of uric acid stone formation do not differ from other types of urolithiasis, except that the stones are usually small and easily passed and, unless secondarily calcified, are radiolucent. Their chemical nature can be established by polarized light microscopy. In subjects liable to uric acid stone formation this can usually be prevented by maintaining a dilute urine (through adequate hydration) and reducing urinary acidity by oral sodium bicarbonate. Failing this, administration of allopurinol (see below) is highly effective.

The process of urinary concentration in the renal medulla also predisposes to the precipitation of urate crystals in the interstitial tissues. This can lead eventually to chronic renal failure. Many patients with severe chronic tophaceous gout show some evidence of 'gouty kidney' in the form of proteinuria, impaired tubular functions of concentration or acidification, hypertension or renal failure. Occasionally this is directly the cause of death. All patients with gout require renal evaluation. Fortunately allopurinol provides not only an effective means of preventing renal damage in those at risk, but will also often improve function in the damaged kidney.

Gout, diabetes, hypertension and vascular disease

Apart from nephropathy attributable to gout, there is also a greater than expected association between gout, hypertension, ischaemic heart disease, diabetes and plasma lipoprotein abnormalities. There is a variety of reasons for this. Genetic association is one. Common aetiological factors such as diet and obesity may play a role. Also, drugs used in the treatment of hypertension may contribute to hyperuricaemia. The important practical point is that there is no evidence that hyperuricaemia itself contributes

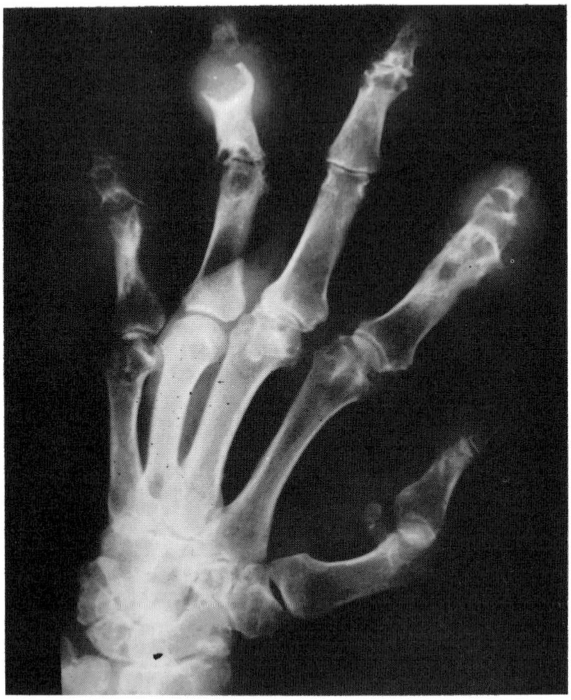

Fig. 39.3 Radiological erosions in gout

directly to hypertension, vascular disease or diabetes. This has to be remembered when considering whether asymptomatic hyperuricaemia requires treatment.

Pathology

Acute gouty arthritis (crystal synovitis)

The central event in an acute attack of gout is the interaction between microcrystals of urate and the polymorphonuclear leucocyte. This has been established beyond all reasonable doubt in experimental animals (Phelps et al 1966). However, the factors which initiate and terminate the attack remain unclear (Dieppe 1984). The solubility of urate in physiological saline at body temperature is about 530 μmol/l (8.8 mg/100 ml). Protein and other components of the plasma allow it to hold a higher concentration of urate than this, but at some point this is exceeded and precipitation of urate crystals occurs into the tissues. The predilection for deposition into joint cartilage may depend on differing rates of diffusion into this avascular structure by urate and other components of the synovial fluid. Possibly also cartilage provides the essential nucleating factor which sets off crystallization. Evidence from 'secondary gout' (see below) suggests that hyperuricaemia has to be present for some years before the first attack of gout occurs. This seems to point to a requirement for a critical load of urate in the tissues.

How trauma or fluctuations in urate levels trigger the attack is unknown. Coating of urate crystals with IgG is probably an essential prerequisite for phagocytosis. Once synovial fluid polymorphs start phagocytosing microcrystals of urate, lysosomal and cytoplasmic enzymes, prostaglandins, toxic oxygen-derived free radicals, and other mediators of inflammation are released by these cells (Platt & Dick 1984). In addition, activation of the complement cascade of enzymes, as well as contributing to the inflammation, provides a chemotactic stimulus drawing more neutrophils from the circulation into the synovial fluid (Russell et al 1982). Because of their surface properties urate crystals have a destructive effect on cell membranes. Thus the phagosomes within which they are ingested rupture and the cell is killed, adding to the release of inflammatory mediators. This amplification scheme accounts for the rapid build-up of the acute attack. It is not clear what causes an attack to end, unless through intervention: aspiration of the fluid removes crystals, while administration of colchicine (a drug without effect on uric acid metabolism) interferes with neutrophil function (Fordham et al 1981).

Predictably, the characteristic finding in the synovial fluid during an acute attack is numerous neutrophils, many containing ingested microcrystals of urate (see below). However it is notable that a few crystals may occasionally be identified in fluid from apparently unaffected joints of gouty patients, while a dusting of urate may be seen on the surface of cartilage from noninflamed joints.

Chronic gouty arthritis

The characteristic lesion is the tophus. Multicentric deposits of monosodium urate crystals grow by further deposition of crystals until each deposit consists of a nidus of radially arranged crystals with an interstitial matrix, and surrounded by a foreign body giant cell reaction. With continued growth these deposits coalesce to form increasingly large chalky concretions which may eventually become secondarily calcified. Starting as a nidus in the joint cartilage, such tophi will expand to destroy the cartilage locally, and also grow inwards to invade subchondral bone (producing radiological erosions) and also grow outwards to appear clinically as periarticular masses (see Fig. 39.1). Necrosis of the overlying skin may then result in the discharge of chalky material. Other periarticular tissues, the helix of the ear (see Fig. 39.2), bursae, tendons, the kidneys and (rarely) almost any other tissue may be the site of tophus formation.

Diagnosis

'When in doubt, think of gout' remains a useful maxim. However, the ready availability of plasma uric acid determinations as part of autoanalyser printouts has now made overdiagnosis of gout an equal hazard. The following points require consideration:

The clinical presentation. The classical picture of acute podagra in a young or middle-aged man with a positive family history is unmistakable. Milder attacks involving other or multiple joints may occasionally cause confusion. Local infections in the foot, particularly cellulitis, may mimic acute gout. Careful examination will usually give the correct answer. With acute crystal synovitis any passive movement of the joint is very painful. In the case of periarticular cellulitis, while extremes of passive movement will cause pain (by distorting the soft tissues), careful testing should reveal some range of painless movement. Other clues may come from the presence of a site of entry of infection such as a skin crack between the toes or lymphangitis.

Plasma uric acid levels. Unless the patient is taking a urate-lowering drug, a persistently normal plasma level of urate almost completely excludes a diagnosis of gout. By contrast an elevated plasma level, especially a single reading, certainly does not establish a diagnosis of gout. As explained below, a single tablet of aspirin may produce hyperuricaemia. Also, many subjects with persistently elevated levels of plasma urate never develop gout. Failure to appreciate this is the cause of much inappropriate prescription of allopurinol.

Crystals in joint fluid (Chayen 1983). Identification of crystals of urate within synovial fluid is the 'gold standard' for the diagnosis of gout. While sparse extracellular crystals may occasionally be found in nongouty fluids, the typical appearance of numerous intracellular crystals establishes the diagnosis beyond doubt. Fluid for this examination should not have anticoagulant added. Aspiration of even a drop or two from a small joint may be sufficient to establish the diagnosis. A drop of fluid, either the centrifuged deposit or a fragment of clot, is examined under a coverslip by polarized light microscopy. Viewed with 'crossed polars' the birefringent urate crystals stand out brightly against the dark background. There are generally needle-shaped, about 2–12 μm in length, and many lie within polymorphs (Fig. 39.4).

More precise identification of the crystals (and differentiation from pyrophosphate crystals) is obtained by rotating the microscope stage with polars crossed. This shows that the bright birefringence of the crystals 'extinguishes' when parallel with the polars. Next a 'first order red'

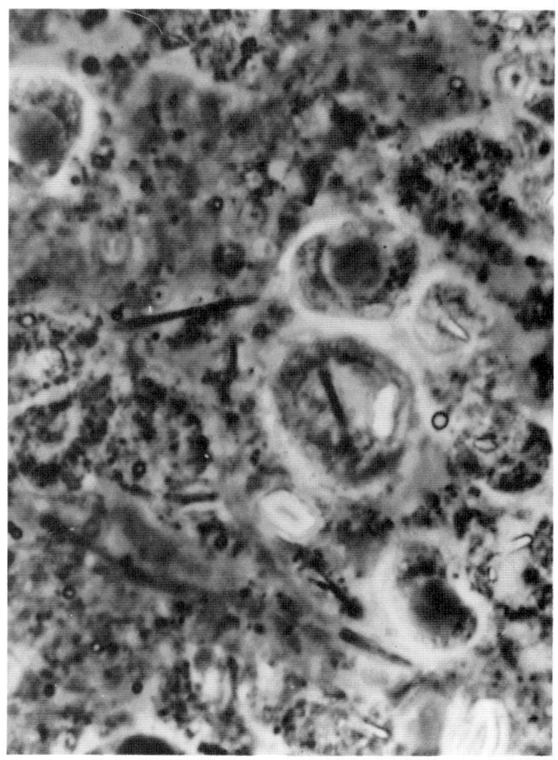

Fig. 39.4 Gouty synovial fluid. Needle-shaped birefringent urate crystals lying amongst polymorphs. Some of the crystals are intracellular. (Partially crossed polars with phase contrast)

quartz compensator is introduced into the optical axis of the microscope. Rotation of the stage now shows the urate crystals to take on a yellow colour (against the red background) when the crystal is parallel with the 'slow component' of the compensator, and a blue colour when at right angles to it. By convention this colour pattern indicates 'negative birefringence'. Further details of the technique of examining synovial fluids for crystals will be found in standard texts (Hartshorne & Stuart 1970).

Examination of tophi and synovial tissue. Solid matter scraped from a tophus with a needle is readily examined by polarized light microscopy. The clusters of needle-shaped crystals are unmistakable (Fig. 39.5). Similarly synovial or any other biopsy material can be examined in this way. However, if such material is to be fixed before examination, it is important to use a nonaqueous fixative (such as absolute alcohol) to avoid dissolving the crystals.

Radiology. Acute gouty arthritis shows no change on X-ray apart from soft tissue swelling. Once tophaceous deposits extend into bone these show as bony erosions (see Fig. 39.3). There may also be loss of joint space and changes of secondary osteoarthritis. Pure urate tophi are radiolucent, but secondary calcification may occur in advanced cases.

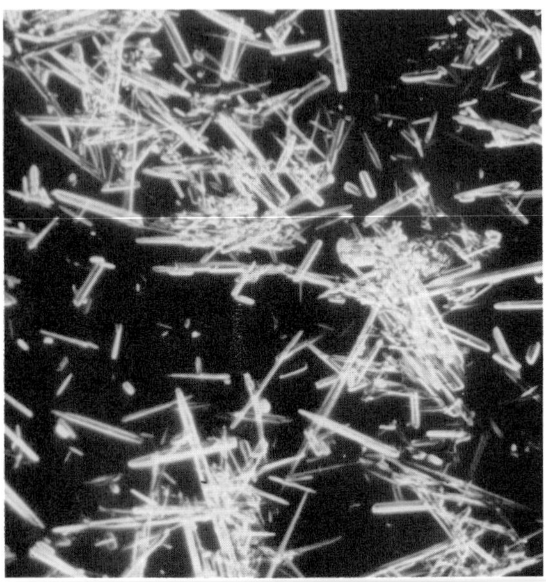

Fig. 39.5 Scrapings from a tophus viewed by polarized light microscopy. Numerous needle-shaped birefringent crystals

While these radiological changes will indicate the severity of joint damage, they are rarely of any value in establishing the diagnosis. This is because the gouty erosions, in contrast to the situation in rheumatoid arthritis, are a late feature. By the time they appear, clinically apparent tophi will almost invariably have made the diagnosis obvious.

Plasma levels of uric acid

Epidemiological surveys show that there is broad correlation between plasma levels of urate and the prevalence of gout. However, as has been pointed out above, the duration of hyperuricaemia is an important determining factor. Short term increases in urate levels in the plasma, even if extreme in degree, seldom lead to clinical gout.

In children, plasma urate levels are low, but rise at puberty, particularly in boys, so that young adult males in general have levels 60 μmol/l higher than females. At the menopause levels in women rise, possibly because of an adrenal androgenic effect, to approach those for men.

Plasma uric acid levels for gouty and nongouty subjects form two separate distribution curves. In an English study (Snaith & Scott 1971) the mean level for normal men was 306 μmol/l (+/- 60), that for gouty men 474 μmol/l (+/- 54). The two distribution curves overlap between 360 and 450 μmol/l. For practical purposes the 'upper limit of normal' for men may be taken as 420 μmol/l (7.0 mg/100 ml), and for women 360 μmol/l (6.0 mg/100 ml). There are racial differences. New Zealand Maoris have higher urate levels as well as a great prevalence of gout.

Uric acid metabolism

Uric acid is a weak dibasic organic acid which exists in two tautomeric forms:

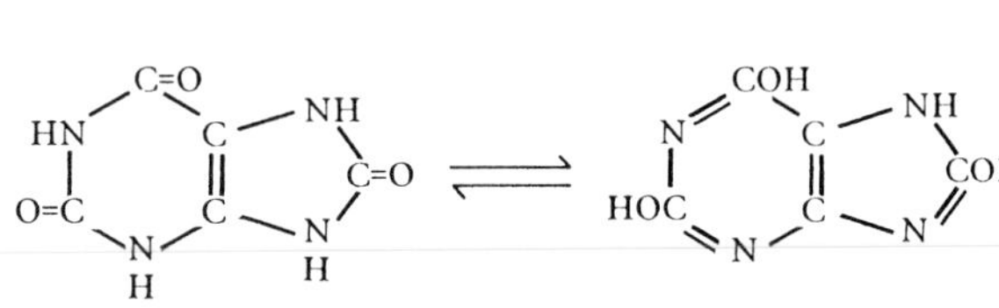

KETO FORM ENOL FORM

At the near neutral pH of the plasma and the body tissues generally it is in the form of the monosodium salt. At the lower pH of the urine much is converted to free uric acid.

Uric acid formation

Uric acid is produced as the end product in the degradation of the purine bases adenine and guanine (constituents of nucleic acids and nucleotides) according to the following (much simplified) scheme:

ADENINE → GUANINE
↓ ↓
HYPOXANTHINE→XANTHINE→URIC ACID

In this respect the purines differ from most other nitrogen-containing body constituents, in that they are not degraded to urea. In lower mammals this degradation is taken one stage further by the enzyme uricase, which converts uric acid to the readily soluble and easily eliminated substance allantoin. Man, however, has suffered an apparently deleterious mutation and no longer codes for uricase. This leaves the relatively insoluble uric acid as the end product to be eliminated.

A complex system of enzymatic reactions controls the synthesis, interconversions and catabolism of purines. Some of these pathways are illustrated in Fig. 39.6. Factors which add purines to the pool (and hence contribute to uric acid formation) are synthesis of new purines (as in cell replication), breakdown of tissue nucleic acids (as in cell death) and dietary intake of purines.

Uric acid elimination

In the mammalian kidney, urate, being a relatively small molecule and bound, if at all, only very lightly to plasma proteins, is filtered freely through the glomerulus. It is then completely, or almost completely, reabsorbed in the proximal tubule by an active transport process. This is a bidirectional

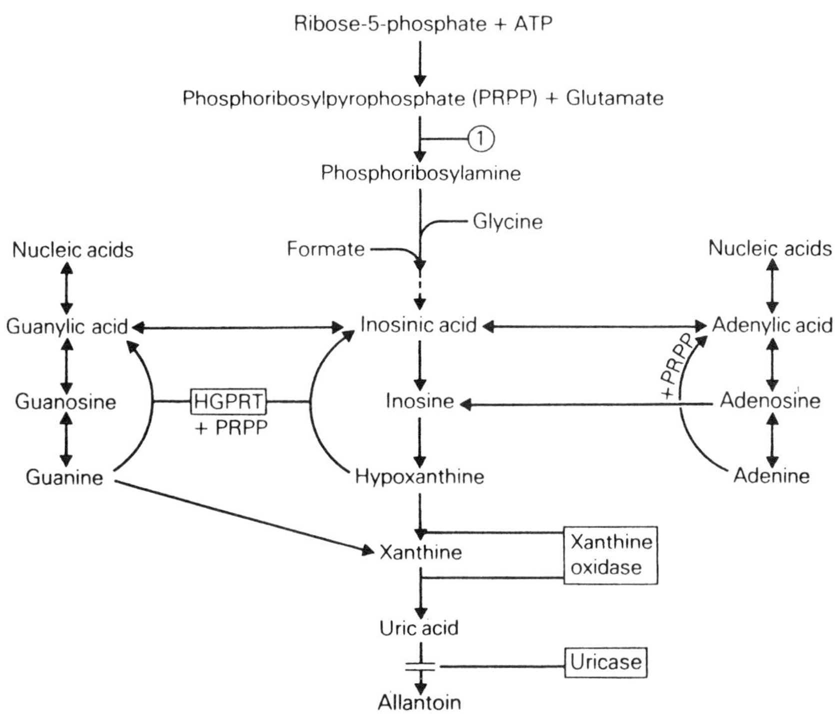

Fig. 39.6 Purine metabolism pathways. Reaction (1) is brought about by the enzyme amidophosphoribosyltransferase, and is the site of feedback inhibition by purines. HGPRT = hypoxanthine-guanine phosphoribosyltransferase, the enzyme missing in the Lesch-Nyhan syndrome. Man lacks uricase. (By permission from Currey 1984)

tubular transport system, and most of the urate eliminated in the urine comes from secretion back into the tubule. Some more distal reabsorption also occurs.

The bidirectional active tubular transport system is relatively nonspecific, being shared by many other weak organic acids. Thus competition at this level by other weak organic acids (e.g. ketoacids or aspirin) may markedly influence the renal handling of urate and hence account for fluctuations in plasma and urinary levels of urate. On a purine-free diet the mean normal 24-hour urinary uric acid is about 2.4 mmol (400 mg) with an upper limit of normal of 3.6 mmol (600 mg).

About 30% of urate excretion takes place into the gut. Within the lumen this urate encounters uricase synthesized by the gut flora. This is therefore the one site of uricolysis in man.

Hyperuricaemia

The factors determining the level of urate in the plasma are illustrated in Fig. 39.7. Clinical gout is represented as a spill-over of urate from the plasma into the tissues by crystallization (and effective treatment with allopurinol as this process in reverse). Plasma levels of urate depend mainly on the balance between synthesis and renal elimination. Gouty patients in whom hyperuricaemia is due to increased synthesis are referred to as 'overproducers', while those in whom renal elimination is defective are 'underexcretors'. Similarly, when hyperuricaemia is clearly due to some environmental factor or other disease process (e.g. overproduction of purines in leukaemia or renal retention due to a drug) it is called 'secondary', while 'primary' gout results from hyperuricaemia attributable mainly to an inherited abnormality in the control of purine metabolism. In practice many cases of gout are multifactorial. The mechanism of the association of other factors with hyperuricaemia remains uncertain.

Increased formation of uric acid

Specific enzyme abnormalities (Nuki 1983). A group of rare inherited enzyme defects has thrown important light on purine intermediate metabolism. Most interest has centered on the Lesch–Nyhan syndrome (Kelly et al 1969). This is an X-linked disorder of boys who develop spasticity, choreo-athetosis, mental deficiency and striking compulsive self-mutilation with biting of fingers and lips.

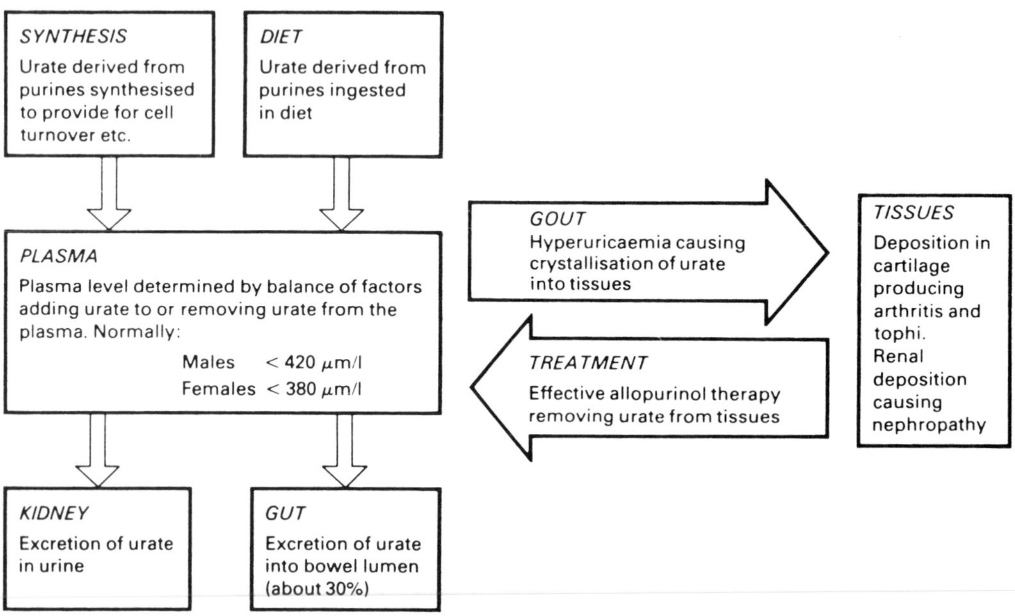

Fig. 39.7 Factors determining the level of urate in plasma and deposition into the tissues (By permission of Currey 1983)

Plasma and urinary urate levels are very high, and may result in gout, urolithiasis and renal failure. The massive overproduction of urate is due to lack of the enzyme HGPRT (see Fig. 39.6).

Increased nucleoprotein turnover. Any proliferative disorder of the haemopoietic system is likely to produce hyperuricaemia. In practice the myeloproliferative diseases (chronic myeloid leukaemia, polycythaemia rubra vera, myelofibrosis, etc.) are the disorders most associated with gout.

High purine diet. The difference between a high and a low purine diet can account for a difference of about 50 μmol/l in plasma urate levels.

Decreased excretion of uric acid

Altered renal function. Severe renal failure results in progressive hyperuricaemia. In practice gout secondary to renal disease is rare, perhaps largely because such patients do not survive long enough for the critical load of urate to be deposited.

Drugs. The bidirectional renal tubular transport mechanism accounts for the paradoxical biphasic action of drugs such as aspirin. Plasma salicylate levels of 10 mg/100 ml or more produce uricosuria, while lower levels cause urate retention. Attention has already been drawn to how easily this can lead to misinterpretation of laboratory results: one or two aspirin tablets taken for a skeletal pain can readily account for a considerable elevation of urate level in the plasma. Other drugs lack this biphasic action. Thiazide and other diuretics cause urate retention and are an important cause both of hyperuricaemia and (secondary) gout. Probenecid and similar drugs are potent uricosurics and are used for this purpose therapeutically (see p. 846).

Lactic acidaemia. Lactic acid competes with urate for renal tubular transport. This contributes to the hyperuricaemia which may accompany physical exercise, type 1 glycogen storage disease and alcoholic intoxication.

Ketoacidosis. Ketoacids such as aceto-acetic acid act like lactic acid at the level of the renal tubule. Thus both starvation and diabetic ketoacidosis cause hyperuricaemia.

Hypertension. The well known association between hypertension and gout is accounted for by various factors, including treatment of hypertension with diuretics, 'gouty kidney', and a genetic linkage between predispositions to both conditions. There is no evidence that correcting hyperuricaemia influences essential hypertension.

Lead poisoning. 'Saturnine gout' results from renal urate retention secondary to tubular damage by lead.

Hypercalcaemia. The hyperuricaemia (and occasionally gout) which sometimes accompanies hypercalcaemic conditions such as hyperparathyroidism may result from altered renal handling of urate secondary to calcium deposition in the renal tubules.

Hypothyroidism. Urate retention has been reported in myxoedema. The mechanism is unknown.

Other factors associated with hyperuricaemia and gout

Genetics. A positive family history is obtained in about 40% of cases of primary gout. Inherited variations in the renal handling of urate and in the 'setting' of feedback controls in the intermediate metabolism of purines probably account for this. Single biochemical defects underlie the inheritance of conditions such as HGPRT deficiency.

Body weight. Obesity is associated with both hyperuricaemia and gout. Correction of obesity results in a fall in plasma urate, a point of obvious therapeutic importance.

Affluence and intelligence. There is some evidence of a positive correlation between gout and affluence, intellectual capacity and 'drive'.

Alcohol. A relatively high proportion of gout patients indulge in alcohol, and a reduction in alcohol intake will predictably reduce plasma urate levels. The metabolic explanation for this effect is uncertain.

Plasma lipids. There is a well established association between hyperlipoproteinaemia and hyperuricaemia (and gout). Again, the metabolic explanation is unclear.

Ischaemic heart disease and diabetes. Attention has already been drawn to the association between coronary artery disease, diabetes and gout. The association is probably a genetic one. Correction of hyperuricaemia does not influence heart disease or glucose metabolism.

Management of gout

Once a diagnosis of gout is established the patient requires investigation to exclude causes of secondary gout, including questioning about alcohol and drugs, particularly diuretics. Splenomegaly may provide the clue to a myeloproliferative disorder. A full blood count, renal function tests, fasting plasma urate determinations, and urinary 24 hour urate (on a low urate diet) should be obtained.

Urate overproducers (over 3.6 mmol (600 mg) urinary urate per 24 hours) should have red cell lysates examined to exclude a deficiency of HGPRT (see page 843).

In planning drug management it is essential to appreciate that terminating an acute attack is an entirely separate issue from introducing long-term (urate-lowering) therapy. The latter must never be started during an acute attack. Lowering urate levels at this stage may both worsen and prolong the attack.

The acute attack

The affected joint will need rest and protection. Most of the nonsteroidal anti-inflammatory drugs are effective in aborting the attack if given early and in large doses. Indomethacin 50 mg four times daily or naproxen 250 mg three times daily are examples of drug regimens which are usually satisfactory. As the attack subsides over the next few days the dose is tapered down. Once an effective regimen is established for a particular patient he should always carry the drug with him to start at the first warning of an attack.

Colchicine, the time-honoured (and specific) remedy for acute gout (1 mg immediately, followed by 0.5 mg 2-hourly until the attack subsides) tends to produce diarrhoea as the effective total dose is reached. For this reason it has largely given way to the newer drugs.

If a gouty joint is aspirated for diagnostic purposes, the opportunity can be taken to inject corticosteroid locally.

Patients on established allopurinol therapy should continue the drug during the acute attack. However, as mentioned above, such therapy should on no account be started during an acute attack.

Long-term management

After the acute attack has subsided a decision will need to be taken about whether urate-lowering treatment should be started. Once started, such therapy should normally be continued indefinitely. Indications for starting this treatment include:

Frequent acute attacks
Tophi
Urate nephropathy
Severe hyperuricaemia (above about 500 μmol/l)

In the absence of one of these indications it is usually advisable to await events. Sometimes the experience of an acute attack and having faced up to the implications of the diagnosis may produce changes in the patient's lifestyle such that he has few or no further attacks.

Allopurinol. If urate lowering treatment is considered necessary, allopurinol is the drug of choice. By competitive inhibition of the enzyme xanthine oxidase (see Fig. 39.6) it reduces urate production and it also has a second action in inhibiting purine synthesis. The result is a predictable reduction in plasma urate levels, which can usually be brought within the normal range. A single tablet of 300 mg is normally sufficient. Occasionally larger doses are needed. For patients in renal failure the dose should be reduced. The final dose should be that which will just maintain a normal plasma urate level. Acute attacks are particularly liable to occur during the period of introducing allopurinol. The chance of this happening is reduced by 'covering' the patient with a small daily dose of colchicine or a nonsteriodal anti-inflammatory drug during the period of urate lowering, and possibly by starting with a small dose of allopurinol. Apart from occasional skin rashes (which unfortunately require stopping the drug) side-effects are uncommon. Once steady-state metabolic control is achieved, attacks of acute gout cease, and tophi begin to get smaller.

Uricosuric drugs. Uricosuric drugs specifically block renal tubular transport of urate, resulting in a net increase in urinary urate. The choice lies between probenecid or ethebenecid (both 0.5–1.0 g twice daily) and sulphinopyrazone (100 mg three or four times daily). These drugs are less effective than allopurinol, particularly in patients with renal failure, and they may actually increase the risk of stone formation. They are used when allopurinol is not tolerated, or in order to get an added effect.

Diet. Strict dietary limitations are not necessary if allopurinol is given, but moderation in the intake of high-purine foods and alcohol are normally advised. Similarly, any obesity should be corrected.

PYROPHOSPHATE ARTHROPATHY (PSEUDOGOUT: CHONDROCALCINOSIS)

In a manner similar to gout, pyrophosphate arthropathy results from the deposition in joints of a crystalline metabolite. The metabolite in this case is calcium pyrophosphate dihydrate (CPPD) (McCarty et al 1965). Being opaque, this material produces a characteristic appearance on X-ray: 'chondrocalcinosis'. Attacks of acute arthritis due to CPPD are referred to as 'pseudogout'. The cause of pyrophosphate deposition is unknown, but it probably differs from urate deposition in that the pyrophosphate is generated locally in the cartilage by the chondrocytes.

Clinical features

Pyrophosphate arthropathy is most common in the middle-aged and elderly. The two sexes are equally affected. A positive family history is uncommon, except in certain geographical localities such as Czechoslovakia (Zitnan & Sit'aj 1963) where familial clustering of severely affected patients at an earlier age represents a more severe form of the disease.

Chondrocalcinosis is a relatively common radiological finding in the elderly, and this is often not associated with evidence of arthritis. When chondrocalcinosis (or CPPD crystals) and arthritis occur together there may — as discussed below — be a 'chicken-and-egg' problem of whether the CPPD deposition is the cause or the result of the arthritis. The present evidence suggests that CPPD deposition can be the cause of:

Episodic attacks of acute arthritis
Chronic 'degenerative' joint damage
Progressive chronic changes punctuated by acute episodes
Subacute polyarthritis mimicking rheumatoid arthritis

The acute attack

The pseudogout attack may mimic acute gout, but is usually somewhat less severe. It generally affects one or a few joints at a time. An important difference is that pyrophosphate arthropathy tends to affect large, rather than small, limb joints. Podagra has been described, but much the most common site is the knee joint, and the hips and shoulder joints are often affected. Acute attacks may be precipitated by trauma, surgical operations, or the taking of a diuretic. Untreated, the acute attack lasts about 10 days, but may grumble on in a subacute form for some weeks. At the height of the acute attack there may be a systemic disturbance, with malaise, fever, leucocytosis and elevated sedimentation rate. The association of these features with an acutely inflamed joint can easily lead to an erroneous diagnosis of septic arthritis, if the tell-tale sign of chondrocalcinosis is overlooked on the knee X-ray, and if the synovial fluid is not examined for crystals (Hamblen et al 1966).

Chronic arthritis

The clinical features of chronic pyrophosphate arthropathy do not differ significantly from those of 'primary' osteoarthritis. This diagnosis is made when a patient with what appears to be degenerative joint disease of a knee or shoulder joint is found to have in addition radiological chondrocalcinosis and/or CPPD crystals in the synovial fluid. In some cases this picture is punctuated by episodes of acute crystal synovitis (see above). In others there may be no such attacks. Usually only a few joints are involved but, particularly in the younger-onset familial cases, there may be widespread polyarthritis, including involvement of finger and spinal joints. Elderly patients with severe destructive changes in one or both shoulder joints are sometimes found to have pyrophosphate deposits in the affected joint(s), and severe destructive lesions are sometimes seen with CPPD deposition in other joints (Richards & Hamilton 1974). It is not known to what extent these are associated specifically with pyrophosphate deposition. Another association with pyrophosphate deposition is carpal tunnel syndrome. Routine examination of material removed at the time of median nerve decompression sometimes reveals unsuspected pyrophosphate deposits.

Subacute polyarthritis

An uncommon presentation of pyrophosphate arthropathy is as subacute polyarthritis affecting many joints. There may be an associated systemic disturbance, with elevation of the sedimentation rate, so that the condition may closely mimic rheumatoid arthritis.

Associated conditions

In most patients with pyrophosphate arthropathy this occurs without any identifiable predisposing cause, except perhaps for advancing years. In a minority, however, there is a general or local associated condition which appears to play a role in determining either the appearance or the distribution of the pyrophosphate deposition. The general conditions include hyperparathyroidism and other causes of hypercalcaemia, hypophosphatasia, haemochromatosis, and Wilson's disease. There may be a slight association also with acromegaly and diabetes. Local predisposing causes include neuropathic (Charcot) arthropathy, previous meniscectomy in a knee joint, and urate gouty arthritis. There may possibly be a tendency for pyrophosphate to be deposited in any badly damaged joint.

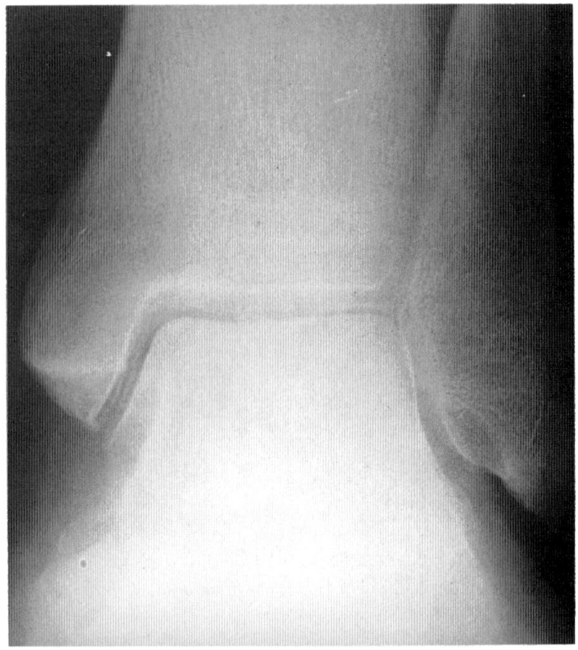

Fig. 39.8 Chondrocalcinosis. The best site to screen for chondrocalcinosis is the knee joint. Only in gross cases can it be identified (as in this illustration) as a thin line of opacification between the ankle and tarsal bones

Radiology (Fig. 39.8)

Chondrocalcinosis is the characteristic radiological sign. In hyaline articular cartilage this shows as a fine stippled line of opacification running parallel to the subarticular bone cortex and narrowly separated from it. In fibrocartilage the calcification shows as coarser opacities in the knee menisci, labrum acetabulare, triangular ligament of the wrist, etc. When degenerative changes result in destruction of cartilage the chondrocalcinosis predictably may disappear. Much the most common site in which to identify chondrocalcinosis is the knee, and this is the joint which should be X-rayed when screening for the condition. The next most common sites are the wrist, shoulder, symphysis pubis, hip, elbow and metacarpophalangeal joints. The last are involved particularly in patients with haemochromatosis. It needs to be emphasized that chondrocalcinosis is an increasingly common finding with advancing years. Amongst the very elderly something like 10% have at least some cartilage calcification. This is often asymptomatic, or associated with no more than the degenerative changes to be expected at that age.

Investigations

In a patient with arthritis the association of chondrocalcinosis and crystals of CPPD in the synovial fluid (or in the synovial membrane) is generally accepted as evidence of pyrophosphate arthropathy. Rarely the chondrocalcinosis is lacking, sometimes because of cartilage destruction (see above). The technique of identifying CPPD crystals by polarized light microscopy is similar to that described above for urate crystals. CPPD crystals exhibit weak positive birefringence and oblique extinction (Fig. 39.9). A diagnosis of pyrophosphate arthropathy, or the presence of radiological chondrocalcinosis, demands investigations to exclude hyperparathyroidism, haemochromatosis and the other conditions listed above.

Pathogenesis and aetiology (Casewell et al 1983)

Acute pyrophosphate arthropathy (pseudogout) seems to be an example of crystal synovitis in which the inflammatory mechanism is similar to that

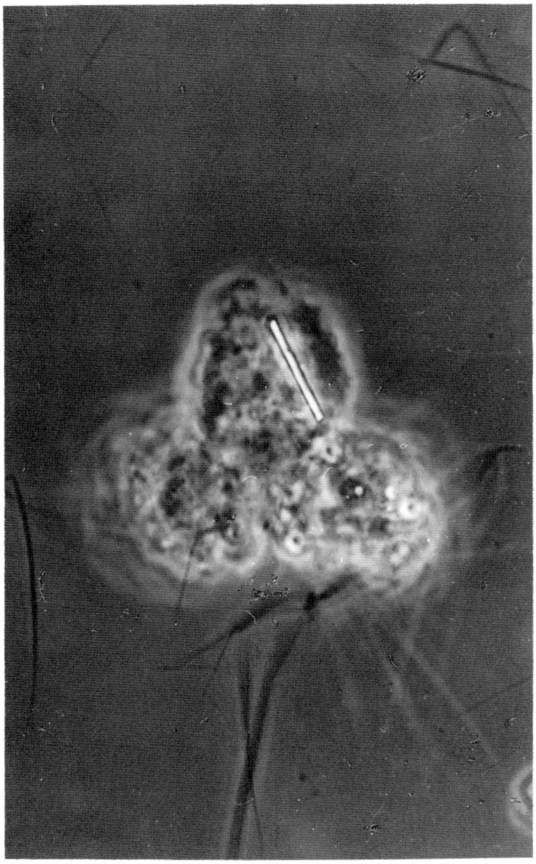

Fig. 39.9 A crystal of calcium pyrophosphate dihydrate lying within a polymorph in synovial fluid from a patient suffering from pyrophosphate arthropathy (phase contrast and partially crossed polars). Photomicrograph kindly provided by Professor B. Vernon-Roberts

described for urate gout. It appears likely that the pyrophosphate originates in the chondrocytes, where it is generated as an intermediate metabolite in the synthesis of macromolecules such as proteoglycan and collagen. What upsets the balance so that it is released in excess to accumulate in crystalline form in the cartilage is unknown. Age-related changes are probably important, but how conditions such as hyperparathyroidism operate is unknown. Some evidence points to cartilage damage from any cause stimulating chondrocytes to overproduce pyrophosphate. From this stems the chicken-and-egg problem of whether, in the case of chronic pyrophosphate arthropathy, cartilage damage causes the deposition of CPPD, or vice versa (Doherty 1983). Familial cases probably have a primary biochemical defect.

Management

An acute attack of pyrophosphate arthropathy is treated in exactly the same way as an attack of urate gout (see pp. 845–847) by the immediate administration of relatively large doses of a nonsteroidal anti-inflammatory drug. The dose is then tailed off as the attack settles. In addition, because pseudogout so often affects larger joints, particularly the knee, it is often easy to drain off the effusion and inject a corticosteroid preparation locally. This usually produces dramatic relief. No effective interval treatment is known (although colchicine has been tried). Treatment of underlying conditions such as hyperparathyroidism does not influence the arthritis.

APATITE ASSOCIATED ARTHRITIS

The description by Dieppe et al (1976) and Schumacher et al (1977) of hydroxyapatite crystals within synovial fluids from osteoarthritic joints raised the possibility that a further type of crystal arthropathy has been identified. This question has not yet been settled. Crystals of hydroxyapatite (the mineral component of bone) are too small to identify by the simple optical microscopy methods which can be used in the case of urate or pyrophosphate crystals. Their identification requires electron microscopy and other elaborate techniques (Paul et al 1983, Crocker et al 1976). Examination of synovial fluid from osteoarthritic joints has shown something like one-quarter of them to contain apatite crystals (Giblisco et al 1982, Dieppe et al 1979). Some fluids contained also crystals of pyrophosphate. The presence of apatite crystals correlated with the severity of the joint damage, but the physical form of the crystals makes it unlikely that they arrived in the synovial fluid through simple grinding away of exposed bone ends. Like urate and pyrophosphate, such crystals are phlogistic in experimental animal models (Glatt et al 1979).

Views about the possible role of apatite crystals have varied widely. At one extreme was the suggestion that they might play a central role in the pathogenesis of the disorder. A more popular view has been that hydroxyapatite crystal synovitis might account for some of the more 'inflammatory' features of osteoarthritis. They might, however, represent no more than an unimportant epiphenomenon. By and large the present evidence seems to point to the presence of apatite crystals being a consequence rather than a cause of osteoarthritis (Nuki 1984).

It is notable that intra-articular apatite crystals are often associated with perivascular calcification in tendons and elsewhere. These calcific deposits also consist of hydroxyapatite, and they may certainly induce soft tissue inflammation (Pinals & Short 1966).

Dieppe and his colleagues (1984) have recently desribed a group of 12 elderly patients with a distinctive type of destructive arthritis affecting predominantly their shoulders and knees. These painful joints progressed rapidly to instability, with very large, cool effusions and noninflammatory characteristics in the synovial fluids. All contained large numbers of ovoid bodies ranging from 0.5 to 5 μm in diameter and consisting of aggregates of apatite crystals. Many of the fluids contained also some crystals of pyrophosphate. The clinical description of these patients is reminiscent of similar case reports from France (de Seze et al 1968) and from North America (McCarty et al 1981). Here again, a pathogenic role for the apatite crystals remains to be proven. At present it appears best to classify these various conditions as 'crystal associated diseases' (Nuki 1984).

OCHRONOSIS (ALKAPTONURIA)

This extremely rare congenital metabolic disorder is mentioned here only to complete the classification of metabolic deposition arthropathies. It is an autosomal recessive defect in which the absence of the enzyme homogentisic acid oxidase blocks the degradation of tyrosine, so that homogentisic acid accumulates. The urine darkens on standing and pigmented metabolites accumulate in cartilage. Arthritis develops in a centripetal distribution and may lead to gross spinal rigidity (O'Brien et al 1963).

REFERENCES

Casewell A, Guilland-Cumming D F, Hearn P R, McGuire M K B, Russell R G G 1983 Pathogenesis of chondrocalcinosis and pseudogout. Metabolism of inorganic pyrophosphate and production of calcium pyrophosphate dihydrate crystals. Ann Rheum Dis 42 (Suppl): 27–37

Chayen J 1983 Polarised light microscopy: principles and practice for rheumatologists. Ann Rheum Dis 42 (Suppl): 64–67

Crocker P R, Dieppe P A, Tyler T, Chapman S K, Willoughby D A 1976 The identification of particulate matter in biological tissues and fluids. J Pathol 121: 37–40

Currey H L F 1970 In: Mason R M, Currey H L F (eds) An Introduction to Clinical Rheumatology. Pitman, London

Currey H L F 1983 Essentials of Rheumatology. Pitman, London

Currey H L F 1984 Crystal deposition diseases. In: Dickson A, Wright V (eds) Integrated Clinical Science. Musculoskeletal Disease. V. Heinemann. London

de Seze S, Babaut A, Ramdon S 1968 L'épaule senile hemorrhagique. In: L'Actualité Rheumatologique Vol 1 Expansion Scientific Française, Paris, pp 107–115

Dieppe P A 1984 Crystal deposition and inflammation. Quart J Med 53: 309–316

Dieppe P A, Crocker P, Huskisson E C, Willoughby D A 1976 Apatite deposition disease: a new arthropathy. Lancet i: 266–268

Dieppe P A, Crocker P R, Corke C F, Doyle D V, Huskisson E C, Willoughby D A 1979 Q J Med 48: 533–553

Dieppe P A, Doherty M, Macfarlane D G, Hutton C W, Bradfield J and Watt I 1984 Apatite associated destructive arthritis. Br J Rheum 23: 84–91

Doherty M 1983 Pyrophosphate arthropathy — recent clinical advances. Ann Rheum Dis 42 (Suppl): 38–44

Fordham J N, Kirwan J R, Cason J, Currey H L F 1981 Prolonged reduction in polymorphonuclear adhesion following oral colchicine. Ann Rheum Dis 40: 605–608

Giblisco P A, Schumacher H R, Sieck M 1982 Studies on the role of synovial fluid apatite and calcium pyrophosphate crystals in osteoarthritis (abstract). Arthritis Rheum 25 (Suppl): S43

Glatt M, Dieppe P A, Willoughby D A 1979 Crystal-induced inflammation, enzyme release and the effect of drugs in the rat pleural space. J Rheum 6: 251–258

Hamblen D L, Currey H L F, Key J J 1966 Pseudogout simulating acute suppurative arthritis. J Bone Joint Surg 48B: 51–55

Hartshorne N H, Stuart A 1970 Crystals and the Polarising Microscope. Edward Arnold, London

Kelly W N, Greene M L, Rosenbloom F M, Henderson J F, Seegmiller J E 1969 Hypoxanthine-guanine phosphoribosyltransferase deficiency in gout. Ann Int Med 70: 155–206

McCarty D J, Kohn N N, Faires J S 1965 The significance of phosphate crystals in the synovial fluid of arthritis patients: the pseudogout syndrome. Ann Intern Med 56: 711–737

McCarty D J, Halverson P B, Carrera G F, Brewer B J, Kozin F 1981 "Milwaukee shoulder" — association of microspheroids containing hydroxyapatite crystals, active collagenase and neutral protease with rotator cuff defects 24: 474–483

Nuki G 1983 Human purine metabolism: some recent advances and relationships with immunodeficiency. Ann Rheum Dis 42: (Suppl): 8–11

Nuki G 1984 Apatite associated arthritis (editorial). Br J Rheum 23: 81–82

O'Brien W M, La Du B N, Bunim J J 1963 Biochemical, pathological and clinical aspects of alkaptonuria, ochronosis and ochronotic arthropathy. Review of the world literature (1584-1962). Am J Med 34: 813-838

Paul H, Reginato A J, Schumacher H R, 1983 Alizarin Red S staining as a screening test to detect calcium compounds in synovial fluid. Arthritis Rheum 26: 191-200

Phelps P, McCarty D J 1966 Crystal-induced inflammation in canine joints II Importance of polymorphonuclear leucocytes. J Exp Med 124: 115-126

Pinals R S, Short C L 1966 Calcific periarthritis involving many sites. Arthritis Rheum 9: 566-574

Platt P, Dick W C 1984 Crystals and inflammation. Ann Rheum Dis (Suppl) 42: 4-7

Richards A J, Hamilton E B D 1974 Destructive arthropathy in chondrocalcinosis articularis. Ann Rheum Dis 33: 196-203

Russell I J, Mansen C, Kolb L M, Kolb W P 1982 Activation of the fifth component of human complement (C5) induced by monosodium urate crystals; C5 convertase assembly on the crystal surface. Clin Immunol Immunopathol 24: 239-250

Schumacher H R, Somlyo A P, Tse R L, Maurer K 1977 Arthritis associated with apatite crystals. Ann Intern Med 87: 411-416

Snaith M L, Scott J T 1971 Uric acid clearance in patients with gout and normal subjects. Ann Rheum Dis 30: 285-289

Zitnan D, Sit'aj S 1963 Chondrocalcinosis articularis I. Clinical and radiological study. Ann Rheum Dis 22: 142-152

The swollen foot

Many, perhaps most abnormalities of the foot cause swelling. Gravitational oedema is usually painless and generalized over the foot and possibly the ankle and lower leg. Temperature and colour are normal. Pitting can be demonstrated on pressure.

Inflammatory oedema may be localized or generalized over the foot but rarely spreads above the ankle. There is usually tenderness, erythema and increased local temperature. It does not pit. Solid swellings are usually localized and may be tender.

Occasionally a patient will present, complaining of his foot being swollen and discoloured, without mentioning that he injured his leg and has bruising higher up the limb. This he has accepted as a result of the injury but he is now worried when the blood has tracked down to the foot.

Similarly although a ruptured knee joint or Baker's cyst usually causes a painful swelling of the calf, if the pain is slight, the patient keeps walking and the fluid spreads down to the foot where he notices swelling and feels concerned.

BILATERAL PAINLESS SWELLING

Interstitial fluid is constantly being recycled. Any tendency to fluid retention will, because of gravity, be more prominent in the foot. Bilateral foot swelling is, therefore, present in right-sided cardiac failure, nephrotic syndrome, inferior vena cava obstruction, in paraplegics and in others confined to a wheelchair. Disabled people unable to walk properly frequently develop foot oedema in later life due to insufficient muscular activity to maintain adequate venous return from the lower limbs. It is common in pregnancy. Except for nephrotic oedema the swelling typically reduces considerably, if not completely, overnight.

Venous obstruction due to the wearing of garters is no longer a problem but elastic knee supports are popular and may hamper venous return from the feet.

Treatment is that of the primary disorder in so far as it is possible, diuretics and possibly compression hosiery.

Chronic oedema may become infected. The resulting cellulitis is painful, red, tender and depending on the organism, may lead to serious spreading infection. Treatment is by an appropriate antibiotic.

UNILATERAL PAINLESS OEDEMA

This is, in most cases, due to proximal limb abnormalities. The commonest are venous insufficiency due to venous valvular incompetence, deep vein thrombosis or pressure on the vein by a tumour — commonly in the pelvis. Lymphatic oedema is more brawny and does not pit on pressure.

Oedema also occurs in a paralysed leg due to inadequate pumping activity by the muscles. Treatment is as for bilateral oedema.

LYMPHOEDEMA

Oedema may result not from inadequacy of the venous drainage system but from insufficiency of lymphatic drainage. This may be congenital. Milroy's disease is a familial lymphoedema of one or both legs.

Acquired lymphoedema is usually due to blockage

of the lymph glands by infection. Filariasis is the commonest cause in the tropics (see Ch. 28). In temperate countries a similar condition may arise, much less frequently, from repeated cellulitis due to streptococci or other bacteria.

Lymphatic insufficiency may follow surgery and the lymphatics may be obstructed by malignant invasion of the glands of the groins, pelvis or para-aortic chains resulting in lymphoedema of the foot.

Lymphoedematous limbs are susceptible to recurrent cellulitis and scrupulous attention should be paid to the skin and any minor injuries or lesions. The patient should be advised to report immediately any pain, tenderness, redness or other evidence of inflammation and antibiotic therapy must be instituted if infection seems to be spreading.

CHRONIC VENOUS INSUFFICIENCY

In a healthy person, the venous presssure at the ankle whilst standing still is about 90 mmHg. Muscle contractions during walking reduce this, provided there is no venous obstruction and the valves are competent, to 25–30 mmHg. With superficial varicose veins the pressure rises to 40 mmHg and in deep vein incompetence to 60 mmHg.

As the plasma protein osmotic pressure is about 25 mmHg return of the interstitial fluid into the veins will obviously be readily impeded by venous insufficiency.

If surgical correction is not applicable, diffusion of interstitial fluid into the veins can be assisted by elastic stockings or tights. 'Light' compression hosiery exerts 12 mmHg at the ankle, 'medium' 20 mmHg and 'strong' 30 mmHg. It is important that the stockings fit the whole leg properly and do not themselves obstruct the venous flow. The size should be chosen according to the ankle measurement in the morning before swelling occurs.

Care must be taken not to injure the skin as ulceration is a serious complication.

VENOUS OR GRAVITATIONAL ULCERATION

Chronic incompetence of the deep veins, usually the result of thrombosis, leads to dilatation of the small venules in the lower leg, ankle and foot, with pigmentation and impaired nutrition of the skin. Minor trauma may then damage the skin which does not heal and a chronic ulcer forms usually on the medial surface of the leg just above the ankle, but possibly on the foot itself.

Casual treatment will not heal a venous ulcer. Therapy has to be determined, careful and persistent. There are a host of local applications to apply to the surface of the ulcer but the essentials of treatment are to remove oedema and promote venous return. Compression hosiery, crepe or elastic bandages, should be worn at all times. A non-stick dressing should be put over the ulcer and covered by a pad under the stocking (or bandaging) to provide extra pressure over the ulcer. Oedema can be removed temporarily by massage or the use of intermittent compression given by means of double-walled boots connected to a pump. Despite these measures, the ulcer may not heal. It is, therefore, often necessary to keep the patient in bed with the leg slightly raised.

With this additional measure, healing usually takes place but it may take several weeks. Allowing the patient to walk about again before healing is complete, leads to a relapse.

LOCALIZED PAINLESS SWELLING

Localized painless swellings of the foot may be tumours (see Ch. 35).

A patient may complain about an enlarged but painless osteoarthritic first metatarsophalangeal joint or of increasing prominence of the bones of the medial border of the foot as a result of degenerative changes. These are best left alone and the patient reassured.

A neuropathic foot resulting from diabetes, occasionally from rheumatoid neuropathy, rarely from tabes and possibly from other neurological disorders may develop infection through wounds or pressure sores without becoming painful. Whereas the swelling is more obvious on the upper aspect, the cause is usually found on the lower surface of the foot.

Nodules

Rheumatoid nodules are less common in the feet

than on the hands or elbows but may be of two types. The classical subcutaneous nodules form at pressure points and typically occur at the back of the heel, under the metatarsophalangeal joints or over other bony prominences. They are usually painless. The second type are intradermal and may be associated with other rheumatoid vasculitis lesions on the toes and nails. The nodules are small and shotty, frequently tender at first, and have small necrotic centres which may ulcerate.

Gouty tophi classically occur around the toes. Since the advent of uricosuric agents and the xanthine oxidase inhibitor, allopurinol, they have become rare. Chalky urate may be seen through the skin or may be discharged if ulceration occurs. The long crystals of sodium biurate can be identified by microscopy or by the chemical murexide test.

Xanthomata form around the heel especially over the Achilles tendon and its insertion. They usually appear slightly yellowish and are firm in consistency. There may be associated elbow xanthomata and xanthelesma on the eyelids.

In neurofibromatosis (Von Recklinghausen's disease) a familial condition associated with cafe-au-lait skin pigmentation, small tumours tend to occur in the feet as well as all over the body. Deeper seated neurofibromata may cause nerve trunk compression and produce numbness and paraesthesiae in the plantar nerve distributions, including the tarsal tunnel syndrome.

BILATERAL PAINFUL SWOLLEN FEET

These are most likely affected by inflammatory polyarthritis. All the systemic inflammatory arthropathies tend to involve the feet. The onset may be bilateral but may initially be unilateral or at least asymmetrical. All the conditions tend to involve the metatarsophalangeal joints but there are various special features more common in, rather than exclusive to, the different pathologies.

Reiter's disease, which can produce considerable pain, swelling and prolonged disability of the foot, is remarkable for its tendency to cause plantar fasciitis with or without arthritis. The sole is tender, sometimes exquisitely tender, particularly under the plantar fascia attachments to the calcaneum and tarsal bones. The interphalangeal joints of the toes tend to be affected and there may be associated keratoderma blennorrhagica of the skin of the soles. The full triad (arthritis, urethritis, conjunctivitis) may be present.

The foot in rheumatoid arthritis is very rarely as acutely tender as it can be in Reiter's disease or gout, but the metatarsophalangeal joints are thickened and tender and careful examination will usually detect similar changes in the hands, whilst questioning will reveal symptoms of pain and morning stiffness in other joints.

Like Reiter's disease, psoriatic arthritis tends to affect the interphalangeal joints and has a tendency to cause sausage-shaped toe swelling in contrast to the more spindle-shaped swelling of rheumatoid arthritis interphalangeal involvement.

Scaling skin lesions should be sought over the knees or elbows, on the scalp, over the sacral region or even in the perianal region, to which it may be localized. Nail dystrophy, in particular punctate pitting dystrophy, is more easily seen in the fingernails than in the toenails.

Particularly in children and adolescents but also in young adults, ankylosing spondylitis may present with pain and swelling of the feet. Sacroiliitis may be found on examination or radiography but it is often absent initially, even when sought by thermography or scintillography (technetium bone scanning). The only evidence of spondylitis may be a minimal lack of the usual free mobility expected at this age. Chest expansion may be less than the expected minimum of 6 cm. A history of sore eyes might indicate an episode of uveitis. The metatarsophalangeal joints may be the most affected but usually symptoms are present in the hindfoot with Achilles tendinitis, pain under the heel or painful joints. The response to nonsteroidal anti-inflammatory drugs is frequently fairly dramatic and more satisfying than in rheumatoid arthritis.

The 'enteropathic arthritis' of ulcerative colitis or Crohn's disease may present in the feet with changes resembling either spondylitis or rheumatoid involvement. The joint changes may precede the bowel symptoms making the diagnosis impossible unless there is also a family history of inflammatory bowel disease alerting one to this possibility. Proctoscopy and sigmoidoscopy with biopsy may reveal minor but diagnostic changes at a stage before the clinical syndrome has developed.

B.27 foot

This is a new concept. The seronegative spondyloarthropathies associated with psoriasis, Reiter's disease and colitis have several features in common besides the absence of rheumatoid factor in the blood. There is the tendency to have skin changes and to be associated with inflammation of the eyes. Sacroiliitis and spondylitis are common and there may be associated urinary or pelvic inflammatory disease.

Tissue typing of HLA antigen studies have shown that these spondyloarthropathies occur more commonly in people who have the B.27 antigen. It is suggested that subjects with these antigens react to infection by various organisms (such as *Chlamydia*, *Shigella* or *Yersinia*) with this rheumatic syndrome.

One of the prominent features of the spondyloarthropathy is the tendency to painful feet with plantar fasciitis or tendinitis as well as arthritis. Several cases have been described with the foot changes typical of this syndrome but without the other features. There was no spondylitis or other joint involvement. However tissue-typing revealed B.27 antigens. It was tentatively suggested that these cases represent a partial form of the spondyloarthritic syndrome occurring in B.27 individuals. The B.27 foot usually responds well to nonsteroidal anti-inflammatory drug therapy.

Acute benign polyarthritis

This is a polyarthritis which may affect both feet. It presents very similarly to rheumatoid arthritis, but tests for rheumatoid factor are negative, the sedimentation rate is usually normal and X-rays do not show erosions. After a few weeks the condition resolves without residue. It is thought that most cases are a form of reactive arthropathy.

The reactive arthropathies

Transient or self-limiting polyarthritides occur after many infections. Most do not show any predilection for the foot but may well involve or event present in the foot. The conditions take various forms and are thought to be autoimmune in nature. Living organisms are not found in the joints. Reactive arthropathy may also occur after enteric infections with *Salmonella*, *Campylobacter* or *Yersinia* organisms. *Salmonella* may invade the joint causing a true infective arthritis. This is usually unilateral.

Rheumatic fever

Rheumatic fever is now uncommon in developed countries. There is fever, carditis and an acute arthritis that moves from joint to joint, including the ankles and feet, following a streptococcal infection. Both the full syndrome and less severe forms are diagnosed by a high serum antistreptolysin titre.

Erythema nodosum

Palpable, raised, reddish-blue skin lesions occurring on the lower legs or forearms and mainly on the anterior surface, are associated with joint pains and swelling. Both the skin nodules and the arthritis may occur in the foot. The syndrome usually follows an infection such as a streptococcal pharyngitis or primary tuberculosis. Sarcoidosis is a common cause and may be identified by hilar adenopathy in a chest radiograph, negative tuberculin testing and a positive Kveim test.

THE SINGLE PAINFUL SWOLLEN FOOT

Most of the conditions described in this volume could present in this way. It may be the beginning of a generalized polyarthritis (Ch. 25) or a stress fracture (Ch. 47), chronic tenosynovitis (Ch. 29) or Sudeck's atrophy (Ch. 54), Madura foot (Ch. 32) or policeman's heel (Ch. 45).

Assessment

Unless various pieces of information make the diagnosis fairly obvious, it is good to proceed by taking the history of the foot condition first, then asking for the general medical history, carrying out a general examination, and finally examining the affected foot (Ch. 13).

Is the foot cool or hot? Are there signs of inflammation? Is there tenderness and if so where exactly and of what? Passive stretching causes pain in inflamed joint capsules, tendons and ligaments.

Resisted contractions cause pain in inflamed tendons or muscles. If there is swelling, pain is most unlikely to be referred and there should be tenderness, but in the tarsal tunnel syndrome (Ch. 10) the pain is felt in the forefoot whilst the pathology is in the hindfoot.

One of the commonest causes of a swollen foot is minor trauma. The foot swells after unaccustomed or excessive walking due to a variable combination of mechanical soft tissue inflammation, tenosynovitis and traumatic synovitis of one or more joints. If there was no actual injury the patient may omit to mention the obvious precipitating activity, particularly if it was spread out over several days. Holiday activities are a common culprit.

A strained ligament is frequently the cause of ankle swelling and can be diagnosed by the combination of local tenderness and pain on passive stretching.

Pain and swelling of the first metatarsophalangeal joint is very common. Hallux valgus leads to bursa formation and a bunion. Hallux rigidus is frequently complicated by acute and/or chronic synovitis (Ch. 21).

Infection is usually indicated by the classical combination of pain, redness, heat, swelling and loss of function. An infected foot usually follows a penetrating injury or direct spread from a septic focus but haematogenous spread is seen in gonococcal or *Salmonella* infections where an isolated arthritis may involve the foot. Isolation of the organism either from the lesion or by blood culture is an urgent necessity. Sensitivity tests will demonstrate the best antibiotic to use (Ch. 31).

Chronic infections such as tuberculosis (Ch. 30) or infestations (Ch. 32) produce more swelling and induration but less pain and erythema. Clinical examination should be followed by X-rays of both feet so that osteoporosis is not missed and suspected abnormalities can be compared with the opposite foot.

If a bone lesion is suspected but not shown on the X-rays a bone scan should be arranged. Routine technetium scans are usually sufficient, but where infection is suspected a gallium scan may give better information. Thermography is a useful noninvasive technique for showing circulatory abnormalities and especially for demonstrating algodystrophic changes. Doppler testing of the main vessels is also valuable in checking blood flow problems.

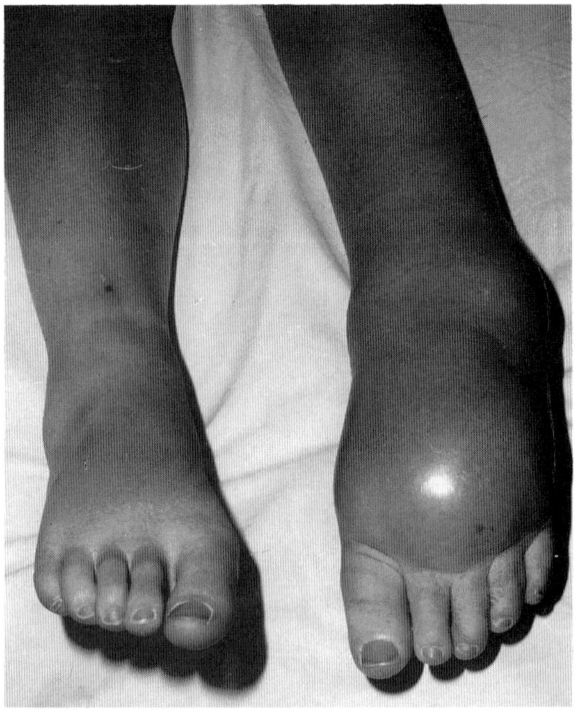

Fig. 40.1 An unusual case of algodystrophy with relapse after sympathectomy

Management

If none of these examinations provides adequate evidence for a positive diagnosis the diagnosis should be kept open. Support insoles, intrinsic muscle exercises and perhaps other physiotherapy can be prescribed and the foot kept under observation.

Where there is uncertainty between gout and acute infection the patient can be given colchicine 0.5 mg orally every 2 hours until diarrhoea commences, or preferably indomethacin 50 mg 6-hourly with food, or diclofenac 75 mg by intramuscular injection at 12 hour intervals, after blood has been taken for analysis. After 24 hours a diagnosis of gout should be confirmed by a raised serum urate and appreciable improvement. If neither are found, gout is unlikely.

If algodystrophy is a possible diagnosis but examination and investigations are inconclusive, the response to a paravertebral sympathetic block is worthwhile trying as a therapeutic diagnostic test. During the first few weeks of the syndrome, a dramatic improvement should occur, although it may only last for 1 to 3 days.

Conditions that are often difficult to diagnose on first presentation

These are:

1. March fracture: The fracture may not show on X-ray but repeat films three weeks later may show callus (Ch. 41).
2. Algodystrophy: This diagnosis is worth considering when there is unexplained pain, swelling, and circulatory change (Ch. 48).
3. Silent deep vein thrombosis: On returning home after being in hospital or on becoming mobile after surgery, swelling of the foot frequently indicates an unsuspected thrombosis.
4. Rheumatoid arthritis: The disease may present with a 'stuttering onset'. Pain and swelling come and go (Ch. 25).
5. Palindromic rheumatism: Episodes of pain and swelling may be severe for 1 or 2 days then clear completely. Attacks can be frequent or at long intervals but no lasting sequelae result.
6. Osteoid osteoma: May give severe pain before physical signs and X-rays are positive.
7. Chronic footstrain: A rather vague entity probably produced by a combination of features. Pain and some swelling develop after standing or walking but all examination and investigations are negative. Sympathetic management with physiotherapy and moulded insole supports usually improve the condition.

MISCELLANEOUS CONDITIONS TO BE CONSIDERED

Polyarteritis nodosa

This is usually a systemic and fatal disease but there is a chronic form that usually remains restricted to the skin and rarely converts to the systemic form. It is more common in the lower limbs and may start in the foot as painful, tender, red, swollen lesions.

Dermatomyositis

Pain and weakness of the proximal muscles is associated with skin changes which may affect the feet. The typical feature of dermatomyositis is the violaceous colour of the erythema on the hands, feet and around the eyes. It can affect young children and in adults may often be associated with malignant disease.

Scleroderma or systemic sclerosis

Although the classical changes are of skin contracture and loss of tissue, in the early stages, the skin of the foot may be thickened, swollen and tight.

Sarcoidosis

The most common musculoskeletal manifestation is erythema nodosum (see above) but the foot may be involved in the polyarticular sarcoid arthritis or sarcoid bone infiltrations. It is more common in coloured than in white people.

Hypertrophic pulmonary osteoarthropathy

Clubbing of the fingers and toes is a recognized manifestation of chronic heart or lung disease. In some cases there is excessive periosteal new bone formation at the wrists and ankles causing painful enlargement. Occasional cases associated with gastrointestinal carcinomas have been reported but chest radiography usually demonstrates the underlying pathology.

Endocrine disease

Myxoedema due to hypothyroidism may cause thickening of the feet and hands as well as of the facial skin.

True overgrowth of the soft tissues of the feet occurs in acromegaly due to adenoma or hyperplasia of growth-hormone producing cells in the anterior pituitary gland.

Diabetes mellitus commonly affects the feet (Ch. 29). Neuropathy and peripheral vascular disease predispose to infection and ulceration.

Angioneurotic oedema (Angiotic odema)

This is an allergic disorder in which exposure to the sensitizing allergen provokes oedema in one or more places. One or both feet may be involved. The swelling is recurrent, tense, painless and non-pitting. It resolves spontaneously after 2 or 3 days.

Tinea pedis

Mycotic infection between the toes may cause swelling of the dorsum of the foot. The patient may be unaware of its presence.

John Foulston

Ingrowing toe nail

INTRODUCTION

The true ingrown nail plate is usually called onychocryptosis and is characterized by the typical signs of concurrent trauma, infection and repair. However, the term ingrown or ingrowing nail is also used loosely for the nail plate that is causing painful pressure onto the nail sulcus. In this case the trauma is as yet without penetration of the soft tissues and the pain experienced may be due to the pressure lesions of corn or callus. Because the use of the term 'ingrown nail' is so widespread, occurs as an *Index Medicus* heading and describes the major result of damage so well, it is proposed to use it throughout this chapter.

There are a number of systemic, dermatological or local disorders of the nails that might cause a patient to seek help. Usually, the worry is caused by pain, discomfort or the cosmetic appearance of the nail region of the foot. Since nail plate is harder than the surrounding tissues it tends to cause damage to those tissues in a number of cases. Crowding of the toes into the toe-box of the shoe leads to mechanical loading which affects both the structure and shape of the toes and of the nail plates.

HISTORY

This painful condition is one that causes much grief to patients. Methods of treatment may vary depending on which part of the medical system is approached for treatment. Surgical techniques often involve the risk of general anaesthetic and require several days of hospitalization. In addition, large areas of the nail are sometimes removed in order to prevent regrowth of nail plate segments or spikes. The resultant damage may not leave a functional or cosmetic nail. Some other methods tend to leave the nail matrix intact which allows the condition to recur as new nail plate germinates and grows forward. Inadequate footwear that was implicated in the aetiology of the original condition may be worn post-operatively by the patient without any adverse comment by the clinician involved.

There has been a dual history of the development of methodologies of treatment of nail conditions by the surgical and chiropodial/podiatric professions. It is rare to find cross references within both sets of literature and only recently has there been a tendency to study the effects of different treatments (Morkane et al 1984).

ANATOMY, PHYSIOLOGY AND HISTOLOGY OF THE NORMAL NAIL

A good detailed description of the anatomy and physiology of the normal nail structure may be obtained from Samman (1978), Zaias (1980) and from Barrin & Dawber (1984). Hashimoto (1971) gives a detailed account of the histology of the nail. These concepts have led to the formation of ideas about the growth and development of nails which are important in the choice of treatment methods. Figure 41.1 shows a typical longitudinal and transverse section through a normal nail.

The nail plate is a hard thermoplastic material formed from keratinized interleaved cells which are derived from the mitosis and differentiation of basal layer cells. A biochemical analysis of nail plate reveals that its keratin contains a higher proportion of sulphur-rich amino acids than skin keratin. The presence of sulphur-rich amino acids in the protein

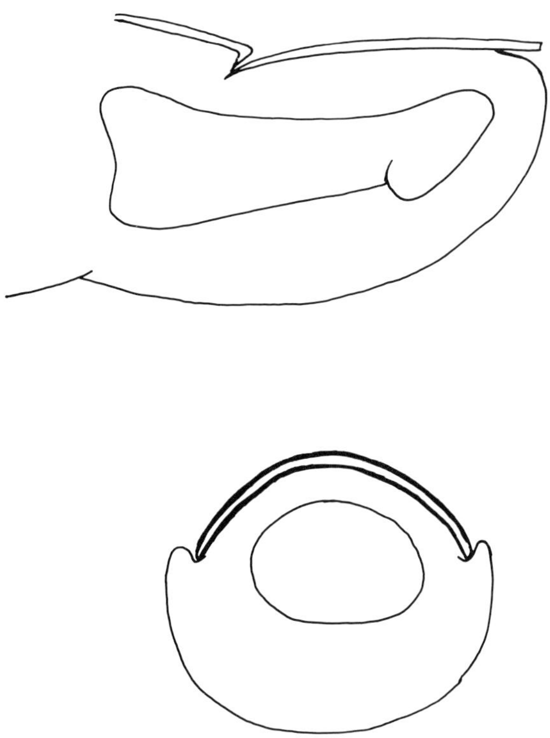

Fig. 41.1 A longitudinal and a transverse section through the distal part of a great toe. The relationship between hard nail plate, the distal phalanx and the soft tissues should be noted

chain leads to the formation of disulphide bonds which cross-link the folded keratin molecules and give the characteristic hardness of nail plate. It is possible to identify three distinct histological layers in the nail plate; thin dorsal and ventral layers form the top and bottom of a sandwich with a thick intermediate layer between.

The nail bed forms an intimate contact between the soft tissues on the dorsal aspect of the distal part of the phalanx and the ventral portion of the nail plate. The nail bed is epidermal in nature with only a couple of cell layers present. As cells keratinize and differentiate from basal cells, they tend to be swept forward and become incorporated into the structure of the ventral portion of the nail plate. There is some debate about the germinating characteristics and position of the matrix (Dawber 1980). Lewis (1954) suggests that the nail bed contributes cells to the ventral nail plate but successful treatment with surgical or chemical destruction of the germinating section of nail is usually confined to the proximal region beneath the eponychium indicating that it is this area alone which contributes to the hard nail plate. If the nail plate is removed or missing, full keratinization of the nail bed cells will tend to take place leading to the production of a normally desquamating epidermis at this site.

The nail bed is tied to the distal phalanx by vertical collagen fibres. The resultant stability of nail on finger or toe tip has functional advantages to the organism and the relationship between nail plate and distal phalanx via the nail bed is an important one when considering or performing surgery to the nail.

The lateral and medial sides of the nail merge into the skin of the digit via the lateral nail fold or sulcus. These join on the posterior aspect of the nail to form the proximal nail fold which is sometimes called the eponychium. On the dorsal aspect of the nail, the cuticle forms an effective posterior seal as the nail plate extrudes from the matrix onto the surface. At the distal end of the nail, the hyponychium is the forward part of the nail bed beyond which the curvature of the end of the digit allows separation of nail bed from nail plate and normal skin keratinization occurs. The hyponychium and cuticle form an effective barrier to the penetration of micro-organisms and foreign bodies into a sensitive and vascular area of the body. Damage to these structures may therefore be followed by an infection of the nail area.

Nail plate pigmentation is determined by melanocytes within the nail matrix and the overall pale pink colour of the translucent nail plate in those with white skins is governed by the vascular nature of the underlying nail bed. The lunula is the whitish 'half-moon' just distal to the cuticle and seems to be of no particular functional significance.

The nail area is very vascular. The medial and lateral ventral digital arteries anastomose within the plantar pad and branch upwards onto the dorsal aspect of the distal phalanx where they form the proximal and distal arcades, the proximal arcade receiving further vessels from a dorsal digital artery.

Medial and lateral digital nerves supply the nail area. These often branch to give rise to sensation from the opposite side of the nail. The practical importance is that in administering local analgesia by means of a ring block to a toe, it is essential that both medial and lateral aspects of the base of the toe are injected.

Barrin & Dawber (1984) list various factors which

influence nail growth rate. Nails tend to grow faster in daytime, finger nails grow faster than toe nails, male nails grow faster than female nails and factors such as immobilization of the digit, fever, denervation, and poor nutrition tend to slow the rate of nail growth. Among factors tending to increase growth rate are psoriasis, hyperthyroidism, medication with L-dopa and minor trauma or nail biting. Barrin & Dawber (1984) also suggest that the various complicated studies of the increase in volume of the nails over time correlate well with simple measurements of increase in length which are satisfactory estimates of nail 'growth'. This is normally at about the rate of 100 μm (0.1 mm) per day. Thus a nail plate of length 25 mm takes about 250 days to grow from one end to the other.

The most important factor to emerge from a study of the anatomy, physiology and histology of the nail is an understanding of the relationship between structure and function. Any alteration to the microanatomy or physiology of the nail production region by disease, trauma or surgery will influence the subsequent growth and development of the nail plate which in turn will affect the soft tissues in its environment. These soft tissue changes may well include the nail production region.

AETIOLOGY, PATHOLOGY AND CLINICAL PRESENTATION

Thick nails

The nail plate may become distorted in thickness through systemic disease, local fungal infection or through long-term trauma. The signs of a thickened, crumbly and discoloured nail plate could result from any of these causes. It is worth noting that the accurate diagnosis of the underlying cause of the nail condition is sometimes difficult. For example, mycological investigation of samples of a fungally infected nail plate is unreliable and often does not give a positive result. It is necessary also to sample surrounding skin, which, if shown to be infected by a dermatophyte, implies that the nail plate with physical signs present is similarly infected.

The increased thickness of the nail plate may in itself lead to extra mechanical loading being applied to the surrounding tissues as well as the tissues being traumatized by the mechanical loading that is responsible for the nail-plate distortion in the first place. If the thickening of the nail-plate is accompanied by a distortion of the nail bed (onychogryphosis) then the condition is more difficult to deal with. Firstly, the nail bed distortion means that the nail-plate will always grow in a distorted manner itself and will, if left for some time, assume the typical 'ram's horn' shape of the well developed onychogryphosis (Fig. 41.2). Secondly, the increase in nail-plate thickness together with the nail bed deformity tends to lead to a pressure being applied to the surrounding tissues which if allowed to continue will develop through the recognizable stages of callus, corn and ulceration. A well thickened nail plate rarely penetrates into the skin of the sulcus to leave the typical ingrown nail unless it has a ragged edge but the anterior edge of the 'ram's horn' has been known to penetrate its own or an adjacent toe causing a secondary lesion for which the patient will seek treatment.

The clinical appearance is that there is an increase in thickness of the nail plate. There may just be simple thickening of the nail plate as in onychauxis. Here there will be no particular symptoms except for subsequent trauma to the sulcus or nail bed because of the thickening. In onychogryphosis, the thickening of the nail plate will be accompanied by a distortion of the nail bed. The nail plate will assume the 'ram's horn' effect that is shown in Fig. 41.2. The nail plate may be discoloured and crumbly if traumatized or if infected by mycotic organisms. It is worth noting that a treated and reduced onychogryphosis is still a potential problem because the distorted nail bed will lead to further distorted nail plate growth.

Nails with excessive curvature

Another way in which the nail plate may become distorted is for it to have an increase in curvature in the longitudinal axis. This increase in curvature is related to forces acting onto the nail from medial or lateral sides. In turn, the sideways pressure is related to the physical space available within the shoe. It has to be noted that even the softest materials used in hosiery, shoe or slipper manufacture will cause crowding of the forefoot if the toe box of the shoe is the wrong shape or if there is inadequate fastening at the instep to hold the foot back in the shoe and thus

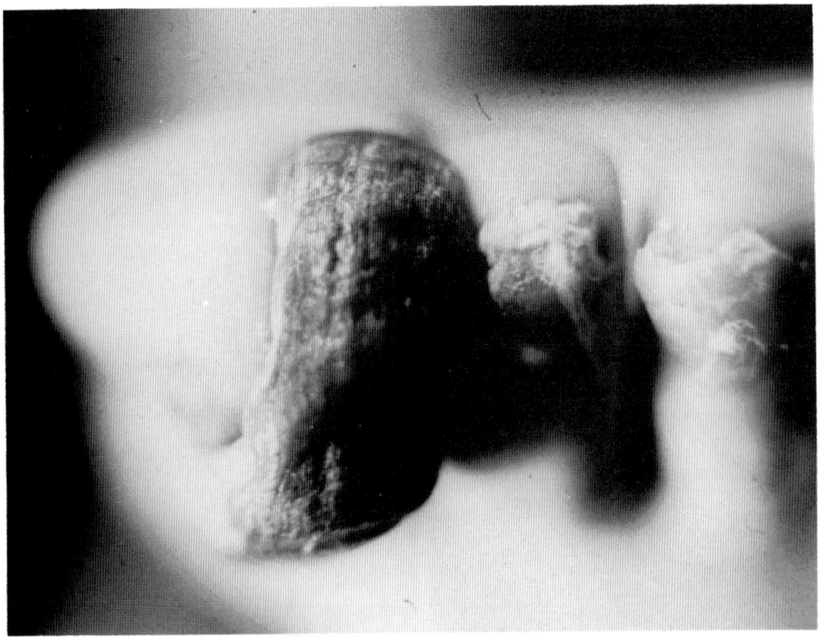

Fig. 41.2 An anterior view of a thickened and distorted nail plate on the great toe, a true onychogryphosis. The nail plate may penetrate the skin and there may be local pressure lesions because of the physical bulk of the nail

keep the toes away from contact with the front. Long-term sideways pressure onto the distal part of the toe will lead to a change of shape of the nail region and potential penetration of nail plate into softer tissues.

These nails show an increase in curvature along the longitudinal axis of the toe. The nail plate borders may be buried deeply in the sulci on one or both sides of the toe. In itself, this condition is not a usual presenting problem but consequent trauma to the soft tissues by the nail plate may be the reason for advice being sought. There is usually a related toe deformity or crowding of toes within the footwear.

Thin nails

There are a number of conditions of the nail where the nail plate is thin or brittle. In these circumstances, the sharp edge to the nail plate easily penetrates into the tissues. If the nail has been cut incorrectly, then a sharp edge or splinter will penetrate the skin as the nail plate grows forward.

Ingrown nails (onychocryptosis)

Onychocryptosis is defined as a condition where part of the nail plate has penetrated into the soft tissues surrounding the nail area (Fig. 41.3). The usual and typical case is where a splinter of nail in the sulcus has become buried as the nail grows forward. Because the penetrating foreign body is of host protein in origin, the tissue reaction tends to be limited to that of reaction to an inert sharp object until early invasion of the wound by pathogenic micro-organisms. The infection together with the presence of the foreign body into a sensitive area tends to make an ingrown nail an extremely painful and worrying condition for the patient. Damage occurs and repair is attempted concurrently. The repair process leads to the formation of an excessive amount of granulation tissue which wells up to cover the affected side of the nail plate and in time this may become organized into fibrous tissue. Unfortunately, because this condition and its treatment have a poor name for successful and pain-free results, patients seem often reluctant to seek help. A limitation of treatment to antibiotic therapy only clears the sepsis for a time but does nothing for the underlying condition.

However, as has been seen from the above list of predisposing conditions, it is possible for the nail plate to penetrate into the soft tissues from a variety

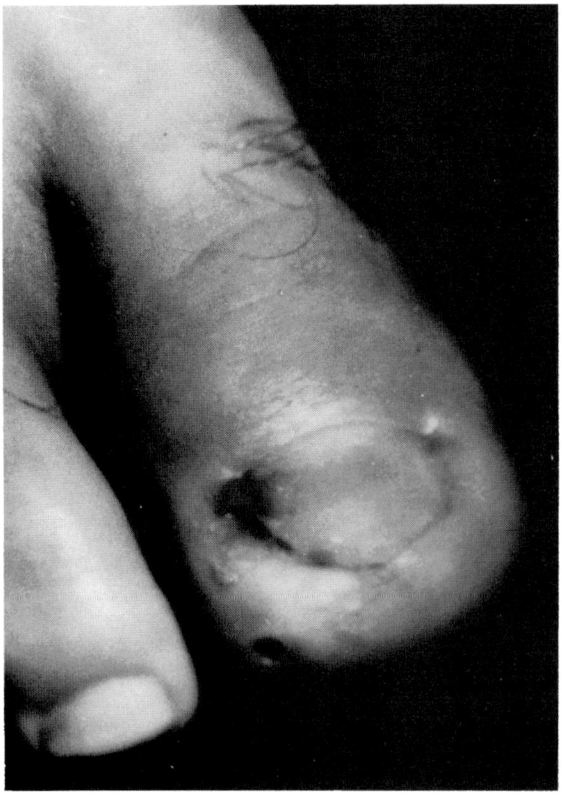

Fig. 41.3 An ingrown great toe nail. There has been penetration of the soft tissues by the nail plate in both the lateral and medial sulcus. The lateral splinter of nail plate has penetrated through the soft tissues to emerge at the apex of the toe. Systemic antibiotics have reduced the usual sepsis which accompanies ingrown nail

of causes. A single major dorsal trauma may drive the nail into both sulci as well as causing damage to the nail bed. Repeated minor trauma from ill-fitting footwear will also lead to a nail plate pressing onto its sulci and if the pressure is enough, the nail plate sharp enough or if the tissues are macerated then penetration will occur. In each case the treatment of the resultant condition tends to be similar.

A nail plate that is traumatizing the soft tissues will give rise to the signs and symptoms of pain and inflammation that increase with the amount of damage being done. A mild onychophosis (corn, callus or skin debris in the sulcus) is at one end of the spectrum and the sepsis, excessive granulation tissue and severe pain of onychocryptosis as shown in Fig. 41.3 with the penetration of nail plate into the tissues, is at the other. Digital neuropathy associated with some systemic conditions such as diabetes, spina bifida, and Hansen's disease may give rise to serious ulceration in the nail region in the absence of pain. Systemic anti-inflammatory medication may mask the inflammatory reaction of the condition and antibiotic therapy to control the infection of an ingrown nail may reduce the symptoms without controlling the penetrating nail plate. A careful history and inspection of the site should always be made. A probe run gently along the length of the nail edge in the sulcus will give an indication of how much nail plate is buried in the tissues. The treated nail is shown in Fig. 41.4.

TREATMENT

Thick nails

It has been shown (Davies 1984) that some chiropodists have antibodies present in their blood

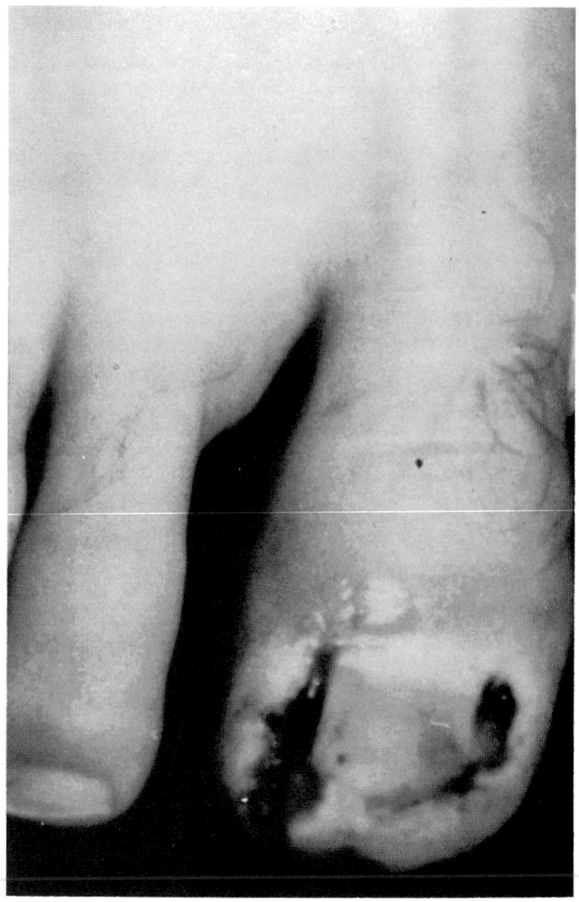

Fig. 41.4 The nail plate from Figure 41.3 immediately after partial avulsion on the medial and lateral sides

raised from skin and nail plate mycological antigenic material. This fact is important when considering the treatment of a patient with a thickened nail. Mechanical nail burrs should not be used routinely without adequate air extraction to remove the nail dust produced and it is likely that the spread of fungal nail conditions in medical surroundings can be reduced by avoiding the production of small nail particles when there is the suspicion or firm diagnosis of nail plate infection with mycotic organisms.

An increase in thickness may just be simple thickening of the nail plate itself (onychauxis) in which case treatment consists of identifying and remedying the underlying cause, which is usually pressure from footwear and reduction of the thick nail-plate, by mechanical means. The sulci may need to be cleared of skin cell debris or of any corn or callus.

The onychogryphotic nail plate may be treated very easily by strong nail nippers and a good file or rasp. The nail plate will fracture along the lines or grooves on the dorsal surface when cut with nippers at one edge. The mechanical nail burr will reduce the thickness to a good cosmetic appearance after the major portion has been cut off. For long-term freedom from the bother of a nail plate that grows to an increased thickness it is possible to perform surgically a total nail plate avulsion but it is absolutely essential to phenolize or destroy caustically the proximal nail-producing cells. This step is not to be taken lightly because the nail plate, although thickened, still protects the underlying soft tissue and because the surgical removal of a nail plate is always liable to leave troublesome spikes of nail from undestroyed matrix cells. The routine conservative treatment described above is extremely easy and quick for an experienced chiropodist to carry out about three or four times a year and the nail is left in such a good cosmetic condition that following the application of coloured nail varnish, it is not possible for an observer standing next to the patient to detect any abnormality, except perhaps for a short nail plate.

Nails with excessive curvature

Treatment for such a condition involves making room for the toes within the footwear. Once this has been done, there is often a flattening out of the longitudinal nail plate curvature with a reduction of sulcus damage. However, if the condition persists and does continue to cause damage, then it is possible to resort to a number of corrective remedies. Nail plate is a thermoplastic material. Heating and correction of the curvature of the distal portion of the nail plate by fairly massive metal pincers at a temperature of 100° Celsius and allowing the cooled nail to achieve an altered shape has been used to achieve a lasting improvement. Small, shaped nail braces made from stainless steel dental wire or plastic nail sulcus inserts have also been successfully used serially to correct the excessive curvature in the longitudinal plane once the causative pressure from footwear has been eliminated. A partial nail avulsion with destruction of the appropriate nail matrix has also been used to reduce the width of the nail plate and thus the potential for lateral pressure of the plate into the sulcus.

Thin nails

In all of these cases, correct nail cutting and care about the medial and lateral edges of the nail plate help to prevent damage. There is no evidence to support the theory that a notch in the centre of the nail plate will deviate the edge from the sulcus. There are cases where the side of this notch itself penetrates the distal part of the toe. Careful smoothing of the nail plate together with a soft packing material such as a sliver of chiropody foam or a plastic gutter into the sulcus (Wallace et al 1979) will lessen the chance of a thin nail penetrating into the skin.

OPERATIVE PROCEDURES

Operative procedures for nails vary from the very simple clearing of a sulcus to radical removal of tissue in the case of severe ingrowing nail.

Surgical techniques may be ranked in order according to the amount of tissue removed:

1. Amputation of the distal phalanx. DuVries (1959) reports that this procedure has been used in the past in order to avoid the possibility of regrowth of nail plate from undestroyed matrix and was simpler than plastic repair of the nail lip.

2. Radical removal of tissue. This technique was described by Zadik (1950) as total matrix removal. The whole nail plate is lifted and removed. A flap of tissue is lifted at the base of the nail and the nail matrix area at the proximal end is ablated down to the level of the distal phalanx and across the whole width of the toe. Sutures are used to close the incisions.

3. Partial matrix removal was described by Winograd (1929). A section of nail plate is lifted and removed. The associated nail matrix area is excised and the tissues sutured.

4. A recent technique has been described by Antrum (1984). Here the nailfold at the side of the nail plate is sliced away from proximal to distal ends and then removed by amputation at the proximal end. The lesion is dressed with topical antiseptic and allowed to heal.

5. Gabriel (1979) has described a careful method of surgical removal of a section of nail plate and the excision of a segment of germinal matrix without cutting the skin and with minimal interference with the nail wall.

6. Total and partial avulsions of nail plate have been carried out followed by chemical matricectomy using phenol or sodium hydroxide. Dagnall (1981) has written an excellent review of the history and development of the phenolization techniques. The method usually involves careful removal of all of or part of the nail plate without any incision into soft tissue followed by the application of the chemical to the germinating matrix cells only. An alternative is the use of a metal probe and negative galvanic current to generate sodium hydroxide on site by hydrolysis of body fluids.

In each case, postoperative management of the condition is to keep the wound drained and clean. Topical antiseptics are applied and antibiotic cover is maintained until any sepsis is reduced.

Criteria for the successful treatment of an ingrown nail may be stated by slightly modifying the list produced by Gabriel et al (1979). These are:

a. The recurrence rate should be minimal

b. Normal footwear of an approved nature should be worn within a couple of days of the operation

c. Painless nail bearing should be the end result

d. The procedure should be simple.

Investigations into the effectiveness of the various techniques have been carried out. Palmer et al (1979) showed in a retrospective study of 245 operations on 208 patients at King's College Hospital in London that the recurrence rate for various techniques was:

Avulsion of a strip of nail	83%
Total nail avulsion	70%
Zadik's operation	28%
Wedge resection	29%

They recommended that immediate avulsion of toenails should not be a routine procedure.

Morkane et al (1984) have shown that in a controlled prospective study of 53 wedge resections as per Winograd (1929) and 54 segmental phenolizations as described by Ross (1969), there was no difference in discomfort after one week but over a fourteen month follow-up there were sixteen spikes of nail growth (30%) in the wedge resection group and only four (7%) in the phenol group. A *Lancet* (1979) comment on the paper by Gabriel et al (1979) praised the low recurrence rate achieved (1.7%) in their 528 patients and suggested that careful work by an experienced surgeon enabled 79% of patients to wear their own shoes after seven days and to lower the recurrence rate to an acceptable level.

PREFERRED METHOD

Partial nail avulsion with phenolization of the appropriate matrix area under local analgesic ring block of the whole toe is the most successful method of treatment of the ingrown nail. Prior control of sepsis is necessary if the infected area of the toe spreads too far proximally and the patient is at risk from the administration of the local analgesia into the base of the toe on both sides. An ankle ring block is also possible in such cases. The surgical technique involves cutting of nail plate only. No incision is made into soft tissue. Postoperative dressing with a topical antiseptic, sterile nonadherent gauze and tubular bandage is all that is required. Most patients return to work on the same day or on the following day and wear their own shoes providing that there is adequate room within them for the toe and dressing. Redressings are necessary at intervals for a couple of weeks until the part is dry. Care must be taken to eliminate at the start of treatment any underlying cause of the condition. This usually means strong advice about adequate footwear and perhaps the treatment of a hyperhidrotic foot in the adolescent. If sepsis is severe or the patient is at risk because of some medical condition, systemic antibiotic therapy may be necessary.

The initial procedure, providing that local analgesia is not contraindicated because of an underlying medical reason, is to administer the local analgesia as a ring block to the toe. The use of about 2 ml of 3% mepivacaine hydrochloride (Scandonest 3%) is found to be quite adequate to produce complete anaesthesia of the toe. Half of the dose is administered to the soft tissues on either side of the base of the toe at the level of the shaft of the proximal phalanx. Because of the danger of distal necrosis, it is absolutely contraindicated to use local analgesia containing vasoconstrictors on the digits. While the local analgesia is taking effect, a decision about the amount of nail plate to be excised is made. This needs to be enough to remove the implanted portion at the side but also needs to be the correct amount to achieve a good long-term cosmetic result with minimal possibility of recurrence of the condition. Careful note is then taken of the proposed line of incision in order to remove the desired portion of nail plate. This line will be parallel to the long axis of the nail plate.

When anaesthesia is complete, the nail plate is loosened gently both under the eponychium and hypernychium at the site of the proposed incision into the nail plate. Exsanguination of the toe and a blood-free operating field is achieved by use of a rubber strip torniquet. Note should be made of the time of application of the torniquet so that a maximum of about 15 minutes is not exceeded.

The nail plate is split gently along the desired line of incision by Thwaite nail nippers. These do not have a large anvil that would damage the nail bed on the lower surface. At the edge of the hyponychium where the nail plate disappears from view, cutting with the nippers is discontinued. From here proximally, the nail plate is split with a narrow-bladed chisel. It should be remembered from the anatomy of the nail area that the nail plate curves gently downwards towards its matrix. This is the line to be followed by the chisel and is shown in Fig. 41.5. With care, the sudden lessening of resistance to the chisel blade is felt as it exits from nail plate into softer tissue. It should be noted that the proximal phalanx is just posterior to the nail matrix area and too

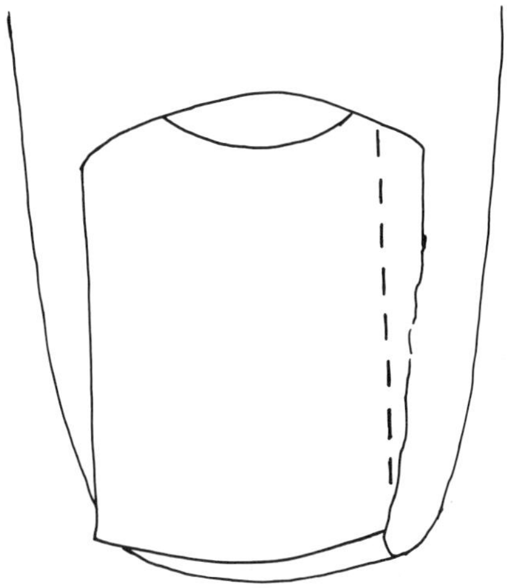

Fig. 41.5 The dotted line shows the line of splitting a nail plate during the operative procedure. The exposed nail plate may be split with a Thwaite nail nipper and the proximal part of nail under the nail fold split with a narrow-bladed chisel. Care is taken to follow the longitudinal curvature of the nail plate (Fig. 1) and to cause the minimum of damage to the underlying soft tissues

enthusiastic pushing with the chisel will damage this bone or its periosteum.

Once the nail plate has been split, the part that is to be removed is grasped firmly with locking artery forceps. These are then twisted gently in order to loosen the part of nail. When rotating freely after a couple of turns, the section of nail may be removed. A careful inspection of this piece of nail should be made. A thin 'feathered' proximal end shows that the whole section of nail plate has been taken out and that nothing remains attached to the matrix.

A further exploration of the cavity formed and the removal of any remaining debris is the next step in the procedure. A long-standing ingrown nail will have quite a lot of fibrous tissue surrounding the penetrating section. This too needs to be taken out at this stage together with any loose excess granulation tissue. The cut part of the remaining nail plate needs to be smoothed with a Black's file or fine rasp so that further damage by the newly exposed sharp edge does not occur.

While still keeping the tourniquet in place, Liquefied Phenol BP is applied by means of a sloping cut wooden applicator stick to the exposed nail matrix, nail wall and roof of the cavity. It has to be ensured that enough phenol undiluted by body fluids reaches and destroys these nail growing cells.

Three or four applicator sticks with about a centimetre or so of their length soaked in the phenol has been found to be enough for each cavity.

The phenol within the cavity is then diluted and flushed out with alcohol. Skin disinfection strength of spirituous Hibitane® has been found to be suitable for this. An excess of solution is applied by dropper or by squeezing a soaked pad of cotton wool. The toe is dried with sterile cotton wool or gauze and the tourniquet removed. Some postoperative bleeding is sometimes experienced but this has never been a major problem. (See Fig. 41.4)

The toe is dressed with a topical antiseptic that does not have a stiff base which will tend to prevent drainage of the site (Ponoxylan® gel, Betadine®), sterile gauze and not too tight tubular bandage. The patient is told to add further dressings to the top of the ones in place should there be any later blood staining through the tubular bandage. A loose shoe or sandal is quite adequate to take the foot with its one or two layers of gauze and tubular bandage on the toe. Redressing and replacement of the antiseptic and gauze is done in about two or three days and then at weekly intervals until the lesion is dry. The foot is to be kept dry during this time. A couple of weeks is usually the time taken before the lesion has closed. The amount of phenol used and the amount of infection present at the time of surgery seem to determine this time interval.

After the nail plate has grown its full length, in about nine months, the new nail sulcus will form on the operative side and a narrower nail plate of perfect cosmetic appearance will be the result. There is no scar tissue because there has been no interference with the skin.

POSTOPERATIVE PROBLEMS

Postoperative problems in partial nail avulsion and matrix phenolization are not common. Pain is controlled by the analgesic effect of the phenol and postoperative discomfort is always less than the pain of the original ingrown nail.

Slow healing of the site of phenolization may sometimes occur. This is related to the chemical tissue destruction effects of the phenol which Rinaldi et al (1982) suggest may be followed by bacterial infection. Dagnall (1981) states that the alcohol used to flush away excess phenol may be responsible for some of the delay in healing. In any case, a good nonclogging topical antiseptic is important to allow for rapid noninfected healing of the site. If healing is longer than two to three weeks, a change in topical antiseptic should be considered. Dry powder Betadine® is a good choice for the patient to apply himself.

In the long term, regrowth of the edge of nail plate is a possibility. The regrowth rate with the phenolization technique has been shown to vary from zero in a random retrospective survey of 30 patients (Siegle et al 1984) to 7% in a randomized controlled study of 54 treatments by Morkane (1984). Sometimes with care of the regrowing nail plate in the sulcus and with adequate room within the footwear, it is possible to produce a healthy nail without further surgery, but a second and more detailed phenolization is usually the answer to regrowth. A more radical surgical technique should be carried out if there is any doubt.

CONCLUSION

The ingrowing or ingrown nail should not now hold the terrors previously associated with this problem. Where there has been, as yet, no penetration of nail plate into the soft tissues, conservative treatment should be undertaken immediately. This is the removal of the cause of the condition, which is most likely to be inadequate footwear, careful treatment of the nail area to reduce the offending nail mass and removal of any associated debris, corn or callus from the sulcus. Where true onychocryptosis has developed, or as a long term solution to poorly shaped nail plates, medication to reduce any sepsis and partial nail avulsion with matrix destruction will leave a good cosmetic result with no scar tissue or possibility of recurrence of the condition.

The most important part of the treatment of all of these nail conditions is the careful investigation into the likely aetiology by both practitioner and patient and the development of a scheme of advice which will prevent any future trouble. Patients who are at risk because of an underlying circulatory or neurological medical condition should be under the regular care of a State Registered Chiropodist.

REFERENCES

Antrum R M 1984 Radical excision of the nailfold for ingrowing toenail. J Bone Joint Surg 66(1): 63–65

Barrin R, Dawber R P R 1984 Diseases of the nails and their management. Blackwell Scientific Publications, London

Dagnall J C 1981 The history, development and current status of nail matrix phenolisation. Chiropodist 36(9): 315–324

Davies R R 1984 Nail dust in chiropody practice. J R Soc Health 104: 1-5

Dawber P R 1980 The ultrastructure and growth of human nails. Arch Dermatol Res 269: 197–204

DuVries H L 1959 Surgery of the foot. C V Mosby Company, St Louis

Gabriel S S et al 1979 The ingrowing toenail; a modified segmental matrix excision operation. Br J Surg 66: 285–286

Hashimoto K 1971 Ultrastructure of the human toenail. J Ultrastructure Research 36: 391–410

Lancet 1979 On not outgrowing the toenail (editorial). Lancet 1(8128): 1223

Lewis B L 1954 Microscopic studies of foetal and mature nail and surrounding soft tissue. Arch Dermatol 70: 732

Morkane A J et al 1984 Segmental phenolisation of ingrowing toenails: a randomised controlled study. Br J Surg 71(7): 526–527

Palmer B V et al 1979 Ingrowing toenails: the results of treatment. Br J Surg 66(8): 575–576

Rinaldi R, Sabia M, Gross J 1982 The treatment and prevention of infection in phenol alcohol matricectomies. J Am Pod Assn 72(9): 453–457

Ross W R 1969 Treatment of the ingrown toenail. Surg Clin N Amer 49: 1499–1504

Samman P D 1978 The nails in disease. Heinemann Medical Books, London

Siegle R J et al 1984 Phenol alcohol technique for permanent matricectomy. Arch Dermatol 120(3): 348–350

Wallace W A et al 1979 Gutter treatment for ingrowing toenails. Br Med J 2(6183): 168–171

Winograd A M 1929 A modification of the technique of operation for ingrown toenail. JAMA 92: 229–230

Zadik F R 1950 Obliteration of the nailbed of the great toe without shortening the terminal phalanx. J Bone Jt Surg 32B: 66–67

Zaias N 1980 The nail in health and disease. Medical and Scientific Books, New York

Ankle injuries

HISTORY

The first description of ankle fractures is ascribed to Percival Pott (1768) who suffered a transverse fracture of his fibula within 2–3 in of its lower extremity. His name is often applied erroneously to all fractures around the ankle.

Dupuytren added his description in 1819 of a fibula fractured by an abducting force allied to damage either of the medial malleolus or deltoid ligament. Maisonneuve in 1840 demonstrated in the cadaver the results of external rotation of the foot on the ankle. He described not only 3° of external rotation fracture when the anterior tibiofibular ligament remained intact, but also the fracture through the neck of the fibula when the anterior tibiofibular ligament tears, that bears his name.

Rochet (1890) demonstrated compression fractures involving the tibial articular surface and showed that the position of the foot influenced the result. With the foot in plantar flexion, the maximum damage occurs to the posterior part of the surface and conversely in dorsiflexion, fracturing is mainly of the anterior surface.

The subject remained rather disordered and fragmentary until Ashhurst & Bromer published their classification of ankle fractures in 1922. They considered that the fracture of the fibula was not associated with a rupture of the tibiofibular ligament in external rotation injuries and that the second degree occurred when the deltoid ligament ruptured or the medial malleolus was avulsed and finally that a third degree fracture involved the posterior tibial margin.

Lauge-Hansen in 1942 produced a more rational classification of ankle fractures in which he drew attention to the foot position in determining the effect on the ankle of forced external rotation. He was of the opinion that the anterior tibiofibular ligament was the first to rupture and that this was then followed by the fracture of the fibula. Next, the posterior tibial elements gave way and finally in a further stage the medial ligament or malleolus. Since Lauge-Hansen's classification was published, opinions have been many and varied as to the exact sequence of changes in external rotation ankle fractures (Yde 1980).

Cedell (1967) has questioned the exact sequence of injuries as described by Lauge-Hansen and demonstrated at operation that the anterior tibiofibular ligament was intact in 4% of cases in association with the distal oblique fibular fracture. Whilst there is, therefore, still some argument as to the combination of ligamentous and bony damage and the order in which they occur with different forces, nonetheless, a classification based on Lauge-Hansen's work gives a good working hypothesis.

GENERAL

Fractures involving the ankle joint are common and often occur with little apparent force. The long lever of the lower limb produces considerable stress on the bones of the ankle when the foot is held and the body weight applied, even when no other external forces are involved. Most patients are unaware of the exact forces that have operated on the ankle resulting in a fracture. Cedell (1967) found that 85% of 417 patients could give no information at all on the mechanism of their injuries. Nonetheless, examination of radiographs will usually indicate what must have happened. The type of fracture is dependent on two factors: the force acting on the joint and, secondly, the position of the foot at the time of the injury. Should the foot be in a position of pronation, this will tighten the soft tissue structures on the medial side so that the maximum damage initially will occur on this side of the joint, while supination will have the effect of stressing the lateral side of the ankle.

Therefore ankle fractures are considered under the following headings:

1. Supination — external rotation
2. Pronation — external rotation
3. Pronation — abduction
4. Supination — adduction
5. Vertical compression

A most important factor in the assessment of these fractures is the question of stability, and for this purpose it is helpful to regard the mortice as a ring. As Neer points out (1953), if only one point in the ring is ruptured, either of bone or ligament, then the complex remains stable. On the other hand, should two points be ruptured, either by two fractures or by a fracture and a ligamentous disruption, then the ring becomes unstable and the necessity of surgery to produce stability is that much greater.

Diagnosis

In order that a clear picture of ankle injuries can be gained, radiographs should be taken in antero-posterior view at 0° of rotation to visualize the joint space between the talus and medial malleolus and in 20° internal rotation to assess the joint space on the outer side of the talus, with a true lateral film. On occasions, stress films will be needed to evaluate the integrity of the ligaments, particularly those of the tibiofibular syndesmosis, so that diastasis may be excluded.

SUPINATION — EXTERNAL ROTATION FRACTURES

These are common and constitute about 65% of all ankle fractures (Cedell 1967). They result from a slip on level ground, which occurred in 40% of Cedell's cases (1967), or from such accidents as catching the forefoot on the edge of a step (17.5%), as the patient turns to one side or makes a sudden change of direction with the foot fixed on the ground. The foot is in supination which tightens the lateral structures. The anterior tibiofibular ligament is ruptured and as the external rotation force continues, pressure falls on the lower part of the fibula, breaking it off so that the line of cleavage starts above from the posterior surface and runs downwards between the anterior and posterior tibiofibular ligaments to the anterior surface of the lateral malleolus just below the tibial articular surface (Figs. 42.1, 2, 3 and 4). The talus remains firmly attached to the lower fragment.

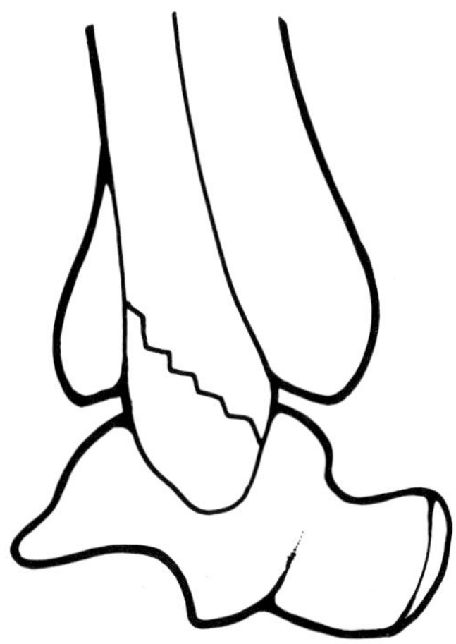

Fig. 42.1 Lateral view of the oblique fracture of the fibula occurring in the supination external rotation fracture

If the rotational force continues, the medial structures tighten so that either a medial malleolus avulsion fracture results or the deltoid ligament ruptures (Figs. 42.5, 6 and 7). The foot with the talus and attached lower portion of the lateral malleolus are now completely free and further progression of the force will carry the talus posteriorly so that finally the posterior tibial articular surface may fracture (Trethowan's third malleolus) allowing the talus to displace backwards and upwards. On occasions the damage to the posterior tibial surface may precede the fracture of the medial malleolus and indeed Lauge-Hansen is of the opinion that this most usually occurs.

The amount of the tibial articular surface which is displaced posteriorly is usually small and should be distinguished from the much larger posterior tibial fragment that is displaced in a compression fracture. It only rarely requires surgical replacement.

Stage I injuries where only the anterior tibiofibular ligament has ruptured are most easily

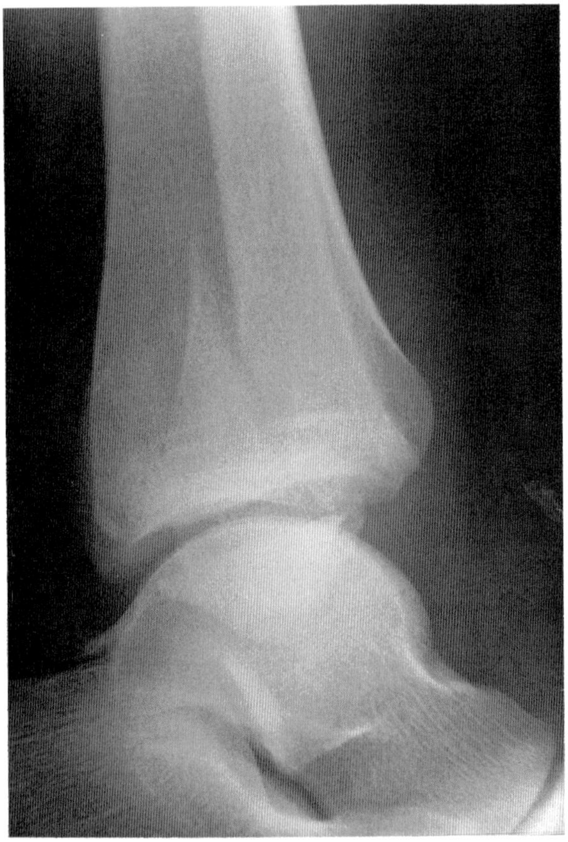

Fig. 42.2 Radiograph of Fig. 42.1

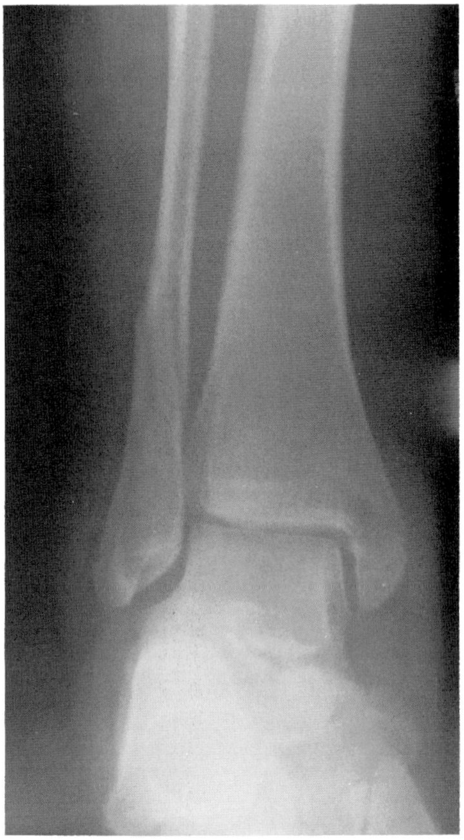

Fig. 42.4 Radiograph of Fig. 42.3

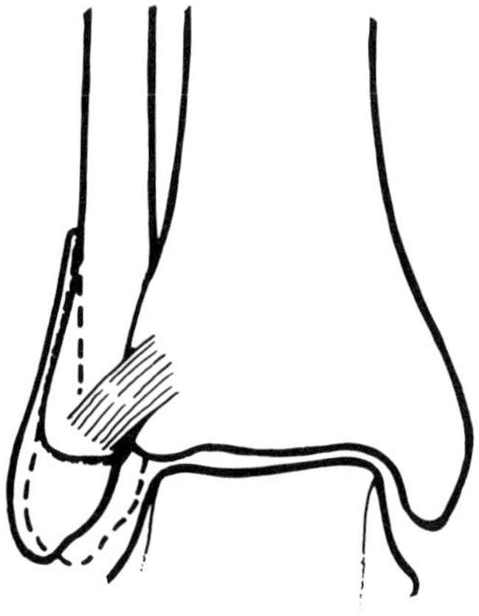

Fig. 42.3 Anteroposterior view of supination external rotation fracture. As the talus moves laterally the dotted line indicates the displaced position of the distal part of the fibula

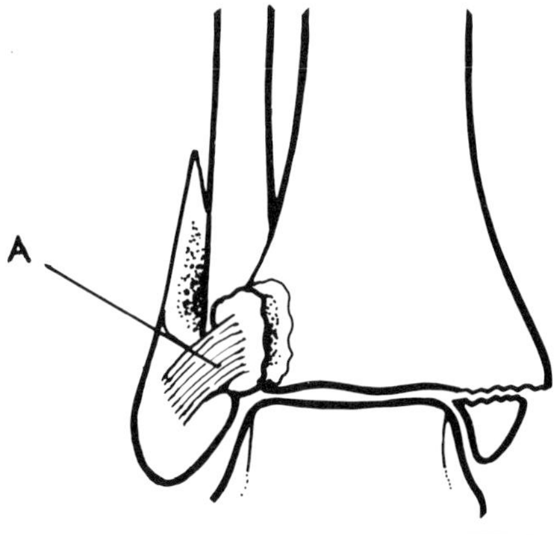

Fig. 42.5 Supination external rotation fracture with displacement. The tibiofibular ligament (A) has avulsed a fragment from the tibia

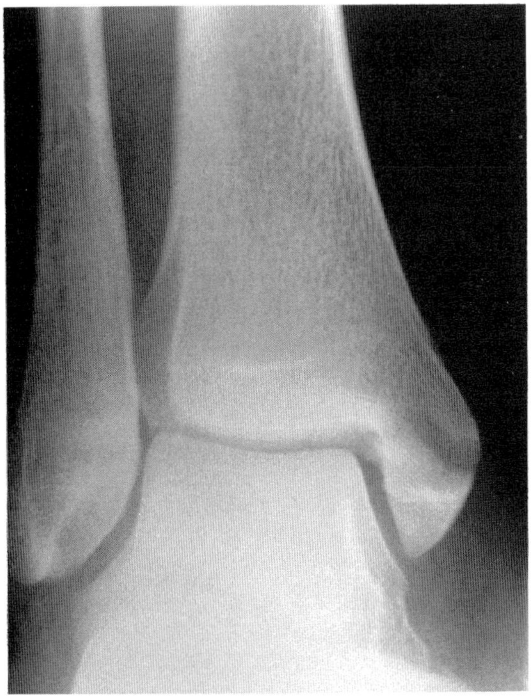

Fig. 42.6 Anteroposterior radiograph of supination external rotation fracture. The fibular fracture is seen with some difficulty

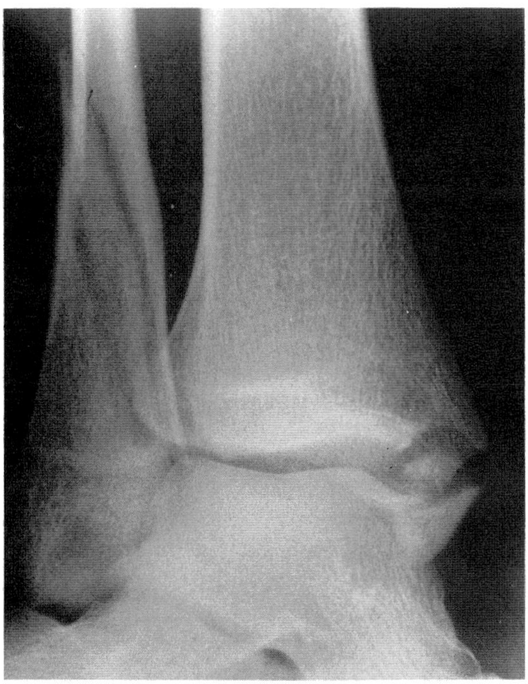

Fig. 42.7 Oblique radiograph of the same ankle showing the fibular displacement more clearly

diagnosed when there is some bone avulsed either from the tibia or the fibula. Clinically, pain may be produced in the area of the ligament either by forced external rotation of the supinated foot or by forced dorsiflexion of the ankle. There is in addition localized tenderness and swelling, but these signs may be obscured by the presence of a haemarthrosis. The more common injury to the anterior talofibular ligament must be distinguished since the two ligaments are in close proximity. The presence of pain on forced pullforward of the foot and if necessary a lateral stress film will establish the diagnosis of damage to the anterior talofibular ligament.

Treatment

The simple rotational fracture of the lateral malleolus is usually stable and the only requirement may be to alleviate the pain. Elastoplast® strapping may be sufficient, but if there is still much pain then a below-knee walking plaster may be required. Some cases of fibular fracture may be unstable especially when associated with rupture of the anterior tibiofibular ligament. Lauge-Hansen was able to demonstrate lateral talar shift of as much as 2–3 mm. When there has been damage to the medial side of the joint it is potentially unstable and more support is required. The necessity for this may be apparent from the radiographs, which may show an avulsion fracture of the medial malleolus or from clinical examination which indicates damage to the deltoid ligament — swelling and local tenderness.

The radiographs may also show lateral displacement of the talus (Fig. 42.8) and this must be corrected; a manoeuvre which requires anaesthesia. With the patient relaxed, firm pressure is applied to the medial surface of the tibia and the outer side of the foot so as to produce a medial rotational force. Over reduction cannot occur. When talar displacement has taken place the limb must be protected from weight bearing for two to three weeks. In those cases in which there is gross swelling a short period of elevation may be required following the initial reduction, until it is safe to apply a well moulded cast. Further radiographs are advisable after changing the cast or after weight bearing to make sure that redisplacement has not occurred.

In those cases in which there is posterior

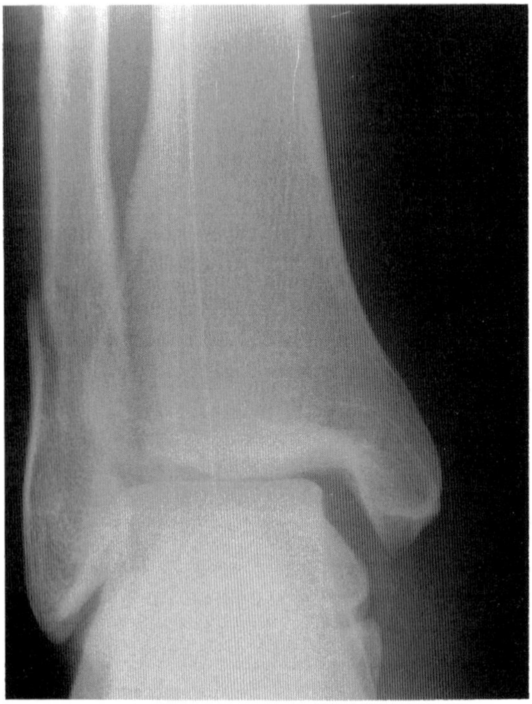

Fig. 42.8 Displaced supination external fracture. The medial malleolus has remained intact, but there is evident lateral displacement of the talus. There is soft tissue swelling over the medial ligament which has ruptured

dislocation with fracture of the posterior malleolus, reduction can only be obtained with the knee flexed to relax the calf muscles. If there is a sizeable posterior fragment which remains less than perfectly reduced, then open reduction may be necessary, since the weight-bearing surface of the tibia is impaired and failure to reduce the fragment and hold it reduced will result in degenerative arthritis. The necessity for open reduction depends on the size of the displaced fragment. If in the lateral view the vertical fracture is placed in the posterior third of the tibial articular surface, the amount of the joint surface damage is small and can be neglected. Cedell (1967) only found it necessary to operate on 15 patients out of 222 ankle fractures; 42 (18%) of whom had a fragment involving one-fourth of the articular surface.

PRONATION — EXTERNAL ROTATION FRACTURES

In this type of fracture the medial structures are tight due to the pronation of the foot. Damage occurs initially to the medial malleolus or the deltoid ligament. Once the rupture of the medial part of the ring has occurred, a continuing torsional force is applied to the fibula which ruptures the anterior tibiofibular ligament with or without avulsing some bone from the tibia. Next, the interosseous ligament gives way so that the fibula takes the force and may fracture (Figs. 42.9, 10a and 10b). The level of this fracture is never less than 2.5 cm above the tibial articular surface, but may be as high as the neck of the fibula (Maisonneuve fracture) if the force applied is purely external rotation. (Fig. 42.11)

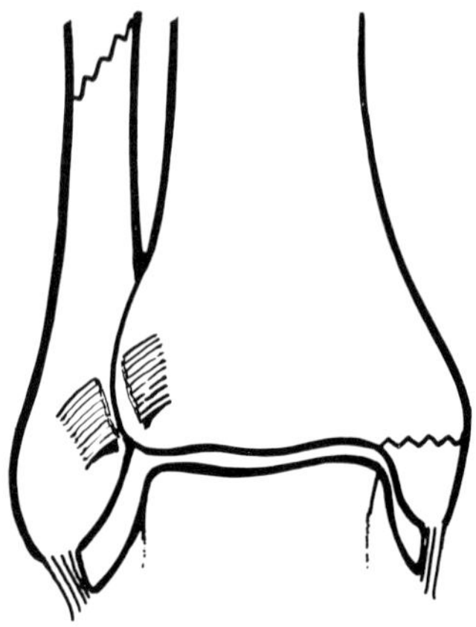

Fig. 42.9 Pronation external rotation fracture

In those cases in which the fracture of the fibula is at a more distal level, there is some degree of abduction force. As a result, the fibular fracture appears to be more transverse, rather than oblique as in the more proximal break. The name of Dupuytren is applied to the more distal fracture.

Diagnosis

In those cases in which there is marked displacement of the fibular fragment there is little difficulty in recognizing that the syndesmosis has been disrupted. On the other hand, when displacement is slight and the fracture has occurred through the fibular neck, it may be missed unless care is taken in the examination. A combination of tenderness over the medial side of the joint and over the syndesmosis should lead to palpation of the whole length of the fibula and radiographs, not only of the ankle, but of the whole length of the fibula should be taken.

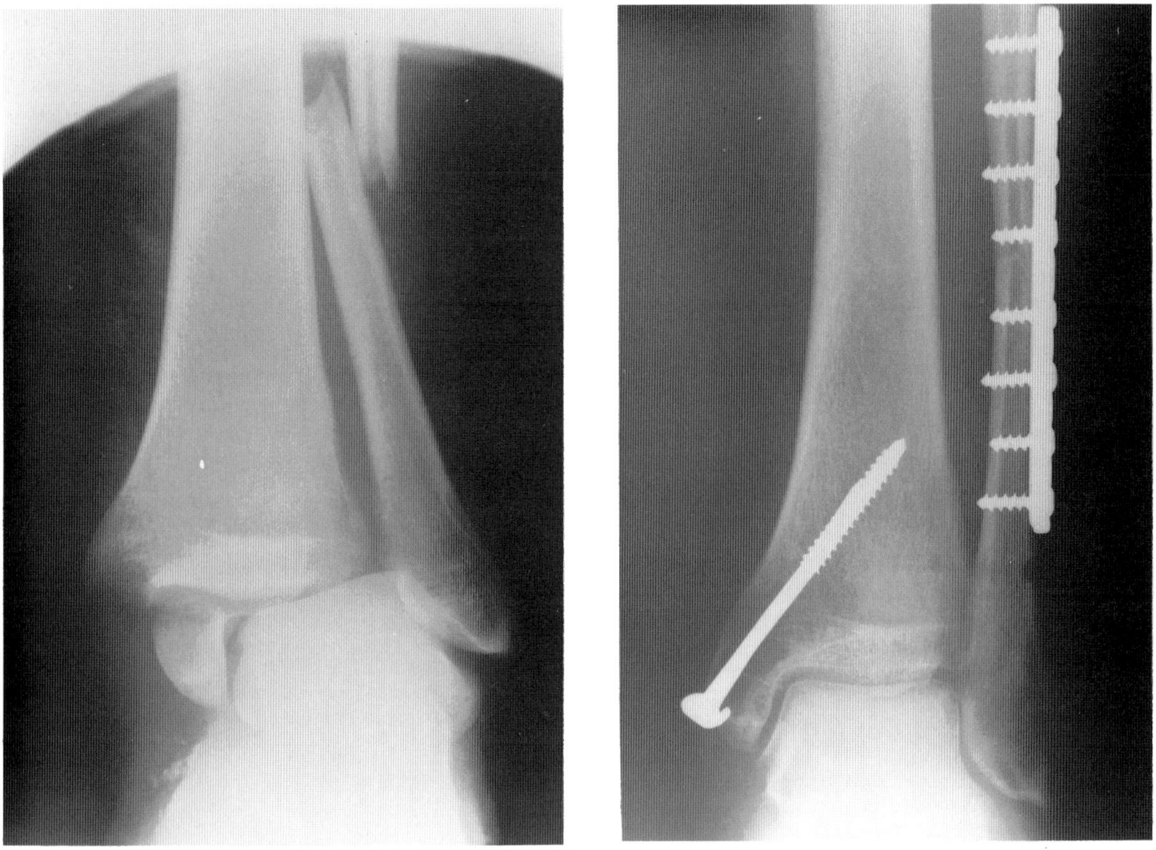

a b

Fig. 42.10(a) Pronation external rotation fracture in which the talus has dislocated laterally. (b), Radiograph following open reduction and fixation of both fractures. A screw to reduce the diastasis which was placed transversely has been removed but this track can still be seen

Treatment

Those cases with only limited diastasis, can be treated conservatively, since the posterior tibiofibular ligament is intact and will act as a stabilizing force as the foot is internally rotated. After reduction, an above-knee plaster is applied to control rotation. Should postreduction radiographs show any doubt as to the position of the joint, then open reduction is advisable, if the patient is fit in other respects.

Surgery is also best carried out if there is gross displacement, since the support of the posterior tibiofibular ligament has been lost. Fixation of the fibula should be carried out so that the bone is reduced and pulled out to length. Stabilization is best obtained by application of a plate long enough to give adequate fixation both above and below the fracture line. Repair of the anterior tibiofibular ligament is possible through the same incision; this is situated over the anterolateral aspect of the fibula and extended downwards as far as necessary. Care should be taken to avoid the superficial peroneal nerve anteriorly and the sural nerve posteriorly and distally. The structures on the medial side should be fixed through a separate incision. It is usually possible to insert a screw through the medial malleolus if a fracture is present, but if too small then compression wiring may be employed.

Finally, when it is certain that the talus has been fully corrected in the ankle mortice a screw is inserted through the fibula into the tibia to stabilize the tibiofibular syndesmosis. Care must be taken where this is inserted, not to narrow the mortice as this will prevent full dorsiflexion of the ankle. The screw should be inserted obliquely passing upwards into the tibia and as it is tightened the foot should be fully dorsiflexed, so that the widest part of the talus is

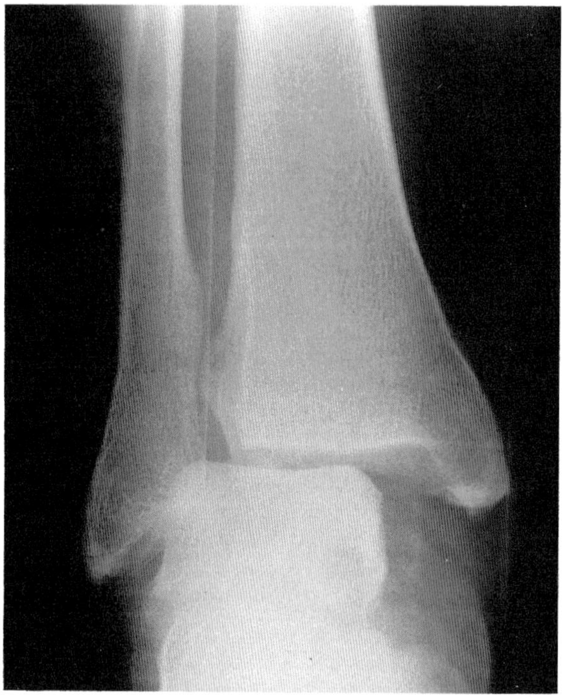

Fig. 42.11 Rupture of the tibiofibular joint. Is there a fracture in the upper third of the fibula?

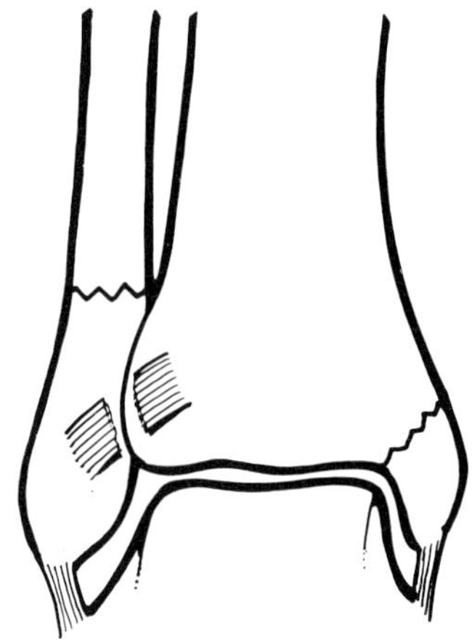

Fig. 42.12 Pronation abduction fracture. The tibiofibular ligament has ruptured and a continuing abduction force on the fibula has broken it transversely above the syndesmosis

engaged in the joint. The screw should be removed when the fracture has united as otherwise it will interfere with the normal tibial rotation.

PRONATION — ABDUCTION FRACTURES

Whilst the foot is in pronation, abduction initially will fracture the medial malleolus or rupture the deltoid ligament. Continuation of an outward force causes the syndesmosis to give way so that further force falls on the fibula, fracturing it (Fig. 42.12). Abduction will produce a transverse fibular fracture not less than 2.5 cm above the tibiotalar joint in contradistinction to the oblique fracture caused by a rotational force. Finally, the posterior tibiofibular ligament may rupture and allow the talus to dislocate outwards.

Treatment

Manipulation under anaesthesia may be satisfactory. Care should be taken to move the foot medially and not only to invert it. A below-knee plaster may be sufficient if there is little swelling, but in those cases in which there has been some rotational element then it should be carried above the knee. Failure accurately to reduce the ankle or any subsequent redisplacement is best treated by open reduction and fixation of the malleolus.

Malunion

Should malunion occur, it is most likely to be with shortening of the fibula and lateral displacement of the talus. Correction can only be carried out if the fibula is brought out to length, so that the talus is then free to move back to its normal position. To correct the deformity it will be necessary first to osteotomize the fibula at the level of the fracture and, having pulled it distally, to fix it with a plate. The syndesmosis can then be held in a corrected position by an oblique screw. This screw should be removed when union has occurred.

SUPINATION — ADDUCTION FRACTURES

If an internal rotation force is applied to the foot the joints of the foot lock in supination and any further force is converted to adduction of the ankle. The fibula is snapped transversely just below the level of the joint surface. The continuing force is thrown on to the medial malleolus which fractures vertically (Figs. 42.13, 14 and 15). Medial displacement of the talus can then freely occur and the ankle may be

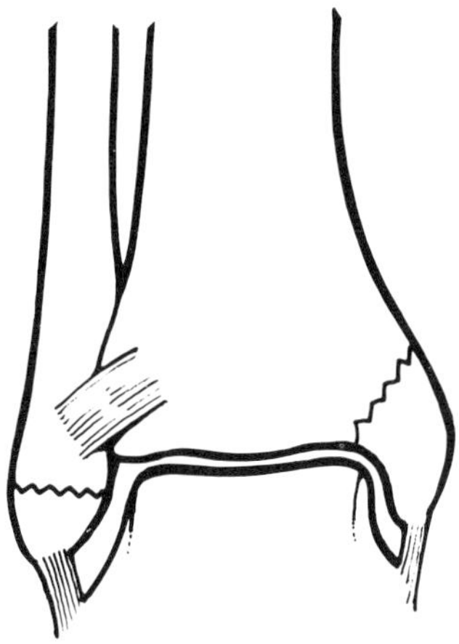

Fig. 42.13 Supination adduction fracture

dislocated with the addition of fracture of the posterior margin of the tibia.

On occasions, the initial force falls predominantly on the medial malleolus, so that an isolated vertical fracture of this bone may occur.

Treatment

The medial malleolar fracture often will not reduce fully as soft tissue may be interposed. Since this will lead to a painful fibrous union, open reduction and

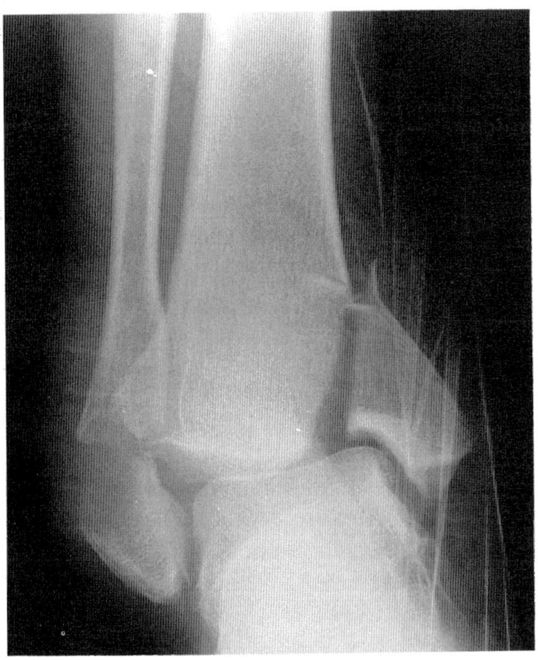

Fig. 42.14 Displaced supination adduction fracture

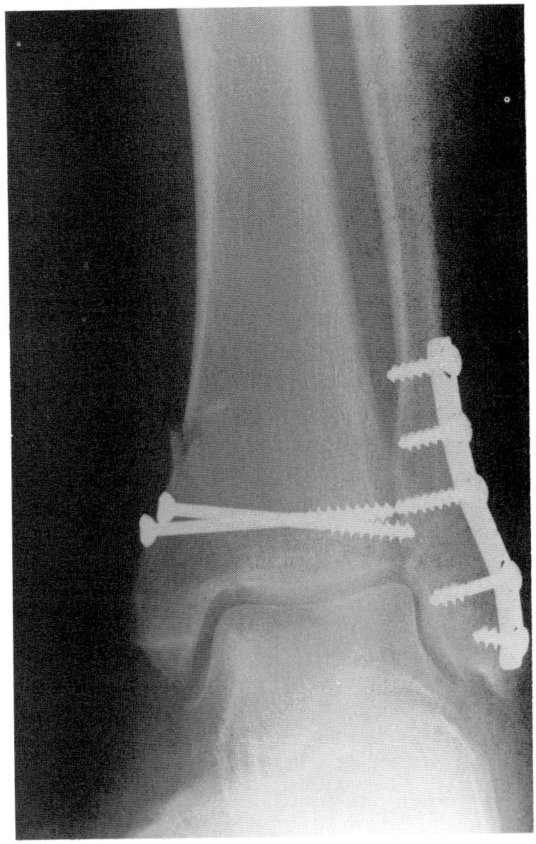

Fig. 42.15 The same fracture after open reduction

screw fixation is the preferred method of treatment. In those cases in which only the fibula is fractured, below-knee fixation in a plaster cast is likely to be all that is needed. Displacement can usually be corrected by an abduction force. Should accurate reduction not be possible, then open reduction and fixation by a vertical screw is advisable.

VERTICAL COMPRESSION FRACTURES

These fractures occur when a vertical compression force is applied to the limb, such as in a patient falling from a height onto the foot. The damage that follows depends on the position of the foot at the moment of impact. Should the ankle be plantarflexed then the force falls posteriorly, splitting off the posterior tibial articular surface and causing posterior dislocation. With the ankle in dorsiflexion, the force is expended on the anterior tibial area, so that a fragment may be split off and the talus carried forwards (Fig. 42.16). Whether the force is anterior or posterior, the tibial surface of the joint is damaged and reposition of the tibial fragments should be meticulously carried out so that minimal irregularity of the joint surface remains. In most cases this will require open reduction and fixation by screws.

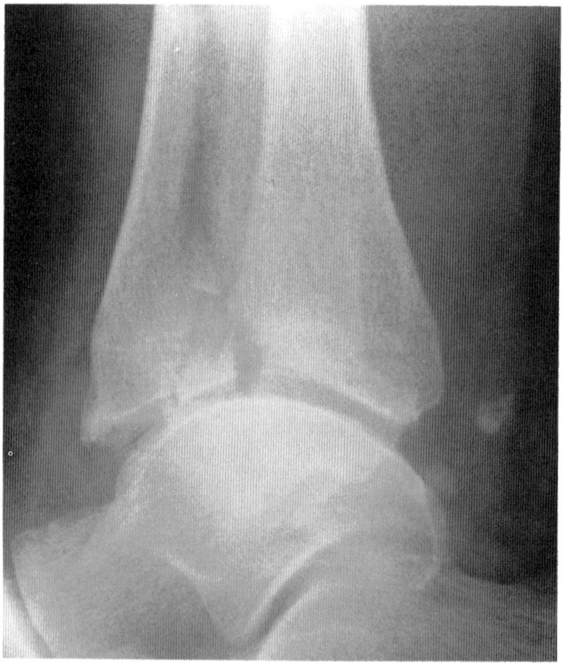

Fig. 42.16 Vertical compression fracture in which the force has fallen predominantly on the anterior part of the tibia, the foot having been in dorsiflexion

In some cases there is considerable comminution of the tibial fracture, so that accurate reduction is difficult, if not impossible. Should this be the case or indeed if the patent is not fit for surgery, then traction should be applied by means of a pin through the os calcis to hold reduction. The limb is most easily nursed on a Braun's frame. Exercises should be encouraged. Within two to three weeks a below-knee plaster can be applied, incorporating the pin. Weight bearing must be prevented for a period of 10 to 12 weeks; by which time union will have occurred. Since a stiff ankle will often result in these more severe fractures, any immobilization should be carried out with the ankle in 5–10° of dorsiflexion. In this position, the patient can walk most easily, rocking on the heel. Occasionally, a painful ankylosis results and arthrodesis may be necessary.

Fixation of posterior tibial fragments has already been discussed when these result from rotational forces. Should the pieces be fairly small then open reduction and fixation is unnecessary. If the vertical fracture visible in the lateral view passes through the posterior third of the tibial surface, in all probability surgery is unnecessary, since the fracture passes obliquely across the tibial surface and only splits off a small area of chondral surface (Fig. 42.17). Those fractures resulting from vertical compression force tend to be larger and require fixation to correct posterior subluxation of the talus and to prevent late onset of osteoarthritis.

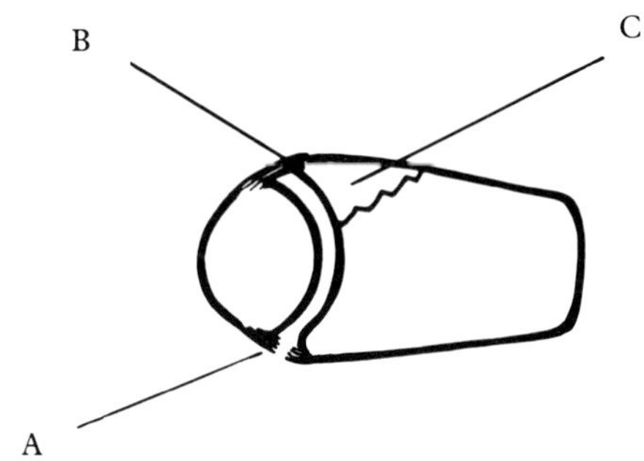

Fig. 42.17 The small area of posterior tibial surface which may be displaced in a rotational fracture. A = Anterior tibiofibular ligament; B = Posterior tibiofibular ligament; C = Fragment of tibial articular surface

The approach to the posterior fragment should be through a posteromedial incision placed parallel to the Achilles tendon. The tendons, posterior tibial vessels and nerves are exposed and can be retracted medially. This allows exposure of the fragment and also the posterior surface of the tibiofibular joint. The fragment must be accurately repositioned before fixation with one or more screws.

In those injuries which result in severe comminution of the tibial surface and in which it is not thought possible to effect adequate reduction so that the tibial surface is reconstituted, it is wise to carry out conservative treatment by traction and exercises and not to proceed to immediate arthrodesis, since on occasions the end result may be reasonably satisfactory. Rarely, if ever, should immediate arthrodesis be advocated, since this can be embarked on at a later date when it is evident that pain and disability warrant joint stiffening.

GENERAL ADVICE ON THE INDICATIONS FOR SURGERY AND ON TECHNIQUE

To some extent the decision to operate on a fractured ankle will depend on the surgeon's view, since many fractures can be treated with satisfactory results both conservatively and surgically and some surgeons will find it easier to control the injury by a well fitting plaster rather than by internal fixation. In general, however, if the fracture is unstable then accurate reduction is more likely to be achieved and held by surgical methods. Clearly the age and the general condition of the patient and the presence of other injuries will play a part in the decision, though with modern anaesthesia there are few patients who cannot tolerate an operation. Beauchamp et al (1983) have drawn attention to the difficulties encountered in patients over 50, particularly women, due to osteoporosis.

Should surgery be employed then fixation of the fracture should be firm enough to allow non-weightbearing exercise in elevation to be carried out initially, so that a good range of movement is regained in the joint and any oedema removed before plaster is applied. This may require a week or 10 days. Once the swelling has disappeared and good movement regained, then plaster can be applied to hold the joint until union has occurred; a period which is likely to be a further four to six weeks.

In the past many surgeons took the view that the structures on the medial side of the ankle were the more important and should be fixed first. Indeed, Cox & Laxson (1952) were of the opinion that the lateral malleolus never requires operative treatment. Since Danis (1949) put forward the view that the lateral components were the more important, others have taken the same view (Weber 1966) and now most surgeons would consider that the fibular fracture should be fixed first since this controls the position of the talus. Indeed, until the fibula is reduced and brought out to length there may be difficulty in reducing the medial side (Figs. 42.18 and 19). Radiographic evidence of the necessity for this can be gained by measuring the talotibial angle and comparing it with that of the uninjured side.

The talotibial angle is measured by drawing two lines — one parallel to the tibial articular surface and another through the tips of the malleoli (Figs. 42.20 and 21). This varies between 8 and 15° (Sarkisian & Cody 1976) but a difference of more than 2° between the two sides indicates a failure to restore the ankle mortice to normal.

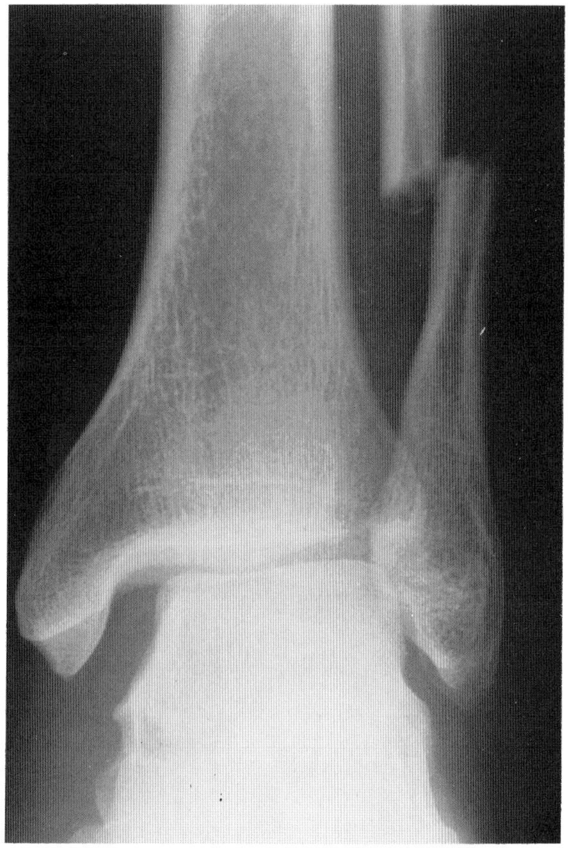

Fig. 42.18 Pronation external rotation fracture with lateral displacement of the fibula and a tear of the deltoid ligament

Convincing evidence has been produced by Yablon et al (1977) of the need to fix the lateral side of the ankle before attention is directed to the medial structures. He and his coworkers showed experimentally that division of the deltoid ligament did not produce instability of the ankle and even resection of the medial malleolus only allowed 10° of rotatory instability and virtually no valgus instability. On the other hand when the fibular collateral ligament was divided there was approximately 30° of external rotatory instability and marked talar instability.

In experimental abduction-external rotation fractures Yablon and his associates found that attempts at reduction were invariably impeded by impingement of the lateral malleolus on the proximal fibular ligament. Fixation of the medial malleolus did not help.

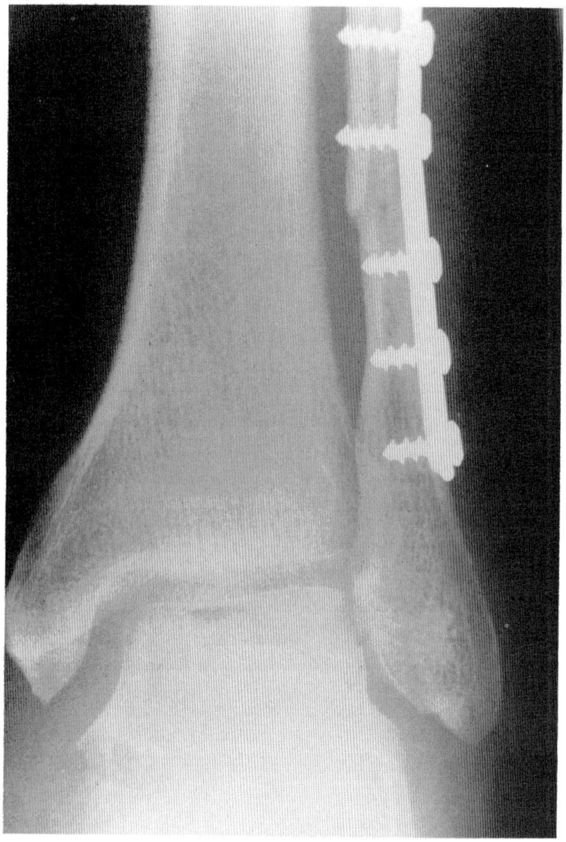

Fig. 42.19 Following open reduction of the fibular fracture. There is slight overlap at the fracture site so that the fibula has not been fully brought out to length. As a result there is still persistent lateral displacement of the talus

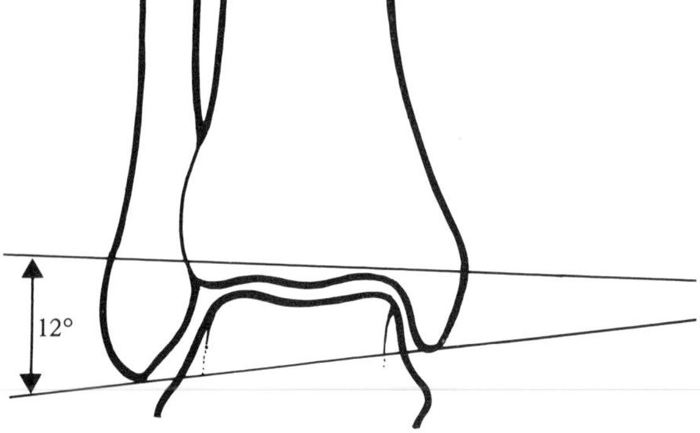

Fig. 42.20 Diagram of the talotibial angle

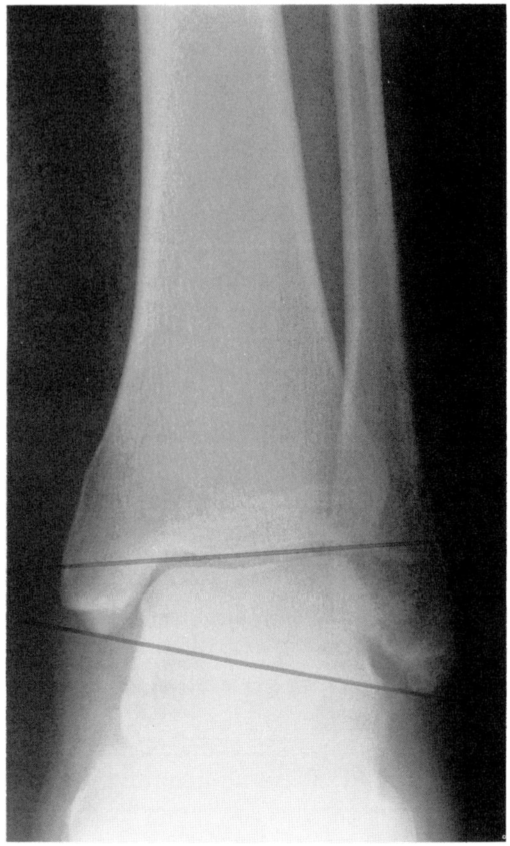

Fig. 42.21 Radiograph of the talotibial angle

Much the same problem emerged from a clinical study. In 17 patients who had primary reduction of the medial malleolus, 14 showed residual talar tilt. In 53 patients on the other hand in whom the lateral malleolus was accurately reduced and fixed, postreduction radiographs showed reduction of the talus. Other authors also have demonstrated that incomplete reduction of the lateral malleolus is the most common cause of residual symptoms and eventually of degenerative arthritis.

Results

A number of factors predispose to poor results, but the most troublesome is poor reduction (Joy et al 1974), in particular the amount of talar displacement. Brodie & Denham (1974) found that of those patients with persistent shift or tilt of the talus 75% had pain, swelling or stiffness of the ankle. Compression fractures also do badly, often resulting in stiffness of the ankle and subtalar joints. 25% may develop osteoarthritis (Brodie & Denham 1974).

Ramsey & Hamilton (1976) have shown that lateral shift of talus of even as little as 1 mm may result in as much as 42% reduction of tibiotalar contact (Fig. 42.22). Since the stress per unit area increases inversely in relation to the total contact area, it is apparent that even minor displacement may be a major factor in producing a poor result. Accurate radiographic evaluation is, therefore, of the greatest importance.

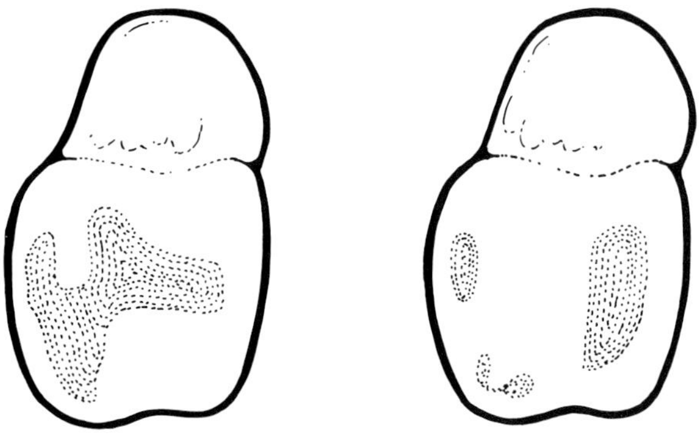

Fig. 42.22 Effect of a 2 mm lateral shift of the talus on the tibial contact area. A = Normal; B = 2 mm shift — the shaded part is the contact area (after Ramsey & Hamilton 1976)

Georgen et al (1977) have pointed to the difficulties of relying on the medial clear space as a measure of talar shift in radiographs which are not properly positioned. Radiographs which are in 15° to 20° of medial rotation will allow the medial articular surface of the talus to become tangent to the X-ray beam. In this position the concave landmark on the posteromedial surface of the talus which represents the insertion of the deep fibres of the deltoid ligament will be seen just lateral to the medial articular surface (Fig. 42.23). Films taken in this position will allow accurate evaluation of the medial joint space.

EPIPHYSEAL INJURIES

Although the forces producing these injuries are similar to those of the adult fractures, the presence of an active growth plate introduces a greater possibility of complications due to damage to the epiphysis. The problems have been well reviewed by Spiegel et al (1978) in their analysis of 184 cases.

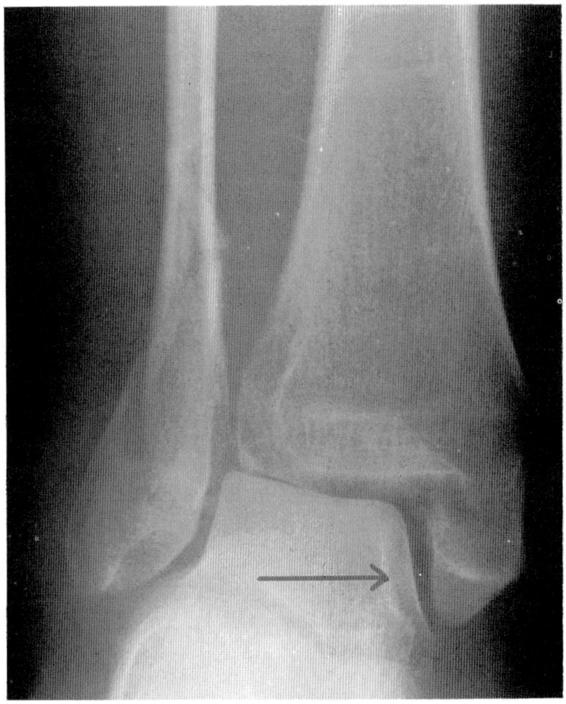

Fig. 42.23 The line (indicated by arrow) representing the insertion of the deep part of the deltoid ligament

Generally speaking, injuries to the fibular epiphysis are not a great problem, since although some shortening of the fibula may occur, angulation and interference with loadbearing does not arise.

Their analysis of the tibial injuries was based on the Salter–Harris (1963) classification of epiphyseal injuries. These groups were distinguished as low risk and high risk. All the fibular and Type I displacements of the tibia fell into the low risk group and also those Type III and IV fractures in which there was 2 mm or less of displacement. In none of these was surgical treatment considered necessary.

The high risk group consisted of Type III and IV injuries in which the displacement was greater than 2 mm and in consequence surgery for reduction was considered necessary. Juvenile Tilleaux fractures affecting the anterolateral corner of the distal tibial epiphysis were also included, although all these were treated conservatively. Finally, compression injuries (Type V) as in the adult did poorly, due to comminution of the weight-bearing surface and triplane fractures, which may be difficult to diagnose.

Triplane injuries were reported by Marmor (1970) as an unusual fracture of the tibial epiphysis and later by Lynn (1972) and Torg & Ruggiero (1975). Cooperman et al (1978) gave the first comprehensive survey of this condition illustrated by 15 cases (Fig. 42.24). They pointed out that a maturing, partially fused epiphysis was probably a prerequisite for the occurrence of this fracture (Figs. 42.25a, 25b, 26a and 26b). They are characterized by sagittal, transverse and coronal components. Part is a Type III Salter–Harris injury and part Type II which projects forwards as in Fig. 42.24. Diagnosis may be difficult, but if suspected, tomography will produce better definition.

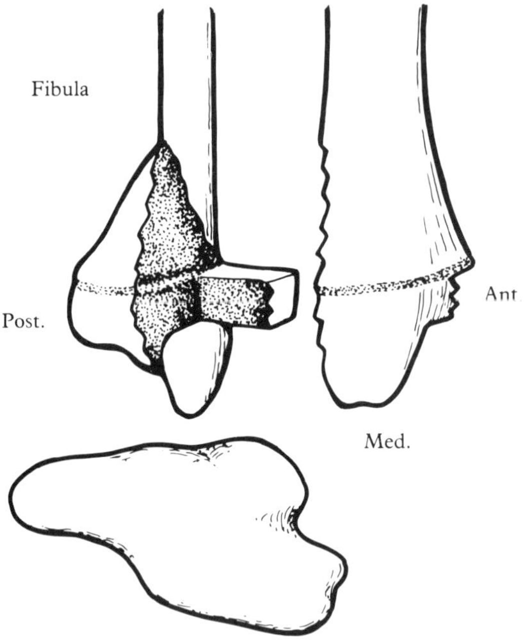

Fig. 42.24 Triplane fracture (after Cooperman et al 1978)

Most of these fractures will reduce with internal rotation of the foot and this should be attempted if more than 2 mm displacement is seen on the routine anteroposterior or lateral radiographs. General anaesthesia is necessary. If not successful, then open reduction and cancellous screws above the epiphysis may be needed.

Finally, Spiegel et al (1978) have a third or unpredictable risk group which remains. These are all Type II tibial fractures (Figs. 42.27a and 27b). Some cases which showed little displacement appeared just as liable to complications as those with considerable displacement. Of 91 patients, six had angular deformities of more than 5° and nine had shortening ranging from 0.4–1.3 cm. None was treated surgically.

REFERENCES

Ashhurst A P C, Bromer R S 1922 Classification and mechanisms of fractures of the leg bones involving the ankles. A M A Arch Surg 4: 51

a

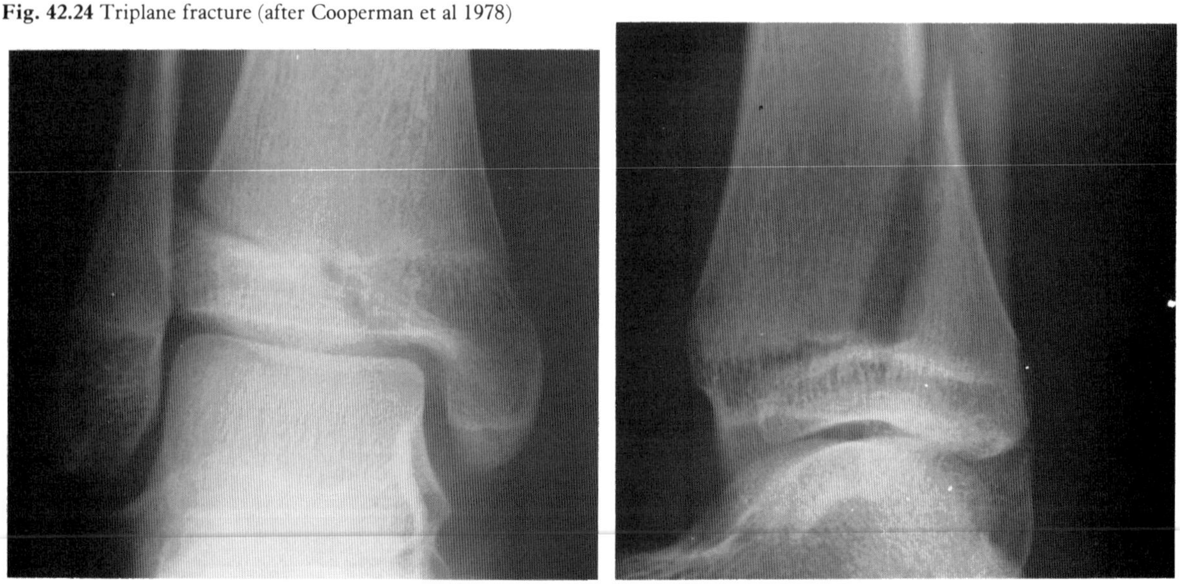

b

Fig. 42.25 Anteroposterior (a) and lateral (b) radiographs of triplane epiphyseal fracture

a

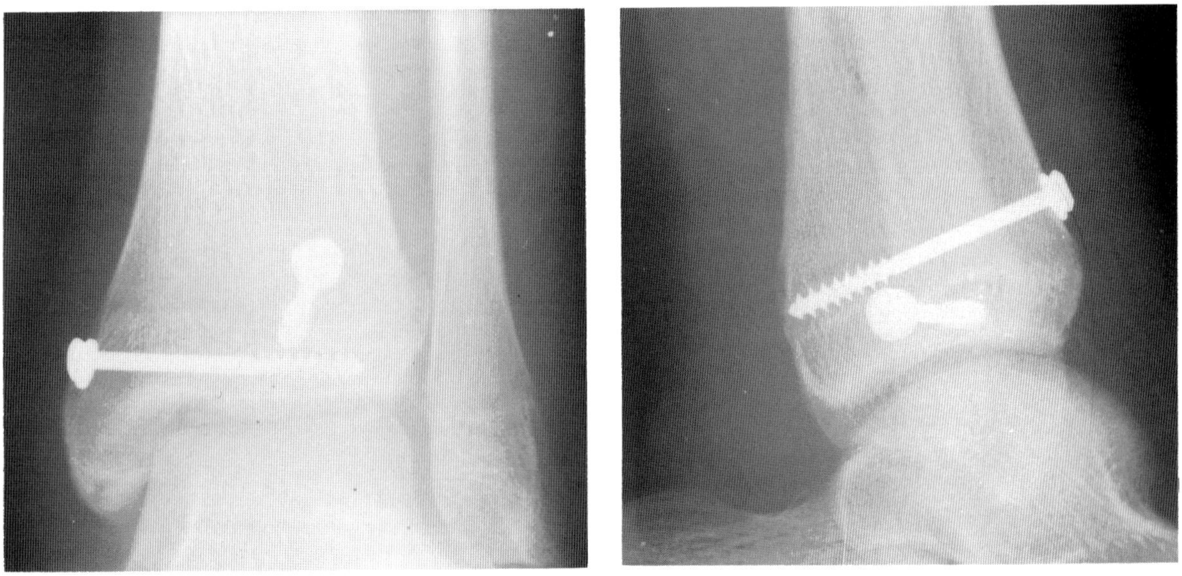

Fig. 42.26 Anteroposterior (a) and lateral (b) radiographs of triplane fracture after open reduction and screw fixation

a

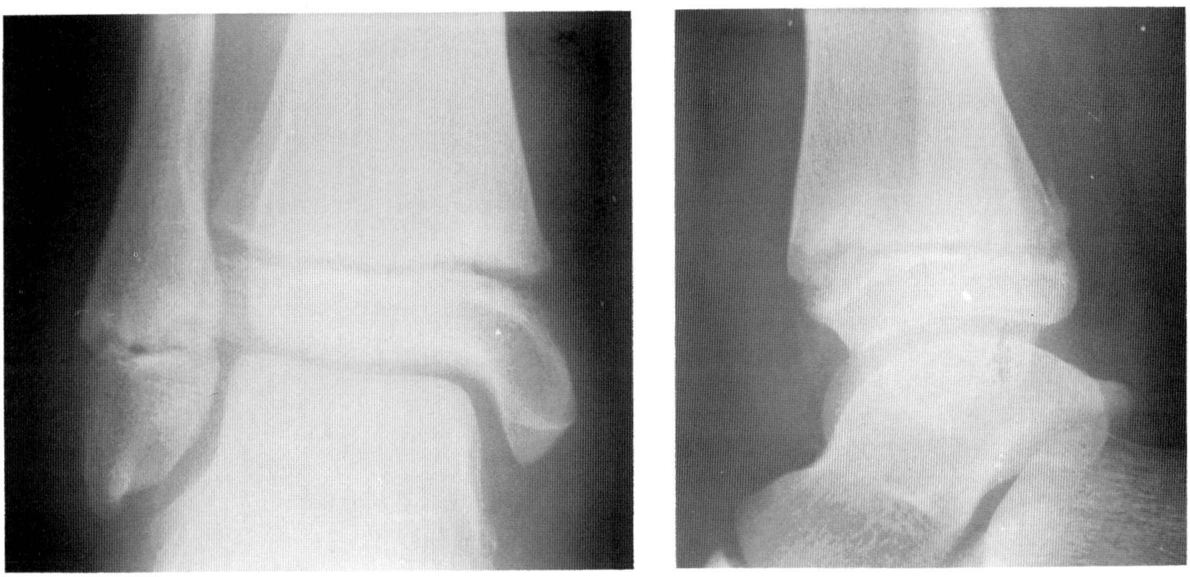

b

Fig. 42.27 Anteroposterior radiograph (a) of Type II epiphyseal displacement. There is also slight displacement of the fibular epiphysis. Lateral radiograph (b) of Type II epiphyseal displacement

Beauchamp C G, Clay N R, Thexton P W 1983 Displaced ankle fractures in patients over 50 years of age. J Bone Joint Surg (Br) 65B: 329–332

Brodie I A O D, Denham R A 1974 The treatment of unstable ankle fractures. J Bone Joint Surg (Br) 56B: 256–262

Cedell C A 1967 Supination outward rotation injuries of the ankle. Acta Orthop Scand (Suppl) 110: Munksgaard, Copenhagen

Cooperman D R, Spiegel P G, Laros G B 1978 Tibial fractures involving the ankle in children. J Bone Joint Surg (Am) 60A: 1040–1046

Cox F J, Laxson W W 1952 Fractures about the ankle joint. Am J Surg 83: 674

Danis R 1949 Les fractures malléolaires. In: Théorie et practique de l'ostéosynthèse. Masson, Paris

Dupuytren G 1819 Of fractures of the lower extremity of the fibula and luxation of the foot. Reprinted in 1939, Medical Classics 4: 151–172

Georgen T G, Danzig L A, Resnick D, Owen C 1977 Roentgenographic evaluation of the tibio-fibular joint. J Bone Joint Surg (Am) 59A: 874–877

Iselin M, De Vellis H 1961 La primauté du péroné dans les fractures du cou-de-pied. Mém Acad Chir 87: 399
Joy G, Patzakis M J, Harvey J P 1974 Precise evaluation of the reduction of severe ankle fractures. J Bone Joint Surg (Am) 56A: 979–997
Lauge-Hansen N 1942 Ankel brud I genetisk diagnose og reposition. Diss: Munksgaard København
Lauge-Hansen N 1950 Fractures of the ankle. Arch Surg 60: 957
Lauge-Hansen N 1953 Fractures of the ankle. Arch Surg 67: 813
Lauge-Hansen N 1954 Fractures of the ankle III. Genetic roentgenologic diagnosis of the fractures of the ankle. Am J Roentgenol 71: 456
Lynn M D 1972 The triplane distal tibial epiphyseal fracture. Clin Orthop 86: 187–190
Maisonneuve J G 1840 Recherches sur la fracture due perone. Arch Gen de Med 7: 165–187, 433–473
Marmor L 1970 An unusual fracture of the tibial epiphysis. Clin Orthop 73: 132–135
Neer C S 1953 II Injuries of the ankle joint — evaluation. Conn St Med J 17: 580–583
Picaud A J 1953 Reflexions a propos d'un traitement chirurgical simple des fractures recentes de la cheville. Rev Chir Orthop 39: 70
Pott P 1768 Some few general remarks on fractures and dislocations. Hawes, Clarke, Collins; London
Ramsey P L, Hamilton W 1976 Changes in the tibio-talar area of contact caused by lateral talar shift. J Bone Joint Surg (Am) 58A: 356–357
Rochet V 1890 Du mécanisme des luxations doubles de l'astragule. Rev Orthop 1: 269
Salter R B, Harris W R 1963 Injuries involving the epiphyseal plate. J Bone Joint Surg (Am) 45A: 587–622
Sarkisian J S, Cody G W 1976 Closed treatment of ankle fractures: A new criterion for evaluation. A review of 250 cases. J Trauma 16: 323
Spiegel P G, Cooperman D R, Laros G S 1978 Epiphyseal fractures of the distal ends of the tibia and fibula. J Bone Joint Surg (Am) 60A: 1046–1050
Tilleaux (reported by Gosselin) 1872 Rapports recherches, cliniques et experimentales sur les fractures malleolaires. Bulletin de l'Académie de Médecine Series 2; 1: 817
Torg J S, Ruggiero R A 1975 Comminuted epiphyseal fractures of the distal tibia. Clin Orthop 110: 215–217
Weber B G 1966 Die verletzungen des oberen sprunggelenkes. In: Aktuelle probleme in der chirurgie 3. Verlag Hans Huber, Bern und Stuttgart
Yablon I G, Heller F G, Shouse L 1977 The key role of the lateral malleolus in displaced fractures of the ankle. J Bone Joint Surg (Am) 59A: 169–173
Yde J 1980 The Lauge-Hansen classification of malleolar fractures. Acta Orthop Scand 51: 181

LIGAMENTOUS INJURIES

Damage to the lateral ligaments of the ankle is one of the most frequent injuries that presents in the Casualty Department; about half occurring as a result of athletic activity (Lindstrand 1976). The majority of these injuries affect the outer side of the joint. This predilection for the lateral ligaments is mainly due to supination of the foot which tightens these structures as the patient turns. There is also evidence that damage to the medial ligament results in very little instability of the ankle (Yablon et al 1977), so that complaints are fewer in comparison with the lateral side.

Stability of the ankle

Bones

The ankle owes much of its stability to the joint geometry. Compared to the knee it is very stable, particularly when in dorsiflexion; a position which brings the widest part of the talus into the tibiofibular mortice and prevents lateral movements. As the ankle plantarflexes, the malleoli remain in close contact with the talus due to rotation of the tibia on the talus and rotation of the fibula. There is enough elasticity in the tibiofibular ligaments to allow an intermalleolar expansion of 1–2 mm.

Ligaments

On the outer side of the joint the collateral ligament is arranged to give protection in all positions of the ankle.

The anterior talofibular ligament runs forwards from the anterior and lower part of the fibula to the neck of the talus and is about 2 cm in length and 1 cm broad (Fig. 42.28). It is tense in all positions of the joint. When this ligament is cut, the talus can be displaced forwards and rotated in a medial direction (Dehne 1933, Anderson et al 1952).

The middle or calcaneofibular ligament (Fig. 42.28) which runs obliquely down and backwards from the tip of the malleolus to the lateral surface of the calcaneum is rather thicker than the anterior part with a diameter of 4–8 mm and is only tense when the heel is inverted, so that mostly it is relaxed. When the ankle is plantarflexed it is almost at a right angle to the fibula. The fibres have a close association with the peroneus tendon sheath (Fig. 42.28) so that its disruption almost always leads to a defect in the

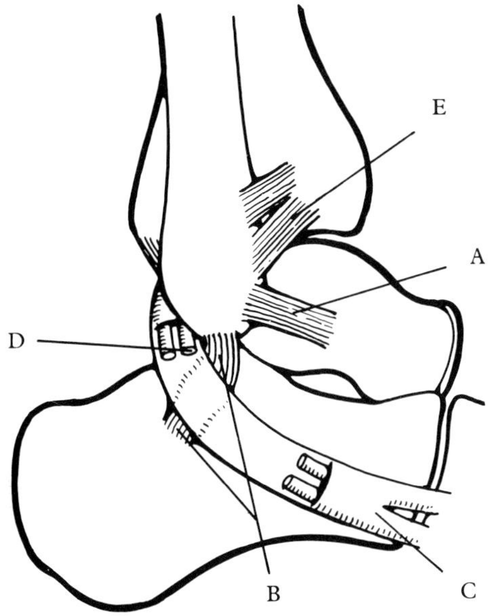

Fig. 42.28 Ligaments on the outer side of the ankle and hindfoot. A = Anterior talofibular ligament; B = Calcaneofibular ligament; C = Peroneal tendon sheath; D = Peroneus longus and brevis tendons; E = Anterior tibiofibular ligament

sheath. When the ligament is tensed by full supination of the foot, it can be palpated.

The posterior component runs horizontally backwards from the malleolus to the posterolateral part of the talus. The ligament is lax when the foot is in neutral position.

The deltoid ligament is fan-shaped and its lower insertion curves downwards and backwards from the navicular bone across the calcaneum to the posterior part of the talus. When cut, it produces surprisingly little instability of the ankle in contradistinction to lateral ligamentous injuries. Brostrom (1964) also stated that partial tears in none of his cases gave rise to any instability.

The tibiofibular ligaments (Fig. 42.28) contribute to the stability of the ankle joint. The anterior component which may be torn by external rotational movements of the foot, particularly when the latter is supinated, has superficial fibres some 2–3 cm in length. The ligament is tensed by dorsiflexion of the foot or by outward rotation of the talus.

The central ligament is in reality the distal part of the tibiofibular interosseous membrane.

The posterior component runs distally from the posterior tibial process to the posterior margin of the lateral malleolus.

Muscles

To a considerable degree the evertors of the foot, the peronei, can contribute to the stability of the ankle. Indeed, Freeman et al (1965) pointed out that lack of muscular control would explain the giving way of the ankle which may occur after injury in those joints which appear to be unstable even when stress radiographs do not demonstrate any ligamentous laxity. Freeman suggested that this was due to a proprioceptive deficit and showed that retraining by a physiotherapist will often restore stability. Furthermore, it is not uncommon to find more laxity in the 'normal' ankle when both are submitted to stress in order to investigate a joint which is continually giving way.

Capsule

This structure will also give some degree of stability and the extent to which it is torn can be correlated statistically with the anterior displacement possible when carrying out stress films — the greater the extent of the capsular lesion, the greater the anterior instability (Lindstrand 1976).

Clinical

97% of all ankle ligament ruptures occur on the anterolateral side (Brostrom 1965). Most ruptures involve the anterior talofibular ligament only, but 25% of these are combined with tearing of the calcaneofibular ligament and 10% also involve the anterior tibiofibular ligament. In Brostrom's series the anterior talofibular ligament was torn in 90 of 99 sprains that were explored and in 24 the calcaneofibular ligament was torn, though this was never in isolation.

Unlike the knee, which when it buckles, may do so in a way which the patient finds difficult to describe, most will appreciate that the supinated foot has gone into varus at the ankle. There is immediate severe pain and in a high proportion of cases the patient may be aware of an audible crack. This latter feature is less common in those cases with a previous history of giving way. Weight bearing is immediately difficult because of pain and more rarely, of a sensation of instability.

Bruising appears within the next 24 hours on the

outer side of the heel extending forwards to the area of the fifth metatarsal and occasionally into the outer toes. In about a quarter of cases the patients have difficulty in putting weight on the injured side.

Examination will reveal tenderness which is maximal over the torn fasciculus, most frequently only the anterior. Any attempt to displace the foot forwards at the ankle or to invert the heel is very painful. Brostrom (1965) found that in 40% of cases the tenderness was diffuse and offered a poor guide to differentiation of the site of the ligamentous tear.

The degree of anterior instability can be investigated by the anterior drawer test. To carry this out the patient lies supine on a couch with the hip and knee flexed. One hand is placed behind the heel to fix it and the opposite hand on the shin. Sudden backwards pressure is then exerted over the shin and, if the test is positive, will cause pain at the site of the torn ligament. In a high proportion of those cases in which the anterior fasciculus has been torn there is visible forward movement of the talus in the tibiofibular mortice. Actual forward movement is, however, often difficult to demonstrate in the unanaesthetized patient.

In a proportion of cases it is also possible to demonstrate increased inversion of the heel on the affected side. This test is best carried out with the patient prone and the feet clear of the lower end of the couch. Forced supination of the feet will invert the heels and the two sides can be compared. This test is most frequently positive in those cases in which the calcaneofibular ligament is also torn. Because of pain it is often difficult to carry out this part of the examination without the help of anaesthesia. Since this adjunct will be needed for producing stress films, it is better to arrange that this part of the clinical examination, if very painful, is only done when radiography has been arranged.

Radiographic investigation

Straight films

Anteroposterior and lateral films should be carried out. These will exclude the presence of any fractures, the presence of fluid in the joint and also record soft tissue swelling. Osteochondral fractures of the talus may be associated with 5% of sprained ankles and should be looked for, since failure to treat them will lead to continuing symptoms. Should the degree of soft tissue injury suggest significant damage to the ligamentous structure, it is wise to proceed to stress radiography even if instability has not been diagnosed on the initial clinical examination.

Stress radiography

This is best carried out with the aid of anaesthesia. In most cases local anaesthetic is sufficient. Up to 10 cc of Marcain® may be necessary and this should be injected into the painful areas until it is possible to manipulate the hindfoot with reasonable comfort. Most will only need to be injected on the lateral side of the joint but the medial side should also be anaesthetized if this has been damaged and is painful. Because of the degree of swelling that is already present in the acutely injured ankle, some care should be exercised to ensure that an excessive amount of fluid is not used.

Stress films will need to be taken in two planes, anteroposterior and lateral, and on both occasions the opposite ankle should be taken as a control. Enquiries as to previous episodes of giving way in this joint should be made, as it is not uncommon for this also to be unstable.

AP inversion stress films (Fig. 42.29)

Care must be taken to have the joint in the correct position as the film is taken, namely about 15° of internal rotation. The patient should be informed as to what is to happen and asked to relax as much as possible. Since despite the introduction of local anaesthetic there may still be some pain in extreme inversion of the heel, it is essential to have the patient's cooperation and furthermore the inverted position should only be held for a few seconds as the film is taken.

Lateral stress films

This should follow immediately after the AP stress film of the anaesthetized ankle. The patient will need to be supine and the hip and knee flexed to about 30° with the aid of support behind the heel and thigh. A load of 4 kg is applied to the shin by means of sandbags laid over it. Once more it is necessary to have the cooperation of the patient so that relaxation

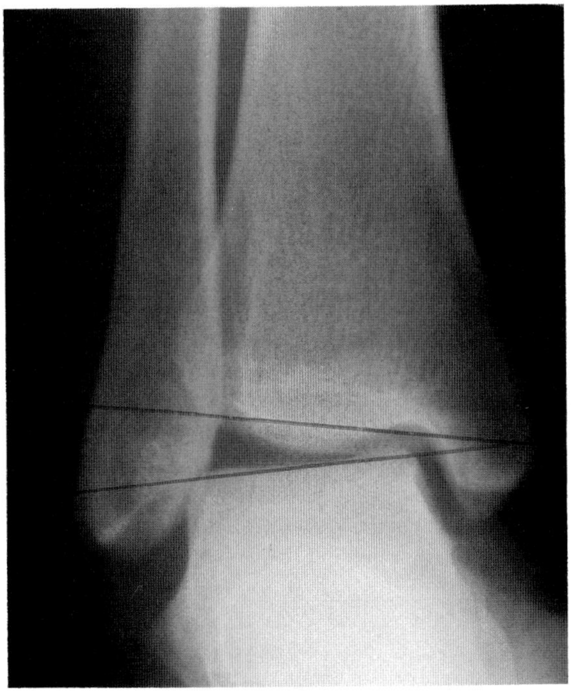

Fig. 42.29 Anterior stress film showing talar tilt

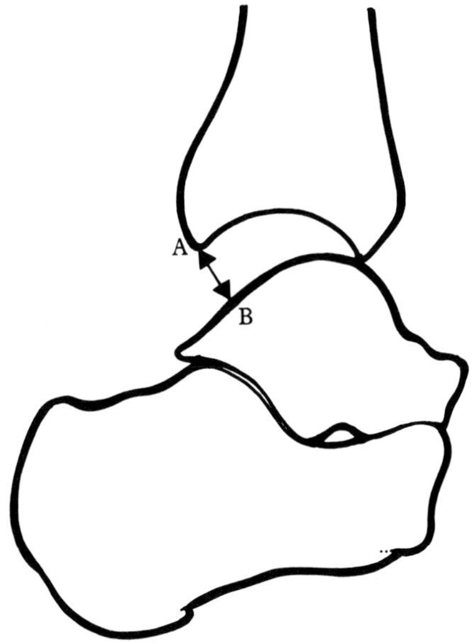

Fig. 42.30 Lateral stress film showing anterior talar subluxation. The arrowed measurement between the most posterior part of the tibial joint surface and the nearest part of the talus represents the amount of subluxation

is obtained. A lateral view of the ankle is taken after the load has been applied for not less than two minutes (Fig. 42.30).

Interpretation of stress films. The lateral stress film is evaluated by measuring the distance from the back of the dome of the talus to the posterior surface of the tibial joint surface as in the diagram (Fig. 42.31). The normal degree of separation has been variously estimated as 4 mm in adults with no history of previous injury (Laurin & Mathieu 1975), 5 mm by Castaing and Delplace (1972) and 2.5–3 mm by Landeros et al (1968). Lindstrand (1976) considered that 3 mm was the upper limit of normal.

After experimental section of the anterior talofibular ligament, Castaing & Delplace (1972) found a displacement of 8–10 mm and in all probability anything over 5 mm is pathological. Laurin & Mathieu (1975) pointed out that forward displacement in the normal ankle was unaltered or even less when the ankle was in plantar flexion. If, however, the anterior talofibular ligament was torn then displacement, if anything, was greater in this position.

Since the anterior talofibular ligament is the first to tear in an acute sprain of the ankle, the anterior displacement is of greater importance than measurement of talar tilt. This latter angle may vary considerably even in 'normal' ankles and Rubin & Witten (1960) found a range from 3–23°. Brostrom (1965), in the ankles in which exploration was carried out and a tear confirmed, found a talar tilt angle of 5–23° in 14 out of 47 cases in which both calcaneofibular and anterior talofibular ligaments were injured and 5–16° in 30 out of 158 cases with isolated rupture of the anterior talofibular ligament. Certainly the angle may be significantly increased in hypermobile ankles and may even be as high as 25° (Bonnin 1944). Examination of other joints in the upper limbs may give some measure of the joint laxity, but nevertheless examination of both ankles should be carried out, so that a direct comparison may be made. The difference is usually less than 10° (Laurin et al 1968).

Stress tenography

Evans & Frenyo (1979) claim that more accurate diagnosis of the degree of collateral ligament damage can be made by tenography of the peroneal tendons. They state that the tendon sheath is almost invariably torn when there is involvement of the

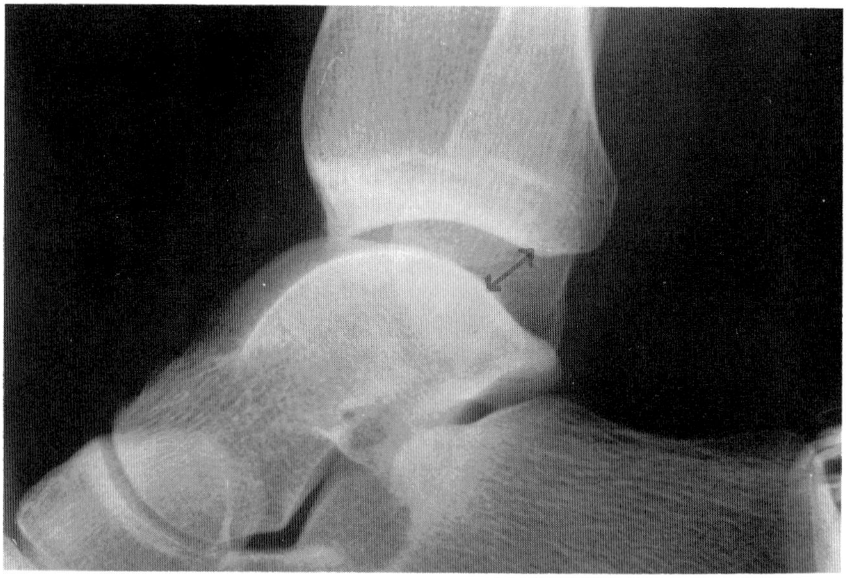

Fig. 42.31 The forward shift of the talus. The distance indicated between the posterior part of the tibia and the nearest part of the talar dome represents the displacement

calcaneofibular ligament (Fig. 42.32). As a result fluid leaks into the joint (Figs. 42.33 and 34). Of 16 cases in which only the anterior fasciculus was ruptured, there was no leakage into the joint. In 12 cases in which the calcaneofibular ligament was ruptured, 11 gave a positive result. All their cases were operated on and the pathology confirmed. The one case that gave a false negative did not appear to have ruptured the peroneal sheath.

Arthrography

This investigation in general gives very little help in the diagnosis of ligament injury. If leakage occurs from the joint, it is almost invariably anteriorly when the anterior fasciculus and adjoining capsule have ruptured and only unusually does fluid get into the peroneal sheath and indicate damage to the calcaneofibular ligament (Fig. 42.35).

Brostrom et al (1965) found that leakage in front of the lateral malleolus was associated with fresh ruptures of the anterior talofibular ligament. Appearance of contrast medium in the peroneal sheath was often related to tearing of the calcaneofibular ligament, but this could be misleading in those cases with a previous history of ankle sprain.

Some leakage in front of the tibiofibular syndesmosis always occurred with acute rupture of the anterior tibiofibular ligament and this lesion was usually complete (Fig. 42.35). Leakage on the inner side of the ankle followed tearing of the deltoid ligament, though this was invariably an incomplete rupture.

On occasions an arthrogram may show up a cartilage fracture or perhaps an osteochondral fragment, which might otherwise have been missed due to the osseous component being small. This is a procedure which should be carried out if the patient continues to have symptoms despite adequate treatment.

Subtalar tomography

This investigation is probably unnecessary in acute ankle injuries. In the unstable ankle, however, when no significant degree of talar tilt is apparent, useful information may be gained. Brantigan et al (1977) reported three cases in which subtalar instability was thought to be the cause of the patient's symptoms. They showed that the subtalar inversion angle averaged 38° with a standard deviation of 6°, whilst in feet that were symptomatic the tilt was 57° with a deviation of 5°. The tests were carried out with the foot in dorsiflexion; a position in which the calcaneofibular ligament is tight.

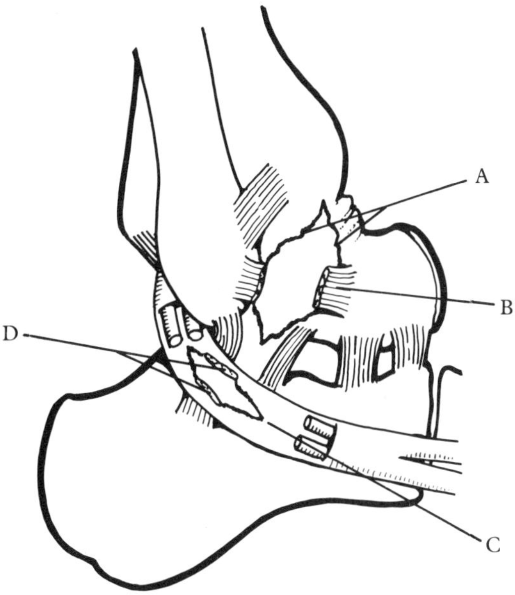

Fig. 42.32 Tear of anterior capsule of the ankle joint, A, with associated tear of anterior talofibular ligament, B. Tear of peroneal tendon sheath C, and tear of underlying calcaneofibular ligament, D

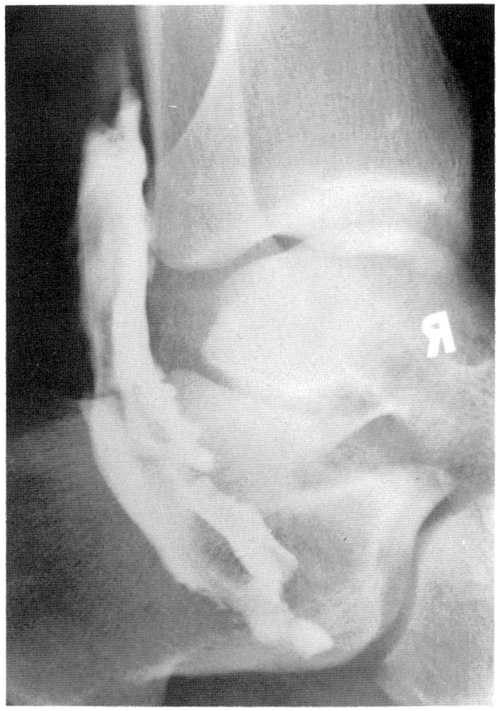

Fig. 42.33 Peroneal tenogram with no leakage, indicating an intact tendon sheath and integrity of the calcaneofibular ligament

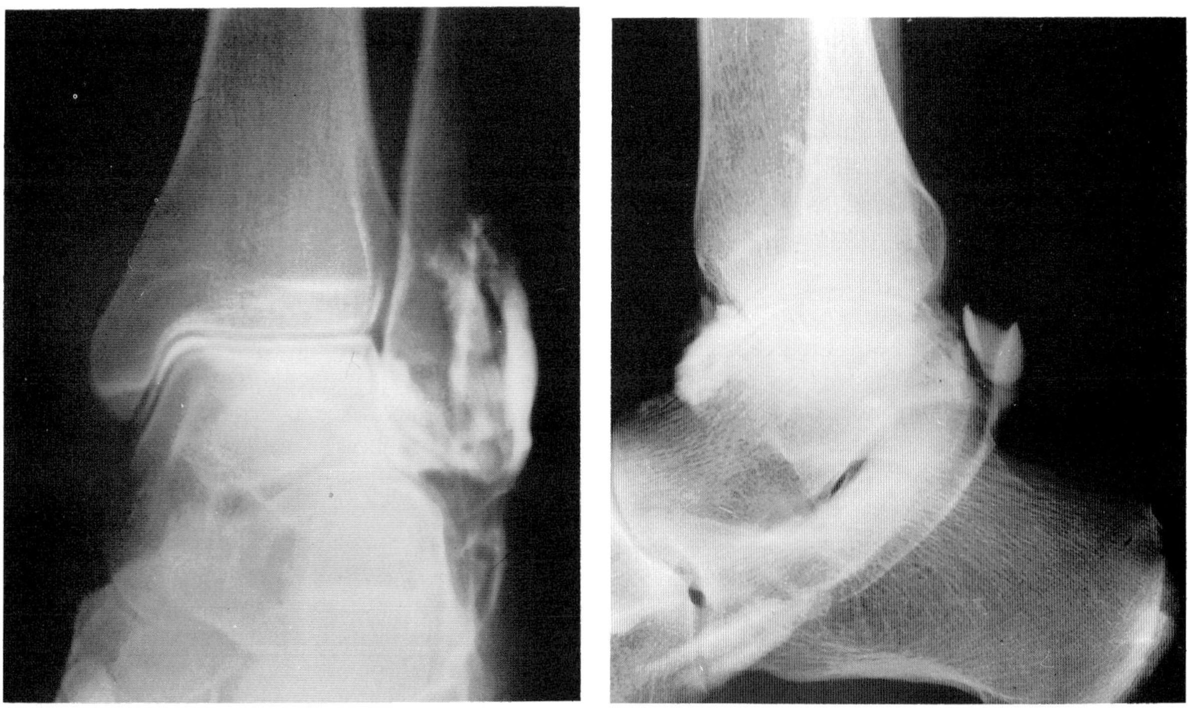

Fig. 42.34 Peroneal tenogram with leakage into the joint space, indicating a tear of the calcaneofibular ligament

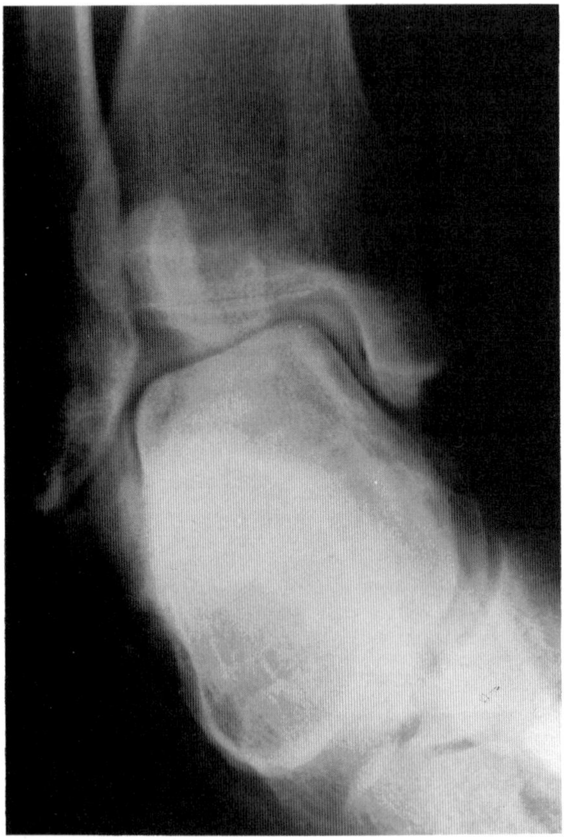

Fig. 42.35 Arthrogram of ankle. The degree of talar tilt indicates that the calaneofibular ligament is probably torn and this would be confirmed by the leak of fluid into the peroneal tendon sheath. There is also some leakage upwards from the syndesmosis, suggesting that the tibiofibular ligament is also torn

Treatment

This will depend on the stability of the joint. If there is no demonstrable instability either clinically or radiographically, then it may well be that no more than symptomatic treatment is necessary. Should there be no obvious bruising, a negative anterior draw sign and only some local tenderness and swelling, then local heat and analgesics may be all that is necessary. The patient should, however, be able to walk without a limp and sometimes the application of strapping with the foot in neutral position will help.

If the joint seems to be more painful even when apparently stable, then two weeks in a brace will accelerate the patient's recovery.

The unstable ankle

If this has been confirmed by radiography, then the choice lies between plaster immobilization (Leonard 1949, Chirls 1973, Gross & MacIntosh 1973), by primary surgical repair (Ruth 1961, Brostrom 1966, Staples 1975), early mobilization (Freeman 1965, Jackson et al 1974) or finally the use of a brace which to some extent combines the advantages of early mobilization with lateral support for the ankle and subtalar joints.

Treatment by plaster cast fixation has been practised by many surgeons (Ruth 1961, Freeman 1965, Chirls 1973, Gross & MacIntosh 1973, Staples 1975) and there is no doubt that it leads in most cases to a fairly acceptable result. Freeman (1965) found that it was as long as a year before the patient was symptomless and this compared with 12 weeks in those patients who had been actively mobilized. The delay in recovery was largely due to persistent stiffness and pain. Ruth (1961) reported that of 72 patients, all regained satisfactory function, but that only two-thirds were stable. Staples (1975) found that 59% had no symptoms after an average folow-up of nine years, but two out of 68 were seriously disabled.

Unfortunately in all the series there is no easy way of making a comparison between the original injuries and no exact criteria of the degree of recovery. It seems probable, however, that most patients obtain a satisfactory result, but the recovery time is at least six months and may be as long as a year.

Most authors favour suture of the affected ligament in the young and athletic since by this means a mechanically stable ankle is thought to be a more likely end result (Ruth 1961, Brostrom 1966, Staples 1975). Desirable as this may be, it should be pointed out that it is only gained at the expense of a much longer convalescent period and also the risks, both general and local of surgery. Indeed, Freeman (1965) pointed out that the advantages over early mobilization were not striking and that there tended to be persistent pain and swelling and some loss of movement.

In Brostrom's large series (1966) which he reported in some detail, he found that immobilization in plaster or by strapping gave residual symptoms in about 20% of cases. In only 5 out of 95 cases were these symptoms of any severity and were all concerned with giving way. On the other hand, surgery was followed by instability in only 3% of cases. The period of time off work was very much longer after operation and averaged 45 days as opposed to 18 days after strapping. Furthermore, operation led to some increased stiffness of the subtalar joint.

Brostrom's conclusions were that surgery was only indicated in the young and athletic and particularly if there was a history of previous episodes which predisposed to more instability after conservative treatment. He further pointed out that there was some increased risk from postoperative infection and scar discomfort and traumatic neuromata. His investigation of the state of ligaments in cases explored even after some years disclosed that they were relatively little changed and that suture at a late stage was quite feasible. Few surgeons appear to have utilized this important possibility and almost all late repairs have been treated by tenodesis or by artificial implants.

Finally, treatment by a brace may be advocated. This method has the advantages that early movement of the ankle is encouraged and in consequence there is more rapid absorption of the haematoma and oedema; the nutrition of the articular cartilage is encouraged from the start of treatment and there is significantly less muscle wasting. Furthermore, there is evidence that ligaments undergo atrophy as a result of immobilization (Noyes 1977), and that they only slowly recover their normal strength. The author is of the opinion that this method has a real advantage over other methods.

The brace, whilst allowing plantar and dorsiflexion of the ankle, gives lateral stability and prevents inversion and eversion of the heel. Immediately it is fitted, in most cases the patient will spontaneously lose his limp and walk with a normal gait. In those cases that continue to limp a physiotherapy session almost invariably will cure it. A period of three weeks will allow stability to be regained and the brace can then be removed. Exercises and training on a wobble board thereafter will allow a rapid return to sporting activities. A review of 42 cases, all sporting injuries, treated in this way showed that, with one exception, all returned to their sport. Most were engaged in soccer. 22 of these cases had instability confirmed by radiography. In the remaining 20, the diagnosis was clinical; lack of time or of radiographic facilities prevented strain films being carried out in these cases. Although some complained of continuing soreness, none was affected by the ankle giving way, with one exception. This patient complained of his ankle giving way occasionally but had been able to resume his sport of hockey. Further stress films in this case failed to show any evidence of mechanical instability.

Although there are claims that suture of the ligament followed by immobilization gives the best hope of producing a mechanically stable ankle (Ruth 1961, Freeman 1965), any form of plaster fixation, particularly if associated with surgery, is likely to be followed by pain, stiffness and swelling in a proportion of cases. Furthermore, the period of rehabilitation is long and at least six weeks are required after removal of the plaster to regain full movement. In those cases treated in a brace, 12 complained of pain, though in none was it serious, and only one complained of stiffness.

A brace has the advantage of allowing the hygiene of the foot to be continued (an important point in athletes), since the heel piece can be removed for this purpose. The period of rehabilitation is rapid, since joint movement is satisfactory when it is removed and there is rarely any serious muscle wasting. Two patients, in both of whom there was radiographic instability, were able to return to first team football in the first division within five weeks of the injury occurring. They have had no further trouble after 28 and 32 months.

The author is of the opinion that all cases, certainly after significant ligamentous tears, are best referred to a physiotherapist when any splinting has been removed since this will allow the redevelopment of proprioception on a wobble board. There seems good reason to think that functional instability of the foot is often due to motor incoordination consequent on articular deafferentation which can be relieved by suitable retraining exercises (Freeman 1965).

Method of application of support

Strapping. Elastoplast® is to be preferred to nonextensible strapping since the risks of skin damage or arterial occlusion are less because of its elasticity. The material should be applied with the foot in neutral or certainly no more than slight eversion. A figure-of-eight is used and the strapping taken across the sole of the foot to the outer side so that it will be reasonably tense as it is drawn upwards and across the front of the ankle joint.

Patients should be advised to remove the strapping themselves if they feel that it is too tight and not to wait until they can return to hospital; should they remove it further advice should be sought urgently.

Plaster. A below-knee plaster is applied with the foot in neutral position and the ankle at a right angle. Light material such as Scotchcast® is preferable since it allows the patient to walk with a more satisfactory gait. Both with strapping and plaster a period of 24 or 48 hours with the leg in elevation may be necessary if the swelling is very severe. Early change of plaster may be advisable if it should become loose due to the resolution of swelling. Provided the patient is comfortable in plaster, weight bearing should be encouraged.

Brace. This needs to be constructed from light materials if the patient is to walk with a normal gait. In practice, Scotchcast® has been found very satisfactory. A well fitting gaiter from below knee to the ankle is applied (Fig. 42.36). This is then followed by the application of a plastic heel piece held by two lateral plastic hinges (Fig. 42.37). A velcro strap across the insole holds the heel piece in position (Fig. 42.38). Initially, this was arranged so that the hinges could be pulled out of the gaiter but it was found that this method was often followed by damage to the brace. In consequence the hinges are now fixed firmly to the gaiter. The hinges are pliable enough to enable the patient to take the heel piece backwards when the strap is undone so that hygiene can be carried out. In most cases only one brace is required but occasionally if the swelling around the joint has been severe, replacement at the end of a week may be necessary. Unusually, the patient walks with a limp and, if so, some instruction by a physiotherapist will correct this. In all cases if there is any sensation of instability, retraining on a wobble board should be advised before it becomes established and further injury occurs.

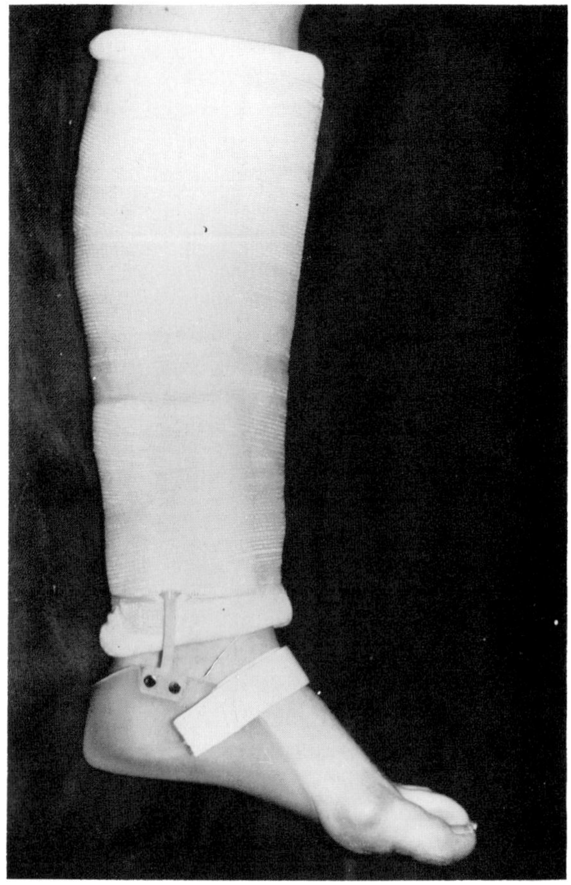

Fig. 42.36 Scotchcast gaiter

Surgery

If it is decided that surgery is necessary, then it should be carried out as soon as possible after the original injury, although a short period of delay to reduce swelling may be advisable if this is excessive.

The skin incision should start in front of the fibula about 5 cm over the tip of the malleolus (Fig. 42.39). It passes downwards and curves backwards just below the malleolus. Care should be taken to identify and preserve the lateral branch of the deep peroneal nerve and the sural nerves. The fascia is divided in the line of the skin incision to expose the anterior talofibular ligament. The calcaneofibular and posterior talofibular ligaments are exposed by incising the peroneal tendon sheath and then retracting the tendon posteriorly and downwards. The joint will have to be opened since there is invariably an associated capsular tear and the joint surfaces should be inspected as far as possible by subluxating the joint by internal rotation of the talus. Any debris should be washed out. Any sizeable

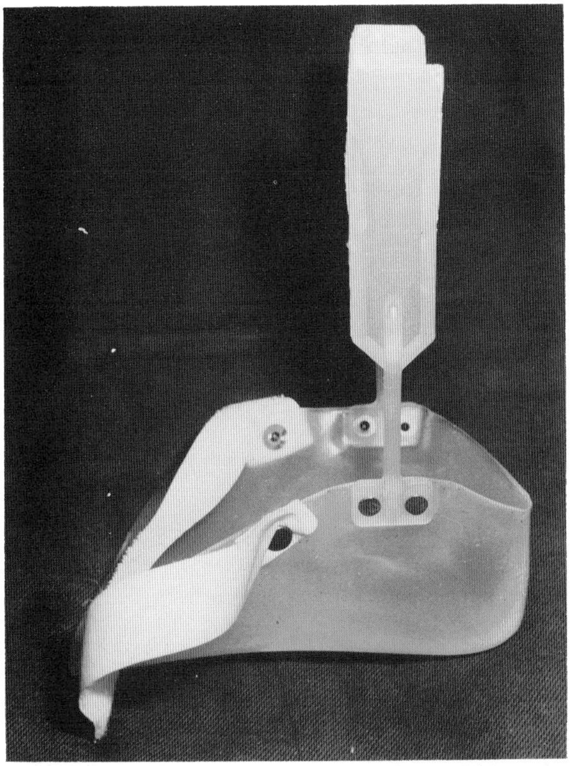

Fig. 42.37 Plastic heel support with lateral hinges which can be slotted into the side of the gaiter

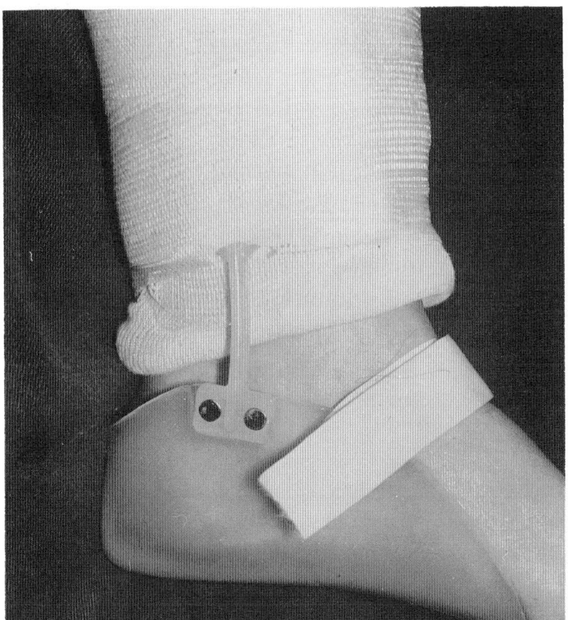

Fig. 42.38 Detail of Fig. 42.36

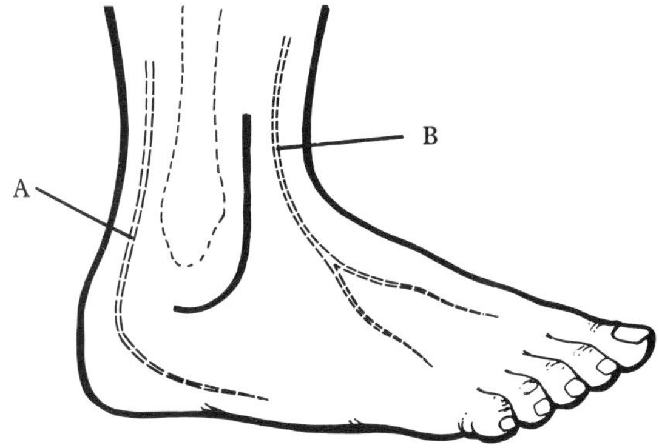

Fig. 42.39 Incision for repair of lateral collateral ligament of the ankle. A = Sural nerve; B = Deep peroneal nerve

osteochondral fracture should be reduced. When the tears have been identified, the ends should be approximated by an absorbable suture material such as Dexon®.

After wound closure a below-knee plaster should be applied with the ankle and foot in neutral position. This should be removed in three weeks and active foot exercises encouraged under the supervision of a physiotherapist.

A return to active sport should not be recommended until virtually full movement has been regained and the ankle feels stable. This period may vary from three to six months.

REFERENCES

Anderson K, Lecocq J, Lecocq E 1952 Recurrent anterior subluxation of the ankle joint. A report of two cases and an experimental study. J Bone Joint Surg (Am) 34A: 853–860

Bonnin J 1944 Injuries to the ankle. William Heinemann Medical Books Ltd, London

Brantigan J W, Pedegana L R, Lippert F G 1977 Instability of the subtalar joint. J Bone Joint Surg (Am) 59: 321–324

Brostrom L 1964 Sprained ankles I: Anatomic lesions in recent sprains. Acta Chir Scand 128: 483–495

Brostrom L, Liljedahl S O, Lindvall N 1965 Sprained ankles II: Arthrographic diagnosis of recent ligament ruptures. Acta Chir Scand 129: 584–599

Brostrom L 1965 Sprained ankles III: Clinical observations in recent ligament ruptures. Acta Chir Scand 130: 560–569

Brostrom L 1966 Sprained ankles V: Treatment and prognosis in recent ligament ruptures. Acta Chir Scand 132: 537–550

Castaing J, Delplace J 1972 Entorse de la cheville intérêt de l'étude de la stabilité dans le plan sagittal pour le diagnostic de granite. Rev Chir Orth 58: 51–63

Chirls M 1973 Inversion injuries of the ankle. J Med Soc New Jersey 70: 751–755

Dehne E 1933 Die klinik der frischen und habituellen adduktions-supinations distorsion des fusses. Deutsch Zschr 242: 40–61

Evans G A, Frenyo S D 1979 The stress tenogram in the diagnosis of ruptures of the lateral ligament of the ankle. J Bone Joint Surg (Br) 61B: 347–351
Freeman M A R 1965 Treatment of ruptures of the lateral ligament of the ankle. J Bone Joint Surg (Br) 47B: 661–668
Freeman M A R, Dean M R E, Hanham I W F 1965 The etiology and functional instability of the foot. J Bone Joint Surg (Br) 47B: 678–685
Gross A E, MacIntosh D L 1973 Injury to the lateral ligament of the ankle: A clinical study. Can J Surg 16: 115–117
Jackson D W, Ashley R L, Powell J W 1974 Ankle sprains in young athletes. Clin Orthop 101: 201–215
Landeros O, Frost H, Higgins C 1968 Post-traumatic ankle instability. Clin Orthop 56: 169–178
Laurin C A, Ouellet R, St. Jacques R 1968 Talar and subtalar tilt: An experimental investigation. Can J Surg 11: 270–279
Laurin C, Mathieu J 1975 Sagittal mobility of the normal ankle. Clin Orthop 108: 99–104
Leonard M H 1949 Injuries of the lateral ligaments of the ankle. J Bone Joint Surg (Am) 31A: 373–377
Lindstrand A 1976 Lateral lesions in sprained ankle. The University Hospital S-221 85 Lund, Sweden
Noyes F R 1977 Functional properties of knee ligaments and alteration induced by immobilisation. Clin Orthop 123: 210–242
Rubin G, Witten M 1960 The talar tilt angle and the fibular collateral ligaments. J Bone Joint Surg (Am) 42A: 311–326
Ruth C J 1961 The surgical treatment of injuries of the fibular collateral ligaments of the ankle. J Bone Joint Surg (Am) 43A: 229–239
Staples O S 1975 Ruptures of the fibular collateral ligaments of the ankle. Result study of immediate surgical treatment. J Bone Joint Surg (Am) 57A: 101–107
Yablon I G, Heller F G, Shouse L 1977 The key role of the lateral malleolus in displaced fractures of the ankle. J Bone Joint Surg (Am) 59A: 169–173

RUPTURE OF TIBIALIS ANTERIOR TENDON

Four patients were reported by Dooley et al (1980) who also reviewed the literature. This tendon ruptures uncommonly and the literature is scanty. Mensor & Ordway (1953) reported two cases and recalled ten more.

Patients are almost invariably over the age of 45 and present with weakness of dorsiflexion and swelling about the ankle. If trauma has occurred, it is usually mild. There may be transient episodes of pain before final rupture occurs.

Patients leading a fairly active life, particularly if rupture has occurred within the last three months, are best treated surgically. The rupture usually occurs within 0.5 cm of the insertion (Dooley et al 1980) and direct suture is often possible. In those cases where there has been excessive tendon retraction, suture to the long extensor of the first toe will help. Following surgery the results are reasonably satisfactory.

RUPTURE OF TIBIALIS POSTERIOR TENDON

Little interest has been shown in the condition until the review published by Mann & Thompson in 1985. Spontaneous rupture was reported by Kettlekamp & Alexander (1969) who stated that it was more likely to occur in association with nonspecific tenosynovitis. Griffiths (1965) reported four cases (three of them traumatic) and emphasized the need for urgent surgery. He found that poor results followed late repair. Mann & Thompson described 17 cases. All were patients presenting with a flat foot deformity, mostly for a long period. In 10 cases there was a specific injury.

The condition is characterized by a progressive collapse of the longitudinal arch, the os calcis going into a valgus position, the talus plantarflexing and the forefoot adducting, so that the foot has a pronated appearance. Pain is felt near or distal to the medial malleolus. Patients find that their walking distance becomes limited and there is increasing difficulty with footwear due to its distortion.

Examination reveals that the deformity is unilateral and the forefoot is adducted. The os calcis does not invert when the patient is asked to stand on tip toe. The tibialis posterior tendon cannot be felt or seen on attempted inversion, though this is not always easy in a normal foot. Finally, radiographs will demonstrate the deformity when compared with the normal side.

Treatment

Surgery is the treatment of choice. Unfortunately, the initial symptoms are not usually severe and the patient may not seek advice until the deformity is well established. If possible the tendon should be sutured, with advancement if necessary. Failing this, tendon transfer should be carried out. Mann & Thompson (1985) advocate the use of the flexor digitorum longus and reported good results for pain relief, although the deformity was not always corrected. The tendon is passed through the tibialis posterior sheath and fixed to a drill hole in the navicular. The distal part of the toe flexor is attached to the flexor of the first toe.

In the event that the deformity is very fixed with osteoarthritic changes in the foot, some relief may be given by a moulded arch support. Arthrodesis of the calcaneocuboid and talonavicular joints may be considered if pain continues. These joints, however, are not always easy to fuse, particularly when there is sclerotic bone, and older patients do not always do well with foot arthrodesis.

Traumatic dislocation of the tibialis posterior tendon has also been reported by Nava (1968). This occurred as the result of a road traffic accident. It was associated with an avulsion fracture of the lateral malleolus. Surgical reduction was carried out and the retinaculum sutured. The final result was excellent.

RUPTURE OF THE PERONEAL TENDONS

This appears to be very rare. Abraham & Stirnaman (1979) recorded a case, but could find no other similar patients after a search of the literature. They do, however, suggest that this condition may be more common than is thought, due to failure of diagnosis.

The case reported was only diagnosed at 3½ years, although a negative exploration was carried out after 18 months: subsequently thought to have been inadequate.

The condition is characterized by weak eversion of the hindfoot and symptoms of pain and ankle instability.

End-to-end anastomosis 42 months after the injury is reported to have given a good result.

REFERENCES

Abraham E, Stirnaman J E 1979 Neglected rupture of the peroneal tendon causing recurrent sprains of the ankle. J Bone Joint Surg (Am) 61A: 1247–1248

Dooley B J, Kudelka P, Menelaus M B 1980 Subcutaneous rupture of the tendon of tibialis anterior. J Bone Joint Surg (Br) 62B: 471–472

Griffiths J C 1965 Tendon injuries around the ankle. J Bone Joint Surg (Br) 47B: 686–689

Kettlekamp D B, Alexander H H 1969 Spontaneous rupture of the posterior tibial tendon. J Bone Surg (Am) 51A: 759

Mann R A, Thompson F M 1985 Rupture of the posterior tibial tendon causing flat foot. J Bone Joint Surg (Am) 67A: 556–561

Mensor M C, Ordway G L 1953 Traumatic subcutaneous rupture of the tibialis anterior tendon. J Bone Joint Surg (Am) 35A: 675–680

Nava B E 1968 Traumatic dislocation of the tibialis posterior tendon at the ankle. J Bone Joint Surg (Br) 50B: 150

G. R. Fisk

Calcaneal fractures

'It shall bruise thy head and thou shalt bruise his heel' (Gen. 3: 15)

INTRODUCTION

Of all fractures in the human body that of the calcaneum has perhaps the most sinister reputation. It is an injury which is feared by the workman and not well understood by the surgeon. The traditional approach to the treatment of fractures, of reduction, fixation and maintenance of function, has been largely ignored or regarded as ineffective in this fracture and most surgeons try by conservative care to make the best of a bad job for their patients. Where treatment has been vigorously pursued it almost seems as though the surgeon had been punishing the patient for having such a difficult fracture. For instance Herman in 1937, developing Böhler's method, first of all pounded the outside of the heel with a padded mallet. Tongs were then passed through the posterior part of the heel and traction commenced. A bone clamp was applied to remould the shape and then the foot was immobilized in plaster with pads below the malleoli for 12 weeks, changing the plaster and pads at fortnightly intervals. The patient was then provided with 'an ambulatory brace,' physiotherapy was started and weight bearing allowed after four-and-a-half months. For those patients who still had the temerity to complain of persisting pain, triple arthrodesis or 'scraping the bone below the lateral malleolus' was advocated.

It is not surprising that the end result of this fracture has traditionally been regarded as melancholy, the effect on working capacity profound and osteoarthritic degeneration inevitable. Cotton & Henderson in 1916 stated 'The man who breaks his heel is done for as far as industrial future is concerned'. Conn in 1926 described the end results as 'incredibly bad' and Bankart in 1942 regarded the result of treatment as 'rotten'. Contemporary textbooks on fractures continue to express pessimism and advocate only conservative care and many authors, bemused by the welter of opinions, fail to advocate any precise regimen for the management of this fracture.

Fracture of the calcaneum is in fact a rare injury and most collected series give an overall incidence of 2.0 to 2.5%. Schofield in 1936 recorded 2025 injuries sustained by workmen building the Boulder Dam in the United States. This would have been an industrial undertaking calculated to expose the workmen to falls or crush injuries, but in fact there were only 52 calcaneal fractures and only 23 (a little over 1% of the total) in Schofield's opinion merited any sort of reduction. It is thus difficult for any one surgeon to collect in a short time a sufficiently large series of cases to understand the pathology of the fracture, to devise a modus operandi and acquire sufficient skill in reduction and splinting. Furthermore, this injury is often treated on an out-patient basis and is largely managed by junior medical officers who are conditioned into believing that hospital beds must be reserved for only the most serious cases and to whom the walking plaster is therefore the mainstay of treatment. This virtually guarantees that the results will be poor, whereas this fracture above all merits in-patient care in the hands of an experienced and senior orthopaedic surgeon.

HISTORICAL SURVEY

Fracture of the calcaneum has been known and recognized for centuries. That the fracture was due to compression was recognized by Norris (1839) and by Malgaigne (1847), while Morestin (1902) first appreciated that the fracture was 'like a seesaw, down in the front and up at the back', but Böhler (1931) was first credited with classifying the types of fracture according to their X-ray appearance.

The first half of the present century saw attempts by authors to classify the fracture into seven or more types but these are often difficult to comprehend and indeed every fracture differs slightly from the others and categorization is almost impossible. There were many attempts, particularly on the continent of Europe, to use complicated methods of traction and instrumentation in order to restore the shape of the calcaneum with little emphasis on restoration of function with a mobile hindfoot. There were also several attempts to restore early function to the foot by primary subtalar arthrodesis.

In Britain conservative methods have largely prevailed (with only half-hearted attempts to reduce the fracture and restore the shape of the calcaneum) by commencing early active and passive movements of the foot without weight bearing, and with progressive rehabilitation. However most of these published series are of relatively small numbers, the assembly of clinical material has been retrospective and follow-up examination and long-term review have been largely unpublished.

AETIOLOGY

Calcaneal fractures are sustained almost invariably by falls from a height. The supposition that the higher the fall the worse the fracture is not borne out in practice and the exact nature of the fall, the weight of the patient and the presence or otherwise of osteoporosis are factors of great importance. It is inevitable that this injury should be commoner in those workmen engaged in the 'vertical trades', such as seamen, dockers, stevedores, riggers, crane drivers, painters, window cleaners, etc. In a mixed civilian practice about 25% of the patients will be female, but in industrial practice the vast majority of the injured are male.

The second variety of injury is that caused by a force exerted from below when the subject is immobile, such as a head-on collision in a motor vehicle when the driver's heels are crushed by the floor of the car. The same mechanism applies in explosions such as land mines, booby traps, torpedoes, etc.

In males the incidence is commonest in the two age groups 30 to 34 and 40 to 49, with 72% of the fractures occurring in patients under 50 years of age, but in females it is commonest in the 65 plus age group, with 38% of the fractures occurring in patients under 50 years of age (Burke 1983).

The exact nature of the fall and the direction of the stresses placed on the calcaneum at the moment of impact bears an important relation to the type and severity of the fracture (Fig. 43.1). Whittaker (1947) using a high speed camera showed that the foot strikes the ground in a pronated position with the tuberosity outwards, backwards and downwards. At the moment of impact, the talus is driven down against the articular condyle, the subject usually falling forwards so that the talus penetrates downwards and backwards into the calcaneum, rotating the articular condyle within it. Body weight is taken upon the inside of the foot so that the

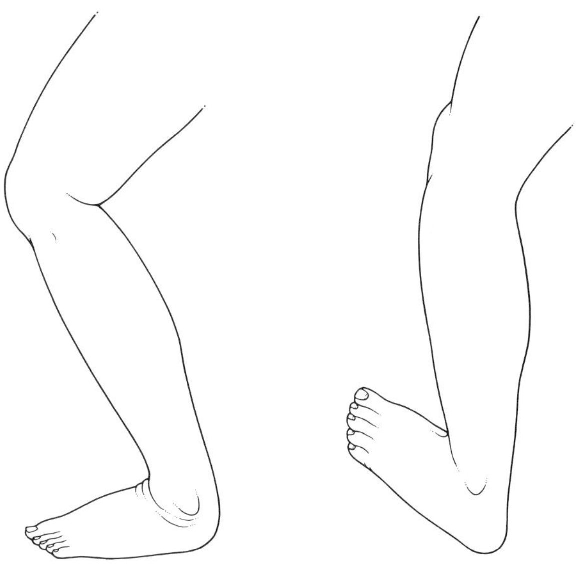

Fig. 43.1 The foot is compressed at the moment of impact with the ground. It goes into valgus and increasing dorsiflexion as the body weight is transferred forwards

longitudinal arch is destroyed, the heel goes into valgus comminuting the inner wall of the calcaneum, and as compression continues the outer wall is burst; the posterior half of the calcaneum goes into valgus and displaces laterally so that the inner concave surface of the bone is reversed into a convex deformity. The crushing effect may be so great as to divide the calcaneum into a number of fragments, the fracture lines passing through to the sole of the foot. The tuberosity may be crushed and distorted upwards, the sustentaculum tali is almost invariably fractured from the body of the bone but rarely displaced. The fracture may pass forwards and enter the calcaneocuboid joint, which in consequence may be subluxated. In this context the calcaneum may be conceived as a rectangular box with a domed lid which is struck by a mallet (Fig. 43.2).

In forces exerted from below the reverse deformity may ensue. The blow again drives the talus against the main articular condyle, the foot goes into equinus (or the patient may fall backwards) so that the condyle is rotated into the opposite direction so as to face backwards and the posterior fragment of the calcaneum rotates into varus.

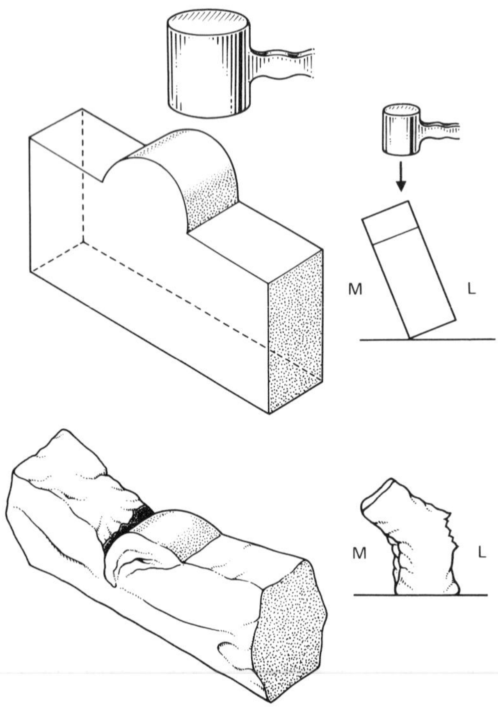

Fig. 43.2 A domed box is struck by a mallet while it is standing upon its inner corner

ANATOMY

The detailed anatomy of the calcaneum is dealt with in Chapter 4 but the internal trabecular pattern is not without relevance (Fig. 43.3). Weight bearing taken on the posterior articular facet is transmitted to the tuberosity partly posteriorly and downwards and partly anteriorly and downwards towards the calcaneocuboid joint. This leaves a divergent area lying immediately below the posterior articular facet and the tarsal canal, which some authors have regarded as an area of weakness (Fig. 43.4). There is heaping-up of the cortex on the inner surface of the bone around the sustentaculum tali, in the floor of the tarsal canal and along the upper border of the articular condyle.

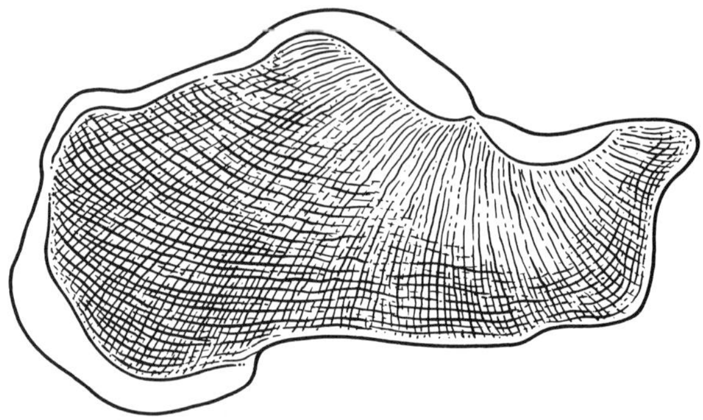

Fig. 43.3 Trabecular pattern within the calcaneum

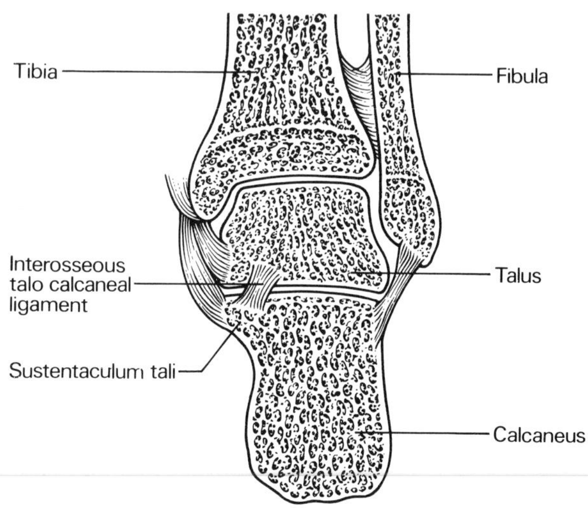

Fig. 43.4 Coronal section through the ankle and hindfoot

The upper surface of the calcaneum carries three articular facets, the two anterior being concerned with tarsal movement at the talocalcaneal-navicular joint (Fig. 43.5). This is very rarely involved in the fracture and indeed gross displacement will take place elsewhere while this complex remains intact.

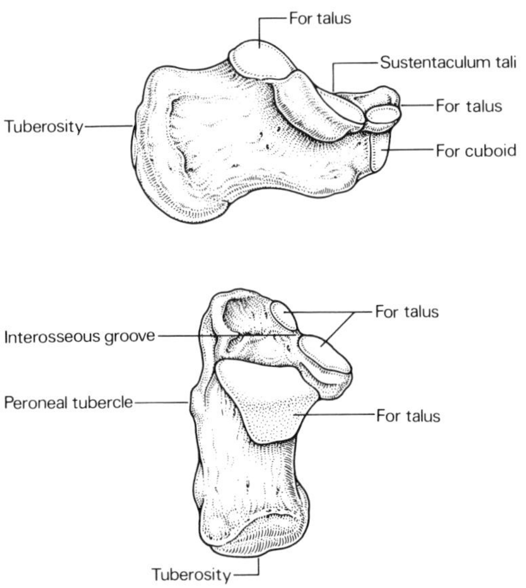

Fig. 43.5 Medial and upper aspects of the calcaneum

The tarsal canal separates this complex from the main condyle which carries the articular facet. It is the damage to and deformity of this main articular condyle which determines the future outlook for the fracture and to which reduction and support is principally directed.

Anteriorly the calcaneum articulates with the cuboid and it is the integrity of this joint which is essential to the free moving of the subtaloid joint and it is often involved in comminuted fracture of the calcaneum. Subluxation here can be observed in many instances and its subsequent stiffness and deformity influences the future function of the foot (Figs. 43.6 and 7).

Although the posterior tuberosity carries the insertion of the tendo Achillis it should be noted that this is attached to the lower half of the bone, the upper being covered by a bursa, although some authorities (Protheroe 1969) suggest that avulsion of

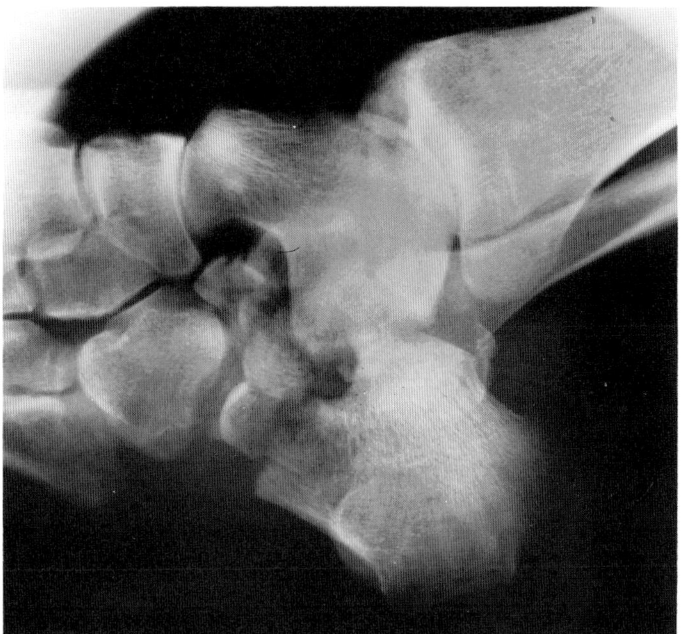

Fig. 43.6 An unusually severe crush injury with comminution of the anterior part and dislocation of the subtaloid joint

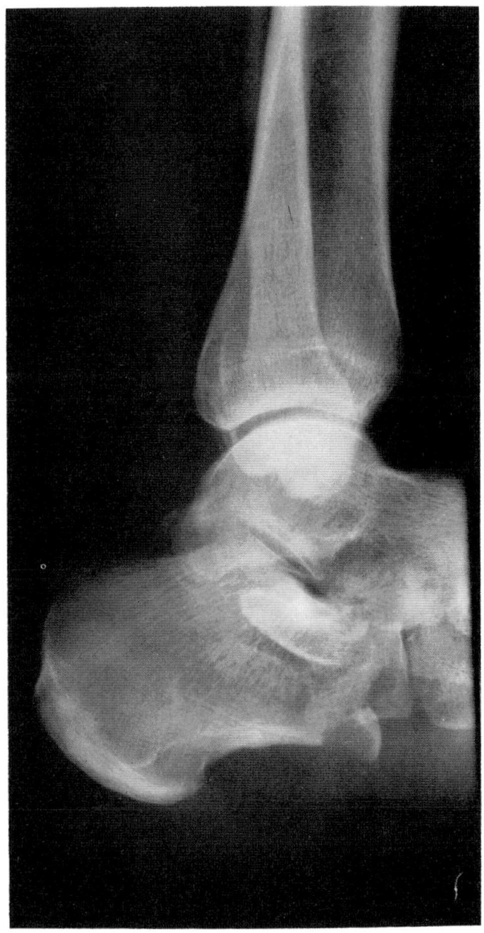

Fig. 43.7 Dislocation reduced

the posterior part of the calcaneum occurs when the tendo Achillis is inserted more proximally.

On the outer side, the peroneal tubercle separates the groove above, in which lies the peroneus brevis tendon, from the lower one carrying the peroneus longus. The tendons are retained in their grooves by a stout retinaculum and the tendon sheaths extend above and below the retinaculum. This is an important anatomical feature since the pain and difficulty following unreduced fractures of the calcaneum are said to be due to involvement of the peroneal tendons in the fracture and result in a characteristic pain which passes along the line of the tendons on weight bearing; however this is not the cause, but rather a referred pain from the subtaloid joint. Repeated observation at the time of many operations, when the fracture has been exposed from the outer side, reveals that the sheaths may occasionally contain a blood-stained effusion but almost invariably the tendons and the peroneal tubercle are floated outwards intact upon the bulging lateral wall.

Finally the integrity of the subtaloid joint, its proprioception and its control by freely moving tendons around the hindfoot, are all designed for balance, climbing and negotiating uneven surfaces. Fractures prejudice this important feature and stiffening of the joint destroys this mechanism which is essential in precisely those who work at heights and who are exposed to calcaneal fracture.

CLINICAL PRESENTATION

Diagnosis of fractured calcaneum should present little difficulty. Nevertheless the injury is not infrequently overlooked, partly because the fracture may not be sufficiently severe to deform the appearance, and secondly it may only be one fracture in multiple injury. The patient may not be capable of complaining of pain and stiffness of the foot or the feet may not have been subjected to routine clinical examination. In addition, such patients are often treated in recumbency, concealing the inability to weight bear which might thereby have drawn attention to the fracture. Between 2 and 10% of fractures of the lumbar spine are associated with a fractured calcaneum and careful examination of the other area should always be carried out in either injury.

The so-called 'Oxford sign', which was in fact described by Böhler in the 1930s, consists of bruising of the sole of the foot on its inner side, which results from blood suffusing under the plantar fascia. This sign is not usually revealed for 24 hours and is by no means invariably present.

The characteristic fracture results in the subtaloid joint becoming disorganized with the calcaneum losing height, the bone bulging under the lateral malleolus, the broadened heel lying in valgus and the longitudinal arch lost. The compression of the bone causes comparative lengthening of the tendo Achillis so that there is an excessive degree of passive dorsiflexion of the foot. Pronation and supination of the hindfoot are of course almost totally lost. It is thus evident that if the fracture is allowed to heal in this deformed position the effect on the function of the foot is profound and indeed this is almost totally destroyed.

CLASSIFICATION

Thorèn in 1964 produced experimental fractures in cadavers in which the limb was clamped to a stand, the tendo Achillis was kept taut by means of a sling, a shoe was applied to the foot and the heel was struck by a 75 kg weight mounted on a pendulum. Only when the stand was allowed to move along the ground as the heel was struck did injuries occur which corresponded to those seen in life. He was able to vary the type of fracture according to the degree of dorsiflexion and pronation of the foot at the moment of impact. In the supinated foot the force was taken principally on the sustentaculum tali whereas in the pronated foot the fracture would pass through or behind the articular condyle. Because of the strong ligamentous attachments to the calcaneum most of the fragments remained in their normal relationship, but the main articular condyle lacking such attachments, would be depressed in various ways depending on the force directed upon it.

Owing to the complex nature of this injury therefore, it is not surprising that different authors have produced their own classifications. These have mostly been based on X-ray appearances and some upon post mortem studies. Schofield in 1936 described five types. Widèn in 1954 described eight types, some of which were again subdivided. Essex-

Lopresti (1952) followed Böhler's classification (Fig. 43.8). He postulated two lines of force: an outer route (Figs. 43.8a, b and c) when the subtaloid joint is forced into eversion and the outer taloid spur is driven into the crucial angle, and an inner route (Figs. 43.8d, e and f) when the residual force shears off the sustentaculum tali with a variable fragment of the articular condyle depressed into the body.

Palmer in 1948 described a primary shearing of the fracture which commenced on the medial aspect of the bone and ran laterally and upwards into the talocalcaneal joint and sometimes anteriorly to involve the calcaneocuboid joint. This divided the calcaneum into two main fragments, the medial one comprising the sustentaculum and the anteromedial aspect of the bone, the lateral fragment comprising the body of the calcaneum with the lateral part or the whole of the main articular condyle (Fig. 43.9).

Palmer's secondary fracture is described as a compression of the lateral main fragment carrying the articular condyle. If the condyle had been involved by a vertical fracture the two or more elements might be unevenly depressed. Essex-Lopresti drew attention to the frequency with which this condyle carries the posterior upper part of the body which has been called the 'tongue' fracture and Allan in 1955 regarded this as a tertiary fracture line.

Warwick & Bremner in 1953 introduced an important new classification of these fractures. They drew attention to the fact that the oblique fracture line may run across or behind the main articular condyle and secondly that the depression depended upon the exact position of the primary fracture line. They did not attempt to discuss the treatment of the fractures that they classified (Fig. 43.10).

The enquiring reader will no doubt become increasingly confused by the many attempts to classify the fracture and the great difficulty in interpreting the various X-ray views, but fortunately from the point of view of treatment, complicated classifications are largely of academic interest.

For the purpose of operative reduction there are only four varieties of deformity (Fig. 43.11). Attention should be directed to the displacement of the articular condyle: most commonly it is depressed straight into the body; less frequently (Fig. 43.12) it

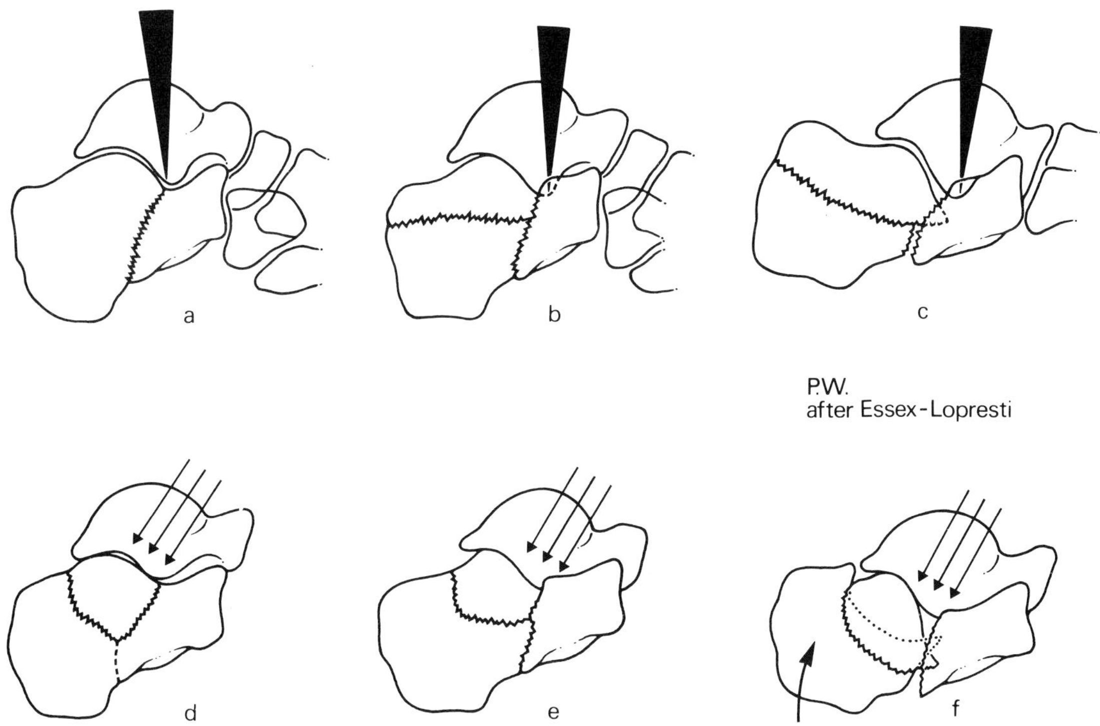

Fig. 43.8 Essex-Lopresti's classification of major fractures

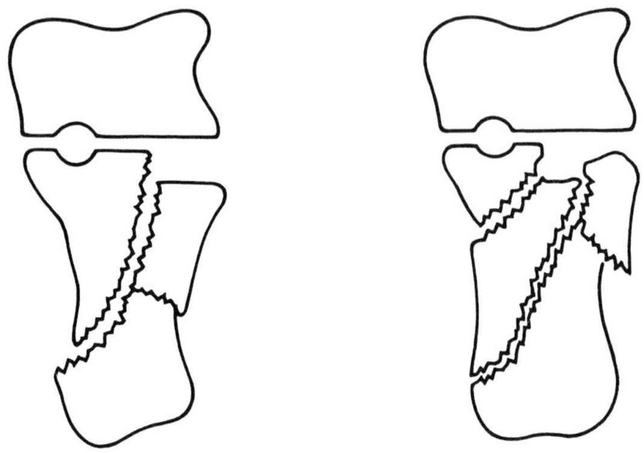

Fig. 43.9 Palmer's primary and secondary fractures viewed in the axial radiograph

is rotated forwards on a transverse axis and if the upper aspect of the calcaneum remains with the condyle it is elevated as a 'tongue' fracture. More rarely a reverse rotation takes place and this is seen when the force is exerted from below.

Group I. Minor fractures

These comprise injuries of the processes, namely the posterior tuberosity, the sustentaculum tali and the anterior articular surface, usually involving the calcaneocuboid joint.

Fracture of the posterior extremity of the calcaneum

This may involve the tuberosity only. It results from a fall onto the heel not serious enough to fracture the body of the bone itself. It is not usually displaced. It is occasionally comminuted or compressed. Only rarely does this injury require internal fixation by a transfixion screw. It is best treated by elevation to reduce the swelling and then immobilization of the lower leg in a walking plaster for about four weeks. Persisting deformity of the tuberosity is of no consequence and does not normally give rise to persisting symptoms. This is said to account for 17% of all fractures of the calcaneum.

Avulsion fracture of the Achilles tendon ('duckbill fracture')

This is rare and accounts for about 1%. It is said to occur when the tendo Achillis is abnormally proximally inserted (Protheroe 1969) but it is more likely that this injury is caused by a direct blow on the back of the heel from a falling object or from forcible equinus injury when the upper aspect of the tuberosity strikes against the back of the talus. These injuries occasionally require open reduction and internal fixation, particularly if strands of the tendo Achillis are attached to them. Spontaneous union is the rule.

Fracture of the anterior end of the calcaneum

This fracture involving the calcaneocuboid joint occurs in some 7% of cases. The fracture usually

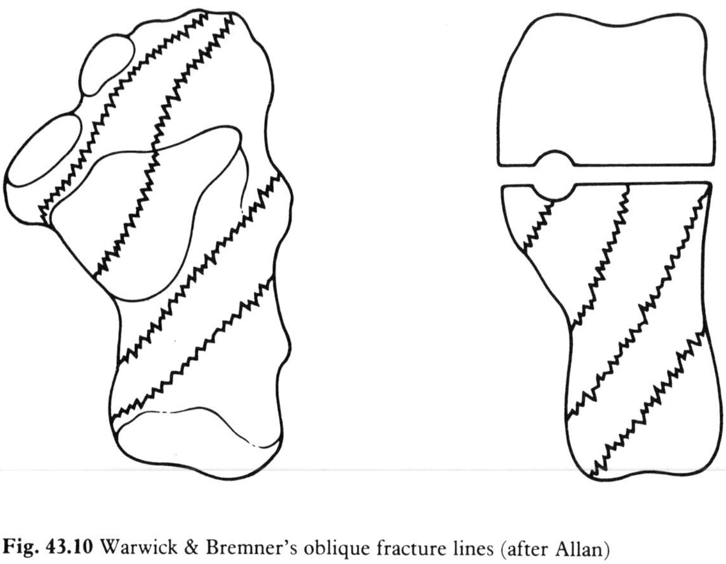

Fig. 43.10 Warwick & Bremner's oblique fracture lines (after Allan)

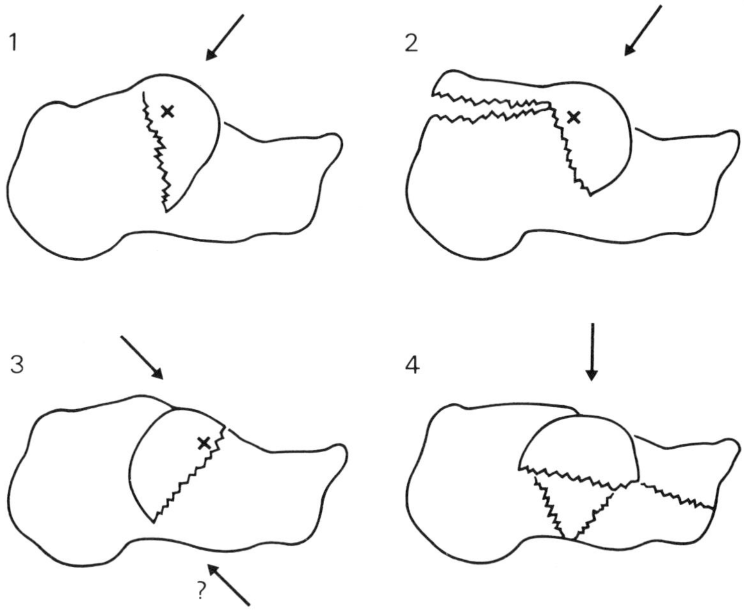

Fig. 43.11 A simple guide to open reduction. x = point of pivot

a

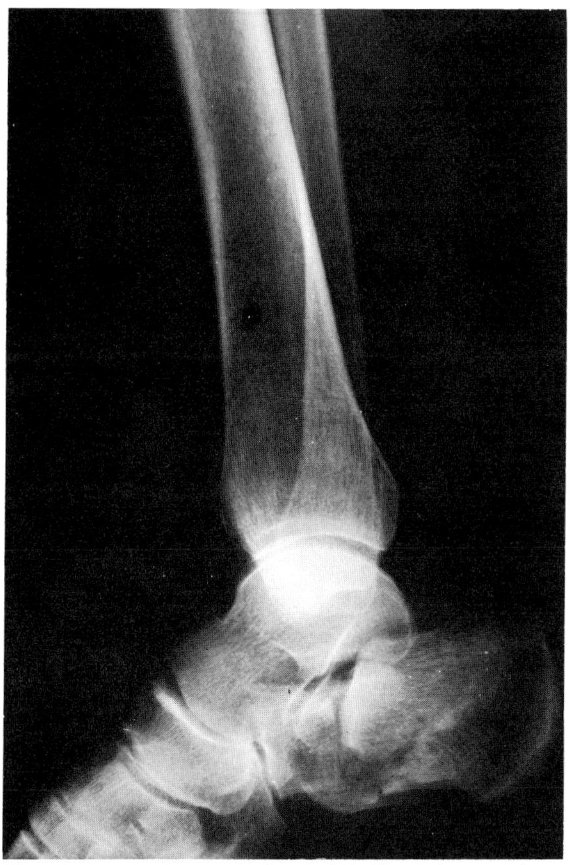

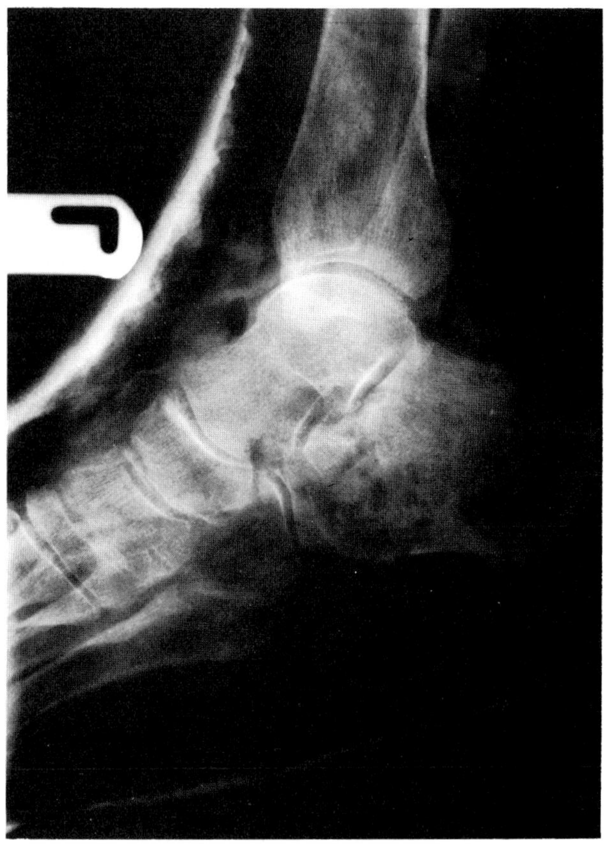

b

Fig. 43.12 (a) A 68-year-old female fell off a chair sustaining a comminuted fracture in which the articular condyle had rotated downwards and forwards. (b) Open reduction and grafting enabled her to return to hill walking one year later occurs by a forced dorsiflexion of the midfoot following a fall by twisting injuries in which the fracture is part of a midtarsal injury or by a direct crush. Full recovery is the rule but some midtarsal stiffening may be permanent.

Fracture of the sustentaculum tali

There is rarely an isolated fracture of the sustentaculum while the rest of the calcaneum remains intact — probably when the foot is supinated at the moment of impact. The fracture may not be easily discerned in the routine radiograph and the patient may complain of severe pain and tenderness along the inner border of the foot. A 'tunnel' X-ray view may be necessary to make the diagnosis, and if symptoms persist screw fixation will be required.

Group II. Fractures of the body

This includes those fractures involving the main body of the calcaneum including the main articular condyle. If the injury consists of undisplaced fractures and fissures of the body, treatment is always conservative. There is invariably a return of almost perfect function although there may be some persisting subtalar stiffness. Fractures of this type account for a little under a quarter of Group II fractures.

Fractures which involve the main articular condyle with displacement constitute a group around which controversy persists and which accounts for the bad reputation of this injury. It is essential to recognize that the articular condyle or part of it is rotated downwards into the body of the calcaneum and that it is the reduction of this rotational deformity upon which success depends. Fractures depressing the main articular condyle frequently continue through the floor of the bone so that it bursts out into the sole but this bony deformity does not seem to give the patient discomfort on weight bearing.

If the fracture passes forwards and enters the calcaneocuboid joint there may be subluxation partly from the fracture line itself and partly from the general deformity of the calcaneum.

It suffices to say that no two fractures are the same, and the only necessary criterion for treatment is to decide whether the articular condyle is depressed or not and whether it warrants reduction and what other associated deformity requires correction at the same time.

RADIOLOGICAL EXAMINATION

There are two standard views normally employed in X-ray departments to display this fracture, the lateral and the axial view. A large number of other views have been described and no doubt they reveal the exact nature of the fracture more clearly. However most busy X-ray departments find it difficult to produce these views with any consistency and the patient with a recent injury is subject to positioning which may give rise to unnecessary pain and distress.

It is not sufficiently emphasized that comparable views of the intact opposite heel should be taken since there is a wide variety in the shape and texture of the normal calcaneum.

The lateral view

The lateral view gives the most valuable information but it requires experience in interpretation. Böhler's angle was first described in 1931 as the 'tuber-joint sign'. It consists of measuring the angle between a line passing from the condyle to the anterior upper tuberosity and another line from the tuberosity to the articular condyle, which would normally meet at an angle of 35° (Fig. 43.13). Many authors adjudge the severity of the injury by the distortion of this angle and its restoration as evidence of reduction of the fracture. Unhappily this does not take into account the rotational deformity of the articular condyle and although it may be a rough and ready guide to the deformity too much reliance should not be placed upon this measurement.

The axial view

This is technically difficult to take. There is a tendency for the radiographer to place the cassette too distally so that the subtaloid joint is not included in the film nor adequately outlined. The foot should be dorsiflexed beyond a right angle and this may be conveniently achieved by the patient himself pulling

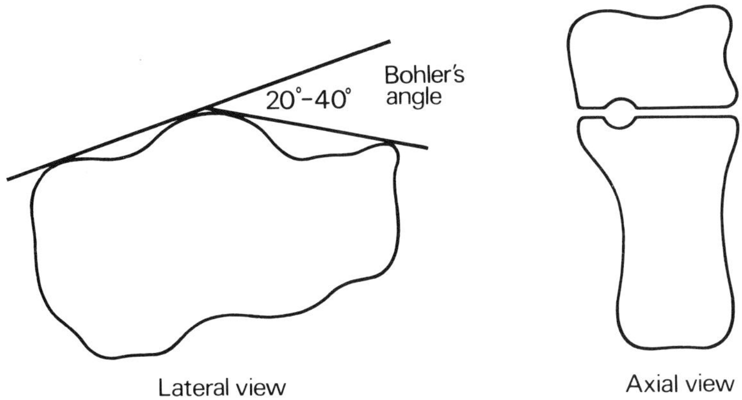

Fig. 43.13 Standard lateral and axial views

on a bandage which is looped around the forefoot. The X-ray tube is placed below the sole and tilted to 45° and directed towards the lateral malleolus. The X-ray obtained is not an accurate anatomical outline but simply a shadow of its composite shape, thus the top of the film is anterosuperior and the bottom of the film outlining the tuberosity is posteroinferior (see Fig. 43.13). The X-ray should outline the main subtaloid joint on the lateral side, while the tarsal canal may be seen as a notch and the anterior joint and the sustentaculum tali should be clearly visible on the inner side.

The general alignment of the body of the calcaneum occupies the rest of the film and its general alignment can be observed but the length of the bone simply depends upon the inclination of the X-rays. The sustentaculum tali is almost invariably sheared off but it is never displaced.

Palmer (1948) drew attention to the varieties of fracture of the main articular condyle which this view reveals and he explained the depression of the central part of the condyle as being due to elastic recoil following the downward depression of all of the upper surface of the calcaneum. The sustentaculum returns to its anatomical position from its capsular attachments and the support of the tendon of flexor hallucis. The main articular condyle remains depressed, and the widening or distortion of the subtaloid joint indicates the degree of depression or rotation. The articular condyle may also be split so that its inner half remains buried deeply within the substance of the body of the bone. Allan (1955) has shown how the primary fracture lines may pass obliquely across the calcaneum forwards from the medial aspect either in front of the condyle, separating the sustentaculum tali, across the condyle or behind it (see Fig. 43.10).

Other views

A large number of other X-ray views have been advocated and although they may provide additional information they will not influence the effectiveness of treatment. London (1967) illustrated a number of these views but only one of them is commonly used and that was described by Anthonsen in 1943 as follows: 'The foot is placed in dorsal flexion with its lateral side towards the film. The central ray is directed against a point just below the medial malleolus with an inclination of 25° in cranio-distal direction and 30° in dorso-ventral direction. The distance of focus is reduced to 25 to 35 cm'. This view outlines the posterior calcaneal articular surface and is useful in checking the completeness of reduction. Other views were recommended by Broden (1949).

TREATMENT

It is generally agreed that fractures of the processes simply require immobilization and occasional internal fixation. Major undisplaced fractures of the articular condyle may be treated by immobilization in plaster for six to eight weeks, weight bearing is permitted if the plaster is well fitting and the patient comfortable. Alternatively this type of injury may be as well treated by pressure bandaging to reduce the oedema, early mobilization and graduated weight bearing. This is undoubtedly more uncomfortable for the patient and requires the use of crutches for two or three months, but the results are probably superior to prolonged immobilization.

There is however no unanimity concerning the treatment of fractures which are displaced. A large number of methods, often diametrically opposed, have been advocated in the literature and the reader cannot fail to be impressed with the celerity which authors have displayed in publishing a new variety of treatment which they have performed on a few cases with very little follow-up examination. Even the larger series, carefully documented and described, fail in this respect. However methods fall into seven main categories:

Immobilization without reduction

This almost always involves prolonged periods in a plaster cast with or without weight bearing. In the worst fractures this means ankylosis of the hindfoot in a position of great deformity and is not to be recommended in any but the mildest cases. It is unhappily the standard treatment provided in most Accident Departments and is based largely on an admission of ignorance of the fracture and its pathology and is, as has already been remarked, a device for treatment of the patient on an out-patient basis. Statistics show that in displaced fractures with or without reduction, prolonged immobilization of more than six weeks leads to ankylosis and an inferior functional result.

Manual reduction

This is at least a gesture on the part of the surgeon in an attempt to restore the general shape of the heel and render it plantigrade but it is not possible by this method alone to restore the depressed articular surface. The same melancholy results follow if prolonged fixation is thereafter employed but some advantage may have been gained by improving the alignment of the heel.

Instrumental reduction

Böhler was largely responsible for popularizing this method and he published his results in 1931. He first attempted to disimpact the fracture with a wooden wedge and then crush it into shape with a 'redressor' and this fearsome instrument used to be seen gathering dust in the store cupboards of many an Orthopaedic Department. Unhappily the kidney-shaped clamps were applied to already damaged and swollen soft tissues in an area where the skin normally has a poor blood supply and ensuing necrosis was a serious hazard. He inserted two pins, one in the lower tibia and the other in the tuberosity of the calcaneum. The fracture was then subjected to traction and the pins immobilized in a plaster cast for three to five weeks. A walking plaster was applied for three months and Böhler claimed restoration of a high degree of function. His published series comprised 100 fresh fractures but there is no follow-up.

Many variations in Böhler's method have been described, but they all suffer from the same disadvantage of producing a stiff and often painful hindfoot. It is likely that the widespread use of this method gave rise to the mistaken belief that relief from symptoms is only obtained when the hindfoot ankyloses.

Essex-Lopresti (1952) gave Gissane (1947) credit for inventing a spike fitted with a handle which was passed into the tongue fracture, elevating it into position, the handle being removed and the spike immobilized in a plaster shoe. The spike and the plaster shoe were removed at the end of four weeks and then a protective below-knee plaster was applied for a further four weeks and weight bearing allowed at eight to 10 weeks. His published figures show that he carried out this reduction on 39 occasions. His patients do not seem to have suffered the complication of infection which is almost inevitable around a transfixion pin and Lindsay & Dewar (1958) reported an incidence of 11% of infections using this device. At best it is only useful when the displaced condylar fragment can be impaled from behind and elevated blindly. In addition this method suffers the disadvantage of other approaches which require fixation until the defect created by the fracture has been filled by new bone.

Primary arthrodesis

Several series have been described in the literature by British, Canadian and American authors, particularly Gallie (1943), who advocated fusion of the subtaloid joint by a posterior approach and the insertion of two tibial grafts. He reported 50 personal cases and 50 others which he had heard about.

It was however pointed out by Conn (1943) in discussing Gallie's paper that this did not correct the bony deformity, the entrapment of peroneal tendons or injuries to the midtarsal joints.

Other authors, particularly Bankart in 1942 and Moberg in 1951 advised triple arthrodesis. It is however important to classify the injury before advocating one variety of treatment. Immediate arthrodesis was recommended by Hall & Pennal in 1960, who carried out primary fusion using Gallie's method on 'severe fractures of the calcaneum with joint comminution and depression'. They claimed excellent or very good results in 23 patients, fair in six and poor in two. 25 out of 29 of them had returned to their full previous employment. Fusion failed in three cases and there were four infections.

Late triple arthrodesis. This has been advocated for those cases of intractable pain or in which other forms of treatment have failed. However the results appear to be generally rather disappointing, probably because the source of the pain lies not only in the damaged subtaloid joint but in the general disorganization of the foot mechanics which inevitably followed a crushed and distorted calcaneum.

Zayer (1969) reviewed 110 fractures of the calcaneum involving the articular condyle. 46 of these had been subjected to triple arthrodesis and he classified them as 23 good and 23 bad. The writer's personal series of six cases undergoing triple arthrodesis after prolonged treatment showed that five of these continued to suffer a permanent disability.

Excision of the calcaneum

Several authors including Pridie (1946) claimed that in extremely comminuted fractures it was possible to excise the calcaneum entirely and allow weight bearing on the fibro-fatty pad which remained. It is difficult to imagine a situation where this operation would be indicated in view of the wide variety of treatment available but it might conceivably be used in cases of tumour or intractable infection. It is unlikely that this operation has ever been performed on more than a few occasions.

Early movement without weight bearing or attempted reduction

This method enjoys a continued vogue in Britain and there is no doubt that remarkably good results can be obtained in a considerable proportion of cases. It has been practised for many years and Roberts & Sayle-Creer (1947) advocated this method in all fractures of the calcaneum whether displaced or not.

Burke has recently reviewed 288 fractures of the calcaneum treated conservatively in Sheffield over the 10-year period 1961 to 1971. He reports that 'The standard method of treatment was with wool and crepe bandage compression and early joint movement'. 25 cases with no displacement of the joint surfaces all returned to work at six months and 85% at three months. None of this group were admitted to hospital on account of the fracture.

The writer's personal series of 38 undisplaced fractures in 33 patients (Table 43.1) were treated either by plaster fixation and physiotherapy or by movement from the start. A high level of recovery was almost invariably obtained with return to preaccident work and activities, the average total disability being about four months. 28 of this series followed up from one to nine years showed that they all returned to their preaccident employment but five of them had ankylosed or partially stiffened subtaloid joints indicating that if this joint is involved in any degree full mobility may never be restored. Essex-Lopresti advocated this method for all patients over the age of 50 but this is altogether too conservative an attitude and only the fracture per se should influence the method of treatment.

Table 43.1 Undisplaced fractures of body of calcaneum at follow-up

38 fractures in 33 patients	
2 female, 31 male	
Average age 48 years	
(increase in average age suggests less exposure to serious injury)	
Average total disability (18 patients)	= 4 months
Average partial disability (16 patients)	= 2 weeks
Permanent disability (one retired)	
Returned to same work	24 = 86%
Returned to lighter work	2 = 7%
Changed occupation	2 = 7%
Total where work recorded	28

Open reduction with bone grafting

Morestin in 1902 advocated elevation of the depressed fragment but Leriche in 1922 is usually credited with the first attempt to reduce the fracture and fix it by screws. Lenormant et al in 1928 were the first to insert bone grafts into the calcaneum after open reduction. Palmer in 1945 and 1948 described open reduction and the insertion of iliac crest grafts using traction by a pin through the tuberosity during the operation. Widèn in 1954 helped to popularize this method when he described Palmer's results in a monograph published in *Acta Chirurgica Scandinavica*.

Allan in 1955 accurately described the pathology of the fracture and the operation. He advocated a non-weightbearing plaster cast for six weeks followed by physiotherapy and weight bearing four weeks later. He made one significant observation: 'If under direct vision one attempts to employ some of the accepted methods of closed reduction it is apparent that the posterior facet is not elevated and rotated back to its normal position and the subtaloid joint is distorted although the tuberosity is pulled down'. He described a series of 16 cases and followed 12 of them for two years. All 12 were carrying out the same work and play as before the injury and 10 out of the 12 were rated as excellent as far as function was concerned.

Soeur & Rémy published in 1975 a series of 58 patients treated by open reduction and Kirschner wire fixation, but not by bone grafting. They exposed the sinus tarsi through an incision above and in front of the peroneal tendons, displaying the deformity of the talus and fixing this firstly to the sustentaculum by a transverse wire and then passing one or more wires obliquely from the lateral to the medial side. Postoperative care involved elevation for four weeks in plaster, four weeks in a walking plaster and then four weeks in a compression bandage. The wires were removed on the average eight months after the operation. They estimated normal subtalar movement in 20, diminished in 13 and absent in 12 cases. All except eight patients had resumed their normal work. Their article does not contain any long-term follow-up although there is little doubt that the results remain excellent.

McReynolds (1976) described a medial approach with reduction of the fracture and internal fixation by staples in 48 cases. Overall results were recorded as 'impressive'.

Author's preferred method

It was decided in 1958 to carry out a prolonged prospective study of major fractures of the calcaneum with displaced fractures treated by open reduction and fixation by a single iliac crest graft. Circumstances were particularly favourable since the patients were largely drawn from maritime workers with whom falls were relatively common from the hazards of their trade. The series consisted almost entirely of men in their active working years and it was possible to provide a high level of rehabilitation and a prolonged follow-up. Two other general hospitals were involved but the final proportion of males to females does not accurately reflect the population at risk.

Minor fractures of processes were not included in this study, as they were treated conservatively. Up to 1971, 252 fractures had been recorded in the hospital files. This figure includes some cases of conservative treatment of unreduced fractures from a fourth hospital. By 1978, a period of 20 years, records were available of some 206 examples of major fracture with 116 open reductions, 51 unreduced fractures and 39 undisplaced fractures, described in a Hunterian Lecture at the Royal College of Surgeons of England (Fisk 1978).

These figures do not accurately portray the relative frequency of these injuries as the primary purpose was to observe and follow up those cases treated by open reduction and grafting. Many of these cases were lost to follow-up by death from unrelated causes, the return of foreign workers, particularly seamen, to their homes, and changes of address. It was the tendency of these patients, having gained an acceptable result, to fail to attend follow-up examination clinics.

All displaced fractures were reviewed on arrival at hospital and considered for open reduction. It became clear quite early on that a fracture seen after three weeks could not be satisfactorily reduced and this was treated in the conservative method outlined above and served as a useful comparison.

Fresh displaced fractures were treated by elevation and compression bandages. No attempt was made to carry out immediate reduction on these fractures, although this would certainly be worth considering in any future study. Surgery was found to be unsafe within the first 10 days because of the intense swelling, contusion and threatened ischaemia of the soft tissues. There was thus a 'window' from 10 to 20 days when the fracture was not sufficiently 'sticky' to prevent full reduction but the soft tissues and particularly the skin had regained sufficient blood supply for primary healing of the wound. Close examination of the X-rays revealed the exact nature of the displacement and the degree of comminution. No fracture was excluded on the grounds of severity since it was felt that much of the benefit of the operation was derived from the realignment of the calcaneum and the restoration of its height, even if the subtaloid joint was so damaged that ankylosis would be almost inevitable.

The operation (Fig. 43.14)

Under general anaesthesia the limb is exsanguinated and a pneumatic tourniquet is placed around the lower thigh. The patient is laid upon the opposite side with a pillow between the knees and a sandbag

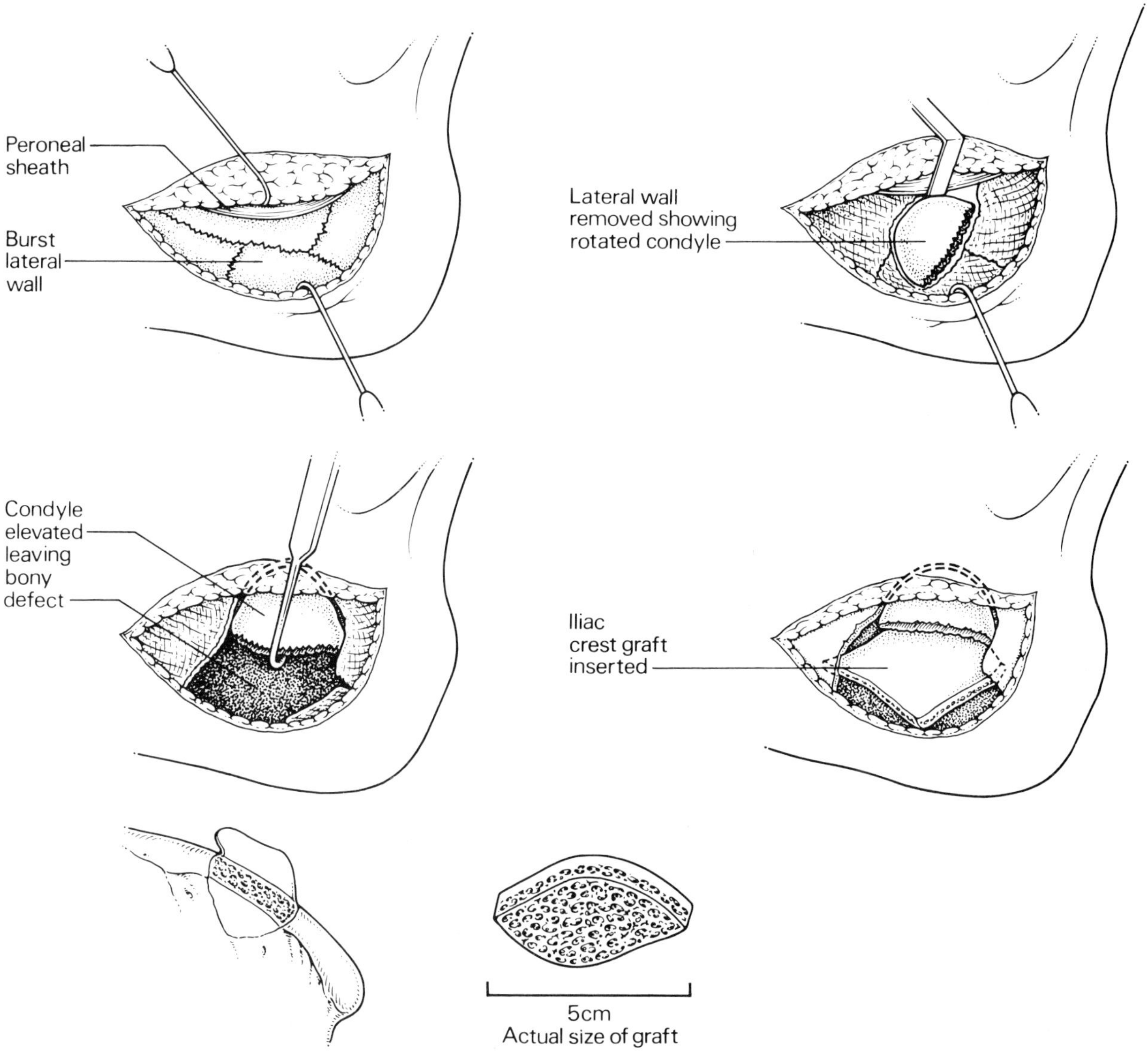

Fig. 43.14 Open reduction of fractured calcaneum — see text for detail

supporting the affected foot. The lower leg, the foot and the iliac crest are prepared. A curved incision some 3 in long is made below and behind the lateral malleolus and midway between the sole and the tip of the lateral malleolus. Great care must be taken to preserve the sural nerve and this may either be identified or included in the upper full-thickness flap. The peroneal tendons and their sheaths are usually exposed and examined and a serosanguinous effusion is occasionally seen within the sheaths. Even in the presence of considerable crushing the relationship of the peroneal tubercle and the tendons is well preserved as these structures ride laterally upon the bulging lateral wall. The ligamentous tissues and periosteum are stripped off the outer wall of the calcaneum and it is occasionally desirable to open and inspect the subtaloid joint, but this is not an essential step in the operation. *Reduction cannot be successfully performed unless the lateral wall of the calcaneum is removed from the surgical field either entirely or hinged on remaining periosteal shreds.*

The surgeon may now look into the interior of the calcaneum. Blood clot and loose bone fragments are removed and the buried condyle recognized when its articular surface comes into view. It becomes abundantly clear at this stage that no manipulation or other closed manoeuvres could possibly have influenced the position of this condyle and the Essex-Lopresti method of elevation by a bone spike is unlikely to succeed. It requires considerable experience and judgement to decide exactly how the depressed condyle should be elevated but when this is achieved by means of bone levers it is held in position by a sharp hook. If there is a tongue fracture it is wise to depress this with a second hook as the condyle is elevated. The general alignment of the calcaneum can at the same time be restored by inverting the heel and rotating the posterior half of the bone towards the midline so that the natural concave surface of the inner wall of the calcaneum is restored and this can be confirmed by palpation. It has not been found necessary to put the calcaneum on traction as advocated by Palmer.

While reduction is being achieved an assistant has removed either an oblong or diamond-shaped graft from the iliac crest some 5 cm long and about 2 cm broad at its widest part. This graft, after some trimming, is now placed under the elevated condyle usually with its long axis in anteroposterior alignment. It is important to obtain a snug fit both at the front and back, otherwise it may protrude through the floor of the bone if serious disruption has already occurred. Occasionally if there are vertical splits in the condyle it is better supported by the graft being placed transversely. The graft may be gently impacted into position by means of a punch and its stability should be sufficient to maintain the condyle elevated in its correct position. As soon as the height of the heel has been restored by the graft, the foot resumes a normal shape and the longitudinal arch reappears. The fragments of the lateral wall may be replaced but it is important *not* to increase the total volume of the bone as this will lead to undue tension on the soft tissues and slow healing of the wound. It is also important for the same reason not to exaggerate the height of the heel by too large a graft. The wound is closed by interrupted sutures and a padded plaster cast is applied to the lower limb with the foot in slight equinus.

If the reduction has been successfully performed and is fully stable, the foot may be supported only by a padded pressure bandage. Postoperatively the leg is kept elevated and when the wound of the iliac crest has settled the patient may be up in a wheelchair, keeping the leg elevated. At the end of 10 to 14 days the plaster or bandage is removed and the wound inspected. Because the skin over the outer side of the heel normally is poorly vascularized there may be a little delay in sound healing. At this stage the leg is supported by a crepe bandage, the patient is allowed up non-weightbearing with the aid of crutches and intensive active and passive movements of the foot are commenced.

At the end of a further four weeks, that is to say six weeks after the reduction, the patient is allowed to commence progressive weight bearing. In none of these cases has redisplacement occurred at this stage as a result of weight bearing although in some cases inadequate reduction and insecure grafting has led to some late deformity. Attempts at late reduction of this fracture is convincing evidence of how very rapidly the bone consolidates and becomes suitable for weight bearing, so that six weeks protection is quite adequate.

The patient is encouraged to wear his ordinary shoe as soon as possible and he receives intensive walking exercises at first using crutches or a walking frame and later with sticks. He must spend a considerable time on tiptoe exercises if his gait is to be restored to normal. The patient will experience discomfort in the foot on weight bearing and with attempts to mobilize the foot, but he is encouraged to persevere in the confident hope that much if not all of his discomfort will eventually disappear.

Aftercare

It cannot be too strongly emphasized that these patients require constant encouragement and must persevere with active exercises for some months. A gloomy or uncaring attitude by the surgeon and his assistants leads only to despair and the abandonment of efforts by the patient to rehabilitate himself. He must be reassured that he will be able to return to earning his living except in the most demanding and hazardous of occupations. On no account must he be sent to languish in those Centres where this injury and its outlook are not fully understood. Retraining and resettlement are very rarely required. The majority of these patients become involved in compensation claims and a gloomy prognosis is often offered by those who do not understand the nature of this injury or misguidedly feel that their obligation to the patient obliges them to take a serious view of the litigant's working capacity. Talk of 'arthritis setting in' is often the death-knell of the patient's hopes, though it may inflate the size of his claim.

In 1968 Qazi followed up 51 fractures treated in my Department by open reduction and grafting in 46 patients for the purposes of his thesis for the Mastership of Orthopaedics of Liverpool University (Table 43.2). Ages ranged from one child under the age of 10 to two cases between the ages of 60 and 70. The average total disability was four months. With the exception of one patient all were back at some work under six months. Only three out of 46 did not return to their preaccident jobs. About 80% of them were back in preaccident work under nine months. Six had no disability at all, 32 had a trivial disability and it was moderate in six. The great majority had symptoms and function stabilized between 18 months and two years, but five out of 46 said that the condition was still improving. Pain of varying intensity was the commonest complaint. 23 patients had occasional mild ache and 10 had pain of short duration. Although 42 out of the 46 patients complained of some stiffness only nine had stiffening of significant degree. One case had a severe disability. Three-quarters of them had a normal gait and could tiptoe normally. Of the remaining 10 only two were unable to tiptoe. Of 39 patients with unilateral fracture, six had normal subtaloid movement, 23 patients had half or more, four patients had only slight movement and in six patients the subtaloid joint was completely ankylosed.

There was a correlation between the function results and the mobility of the subtaloid joint and also in the restoration of Böhler's angle (which implies that the best results were obtained in those that were accurately reduced). None of these cases came to subtaloid or triple arthrodesis because of persisting disabling symptoms. There had been no delayed onset of pain or late exacerbation of symptoms.

Long-term results

This section records a personal series of 114 cases of long-term results in which incomplete records were present in 11 patients, leaving 105 cases for detailed review (Table 43.3). At the same time a follow-up examination of a comparable series of 51 displaced fractures which had not been reduced (Table 43.4) was similarly examined. Untreated displaced

Table 43.2 Preliminary results of open reduction (Qazi) (46 patients)

Subtaloid movement	
Normal	15.5%
Half or more	59%
Slight	10%
Nil	15.5%
Normal gait and tiptoe	36 (32 nil or trivial disability)
2 unable to tiptoe 7 difficulty on tiptoe	} 9, but normal gait

Table 43.3 Open reduction (114 in 94 patients)

Women 6	
Ages ranging from 6–74 years	
Average age (77 patients)	= 41.2 years
Average follow-up (67 patients)	= 3.7 years
Types where recorded	
a. Compression of condyle	42 = 54%
b. Rotated	25 = 32%
c. Comminuted	11 = 14%
	78

Table 43.4 Unreduced displaced fractures

1 female; 41 males with 51 fractures	
Age range 20–65 years, average 45.3 years	
Average follow-up = 4.6 years in 37 patients	
Total disability in 38 patients	= 7 months
Partial disability in 19 patients	= 15½ months
Permanent disability where followed up	= 14 patients
Where work was recorded in 37 patients:	
Returned to same work:	20 = 54%
Returned to lighter work:	14 = 38%
Changed occupation:	3 = 8%
Triple arthrodesis: 6 patients, but persistent disability in 5!	

Table 43.5 Comparative results in reduced and unreduced displaced fractures

	Reduced	Unreduced
Total numbers	114 (6 females)	51 (1 female)
Average age	41.2 years	45.3 years
Average follow-up	3.7 years	4.6 years
Total disability	4.8 months in 73 cases	7.0 months in 38 cases
Partial disability	6.7 months in 63 cases	15.5 months in 19 cases

fractures of the body of the calcaneum involving the articular condyle on the whole produced valgoid stiff feet (Table 43.5).

There have been a few cases in which the comminution has been so severe as to render attempts at restoring the articular surface impossible. No age limit has been placed upon this operation and although in the older age group recovery has been slower, many of them have gained quite a high order of recovery. The indication to carry out open reduction does not depend on age but on the state of the foot at the time of the injury, the occupation of the patient, the bodily habitus and the general level of morale. The light, active and well motivated, elderly person is quite capable of producing advanced recovery whereas the sluggish, overweight, poorly motivated subject will probably not work again whatever is done.

Ankylosis of the subtaloid joint is quite compatible with a high measure of recovery of function and comfort but the balance and power of the foot is never fully restored and the patient may be reluctant to resume climbing ladders or working on uneven surfaces. Restoring half or more of the range of the subtaloid joint is perhaps the most important goal of treatment.

Speaking generally therefore, the prognosis depends on two factors: firstly the restoration of shape and height of the calcaneum. The orthograde attitude of the bone does much to restore the mechanics of the foot and this by itself makes open reduction worth while. Secondly, there is the preservation of subtaloid movement. Figures suggest that the range of residual subtaloid movement bears some relationship to the ultimate result, but quite a high degree of agility is attained with less than half the normal range of subtaloid movement.

In 84 cases where the age of the patient and the range of movement was recorded at follow-up, 17% had regained virtually full movement, 31% half or more, 28% less than half and 24% had the subtaloid joint ankylosed. There was no significant age difference in any of these categories (Table 43.6). No late painful degenerative change was observed except where there was involvement of the calcaneocuboid joint. The series contains six patients who underwent late triple arthrodesis and only in one of them was the clinical state improved. Primary subtaloid fusion is only effective where the shape and position of the calcaneum has not been seriously disturbed, and in any event these are best treated conservatively. The conclusion must be reached that subtaloid fusion in the absence of reduction is comparable to that of the totally untreated fracture.

Table 43.6 Residual subtaloid movement in reduced displaced fractures where age and range of movement recorded at follow-up

	Full or nearly full	Half or more	Less than half	Ankylosed
Number	14	26	24	20
%	17%	31%	28%	24%
Average age (years)	41	39	43	41

LATE SURGERY

Calcaneofibular abutment and peroneal tendon entrapment

Isbister in 1974 reported excision of the tip of the fibula as an effective method of relieving intractable pain occasioned by the bulging lateral wall of the calcaneum. He reported relief of pain in five cases. He drew attention to the unreduced state of the bone, the lateral bulge of the calcaneum in actual bony contact with the tip of the fibula or compression of the peroneal tendons in the narrowed gap between the bones. He makes the significant remark that 'The patients reported here would probably have avoided this complication if the lateral displacement of the calcaneum had been reduced at the time of the injury'. Previous attempts at relieving this discomfort had been by excision of the bulging lateral wall (Cabot & Binney 1907, Cotton 1921, Magnuson 1923). Evans (1968) decompressed the peroneal tunnel by 'removing functionless tendons'. It can be readily understood therefore that such operation is only necessary where the fracture has not been reduced, when it is undoubtedly beneficial, but after successful reduction this complication is hardly ever seen and the operation rarely necessary.

Is late salvage surgery ever necessary?

Recovery of function and relief of pain after any fracture of the calcaneum is a long and gradual business and many subjects continue to improve up to two or three years after the injury. It is therefore unwise to attempt the surgical relief of symptoms before such a period has elapsed. Much is written about a slow ankylosis of the subtaloid joint and the gradual onset and inexorable increase of 'osteo-arthritis'. Prolonged follow-up of this large personal series of cases, extending over 20 years, has shown that late degenerative change is almost nonexistent and the reader is invited to recall whether he has ever encountered an old case of fractured calcaneum in a patient who has returned to hospital complaining of recent onset or aggravation of pain and demanding treatment. Many patients continue to complain of severe disability for a long period but among these there is a significant proportion of patients involved in litigation, whose morale is low, or who are seeking an excuse for a less arduous life. This is especially true if the surgeon has not maintained an encouraging and hopeful attitude to the patient or when the gravity of the injury has been inculcated in a patient and he becomes convinced that he is 'crippled for life'.

It can be confidently claimed that steady improvement in comfort and function can be anticipated for two or three years until a plateau is reached and the level of this depends on many factors, but thereafter there is no significant decline and late salvage surgery is hardly ever indicated.

A recent review by Pozo et al (1984) of the long-term results of conservative management of severely displaced fractures of the calcaneum confirms these views. 21 patients with an average follow-up of 15 years revealed that three-quarters of the patients achieved a good result with minor symptoms, two-thirds of the patients had reached a point of maximum recovery at two or three years, but a further quarter continued to improve for six years. None of the patients thereafter experienced any deterioration. They make the further observation that neither the degree of clinical stiffness nor the degeneration of the subtalar joint assessed radiographically correlated with the severity of symptoms or functional disability. However if three further cases which had undergone late arthrodesis and which would be considered failures of conservative treatment are included, the good results are reduced to 67%.

COMPLICATIONS

Bilateral calcaneal fracture

This occurs in about 15% of cases and represents a disability more than twice as grave as a unilateral injury. The patient is obliged to be off his feet for not less than two months; he requires crutches and later sticks for several more months, and without one normal foot as support, gait and tiptoeing are slower to recover. However there is no reason to suppose the final result is any more inferior than for a single-sided injury (Figs. 43.15, 16 and 17).

Associated injuries

These may include fractures around the ankle or midtarsus and will seriously limit restoration of movement and mobility.

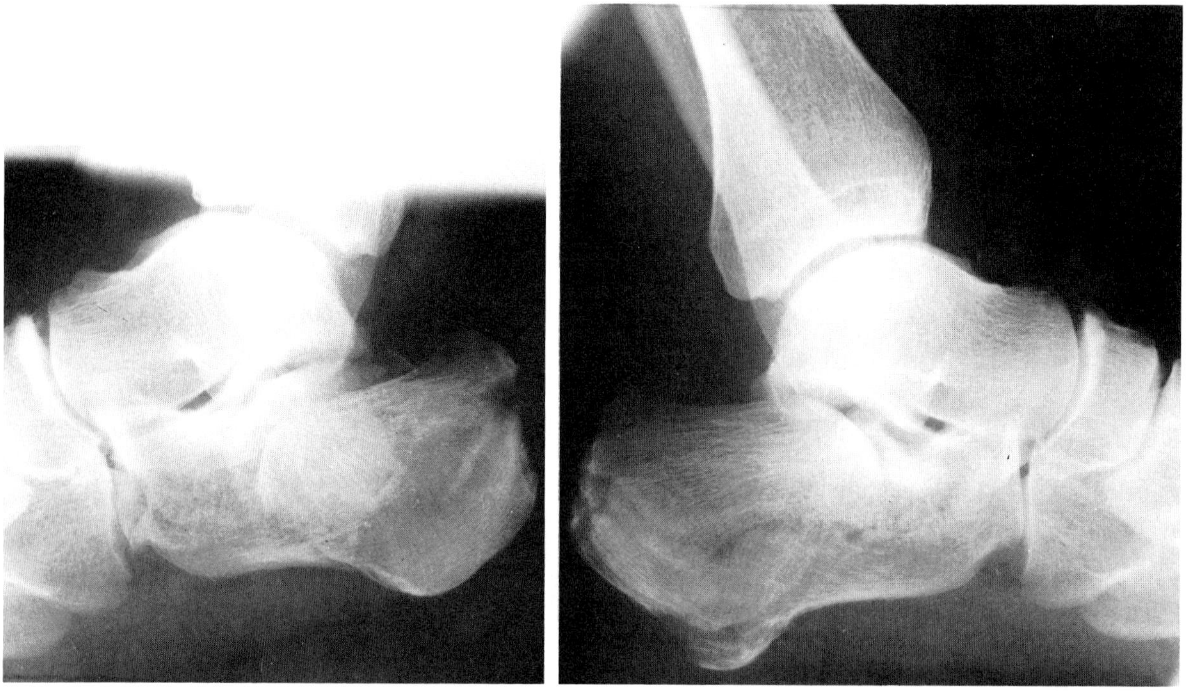

Fig. 43.15 Steeple-jack aged 41 sustained bilateral 'tongue' fractures

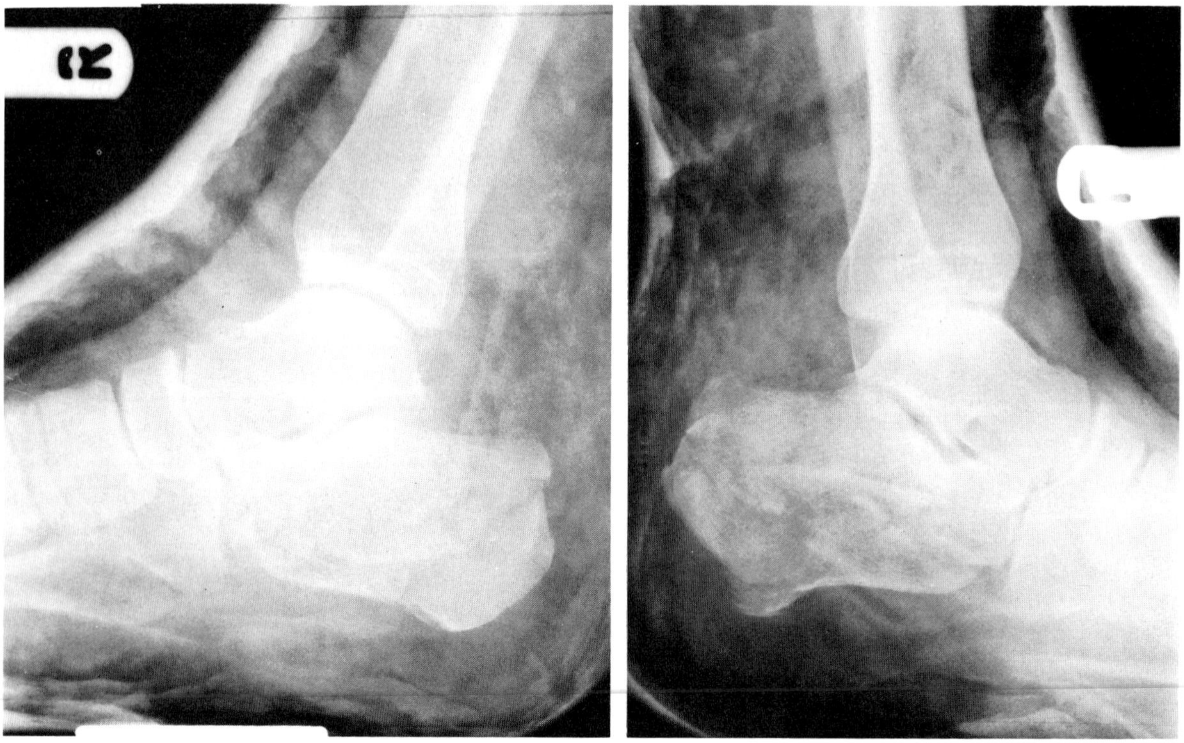

Fig. 43.16 Open reduction and grafting enabled him to return to his full duties at six months.

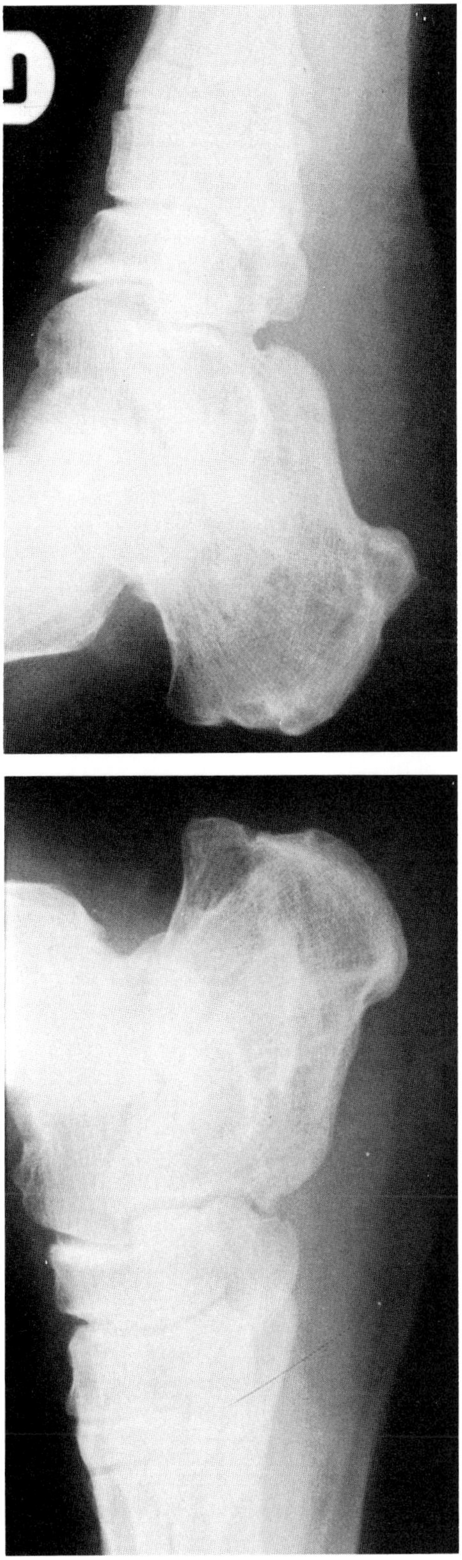

a b

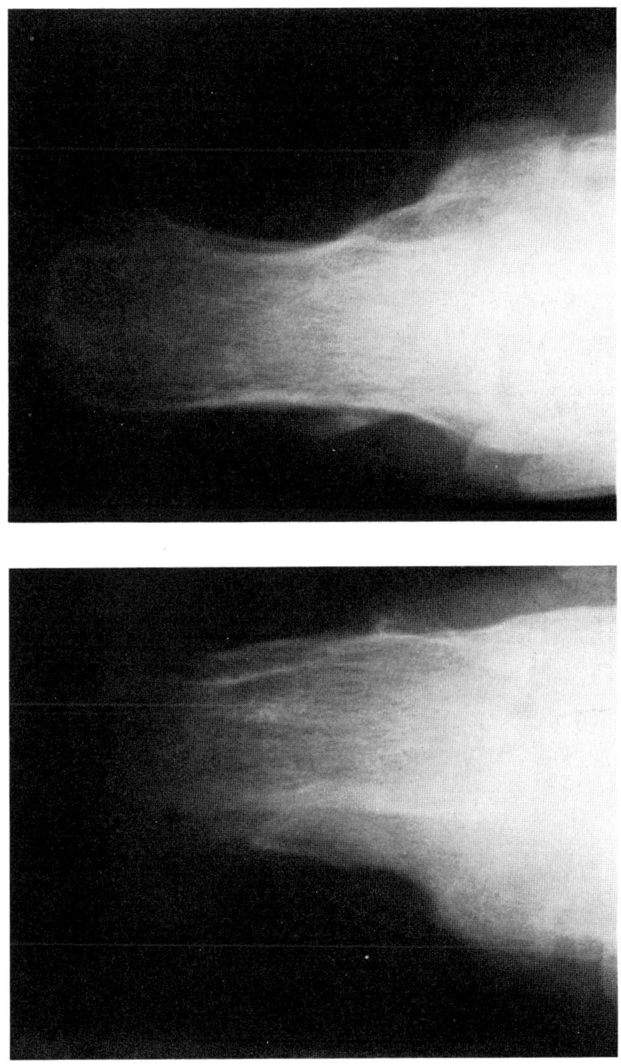

c d

Fig. 43.17a–d Seven year follow-up. Right subtaloid joint (c) probably ankylosed

Persistent pain and tenderness

This is seen chiefly in unreduced fractures and is partly due to bulging of the lateral calcaneal wall (see p. 911) and entrapment of the peroneal tendons but more importantly is due to the destruction of height and posture of the heel with apparent lengthening of the tendo Achillis and valgus deformity of the foot. Many clinics routinely supply their patients with surgical shoes or some variety of support but this simply indicates the ineffectiveness of the treatment provided.

Infection

Infection of the soft tissues and of the bone itself is a serious hazard in those feet which have been impaled by pins or wires and there is always the danger of wound infection after ill-timed or hazardous open surgery. Chronically discharging sinuses may need curettage with some form of soft tissue surgery to achieve healing.

Involvement of the sural nerve

In open reduction of the fracture from the outer side, this nerve or its branches may be involved in the scar. This may lead to permanent tender points, numbness or unpleasant paraesthesia along the outer border of the foot.

Avascular necrosis

It has been claimed that the danger of avascular necrosis of part or the whole of the fractured calcaneum militates against open reduction but in the personal series already cited only one example has been observed and this showed steady revascularization. Indeed the calcaneum is normally so plentifully nourished from multiple sources that bone union is sufficiently advanced within three weeks of the fracture as to make open reduction well nigh impossible.

Osteoarthritic degeneration

All damaged weight-bearing joints must undergo some mechanical changes of wear and tear but although X-ray appearances may indicate osteoarthritis by narrowing of the subtaloid joint with subchondral sclerosis, such changes are not indicative of deteriorating function.

An unusual opportunity has been afforded the writer to carry out postmortem examination in two cases of bilateral fracture of the calcaneum in subjects dying from other causes. The first was a female aged 69 who sustained bilateral fractures some nine years previously. Open reduction and grafting in both heels had been performed. Two years later she had half the range of subtaloid movement in both feet, she could walk well, tiptoe, jump and hop without pain. On exposing the hindfoot at autopsy, the peroneal tendons in both feet were freely mobile with shiny surfaces. The subtaloid joints had smooth articular cartilage but with some fissuring and thinning at the margins. The calcaneocuboid joints were unaffected.

The second case was a male aged 50 who had sustained bilateral fissure fractures some seven years previously. He had been treated conservatively. He had returned to climbing in four months and his full work as a window cleaner six months after the injury. Six years later the feet showed excellent function, normal subtaloid movement and he was able to run and play football in soft sand. Postmortem inspection of the subtaloid joints showed them to be well preserved, but again there was some fibrillated articular cartilage.

CONCLUSION

Fracture of the calcaneum, although a relatively rare condition, continues to be a source of much disability. It is a fracture that is not well understood and it responds poorly to a casual attitude or a counsel of despair by the surgeon. It is evident that intensive treatment, early movement and physiotherapy can produce good results, even if the foot remains permanently deformed. Treatment by plaster fixation for longer than six weeks leads inevitably to a much greater proportion of poor results. An enlightened attitude by Orthopaedic Surgeons, General Practitioners, lawyers and employers and trades unions is essential. These patients are not 'done for' or to be 'written off' as manual workers and the tradition must be broken where authors writing on this condition perpetuate an attitude of gloom which is communicated to young surgeons in training. Full potential of recovery after this injury may take two years or more; late degenerative changes are almost unknown despite X-ray appearances; and there is little or no indication for joint fusion. Late release of peroneal tendon entrapment may occasionally be necessary in those cases which have not been reduced, but early vigorous and enlightened treatment will in the vast majority of cases result in long-lasting and satisfactory function.

ACKNOWLEDGEMENTS

I am grateful to my ex-Registrar Mr. A. A. Qazi for allowing me to quote freely from his MCh. Thesis and to Mr. J. Burke for making his findings available to me of his unpublished retrospective analysis from Sheffield.

REFERENCES

Allan J H 1955 The open reduction of fractures of the os calcis. Ann Surg 141: 890
Anthonsen W 1943 An oblique projection for Roentgen examination of the talo-calcaneal joint particularly regarding intra-articular fracture of the calcaneus. Acta Radiol 24: 306
Bankart A S B 1942 Fractures of the os calcis. Lancet 2: 175
Böhler L 1931 Diagnosis, pathology and treatment of fracture of the os calcis. J Bone Joint Surg 13: 75
Broden B 1949 Roentgen examination of the subtaloid joint in fractures of the calcaneus. Acta Radiol 31: 85
Burke J 1983 Review of 288 fractures of the os calcis seen in Sheffield 1961–71. Personal communication
Cabot H, Binney H 1907 Fractures of the os calcis and astragalus. Ann Surg 45: 51
Conn H R 1926 Fractures of the os calcis. Diagnosis and treatment. Radiology 6: 228
Conn H R 1943 Discussion on arthrodesis in fractures of the os calcis. J Bone Joint Surg 25: 73
Cotton F J 1921 Old os calcis fractures. Ann Surg 74: 294
Cotton F J, Henderson F F 1916 Result of fractures of the os calcis. Amer J Ortho Surg 14: 290
Essex-Lopresti P 1952 The mechanism, reduction technique and results in fractures of the os calcis. Br J Surg 39: 395
Evans D 1968 Fractures of the calcaneus. J Bone Joint Surg 50B: 884
Fisk G R 1978 Fractured calcaneum treated by bone grafting. Hunterian lecture RCS Eng
Gallie W E 1943 Subastragular arthrodesis in fractures of the os calcis. J Bone Joint Surg 25: 73
Gissane W 1947 Discussion. Fractures of the os calcis. Annual meeting of Brit Orthop Assoc London 18–19 1946. J Bone Joint Surg 29: 255
Hall M C, Pennal G F 1960 Primary subtalar arthrodesis in the treatment of fractures of the calcaneum. J Bone Joint Surg 42B: 336
Herman O J 1937 Conservative therapy for fractures of the os calcis. J Bone Joint Surg 19: 709
Isbister J F St. C 1974 Calcaneo-fibular abutment following crush fracture of the calcaneum. J Bone Joint Surg 56B: 274
Lenormant C, Wilmoth T, Lecoeur 1928 A propos de traitement sanglant des fractures du calcaneum. Bull Mem Soc Anat Chir 13: 53
Leriche R 1922 Synthese primitive pour fracture par écrasement du calcaneum. Lyon. Chir 19: 559
Lindsay W R N, Dewar F P 1958 Fractures of the os calcis. Am J Surg 95: 555
London P 1967 A practical guide to the care of the injured. Livingstone, Edinburgh. pp. 523–527
McReynolds I S 1976 Fractures of the os calcis involving the subastragalar joint. Treatment by open reduction and internal fixation with staples using a medial approach. J Bone Joint Surg 58A: 733
Magnuson P B 1923 An operation for relief of disability in old fractures of the os calcis. JAMA 80: 1511
Malgaigne J 1847 Traité des fractures et des luxations. Paris
Moberg E 1951 Comminuted fractures of the calcaneus with joint injuries. Congrès International de Chirurgerie Orthopédique et de Traumatologie: 632
Morestin H 1902 Traitement opératif de l'écrasement du calcaneum. Bull Mem Soc Anat Paris 225
Norris G 1839 Fracture of the os calcis, delirium tremens, gangrene. Am J Med Sci 23: 278
Palmer I 1945 Forstag till operativ behandlung av vissa kalkaneus fracturer. Nord Med 26: 869
Palmer I 1948 Mechanism and treatment of fractures of the calcaneum. J Bone Joint Surg 30A: 2
Pozo J L, Kirwan E O'G, Jackson A M 1984 J Bone Joint Surg 66B: 386
Pridie K 1946 A new method of treatment for severe fractures of the os calcis. Surg Gynecol Obstet 82: 671
Protheroe K 1969 Avulsion fractures of the calcaneus. J Bone Joint Surg 51B: 118
Qazi A A 1968 Open reduction and bone graft as treatment of displaced intra-articular fractures of the os calcis. Thesis MCh (Orth), Liverpool
Roberts N W, Sayle-Creer W 1947 Fractures of the os calcis. Lancet 252: 65
Schofield R O 1936 J Bone Joint Surg 18: 566
Soeur R, Rémy R 1975 Fractures of the calcaneus with displacement of the thalamic portion. J Bone Joint Surg 57B: 413
Thorèn O 1964 Os calcis fractures. Acta Orthop Scand Suppl 70
Warwick C K, Bremner A E 1953 Fractures of the calcaneum. J Bone Joint Surg 35B: 33
Whittaker A H 1947 Treatment of fractures of the os calcis by open reduction and internal fixation. Am J Surg 74: 687
Widèn A 1954 Fractures of the calcaneus. Acta Chir Scand, Stockholm, Suppl 188
Zayer M 1969 Fracture of the calcaneus. A review of 110 fractures. Acta Orthop Scand 40: 530

Talar and peritalar injuries

HISTORY

Originally the astragalus was a rounded piece of bone, used as a die in gambling. It was oblong with two sides curved and four flat. The flat surfaces were numbered 1, 3, 4, 6. The game was played with four astragali — or tali — and the best cast was that which offered different numbers of the four tali — a so-called Venus. The worst was a dog — canis — with the number of one only on each talus.

TALAR ANATOMY AND FUNCTION

The connection between the lower leg and the foot is maintained by the astragalus, or as it is more commonly called, the talus. It is enclosed between the lateral malleolus, the lower articular surface of the tibia and its malleolus, the calcaneus and the navicular bone. It forms the keystone for movements between the foot and the lower leg. It thus has the combined function of stability and mobility in the ankle joint.

The talus consists of the neck and head articulating against the navicular bone, the trochlea against the tibia and fibula, and the body against the calcaneus (Figs. 44.1 and 2).

During the growth period the talus changes its internal direction in two aspects. In infancy the neck is directed some 30° medially. With increasing age this direction diminishes to some 15–20°. Furthermore, in infancy the neck is longitudinally rotated more laterally than in adulthood when it straightens up.

The neck and head

The neck continues into the head which articulates

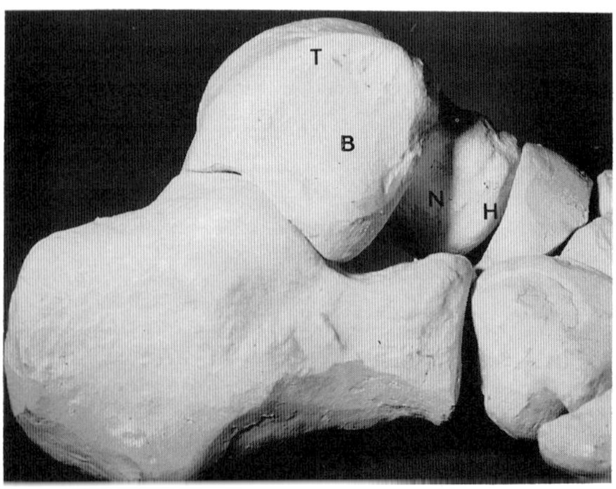

Fig. 44.1 Model of talus and surrounding bones from the lateral aspect. T = Trochlea tali; B = Body; N = Neck; H = Head

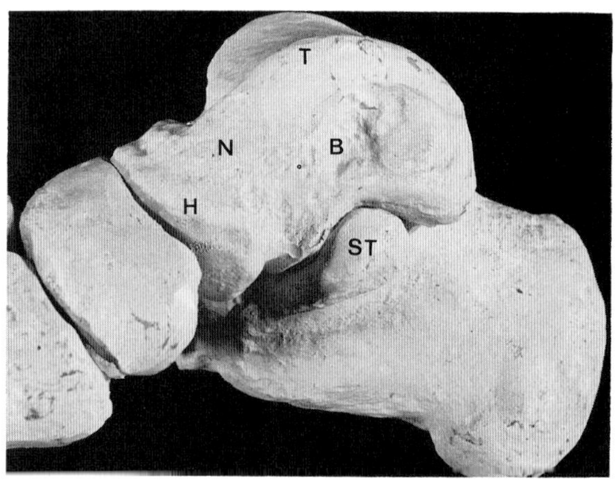

Fig. 44.2 Model of talus and surrounding bones from medial aspect. T = Trochlea; B = Body; N = Neck; H = Head; ST = Sustentaculum tali

against the navicular bone. This joint forms the medial part of the Chopart's joint. The head also articulates against an anterior facet of the calcaneus. Further, it articulates against a ligament which joins the sustentaculum tali of the calcaneus with the tuberosity of the navicular bone. This is the spring or calcaneonavicular ligament. Part of pronation-supination or eversion-inversion occurs in this multiaxial joint (Fig. 44.3).

The trochlea

The trochlea is enclosed in the malleolar mortise giving the lower leg — and consequently the whole body — stability during the stance phase in gait. It is covered by cartilage on the superior aspect articulating against the tibial plafond and on both sides articulating against the medial and the lateral malleoli respectively. The radius of the trochlear curve is some 20 mm and the circumference represents one-third of a circle. The radius of curvature of the talus is less on the medial side than on the lateral. This means that the trochlea is not a section of a cylinder, but rather a frustum of a cone converging medially (Fig. 44.4).

There is a difference in the anterior and posterior transverse dimensions of the trochlea, the range extending from 0 to 6 mm. In most tali there is a wedging of the trochlea with the posterior width as much as 25% less than the anterior (Fig. 44.5). The talar sides are parallel to the articular facets of the malleoli.

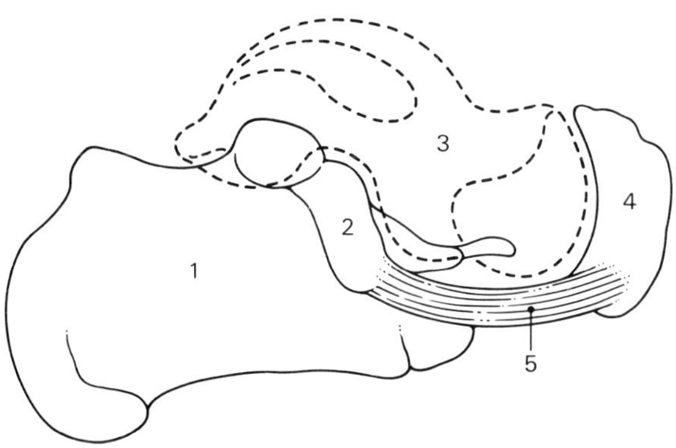

Fig. 44.3 Schematic drawing of calcaneus navicular bone and talus to illustrate the calcaneonavicular ligament. 1 = calcaneus; 2 = articular facet; 3= talus; 4 = navicular bone; 5 = calcaneonavicular ligament

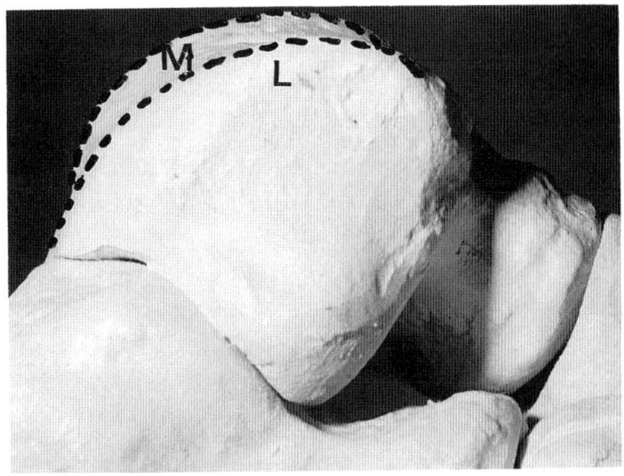

Fig. 44.4 Dotted lines on trochlea illustrate the curvature of the lateral (L) and medial (M) sides respectively. The radius is less on the medial side

The question of stability on plantar flexion, considering the narrowness of the posterior aspect of the trochlea has to be related to the axis around which the trochlea rotates. If the axis is transverse either the distance between the malleoli will change during movement or it will remain stationary and instability will follow on plantar flexion, when the narrower part of the trochlea occupies the mortise.

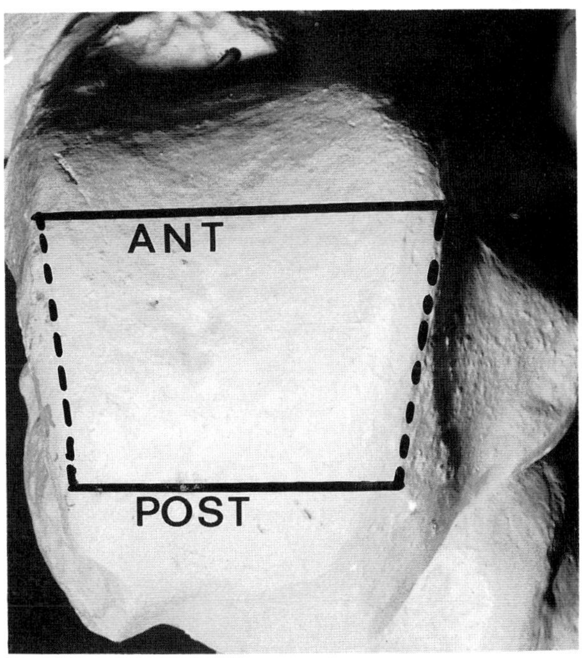

Fig. 44.5 Superior aspect of the trochlea. The anterior transverse dimension is larger than the posterior

Relative to trochlear movement there is a play of the lateral malleolus from 0 to 2 mm. On dorsiflexion of the talus the lateral malleolus is displaced in a straight proximal direction. However, ankle mobility does not become restricted by the absence of mobility of the mortise. In other words a 'stiff' ankle does not limit mobility.

The axis for the rotation of the trochlea is constantly changing within a narrow limit. In the coronal plane the axis runs at an inclination downward from the medial malleolar tip to just distal to the lateral malleolar tip, but deviates posteriorly from the coronal plane.

The body

By its connection with the navicular bone the talus has an important influence on the function of the forefoot.

The hindfoot of which the talus forms a part has a substantial component, the calcaneus. The superior part articulates against and supports the talus by its posterior, middle and anterior articular surfaces. Between the posterior and middle articular surfaces there is a groove, the sulcus calcanei, which together with the sulcus tali forms the sinus tarsi. An artery (arteria sinus tarsi) of some importance to the nutrition of the talus runs through this groove.

The movement of the subtalar joint occurs around an axis inclined in two planes, one running in the sagittal plane at an inclination of 42° and the other in the horizontal plane from posterolateral to anteromedial at an angle of 23° from the midline of the foot. Thus, the motion of the subtalar joint is rotatory in a way corresponding to the movement produced in a 'mitred hinge', which has been suggested as an explanatory term for the complex motion in the subtalar joint. The range of motion varies markedly and values from 10 to 60° have been reported.

TALAR AND PERITALAR INJURIES

Injuries to the talus mostly involve fractures. Peritalar injuries are ligament strains which may turn into ruptures and consequently lead to dislocation of the talus.

Talar injuries

Fractures of the talus occur in the neck, head, body, posterior process and trochlea (so called osteochondral fracture).

Fracture of the neck

More than 30% of talar fractures are sustained in the neck.

Fracture mechanism

In 1952 Coltart reported on a total of 25 000 fractures in patients who had served in the Royal Air Force during World War II. In this material he found 4000 fractures of the foot and of these 228 involved the talus. 106 of these were fractures of the neck and in 69 there was a displacement, the remainder being nondisplaced. Thus, fractures of the neck in this material were encountered in about 45%.

The fracture has been called aviator's fracture as in earlier times it was seen mostly in aviation accidents where no mortalities were recorded. It is evident from most studies that the fracture is produced as a result of motor vehicle accidents, or falls from heights and off falling objects. It has also been believed that the fractures occur when the foot is forcefully pressed in dorsiflexion and the sharp anterior margin of the tibia cuts into the talus.

Coltart (1952) explained the fracture mechanism: 'In an accident dorsiflexion of the foot and impaction of the tibia against the talus occur together. The former ruptures ligaments, the latter fractures the neck. The body of the talus is pressed backwards by the approximation of the wedge-like lower end of the tibia to the calcaneus'. This has been a concept on which most authors have agreed. Some serious criticism, however, was offered on the assumption that if the tibia actually fractured the neck of the talus, it could be argued that more damage to the anterior margin of the tibia and of the cervical cortex of the talus should occur.

In 1974 Peterson studied the fracture mechanism of talar neck fractures and observed that no abnormalities could be demonstrated in the osseous structure of the anterior margin of the tibia. This prompted the question of whether a talar neck fracture may be the result of forces which need not necessarily include involvement of the tibia.

In laboratory experiments the idea was supported that in clinical fractures there is a pretension of the foot, brought about either by extending the leg (contracting the quadriceps and the triceps surae muscles and thus straining the Achilles tendon) or by pressing the heel against a surface. A simultaneous counteracting force must be exerted on the forefoot to produce the fracture.

The assumption was made that force and deformation occur in one plane. Tissues are expected overall to have equal elastic properties and the ligaments to be of secondary importance.

The talus can be assumed to act as a cantilever between the tibia and the calcaneus. At its rear end the talus is clamped in the ankle mortise by a pretension force (P_2, see Fig. 44.6). For external equilibrium a force (P_1) is required for the forefoot. An impact (P_p) is applied to the midfoot and in the experiments this was supplied by a pendulum hammer. As this impact increases in force P_1 will decrease and P_2 will increase. When $P_1 = 0$, equilibrium exists about a fixed axis B, running in the horizontal plane, and $P_p \cdot a - P_2 \cdot b = 0$. If $\frac{a}{b}$ is considered constant during the impact, P_2 will increase proportionally to P_p, i.e. $P_2 = \frac{a}{b} \cdot P_p$. The ultimate strength of the talar neck will at some point be exceeded and the fracture will occur, as during the impact both bending and shear stresses develop.

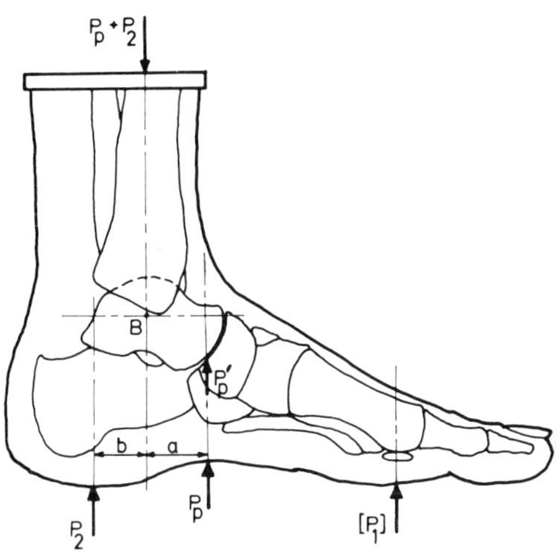

Fig. 44.6 The forces acting on the foot during the impact. For further details see text

These, however, depend on the cross-section of the bone and decreasing cross-sections will give increasing shear stresses. In this manner the collum tali will be exposed to a compound stress with the maximum occurring between the head and the clamped part.

As illustrated in Figs. 44.7a and b, the experiments were carried out by having a pendulum hit the foot at the point expected to be the most likely to convey stresses resulting in a talar neck fracture. The foot was placed in an ordinary shoe to the sole of which two transverse steel bands were rivetted firmly, one under the heads of the metatarsals and one under the heel. In those bands four rigging screws were attached and anchored to the stand by chains, two medially and two laterally. This gave full control of the inversion-eversion and the degree of dorsiflexion. It also allowed the possibility of applying varying pretension to the foot. The striking point and the direction of the pendulum was checked with X-ray in lateral and anteroposterior view and adjustments were made.

The following conclusions could be drawn:

1. Fractures of the talar neck could be produced by an impact on cadaveric feet.
2. The fractures were similar to those seen clinically.
3. The fracture mechanism did not demand a direct contact between the talar neck and the anterior margin of the tibia, which thus did not necessitate a maximal dorsiflexion of the foot as had previously been suggested.
4. The theory of the talus being fixed as a cantilever explained some of the clinical talar neck fractures.

In six experiments fractures were consecutively produced of the talar neck. In another three experiments failures were due to mishaps during the experimental procedure, such as rupture of the heel-coat of the shoe and fractures of the tibia at its insertion in the epoxy-plast due to improper alignment of the forces transferred by the pendulum.

As an example, Peterson reported on a 27-year-old nurse who was driving a car. She noticed at some distance a car approaching which suddenly started skidding towards her. It became obvious to her that a head-on collision was inevitable. Realizing this she instantly pressed her left foot against the clutch and her right foot against the brake. At the same time she

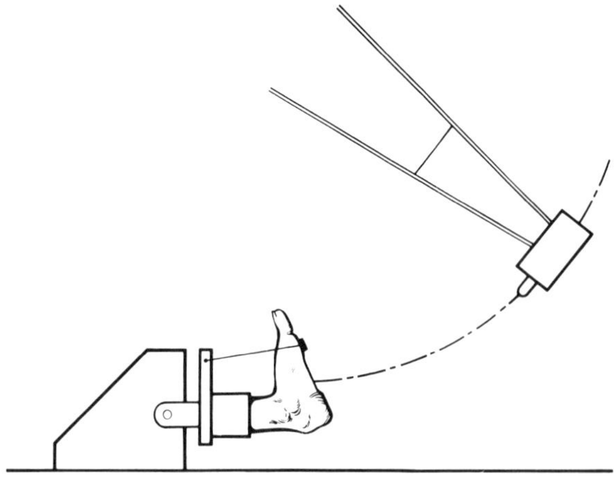

Fig. 44.7a The testing set-up consisting of a pendulum and a foot on a stand. The foot is held in maximal dorsiflexion

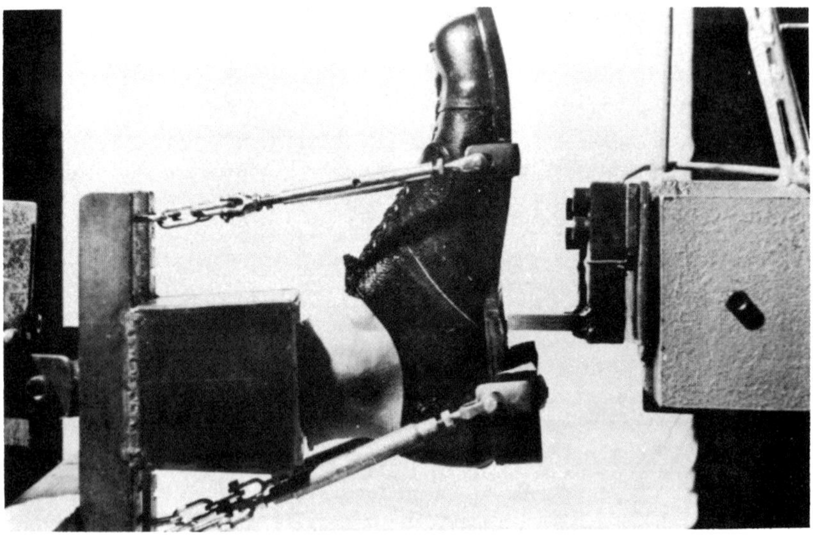

Fig. 44.7b Close-up view of pendulum hammer and foot in shoe strained by rigging screws

stretched out her arms and pressed her hands against the wheel. At the collision the nurse sustained a talar neck fracture in her right foot and a medial malleolar fracture in her left foot. The clutch went down with the foot flat on the floor. The brake, however, stopped at a distance from the floor and acted as an impact body at the moment of collision, thus creating conditions (stretched leg and counteracting force on the forefoot) which Peterson had found in his experimental model to produce talar neck fractures.

Grading

In 1970 Hawkins suggested a grading into three groups of talar neck fractures:

Group I: Vertical fracture of the neck of the talus without displacement (Fig. 44.8).

Group II: Vertical fracture of the neck of the talus with displacement of the body from the subtalar joint but not from the talocrural joint (Fig. 44.9).

Group III: Vertical fracture of the neck of the talus with displacement of the body from both the subtalar and talocrural joints (Figs. 44.10a and b). In material described by Peterson & Goldie (1974) 46 patients were reported. 13 belonged to Group I, 22 to Group II, and 11 to Group III. The age range varied from 15 to 68 years. The majority of patients had sustained their fractures in motor vehicle accidents. Falling from heights was also a common cause.

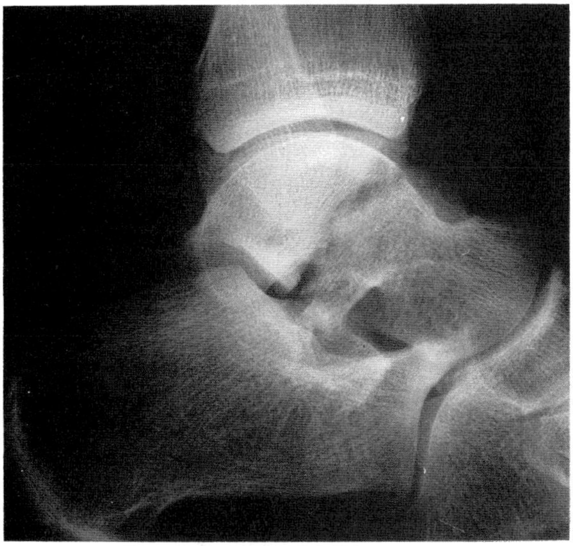

Fig. 44.8 Group 1 fracture of talar neck (Hawkins). No displacement but fracture runs partly into the body

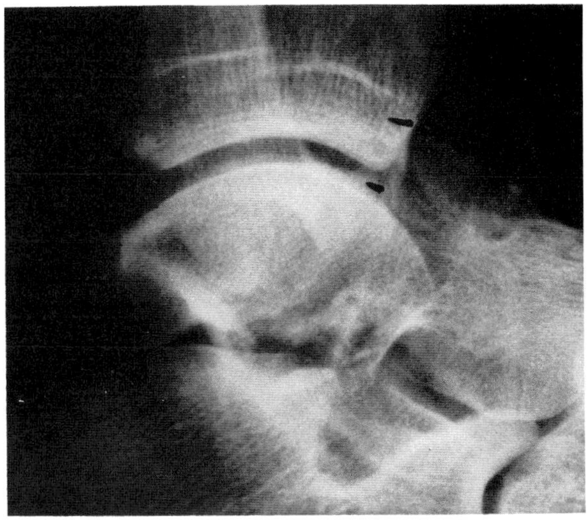

Fig. 44.9 Group 2 fracture of the talar neck (Hawkins). Dislocation

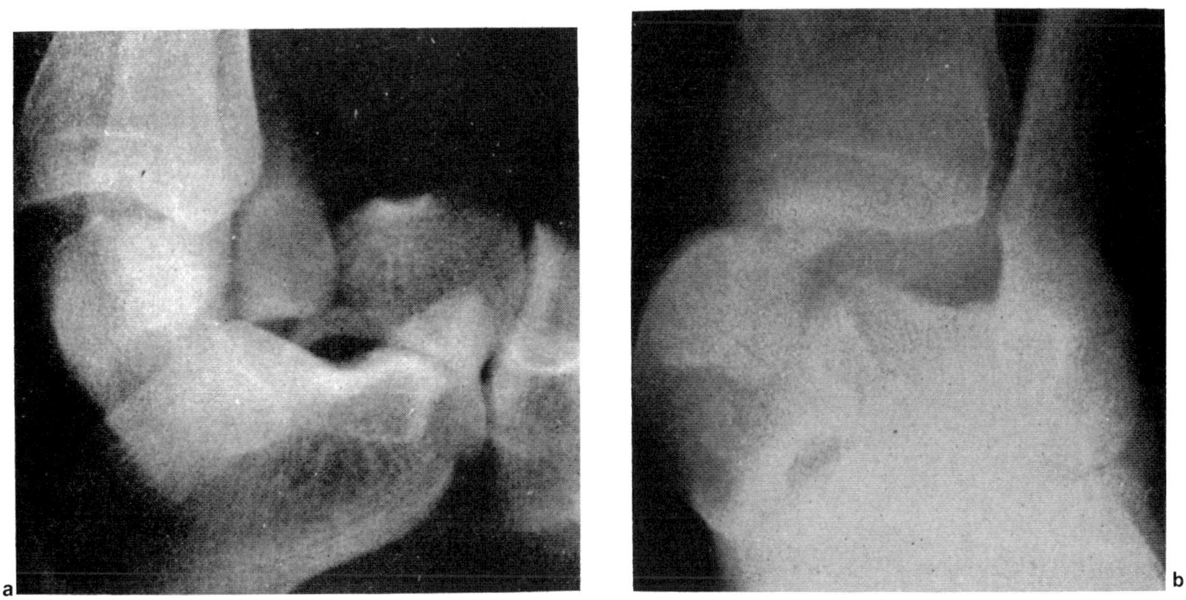

Fig. 44.10 (a) Group 3 fracture of talar neck (Hawkins) severe dislocation and fragmentation. Lateral view. (b) In A-P projection

Symptoms

Symptoms are swelling, at times bruising, around the ankle but also diffusely in the foot, and pain, both at rest and on motion. Passive motion will cause great pain.

Treatment

Treatment depends on the type of fracture. When the fracture is undisplaced, a plaster should be applied from the toes to the knee joint. The foot should preferably be in the neutral position. If, however, reduction is difficult to maintain, plantar flexion may facilitate the maintenance of the reduced position. Immobilization of the foot and non-weight-bearing are maintained for 6–8 weeks. Following this an elastic bandage replaces the plaster for two weeks during which time the patient starts progressively increasing weight bearing. At 10–12 weeks full weight bearing is permitted.

Dislocated fractures must be reduced and this can be done either by closed or open means. If a dislocated fracture can be reduced closed and reduction maintained, a plaster is applied and the same regime followed as for the undisplaced fractures. If the reduction by closed means cannot be maintained, two Kirschner wires should be passed percutaneously through the navicular bone into and through the talus. The same regime is then followed as for undisplaced fractures.

When attempts at closed reduction are unsuccessful, open reduction should be carried out. A medial longitudinal incision is made. The medial malleolus is osteotomized. An excellent exposure of the talus is now offered, facilitating the inspection of the fracture as well as the manipulation of fragments and osseous fixation. This is most easily achieved by one or more Kirschner wires. The same regime as for undisplaced fractures is then followed. With a mean observation time of 6 years, Peterson (1974) could demonstrate excellent results in 30 of 35 patients in Groups I and II and in 6 out of 8 patients in Group III.

Complications

The dreaded complication especially in displaced fractures is the development of avascular necrosis. This is thought to be brought about by the influence the fracture has on the vascular supply to the talus. Once destroyed it appears that the reparative capacity of the vascular network is so poor that it is unable to restore a circulation satisfactory enough to permit normal healing of the fracture. Avascular necrosis on X-ray is interpreted as sclerosis affecting part or all of the talar body. According to Brinkman (1973) this occurs in 2–7% depending on the degree of displacement and in 2% in undisplaced fractures.

Avascular necrosis need not necessarily yield clinical symptoms. The reason for avascular necrosis is nevertheless obscure and becomes more confusing as it has been shown that the talus is in the midst of an arterial network with vascular sources like the arteria canalis tarsi, the anastomosing arteria sinus tarsi, the rami deltoidei from the arteria canalis tarsi, branches from the arteria dorsalis pedis entering the neck of the talus and finally the small arteries in the capsules and ligaments which connect the talus with the surrounding bones.

In a study of the arterial supply of the talus (Goldie et al 1974) it was shown that, apart from the above, there are rich vascular connections between the tibial and the talar marrow spaces by way of the interconnecting capsules and ligaments. It thus appears that the risk of avascular necrosis is minimal if regard is paid to the amount of vessels surrounding and entering the talus. If, on the other hand, these connections become destroyed and are not given a chance to be reestablished by failure in the reduction of a talar neck fracture, the circulation may become impeded giving rise to talar necrosis. In Figs. 44.11a, b, c, and d, the arterial supply is demonstrated after injection of the vascular tree with Micropaque and with the specimens prepared according to the Spalteholtz method, which makes organic tissues transparent.

It has been shown experimentally that fractures without displacement generally rupture ascending

Fig. 44.11a Intraosseous vascularization of the talus and interosseous anastomoses. Medial aspect of a section through the left foot in a 38-year-old woman. The contour of the calcaneus (C) is partly obliterated by the tendon of the flexor hallucis longus (FHL). Large arrow indicates branch from the arteria dorsalis pedis entering the talus. Small arrows indicate the continuation of the penetrating branches from the ramus deltoideus. Black dot at cut arteria canalis tarsi

Fig. 44.11b Intraosseous vascularization of the talus and interosseous anastomoses. Medial aspect of a section from the left foot in a 38-year-old woman. Arrow at arteria canalis tarsi. C = calcaneus; N = navicular bone; T = tibia

Fig. 44.11c Medial aspect of right talocrural joint in 13-year-old girl. Rich anastomotic vascular network in anterior and posterior ligaments and joint capsule between tibia and talus. Marked area is enlarged in Fig. 44.11d. The darker areas in the tibia and the talus are due to insufficient decalcification

Fig. 44.11d Angiography with higher resolution of marked area in Fig. 44.11c. Vascular connections between the tibia and the talus (TA) via the ligaments and the joint capsule

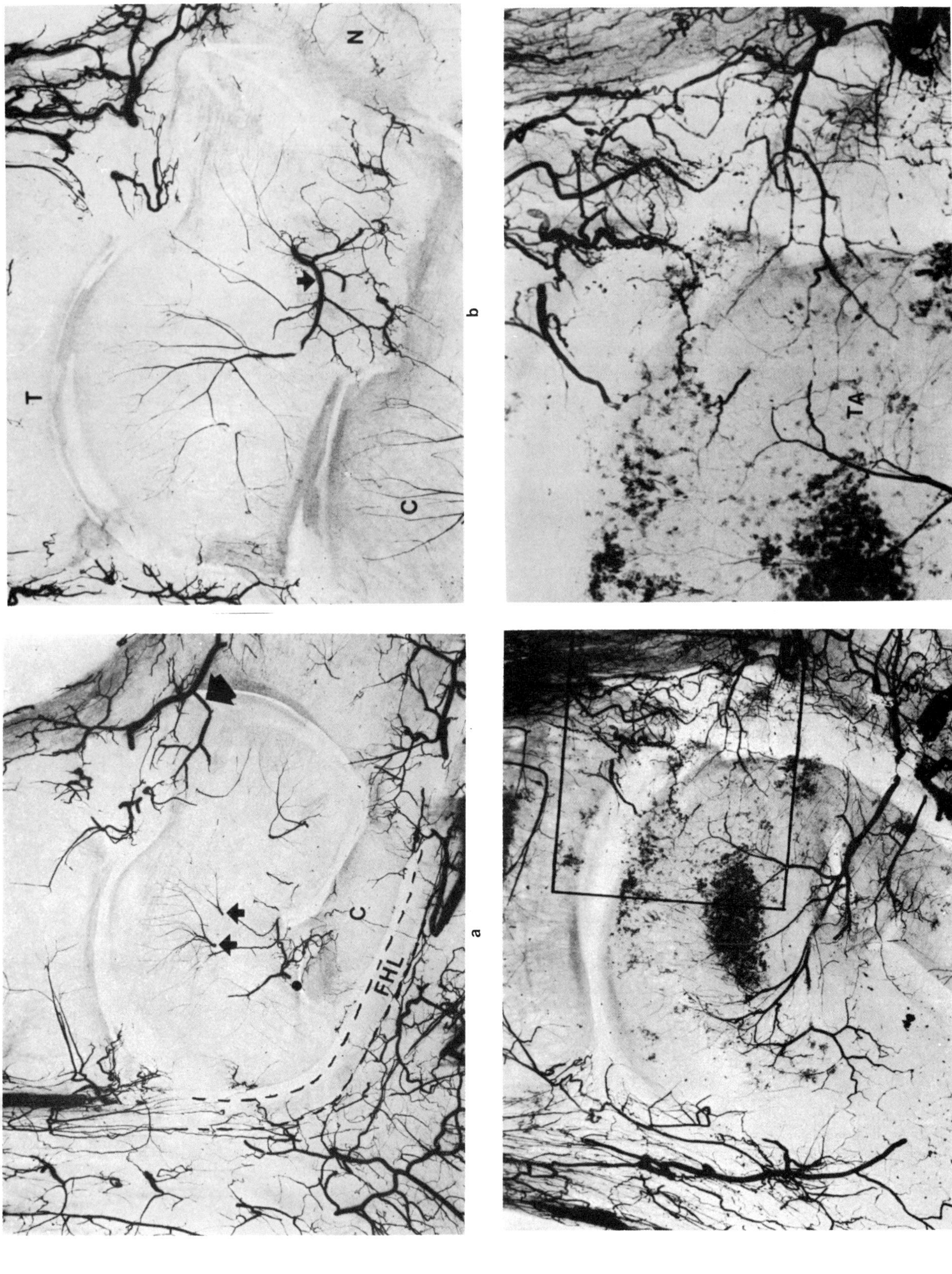
T
N
C
b
C
FHL
a
TA
d
c

branches from the arteria canalis tarsi as well as descending branches from the arteria dorsalis pedis in the fracture area. With displacement of the body of the talus from the subtalar joint the arteria canalis tarsi itself generally ruptures.

How the talus survives and how prominent avascular necrosis becomes is probably dependent on the numerous sources of vessels mentioned above, and it therefore appears obvious that a prompt, exact, and stable reduction should be achieved and maintained in order to restore the best possible circulation to the talar neck. Despite this, some confusion exists as to the best initial handling of these fractures to avoid this possible future complication. Procedures have been suggested like talectomy, amputation, arthrodesis and reduction either by closed or open means. Irrespective of method the aim has been to restore as acceptable as possible a function. Whether the reduction is closed or open does not seem to have any clinical significance as long as the fracture is reduced. In Peterson's material (1974) avascular necrosis occurred in 6 of 16 patients, all in the displaced fracture group. Avascular necrosis seems to be a radiographic diagnosis and need not necessarily yield any clinical symptoms.

Subchondral atrophy seen as a radiolucent line under the cartilage was seen in 18 patients with displaced fractures and was regarded as a good prognostic sign in the prediction of sparing from avascular necrosis (Hawkins 1970). This is in contrast to the femoral head in which a subchondral radiolucent line, the crescent sign after a subcapital fracture, predicts a bad prognosis.

Another complication in the talar neck fracture is delayed union. In Peterson's material (1974) this occurred in 6 patients who, however, had all united at the time of follow-up. A purely mechanical complication may follow a less successful reduction of talar neck fractures. A malunited fracture may block function by limiting dorsiflexion. Degenerative changes were apparent in 35 of 36 patients.

Fracture of the head

Fractures of the talar head are seen in 10% of talar fractures.

Fracture mechanism

A fall on the dorsiflexed foot may cause a fracture of the talar head. It is believed that the fracture is caused by the talar head being compressed against the anterior edge of the tibia and force then being transmitted from the forepart of the foot to the navicular bone dissipating in the talar head and causing the fracture.

Symptoms

There is swelling over the foot with a haematoma. There is tenderness of the talus and eversion and inversion cause pain. There is, nevertheless, motion in the talonavicular joint which can be moved with surprising ease.

As illustrated by radiography, the fractures are very seldom displaced. The fragments are kept in place by the strong intertarsal ligaments.

Treatment

Treatment is conservative with a plaster cast over the foot and lower leg up to the knee. This is changed as the swelling disappears. In all, the cast should be kept on for 8 weeks. Mobilization after removal of the cast might be facilitated by fitting an arch support into the shoe for some time.

Generally, fractures of the talar head heal uneventfully, but an occasional complication is osteoarthritis of the talonavicular joint. If this causes considerable pain an arthrodesis of the joint could be suggested. Before this is done, however, injections of steroid compounds can be offered with a stabilizing orthosis.

Fracture of the body

Fractures of the talar body occur in 20% of injuries involving the talus.

Fracture mechanism

A fall on an extended foot and ankle may cause talar body fracture. It is the result of a significant compression force. As a rule, the force is so considerable that it involves the ligaments and may cause a dislocation of the fragments as well as of the talocalcaneal joint.

Symptoms

There is swelling over the anterior aspect of the ankle joint and moving this causes excessive pain. There is tenderness over the talus and pain on pronation and supination as the talocalcaneal joint is commonly involved.

Treatment

Undisplaced fractures should be treated conservatively with a plaster cast to the knee for 8 weeks. The prognosis is very good and only some 10% have been reported to develop avascular necrosis.

Displaced fractures can be reduced by either closed or open methods. If attempts at closed reduction are not successful, open reduction should not be delayed.

Access to the fracture is most easily accomplished by a medial incision with an osteotomy of the medial malleolus. This provides a good overall view of the talus and also facilitates reduction and the insertion of devices for internal fixation, which should be the simplest possible, e.g. Kirschner wires or screws. The foot is put into a plaster for 8 weeks and should be placed in a neutral position.

The prognosis is good; a favourable prognostic sign is a lucent zone in the subchondral area of the talus (compare talar neck fracture) (Hawkins 1970).

An open fracture is best treated by wound debridement and covered with saline soaks for some 48 to 72 hours after which the wound is reexamined. If it is found necessary, renewed debridement should be carried out and at the same time the fracture reduced and fixed with Kirschner wires. If possible the wound is closed. If there is a risk of tight tension developing it is better to apply a skin graft.

In severely comminuted fracture, opinions vary as to whether a talectomy or an arthrodesis should be carried out. In our own experience arthrodesis has proved a satisfactory procedure, though the patient may experience discomfort for quite some time following the healing of the fracture.

Fracture of the posterior process

Fracture mechanism

The posterior process may become impinged between the posterior lip of the tibia and the calcaneus on extreme flexion of the ankle. When a strong force is applied in this position a fracture may develop.

Symptoms

The patient complains of pain over the posterior aspect of the ankle and there is tenderness posterior to the lateral malleolus over the ankle mortise. Movements in the ankle joint cause pain.

Radiography will disclose the fracture. (The presence of an os trigonum which is an accessory bone has to be remembered). The fragment is hardly ever displaced and treatment can be limited to a stabilizing bandage. When the patient feels no more discomfort, full weight bearing may be permitted. If pain should remain after a long time and there are no signs of healing the fragment should be removed.

Osteochondral fractures (osteochondritis dissecans)

Osteochondral fractures occur in 14% of all fractures of the talus.

Fracture mechanism

It has been reported that in 80–92% of cases significant ankle trauma preceded the development of a talar dome lesion which in location and appearance was similar to that of osteochondritis dissecans.

Experimental evidence has been produced that the talar dome lesion is traumatic in origin and the term ‘transchondral talar fracture’ has been suggested. In 1959 Berndt & Harty presented an extensive review of previously published literature on transchondral fractures of the talar dome as well as their own practical experience, which amounted to 24 patients. In order further to analyse the mechanism of osteochondral fractures of the talar dome, they conducted an experimental investigation on 15 cadaveric feet, which were placed in either inversion and dorsiflexion or inversion, plantarflexion and rotation. By exerting body-weight over the ankle they produced in the first instance fractures of the lateral border of the talus and in the second fractures of the medial border. With this convincing practical and experimental experience it seems appropriate now to discard the term osteochondritis dissecans and consider the talar dome lesion as a fracture, consequently calling it an 'osteochondral fracture'.

The cause of osteochondral fracture is a heavy single compression load on the ankle joint with the foot either in inversion or eversion. However, it has also been suggested that repeated loading may cause fatigue fractures. Medial lesions are produced by compression of the trochlea against the tibia with the foot in plantar flexion and the ankle inverted, and occur in 56–85% of cases (Fig. 44.12). Lateral lesions are caused by the talus being compressed against the lateral malleolus with the ankle everted in dorsiflexion and occur in 20% (Fig. 44.13). The fracture mechanism can thus explain the localization of the respective lesions.

Localization and staging

The fracture appears either on the medial or the lateral border of the talar trochlea. When medially located the lesion generally is more posteriorly situated. Laterally the localization is more anterior. An attempt at staging the fractures has been made on their appearance and with the object of serving as a basis for treatment:

Stage I is a compression of the talar dome with intact articular cartilage but subchondral fracture (Fig. 44.14).

Stage II is an incomplete fracture of both articular cartilage and subchondral bone. The anterior fibulotalar and fibulocalcaneal ligaments are generally ruptured (Fig. 44.15).

Stage III is a complete fracture through both articular cartilage and subchondral bone, but without displacement of the fragment (Fig. 44.16).

Stage IV is the same as Stage III, but with a displacement of the fragment (Fig. 44.17).

Symptoms

The symptoms of osteochondral fractures are pain, sometimes swelling, a sensation of instability and a feeling of arrest during motion. The symptoms may be insidious or spontaneously abrupt. It is not uncommon that the symptoms are misinterpreted as a single ankle sprain.

Treatment

In treating osteochondral fractures of the talus the above staging can be of some help. It has been suggested (Canale & Belding, cited by Stauffer 1983) that the following plan of treatment be followed:

Stage I lesions: nonsurgical treatment
Stage II lesions: nonsurgical treatment
Stage III (medial) lesions: nonoperative treatment initially, then surgical treatment only if symptoms persist
Stage III (lateral) lesions: surgical treatment
Stage IV lesions: surgical treatment

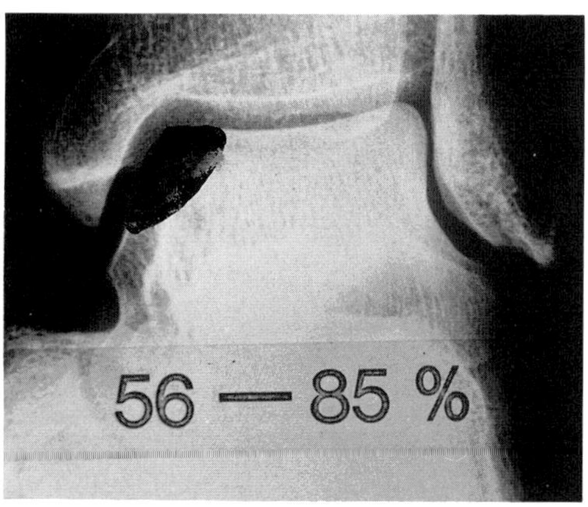

Fig. 44.12 Osteochondral fracture of medial side of trochlea

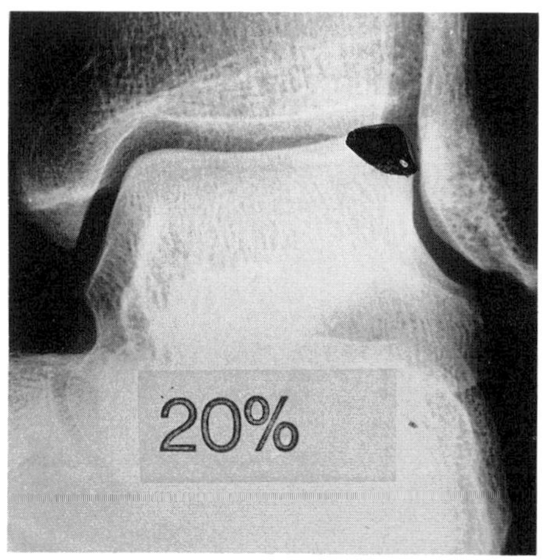

Fig. 44.13 Osteochondral fracture of lateral side of trochlea

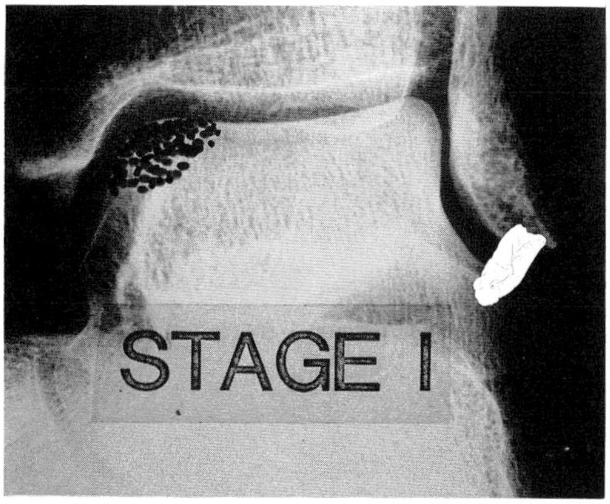

Fig. 44.14 Osteochondral fracture of trochlea. Stage I: Intact articular cartilage. subchondral fracture, intact lateral ligament

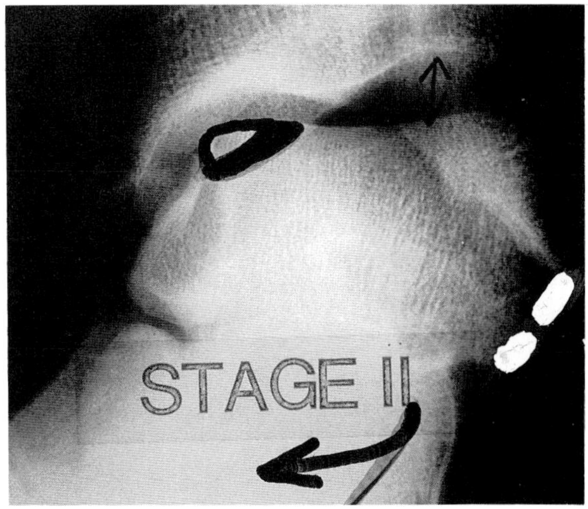

Fig. 44.15 Osteochondral fracture of trochlea. Stage II: Incomplete fracture of articular cartilage and subchondral bone; lateral ligament ruptured

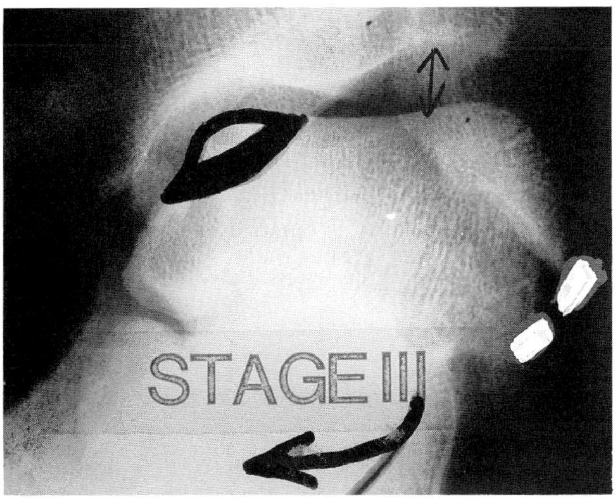

Fig. 44.16 Osteochondral fracture of trochlea. Stage III: Fracture through articular cartilage and subchondral bone. No displacement. Rupture of lateral ligament

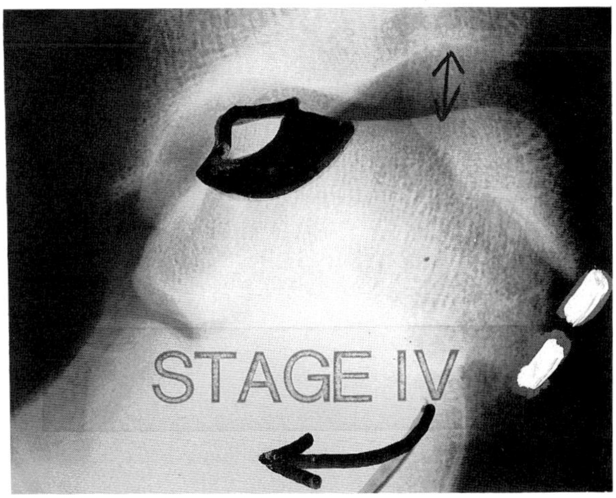

Fig. 44.17 Osteochondral fracture of trochlea. Stage IV: Same as Stage III but displacement of fragment and rupture of lateral ligament

The conservative — or nonsurgical — treatment implies cast immobilization for 8 weeks with a cast from the foot up to the knee.

In the Stage III and IV lesions it is suggested that the osteochondral fragment be surgically excised. The defect can be drilled to facilitate the development of fibrocartilage.

The medial lesion is approached through a curvilinear incision over the medial malleolus which is osteotomized. It is advisable before the osteotomy to drill a hole for and insert a screw, which, after its removal, will leave a canal facilitating its final insertion to fix the osteotomized malleolus.

The lateral lesion is assessed through a straight longitudinal incision anterior to the lateral malleolus.

Following surgery a plaster cast should be applied for 8 weeks. Weight bearing may be resumed four weeks after operation.

In many centres it is routine to fix the fragment with either a small screw, pin or bone peg. However, as the fragment most often is avascular, necrotic or divided into small pieces, this procedure is hardly advisable. There is the exception that when the fragment is large (i.e. about or more than 2 cm) an attempt can be made to fix this fragment with either a bone peg or a pin. Before fixation, however, it is necessary to remove all fibrous tissue between the fragment and the base (Figs. 44.18–23).

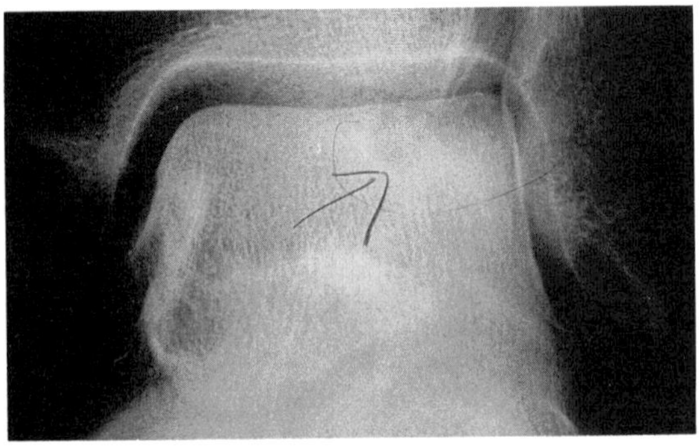

Fig. 44.18 Osteochondral fracture through lateral aspect of left talar dome. 21-year-old man who sustained fracture in December 1982 being operated with bone peg

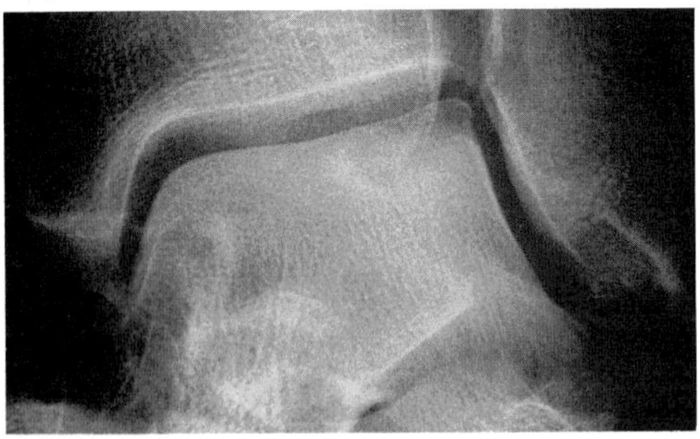

Fig. 44.20 Same as Fig. 44.18 but with foot in supination

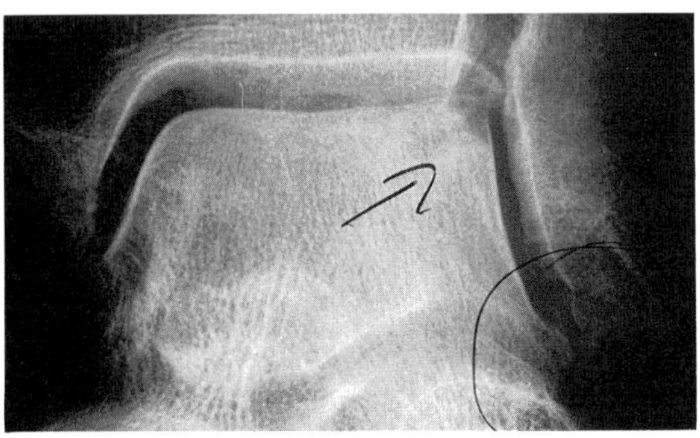

Fig. 44.22 Same as Fig. 44.18 but in October of 1984 still demonstrating the same lesion of the left talar dome. Clinically the patient was completely symptom free. Osteophytes have appeared at lateral malleolus

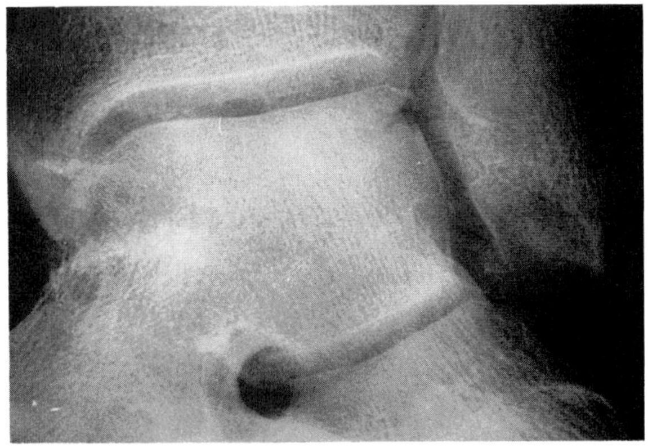

Fig. 44.19 Same as Fig. 44.18 but with foot in pronation

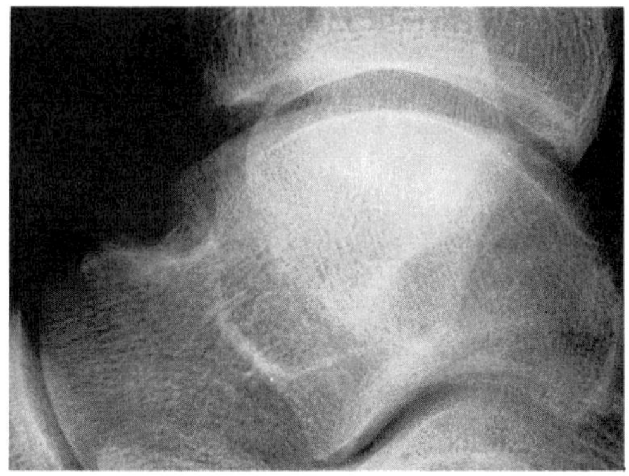

Fig. 44.21 Lateral aspect of talus in patient in Fig. 44.18. It is difficult to distinguish the talar dome lesion

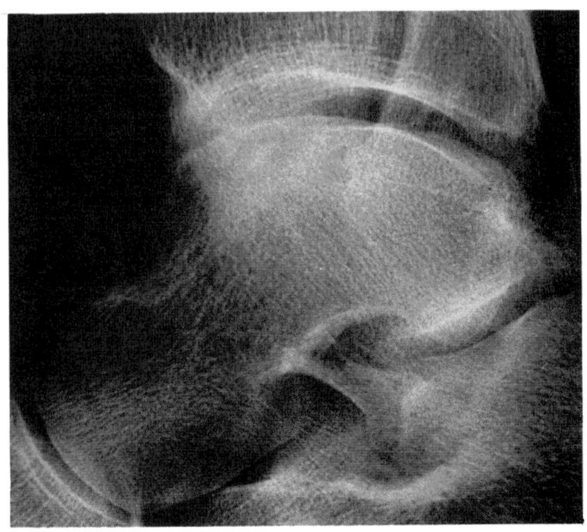

Fig. 44.23 Lateral view of Fig. 44.22. A slight irregularity of the anterior aspect of the talar dome discloses the site of lesion which still remains radiographically but does not give any symptoms clinically

Peritalar injuries

Localization

Peritalar injuries involve the ligaments surrounding the talocrural, talonavicular and subtalar joints. The ligaments of interest are on the *lateral* aspect: the anterior talofibular ligament, the talocalcaneal ligament and the posterior talofibular ligament.

On the medial aspect are the anterior tibiotalar ligament, tibionavicular ligament, the plantar calcaneonavicular ligament, the medial talocalcaneal ligament, the tibiocalcaneal ligament, the posterior tibiotalar ligament and the talonavicular ligament.

Ligament injury mechanism

The most commonly identified ligament injury is that of the anterior talofibular ligament. Also the calcaneofibular and talocalcaneal ligaments may be injured. The injury arises after inversion and plantar flexion movement under load. If the ligament injuries are severe there may be dislocation of the talus. This may occur after hyperflexion of the foot which involves a protrusion of the talus antero-laterally. It is not uncommon that the subtalar joints also become displaced. As a rule the violence which causes this type of dislocation is so severe that open wounds result, and it is not uncommon for the talus to become dislodged completely from its natural place.

Symptoms

In closed dislocations the signs are an obvious protrusion anteriorly of the talus with the foot plantarflexed and most often there is an exaggerated eversion of the foot. With an open wound the injury is more than obvious.

Irrespective of the trauma having caused a closed or open dislocation of the talus there is no great advantage in taking radiographs before a reduction has been completed.

Treatment

In the closed injury it is essential as soon as possible to save the skin and under light anaesthesia reduction can most often be easily achieved. It is most important at this time not only to observe the condition of the skin, but also to observe sensation and circulation distal to the injury.

Once reduction has been achieved, radiography can be carried out further to diagnose the individual injuries of the ankle joint and the patient can then be transported to the operating theatre for appropriate treatment. Despite the various procedures employed in dealing with the surrounding injuries of a displaced talus, it may be difficult to retain the talus in the mortise postoperatively. A simple procedure to maintain the reduction is to drill one or two Kirschner wires through the calcaneus and the talus into the tibia before applying the plaster cast. The wires can be kept in place for some 3–4 weeks after which time the risk for redislocation is minimal. A plaster cast should, however, be kept for 8 weeks after which time non-weightbearing mobilization can be instituted and after another 2 weeks, successive increase in weight bearing can be carried out.

In the treatment of open injuries wound debridement is mandatory. As a rule skin conditions will not permit primary closure and immediate skin grafting is not advisable. Following wound debridement a reduction of the dislocation should be done and if this is difficult to maintain, the use of one or two Kirschner wires through the calcaneus and talus into the tibia is recommended. Surrounding injuries are repaired by the means best suitable for the situation and it is suggested that associated fractures be stabilized internally if this is possible. Failing this, external fixation can be employed. Once conditions permit, skin grafting is carried out. A plaster cast is applied (if external fixation has not been used) for some eight weeks after which time mobilization is instituted, and after another two weeks successively increasing weight bearing.

Complications

There are two complications in the treatment of dislocated talus which have to be considered, one being infection and the other avascular necrosis of the talus. Due to the skin problem, which arises both in closed and open dislocation the rate of infection is considerable. Detenbeck (1969) reported infection in 8 out of 9 patients. The use of prophylactic antibiotics should therefore be seriously considered. In the open wound with talar dislocation prophylactic administration of antibiotics is strongly suggested.

A not uncommon complication in dislocation of the talus is skin necrosis. Once this has occurred, the risk of infection increases considerably. As mentioned above, prophylactic antibiotic measures are most important, but if necrosis has developed it is important to carry out a surgical debridement. It is suggested that the wound be left open and closed secondarily. If infection can not be brought under control and the talar body has become involved, sequestrectomy should be carried out. The removal of only the talus leads to poor results. When the infection has ceased, function is poor in the remainder of the talar and peritalar joints. The best results have been achieved with removal of the remaining talus and fusion of the tibia with the calcaneus.

In 1973 Giannestras reported the personal communication of Brady that in a follow-up study in 24 patients, with total or subtotal dislocation of the talus, avascular necrosis developed in every single case. However, the patients did surprisingly well and it was therefore believed that the consequences of avascular necrosis were overrated. For this reason it was suggested that the long term immobilization following surgery should be shortened considerably and that active mobilization should be instituted as early as possible, i.e. after 10–12 weeks, irrespective of avascular necrosis being present or not. The recommendations of Brady (Giannestras 1973) may be summarized as follows:

> Immediate surgery with internal fixation is advocated if closed reduction is unsuccessful. Kirschner wires insertion at the fracture level of the neck of the talus as well as through the calcaneus into the talus is a recommended form of internal fixation. It is important that the foot be in neutral position at the ankle when these wires are inserted.
>
> If the body is severely comminuted and cannot be realigned tibiocalcaneal fusion is recommended.
>
> The timing of delayed surgical procedure is important. Too often a decision for surgical treatment is made on the basis of X-ray findings, while the patient is still in a cast on a non weight-bearing regimen. It is suggested that surgical treatment be considered only after the foot has been thoroughly tested on a weight bearing programme even in the presence of an avascular necrotic talus.
>
> In total dislocation of the talus surgical treatment is invariably necessary. Astragalectomy for this type of injury leads to a poor result and is not recommended.

Talar tilt

Tilting mechanism

As has already been pointed out the talus and the transverse part of the ankle mortise are parallel and horizontal. Occasionally, however, the talus might become tilted in the horizontal mortise. This is either due to a true tilting of the talus or a tilting of the ankle mortise. The reason for talar tilt is still unknown.

It seems as if the strong plantarflexors of the ankle remain in action after the foot has left the ground and pull the foot into varus which tilts the talus into the same position. However, on radiography the talus seems to retain its normal position so that the varus will not show on the radiograph. Due to increased activity among the population who enjoy long-term athletic endeavours, the ankle joint becomes subjected to continuous exertion, which may result in lateral instability. Patients will complain that they have recurrent pain on the outside of the ankle following activity and also that they feel a giving way of the ankle. On physical examination the patient may exhibit an increased inversion and also a slight anterior drawer sign, which can be verified by stress X-rays on which the degree of talar tilt can be estimated. More than 10° of talar tilt is regarded as abnormal. This type of talar tilt is due to a laxity of the ligament and thus illustrates a 'true' tilting of the talus.

Occasionally, not only the talus but also the tibia is tilted into varus. The reason may be irregularity of growth following a fracture separation of the epiphysis. The mortise thus tilts into varus secondary to a tibia vara.

Symptoms

The symptoms are pain and limping.

Treatment

Talar tilt with lateral ankle joint instability lends itself well to operative procedures. Despite strengthening of the muscles the instability may remain and strapping or heel wedges only give temporary relief.

As for surgical treatment, many operations have been suggested for instability of the ankle joint. One method which has gained great popularity is that of Broström which takes into consideration whether there is a rupture of the lateral ligaments only, or if this is combined with avulsion of bone. When the anterior talofibular ligament is ruptured near its mid portion, the torn ends of the ligament are sutured. If the ligament is thin and weak it can be strengthened with a flap from the lateral talocalcaneal ligament.

In a rupture of the lateral ankle ligaments with avulsion of bone, the proximal end of the ligament is anchored to the anterior margin of the lateral malleolus with interrupted sutures which are pulled through drillholes in the lateral malleolus. The anterior malleolar margin is trimmed to improve healing of ligament to bone. Avulsed bone fragments are removed.

In elongation of the lateral ankle ligaments with scar tissue and no true rupture, the scar tissue is excised and the ligaments sutured end to end.

Following surgery a below-knee cast is applied with the foot in neutral position. The patient is kept in bed for two days with the leg elevated after which time mobilization with full weight bearing is instituted. The plaster is removed after three weeks and the patient is then continued on full weight bearing.

In his series of 60 patients, Broström recorded improvement in 58 patients. In one there was slight improvement and in one no change. One patient became infected (Broström 1966).

In cases of tibia vara with disabling symptoms the surgical procedure should be to return the ankle to normal alignment which can only be achieved by a wedge osteotomy, slightly proximal to the talocrural joint. However, the degree of varus has to be correlated to the symptoms. All varus positions do not necessarily give disabling symptoms!

REFERENCES

Brinkman W H, Fischer H J, Jung H 1973 Diagnose und therapie von talusfrakturen. Bruns Beiter Klin Chir 220: 194

Broström L 1966 Sprained ankle. VI Surgical treatment of "chronic" ligament ruptures. Acta Chir Scand 132: 551–565

Berndt A, Harty M 1959 Transchondral fractures (osteochondritis dissecans) of the talus. J Bone Joint Surg 41A: 988–1020

Coltart W D 1952 Aviators astragalus. J Bone Joint Surg 34B: 545

Detenbeck H 1969 Personal communication

Giannestras N 1973 Foot Disorders. Lea & Febiger, Philadelphia

Goldie I, Peterson L, Lindell D 1974 The arterial supply of the talus. Acta Orthop Scand 45: 260

Hawkins L 1970 Fractures of the neck of the talus. J Bone Joint Surg 52A: 991–1002

Peterson L, Goldie I, Irstam L 1974 Fracture of the neck of the talus. An experimental and clinical study. Thesis, Göteborg

FURTHER READING

Evarts C (ed) 1983 Surgery of the Musculoskeletal System. Volume 3, Section 8. Churchill Livingstone, New York

Harries N 1983 Clinical Orthopaedics. Wright, Bristol

Inman V T 1976 The Joints of the Ankle. Williams & Wilkins Co., Baltimore

Kiene R, Johnson K 1983 Symposium on the Foot and Ankle. American Academy of Orthopaedic Surgeons. Mosby Co., Toronto, London

McMinn R M H, Hutchings R T, Logan B M 1982 A Colour Atlas of Foot and Ankle Anatomy. Wolfe Medical Publications Ltd

Rockwood C, Green D 1984 Fractures in Adults. Lippincott Co., Philadelphia

Stauffer R N 1983 Intraarticular ankle problems. In: Evarts (ed) Surgery of the musculoskeletal system. pp 115–117

Geoffrey Hooper and Sean Hughes

Midfoot and navicular injuries

INTRODUCTION

In this chapter we shall discuss injuries of the midtarsal joint (the talonavicular and calcaneocuboid articulations) and the navicular, cuboid and cuneiform bones. Injuries of the talus and calcaneus will be considered only insofar as they are involved in injuries to the midtarsal joint. Injuries to the tarsometatarsal joints will not be discussed in this chapter and are dealt with in Chapter 46. Stress fractures which can affect the navicular (Torg et al 1982) and cuneiform (Meurman & Elfving 1980) bones are described in Chapter 47.

The midfoot is usually damaged by major violence attributable to falls from heights, road traffic and air accidents, or crushing or trapping between objects. However, quite major injuries of the midtarsal joint can be caused by simple stumbles (Dewar & Evans 1968) and progressive subluxation in the absence of any major injury has also been described (Jensen 1963, Jacobs 1964).

Injuries of the midfoot are relatively uncommon and account for 0.5% of all fractures and dislocations (Wilson 1933). The infrequency of midfoot injuries is explained by the great strength and stability of this part of the foot. Forces applied to the foot are likely to cause structural failure elsewhere before the midfoot is involved. This might also explain why midfoot injuries are commonly accompanied by injuries elsewhere in the foot.

Little has been written about midfoot injuries. Apart from the major review of 69 patients with 71 injuries by Main & Jowett (1975), the 10 midtarsal injuries described by Kenwright & Taylor (1970) and the review of 67 patients with navicular fractures by Eichenholtz & Levine (1964), these injuries have been discussed as small subgroups of talar fractures and dislocations, or presented as case reports. It is therefore reasonable to acknowledge that statements about the management and prognosis of any one type of injury are largely anecdotal; even in the series of Main & Jowett the number of patients in each subgroup of midtarsal injuries was small. Our opinions are based on the views of others and supported by a review of 65 midtarsal injuries treated at the Royal Infirmary of Edinburgh.

CLINICAL FEATURES

In our own experience, and this is supported by a review of the literature, it is striking how often injuries of the midfoot are overlooked initially, even when the foot is the only site of injury and adequate radiographs have been obtained. For example, there was a delay in diagnosis in 30 of the 71 injuries described by Main & Jowett and a quarter of those in Eichenholtz & Levine's series. Quite often a major injury is dismissed as a sprain. There is even more risk of missing a major foot injury when the patient has multiple injuries, for swelling of the foot may not appear of great significance in comparison to other injuries and radiographic examination may be inadequate because of difficulties in positioning the foot.

Clinical examination is usually unhelpful in indicating the exact nature of midfoot injuries; the foot is painful and swollen but swelling may, and usually does, obscure any palpable abnormality. Occasionally the foot may be locked in an obviously abnormal posture, but it is of great importance to realize that rather nonspecific swelling and tenderness may indicate a severe midfoot injury and that adequate radiographs must be obtained and scrutinized with the utmost care to avoid missing such an injury. Antero-posterior, lateral and oblique films of the whole foot, and often of the other foot for comparison, should be obtained. London (1973) has described a special radiographic projection for elucidating the nature of midtarsal injuries, in which the central ray is directed at the talonavicular joint in the plane of the base of the metatarsus and at right angles to the long axis of the foot.

CLASSIFICATION

A classification of injuries affecting a particular anatomical region is desirable for it encourages accurate description, aids prognosis and allows comparison of the results of different forms of treatment. Unfortunately it has proved difficult to produce a satisfactory classification of midfoot injuries. Isolated fractures and dislocations of the bones and joints in the midfoot are uncommon and combined patterns of injuries such as fracture-subluxations and dislocations affecting several bones are more usual. A classification of midfoot injuries in terms of the anatomical structures involved is therefore rather cumbersome. Main & Jowett based their useful classification on the direction of the force involved in the injury, which can usually be inferred from the radiographic appearance. Their 71 injuries fell into five groups: 1. Medial, 2. Longitudinal, 3. Lateral, 4. Plantar and 5. Crush (Fig. 45.1). The first two types were often combined. There were no pure dorsal dislocations of the midtarsal joint in their series, although three of the 10 dislocations reported by Kenwright & Taylor were dorsal.

Common to all such classifications based on the presumed directions of injuring forces, Main & Jowett's classification has the theoretical disadvantages that, a) the direction of a force cannot always be decided with confidence and b) sometimes multidirectional forces may be involved. One specific objection to the classification of Main & Jowett is that it excludes forced plantar flexion of the forefoot, which has been thought to be an important mechanism in causing injuries of the navicular bone (Lehman & Eskeles 1928, Eftekhar et al 1969). Main & Jowett agreed with Wiley (1971) and Wilson (1972) that a plantar strain applied to the forefoot tended to produce an injury at the tarsometatarsal joint, and attributed the majority of the navicular fractures in their series to longitudinal forces. Most

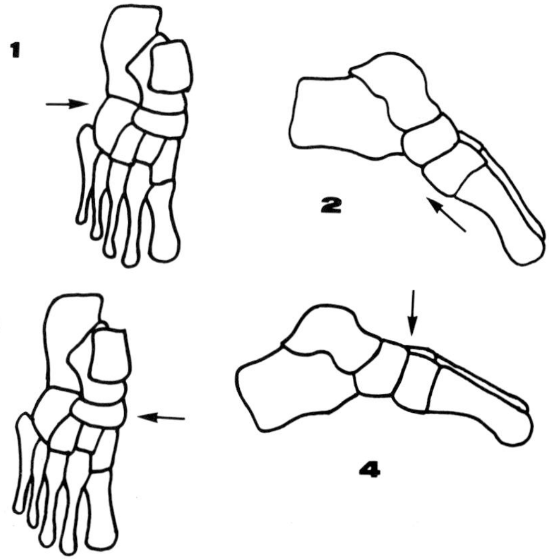

Fig. 45.1 Directions of forces producing injuries of the midfoot. 1) Medial, 2) Longitudinal, 3) Lateral, 4) Plantar. The midfoot may also be injured by crushing and multidirectional forces

of the injuries that we have encountered can fairly readily be fitted into the five groups described by Main & Jowett, but we have added a sixth group to include the few injuries that are not easily classified (Table 45.1).

Table 45.1 Classification of injuries to the midfoot (after Main & Jowett 1975)

Group	Direction of force	Type of injury
1	Medial	Sprain of midtarsal joint Fracture-subluxation or dislocation of midtarsal joint Medial swivel dislocation of midtarsal joint
2	Longitudinal	Fractures and fracture-dislocations of the navicular bone ? Fractures and dislocations of the cuneiform bones
3	Lateral	Fracture-sprain of midtarsal joint Fracture-subluxation of midtarsal joint Lateral swivel dislocation of midtarsal joint
4	Plantar	Fracture-sprain of midtarsal joint Fracture-subluxation and dislocation of midtarsal joint ? Plantar dislocation of cuboid bone
5	Crush	Various
6	Uncertain	Various

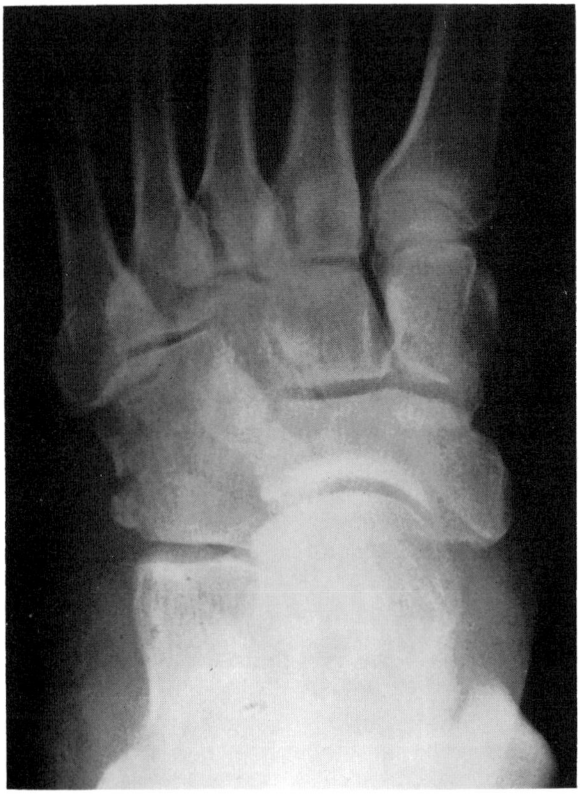

Fig. 45.2 A medial fracture-sprain. A fragment has been avulsed from the cuboid bone

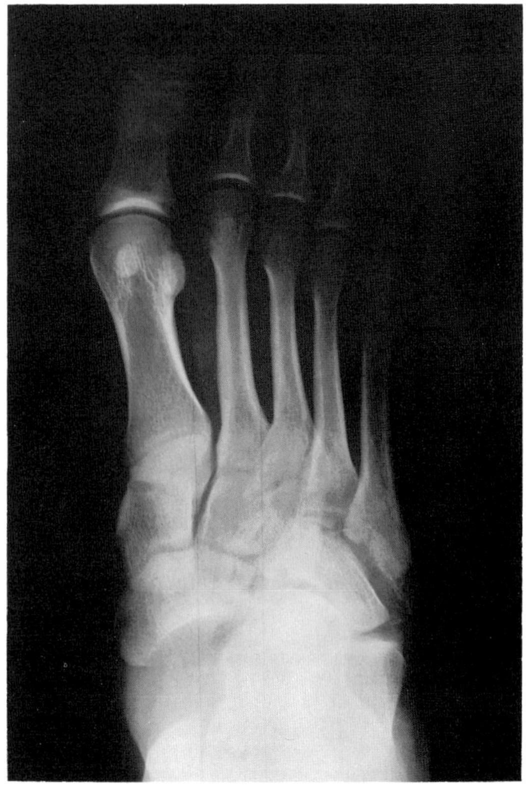

Fig. 45.3 A medial fracture-dislocation. The talonavicular joint is dislocated but the cuboid bone is also crushed, indicating that there has also been a longitudinal force applied to the lateral border of the foot

Group 1: Medial

Medial forces cause sprains, fracture subluxations or dislocations, or swivel dislocations of the midtarsal joints.

Sprains

An inversion strain of the foot can result in damage to ligaments on the dorsum and lateral border of the foot. The clinical features are local tenderness and discomfort on walking. Radiographs will show flake fractures of the dorsal margins of the talus or navicular bone or of the lateral margins of the calcaneus or cuboid (Fig. 45.2). The injury must be distinguished from the more common sprained ankle, and probably many such injuries are missed because a radiograph is taken of the ankle rather than the foot.

Treatment. Symptomatic treatment by strapping or a below-knee walking plaster until discomfort has settled is all that is required. This should be combined with elevation of the foot and foot and ankle exercises. The results of treatment are good.

Fracture-subluxations and dislocations

The forefoot is displaced medially with respect to the hindfoot, which remains in its normal alignment relative to the tibia. Damage to the articular surfaces of the midtarsal joint is common. A pure medial displacement is rather rare and injuries due to a combination of medial and longitudinal forces are common (Fig. 45.3). Medial injuries account for 3 of the 71 injuries in Main & Jowett's series and 5 of the 10 midtarsal dislocations reported by Kenwright & Taylor.

Treatment. A congruent reduction must be obtained by open or closed means and stabilized by Kirschner wire fixation. Open reduction should be carried out through a dorsal longitudinal incision if a satisfactory closed reduction is not obtained. A below-knee plaster is applied and is usually retained for two months. The patient should be non weight-bearing for the first month, after which the K-wire may be removed.

Poor results follow inadequate reduction (Main & Jowett 1975) and late pain and stiffness may require treatment by a triple arthrodesis.

Swivel dislocation

A medial force applied to the forefoot may disrupt the talonavicular joint but leave the calcaneocuboid joint intact. The foot then rotates medially about the axis of the talocalcaneal ligament which remains intact. There is no inversion or eversion of the hindfoot, in contrast to subtalar dislocations in which the talocalcaneal ligament is disrupted. A true lateral radiograph of the foot will show the talus and ankle to be in an oblique plane relative to the foot, indicating that the calcaneus has swivelled beneath the talus (Main & Jowett 1975). There is usually no difficulty in recognizing the talonavicular dislocation and the congruency of the calcaneocuboid joint in an oblique film (Fig. 45.4).

Treatment. Early closed reduction is usually straightforward and the reduction completely stable. We have never had to resort to an open reduction in an early case but open reduction would certainly be indicated if the dislocation could not be reduced closed and might be necessary if the injury were not recognized initially. After reduction a below-knee cast is worn for 4–6 weeks. The results of treatment are good.

Group 2: Longitudinal

This is the most common type of midfoot injury, accounting for 29 of the 71 injuries described by Main & Jowett (1975). Longitudinal forces transmitted through the metatarsal bones result in fractures and fracture-dislocations of the navicular bones and more rarely fractures and dislocations of the cuneiform bones.

Navicular injuries

The pattern of injury is probably dictated by the degree of plantar flexion at the moment of impact. If the foot is in equinus the navicular bone is compressed between the cuneiform bones and the head of the talus and fractures vertically along shearing planes in line with the intercuneiform joints (Fig. 45.5). Minor forces produce undisplaced fractures between segments A and B or B and C. Greater forces usually result in crushing of a segment with some displacement of the rest of the bone, e.g. forces along the third ray crush segment A and displace B, C and D medially (Fig. 45.6). Forces transmitted along the lateral rays are often associated with a medial strain applied to the forefoot and there may be an injury to the cuboid bone associated with medial dislocation of a medial segment of the navicular bone (Penhallow 1937). However, if there is a lateral strain applied to the plantarflexed forefoot the lateral segment of the navicular bone may dislocate dorsally (Eftekhar et al 1969, Nadeau & Templeton 1976).

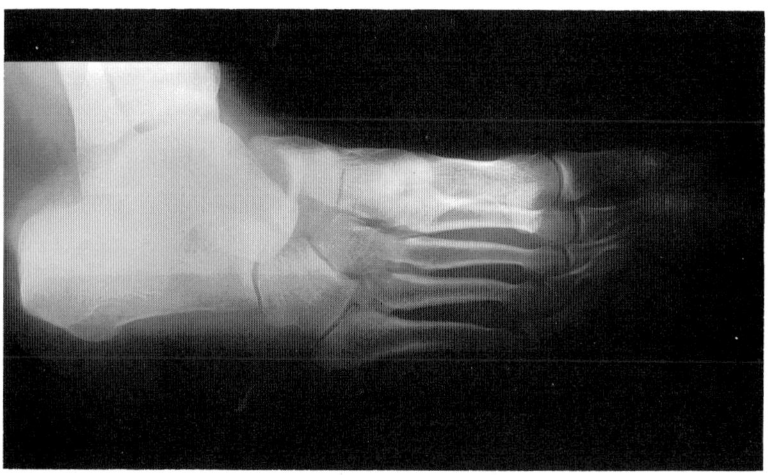

Fig. 45.4 A medial swivel dislocation

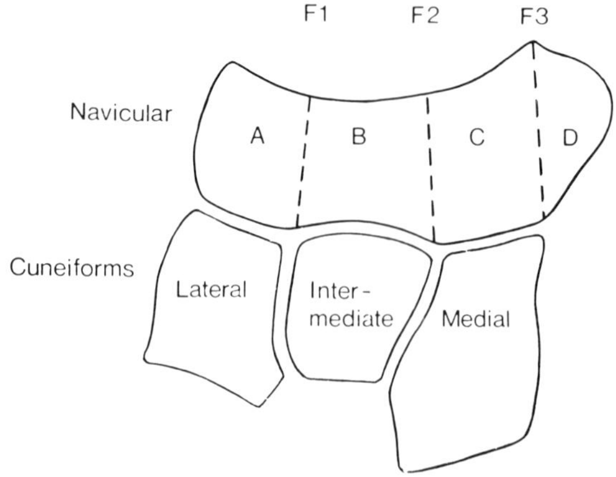

Fig. 45.5 The lines of fracture in the navicular bone caused by longitudinal forces across the cuneiform bones. From Main & Jowett 1975, by kind permission of the Editor

If the forefoot is less plantarflexed, there may be a dorsiflexion component at the midtarsal joint in addition to the longitudinal force. A transverse navicular fracture can then be caused by compression of the inferior aspect of the articular surface of the navicular bone against the head of the talus. The dorsal part of the navicular bone is usually displaced dorsally (Fig. 45.7). Lehman & Eskeles (1928) believed that this pattern of injury can sometimes be the result of forced plantar flexion of the forefoot causing rupture of the dorsal naviculocuneiform ligaments, followed by crushing of the inferior part of the navicular bone by the inferior edge of the medial cuneiform bone.

Treatment

Undisplaced fractures may be treated symptomatically in a below-knee walking type of plaster and the results of treatment are good.

Displaced fractures require more vigorous treatment. The navicular bone is an important component of the mobile medial arch of the foot and displaced fractures can result in severe disability, since a secondary degenerative osteoarthritis will cause a stiff, painful foot. For this reason some authors have recommended primary or early talonavicular or talocalcaneonavicular arthrodesis (Dick 1941, Wilson 1982) for displaced fractures. This is probably unnecessary if the bone can be reduced accurately, since poor results are associated with inadequate reduction (Main & Jowett 1975). Although it may be possible to reduce the navicular bone by closed means, the reduction is seldom

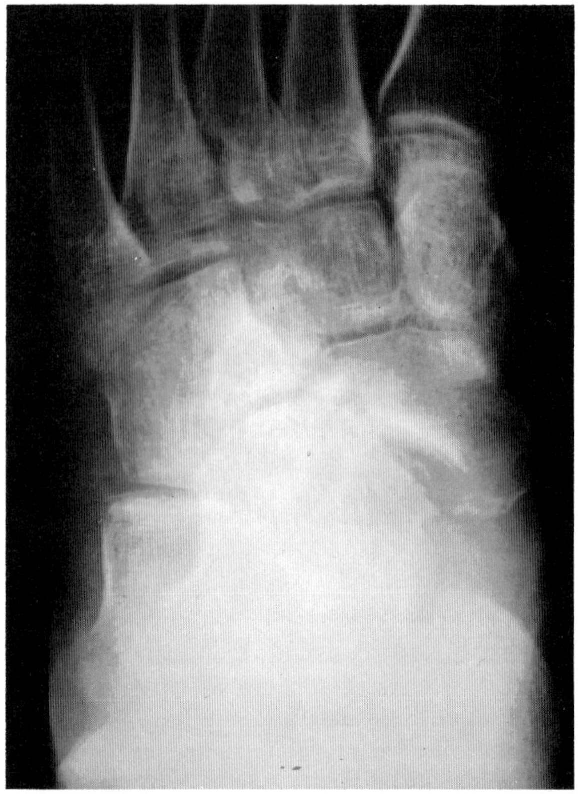

Fig. 45.6 Medial displacement of the medial segment of the navicular bone caused by longitudinal force

accurate or stable and we prefer to carry out open reduction through a dorsal longitudinal incision. The reduced fragments are stabilized by temporary K-wire fixation to the cuneiform bones or, in the case of vertical fractures, internal fixation of the

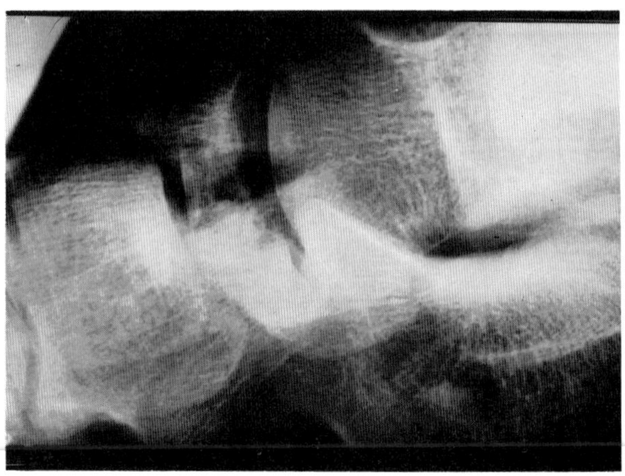

Fig. 45.7 A transverse fracture of the navicular bone with dorsal displacement of a fragment

navicular bone with a compression screw may be possible (Eftekhar et al 1969, Nadeau & Templeton 1976).

Triple arthrodesis is indicated in late untreated cases, or where primary treatment has failed and a stiff painful foot is the result (Eichenholtz & Levine 1964). Triple arthrodesis appears to give better functional ability and relief of pain than talonaviculocuneiform or midtarsal arthrodesis (Main & Jowett 1975). Naviculocuneiform fusion in addition to the triple arthrodesis has been recommended by some (Day 1947, Friedmann 1958) but should probably be reserved for patients in whom there is definite evidence of damage to the naviculocuneiform articulations.

Injuries to the cuneiform bones

These rather uncommon injuries are included here as they are probably caused by longitudinal forces through the medial metatarsal bones; it must be accepted however that they are sometimes difficult to classify in terms of the forces involved.

An isolated crush fracture of the medial cuneiform bone is probably the most frequently encountered of these injuries (Fig. 45.8). Symptomatic treatment is all that is needed.

Dislocations and fracture-dislocations of the medial cuneiform bone are usually associated with tarsometatarsal injuries and are probably best regarded as a variation of dislocations at Lisfranc's joint (Holstein & Joldersma 1950, Brown & McFarlane 1975). Dislocation of the medial cuneiform bone together with the first ray has been described by Schiller & Ray (1970) and Giannestras & Sammarco (1975), and we have also encountered a similar injury in a young motorcyclist (Fig. 45.9). Such a displacement can only occur if the naviculocuneiform ligaments and the strong ligament between the medial cuneiform bone and the base of the second metatarsal bone are disrupted. In the patient described by Schiller & Ray (1970) the first ray was displaced in a plantar direction but in our patient the first ray was displaced proximally with damage to the articular surface of the navicular bone.

Treatment is by reduction, open if necessary, and temporary stabilization with K-wires. Schiller & Ray (1970) recommended naviculocuneiform

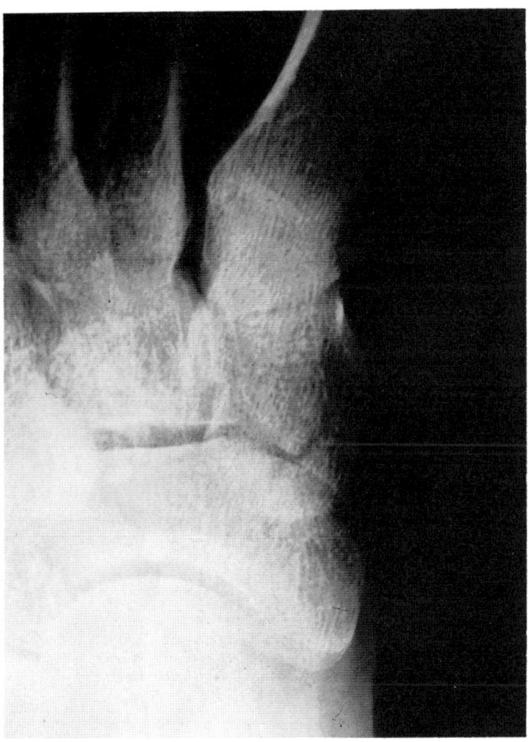

Fig. 45.8 An isolated crush fracture of the medial cuneiform bone

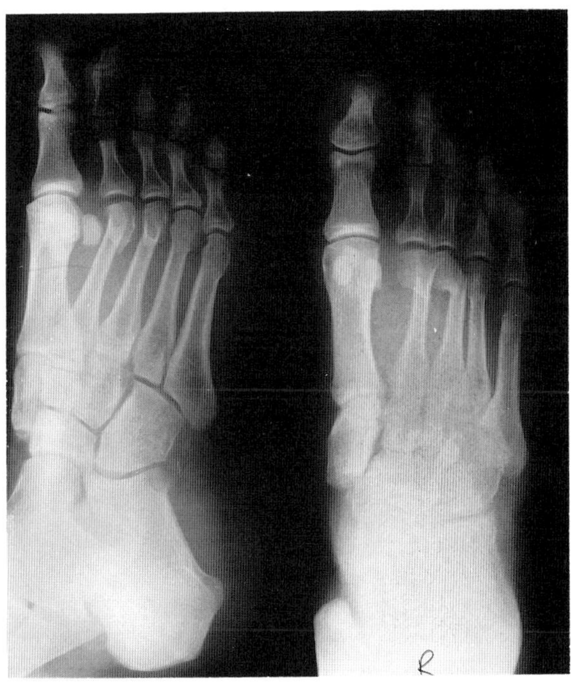

Fig. 45.9 A dorsomedial dislocation of the first ray with the medial cuneiform bone

arthrodesis if the joint was damaged, but this is probably unnecessary as a primary procedure. In carrying out reduction it should be remembered that the tendon of tibialis anterior can become interposed between the first and second rays, making closed reduction impossible (Holstein & Joldersma 1959).

Group 3: Lateral

Lateral forces, usually a result of abduction strains on the forefoot, cause fracture-sprains, fracture-subluxations or lateral swivel dislocations of the midtarsal joint.

Fracture-sprains

These are caused by relatively small forces such as may be involved in a stumble from a kerb or step. The patient is most often a middle-aged woman and the injury may be associated with the wearing of high-heeled shoes (Eichenholtz & Levine 1964). In its most minor form there is an avulsion of a flake of bone from the dorsum of the talus or navicular bone. With greater force the tuberosity of the navicular bone may be avulsed (Fig. 45.10). An avulsion of the tuberosity must be distinguished from an accessory ossicle, the os tibiale externum. The os tibiale externum is usually larger, the line of separation is smoother and the bone is usually present in both feet (Fig. 45.11).

A much more significant injury, and one that can easily be overlooked, can be produced by the same force. The avulsion injury is accompanied by an impaction fracture of the cuboid bone, or the calcaneus, or both bones (Fig. 45.12). This is the 'occult fracture-subluxation' of Dewar & Evans (1968) or the 'nutcracker fracture of the cuboid' (Hermel & Gershon-Cohen 1953). If it is overlooked it can result in severe disability and it must be stressed that any patient who has an avulsion fracture of the navicular bone must have good quality films taken of the calcaneocuboid joint (Fig. 45.13).

Treatment. Minor avulsions from the medial side of the foot require only symptomatic treatment by strapping or a below-knee plaster and a full recovery can be expected.

When there is an injury involving the calcaneocuboid joint, treatment is more controversial. Dewar & Evans (1968) recommended early calcaneocuboid arthrodesis, but this view was based on their experience with patients who had received no, or inadequate, early treatment. Their recommendation was disputed by Stark (1973) who believed that early treatment in a below-knee cast would produce good results. This view is supported

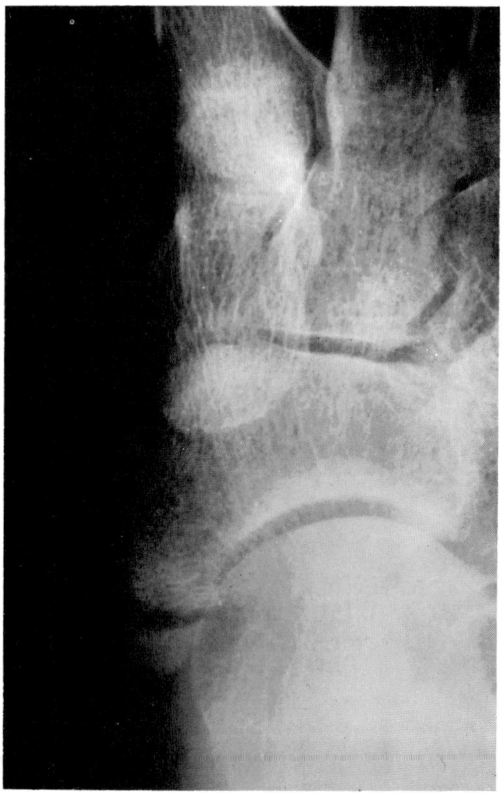

Fig. 45.10 An avulsion of the tuberosity of the navicular bone

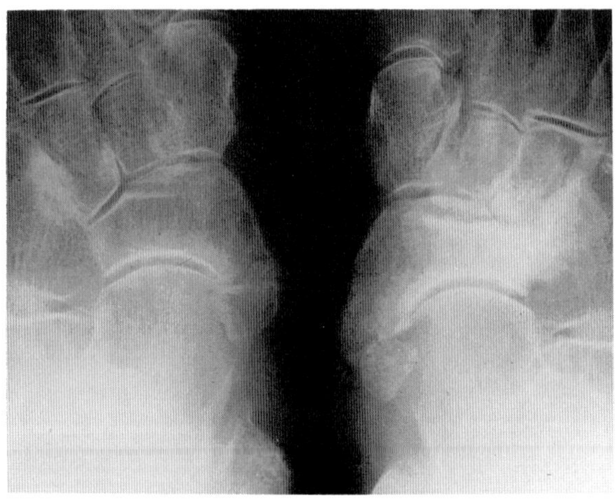

Fig. 45.11 An os tibiale externum is present in each foot

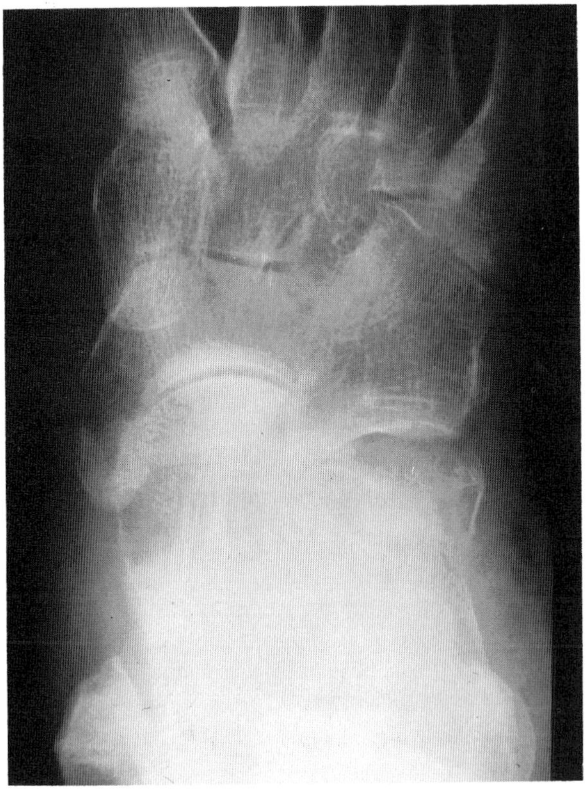

Fig. 45.12 An avulsion of the navicular tuberosity associated with a fracture involving the calcaneocuboid joint. This is the 'occult' fracture-subluxation of the midtarsal joint

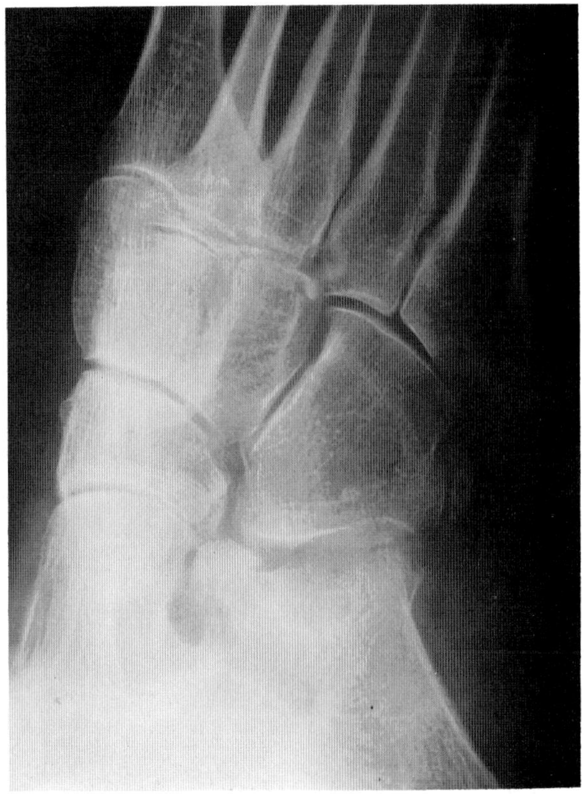

Fig. 45.13 The crush fracture of the anterior part of the calcaneus is best seen on a film centred on the calcaneocuboid joint

by the results of Main & Jowett (1975). On review of our patients with this injury we have also found that those who were treated early in a below-knee cast did not come to later surgery. We therefore recommend that treatment of this injury is by a below-knee cast for 4–6 weeks and that calcaneocuboid arthrodesis is reserved for the patient who is seen with late degenerative osteoarthritis because of inadequate or failed early treatment.

Fracture-subluxation

A stronger, laterally directed force can produce severe comminution of the cuboid or anterior part of the calcaneus in association with lateral subluxation of the navicular bone on the talus. Characteristically this injury is caused by a fall from a height or a road traffic accident, in contrast to the stumble or trip that causes the occult fracture-sprain of the midtarsal joint.

The lateral border of the foot is much more rigid than the medial border (Wood Jones 1944). It has been compared to a rigid oak which breaks before the force of the wind, whereas the medial border bends like a reed (Hermel & Gershon-Cohen 1953). Because of its rigidity, fractures and fracture-dislocations of the lateral column of the foot are much more common than pure lateral dislocations. We have encountered two pure lateral dislocations, both of which occurred in children (Fig. 45.14). Interestingly, in both cases the talonavicular joint appeared to be intact and the forefoot was displaced at the naviculocuneiform and calcaneocuboid articulations.

Treatment. In common with other dislocations and fracture-dislocations involving the midtarsal joint, accurate reduction is a prerequisite for a satisfactory outcome. However, even if the talonavicular joint is reduced and accurately held with K-wires it is almost certain that the associated severe damage to the lateral column of the foot will require treatment

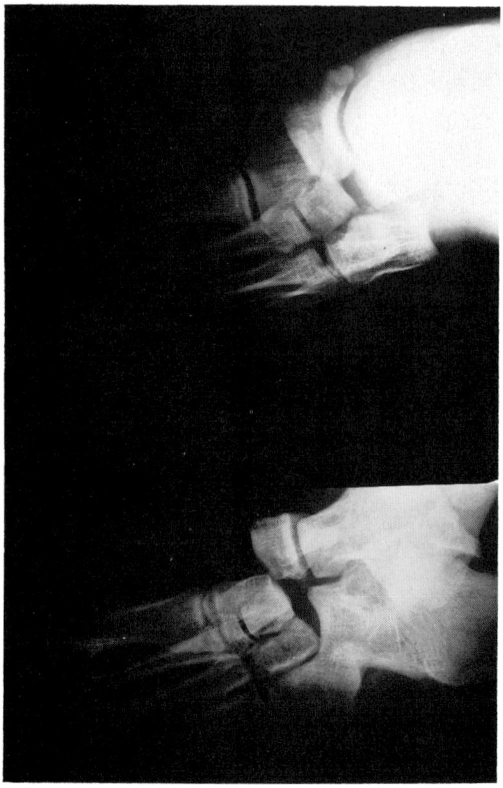

Fig. 45.14 A pure lateral dislocation. The talonavicular joint appears intact but the navicular bone may have been completely dislocated momentarily

by an early calcaneocuboid arthrodesis. None of the four patients with this injury in Main & Jowett's series had a good result and two later had a triple arthrodesis; it should be noted that none had an open reduction as a primary treatment.

The rare lateral dislocation without fracture can be treated by closed reduction and temporary K-wire stabilization.

Lateral swivel dislocation

This is an exceptionally rare injury, one case having been described by Main & Jowett (1975) in a patient who had landed awkwardly when stepping off a train. The talonavicular joint was dislocated laterally but the calcaneocuboid joint was intact. The calcaneus swivelled laterally without eversion of the hindfoot. Treatment by closed reduction and rest in plaster gave a good result.

Group 4: Plantar

Plantar forces can cause fracture-sprains or fracture-subluxations. These injuries are rather uncommon and account for five of the 71 injuries in Main & Jowett's series.

Fracture-sprains

Fragments are avulsed from the dorsum of the talus or navicular bone, or from the anterior process of the calcaneus.

Treatment. Symptomatic treatment only is required.

Fracture-subluxations and dislocations

These occur in falls in which the foot is trapped, or in motorcycle accidents. They can be distinguished from the more common subtalar dislocations because the talus remains in its normal relationship to the calcaneus and the mid-tarsal joint is disrupted. There may be an associated fracture of the inferior part of the calcaneocuboid joint. We have seen such an injury in association with a subluxation at the tarsometatarsal joint in a patient who fell from a height (Fig. 45.15).

Drummond & Hastings (1969) reported a patient who sustained a plantar dislocation of the cuboid, together with the lateral two metatarsal bones at the calcaneocuboid joint in a fall from a roof. As noted previously, calcaneocuboid dislocations are rare because of the rigidity of the lateral column of the

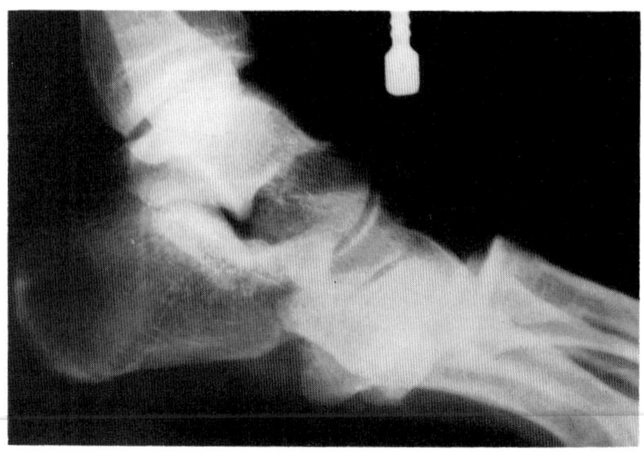

Fig. 45.15 A plantar subluxation of the midtarsal joint associated with a subluxation of the tarsometatarsal joint

foot. We believe that the type of injury described by Drummond & Hastings (1969) is more likely to be the result of a plantar directed force, rather than a laterally directed force, which would tend to produce a lateral column fracture rather than an extrusion of the cuboid bone.

Treatment. The displacement is reduced by closed or, if necessary, open means and the affected joints stabilized by temporary K-wire fixation.

Group 5: Crush

As might be expected, when the foot is crushed beneath a heavy weight there is no constant pattern to the type of injury that may occur and open injuries are quite common. Satisfactory results can follow wound debridement, skeletal stabilization and provision of skin cover, provided that the distal part of the foot is not avascular and sensation is preserved.

Group 6: Others

Although the midfoot injuries that we have encountered can almost always be placed in one of the foregoing categories, occasionally difficulties are encountered. The unclassifiable injuries account for a small proportion of the total. We believe that it is an exercise in futility to be too rigorous in attempting to classify these injuries, which have almost always resulted from the kind of multidirectional forces that might be expected in falls from heights and in road traffic accidents.

Examples of such injuries may be given. Plantar dislocation of the cuboid bone has already been mentioned; probably it is secondary to plantar or plantar and longitudinal forces. Pure navicular dislocations without significant bony damage are sometimes encountered; most often they are dorsal (Fig. 45.16) but may be medial and occasionally plantar (Berman 1924). The direction of the force, or forces, involved is a matter for speculation.

COMPLICATIONS

The most common complication of a midfoot injury is due to the failure to recognize the injury and deal with it; the patient is then seen some time after injury with a stiff, painful foot and it may be impossible to obtain a satisfactory result.

Immediate complications are relatively uncommon; we have not encountered nerve or vessel damage although these should of course always be sought. Damage to the medial and both the medial and lateral plantar nerves has been reported in association with midtarsal dislocations (Kenwright & Taylor 1970, Wilson 1982). Complete paralysis of

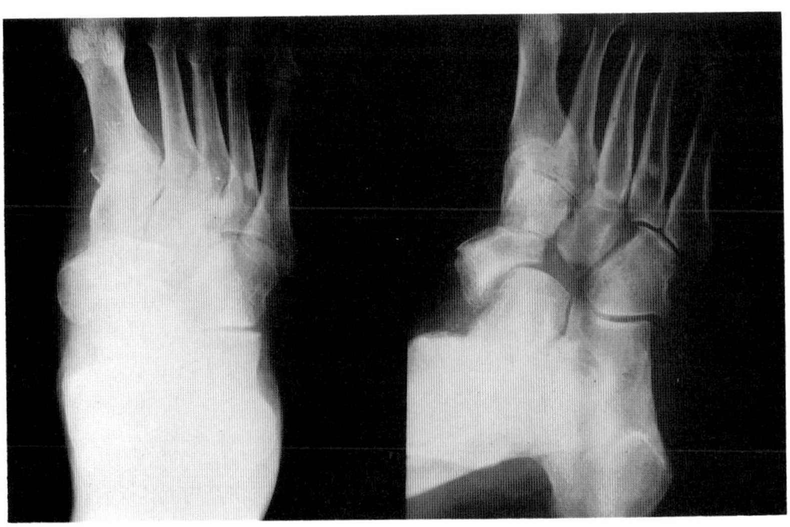

Fig. 45.16 A complete dorsal dislocation of the navicular bone

the medial and lateral plantar nerves causes a 'pied en griffe' deformity, analogous to the deformity seen when there is total intrinsic paralysis in the hand. In common with other fractures and dislocations in which there is nerve or vessel damage, early reduction is essential, followed by exploration of vessels in the region of the injury if impairment of the circulation persists.

Late complications of midfoot injuries are fairly common, but provided the injury has been recognized and treated adequately they should not be disabling. Soft tissue thickening, loss of motion and a tendency for the foot to swell are relatively frequent complaints. The thickening and loss of movement are usually permanent but not severe handicaps. The tendency for the foot to swell usually settles over the course of a few months, provided the foot is not overprotected.

Bony damage to the medial or lateral borders of the foot may however cause much more severe problems. Inadequate or unsuccessful treatment of navicular injuries can severely compromise the functioning of the mobile medial border of the foot. Painful degenerative osteoarthritis may require treatment by triple arthrodesis. A more limited arthrodesis is usually unsuccessful, possibly because degenerative changes may be aggravated in the other joints. Main & Jowett (1975) reported no additional advantage in adding naviculocuneiform arthrodesis to the triple fusion, but this would seem advisable if there is evidence of damage to this joint. When the lateral border of the foot has been severely damaged then calcaneocuboid arthrodesis is likely to be necessary. A more extensive arthrodesis is only needed if the mobile medial border of the foot is also damaged.

Recurrent midtarsal subluxations are rare (Janik 1949, Hooper & McMaster 1979). The reported examples have occurred in young women and the direction of displacement has been in a plantar and medial direction (Fig. 45.17). The initial subluxations have been due to minor stumbles or falls, followed by repeated episodes after trivial trauma. The underlying reason for these repeated episodes is unknown but may be due to some abnormality in the ligaments of the midtarsal joints. Midtarsal arthrodesis may be necessary if symptoms are very disabling.

Curiously enough avascular necrosis does not seem to be a frequent complication of navicular dislocations and fracture-dislocations. It has been reported in a patient who had a plantar dislocation of the midtarsal joint that was satisfactorily reduced (Kenwright & Taylor 1970). Revascularization occurred and the patient had a good result at follow-up four years after injury.

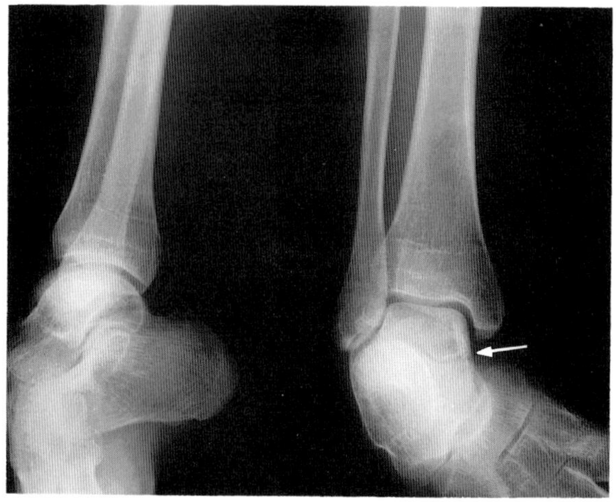

Fig. 45.17 A recurrent subluxation of the midtarsal joint. The arrow indicates the posterior talocalcaneal articulation which is congruent. From Hooper & McMaster 1979, by kind permission of the Editor

AUTHORS' PREFERRED METHODS OF TREATMENT

Acute injuries

Sprains and fracture-sprains

These are treated symptomatically with strapping or a below-knee walking plaster cast. A plaster is necessary if there has been damage to the articular surface of the calcaneocuboid joint.

Dislocations

Closed manipulation is performed but if a congruent reduction is not obtained open reduction is necessary. If the reduction is unstable the bone should be transfixed with Kirschner wires which are retained for 4–6 weeks. A below-knee plaster is worn for 4–6 weeks. Foot exercises and a support insole are necessary after removal of the plaster.

Fracture-dislocations

As above, but open reduction and Kirschner wire fixation is almost always necessary, and a longer period of plaster support (6–8 weeks) is required. Early arthrodesis is not recommended.

Late injuries

Individual treatment is directed to relief of swelling, discomfort and stiffness. If degenerative arthritis is disabling, arthrodesis of the affected and adjacent joints may be necessary.

ACKNOWLEDGEMENT

We are grateful to Colin Howie FRCSE for supervising the review of patients treated at the Royal Infirmary, Edinburgh.

REFERENCES

Berman S 1924 Complete dislocation of the tarsal scaphoid. JAMA 83: 181–182
Brown D C, McFarlane G B 1975 Dislocation of the medial cuneiform bone in tarso-metatarsal fracture-dislocation. J Bone Joint Surg (Am) 57: 858–859
Day A J 1947 The treatment of injuries to the tarsal navicular. J Bone Joint Surg 29: 359–366
Dewar F P, Evans D F 1968 Occult fracture-subluxation of the mid-tarsal joint. J Bone Joint Surg (Br) 50: 386–388
Dick I L 1941 Impacted fracture-dislocation of the tarsal navicular. Proc Roy Soc Med 35: 760
Drummond D S, Hastings D E 1969 Total dislocation of the cuboid bone. J Bone Joint Surg (Br) 51: 716–718
Eftekhar N M, Lyddon D W, Stevens J 1969 An unusual fracture dislocation of the tarsal navicular. J Bone Joint Surg (Am) 51: 577–581
Eichenholtz S N, Levine D B 1964 Fracture of the tarsal navicular bone. Clin Orthop 34: 142–157
Friedmann E 1958 Key graft fixation in mid-tarsal fracture-dislocation. Am J Surg 96: 81–83
Giannestras N J, Sammarco G J 1975 Fractures and dislocations in the foot. In: Rockwood C A, Green D P (eds) Fractures. Lippincott, Philadelphia
Hermel M B, Gershon-Cohen J 1953 The nutcracker fracture of the cuboid by indirect violence. Radiology 60: 850–854
Holstein A, Joldersma R D 1950 Dislocation of the first cuneiform in tarsometatarsal fracture-dislocation. J Bone Joint Surg (Am) 32: 419–421
Hooper G, McMaster M J 1979 Recurrent bilateral midtarsal subluxations. J Bone Joint Surg (Am) 61: 617–619
Jacobs P 1964 Chronic progressive dislocation of the talonavicular joint. J Bone Joint Surg (Br) 40: 214–217
Janik B 1949 Ueber Verrenkungen und habituelle Luxationen im unteren Sprunggelenk (luxatio pedis sub talo). Beitr Klin Chir 178: 363–378
Jensen M K 1963 Bilateral dislocation of the talus of unknown aetiology. J Bone Joint Surg (Br) 45: 148–149
Kenwright J, Taylor R G 1970 Major injuries of the talus. J Bone Joint Surg (Br) 52: 36–48
Lehman E P, Eskeles I H 1928 Fracture of the tarsal scaphoid. With notes on the mechanism. J Bone Joint Surg 10: 108–113
London P S 1973 A special view for midtarsal fracture-subluxation. Injury 5: 65–66
Main B J, Jowett R L 1975 Injuries of the midtarsal joint. J Bone Joint Surg (Br) 57: 89–97
Meurman K O A, Elfving S 1980 Stress fractures of the cuneiform bones. Br J Radiol 53: 157–160
Nadeau P, Templeton J 1976 Vertical fracture dislocation of the tarsal navicular. J Trauma 16: 669–671
Penhallow D P 1937 An unusual fracture-dislocation of the tarsal scaphoid with dislocation of the cuboid. J Bone Joint Surg 19: 517–519
Schiller M G, Ray R D 1970 Isolated dislocation of the medial cuneiform bone: a rare injury of the tarsus. J Bone Joint Surg (Am) 52: 1632–1636
Stark W A 1973 Occult fracture dislocation of the midtarsal joint. Clin Orthop 93: 291–292
Torg J S, Pavlov H, Cooley L H et al 1982 Stress fracture of the tarsal navicular. A retrospective review of 21 cases. J Bone Joint Surg (Am) 64: 700–712
Wiley J J 1971 The mechanism of tarsometatarsal injuries. J Bone Joint Surg (Br) 53: 474–482
Wilson D W 1972 Injuries of the tarsometatarsal joints. J Bone Joint Surg (Br) 54: 677–686
Wilson J N (ed) 1982 Watson-Jones Fractures and Joint Injuries. 6th edn. Churchill Livingstone, Edinburgh. p 1196
Wilson P D 1933 Fractures and dislocations of the tarsal bones. South Med J 24: 833–845
Wood Jones F 1944 Structure and function as seen in the foot. Baillière, Tindall and Cassell, London. p 247

Fractures of the metatarsals and phalanges

In many textbooks devoted to fracture treatment little attention is paid to injuries of the forefoot. This is surprising when one considers the high morbidity which can result from some of these injuries — a morbidity which is not uncommonly due to lack of recognition of their serious nature and surely reflects how little interest is shown in their management. This contrasts markedly with the considerable attention given to injuries of the hindfoot. In one classic textbook there are 58 pages devoted to fractures of the os calcis and barely two pages to the serious and sometimes dangerous fracture dislocation of the tarsometatarsal joint (Böhler 1958a); while in another popular fracture textbook for medical students this particular injury receives no mention (Adams 1983). Is it small wonder that the importance of sprains, fractures and fracture-dislocation of the tarsometatarsal is so commonly overlooked, not only by general practitioners but also by orthopaedic surgeons?

It is a paradox that so much has been written on the os calcis, fractures of which are easily recognized and where treatment has little effect on the outcome, and so little about forefoot fractures which are poorly understood and where correct early treatment can mean the difference between a normal foot and one which is severely crippled. It is no excuse that because many fractures of the forefoot recover completely with the minimal amount of treatment, the whole can be treated in the same cavalier fashion. There are many such injuries which require very careful assessment if a lasting foot deformity is not to ensue. This chapter is mainly concerned with the latter and is written with a view to establishing an awareness among orthopaedic surgeons of the importance of correct diagnosis and treatment.

FRACTURES OF THE METATARSALS

Fracture-dislocations of the tarsometatarsal joint

This is by far the most important injury to the forefoot. It is said to be 'hallowed in history at Waterloo' (J. N. Wilson 1982). Here Lisfranc developed his forefoot amputation for closed injuries of the foot, appreciating the perils of gangrene at this particular site long before the mechanism of traumatic ischaemia was fully understood. In modern times Gissane (1951) highlighted the danger of the injury by showing that not only the dorsalis pedis artery may be damaged but, as the result of forefoot displacement, the posterior tibial vessels may be put on stretch.

Much work has been done in an attempt to establish the mechanism of the injury, but to understand this it is important to be aware of two anatomical facts. Firstly, it must be appreciated that the stability of the tarsometatarsal complex depends upon the recessed nature of the second metatarsal base within a socket formed by the medial, intermediate and lateral cuneiform bones (Fig. 46.1). Secondly, there is no intermetatarsal ligament between the first and second metatarsal bases thus allowing displacement at the first metatarsocuneiform joint independently of the rest of the metatarsus, whereas the second metatarsal is firmly anchored to the medial cuneiform (Lisfranc's ligament) (Jeffreys 1963).

Mechanism of the injury

There is general agreement that this fracture dislocation can be caused by a direct crushing injury — in which case the displacement is dependant on

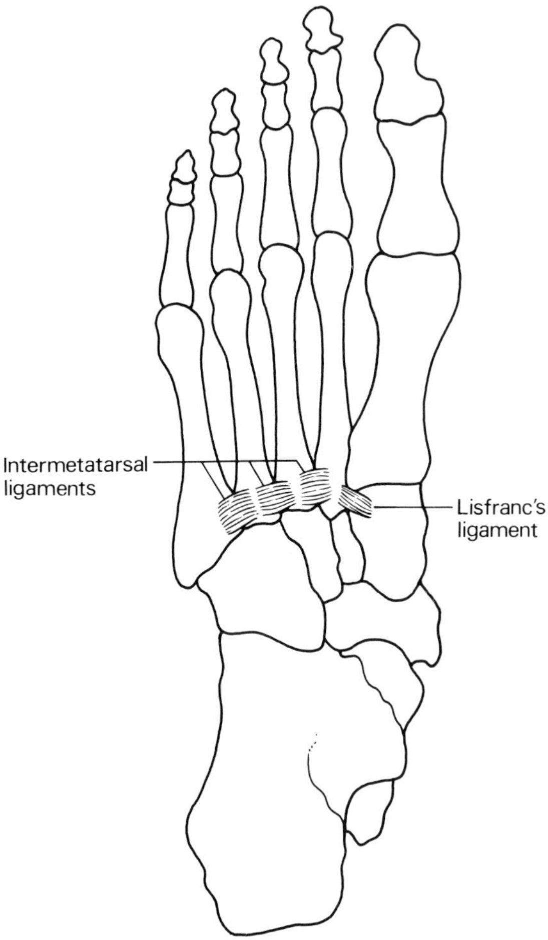

Fig. 46.1 A drawing showing the anatomical arrangement of the tarsometatarsal joint. Note that the base of the second metatarsal is firmly held within a socket formed by the three cuneiform bones, and that the lateral metatarsals cannot displace without disruption of this joint. Also, all the metatarsal bases except the first are held together by intermetatarsal ligaments, thus sometimes allowing the base of the first metatarsal to dislocate independently of the rest of the forefoot

the line of force — or it can be caused by an indirect injury when the displacement follows the pattern set by the anatomical structure already outlined. Most investigators agree that the basic injury produced by an indirect force is a dorsal dislocation of the tarsometatarsal joint. This is produced either by a longitudinal force passing through the acutely plantarflexed foot, or by sudden angulation of the forefoot into acute flexion such as could occur if one foot is trapped in the stirrup while falling from a horse.

Although it is possible that the high incidence of the injury at the Battle of Waterloo was due to cavalry accidents, probably the most common cause in modern times is the car accident where a head-on collision applies forces to the braced plantarflexed foot sufficient to displace the metatarsals dorsally at the tarsometatarsal joint. It is significant that in one series all cases occurred in front seat passengers (Badger 1967).

Fracture patterns. The form of dislocation which follows is probably dependant upon the associated torsion forces. It has been shown experimentally that pronation of the hindfoot on the fixed forefoot will produce lateral dislocation of the whole metatarsus, while supination of the hindfoot will dislocate the first metatarsal and may then proceed to fracture of the base of the second, eventually progressing to the classic displacement of the rest of the metatarsus (Jeffreys 1963, D. W. Wilson 1972).

Although there are a number of minor variations there are only two basic displacements (Fig. 46.2a). Firstly, the homolateral dislocation where, after fracture of the base of the second metatarsal, all the metatarsals dislocate laterally. This injury can be produced experimentally by a pure abduction strain, and in these circumstances it may be associated with a fracture of the cuboid and fractures of the necks and bases of the other small metatarsals (Wiley 1971).

Secondly, there may be a divarication displacement with medial displacement of the first metatarsal and lateral subluxation of the rest of the forefoot (Fig. 46.2b).

Diagnosis

In most instances the severity of the soft injury and the possible addition of circulatory embarrassment should lead the clinician to suspect a tarsometatarsal dislocation. In the acute stage it may be difficult to appreciate clinical deformity because it can be obscured by swelling. This may also be so in minor subluxations, and it is important to correlate an exact description of the trauma with the unusual degree of disability which is always present in this injury.

Radiological diagnosis. Although major disruptions of the tarsometatarsal joint are unlikely to be missed the radiographs can be difficult to interpret. However it is the minor displacement which may be

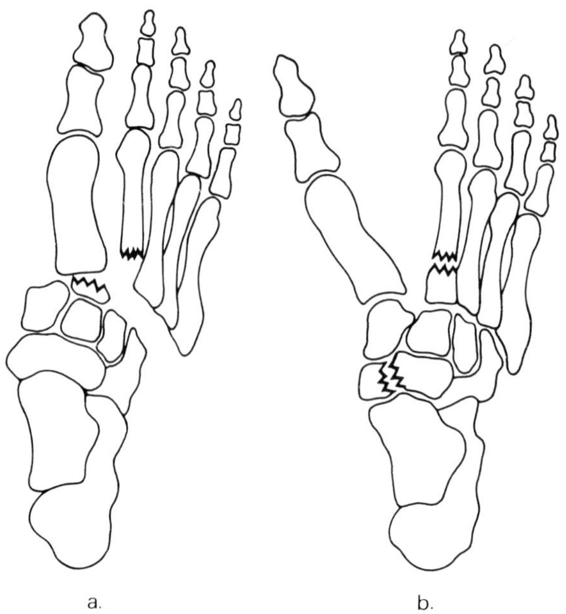

Fig. 46.2 There are two basic fracture patterns in Lisfranc's tarsometatarsal dislocation. Figure 2a shows a lateral shift of all five metatarsals, with the fracture through the base of the second metatarsal which must occur first to unlock the tarsometatarsal joint. Figure 2b shows the divarication injury which probably begins as an isolated medial displacement of the first metatarsal, usually associated with a fracture of the medial cuneiform or scaphoid. It is followed by lateral subluxation of the rest of the metatarsals only if the base of the second metatarsal fractures. (Redrawn with permission from Wilson J N 1982)

overlooked and if treated as a simple sprain can result in permanent deformity, pain and functional disability (Fig. 46.3).

A careful comparison of the radiographs of the affected and normal sides must be carried out. In a study of 200 normal foot radiographs three important anatomical signs have been demonstrated (Foster & Foster 1976). First, in the anteroposterior view of the foot the medial edge of the second metatarsal base should be in a continuous straight line with the medial edge of the middle cuneiform; second, the medial edge of the fourth metatarsal is usually in line with, or within 2 mm of the medial edge of the cuboid; and third, in the lateral view the metatarsal bases are never more dorsal than their corresponding tarsal bone (Fig. 46.4).

Treatment

As it has been shown that most cases ending up with residual deformity complain of pain (D. W. Wilson 1972) the displacement should be accurately reduced (Rockwood & Green 1984). It has also been shown by several workers that it is unusual to obtain a perfect reduction by closed methods and that open reduction and internal fixation should be carried out promptly if a satisfactory position is not achieved by manipulation. Gissane (1951) emphasized the urgency to reduce the displacement early in order to relieve strain on the vascular supply, not only from the vulnerable dorsalis pedis vessel but also from the posterior tibial artery which is put on stretch. He describes three cases which ended up in amputation.

Closed reduction. Preliminary elevation of the limb to reduce swelling has little to commend it, except while awaiting the opportunity for definitive reduction and prolonged delay is certainly contraindicated, particularly when there is any embarrassment of the peripheral circulation. Reduction should be carried out under general anaesthesia by applying traction to the forefoot while rotating into eversion or inversion according to the fracture pattern.

Although continuous traction to the toes has been advocated by some (Böhler 1958a, Rockwood & Green 1984) it is wiser to be prepared immediately to resort to open reduction if a satisfactory reduction cannot be obtained by manipulation. Even if closed reduction is successful it may be unstable and in these circumstances the surgeon should have no hesitation in stabilizing the metatarsals by driving Kirschner wires across the joint into the bones of the tarsus (Fig. 46.5).

Following reduction a well padded below-knee plaster cast should be applied and the limb kept elevated for 5–7 days before allowing the patient up with crutches. This cast should be changed at two weeks when a weight-bearing plaster can be applied. Check radiographs should be taken at the time of plaster change to exclude loss of position. The plaster and the Kirschner wires should remain in position for six weeks.

Open reduction. The key to successful open reduction is to reduce the displaced second metatarsal (Aitken & Poulson 1963). This should be carried out through a longitudinal dorsal incision lying between the first and second metatarsal bases. Where the maximal deformity is at the first metatarsocuneiform joint it must be remembered

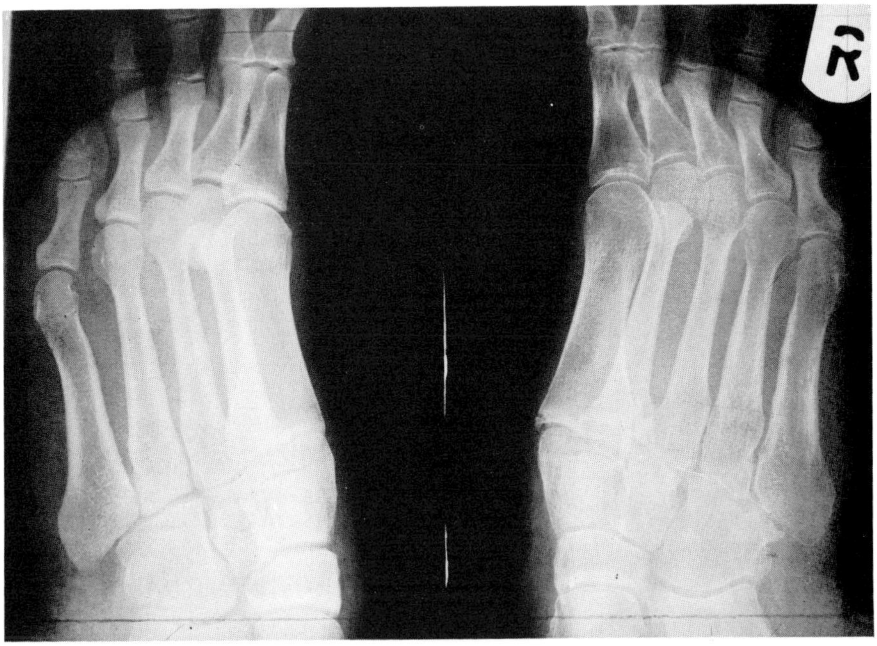

a

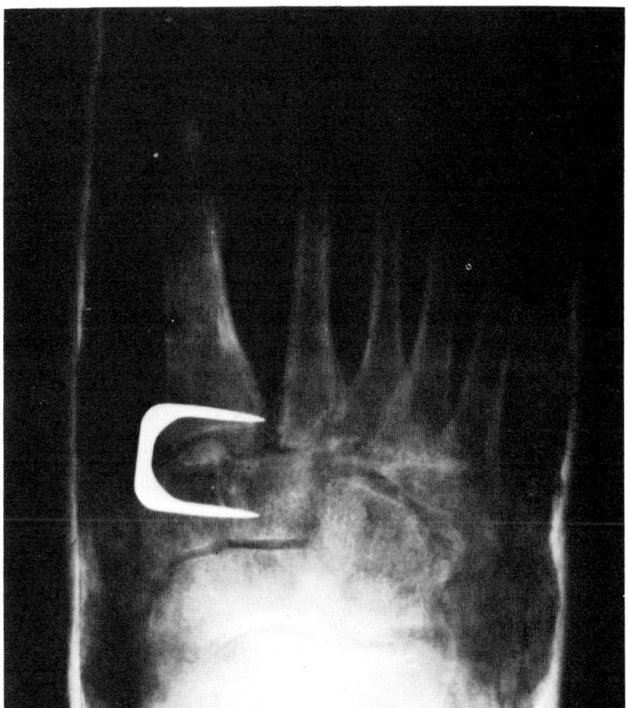

b

Fig. 46.3 A 20-year-old female patient fell only a few feet to sustain this Lisfranc fracture-subluxation of her right foot. The true nature of the injury was not recognized until many months later when she presented with persisting pain in the foot and an abduction deformity of the metatarsus. Comparison X-rays taken at that time (Fig. 3a) clearly show a disruption of the right tarsometatarsal joint (c.f. Fig. 46.4). A wedge resection of bone was necessary to correct the deformity (Fig. 3b)

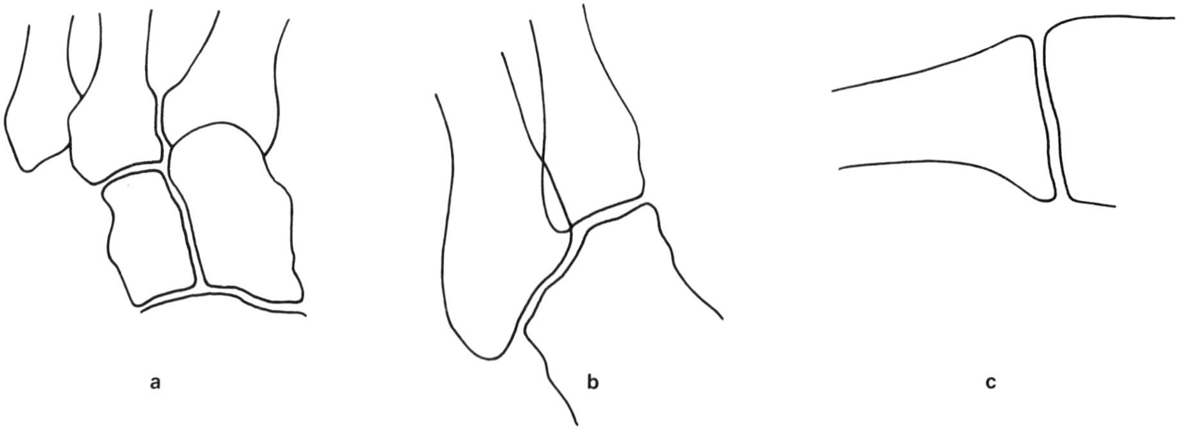

Fig. 46.4 The three anatomical signs of a normal tarsometatarsal joint: Figure 4a shows the medial border of the base of the second metatarsal is in line with the medial border of the middle cuneiform bone; Figure 4b shows that the medial border of the base of the fourth metatarsal is in line with, or within 2 mm of the medial border of the cuboid; and finally, in the lateral view (Fig. 4c) the bases of the metatarsals are never more dorsal than their corresponding tarsal bone

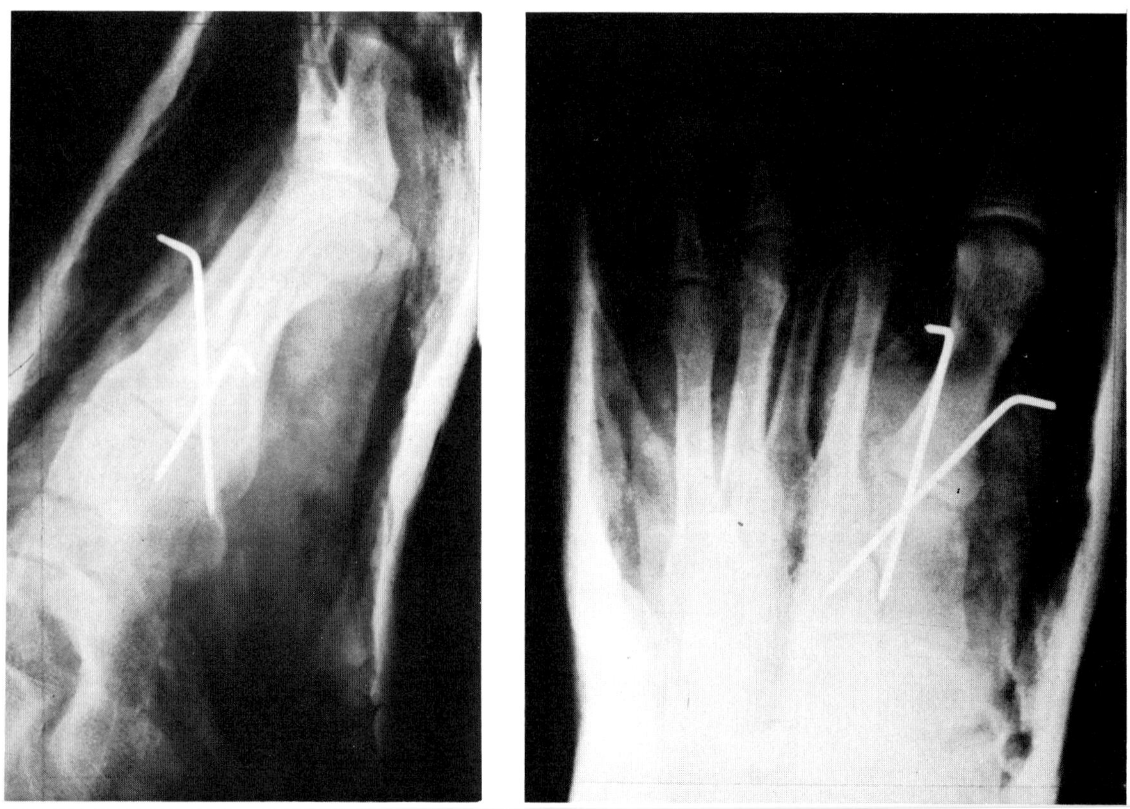

Fig. 46.5 This patient sustained a divarication type of dislocation of the first tarsometatarsal joint without significant displacement of the rest of the metatarsals. Closed reduction was possible but was unstable. The percutaneous Kirschner wire fixation gave excellent stability, the wires being maintained throughout the six weeks that the foot was immobilized in plaster

that the tibialis anterior tendon can be trapped between the cuneiform bones and act as a block to reduction of the first metatarsal (Lowe & Yosipovitch 1976). Having obtained an accurate reduction and confirmed it by X-ray, it is essential to stabilize the reduction by inserting crossed Kirschner wires percutaneously. Thereafter the treatment is as for conservative management by immobilization for six weeks in a below-knee plaster cast.

Late results

As the Lisfranc fracture-dislocation is uncommon there are no reports of the long term follow-up of a large series. In one study of 22 fractures, of the 15 which had been treated conservatively only two were completely free of pain at the time of follow-up and only one had a perfect reduction; whereas six patients with an anatomical reduction were virtually pain free (D. W. Wilson 1972). It is important therefore to strive for as perfect a reduction as possible (if necessary by open reduction) and to maintain this by some form of internal fixation.

Cases presenting with a late valgus deformity, either as a result of imperfect reduction, or because the injury was missed initially, can be improved by bony resection taking an appropriate wedge of bone based medially (see Fig. 46.3). This must be followed by plaster immobilization for at least three months, allowing weight bearing for only the last month. A soft longitudinal insole may be useful as a permanent appliance in such cases.

Fractures of the metatarsal bases

A basal fracture may occur in any metatarsal, but it is only in the case of the first and the fifth metatarsal that problems of treatment may sometimes occur.

Fracture of the base of the fifth metatarsal

This has been given the name of Jones' fracture because it was first described by Sir Robert Jones as a result of sustaining the injury himself while dancing. Previously this injury had always been attributed to a strain of the peroneus tendon and it was only the availability of X-rays which brought to light its true nature (Jones 1902).

Two quite different fractures can occur at the base of the fifth metatarsal and in later literature there seems to be some misinterpretation over the exact nature of Sir Robert's own injury (Torg et al 1984, J. N. Wilson 1982). The common fracture is an avulsion of the tip of the bone due to an inversion strain, which may sometimes involve the articular surface (Figs. 46.6 and 7). This fracture unites with the minimal amount of immobilization and leaves no longstanding disability. Patients are often more comfortable if the foot is immobilized in a below-knee walking plaster for the first three weeks, and then followed on with two or three weeks in an elastic support. However, the fracture will unite equally well if the foot is merely strapped, and some patients prefer this to the inconvenience of a plaster cast. In children this fracture must be distinguished from the normal basal epiphysis by X-ray of the other foot.

The less common and the more disabling injury of the fifth metatarsal is that described in detail by Sir Robert Jones and is a transverse fracture through the shaft of the bone just distal to the tarsometatarsal joint and the insertion of peroneus brevis (Fig. 46.8). It not uncommonly occurs in athletes and because of its tendency for union to be delayed, and the possibility of refracture, special measures may be necessary in treatment.

The mechanism of this injury is thought to be quite different to that causing the tuberosity fracture. Force plate studies and high speed photography have shown that the fracture is probably caused by a vertical force, with a medial or lateral component, acting on the foot with the heel elevated (Kavanagh et al 1978). As already stated these fractures are liable to develop delayed, or even nonunion and in one series of 20 fractures although 75% united with simple conservative measures, 25% required bone grafting for nonunion (Torg et al 1984). In the acute fracture, primary bone healing is more likely if plaster of Paris immobilization is used and more than half the cases can be expected to go on to delayed union if treated by strapping, or a simple supporting bandage (Dameron 1975). Refracture is also not uncommon, particularly in athletes. The injury must therefore be treated with considerably more respect than the tuberosity fracture.

A below-knee plaster cast should be used in all acute injuries and maintained for six weeks, with no weight bearing for the first half of that period. If

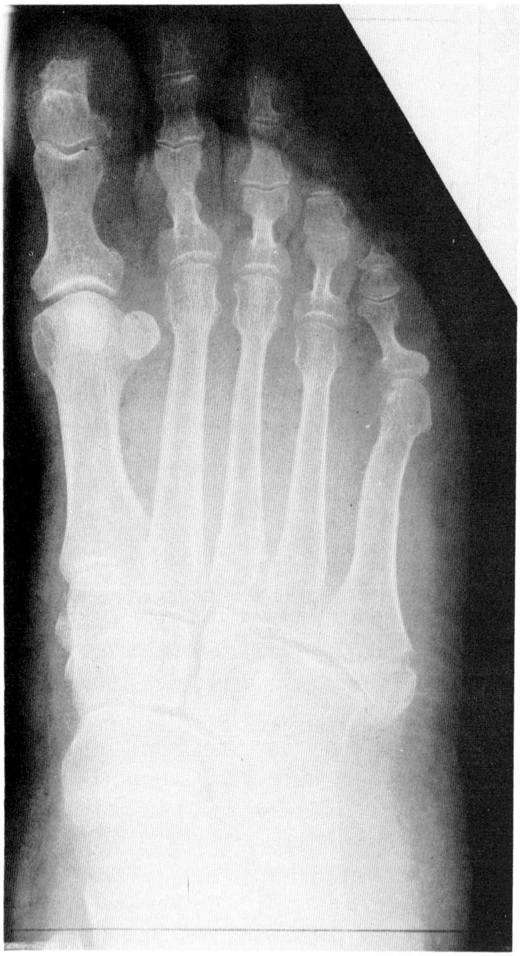

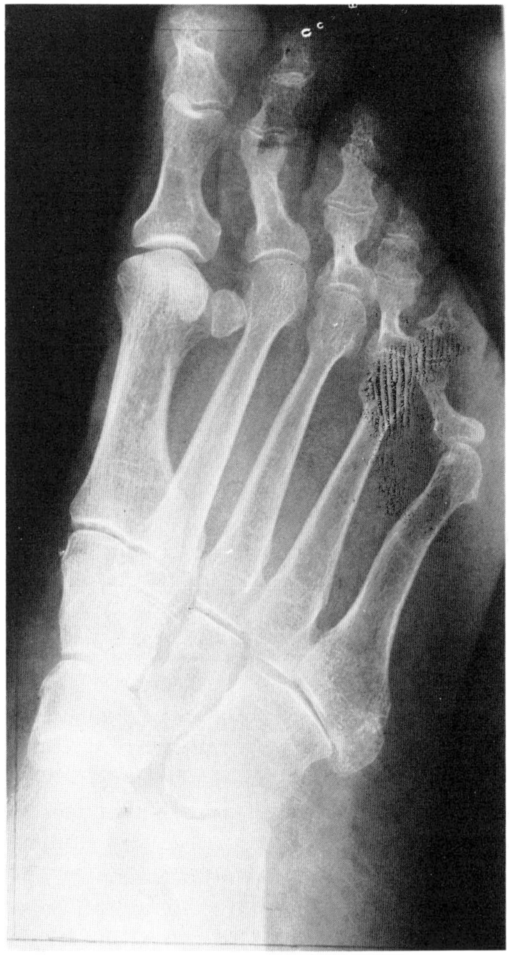

Figs. 46.6 and 7 Figure 6 shows an avulsion type of fracture of the base of the fifth metatarsal. This is caused by inversion of the foot and never results in any permanent disability even though it may involve the joint. Union occurs with only the minimum of immobilization (Fig. 7)

union is delayed, and particularly in a patient who is a keen athlete, bone grafting, using a cortico-cancellous inlay graft may be necessary.

Fracture of the base of the first metatarsal

Simple fractures through the base of the first metatarsal distal to the joint, unless associated with a Lisfranc type of injury, rarely present as a problem. They are usually caused by direct violence and are nearly always transverse and undisplaced. Because the first metatarsal is an important weight-bearing part of the foot the fracture must be treated in a below-knee cast if pain is to be avoided. This should be maintained for six weeks, with weight bearing for the last four weeks of this immobilization.

There is however a more rare injury in the form of a fracture-dislocation of the first tarsometatarsal joint similar to a Bennett's fracture of the first metacarpal base (Fig. 46.9a). This fracture is probably caused by a combination of forces resulting in an acute angulation into plantar flexion. Although accurate reduction can be achieved by manipulation the fracture is potentially unstable and will usually require transcutaneous Kirschner wire fixation to prevent redisplacement while in plaster (Fig. 46.9b). A below-knee walking plaster should be worn for six weeks and the wires should remain in situ until the plaster is finally removed.

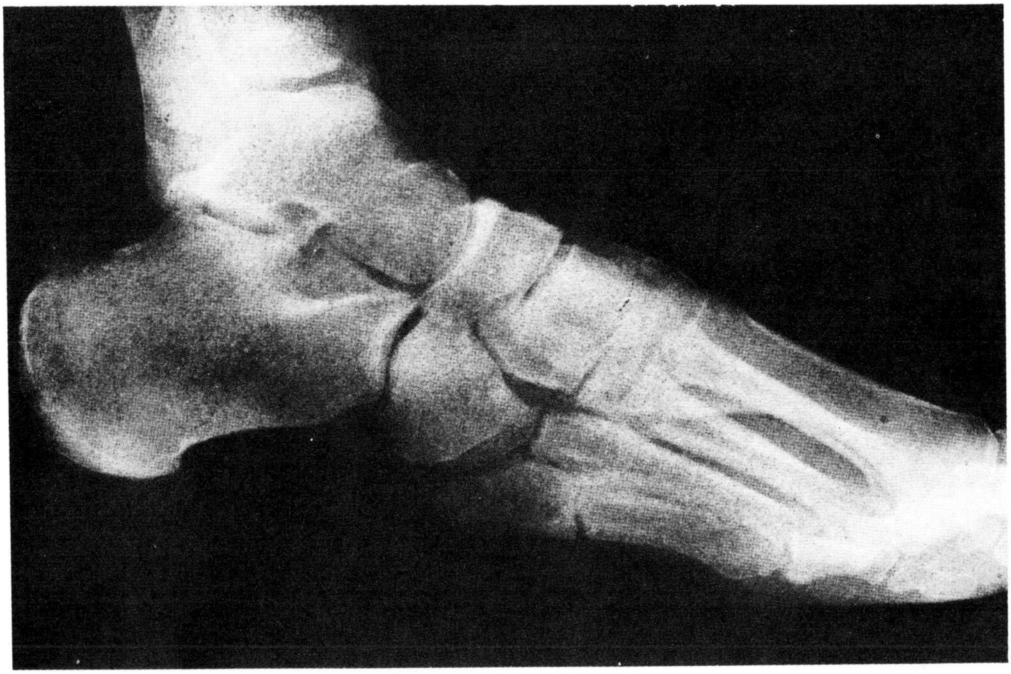

Fig. 46.8 A transverse fracture through the base of the fifth metatarsal distal to the joint should be treated with respect. This fracture may occur in athletes and has a reputation for delayed union and refracture (Reproduced with permission from Jones 1902)

A third isolated fracture-dislocation of the first metatarsal may be associated with a crush fracture of the medial cuneiform bone disrupting its strong plantar ligament attachments and allowing the base of the first metatarsal to displace plantarwards (Fig. 46.10). This injury is produced by an adduction-dorsiflexion strain on the forefoot and is not uncommonly associated with fractures of the proximal shafts of other nearby metatarsals (Fig. 46.10). The treatment by closed reduction under anaesthetic is usually successful and open reduction is rarely needed, but transcutaneous Kirschner wires may be required to prevent redisplacement. A below-knee walking plaster should be applied for six weeks, allowing weight bearing for the last three weeks.

Fractures of the shafts and necks of the metatarsals

Fractures of the shafts and distal ends of the metatarsals are almost exclusively confined to the lateral bones — the thicker and much stronger first metatarsal being rarely involved. The cause is usually a direct injury, such as from a heavy weight falling onto and trapping the forefoot. Commonly, more than one bone is involved, and because of the nature of the trauma the fracture may be compound. Fortunately in the majority of cases there is no gross displacement and the most that is required in the form of treatment is the application of a well padded below-knee plaster which should be moulded to restore the anterior and longitudinal arch. Although some authors have described the use of small fragment screws and plates for internally fixing these fractures (Muller et al, 1979, Schanwecker 1982), this is rarely ever required despite the plea that 'metatarsal fractures of the first and fifth metatarsals must be stabilized in every case because they form the pillars of the plantar arch'. Provided these fractures are in reasonable alignment they will unite and give no residual functional disability (Fig. 46.11). It is therefore wise to beware of overenthusiastic exponents of internal fixation when choosing the best form of treatment for forefoot fractures, and remember that one 'authority' has even described tension wiring for fractures of the tuberosity of the fifth metatarsal base!

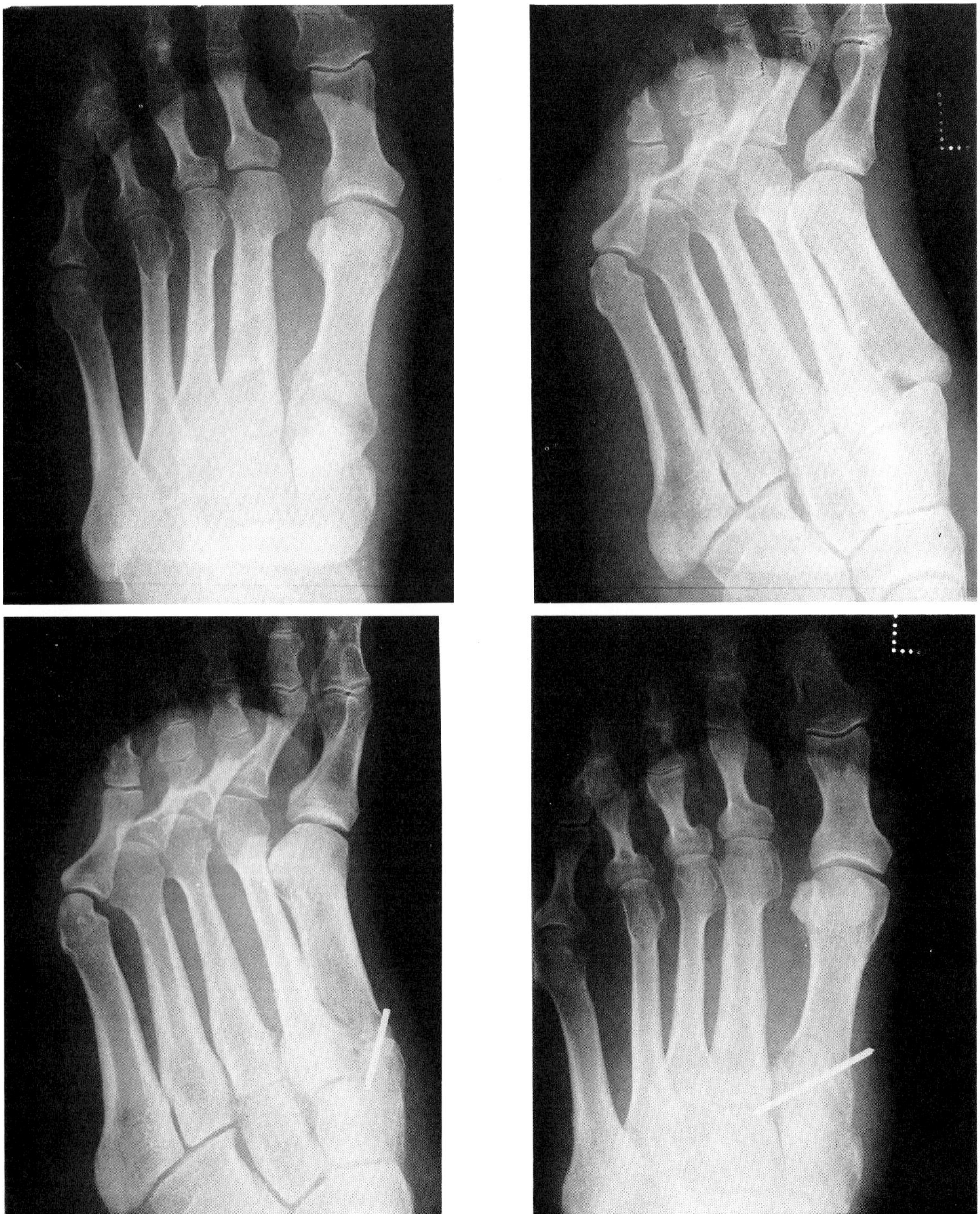

Fig. 46.9 An isolated fracture-dislocation of the first tarsometatarsal joint is the equivalent of a Bennett's fracture dislocation in the hand. The strong plantar ligaments remain intact along with a small fragment of bone, the rest of the metatarsal base displacing dorsally (Fig. 9a). This fracture demands accurate reduction and transcutaneous Kirschner wire fixation (Fig. 9b)

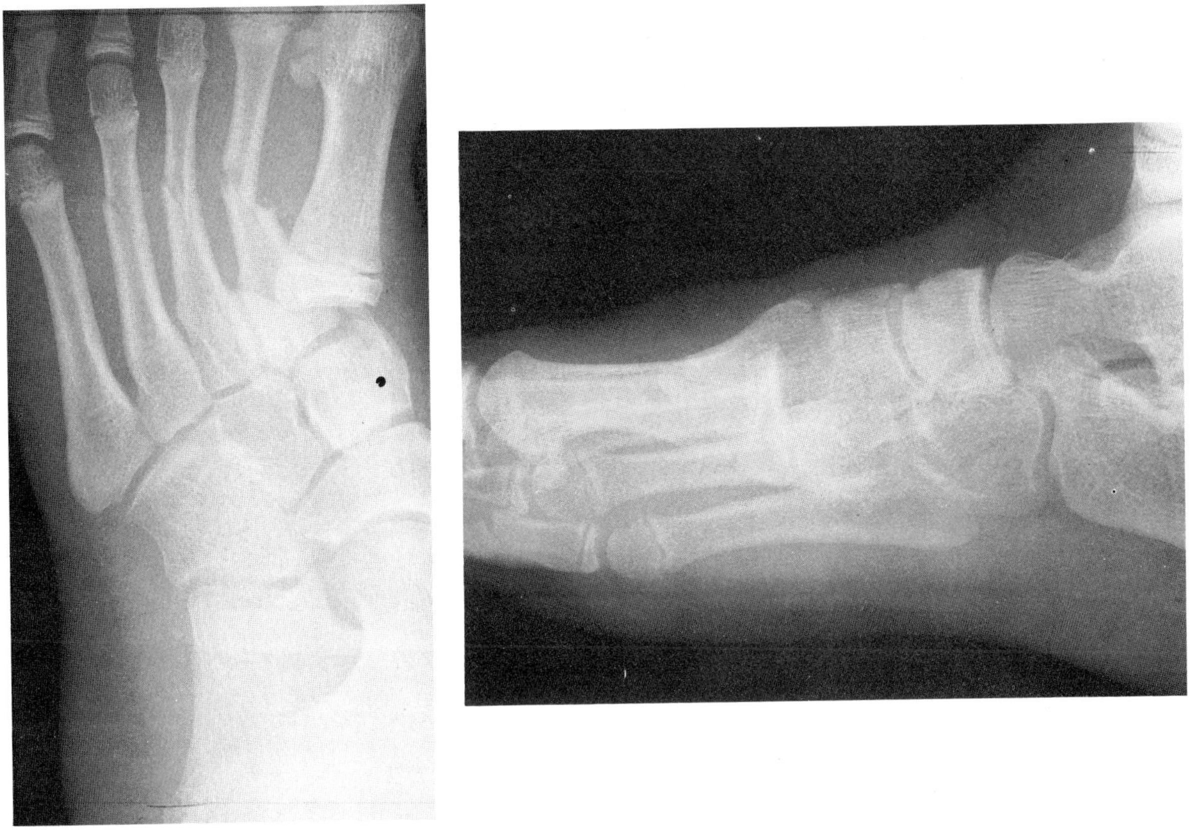

Fig. 46.10 An isolated fracture-dislocation of the base of the first metatarsal associated with a crush fracture of the medial cuneiform may disrupt the plantar ligaments and allow the metatarsal shaft to displace to the plantar aspect. The accompanying fractures of the shafts of the adjacent metatarsals indicate the severity of the force producing the injury

However, if there are multiple shaft or neck fractures in a compound fracture with a skin loss problem, simple alignment of the bones using a retrograde Kirschner wire technique is a simple method of neutralizing the bony injury (Fig. 46.12). Wherever possible this fixation should be supplemented by plaster. There is little place for the external fixateur in the treatment of fractures of the forefoot. The intramedullary wire fixation is equally applicable to the management of displaced metatarsal neck fractures, although it must be emphasized that very few of these fractures give permanent disability unless there is marked plantar displacement of the metatarsal head.

Stress fracture of the metatarsals (march fracture)

Stress fractures are not uncommon in the distal third of the metatarsal shafts, usually affecting the second and third although they have been reported in all five bones (Manu 1978). Although the condition was first described as a complication of route marching by army recruits (hence the term 'march fracture'), it is not uncommon in all walks of life — often associated with unusual exercise such as excessive walking on holiday, or intensive athletic activity; middle-aged 'joggers' are particularly vulnerable! The fracture is rarely seen in the first decade of life and except in high class athletes, it is unusual for it to occur in teenagers.

The history of forefoot pain, possibly over a prolonged period and associated with local tenderness and fullness over the distal third of the middle metatarsals, should immediately alert the clinician to the possibility of a stress fracture. If these findings are accompanied by the history that the onset followed an excessive amount of walking in a

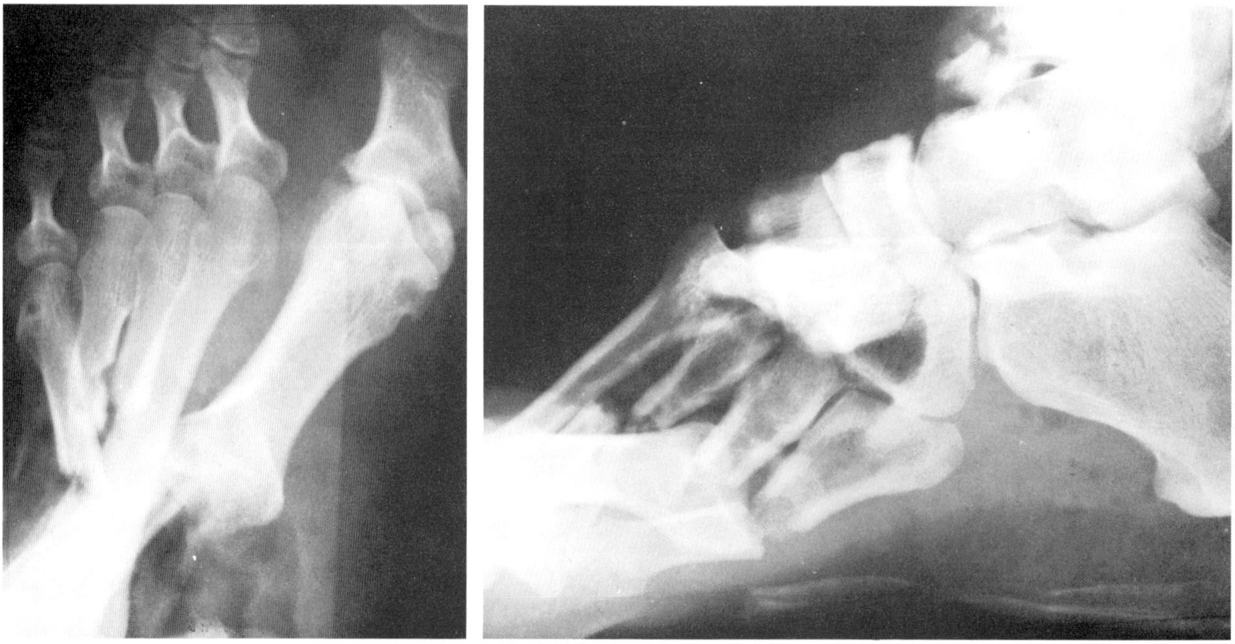

a

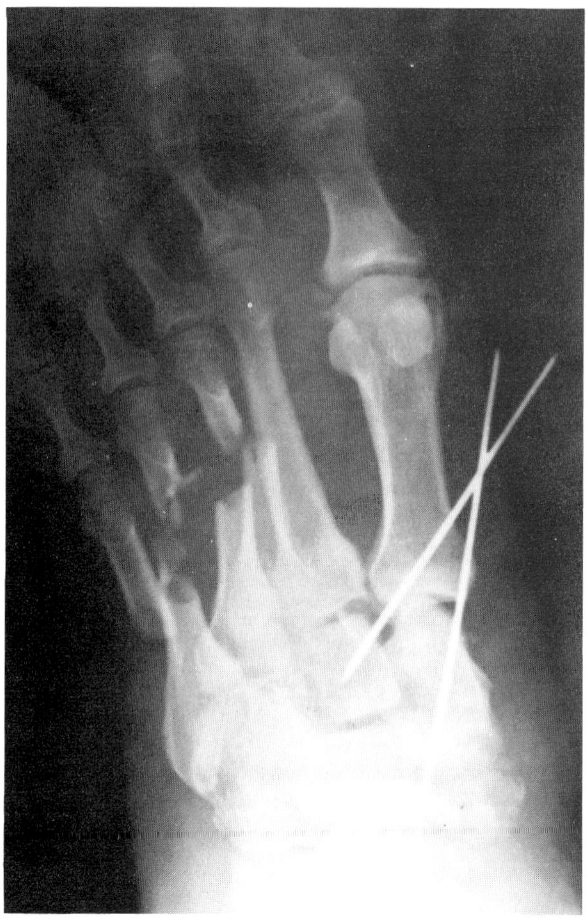

b

Fig. 46.11 The patient who sustained this multiple fracture of the bones of the forefoot was also suffering from a complicated and compound fracture of the ankle (Fig. 11a). The fractures of the metatarsals were pulled into reasonable alignment and the unstable fracture-dislocation of the first tarsometatarsal joint was temporarily fixed with transcutaneous Kirschner wires (Fig. 11b). The final result was an excellent plantigrade foot with all fractures united

usually sedentary person, the diagnosis is almost certain. However, there are three other conditions which can be confused with stress fracture and to the unwary may present with much the same clinical findings.

Firstly, in older people degenerative dorsal subluxation of the second and third metatarso-phalangeal joints can present with a very similar history, but on careful examination it will be found that the major tenderness and swelling is over the dorsum of the metatarsophalangeal joint rather than the neck of the metatarsal; in addition, flexion of the affected toe will be restricted and painful, and is sometimes felt to be dorsally displaced.

Secondly, in children, a common cause of forefoot pain is from osteochondritis of the second, third and sometimes fourth metatarsal head (Freiberg's disease). The clinical findings may be very similar to those of metatarsophalangeal subluxation, but the age group and the fact that the toe is not subluxed should lead to the correct diagnosis.

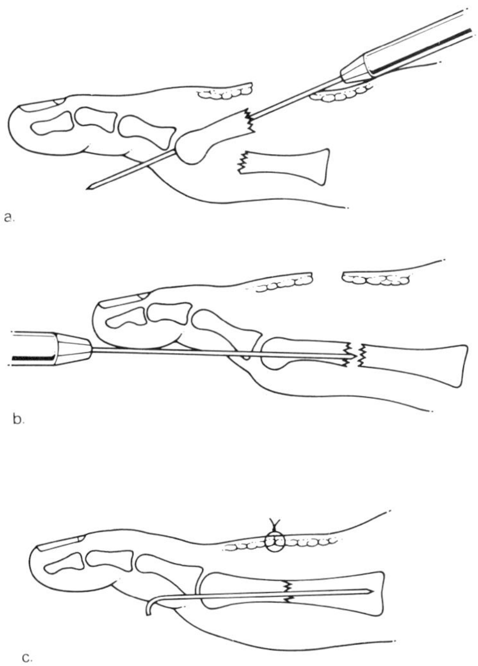

Fig. 46.12 Diagrams to illustrate the technique of retrograde Kirschner wire fixation for displaced fractures of the shafts of the metatarsals

The third condition in the differential diagnosis is that of Morton's metatarsalgia due to a plantar neuroma. However, this condition has the characteristic symptom of sharp pain *under* the metatarsal heads and may be associated with pain and clicking on forefoot compression and sensory loss in the toes supplied by the affected nerve.

X-ray findings

Usually by the time a patient with a stress fracture presents at the hospital the X-ray appearance is characteristic, but occasionally nothing may be seen, even though the diagnosis is strongly suspected from the clinical signs. In these circumstances it is wise to assume that a stress fracture is present and treat accordingly. Further X-rays after an interval of a few weeks will almost certainly show the diagnostic periosteal callus at the site of the fracture (Fig. 46.13).

Treatment

Although these fractures will unite with a minimal degree of immobilization, morbidity from pain can be prolonged and therefore protection in a below-knee walking plaster for six weeks is recommended. Following the removal of the plaster the patient should be warned of the possibility of further stress fractures and advised to wear a metatarsal pad for a period of four to six weeks.

Dislocation of the toes

Degenerative subluxation of the metatarso-phalangeal joints associated with flattening of the anterior metatarsal arch has already been mentioned. Traumatic dislocation of this joint is less common, as most injuries at this level result either in fractures of the metatarsal necks, or fractures of the phalanges. When traumatic dislocation does occur at either the metatarsal or the interphalangeal joints it is almost invariably dorsally displaced and if it is recognized early, it is easily reduced.

Unfortunately, some of these injuries are neglected because they are not uncommonly associated with serious injuries elsewhere in the body. Late, open or closed reduction is a useless exercise and proximal hemiphalangectomy for the metatarsophalangeal joint, with excision arthrodesis for the interphalangeal joints, are the treatments of choice.

There is, however, a more complex dislocation of the first metatarsophalangeal joint which has similarities to the equivalent dislocation of the metacarpophalangeal joint of the thumb. This rare injury, which is basically a dorsal dislocation, has been divided into two types (Lewis & De Lee 1984, Jahss 1980). The first is a dorsal dislocation of the proximal phalanx without disruption of the sesamoid complex. This is usually irreducible by closed methods. The second type is again a dorsal dislocation but with either disruption of the intersesamoid ligament, or a fissure fracture of one or other sesamoid. This type is usually reducible by manipulation because the split through the sesamoids allows free movement of the metatarsal head through the complex, thus restoring normal joint relationship.

The more rare type 1 injury usually demands open reduction. It is recommended that this should be carried out through a dorsal longitudinal incision just to the lateral side of the joint (Lewis & De Lee

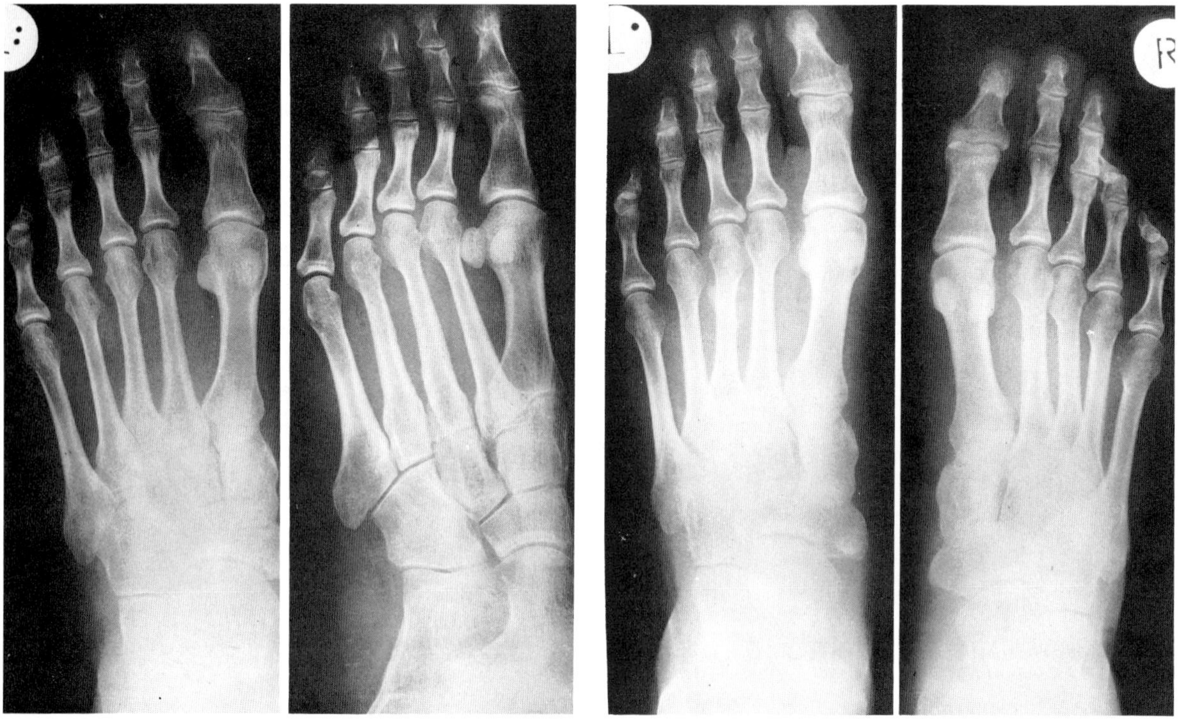

a b

Fig. 46.13 This patient presented with a history of pain in the left forefoot for three weeks, coming on without injury. Although X-rays at that time (Fig. 13a) showed no abnormality the tenderness and local swelling over the neck of the third metatarsal raised the suspicion of a stress fracture. Films taken three weeks later showed an area of ensheathing callus around the metatarsal neck confirming the clinical diagnosis (Fig. 13b)

1984). Under direct vision it will be seen that simple traction on the great toe will tighten up the stranglehold exerted on the first metatarsal neck by the short muscle attachments to the sesamoid, and it is necessary to relieve this by dividing the attachment of the intermetatarsal ligament and the lateral head of flexor hallucis brevis to the lateral sesamoid. If necessary, the intersesamoid attachments forming the flexor cartilaginous plate can be divided longitudinally. Following this soft-tissue release the proximal phalanx can be reduced easily by plantarflexion. Reduction is usually stable, but a period of immobilization for three weeks in a below-knee walking plaster is advisable.

FRACTURES OF THE PHALANGES

The most common of these fractures is that of the proximal phalanx of the fifth toe, sometimes referred to as the 'night walker's fracture' because of its association with a stubbing injury sustained when walking barefoot to answer calls of nature (Jahss 1982)! A fracture may occur in any phalanx but is more common at the base or neck of the proximal phalanx. In children there can be a fracture separation of the basal epiphysis necessitating manipulative reduction under general anaesthesia, but usually there is no necessity, for the correction of deformity and immobilization by strapping adjacent toes together for a week or two is all the treatment that is needed.

Fractures of the terminal phalanges, particularly of the great toe, are often due to a heavy weight falling on the tip of the toes, resulting in an excessively painful subungual haematoma. If this occurs it should be decompressed by burning a hole through the raised nail using the wire of a red-hot paper clip.

Where fractures are multiple (Fig. 46.14) it is kinder to the patient to immobilize the foot and ankle in a below-knee walking plaster for a period of three

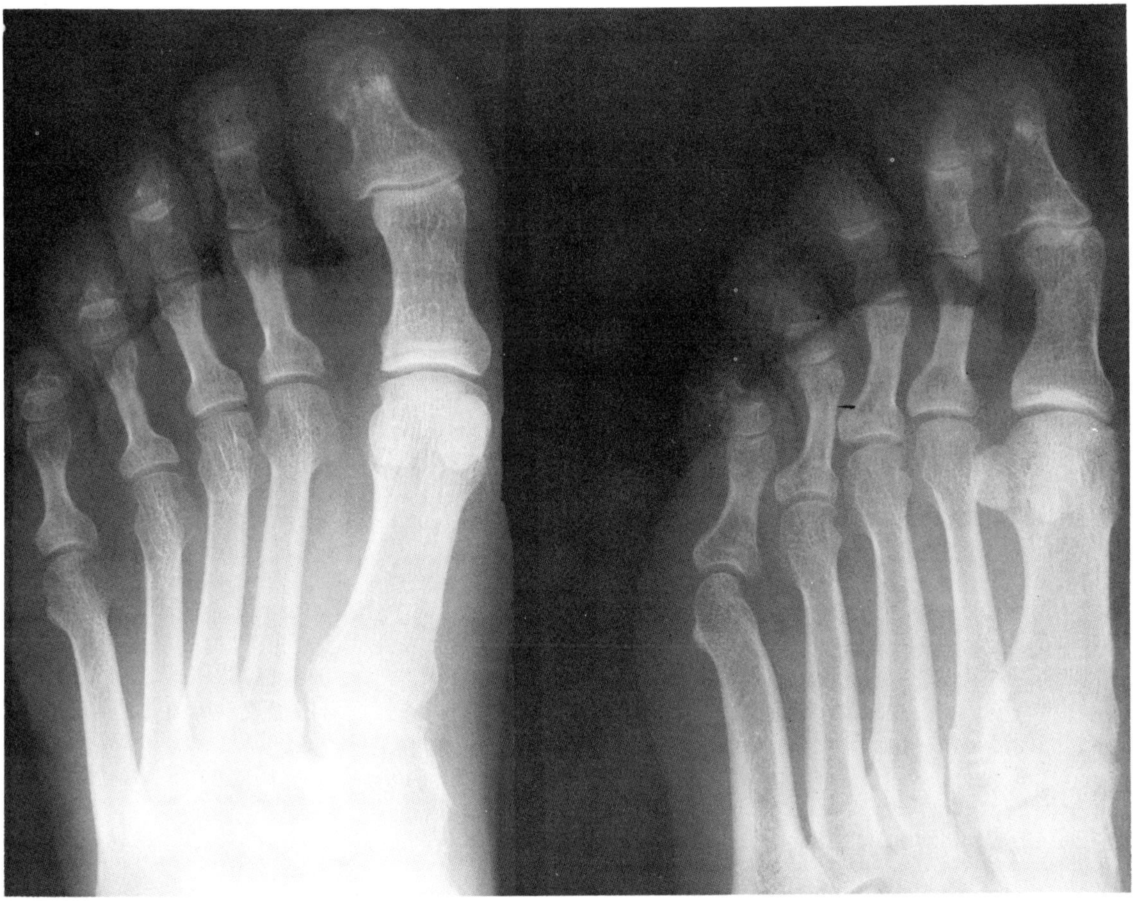

a

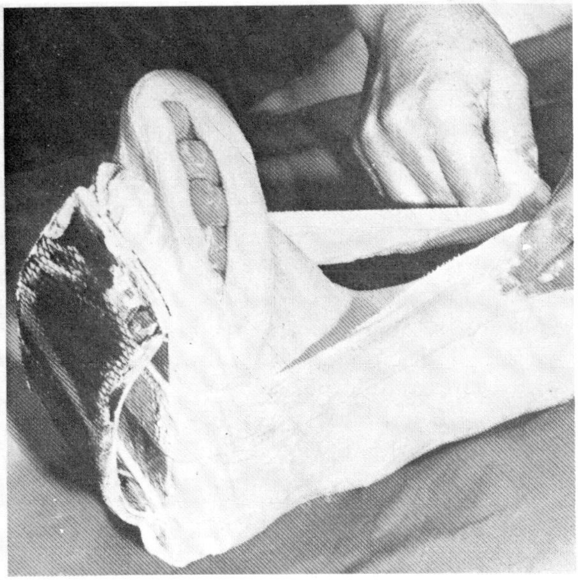

b

Fig. 46.14 Multiple crush fractures of the terminal phalanges can be very disabling. The patient with this X-ray was completely unable to walk when first treated in a compression bandage alone. After three weeks walking pain free in a below-knee plaster the fractures were clinically healed and all immobilization was removed. If plaster is used in the treatment of this injury it must extend to the tips of the toes and a rocker used for weight bearing (14b; Fig. 14b is reproduced with permission from Wilson J N 1982)

weeks, remembering to extend the plaster to the tips of the toes to protect them from minor trauma during the acute stage. Plasters which extend only to the metatarsophalangeal joints are worse than useless.

Fractures of the sesamoid bones

Fractures of the sesamoids are fairly rare and when they occur they are not uncommonly due to an athletic injury. They are typically produced by a fall from a height (as in ballet), or by forced dorsiflexion of the great toe (as may occur to a player lying prone in a football pile-up). The injury to the footballer has possibly been made more likely by the use of the soft type of playing shoe which has become so popular in recent times.

The diagnosis should be suspected when there is localized tenderness (and sometimes swelling) under the ball of the great toe, usually affecting the medial (tibial) sesamoid. Pain is always aggravated by forced dorsiflexion of the first metatarsophalangeal joint even though the toe may still dorsiflex through its full range. Although the fracture is more common on the medial side either sesamoid can be injured. Skyline anteroposterior X-rays of the forefoot, with the great toe hyperextended, should establish the nature of the fracture.

It is important to take comparison views of the normal foot to exclude a bifid sesamoid (Fig. 46.15), but it must be remembered that even though there are similar changes on the other side this does not exclude a sesamoid injury, as a bifid sesamoid is more prone to give trouble than a one-segment bone.

Treatment for the condition varies from the application of a protective felt crescent around the neck of the first metatarsal, to immobilization in a below-knee plaster using a similar felt pad to protect the tender area and a walking rocker to remove all flexion strain on the forefoot. This cast should be worn for three weeks, followed by a metatarsal pad for six weeks or more.

In some cases persistent pain will eventually demand excision of the damaged bone. In the common medial sesamoid fracture this is best achieved through an incision on the plantar aspect, but in lateral sesamoid fractures some authorities advise a dorsal approach (Jahss 1982).

THE MANAGEMENT OF COMPOUND FRACTURES AND LATE DEFORMITY

These are considered together because so often the one leads to the other.

Compound fractures of the toes

Fractures of the phalanges, and particularly those of the terminal phalanx, are always associated with marked soft tissue injury and are therefore not uncommonly compound. Usually the soft tissue involvement can be treated by simple dressings, prophylactic antibiotic therapy, and protective immobilization. Sometimes it may be necessary to decompress a nail bed, but usually the compound wound will carry out its own decompression. In severe contusions circulatory problems can occur and may sometimes result in gangrene. Böhler (1958b) has pointed out the danger of such a fracture occurring in the great toe and quotes a report from pre-Listerian days by Malgaigne of seven deaths resulting from the complications of this injury. Although (as Böhler hastens to add) such drastic consequences should never occur with modern treatment, compound fractures of the toes are not always minor in nature; they should be treated with the respect that they deserve for they can sometimes result in a considerable morbidity.

Compound fractures of the metatarsus

Variations of Lisfranc's fracture-dislocation and multiple fractures of the metatarsals are all too often associated with severe skin loss, sometimes extending to the ankle, and may be accompanied by other more demanding problems from injuries elsewhere (Fig. 46.16). The immediate treatment should be as for any compound fracture — i.e. full debridement and closure of the wound *only* if the skin flaps are viable, there is no tension and no gross loss of soft tissue. When in doubt the wound should be left open, and where the injury is due to gunshot wound or shell splinters the skin should never be closed as a primary treatment. Secondary skin closure may sometimes be possible at five to 10 days after injury, but it is more usual to require split skin grafts to obtain skin cover. It is surprising how effective these grafts can be even in the presence of exposed tendon and bone. Full thickness pedicle, or free flap grafts are not applicable at this stage.

It is important at the time of initial treatment to make every effort to restore and maintain a plantigrade position of the foot, using if necessary transcutaneous Kirschner wires to hold the reduction of any unstable fracture (Fig. 46.17). It must be remembered that the restoration of a plantigrade position of the foot will become progressively more difficult to achieve as the days

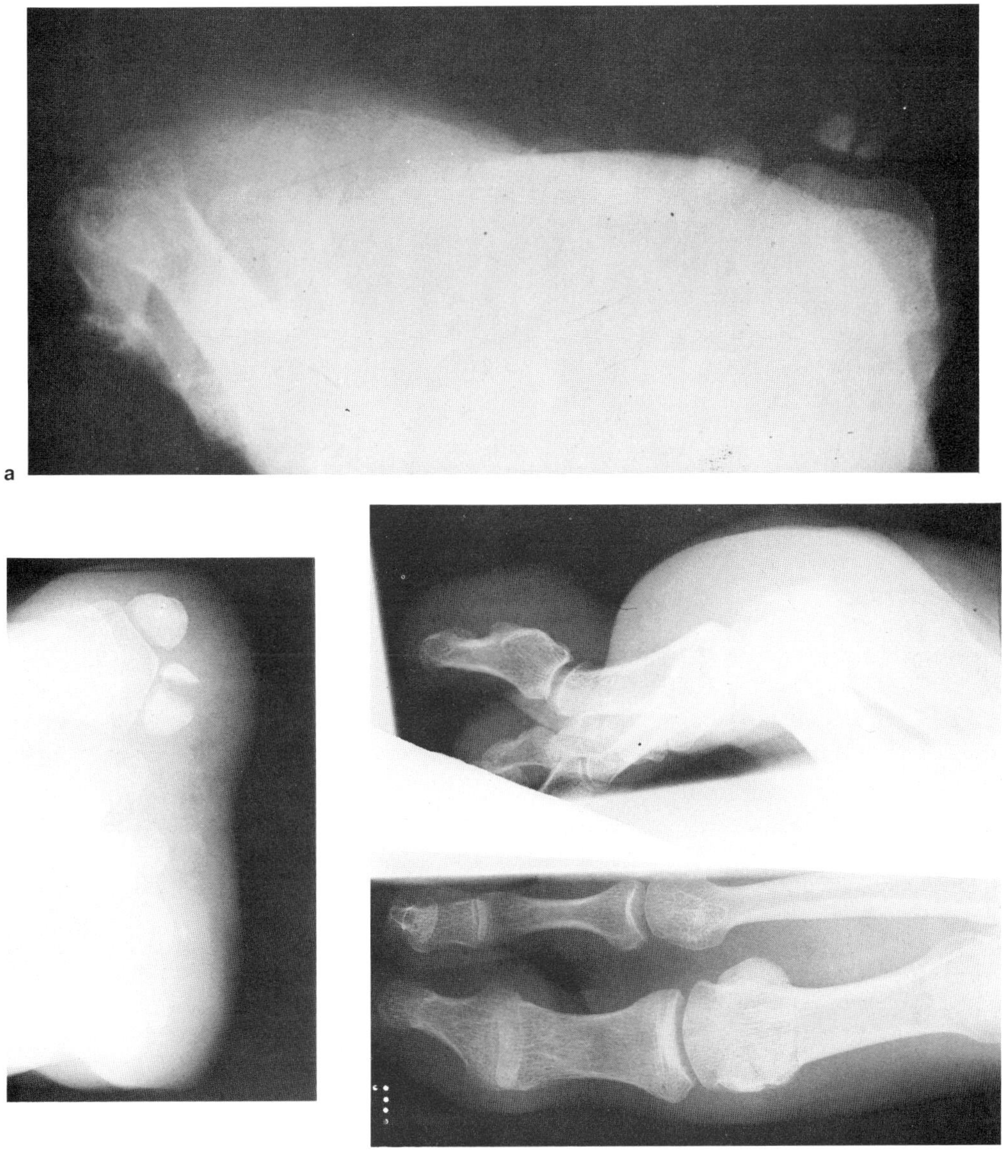

Fig. 46.15 Fractures of the sesamoids usually affect the medial (tibial) bone and can be seen most easily in the skyline view (Fig. 15a). More rarely the lateral sesamoid is injured (Fig. 15b). In this latter case a bifid sesamoid is seen on the medial side. Note the more irregular features of the true fracture, which is usually longitudinal, compared with regular features of the transverse bifid defect

pass and that in these severe crush injuries there may be an element of ischaemia in the foot or lower leg which may obstruct reduction even within a few hours of the initial injury. Because of this possibility plaster immobilization, in addition to Kirschner wire fixation, is essential. There is no more difficult deformity to treat than an equinovarus due to an injury to the forefoot associated with calf ischaemia.

The management of late deformity

Although malunion of the metatarsals and phalanges may cause residual problems (usually in the metatarsal arch) these are unusual and can be easily treated by local surgery such as excision of a metatarsal head or fusion of an interphalangeal joint. It is the deformity resulting from malunion of a

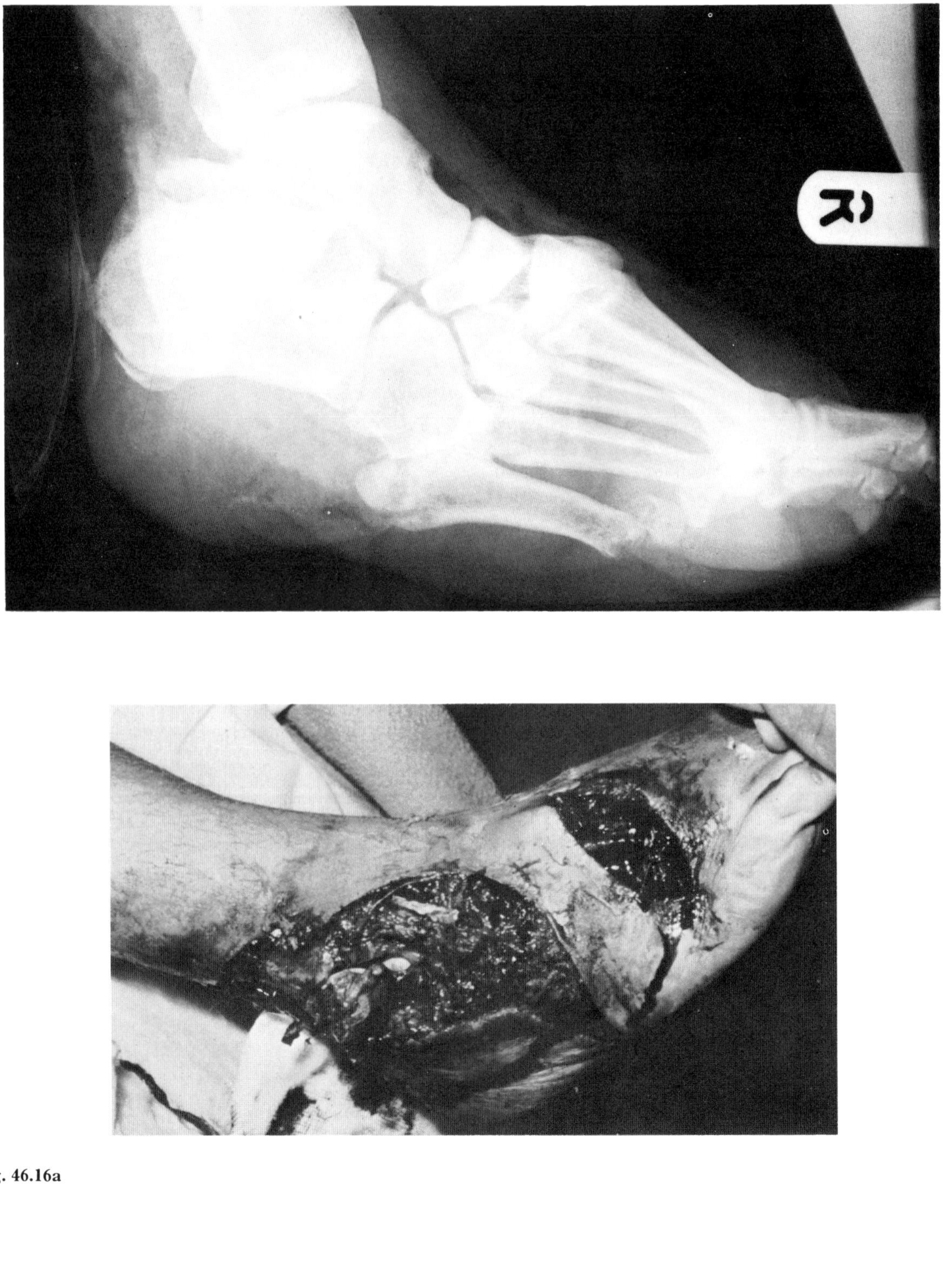

Fig. 46.16a

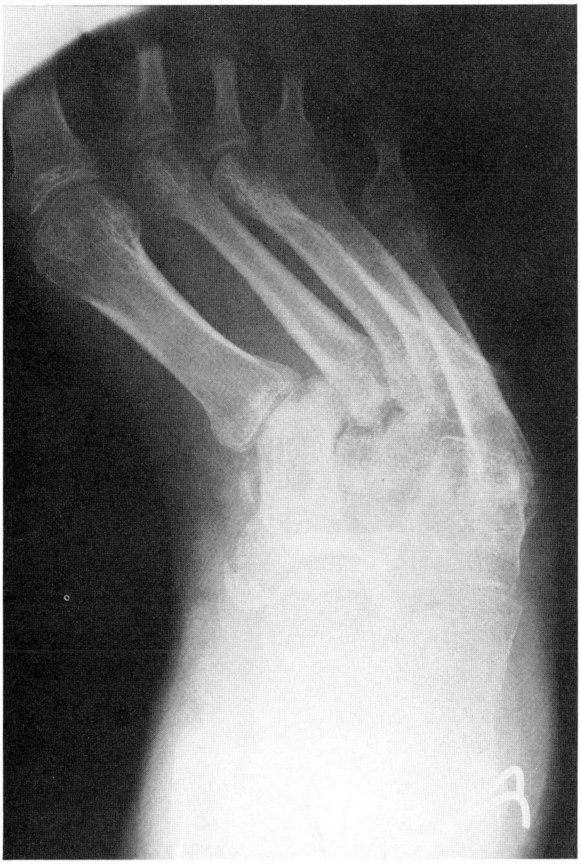

b

Fig. 46.16 The patient who sustained this compound fracture of the metatarsus (Fig. 16a) also suffered from a compound ankle injury, a fracture of the femur, a fracture dislocation of the pelvis and fractures of both forearms. Because of the severity of his injuries the foot fracture was considered of low priority as far as treatment was concerned, and as a result caused more longstanding morbidity than any of the other injuries (Fig. 16b). Wherever possible a displaced compound fracture of the foot should be reduced as early as possible

Fig. 46.17 Transcutaneous Kirschner wires are valuable in maintaining the general alignment in severely displaced multiple forefoot fractures, such as is seen in this compound fracture-dislocation of the tarsometatarsal joint. The dislocated toes were then reduced easily by closed manipulation

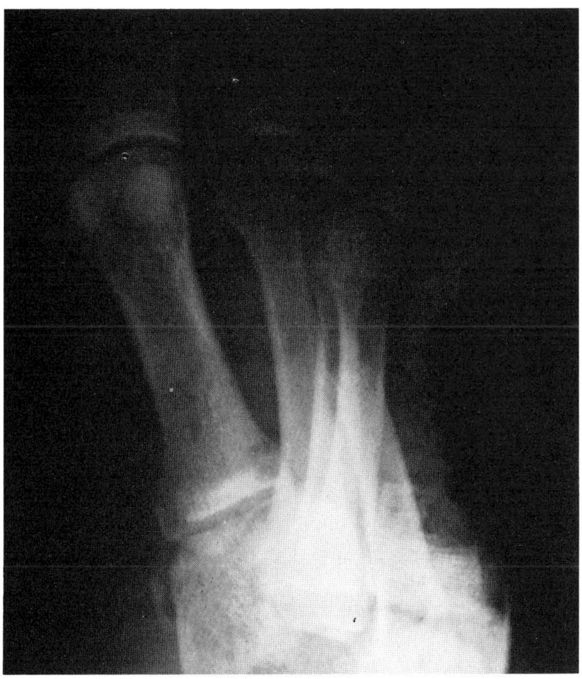

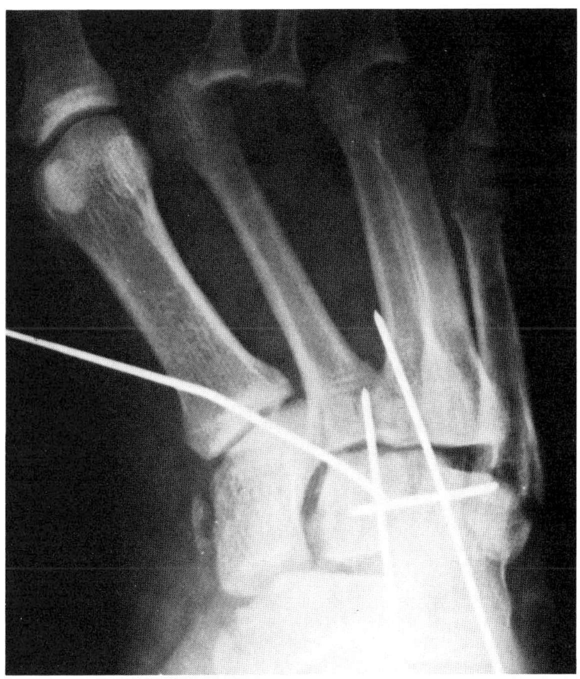

fracture-dislocation of the tarsometatarsal joint which can prove difficult to correct and is the main concern of this last section. Such deformity may be caused by the severity of the injury itself; in other cases it may be due to the injury being unrecognized; or it may be due to inadequate treatment because of lack of appreciation of its serious nature.

Many such injuries have been initially compound with severe skin loss, and before any corrective bone surgery can be performed unstable scars will require replacement with full thickness skin cover. Where the facilities exist, and where the local conditions permit, this can be very satisfactorily achieved by a free vascularized skin graft. But this is a time-consuming operation, usually requiring the expertise of a plastic surgeon skilled in the technique. The simpler, although more cumbersome technique of cross-leg flap is still a useful procedure and ideally suited to the foot (Fig. 46.18).

Correction of the deformity should be carried out

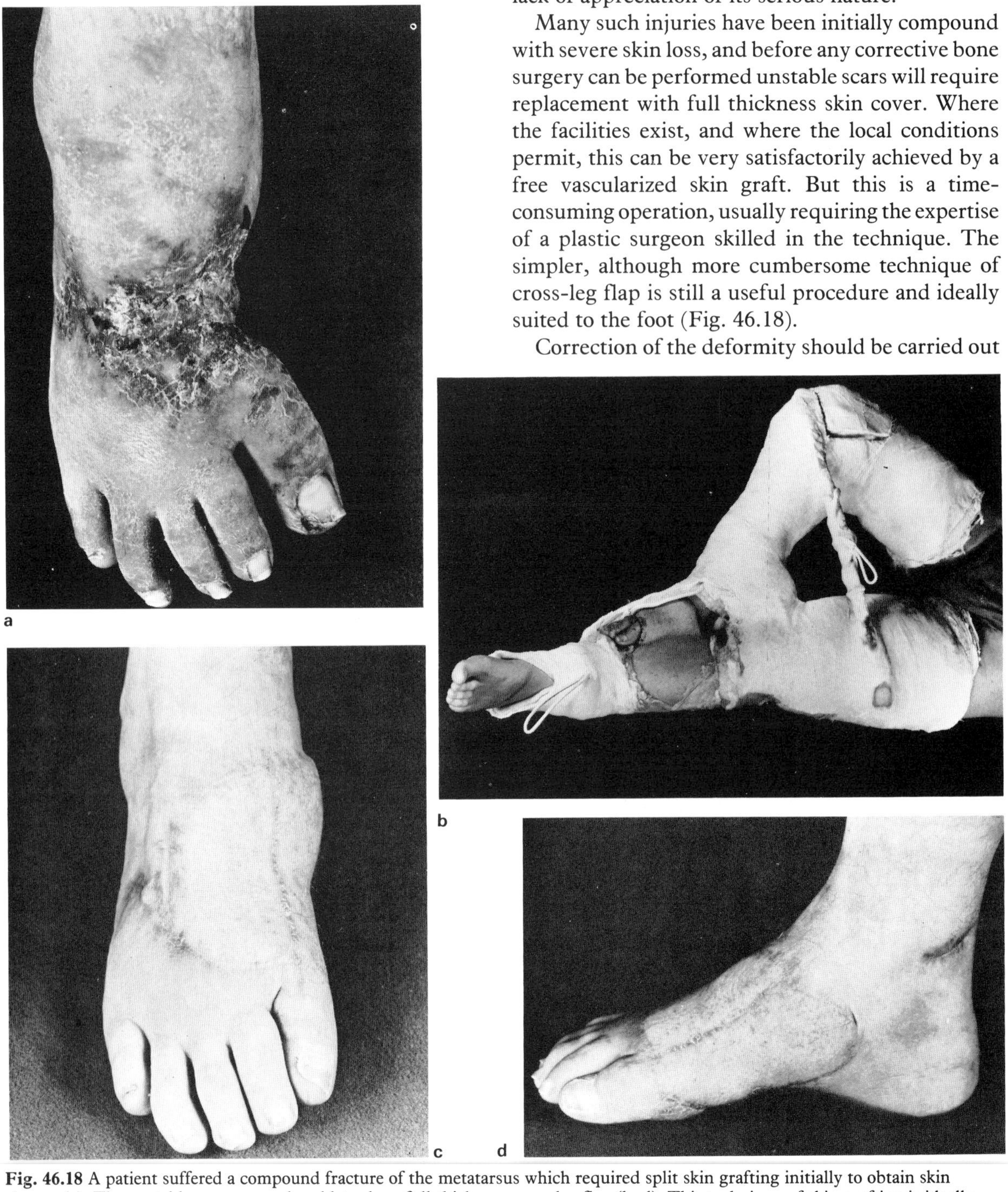

a b c d

Fig. 46.18 A patient suffered a compound fracture of the metatarsus which required split skin grafting initially to obtain skin closure (a). The unstable scar was replaced later by a full thickness cross-leg flap (b–d). This technique of skin grafting is ideally suited to the forefoot and does not require the expertise and equipment necessary for vascularized flaps by the excision of an appropriate wedge of bone — removed without regard to joint planes — the base of the wedge being sited at the apex of the deformity on its convex side. Once the wedge has been removed and the adduction or abduction of the forefoot corrected, any residual pronation or supination deformity can be easily dealt with by rotating the forefoot at the osteotomy site. However, it must be remembered that forefoot trauma of this magnitude may also be associated with displacement at the

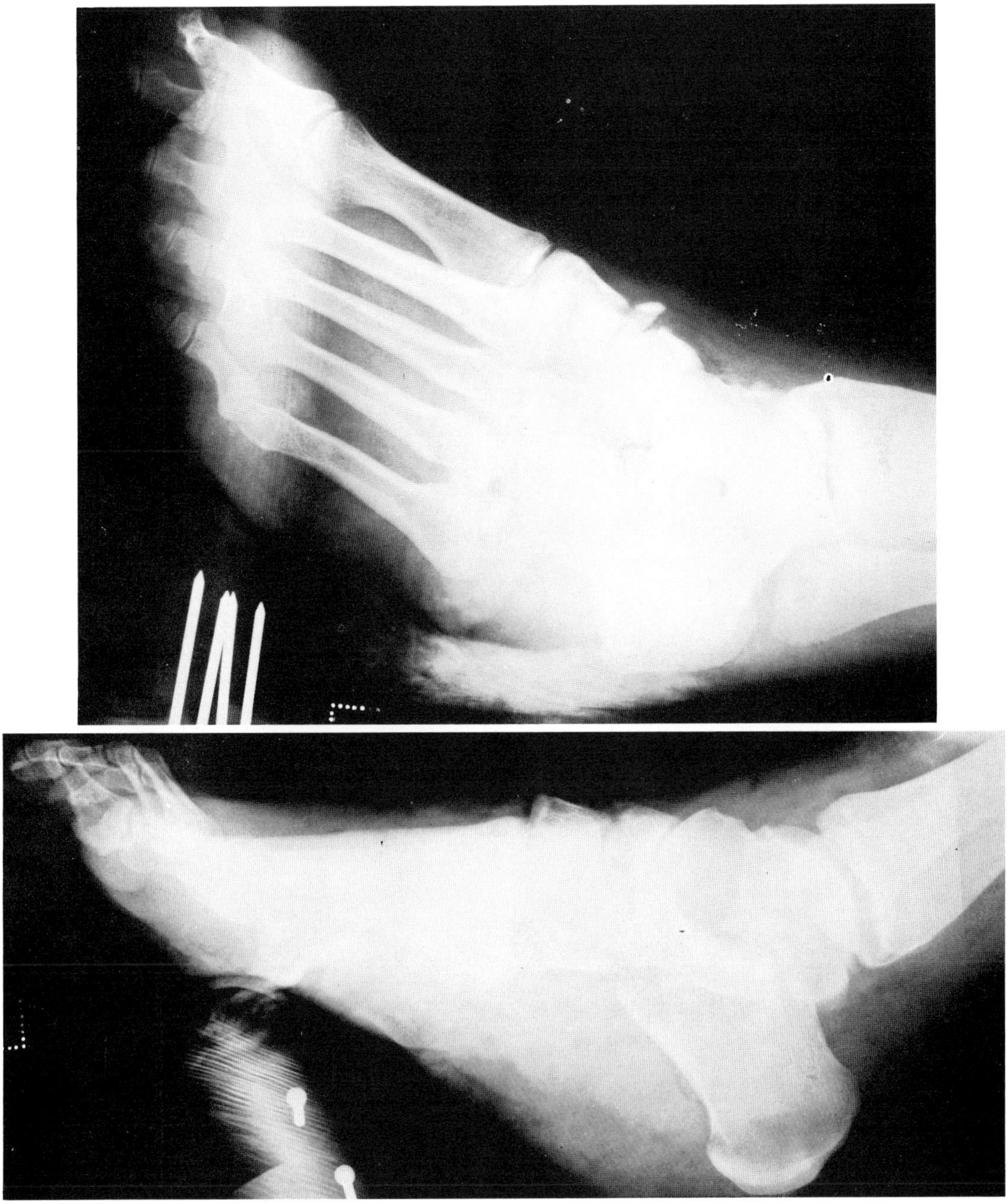

a

Fig. 46.19 Fixed bony deformity of the forefoot from tarsometatarsal injuries may be associated with injury to the midtarsal joint (Fig. 19a). It may be possible to correct the deformity more easily by wedge resection of the midtarsal joint than by tarsometatarsal resection (Fig. 19b, over)

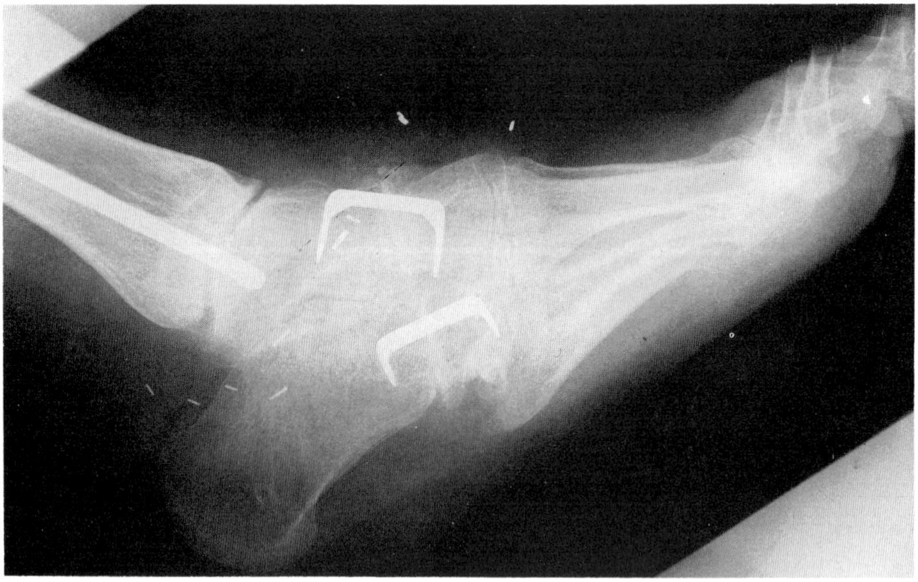

b

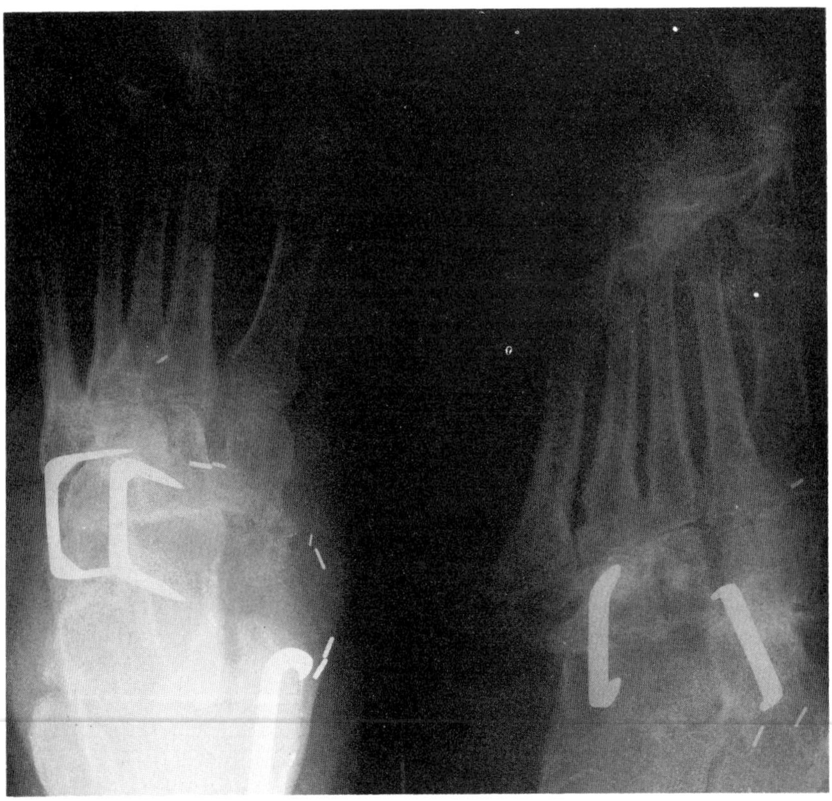

midtarsal joint and that in such cases it can sometimes be easier to correct any forefoot imbalance by removing suitable bone wedges when carrying out a formal, triple arthrodesis (Fig. 46.19).

The use of surgical shoes and orthoses

In conclusion, one should not forget the value of a surgical shoe and suitable insole in the management of the deformed forefoot (Fig. 46.20). These can be used either as a conservative measure alone, or combined with surgery. No surgical correction for marked deformity can be expected to produce a perfectly plantigrade foot, for it will almost certainly result in one which is smaller than on the normal side. This in itself may demand the use of a surgical shoe. If such footwear is combined with a well made insole, distributing overall bodyweight evenly throughout the plantar surface and removing all high-spots, the patient can be restored from being a foot cripple to someone who almost has a normal gait. It is hoped that at least some of the information contained within this chapter may prove useful in achieving this end result.

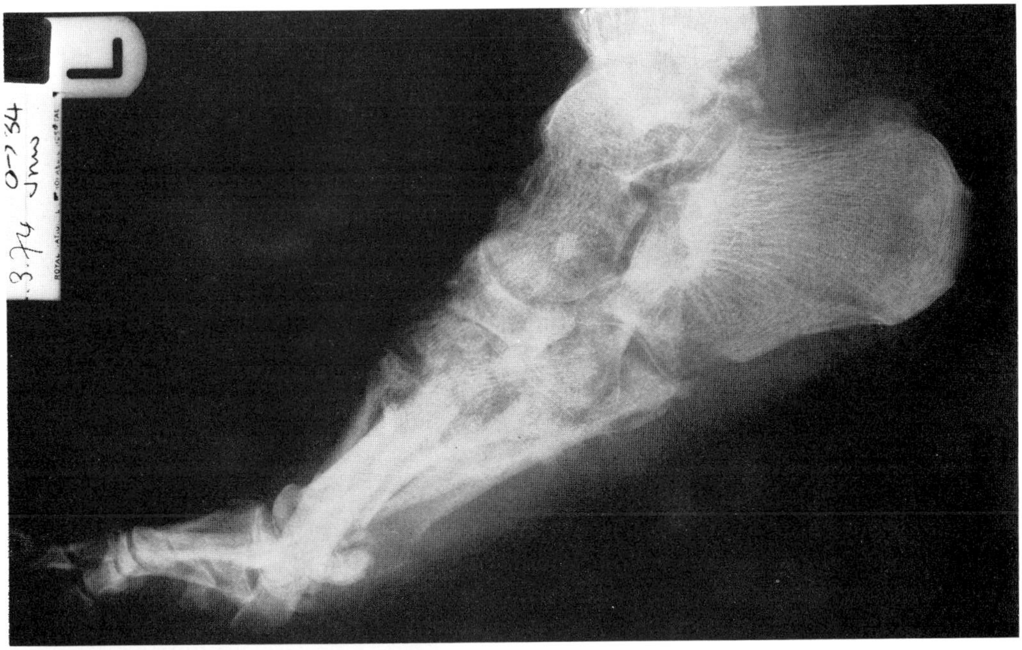

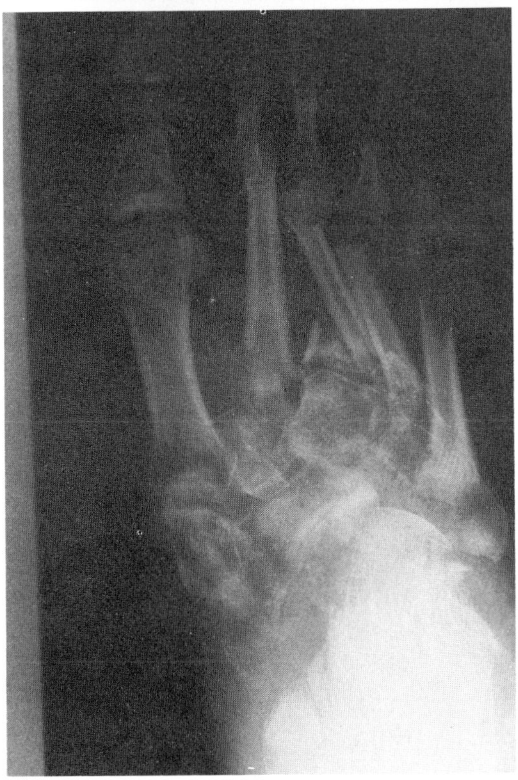

Fig. 46.20 The residual deformity in this patient's severely crushed forefoot was treated successfully by local removal of prominent metatarsal heads and the fitting of a surgical shoe and suitable insole. One must not forget the value of surgical footwear in the treatment of late deformity

REFERENCES

Adams J C 1983 Outline of Fractures, 8th edn. Churchill-Livingstone, London. pp 283–286

Aitken A P, Poulson D 1963 Dislocation of the tarso-metatarsal joint. J Bone Joint Surg 45A: 246

Badger F G 1967 Causes of injury in road accidents. Image and Medical Illustrated, Roche. pp 21, 19

Böhler L 1958a The Treatment of Fractures, Vol. III, 5th edn. Grun & Stratton, New York. pp 2045–2113

Böhler L 1958b The Treatment of Fractures. Vol. III, 5th edn. Grune & Stratton, New York. p 2159

Dameron T B 1975 Fractures and anatomical variations of the proximal portion of the fifth metatarsal. J Bone Joint Surg 57A: 788

Foster S C, Foster R R 1976 Lisfranc's tarso-metatarsal fracture-dislocation. Radiology 120: 79–83

Gissane W 1951 A dangerous type of fracture of the foot. J Bone Joint Surg 33B: 535

Jahss M H 1980 Traumatic dislocations of the first metatarsophalangeal joint. Foot Ankle 1: 15–21

Jahss M H 1982 Disorders of the Foot. Vol 2, W. B. Saunders Company, Philadelphia. p 1585

Jeffreys T E 1963 Lisfranc's fracture-dislocation. A clinical and experimental study of tarso-metatarsal dislocations and fracture-dislocations. J Bone Joint Surg 45B: 546

Jones R 1902 Fracture of the base of the fifth metatarsal bone by indirect violence. Ann Surg 35: 697

Kavanagh J H, Brown J D, Mann R V 1978 The Jones' fracture revisited. J Bone Joint Surg 60A: 776

Lewis A G, De Lee J C 1984 Type 1 complex dislocation of the first metatarso-phalangeal joint — open reduction through a dorsal approach. J Bone Joint Surg 66A: 1120

Lowe J, Yosipovitch Z 1976 Tarso-metatarsal dislocation: a mechanism blocking manipulative reduction. J Bone Joint Surg 58A: 1029

Manu R A 1978 Du Vries' Surgery of the Foot. 4th edn. C. V. Mosby Company, St. Louis. p 195

Muller M E, Allgöwer M, Schneider R, Willenegger H 1979 Manual of Internal Fixation, 2nd edn. Springer-Verlag, Berlin. pp 302–303

Rockwood C A, Green D P 1984 Fractures in Adults, 2nd edn. J. R. Lippincott Co., Philadelphia

Schanwecker F 1982 Practice of Osteosynthesis. Georg Thieme Verlag, Stuttgart. pp 308–309

Torg J S, Baldnini F C, Zelko R R, Pavlov H, Peff T C, Das M 1984 Fractures of the base of the fifth metatarsal distal to tuberosity. Classification and guidelines for non-surgical and surgical management. J Bone Joint Surg 66A: 209

Wiley J J 1971 The mechanism of tarso-metatarsal joint injuries. J Bone Joint Surg 53B: 474

Wilson D W 1972 Injuries of the tarso-metatarsal joints. Etiology, classification and results. J Bone Joint Surg 54B: 677

Wilson J N 1982a Watson-Jones' Fractures and Joint Injuries, 6th edn. Churchill-Livingstone, Edinburgh. p 1196

Wilson J N 1982b Watson-Jones' Fractures and Joint Injuries, 6th edn. Churchill-Livingstone, Edinburgh. p 1200

M. Devas

Stress fractures

This chapter will deal with stress fractures in the foot and also those in the lower tibia and fibula which may give rise to diagnostic problems because of referred pain.

DEFINITION

A stress fracture occurs in the normal bone of a normal individual with normal activity and no injury. Because stress fractures are very common in the leg and foot of athletes, who are usually considered to be in peak condition, it is very unlikely that there can be any inherent abnormality in the bone that sustains a stress fracture. It is to be noted that normal activity may at times be unusual and if, for example, an athlete out of training suddenly exerts himself, this would be unusual, but not abnormal, and he might sustain a stress fracture as a result. Any form of rest or immobilization followed by intensive activity may well produce a stress fracture, so that anybody, for example, who has a foot encased in plaster and then reverts to heavy exercise too rapidly is at risk of a march fracture.

Patients with rheumatoid arthritis have a propensity to stress fractures and although it cannot be said that the individual is normal, their bones sometimes being osteoporotic and particularly if they have had steroid treatment, the stress fractures that are sustained are identical to those in the otherwise normal person.

A bone that is in any way diseased, such as by metastatic deposits from a carcinoma, cannot ever be considered to have a stress fracture.

History

Stress fractures have been known for a long time, even before radiography; the march fracture was the first to be described in 1855 by a German military surgeon called Breithaupt, but in 1773 Gooch made a good description of a cough fracture of the rib. Probably the first radiograph of a stress fracture of a metatarsal bone was that taken by Stechow in 1897. It must be recalled also that in 1855 Lane described the effects of pressure on bony skeleton, but it was not until 1917 that Koch published his laws of bone architecture. Alamen in 1929 published an important work which shows that he well understood how stress affected bone. That animals also get stress fractures is well documented, but the greyhound and horse suffer from them in particular.

Types of stress fractures

The best way to classify stress fractures is radiologically: oblique, transverse, compression and longitudinal (Figs. 47.1 to 4).

The oblique variety is the most common and is seen particularly in long bones and in the metatarsal bones. The transverse stress fracture carries with it a grim prognosis because often the bone will break completely and, having broken, displacement may be considerable and disability severe. It is seen in particular in the tibia and also occurs in the fifth metatarsal bone. The compression stress fracture can occur at any age, but is usually seen in children and older people, but does occur in the first metatarsal bone in the young adult. The longitudinal variety is probably merely an extension along the length of a bone of an oblique stress fracture and is common as a variety of the march fracture.

Clinically, stress fractures can be considered in children (Fig. 47.5), adolescents, young adults and athletes, the middle aged and the elderly (Fig. 47.6).

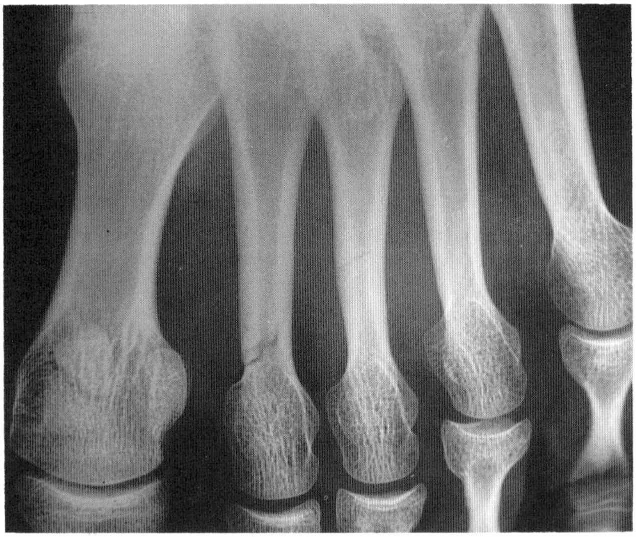

Fig. 47.1. The classical stress fracture in the second metatarsal bone in which the crack can be seen to be running proximally and laterally. The fracture has become complete, so that the fracture line can be seen easily, even though no callus has, as yet, formed

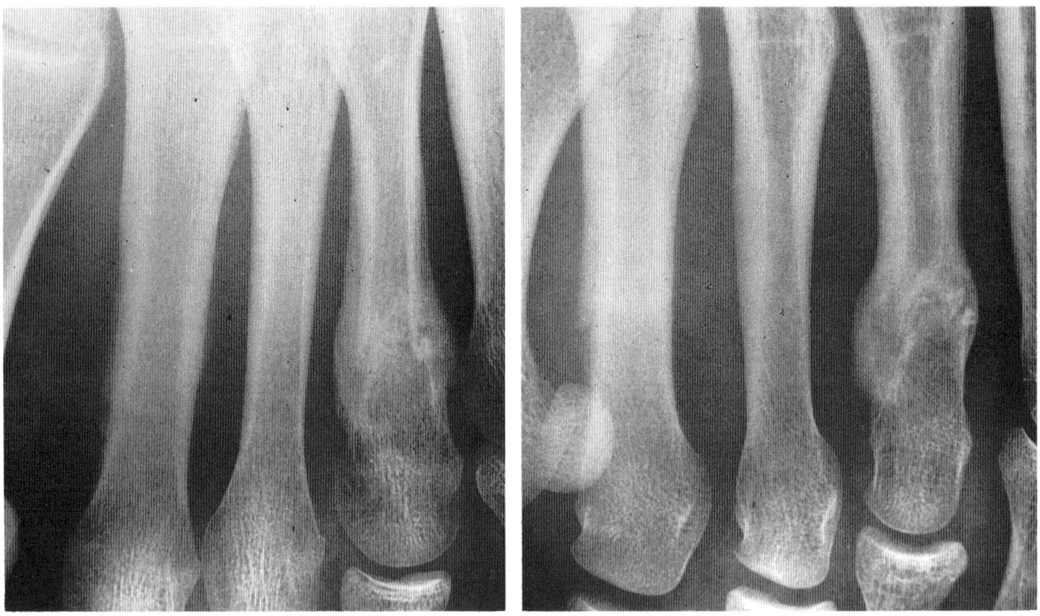

Fig. 47.2 Stress fractures can be multiple. This athlete of 23 had previously had a stress fracture of the lower left fibula. When he got back to training he developed pain in the left forefoot and he has a well established and healing march fracture of the fourth metatarsal bone. He also has a much earlier fracture in the second metatarsal bone, which can be seen best in the oblique view

Stress fractures in children develop very quickly and the whole episode is over within a few weeks, whereas for the adult it may take a few months for symptoms to subside completely. The adolescent can be most interesting in that the fracture may be of the child's variety, but it may also be adult in type and this does not seem to bear any relationship to the activity of the youth concerned, but is probably

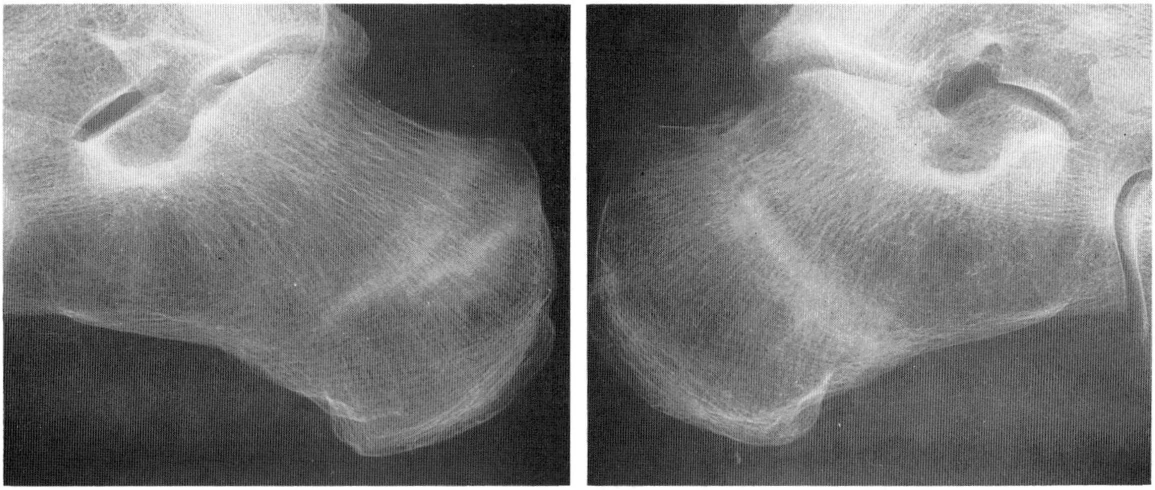

Fig. 47.3 Compression stress fractures of the calcaneus are often bilateral, but one develops faster than the other and rest occasioned by the pain allows the less developed side to start healing. This patient was 71 and had done a lot of extra walking. On the right side there is a double stress fracture following the line of the tuberosity, as does the fracture on the opposite side, which also shows a little external callus at the top of the fracture line

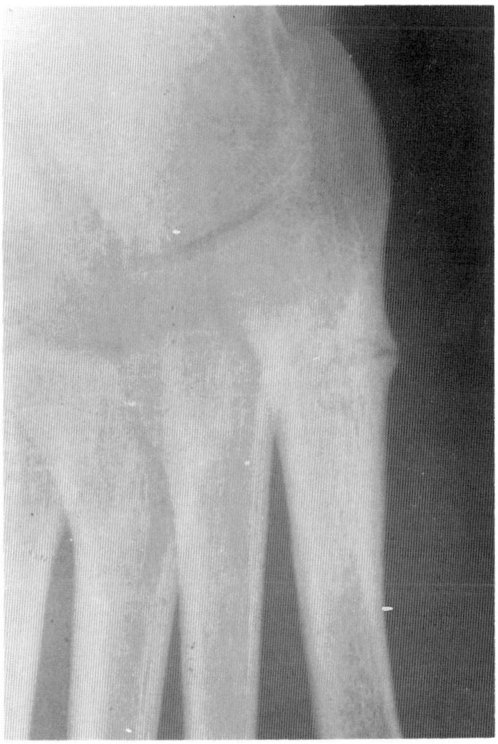

Fig. 47.4 A fencer aged 18 complained of pain in the left foot and a transverse stress fracture of the base of the fifth metatarsal was noted. That it has been present for some while is indicated by the heaping up of the bone on each side of the fracture line. Despite full and proper treatment, the fracture did not unite and a bone graft was necessary. The right fifth metatarsal also sustained a similar fracture, but healed uneventfully

inherent on the extent of development of the skeletal system. Thus, the upper tibia is a common site in children for a compression stress fracture, whereas the adolescent may have that type or the more common oblique stress fracture, seen in the adult. In children and adolescents stress on apophyses and other parts of bone often gives rise to 'osteochondritis', which is a reaction of cartilage and bone to stress, giving rise to Sever's and Kienbock's diseases.

The middle aged sustain any form of stress fracture and it is, of course, of the adult type, but often fairly slow in onset and equally slow to heal. Perhaps this is because the activity is less and is often associated with one or another particular episode of normal but unusual activity, such as an intensive shopping expedition or an extrastrenuous round of golf. In the old person the pattern tends more to that of the child, but with certain definite varieties such as the compression stress fracture of the lower end of the tibia. This gives rise to pain in the foot and ankle; a preliminary radiograph will show nothing (Fig. 47.7) and, not being repeated, the pain continues for many months as an undiagnosed chronic condition.

RADIOLOGY AND SCANNING

The radiology of stress fractures is very important, because if too much faith is placed in the early

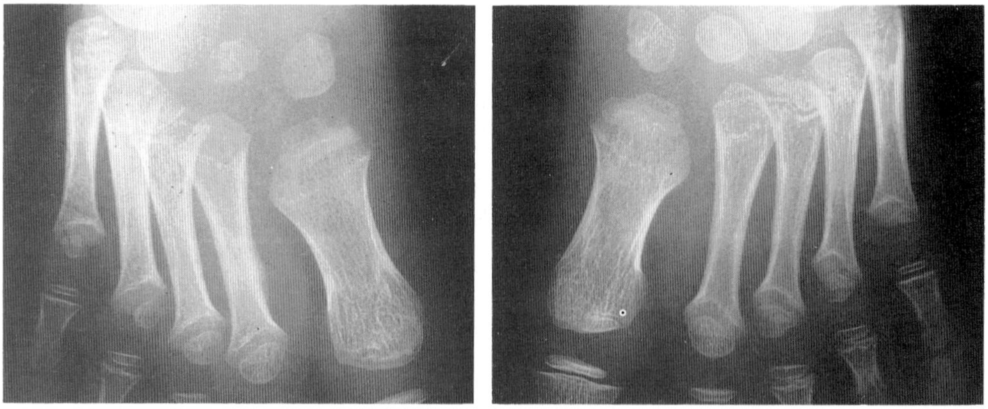

Fig. 47.5 Children do not escape march fractures and these radiographs show the right forefoot of a boy of 4 with the left forefoot for comparison. The callus on the medial side of the second metatarsal shaft is easily seen. Children recover quickly and he was symptom free in two weeks

radiographs the diagnosis may not be made. It must always be remembered that radiology lags far behind the clinical symptoms, thus pain in a forefoot may have been present for three weeks, but there may be no evidence of X-ray changes until five or six weeks.

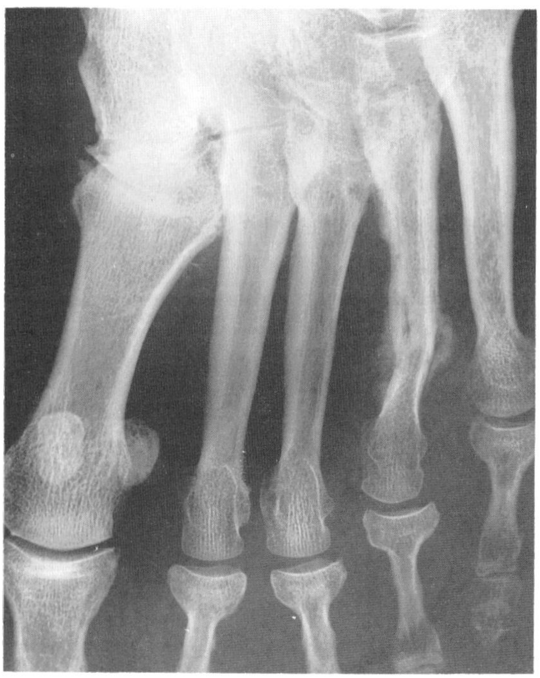

Fig. 47.6 A woman of 76 who was overweight, had a sudden pain followed by swelling on the outer aspect of the right foot one month before attending. The fourth metatarsal march fracture is already healing, but, although only one bone has been affected, there has been angulation

The stress fractures of the calcaneum are particularly difficult in this respect, at times taking three months to show. This also can apply to the stress fractures of the lower tibia, which again may take two or three months before radiographs confirm the lesion. Further, it is important to have very good technique, so that the fine bone detail is shown and to have the positioning accurate so that, if necessary, not only the normal two anteroposterior and lateral views are taken, but also the necessary obliques or tangential views.

Technetium 98 scanning is, however, a very much quicker method of diagnosing a bony lesion and, although a hot spot in a bone is not diagnostic of a stress fracture, if it is combined with the proper history, then this may be taken as confirmatory evidence. Most stress fractures will show on a technetium scan, properly and carefully done, at the same time as the clinical symptoms occur. The use of the scan is not normally necessary if a clinical diagnosis can be made, but there are occasions when the delay of normal radiography as confirmatory evidence has to be bypassed, or in the case of an early lesion in an athlete to whom an immediate and firm diagnosis is essential.

When scanning is not available the patient must be treated on clinical grounds and especially important is the enforcement of rest. The radiographic changes vary with age, not only in the type of stress fracture that may occur, but also with the speed of confirmation; a stress fracture of the fibula in a child will develop so rapidly that within a week

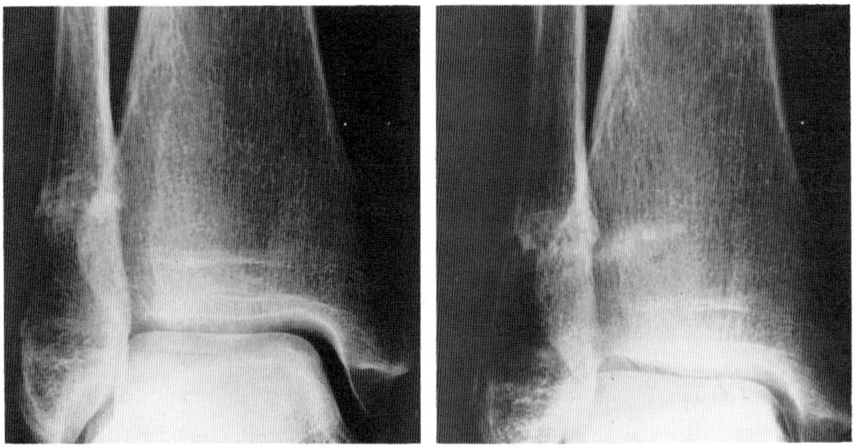

Fig. 47.7 Compression stress fractures can affect both bones of the lower leg just above the ankle. This woman of 62 had pain for six weeks in the right ankle which was thought to be due to a simple stress fracture, but six weeks later the tibia shows a compression stress fracture which emphasizes how long it may take for these fractures to show

radiographic changes will be confirmatory. This is also useful should there be any doubt about the differential diagnosis in a child because within a few days the early changes will have developed into the full picture of a stress fracture.

AETIOLOGY

The cause of a stress fracture is bending of the bone concerned and, whereas long bones will bend in all directions, it must be remembered that bones also will compress and this is what happens to the cubical bones of the foot, such as the calcaneum, which suffers from compression stress fractures in particular.

With bending of a bone it might be considered that eventually the bone would break if the bending strains were continued long enough, like breaking a piece of wire, but the actual cause of the stress fracture is probably molecular change. Any force that is absorbed by the bone, such as a bending or a compression strain, produces a denaturing of the hydroxyapatite crystals which are present in bone to give the otherwise elastic collagen ground substance rigidity. However, this rigidity still maintains a modulus of elasticity and so, with each periodic muscular activity of the part, the bones will bend to a greater or lesser extent. It is not the hitting of the heel on the ground that causes the bone to bend (Figs 47.8 to 10), — it is the muscular activity that goes with it; thus when a runner lands on his forefoot the muscles contract at the moment of impact to maintain plantar flexion, for otherwise the foot would collapse. It is this pull of the muscles on their origins and insertions which will cause the bone to bend and the stress fracture to occur. For example, if we look at the usual type of stress fracture that is seen in the calcaneum, we find that the fracture line is curved, following the line of the surface of the tuberosity at the posteroinferior aspect of the calcaneum. The pull of the calf muscles when they contract puts a stress on the bone at the insertion of the Achilles tendon, which is resisted by the pull of the long plantar ligament. These will give a resultant force going upwards and forwards, or antero-superiorly, thus causing the compression stress fracture in that shape.

If a forefoot is severely and violently dorsiflexed against the resistance of the calf muscles, a similar shaped fracture will occur. If, however, the compression is a result of jumping from a height and landing on the heels, the line of the fracture is transverse, parallel with the ground (see Figs. 47.8 to 10). Thus compression stress fractures are caused by muscular pull and not by rhythmic banging of the heel or foot on the ground.

The strength of bone obviously indicates the amount of stress it can absorb before the hydroxyapatite crystals are so denatured and the microscopic area becomes so weak that with further activity a physical crack occurs through the bone. At

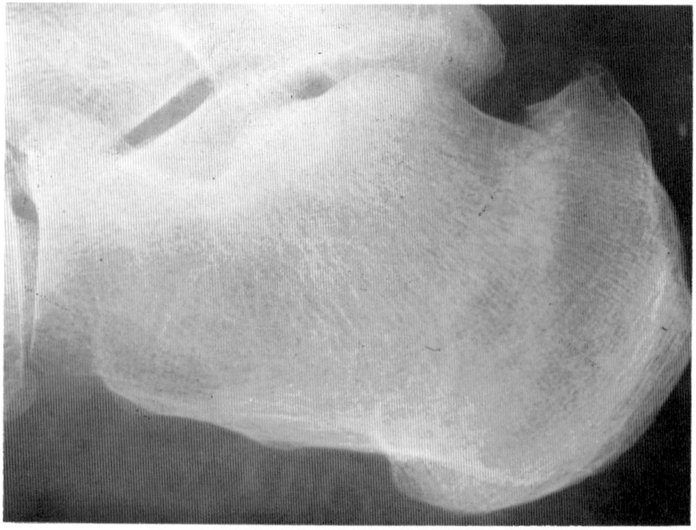

Fig. 47.8 A man was kick-starting a motor when it backfired and forcibly extended the ankle against the pull of the calf muscles. The resulting muscle violence fracture follows the pattern of a compression stress fracture

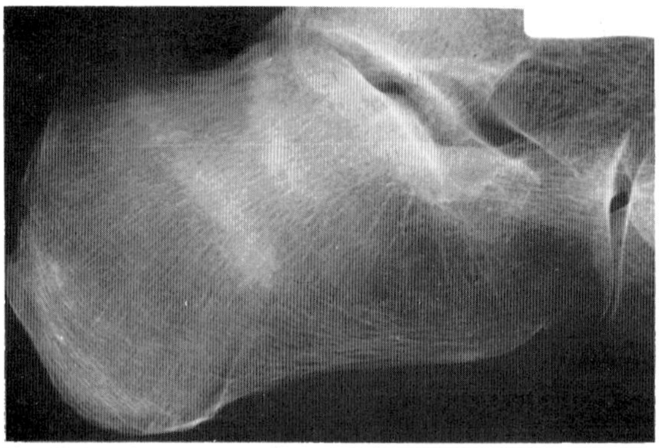

Fig. 47.9 A double stress fracture of the calcaneus in a woman of 80. Compare the line of the fracture with that shown in Fig. 8 and note that the compression and internal callus occurs at right angles to the trabeculae in the tuberosity of the bone

first this crack will be microscopic, but as soon as it occurs and has entered an osteon system a physical inflammatory reaction will start. Once this happens more blood vessels will develop into the part, which will show at first microscopically as an inflammatory process, but which will rapidly increase especially on the surface where the periosteum will have been at least disrupted and at the worst torn. After a short while there will be a palpable swelling if the bone is subcutaneous, such as the lateral malleolus (Figs. 47.11 and 12).

If a bone is immobilized it becomes osteoporotic and the longer the immobilization the worse the

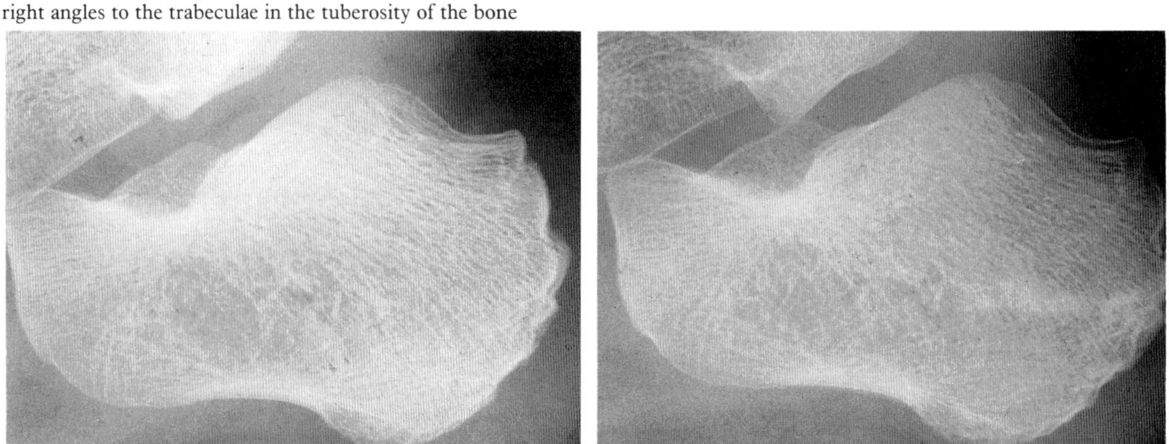

Fig. 47.10 A boy fell off a roof and landed on his heels. The initial X-ray showed no abnormality, but three weeks later a line of internal callus indicates where a compression stress fracture occurred. This is at right angles to the impact force created by landing on the heels and is quite different in direction from that of a stress fracture

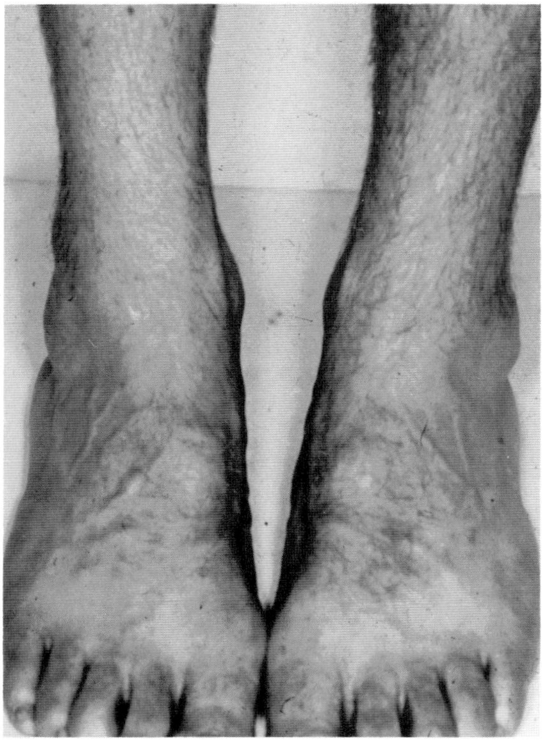

Fig. 47.11 It is very rare to be able to discern swelling on visual examination, but occasionally subcutaneous bones do show it, such as that of the lower right fibula of an athlete, shown above. His radiograph can be seen in Fig. 47.12

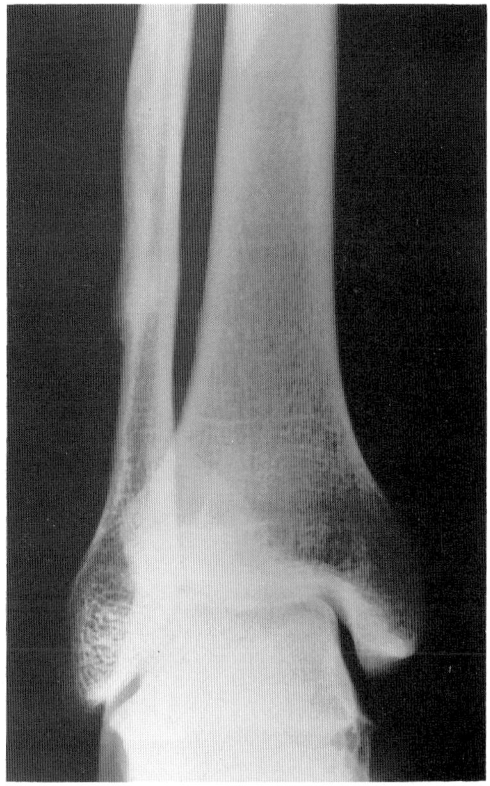

Fig. 47.12 A moderately well advanced stress fracture of the lowermost part of the right fibula. The soft tissue swelling can be felt long before the callus is seen radiologically

osteoporosis. This is because there is a fundamental distaste in nature of keeping any bone stronger than it needs to be. As soon as muscular activity is limited the normal stresses on the bone disappear and calcium is removed, decreasing the strength of the osteons. This process is particularly important when treating athletes because, after immobilization, training may be overdone to an extent which will allow a stress fracture to occur.

It is this fundamental problem of bone strength that first gave rise to the march fracture, because it occurred in recruits. Often ill-fed and poorly developed before they were enrolled into the Armed Forces, muscular strength and weight increased rapidly under their new conditions, but the intensive training produced fractures because muscle strength can be increased far more rapidly than can the strength of bone. Therefore, the overtraining of recruits or athletes in a similar way may contribute considerably to stress fractures, particularly in the lower leg and particularly again in the foot.

Once it has occurred the stress fracture may so weaken the bone that, with further use, the break becomes complete. Sometimes a patient will complain of a mild, dull ache in the foot which quite suddenly gets worse; this is when the fracture has become complete. In others, the early symptoms may be ignored or so slight as not to be noticed until again a sudden and severe pain occurs. This is the mechanism by which a 'sudden' onset is produced.

It is to be expected that stress fractures should be bilateral and they often are. However, it is unlikely that in every person the fractures would develop at exactly the same rate, because as soon as symptoms on the worst side occur, activity lessens and the less advanced stress fracture can start to heal. Nevertheless, the opposite limb must always be carefully examined. In the foot two or more march fractures are often found, sometimes with the fracture in one bone far further advanced than the other (Fig. 47.13).

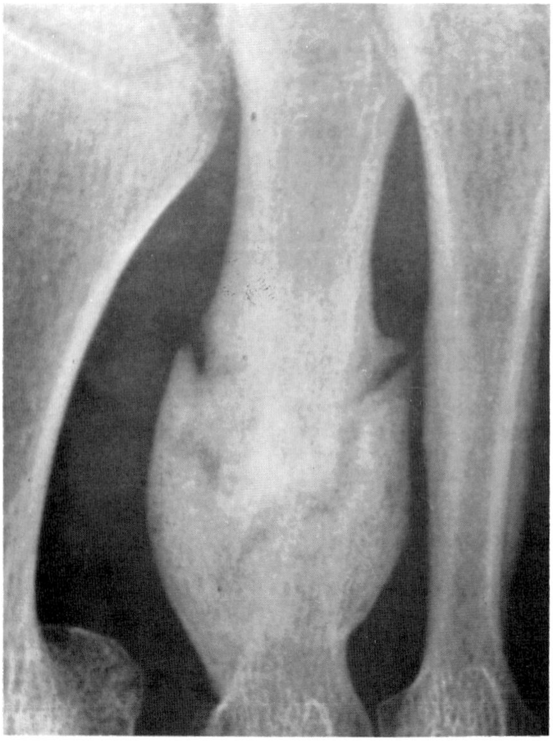

Fig. 47.13 A 52-year-old woman developed pain in her left foot, which had been present for eight months. The radiograph shows nonunion of the second metatarsal bone and a more recent stress fracture of the third metatarsal bone. The callus in the latter fracture can be seen extending all the way up the shaft, so it was probably a longitudinal crack

Stress fractures may also occur in sequence, perhaps with a year or more between them and the runner may have a stress fracture of the lateral malleolus, only to be followed by another in a metatarsal bone.

TREATMENT

In general, rest from the activity causing the pain is sufficient. In the foot, this can often be aided by elastic adhesive strapping, foam inserts or insoles. Usually about three weeks is sufficient to allow healing to start, but restriction on activity must not be lifted for another three weeks and even then with caution. Any resumption of the pain from the stress fracture indicates the need for further rest.

In particular, athletes and other energetic people must get back to training or activity with great care for an overstrenuous training session may not only restart symptoms in the original lesion, but may initiate a new stress fracture in the part already a little weaker (from disuse secondary to the rest) than it was before any symptoms were seen.

PREVENTION

The foot, until a few hundred years ago, was developed for walking or running on earth; it was not designed to walk with hard leather soles, on hard concrete pavements. Therefore, it is wise to ensure that shoes, especially for sport, have thick, soft soles to absorb some of the foot impact and thereby lessen the muscle pull necessary to hold the foot correctly, whether at footfall or take off.

The importance of training cannot be emphasized too much, particularly in the service recruit and the athlete, whether amateur or professional. It has been mentioned that the musculature in the service recruit will develop faster than the strength of bone, so initially, heavy and violent exercises should give way to general toughening up of muscles, with exercise such as swimming.

The athlete who has been out of sport for any length of time is at risk if training is not progressive afterwards and especially at risk is the leg that has been encased in plaster.

STRESS FRACTURES OF THE CALCANEUM

Stress fractures of the calcaneum occur at any age in adults, but are perhaps most common in late middle age. They also occur in children in the form of an apophysitis, or Sever's disease. This stress fracture often accounts for the painful heel which is slow to be diagnosed because of the vagueness of the symptoms and particularly because radiological confirmation is always lacking in the initial stages.

Symptoms and signs

The patient may indicate that there has been an increase in activity, an alteration in footwear, a different habit in walking or some similar alteration in the pattern of life. Sometimes symptoms start abruptly and the patient may complain that the foot, or particularly the heel, has become swollen. Figures 47.14 and 15 show the radiographs of such a patient and the development of the internal callus can be seen. The tangential views also show the callus and may be very helpful in diagnosis.

Examination occasionally reveals some swelling of the hindfoot, but it always shows considerable tenderness in and around the heel, especially on the plantar surface and this, because it is localized at the centre of the heel, may give rise to the mistaken diagnosis of a plantar fasciitis; however the greatest tenderness will be found on each side of the calcaneal tuberosity; otherwise movements of the foot and ankle are found to be free and full, but the patient may not be able to stand on the bare heel and certainly not able to stamp on the ground. Examination must be painstaking to exclude all other local lesions including stress fractures at the lower end of the tibia or fibula and to make sure that there is no lesion of the calcaneal tendon or its bursa or plantar fasciitis.

Other conditions which can mimic the symptoms

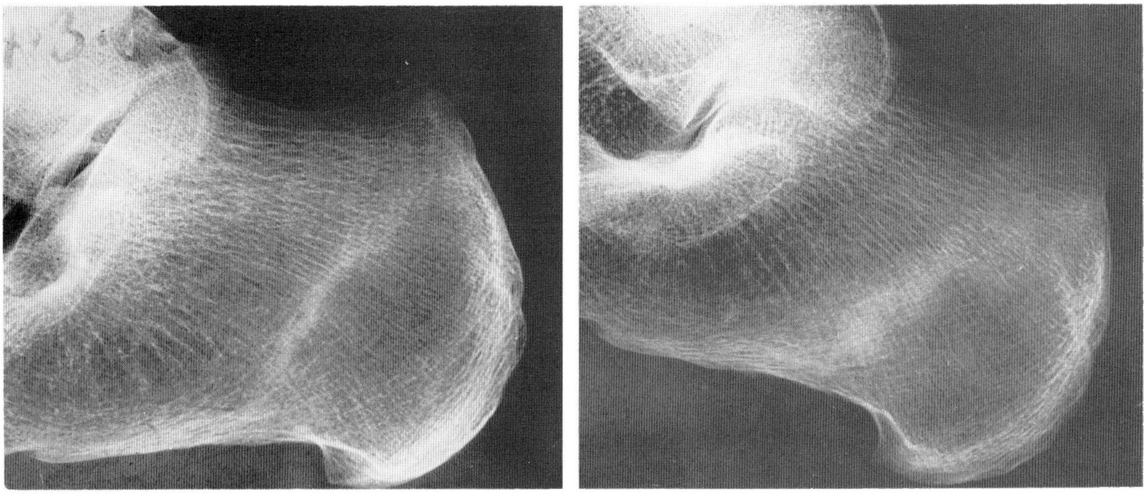

Fig. 47.14

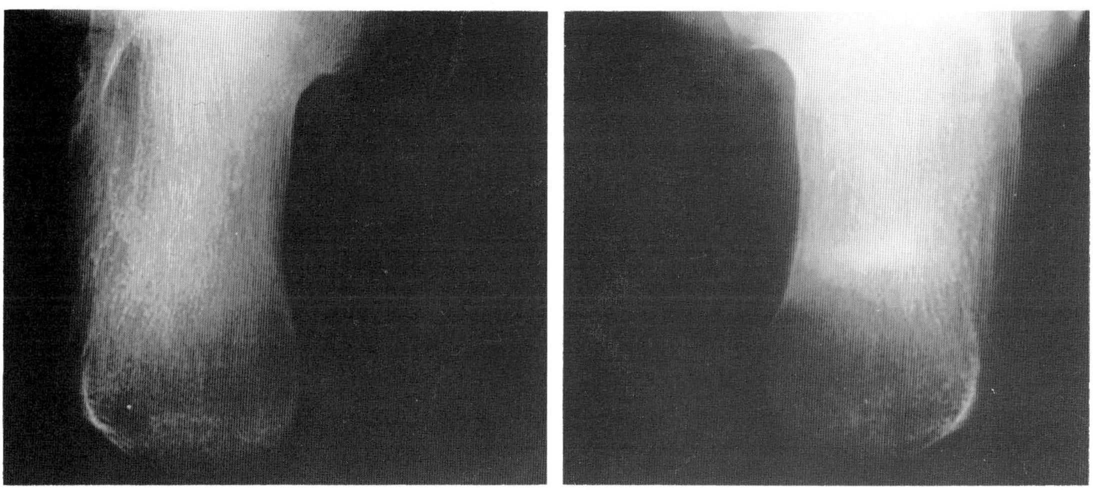

Fig. 47.15

Figs. 47.14 and 15 A stress fracture of the calcaneus when it starts may well be missed, because the radiograph need only show a very faint haze of internal callus. This patient—a woman of 47—had been for a long walk and had developed pain in the ankle with swelling. She was first examined three weeks later, when the faint haze of internal callus could be seen. This developed and was seen more clearly two weeks later. Fig. 15 shows the tangential views of both calcanei, which can be very valuable in the radiological diagnosis of this stress fracture are the medial or lateral nerve compression syndrome and tenosynovitis. It must be realised that the symptoms of a stress fracture can be very long, chronic and drawn out and sometimes not cause great disability. The patient will cut down activities only to an acceptable level of discomfort, which both prevents healing and maintains the fracture, hence the length of history that is often found.

Radiology

The confirmation of a stress fracture of the calcaneum may be very long delayed and this must always be borne in mind. Clear bone detail must be obtained in the lateral and tangential radiographs to ensure that the earliest disruption of the trabeculae and the earliest haze of internal callus are easily seen. In older patients, who are often osteoporotic, compression may actually show in the bone, as in Figure 47.3; this woman of 71 had done a lot of extra walking and had developed pain in both heels over several months.

Sometimes the fracture appears to be double with two lines of callus visible which may not be always concomitant in time (Fig. 47.16). It makes no difference to the diagnosis or to the outlook, as both heal well in due course. If one heel is to be radiographed the other heel should always be done also, because subclinical stress fractures often exist in the opposite limb.

Differential diagnosis

A stress fracture in the calcaneum may be difficult to confirm, but should not be misdiagnosed provided the condition is remembered when the patient is first seen, so that the radiographs may be repeated in due course, thus confirming the diagnosis. The history may not always give a period of increased or different activity. Swelling of the hindfoot is important, but not usual by the time the patient seeks advice. However, if the patient is asked to stand on tip toe and to move in this position, pain is almost always reproduced in the heel because it is this action that has produced the stress fracture. Next in importance is the palpation of the tuberosity of the calcaneum and if this is done with care and gentleness the tenderness will be found to follow the line of the stress fracture down both sides of the bone as well as underneath on the plantar surface. If the plantar surface only is examined and pressed heavily the patient may be rather resistant to further examination because of the intense pain that can be produced and further (and perhaps lesser) tenderness may then be missed.

The differentiation between an acute plantar fasciitis and a compression stress fracture of the calcaneum may be difficult, but it is of tremendous

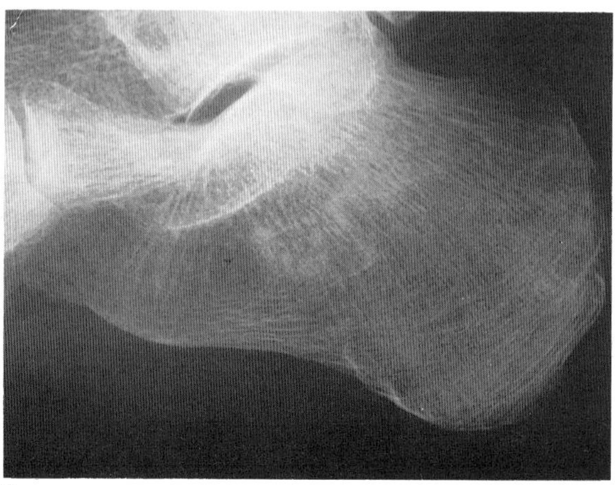

a

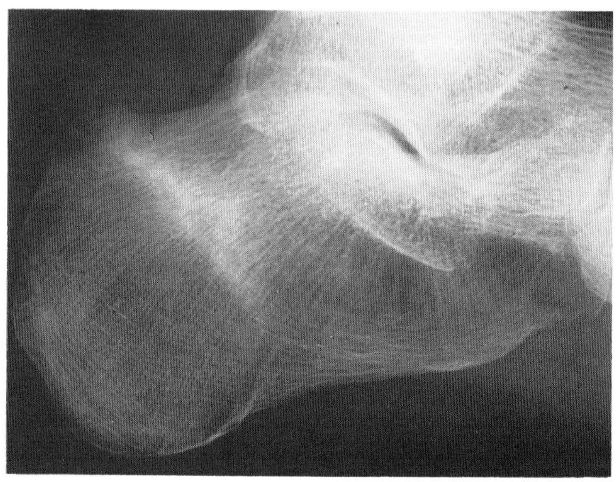

b

Fig. 47.16 A woman of 67 had three weeks pain in her left heel (b), but she had developed a similar but less severe pain in the right heel (a) five weeks before this. The left heel presumably took the weight when the right heel began to hurt and developed more quickly. Both stress fractures are clearly seen. The patient was a diabetic, but otherwise healthy importance because the local injection of an insoluble steroid will have no effect on the stress fracture, but, of course, may be curative for the plantar fasciitis. If there is still difficulty in the early stages, it is better to treat conservatively, because this will soon differentiate the two and will allow time for radiological (or scanning) confirmation. The tenderness of plantar fasciitis is very localized, whereas the tenderness of the stress fracture is much more general and goes round the sides of the bone.

The general conditions that may mimic the stress fracture of the calcaneum are gout, rheumatoid arthritis and even early symptoms of a prolapsed intervertebral disc affecting the first sacral nerve root can produce pain in the heel. In the differential diagnosis of the radiographs there is one condition which may confuse and that is calcification in the posterior tibial artery as it passes down the posteromedial side of the ankle, because if calcified the shadow may resemble that of a stress fracture. However, the tangential view will show no abnormality within the bone.

Treatment

The heel should be raised and padded: this both absorbs the impact of the footfall (which is resisted by muscular contraction causing the stress fracture) and relaxes the calf muscles and the long plantar ligament. Wearing such a pad within a shoe with a soft, rather than a leather, heel and a similar sole will give the patient immediate comfort, if not total relief. However, the treatment must be continued for several weeks and the patient must be warned that if the pad is removed too soon the symptoms will recur. In the older patient at least two or three months are needed.

STRESS FRACTURES OF THE CALCANEUM IN CHILDREN

The stress fracture that occurs in the apophysis of the tuberosity of the calcaneum is known as Sever's disease and characteristically it is described as an 'osteochondritis' or an 'apophysitis'. It is, in fact, identical in aetiology to Osgood–Schlatter's disease and other so-called osteochondritides and is the reaction of the apophysis to stress. Instead of getting the compression stress fracture within the bone the apophysis, which is buffered between itself and the calcaneum by its cartilaginous growth plate, becomes both compressed and distracted by the excess stress that has been imposed upon it. The pain of which the child complains is characteristic of a stress fracture. It comes on in the evening or after a bout of exercise, but rarely does it completely stop the child playing or give rise to a very severe complaint of pain. Examination will show that the tenderness is more at the back of the heel than underneath. Treatment is reassurance of the parents, the forbidding of those activities that cause pain, a soft pad under the heel in shoes that have soft heels themselves and with this the symptoms should subside within two or three weeks.

The radiographs show fragmentation in one or other plane of the apophysis, but occasionally an actual fracture line can be seen through the apophysis (Figs. 47.17–20).

STRESS FRACTURES OF THE NAVICULAR BONE

These are very rare, but when they occur are very distinctive. So far they have been seen in early middle age in active people playing golf. The cause of a stress fracture of the navicular bone is the resistance to the pull of the muscles by the bone when the forefoot is flexed or when weight is taken on the ball of the foot. The form the fracture takes in the adult is that of a transverse type of stress fracture. However, owing to the shape of the bone, the line of the fracture is, in fact, not transverse but longitudinal down the bone (Figs. 47.21–22) and is in the line of the first metatarsal bone. In children the condition known as Kohler's disease is occasioned by the same causes and may be a compression stress fracture leading to avascularity (Fig. 47.23). Ultimately the bone will regenerate if the foot is treated correctly.

Symptoms and signs

Pain in the middle of the foot, which is worse after exercise and towards the end of the day is the usual history and if there is a special activity this may gradually have to stop earlier than would otherwise

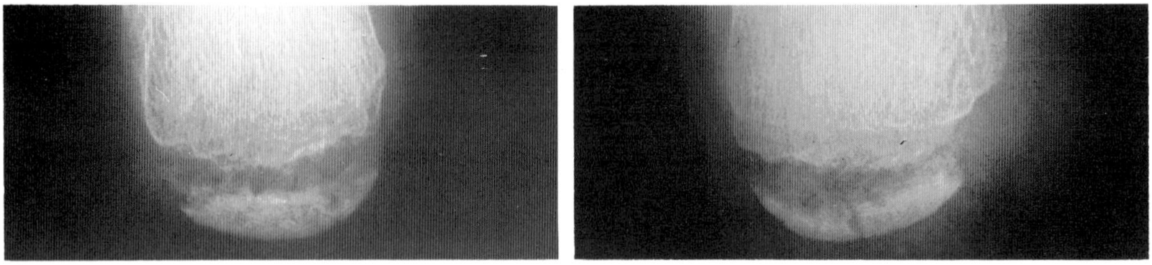

Fig. 47.17

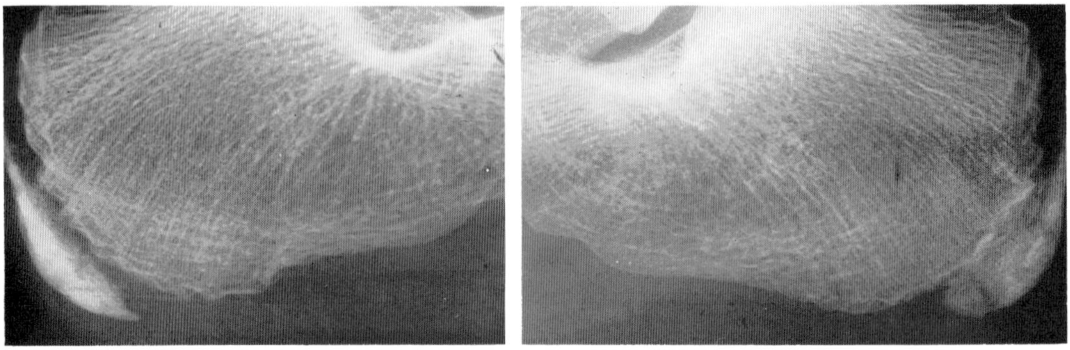

Fig. 47.18

Fig. 47.19

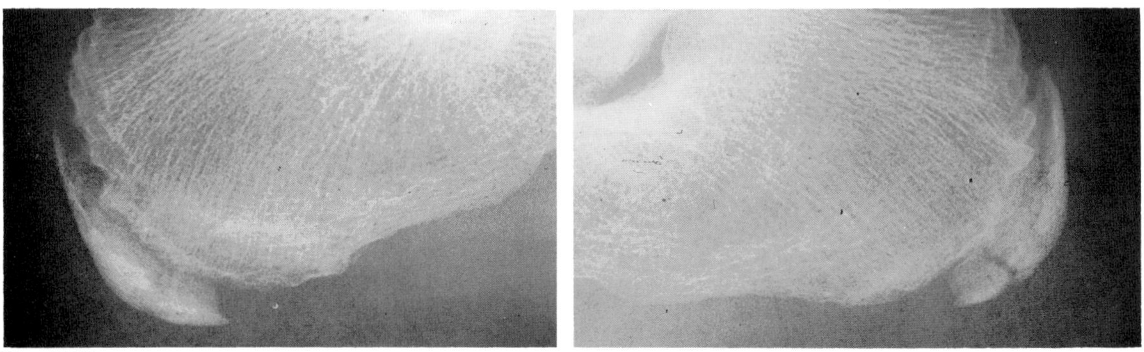

Fig. 47.20

Figs. 47.17–20 This series of X-rays shows the progress of so-called Sever's disease of the apophysis of the calcaneus, which is a stress fracture of the apophysis. In Figure 17 the right apophysis has a fracture line in it, but the left is going dense. Two weeks later, in the lateral view (Fig. 18), the left apophysis is very dense and two fractures can be seen in the right apophysis. Figure 19 shows the tangential views at this time. Figure 20 shows healing three months later.

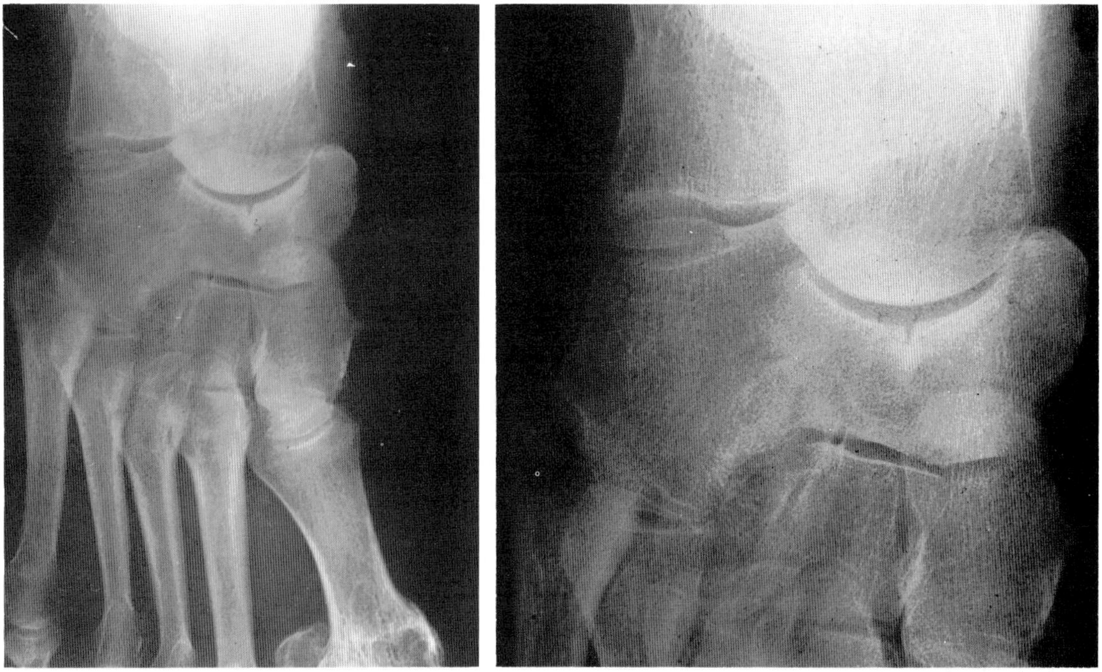

a b

Fig. 47.21 The forefoot of a woman who played a lot of golf at the age of 60, shows a transverse type of stress fracture in the navicular. The crack can be seen clearly in (a) with internal callus lying around and distal to it. This fracture took a long time to become symptom free, but rest with support was all that was needed

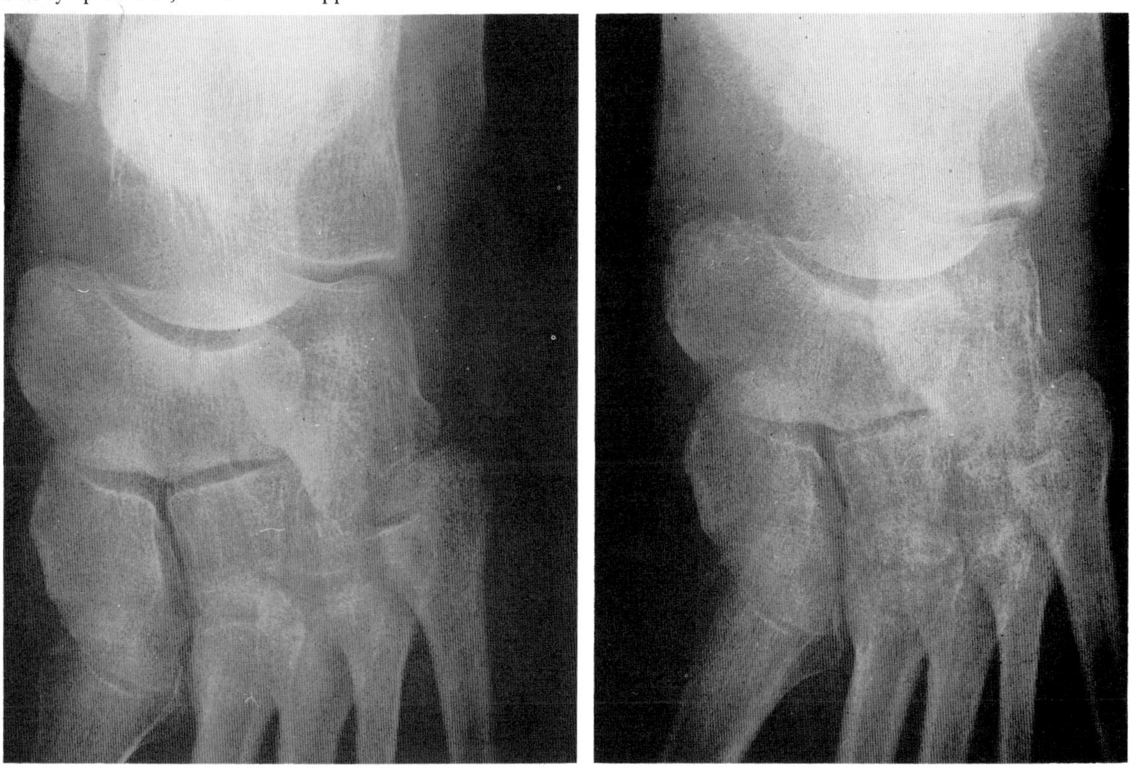

a b

Fig. 47.22 A 66-year-old woman who also played golf, developed pain in her foot. She had a similar stress fracture of the navicular bone (a) which healed rather more rapidly, as shown in b taken five weeks later

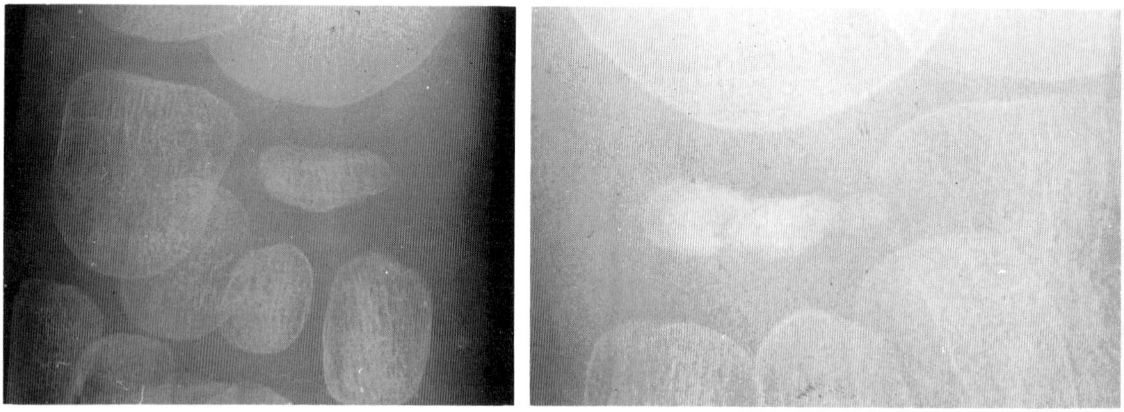

Fig. 47.23 Köhler's disease of the left navicular bone in a boy of 6. This condition is a stress fracture causing avascular necrosis of the navicular bone. The fracture line runs in the same direction as those in the adult patients in Figures 21 and 22

be the case, as occurred to a woman aged 60 (Fig. 47.21.) She was a keen golfer and found that pain was preventing her continuing to play; after several weeks she attended for advice. Examination showed her to be normal within the limits of her age but she was extremely tender over the navicular and there was pain on standing on the ball of the foot and on tip toe.

The history of pain in the foot is so common in middle age that the connection between a stress fracture and rather vague histories will be missed unless emphasis has always been placed on asking the relationship of pain to activity. This particular patient exemplified it well by having her pain come on earlier each day when she played golf, so that she could manage less and less of her round.

Differential diagnosis

The differential diagnosis is of all the usual conditions causing pain on the medial side of the foot and which must be eliminated. Careful and gentle palpation of the medial arch will show that the maximum tenderness is in the navicular bone. A stress fracture of the base of the first metatarsal will, of course, have to be considered, although this is seen at an earlier age.

Radiology

The fracture appears to run caudally through the centre of the navicular bone, almost as though the talus was trying to force its way through. The fracture line develops slowly and stops developing as soon as rest occurs and some internal callus can be seen around the crack (see Figs. 47.21 and 22). The initial lesion is difficult to see early and must be looked for with great care in good radiographs.

Treatment

It may be difficult to relieve the patient of pain whilst partaking of normal activity, in which case a below-knee walking plaster may be applied for three or four weeks to start the healing process. Thereafter firm support with elastic adhesive bandages is sufficient and a stiff sorbo valgus support in soft soled shoes will complete the cure.

AVASCULAR NECROSIS OF THE NAVICULAR BONE IN CHILDREN

If a child attends with pain in the foot and limping and the tenderness is looked for very carefully without frightening the child, it can be localized to the navicular bone. Usually by the time the child attends fragmentation has occurred radiologically (see Fig. 47.23). The opposite foot must also be examined carefully, for the condition is often bilateral, but the limp will be on that side which has developed the most. Provided the child is kept at rest so that pain does not occur and proper support given to the foot until radiological healing is apparent (Fig. 47.23), the bone will develop apparently normally and hopefully give rise to no further problems in adult life.

OTHER TARSAL BONES

Stress fractures have not been seen in the other tarsal bones, but rare though they may be it is possible they could occur and this diagnosis should always be considered in a lesion that causes pain in the typical manner, but which cannot be otherwise explained.

MARCH FRACTURE

This is the commonest stress fracture of all and those that occur in the second or third metatarsal shafts are the most frequent. It is not nowadays possible to give accurate statistics on the number of march fractures that occur except in closed communities such as an Armed Forces Camp, because the condition is so well known that many patients are treated for the condition without ever being referred to hospital or an orthopaedic surgeon. The symptoms of pain and aching in the forefoot are soon relieved by rest and support to the foot, usually in the form of elastic adhesive strapping. Many patients will give a history of having had a march fracture or apparently such a condition which responded to simple restriction of activity and avoidance of those particular conditions which caused pain without ever attending for treatment. Nevertheless, there are certain march fractures which can cause extreme trouble and even severe disability.

After the single march fracture, multiple forms are the most common. Sometimes the outer three metatarsal bones will sustain stress fractures either together or in sequence (Figs. 47.24 and 25). Bilateral march fractures occur, but are rare because (even if both feet sustain a march fracture at the same time) the slight limitation of activity, with the more advanced side giving rise to symptoms first, allows the opposite lesion to heal before it becomes apparent clinically or radiologically. However, multiple march fractures involve the third metatarsal bone more often than not, followed closely by the fourth metatarsal bone.

The site of the stress fracture in the metatarsal bone may be at the base, the shaft or the neck and in children the actual metatarsal head may be involved, giving rise to avascular necrosis and the so-called Frieberg's infraction (see Fig. 47.25). Usually, however, there is an oblique stress fracture in the metatarsal neck and this may start either medially or

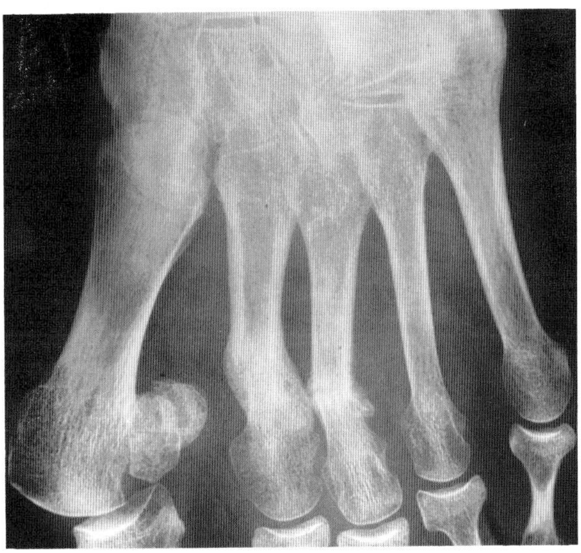

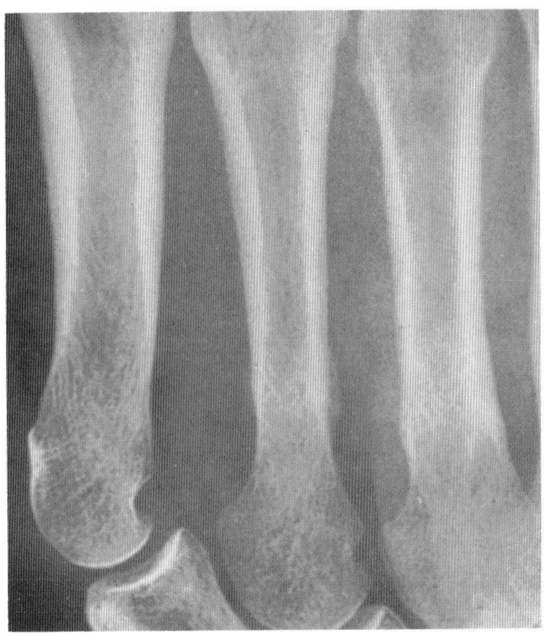

Fig. 47.24 This patient developed two metatarsal stress fractures, which healed with some deformity. One year later the opposite foot developed a stress fracture of the fourth metatarsal bone

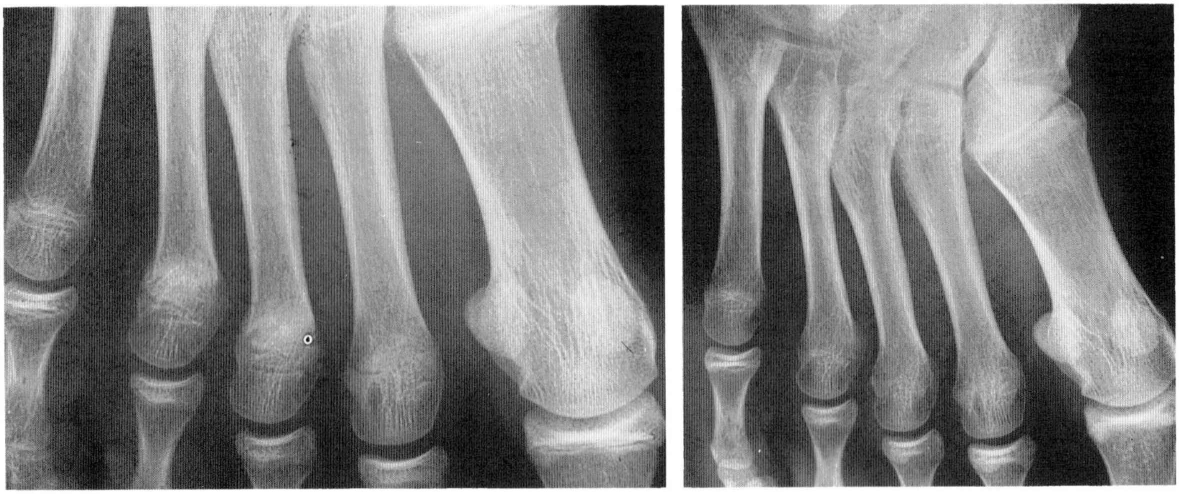

a b

Fig. 47.25 A youth aged 14 developed two stress fractures far distally in the third and fourth metatarsal necks (a), but they healed with no further problem, as shown in the adjacent radiograph taken one year later (b). This sort of stress fracture, if a little more distal, may cause Freiberg's infraction

laterally (Fig. 47.26). No reason for the laterality has been found. In children the fracture tends to be more longitudinal in type, as shown by the length of callus up and down the bone, although this can also occur in adults (Fig. 47.27).

Unless the X-ray beam passes directly through the

Fig. 47.26

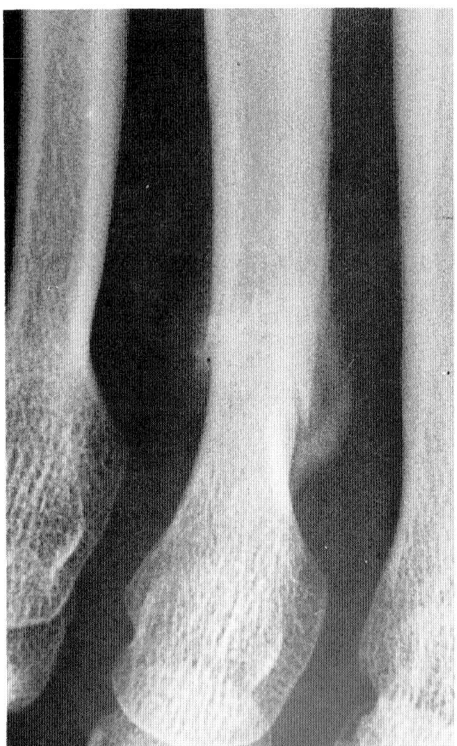

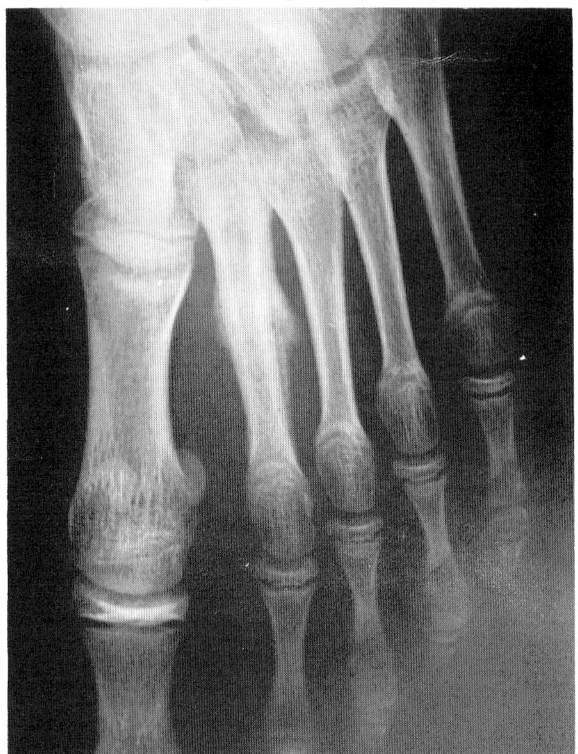

Fi

Figs. 47.26 and 27 The classical march fracture is shown in good detail in Figure 26, which illustrates that initially the crack was on the medial side and that it goes proximally and laterally. Callus is developing well on the medial side and healing is well advanced. Figure 27, of a 12-year-old boy, shows that the younger the patient the longer the callus appears to be plane of the fracture it is not easily seen and only the callus that occurs on the outside of the bone indicates that the lesion exists. This particular type of stress fracture occurs in the tibia and may cause aching in one or both feet (if it is bilateral) (see Fig. 47.40).

It has been said that march fractures occur more commonly after operations, particularly those for hallux valgus, but this is not accepted and there seems to be no reason why a foot which has undergone some reconstructive or other procedure should develop stress fractures any more readily than a normal foot provided the patient does not take too much excessive exercise too quickly after prolonged immobilization.

The march fracture is most common in the middle aged adult, but, of course, was first diagnosed in and is common in the Service recruit and the athlete, for which the explanation has been given above. The march fracture has also had many names applied to it, but it is considered that repetition of these names would only contribute to their unnecessary perpetuation. Even when standing apparently at rest, there is considerable tone so that if under these conditions slight symptoms are present, active treatment is indicated.

Stress fractures of the first and fifth metatarsal bones are often different in pattern, the first showing the compression stress fracture and the fifth the transverse, which has a poor prognosis.

STRESS FRACTURES OF THE SECOND, THIRD AND FOURTH METATARSAL BONES

The march fracture is well known and is extremely common at all ages. There appears to be no definite cause other than activity (see Fig. 47.26). There are many different varieties of stress fractures in the metatarsal bones, either when affected singly or together. The second and third metatarsal bones are probably affected equally, with far fewer fractures being seen in the fourth.

Symptoms and signs

An ache or pain in the forefoot is the usual presenting feature, which may have been related to some special activity (classically a 'march') such as a day's outing, an extra long walk or a rather tiring game of golf. The pain gradually increases in intensity each day, but it is possible for the patient to continue walking, sometimes limping, sometimes flat-footed (taking all the weight on the heel) and sometimes hobbling on the inner or outer border of the foot. Running will be most painful.

In a few patients the pain comes on abruptly, sometimes as a severe exacerbation of a trivial ache (Fig. 47.28). This indicates that the initial crack has become complete.

The child may complain that there is aching which produces a limp. The child whose radiographs are shown in Figure 47.5 was only aged 4, but he complained that his foot hurt on a long walk although not on a short one. The radiograph shows very clearly the stress fracture of the second metatarsal bone of the right foot; it was already healing at two weeks when the child first presented. The older child takes longer to heal, but as is shown in Figure 47.27 healing is occurring at three weeks in a boy aged 12 years who had 'strained' his foot.

Inspection of the foot will show that swelling of the forefoot may or may not be present, but it is rare to find swelling only over the affected bone. In the old person the whole foot may swell.

Palpation will reveal tenderness localized in the metatarsal shaft. It is difficult to be sure which shaft is tender so gentle palpation is essential. Pressure under the forefoot may cause pain and manipulating the bone by holding its head gives rise to pain. Standing on tiptoe is painful. Swelling at the fracture site may not be felt even at the start. Figure 47.29 is the radiograph of the foot of a 20-year-old girl who had had symptoms for 10 days. The distal part of the second metatarsal shaft has a stress fracture, slightly comminuted and displaced, but no swelling could be felt clinically.

Radiology

The radiological confirmation may be late, and the appearances do not bear much relationship to the signs and symptoms (see Fig. 47.28). Sometimes the stress fracture will have a long fracture line running the length of the shaft (Fig. 47.30), or it may show a haze of bone only (Fig. 47.31).

Despite the differences in the radiological findings, it is not possible to correlate these findings

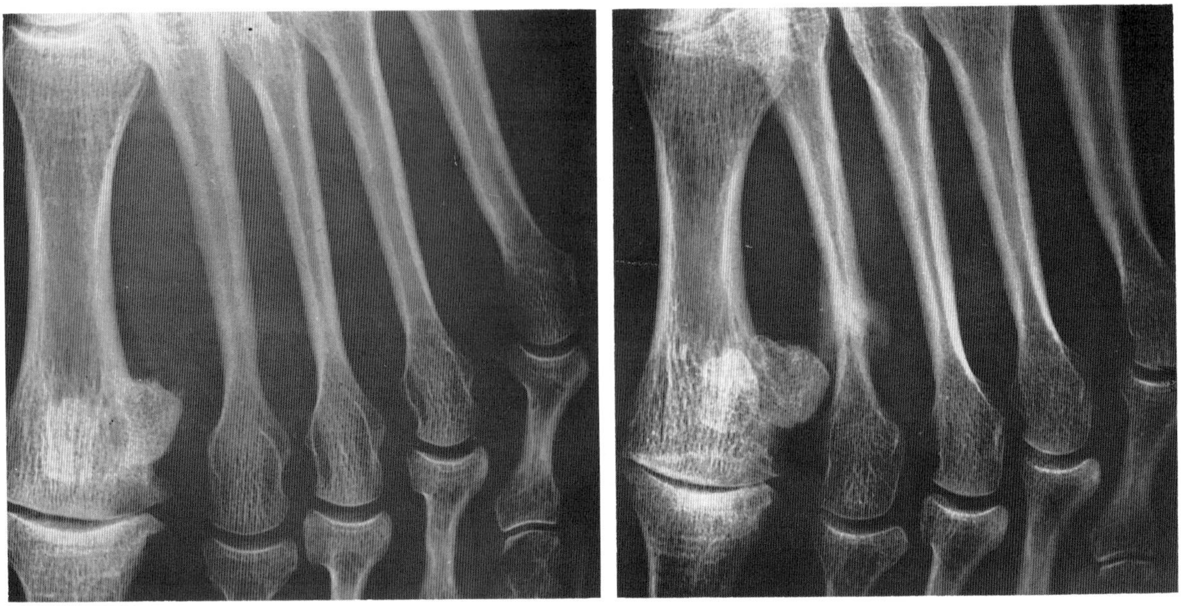

Fig. 47.28 A patient of 57 had a normal foot one morning, but pain that evening. She had recently put on weight. She also had osteoarthritis of the first metatarsophalangeal joint. A few days later the fracture can just be discerned in the lateral cortex of the second metatarsal shaft, but five weeks later it is not only obvious but beginning to heal

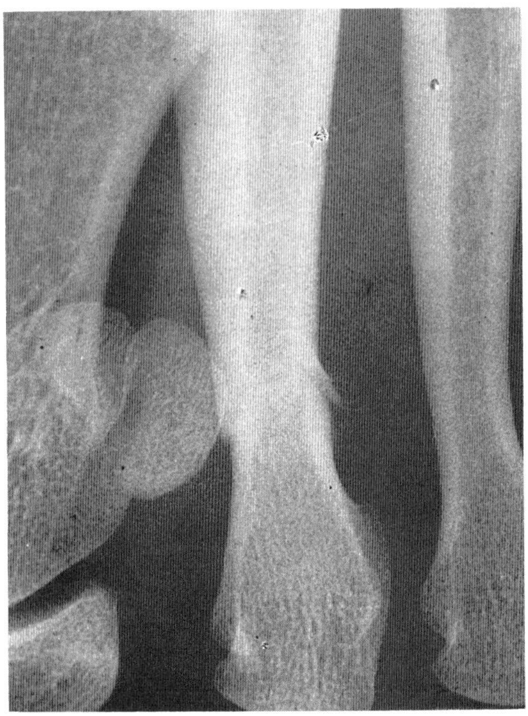

Fig. 47.29 The early radiograph of a march fracture which occurred with simple activity in a girl of 20. There is slight comminution, although it is emphasized there had been no injury

with a clinical prognosis. Sometimes the early radiological changes show little callus, at other times a large amount, and this may relate to the level of movement that is allowed to occur at the fracture site early on, and in turn may be associated with the pain threshold. If the fracture line is seen in the callus it indicates that there is still movement at the fracture site during healing.

There is some connection between the site of the fracture and the length of history and the more proximal the fracture is in the shaft the longer severe symptoms have been present.

Stress fractures of the third metatarsal bone are common, but a little less so than those of the second metatarsal bone. They can occur at most ages and they are more commonly involved in multiple stress fractures of the metatarsal bones than those of the second. One out of every two patients with a stress fracture of the third metatarsal bone will have one or more other metatarsal stress fractures. This characteristic is shared to an even greater extent by the fourth metatarsal, which is more often involved with another metatarsal than it is singly. Usually the other metatarsals involved are either the second or the third. In other words, the first and the fifth metatarsal bones do not share in this multiplicity of

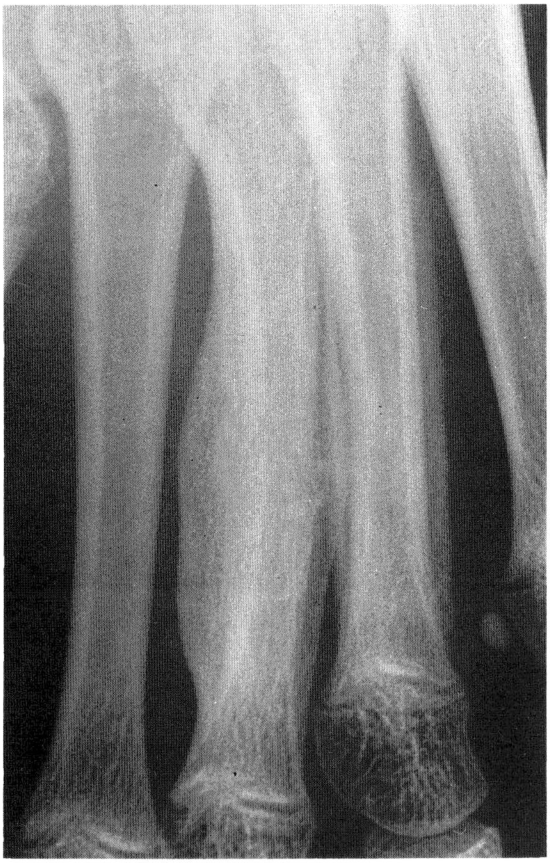

Fig. 47.30 A boy of 16 had three weeks pain in his left foot, but no injury. He has a well developed stress fracture of the third metatarsal bone, but there is also one in the fourth, which is much more recent. Note how the callus in a young person goes almost the whole length of the shaft

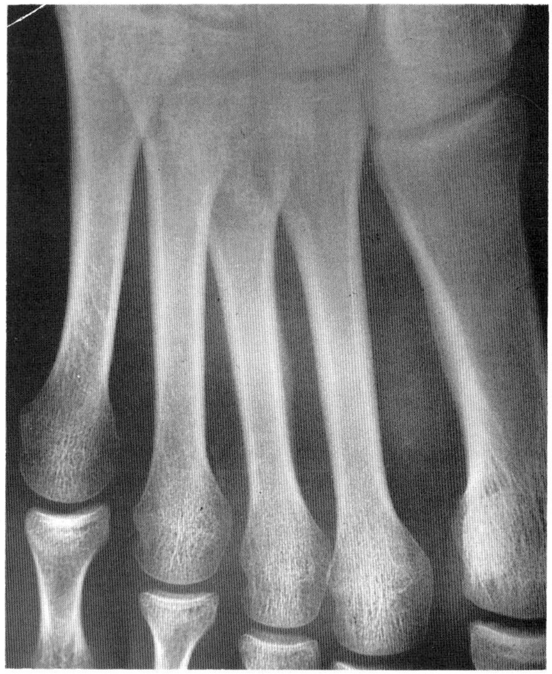

Fig. 47.31 A 19-year-old youth who had had a previous stress fracture of the fibula, had one week's pain in his right foot. Very early haze of new bone is all that shows at this time of his march fracture of the third metatarsal shaft

fractures and if the fifth metatarsal is in fact implicated, it is not at its base but in the shaft that the fracture occurs.

The fourth metatarsal bone does not have nearly so many stress fractures as do the second and third, but, apart from the symptoms and signs being more on the outer side of the foot, there is little difference in presentation.

STRESS FRACTURES OF THE FIRST METATARSAL BONE

The base of this bone is affected by a compression stress fracture and, being in line with the navicular bone, this is to be expected.

Symptoms are slow to occur as are those of most compression stress fractures. The usual complaint is of the gradual onset of pain with activity, which comes on earlier and earlier and gets more and more severe until the patient seeks advice. Usually at this time the early haze of internal callus can be seen (Fig. 47.32). The lesion will have been localized by careful palpation and it may be possible to feel some local swelling, because the anteromedial side of the first metatarsal base is subcutaneous. Treatment is either by restricting activity with or without strapping or with severe symptoms, a below-knee plaster cast for some time.

STRESS FRACTURES OF THE FIFTH METATARSAL BONE

This bone sustains a transverse stress fracture at its base as well as the more ordinary oblique type in its shaft. The former is dangerous to the extent that nonunion occurs even if properly treated, so it is important that any lesion of this particular nature

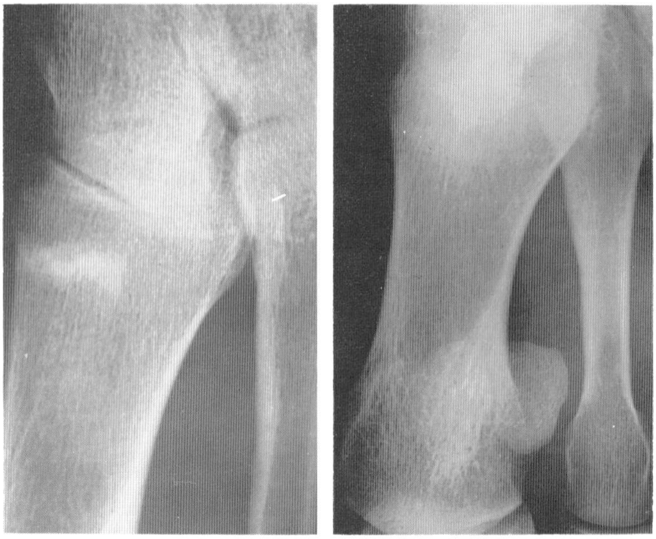

Fig. 47.32 A girl of 20 did much walking in her job and developed pain in the medial border of her right foot. She was very tender at the base of the first metatarsal bone in which the radiograph shows a compression stress fracture

must be given treatment immediately as an emergency (see Fig. 47.4).

It is considered that this transverse type of stress fracture is caused by the tremendous muscular pull that can occur at the base of the fifth metatarsal in activity, such as squash (Fig. 47.33). Again, the opposite foot must be looked at carefully to make sure there is not a similar stress fracture on that side. The traumatic or muscular avulsion fracture of the base of the fifth metatarsal bone is also well known and must be differentiated, but the typical history of pain after sport or activity, gradually coming on earlier and earlier, is usual. Not infrequently there may be an insidious history leading up to a sudden onset of severe pain, indicating that the whole of the metatarsal base has now been broken off. The period of immobilization must be sufficient to allow complete healing or symptoms will recur and may then lead again to nonunion.

The fifth metatarsal shaft oblique fractures are much the same as those of the neighbouring bones.

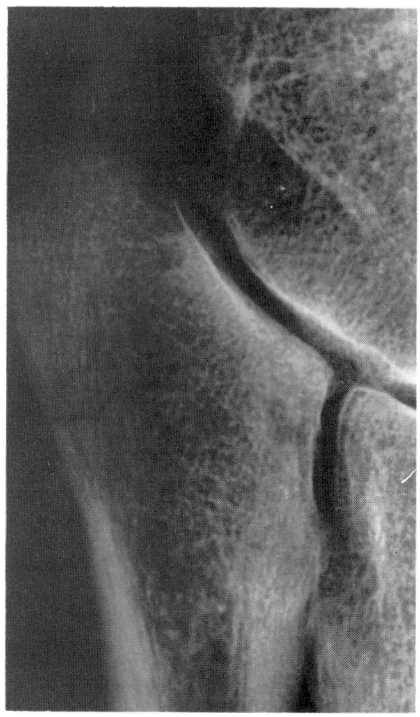

Fig. 47.33 A patient of 57 had long standing rheumatoid arthritis treated by steroids and previously had suffered a compression stress fracture of the tibia. He developed pain in his right foot and the stress fracture at the base of the fifth metatarsal can be seen (compared to that in Fig. 4)

STRESS FRACTURES OF THE SESAMOID BONES OF THE HALLUX

Stress fractures are difficult to diagnose in the sesamoid bone because at the beginning the pain is mild and it may take a long time for the patient to attend for advice; secondly a bipartite sesamoid may have a bursitis or a form of inflammation which may masquerade as a stress fracture. The counterpart in the patella is not uncommon in its various forms but in the sesamoid only the transverse stress fracture has been seen.

Diagnosis is made on clinical examination and history, confirmed by radiography. Scintillography may be difficult to interpret. The lesion, even if seen early, will show a separation of the two parts and this will develop further (Fig. 47.34).

Treatment is by the usual methods of rest and support, but a metatarsal bar to take the weight behind the first metatarsal head may be advantageous. It can be discarded at leisure. A custom-made first metatarsal neck support may also be effective. It is not possible to secure union of the sesamoid, which should be allowed to remain bipartite. Gradually symptoms resolve and the foot becomes fully functional.

STRESS FRACTURES AT THE ANKLE AND LOWER LEG

Stress fractures in the lower leg are included because they can cause a difficulty in diagnosis in those patients in whom the symptoms are only slowly progressive and of a dull, aching nature. The latter is often referred to the foot, either in fact or because aching feet are so common that the patient is self-indoctrinated as to the site of the pain.

After the march fracture, the commonest site for a stress fracture is the lower third of the fibula just at or above the lateral malleolus. This is particularly common in athletes and has been termed 'the runner's fracture', but it also often occurs in middle aged people and following an unusual, but not abnormal, activity, such as a visit to a town on a lengthy shopping expedition.

Symptoms and signs

At first there is a dull ache towards evening in the outer side of the ankle, often referred to the foot and if so it will be on the outer side. The pain will come on earlier and earlier with exercise and, in the case of an athlete, sport eventually has to be abandoned. Usually it takes about two to three weeks for the patient to attend for treatment. By then there is often a little swelling, pain is localized to the lower fibula above the lateral malleolus and walking is painful.

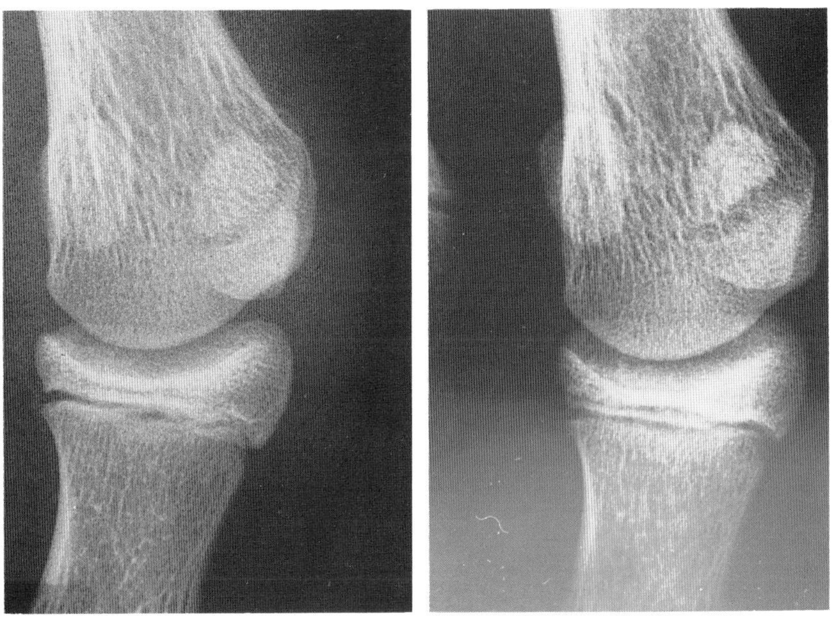

Fig. 47.34 A stress fracture of the sesamoid is difficult to diagnose, but this girl of 12 developed a swollen and painful first metatarsophalangeal joint on the right and the sesamoid itself was extremely tender. The fact that over a period of time it had become more widely separated, suggests that this was, indeed, a stress fracture

Examination will show that a swelling can be seen in most patients (Fig. 47.11). This is, of course, unusual, but the lower end of the fibula is subcutaneous and, therefore, like the base of the first metatarsal bone, swelling can be seen. The swelling will be tender to the touch and springing the fibula may cause pain at the site of the swelling (Fig. 47.35). However, the radiograph may still show no

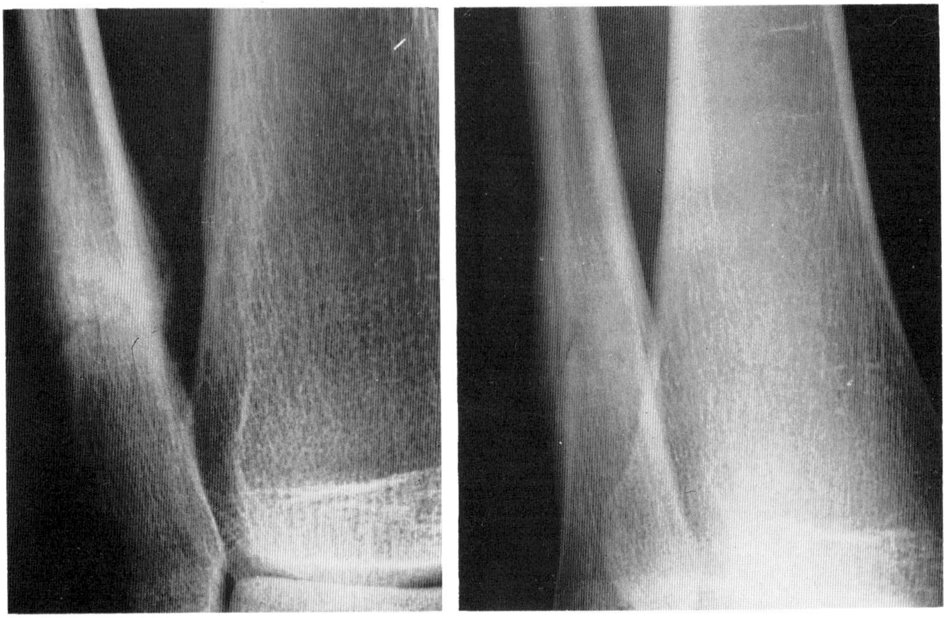

Fig. 47.35 An athlete developed a very painful ankle and foot and had to give up sport. The first radiograph shows a haze of callus, but the second, taken two months later, shows good healing in the initial crack through the lateral cortex which is still clearly seen

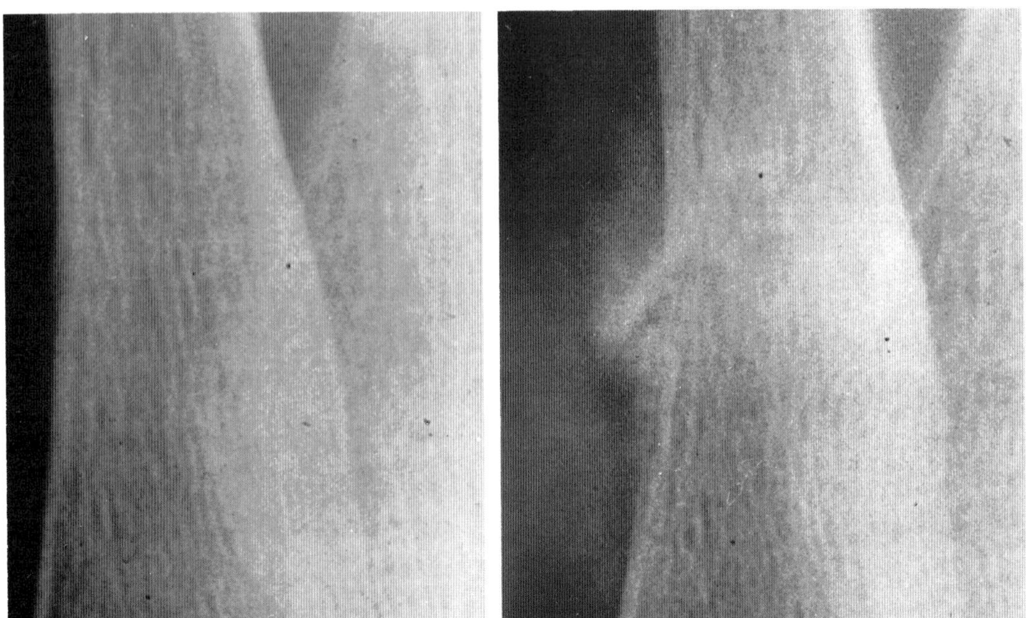

Fig. 47.36 A woman of 57 attended with pain after suffering a stress fracture of the left fibula the year before. She had been told then of the possibility of fracture in the opposite fibula and asked to attend immediately if she felt pain. Careful radiography shows the minute crack in the lateral cortex of the fibula, which needed several oblique views to get the X-ray beam to pass through it. Five weeks later the fracture is healing nicely

abnormality unless it has been taken with extreme care and not overexposed (Fig. 47.36). The cause of the stress fracture in the fibula cannot be weight bearing, because it is not a weight-bearing bone, but it has been shown that during muscular contraction of the calf muscles the fibula is pulled towards the tibia and the maximum bend occurs at the site of maximum occurrence of stress fractures; that is about 1 to 2 cm above the lateral malleolus.

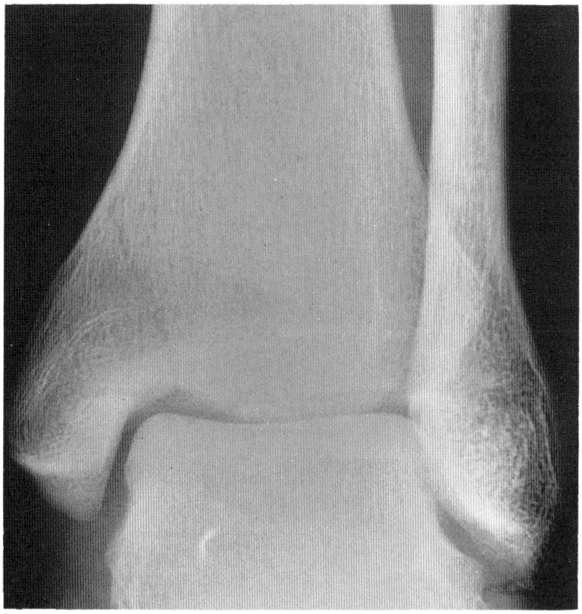

Fig. 47.37 The medial malleolus can sustain a stress fracture, as shown here in the ankle of a boy of 17. It took three months for the fracture to show radiologically

Radiology

The radiographs do not show any lesion for some three weeks in the usual course of events, but a scan will normally show a hot spot at the fracture within a week of the onset of symptoms. In the ordinary course of events the oblique stress fracture may become complete and this is usually signalled by a sudden increase in the pain.

The treatment is the same as for stress fractures in the foot — that is rest from the sport or activity that has caused the problem — and elastic adhesive bandaging. However, in the excessively keen sportsman it may be necessary to add a below-knee

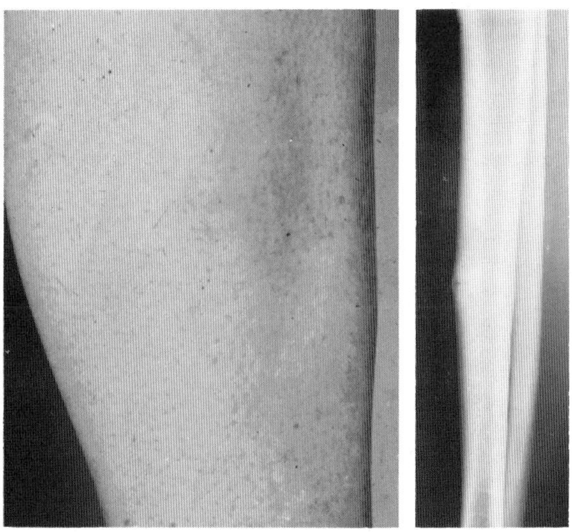

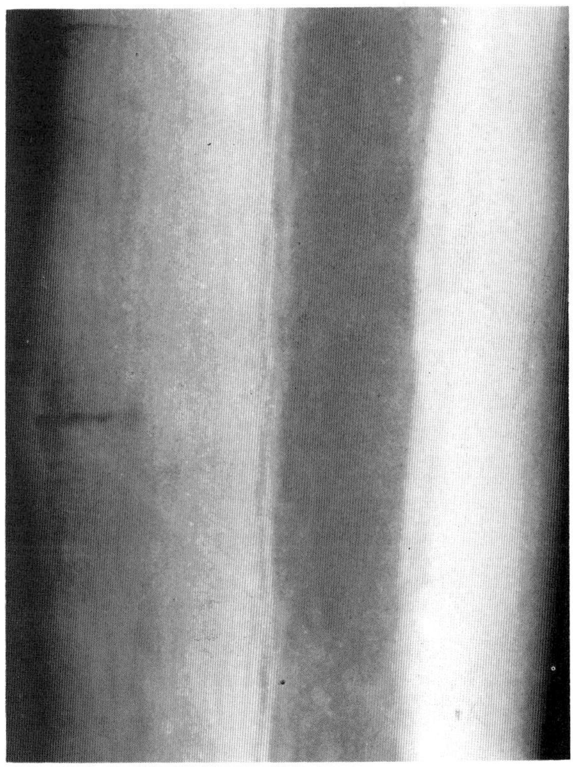

Figs. 47.38 and 39 A ballet dancer developed pain in the shin, which went down the leg into the foot. Clinical examination showed only a very little swelling of the front of the shin and the radiographs show what appears to be a little insignificant crack in the anterior tibial cortex. This is a transverse fracture, the most dangerous type that occur. A magnified view is shown in Figure 39. If ballet dancing, or any other exercise of a similar nature was continued, the fracture would break completely and displace and perhaps ruin a promising career.

walking plaster to curb enthusiastic attempts at returning to excess activity too soon.

Any return to a painful activity means that the healing has been delayed and union will take longer to become solid.

STRESS FRACTURES OF THE MEDIAL MALLEOLUS

These are extremely rare and have been seen in runners (Fig. 47.37). The symptoms are very similar to those of a stress fracture of the fibula, but the symptoms are on the medial side of the ankle and the time lag between diagnosis and X-ray confirmation may be considerable. Local examination will reveal tenderness around the medial malleolus, but it may not be possible to see swelling.

STRESS FRACTURES OF THE LOWER TIBIA

Any lesion in the lowermost third of the tibia may give rise to pain felt in, or going down into, the foot. The very dangerous transverse stress fracture seen in ballet dancers and others who do much jumping, such as in basketball, may also give pain referred to the ankle and foot. The physical signs of tenderness and swelling are present, but they must be looked for carefully (Figs. 47.38 and 39).

The shin soreness type of stress fracture of the athlete is very common in the lowermost third of the tibia and has been named 'shin splints' by athletes. Suffering a chronic continuing pain in the ankle and foot, athletes may blame their running style and foot placement (Figs. 47.40 and 41). It is of interest to

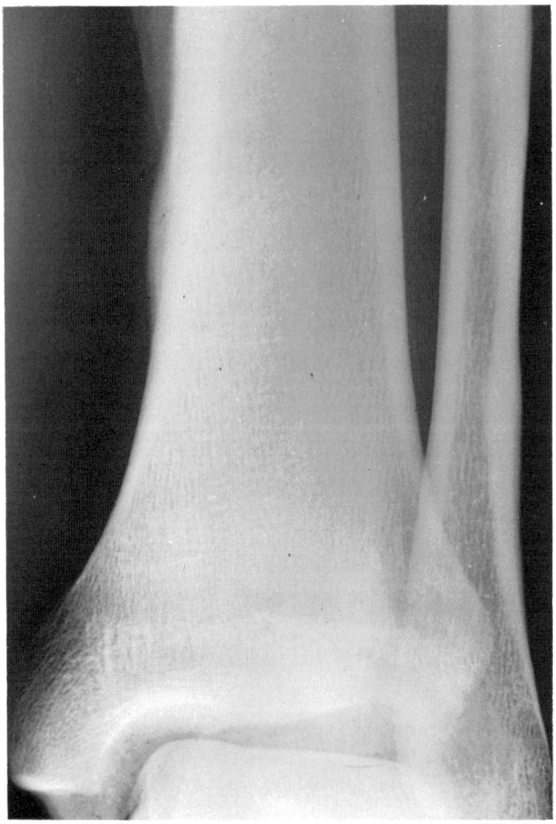

Fig. 47.40 Shin soreness is the bane of the athlete and causes pain in the shin which involves the ankle and foot, quite frequently being referred downwards. Sometimes all that can be seen is a haze of periosteal new bone, but if proper treatment is not instituted the patient will lose a whole season from sport

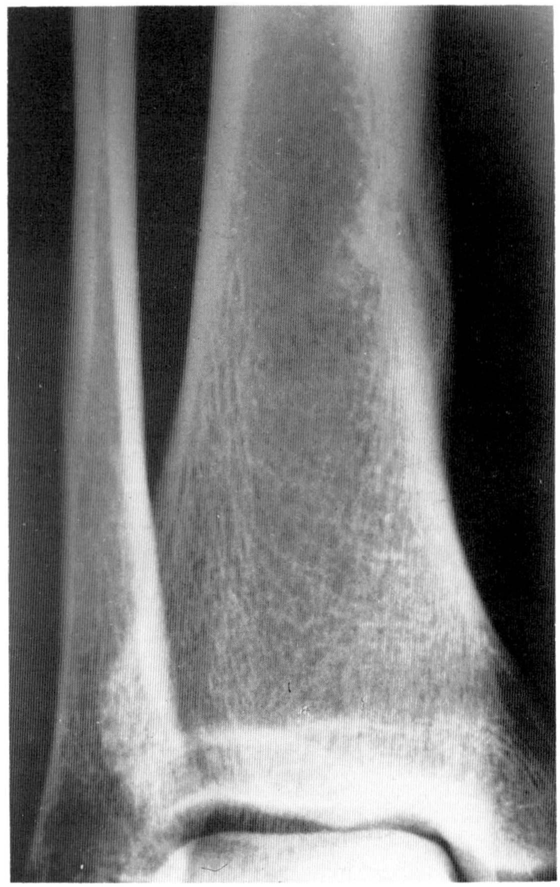

Fig. 47.41 Another variety of shin soreness shows that the stress fracture line goes proximally and laterally through the medial cortex of the lower tibia. This fracture very rarely gives rise to severe complications, but its symptoms can be of very long duration

note that shin soreness, or shin splints, has its counterpart in the horse in which the stress fracture is in the second metacarpal bone which is described below. The longitudinal stress fracture of the lower tibia gives very similar symptoms to the oblique type, of which it may be a variant (Fig. 47.42). The compression stress fracture however is most common in the older person, and sometimes actually 'spreads' into the fibula (Fig. 47.43). The history of these fractures is usually very long and it may take up to three months for the radiograph to show the first haze of internal callus.

COMPARATIVE STRESS FRACTURES

The greyhound gets a stress fracture of what is called the tarsal scaphoid or the navicular bone and it is of interest that this is always on the right side, because that is the leg that takes the greatest thrust in racing counter-clockwise round the course. The right tarsal scaphoid of the racing greyhound when examined macroscopically will show blood staining within the bone caused by stress fractures which did not cause complete disruption. However, sometimes the bone will break completely and the dog limps out of the race. It is of interest to note that for many years the scaphoid in the greyhound was replaced with

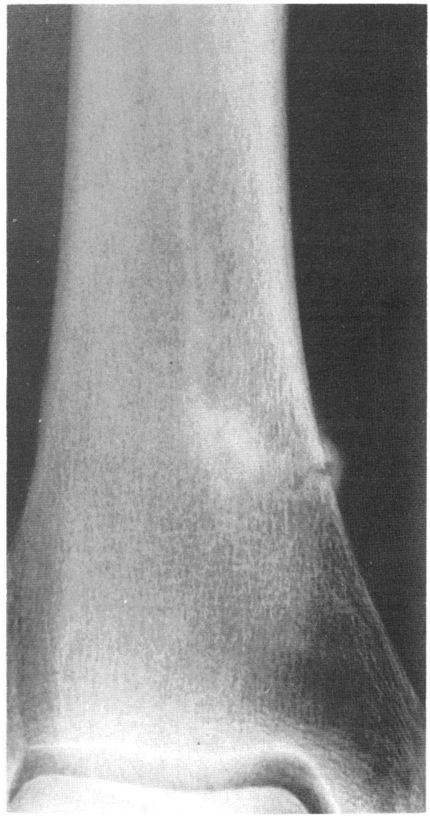

Fig. 47.42 A longitudinal fracture of the lower tibia, which can cause pain and disability, often attributed to the ankle by an athlete

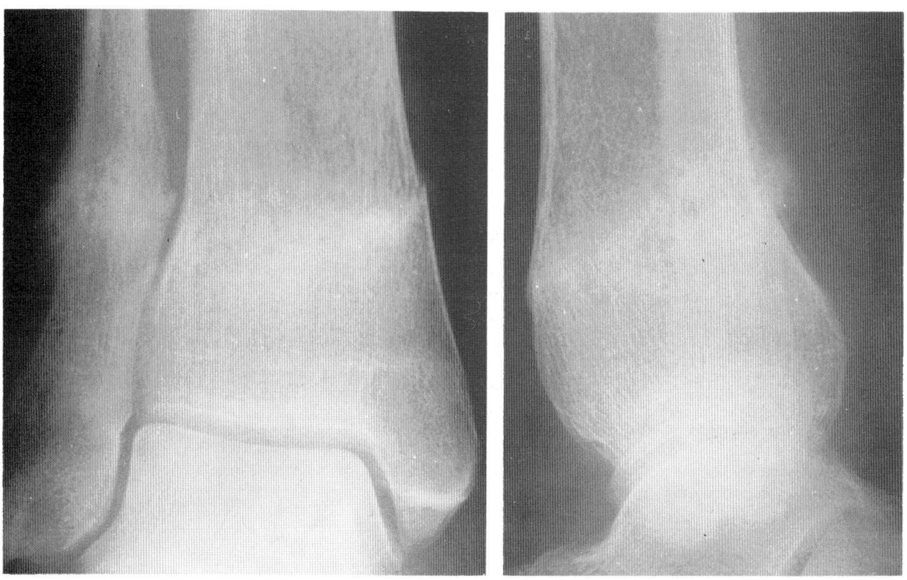

Fig. 47.43 The double stress fracture of the tibia and fibula may cause an elderly person to hobble, and complain of pain in the foot and ankle. This patient was 61, somewhat overweight and had a two months history. She had remained walking throughout and there is slight angulation of the tibia and fibula, but the latter seems to be healing already

successful results by a plastic prosthesis enabling the dogs to return to racing, albeit in slower heats.

Stress fractures occur in horses and there is a condition in yearlings and two-year-olds known as splint disease or 'a splint'. The 'splint' is a small swelling visible on the medial side of the third metacarpal or canon bone. The second and fourth metacarpal bones are remnants which run down each side of the canon bone and are called splint bones. At first this condition was thought to be an inflammation of the splint bone and was treated by cupping and other means including antibiotics. However, with the advent of radiography it became obvious that a splint is merely the swelling of a stress fracture (Figs. 47.44a and b) comparable to that seen in the tibia in athletes. Treatment should consist of rest with a soft litter until the tenderness has completely gone, even if the swelling remains.

CONCLUSIONS

Stress fractures occur in healthy bone and provided the sequence of events is remembered, the diagnosis should not be difficult, even though physical signs are limited and radiographical confirmation is late. Early confirmation of the diagnosis can be achieved by technetium scanning. Treatment is usually rest from painful activity combined with support.

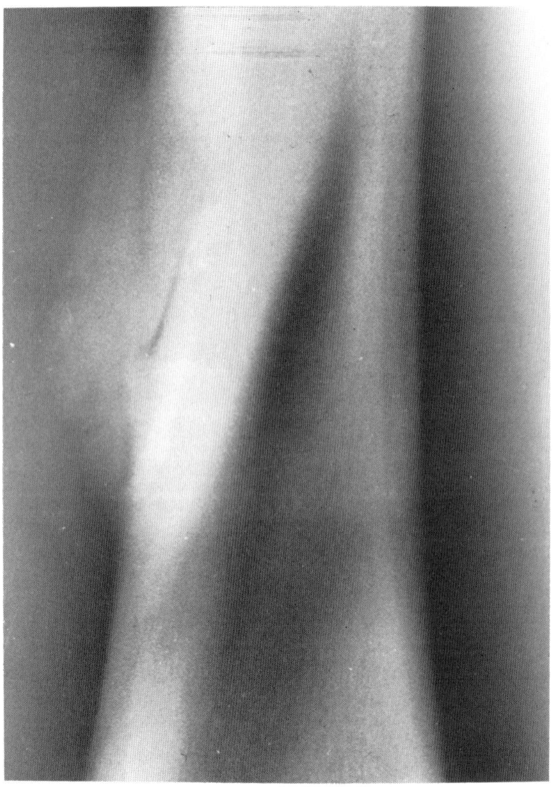

a

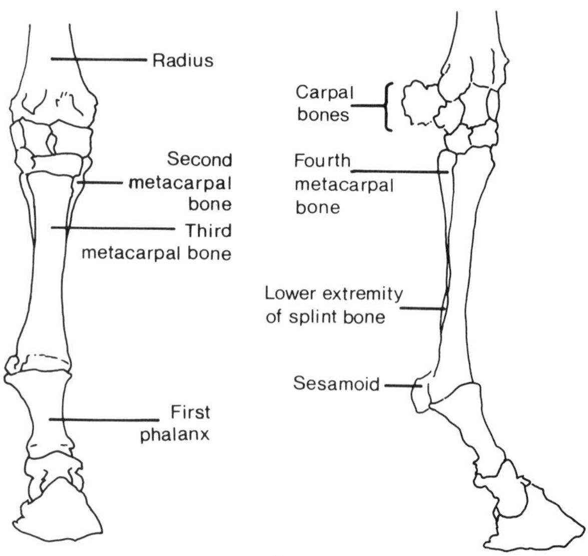

b

Fig. 47.44 (a) The radiograph of the canon, or third metacarpal bone, of the horse shows a stress fracture just beneath the splint bone, which is pushed medially by the swelling. This condition, known as splint disease, occurs in two-year-olds, which is equivalent to the late teens in man. (b): the anatomy of the region

REFERENCES

Aleman O 1929 Omsk marchschalst (syndesmites metatarsea) Tidskrift i Militar Halsovard 54: 191–208

Breithaupt 1855 Zur Pathologie des Menschlichen Fusses Med Zeitung Berlin 24: 169

Koch J C (1917) The laws of bone architecture. Am J Anat 21: 177
Lane W A 1855 Some points in the physiology and pathology of the changes produced by pressure in the bony skeleton of the trunk and shoulder girdle. Guy's Hospital Reports 43: 321
Stechow 1897 Fussodem und Rontgenstrahlen. Deutsche Militärärzliche Zeitschrift 26: 465

FURTHER READING

Devas M 1975 Stress Fractures. Churchill Livingstone, Edinburgh

Sports injuries

The foot serves as the initial interface to the external environment in many sports. The individual who engages in any sport which is not upper extremity related is susceptible to injury of the foot. There are broad classifications of injuries which occur in these sports and these injuries are unique to the specific sport, an example being that of racquet sports in which the player rarely develops the stress fractures seen in runners. Conversely, runners have a much lower incidence of ankle ligament injuries than do players of racquet sports.

Classifications of sports related to the surface impact can be formulated, the unique aspects of each sport being seen in terms of the impact loading present in the foot during performance of the activity. High impact sports are running, aerobics, volleyball, basketball, soccer, and field hockey; medium impact sports are racquet games and handball; low impact sports are walking, skiing, swimming, and cycling.

In addition to the magnitude of impact, the direction of the force is important. Jogging involves an anterior-posterior motion with rotatory forces less important, racquet sports have a medial-lateral component of force, whilst soccer and basketball have a combination of both anterior-posterior and medial-lateral component.

In addition to the amount of force, one must consider how the force is applied. Prolonged, low grade trauma occurs throughout any sport and overuse injuries tend to occur in sports in which the foot is subjected to low level, repetitive, cumulative stress. Obviously, acute trauma occurs in certain more intense sports.

LABORATORY TESTS

The use of routine X-rays is necessary in primary evaluation. When the lesion is obviously of soft tissue, radiographs need not be ordered. Standing anterior-posterior and lateral radiographs are helpful and should be used to evaluate the long arch and pronation (Gould 1983). Special views such as obliques and Harris views are warranted to detect tarsal coalition or internal structural abnormality.

Video taping the individual running or cycling towards the observer gives information about the ankle and foot which cannot otherwise be obtained (Gould 1983). There are other tools available for special evaluation such as pedotopography, crystal impacting and track impacting. These have unique and specific aspects depending on what one is attempting to evaluate.

INDIVIDUAL SPORTS

Soccer

Ligament injuries are the most frequent injury (70%) in soccer players (Simon 1979). These are discussed in another section and no unique distribution of ankle ligament injuries occurs in soccer players compared to the average nonathletic population.

Microtrauma syndrome of soccer players falls into three categories: posterior ankle difficulties, anterior exostoses and diffuse articular arthritis.

Posterior ankle trauma and pain, caused by contact of the posterior talus and the tibia, is present in 80% of all soccer players after several years (Simon 1979). The mechanism of kicking with the foot in forced plantar flexion forces the os trigonum or posterior talar structures against the posterior tibia. Radiographs may show degenerative changes and a 'parrot beak' change at the posterior tibial area. Treatment by infiltration of steroid and local anaesthetic, anti-inflammatories and exercises into hyperflexion are helpful. If recalcitrant, occasionally exploration of the area with removal of the os trigonum or a bone spur is helpful.

Anterior ankle exostoses are present in approximately 7% of soccer players. Treatment is generally conservative but occasionally an arthrotomy and removal of the exostosis is necessary.

Diffuse arthritis occurs with increased frequency around both medial and lateral malleoli in soccer players in the sport for long periods of time (Simon 1979).

Tennis

Foot injury rates in tennis are low. Approximately 2.5% of a large group of tennis players had some type of foot or ankle injury. Acute injuries are obviously those associated with direct or rotational foot trauma. There are three types of chronic injuries: hyperkeratosis, most often in the medial portion of the first metatarsal, chronic swelling of hallux valgus and subungual haematomata.

Volleyball

Posterior tibial tendon inflammation or possible rupture is a problem specific to this sport.

Running

There are numerous injuries associated with running, for the most part of the overuse and not of the acute type. They will be discussed later.

GENERALIZED INJURIES

Distribution of injuries in high impact airborne sports is higher than in medium or low impact sports. In the highest group of sports injuries 50% are to the midfoot, 30% to the forefoot and 20% to the hindfoot. Of all injuries noted in the high impact population, 77% were related to the foot. This includes injuries of the knee, thigh, hip and back which were correlated with the foot abnormality.

GENERALIZED TREATMENTS

Activity modification

The hardest in which to modify activity are individuals involved in the high and medium impact sport groups. Generally they have a definite commitment to a life style in association with their sports and are unwilling totally to give it up. Consequently, an alternative programme needs to be designed around such sports as skiing, walking, swimming or cycling. Specific goals should be set for them in terms of their return to higher level sport. A return to activity sheet is a method of moving an individual back into activities which involve some running and other high impact sports.

Inflammatory management

Inflammatory components are present in any sports injury.

Cold application produces constriction of the vessels, decreasing blood flow and therefore reducing swelling. When the athlete has ceased any specific activity the application of cold compresses in the form of an ice bag or cold gel bag reduces the inflammatory reaction (Mann 1981). Ice is not applied directly to the skin, but is wrapped either in an elastic bandage or a towel. Application may be for approximately 10 minutes at 10 minute intervals. Three applications of 10 minutes each may be given immediately after activity. Once the skin temperature drops below 59°F (15°C) an increase in blood flow occurs. At this point there is redness and burning and continued application of cold will produce increased swelling. The blood flow decreases for 10 to 15 minutes with cold and therefore cold application should not be for more than 10 minutes at any one time.

Heat may be applied to the foot at a time when there is no acute swelling. The heat can be in the form of moist heat, whirlpool, or by ultrasound machine. The skin should not be subjected to temperatures greater than 112°F (44°C). Heat should not be applied for longer than 20 minutes. In the exercising athlete, heat is often applied at a time after the inflammatory reaction from the activity has subsided. In the minimally injured foot this may be 8 to 12 hours after activity, but in the foot that is markedly inflamed heat should not be applied until several days after the initial injury. Application is for approximately 20 minutes, when the physiological responses are vasodilation and increased circulation, which help to decrease much of the spasm and seem to increase the flexibility of the foot.

Medication

The use of salicylates to produce a serum level between 40 to 60 mg/dl is appropriate. For the 70 kg individual, salicylates four times a day in the range of 600 to 900 mg is usually appropriate. The obvious compliance difficulty is that any adult who is active will miss several doses. Because of the compliance problem in adults, nonsteroidal anti-inflammatory drugs have been used. Dosage can be once or twice a day. They do not appear to be any more affective than aspirin. Gastrointestinal upset has been a major side effect, but may be attenuated by the use of some of the newer gastrointestinal medications.

Injectable steroids are never used as a primary treatment of injuries about the foot from sport. They are not used in any area where the steroid might enter a tendon sheath (Lutter 1980). Great care must be taken when they are injected into fatty areas, since the possibility and problem of fat necrosis is high. The shorter acting steroids in conjunction with Xylocaine® have been found to be more effective and less problematic in terms of fat necrosis.

Physical therapy modalities

Although specific stretching and strengthening activities are not often necessary about the foot, on occasion the use of Achilles tendon stretches and foot dorsiflexor strengthening are warranted for foot problems. The efficacy of attempting to stretch the plantar fascia is questionable.

Orthoses and shoes

Orthoses are used in high and medium impact sports. They are generally not necessary in low impact sports, except occasionally cycling. An orthosis has specific biomechanical effects that have been shown to decrease the amount of heel eversion and subsequently pronation of the longitudinal arch. The velocity of pronation can be controlled also by appropriate orthoses. They have been shown significantly to decrease medial and lateral shear (Baker 1979) which obviously has implications where a foot has forward progression or medial-lateral shear as seen in medium and high impact sports.

Orthoses can be categorized into rigid, semi-flexible, and soft. Many sports individuals can make soft types for themselves to use initially. They are essentially a combination of orthopaedic felt, semiflexible cork or leather. Many can be bought as 'over the counter orthoses' and will serve well if the individual does not have a serious requirement for controlled pronation.

Semiflexible orthoses (Fig. 48.1a) can be easily fabricated in the clinic by anyone who understands the biomechanics of the foot. Two materials available are Orthoplast® (Johnson and Johnson, New Brunswick, New Jersey) and Plastazote® (Xylonite Ltd., distributed by Apex Foot Products New York, New York). The materials are heat sensitive, semiflexible and are more pliable when warmed. After the materials are heated, they can be moulded on the foot with the foot held in a neutral position. Appropriate lifts and posts can be placed for additional control as needed. This can serve as an excellent low cost, functional orthosis for a great number of high and medium impact sports.

Rigid orthoses are fabricated over a plaster mould. A negative mould of the foot is made and a positive mould made from this. The thermoplastic material is poured over the plaster. Posting bars and modifications are added later. The cost and time required for this type of orthosis is much higher than for the previous two.

Indications for sport orthoses are foot conditions which anatomically require prevention of specific motion, need pressure transferred to a specific area or need relief of pressure from an area.

The most effective component of an orthosis is its use in controlling a hypermobile flat foot. The orthosis prevents eversion inversion of the subtalar joint. The use in a supinated-varus foot is more difficult since the rigidity of this foot counters the beneficial aspect of the orthosis. Using an orthosis for weight-relieving effect means placement of a pad under the metatarsal head or plantar fascia area.

Selections of the types of orthoses are based upon the length of time for which the individual will need them. The individual with the markedly abnormal

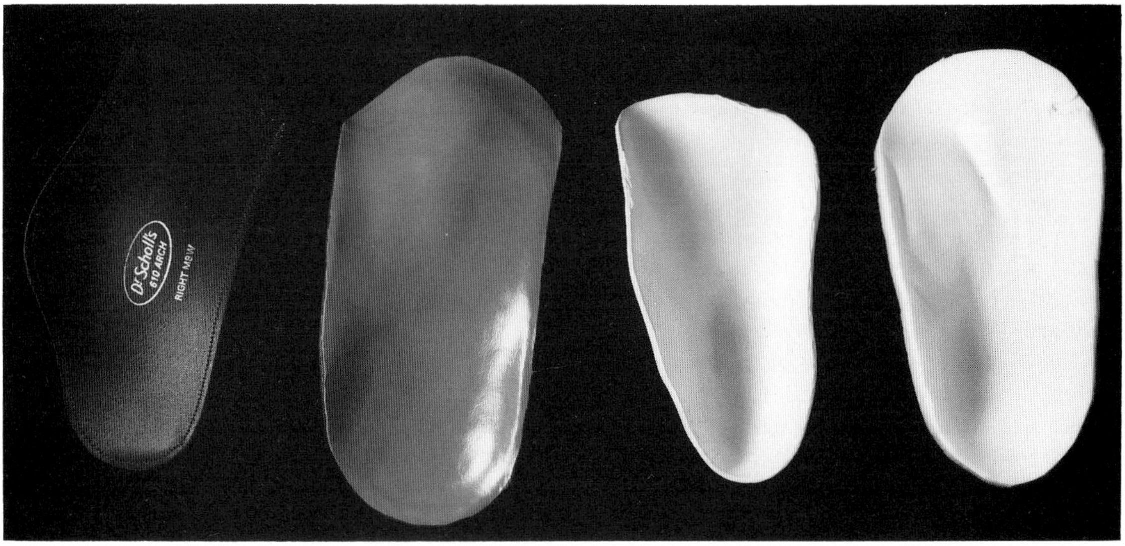

Fig. 48.1a Various types of orthoses available: 1. Far left 'over the counter type'. 2. Cork and Leather. 3. Orthoplast, moulded on the foot, semiflexible. 4. Plastazote, moulded on the foot, semiflexible

foot in either supinated-varus or significant pronation will most likely need an orthosis throughout his sporting life. Soft or semi-soft orthoses will not have a long life span and consequently some of the firmer materials are more appropriate. The semi-rigid materials are generally preferable because they afford some cushioning as well as control of the abnormal rotation. They may last 1½ to 2 years and require moderate servicing.

Rigid orthotic devices are avoided if possible since in high impact they produce problems such as nerve impingement, metatarsal head irritation, neuromata, or stress fractures, due to the inflexibility and lack of shock absorption.

Sports Shoes. Specific modifications to a sports shoe can be made by the skilful and knowledgeable orthopaedic shoe technician. The use of metatarsal bars or sole wedges can help the individuals who have difficulty only during sport. Metatarsal padding or metatarsal bars can be incorporated easily into a sports shoe without changing the configuration or function of the shoe. SACH (solid ankle cushion heel) material also has its use in terms of specific heel injuries. This material is available in soft, medium and firm densities and can be incorporated into a sports shoe quite easily (Edwards 1981). Specific modifications in the wedge and midsole of the shoe must be viewed in terms of variations of the foot and the injury which is present. These will be covered in other sections of the chapter.

SPECIFIC INJURIES

In treating specific injuries anatomic diagnosis is the cornerstone. Symptomatic treatment of most injuries of the foot does not work, since the individual returns with the exact problem that he or she had. Treatment must be designed to change the mechanics of the process.

Sports injuries of the overuse type force a physician to return to traditional thinking processes with emphasis on pathogenesis of the injury and away from systematic treatment. Minimal abnormalities in foot function combined with repetitive stress lay the basis for most injuries. The biomechanics of the injury process must be appreciated and only by applying this understanding to the anatomical variations can a reasonable long-term solution be obtained in more specific injuries.

FOREFOOT

This area receives highest stress in any sport with medium or high impact. The injury to the forefoot therefore constitutes a higher percentage of foot injuries in jogging, running and 'airborne' sports such as basketball and volleyball.

Hammertoe and bunions

Pain in these areas are usually secondary to direct contact and not to biomechanical problems.

Treatment of the shoe with localized stretching by a shoemaker can solve most of these problems. Strict attention to shoe wear and shoe box size is important.

Black toenail

The black toenail is a subungual haematoma which presents in any sport in which the individual is doing repetitive running or rotation (Fig. 48.1b). It is not solely related to abnormal shoe fit, since many runners may develop it with adequate toe room as the toe repetitively taps against the undersurface of the toe box.

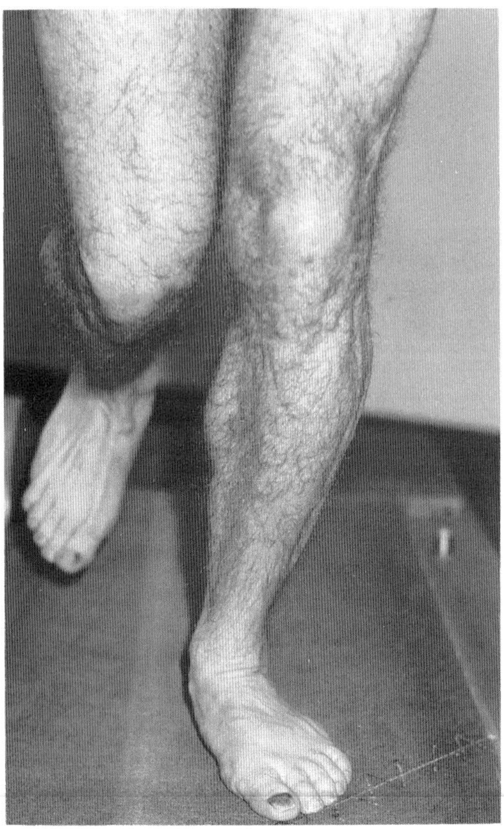

Fig. 48.1b Significant foot pronation: subungual haematoma great toe

Treatment should be by taping the toe to the next to prevent dorsiflexion. Padding the plantar area of the toe will prevent some of the hyperextension.

Nonspecific metatarsophalangeal pain

Physical examination

The pain occurs at the top of the metatarsophalangeal joint of the great toe and generally occurs at toe dorsiflexion. Often it is associated with swelling and a small mass. There is often loss of toe dorsiflexion of more than 20% and there may be early hallux rigidus which could be associated with a palpable osteophytic spur.

Biomechanics

Degenerative changes decreasing the range of motion of the toe put additional stress through the joint.

Treatment

Initial treatment is to place a metatarsal pad at the midsole of the shoe, serving as a rocker bottom and allowing the foot to become airborne without dorsiflexion. This is particularly effective for cross country skiing or sports with a significant amount of lateral motion. On occasion anti-inflammatory medications are useful. Rarely is an operative approach needed and, if so, debridement of the area instead of fusion is performed. Implants have not been used in athletes.

Metatarsal head pain

Metatarsal head pain occurs in a variety of sports and generally in any sport from high to low impact.

Physical examination

Pain is present on the plantar surface of any metatarsal head, but rarely under the first. Often callus build-up is present and highlights the area of most pain. Palpation of the painful area shows it to be localized to the plantar surface directly under the metatarsophalangeal joint. This pain is anatomically distinct from an interdigital neuroma. Other findings may be flatness of the metatarsal arch and related medial longitudinal arch flatness (Fig. 48.2a). Hammer toe of any degree will increase the problem below the metatarsophalangeal joint.

Biomechanics

Any attenuation in forefoot support which changes the normal relationship of the first metatarsal to the lateral four will increase the pressure under specific metatarsal heads. One sees this more frequently in a relaxed foot or one in which there is alteration in the midfoot.

Treatment

Identification of the specific abnormality allows appropriate treatment. In high impact, forward motion sports (running) a simple metatarsal pad placed in the sports shoe may be all that is needed. In high impact, lateral motion sports (basketball and soccer) support of the medial or longitudinal arch is necessary. Appropriate shoes for each sport are necessary, since the use of a running shoe for aerobics or tennis will not provide adequate lateral support making the individual susceptible to problems.

A rocker bottom sole can be applied in conjunction with a metatarsal pad if the latter alone is not adequate. Taping across the metatarsal arch is useful for a short time when competition or training is going on. Supplementation of a soft foam pad taped behind the painful metatarsal head is useful.

Sesamoiditis

This affects most frequently the sesamoids of the great toe. Occurrence is rare when compared to other forefoot sports injuries. It generally occurs in the gait cycle just before toe-off (Figs. 48.2b and c). Often the individual will develop a 'compensatory' injury because of shift of weight to the lateral four toes. It is not unusual for the initial complaint of sesamoiditis to be followed by lateral forefoot pain or metatarsalgia in one of the lateral four metatarsophalangeal joints.

Physical examination

The differentiation from metatarsophalangeal pain

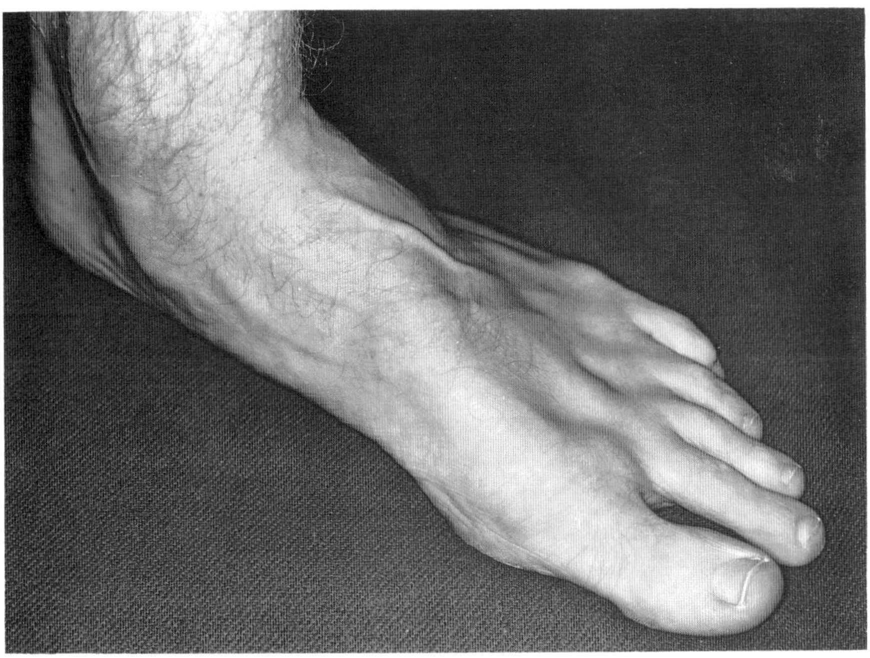

Fig. 48.2a Note the flatness of forefoot, metatarsal arch. Fullness at 1st and 2nd web space associated with metatarsal phalangeal spur

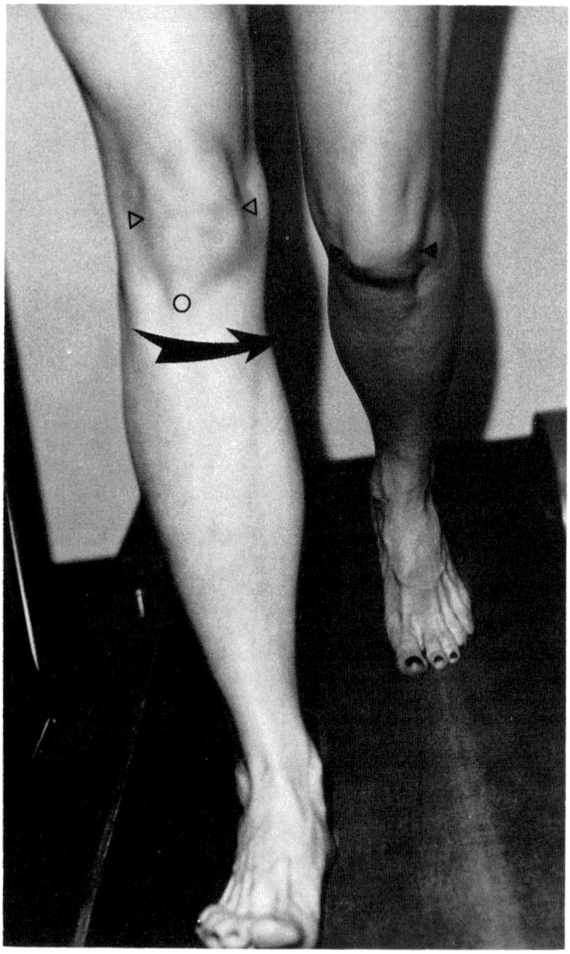

Fig. 48.2b Right foot at heel strike with knee beginning internal rotation. Note internally rotated patella; left knee at toe off

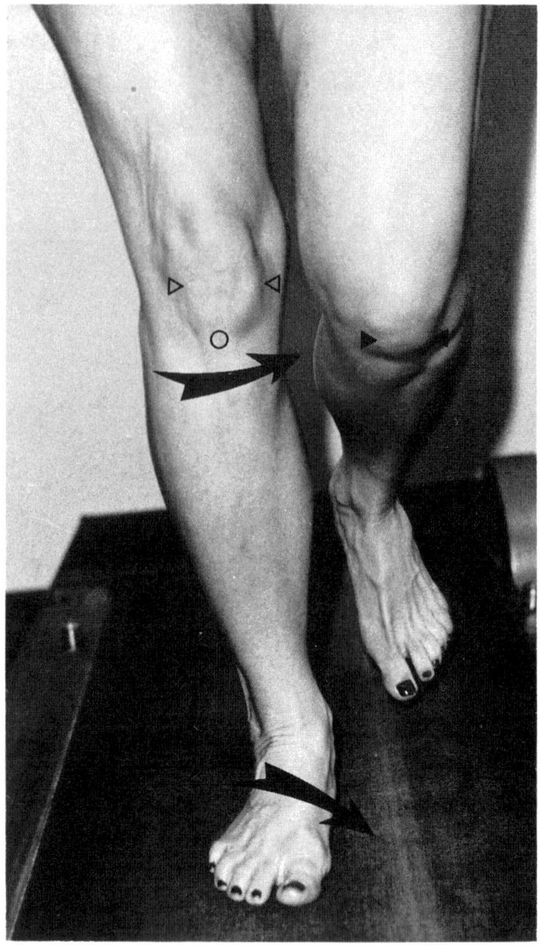

Fig. 48.2c Right foot at full weight bearing. Pronating foot is causing inward rotation of tibia and patella (compare to 2b) Note left tibia and patella beginning external rotation

can be made by direct palpation and grasping the sesamoid. Metatarsophalangeal joint pain will be more distal and not so well localized. A hallux valgus is often present. A foot which hyperpronates is often seen at examination. Radiographically there may be evidence of degenerative changes on a sesamoid view. The diagnosis of stress fracture must always be made cautiously, since the presence of a bipartite sesamoid is very frequent.

Biomechanics

The specifics of this are related to increased pressure over the first ray. Most frequently this is in a foot which hyperpronates, placing excessive pressure on the first metatarsal prior to toe take-off. Hallux valgus abets this by allowing increased rotatory and medial shear force through the first metatarsal.

Treatment

Direct padding under the metatarsal head usually is not helpful except in the early stages. A firm metatarsal pad placed proximal to the sesamoids is most helpful. Control of pronation is necessary if it is present to a significant degree. When a stress or traumatic fracture is identified, taping and a firm sole shoe will allow a return to sport after the initial symptoms have become quiescent. With degenerative changes, occasional injection of the specific joint with a short acting steroid and Xylocaine® has been useful. Surgical excision of a sesamoid has not been done if the goal is to return the individual to anything but a very low impact sport.

Interdigital neuroma

This occurs in a sufficiently high percentage to warrant consideration in the differential diagnosis of forefoot pain. The symptoms are generally not different from interdigital neuroma in the nonathletic population. They may come on earlier in sport than in a nonsporting activity, due to increased stress along the foot. Sports with increased lateral motion (racquet sports, soccer, aerobics) may have symptoms before any pain is present with routine walking. Often the pain is sharp enough to stop sporting activity, which is rare with metatarsalgia.

Physical examination

This condition needs to be separated from metatarsalgia and it can be done so easily. Palpation anteriorly in the interdigital space produces pain, usually in the third and fourth interdigital space, but space two and three can be affected. Often compression across the metatarsal arch produces pain. Direct palpation of the metatarsal head is not painful.

Biomechanics

In the sporting population the mechanics are much the same as in the nonsporting. Entrapment of the nerve and the secondary neuroma produces pain with increased frequency as the individual is active.

Treatment

A firm soled shoe which supports the forefoot may be helpful, but usually is not sufficient. Metatarsal padding to elevate the metatarsal head is generally necessary. Steroid and Xylocaine® injection will give temporary relief, but most often a return to activity causes pain recurrence. Interdigital neuroma excision can be done successfully, with the individual returning to high level sport.

MIDFOOT

The biomechanics of this area have been discussed elsewhere. Throughout the foot cycle the area functions in the changes from a rigid to a flexible foot. A great deal of stress must be dissipated through this area and because of this many injuries may occur. The major problems that occur are in soft tissue instead of bone.

Medial longitudinal arch pain

This is the most frequent complaint in the midfoot area. It has been seen in all types of impact sports. The complaint is usually of pain in the weight bearing portion of the cycle, often prior to pushoff as the individual is accelerating or cutting off the medial border of the foot. A combination of fasciitis, myalgia, or intertarsal ligament pain may be present.

Physical examination

There is pain at the medial border of the foot which is diffuse in nature, extending from the metatarsal heads to the plantar fascia insertion on the calcaneus.

Biomechanics

Related to pronation as noted above.

Treatment

Generally a longitudinal arch support is all that is necessary.

Posterior tibial tendon (Tibial periostitis, shin splints, tibial tendinitis)

This involves three areas, two of which (the tendon insertion and the tendon sheath) are in the foot, (Fig. 48.3). The pain at the insertion generally occurs at the plantar area. The tendon sheath pain may occur anywhere along the course of the tendon.

Physical examination

The individual usually has a pronated foot of significant degree. If the area of pain is at the tibial border, this usually occurs 6 to 8 cm from the medial

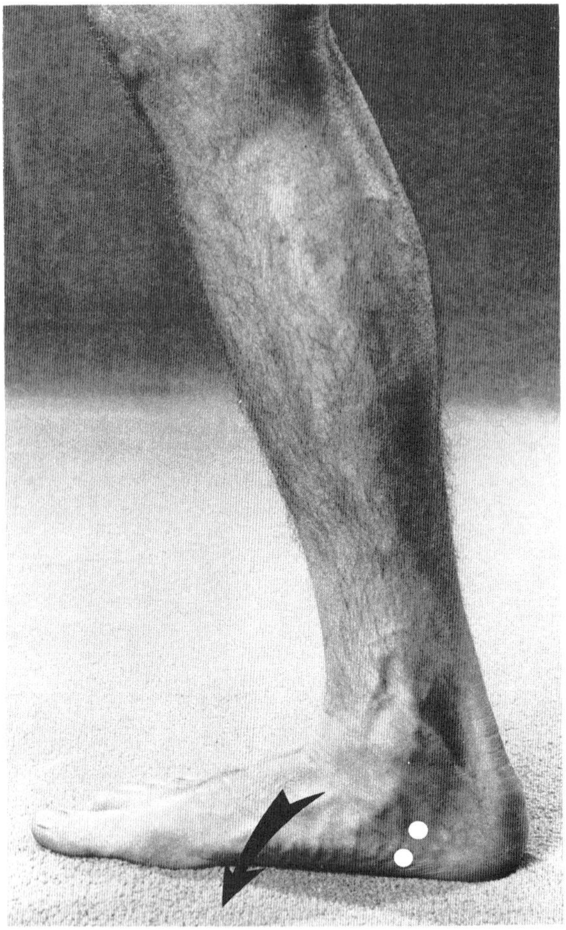

Fig. 48.3 Midstance position. Most heel stress dissipated at this stage. Medial calcaneal neuritis (dots) occur due to pronation (arrow)

malleolus. There is often blunting of the contour of the medial border of the tibia and the individual experiences pain with palpation. There may be crepitus or fullness along the tendon sheath.

Biomechanics

During the support phase of any running component (see Fig. 48.2c) the posterior tibial tendon serves as the primary tendon for external support to the medial longitudinal arch. If the bony configuration of the foot is such that the foot hyperpronates as the centre of gravity moves anteriorly there is increased pull on the posterior tibial tendon, producing irritation anywhere along the tendon.

Treatment

Orthotic control of the hyperpronation must be provided, in addition to which, the previous four general treatments are appropriate.

Peroneal tendinitis

This is a fairly rare problem in sport injuries, but can occur in lateral motion sports.

Physical examination

Generally the individual has a cavus foot configuration with pain along the peroneal tendon. Occasionally there is crepitus and swelling. Often peroneal subluxation occurs and can be identified by palpation of the tendon sliding over the fibula when the foot is plantarflexed and the forefoot is inverted.

Treatment

The irritation can usually be controlled by a lateral sole wedge supplemented by taping to prevent excessive motion of the peroneal tendon.

Midtarsal pain

This generally occurs as an inflammatory process, probably secondary to mild synovitis or capsulitis.

Physical examination

There are no specific examination findings of this other than the localized tenderness. If the athlete has recently finished a brisk workout and is sore, the pain can be elicited by grasping the heel and pronating and supinating the forefoot.

Biomechanics

This may occur in any foot which has ligament laxity. If the 'cutting' motion or lateral motion produces increased mobility at the midtarsal joints (either Lisfranc or Chopart), a capsulitis or synovitis may occur.

Treatment

Anything which decreases motion at the midfoot

area will be adequate. Some athletes prefer to support the foot with circumferential taping of the longitudinal arch. A rigid sole in the athletic shoe or semiflexible orthoses will also solve this problem.

HINDFOOT

A large number of problems associated with the hindfoot are caused by various sporting activities. In our general orthopaedic clinic the heel complaints caused by sports injuries accounted for 39%. Running constituted the greatest number at 76%, while racquet sports caused 9%, basketball 5%, soccer 4% and the remaining sports 6%.

The major problems in the hindfoot fall into a series of well defined groups: plantar fasciitis, calcaneal bursitis, median calcaneal neuritis, fat pad shear syndrome, Achilles tendinitis, Achilles bursitis and calcaneal apophysitis. A series of other terms which are less distinct and anatomically less definable should be discouraged in literature; they include terms such as heel spur, runners' heel, calcaneal exostosis and calcaneal spur.

Plantar fasciitis

The pain in this area is generally well defined (Fig. 48.4). Individuals usually have pain with sport which may be worse after the activity is completed. In the early stages the only problem may be difficulty early in the morning when first stepping on the floor. The complaints are similar anatomically to the heel pain seen in nonathletes.

Physical examination

A hyperpronated foot was present in 52% of the people with these problems and a supinated foot (cavovarus) in 42%. A neutral foot was present in only 6%. Examination showed a very distinct area of pain localized at the plantar fascia insertion to the calcaneus, usually on the medial side.

Biomechanics

A combination of hindfoot rigidity and excessive forefoot supination can account for the problem in the cavus foot, in which there is additional pull on the plantar fascia through the 'windlass effect'

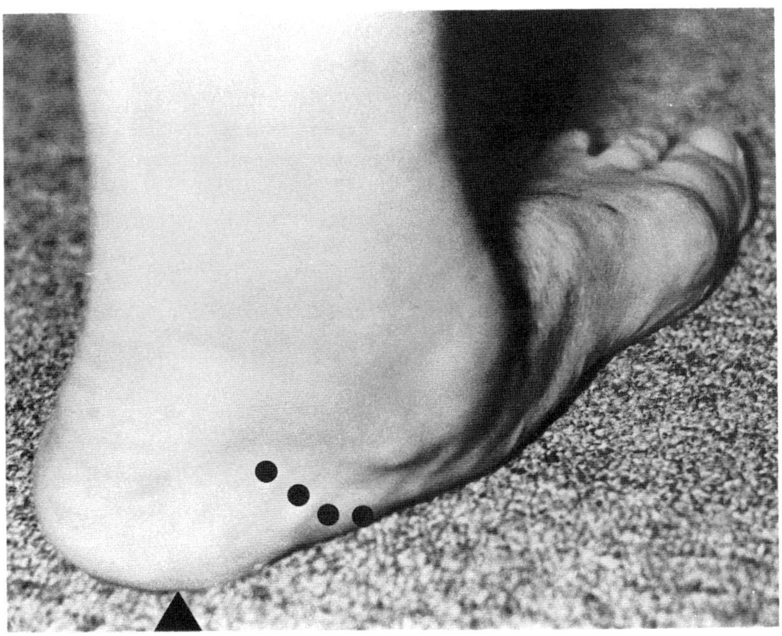

Fig. 48.4 Hyperpronated foot. Dotted line shows medial calcaneal neuritis pain. Triangle is approximate area of plantar fasciitis

producing an inflammation at its bony insertion. In the pronated foot the same mechanics apply.

Treatment

The use of an orthosis to prevent forefoot supination or pronation is necessary. Merely placing a soft pad, even when cut out, under the painful area will not solve the problem, but Sorbothane (polyurethane) shock absorbent pads have been helpful in plantar fasciitis.

Calcaneal bursitis (tuber calcaneal pain)

Most athletes with this problem have a supinated foot (46%), but 30% have a hyperpronated foot.

Physical examination

Examination most often reveals pain at the base of the heel over the tuber calcanei (Fig. 48.5). This is usually very well localized and extremely painful to touch, and is very frequently in a rigid foot with a forefoot which has limited supination.

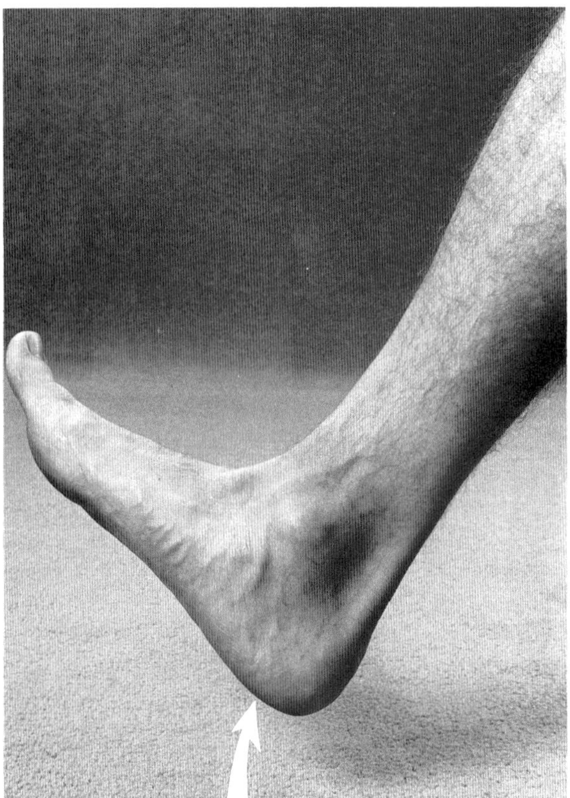

Fig. 48.5 Heel prior to impact. Arrow points to area of calcaneal bursa (tuber calcanei) pain

Biomechanics

The ability of the foot to pronate allows some of the force to be absorbed in the midtarsal joints and ligaments. When something is present which hinders the mechanics, an undue amount of stress is passed to the heel. The heel pad is an intricate biomechanical organ which is designed to dissipate stress. In a foot which is not supple, the force distributing effects of the heel pad do not work. This is especially important when one realizes that at each heel strike, 2½ times body weight passes through the foot.

Treatment

Treatment for this type of heel pain is by the addition of something which will absorb stress. A sports shoe with additional padding is sometimes all that is needed. The time honoured treatment of a heel pad with cutout will often be all that is needed.

Median calcaneal neuritis

Pain is felt along the line of the median calcaneal nerve on the inner side of the heel (Fig. 48.4). The injury can occur in any sport, but straight running produces it most often. Lateral motion or medium impact sports do not produce the injury with the same frequency because the number of heel strike repetitions is less.

Physical examination

There is pain along the median calcaneal nerve which may have an associated positive Tinel's sign. Most individuals have some foot hyperpronation and it is rarely seen in a cavovarus foot.

Biomechanics

During pronation a traction process occurs in which the tissue of the medial side of the foot is pulled downward. It is felt by some that there is an entrapment phenomenon in the abductor hallucis as the nerve penetrates to the depth of the foot.

Treatment

Initially, treatment should prevent abnormal motion by an orthosis. A medial longitudinal arch support is usually all that is needed. Injection of steroids along the course of the nerve is warranted occasionally and only rarely is a surgical release needed. Surgery entails neurolysis of the nerve and myotomy of the abductor hallucis.

Fat pad syndrome

The initial symptom is a diffuse pain occurring early in sporting activity when the individual is not fit. It occurs in high and medium impact sports. Diffuse pain is present over the entire heel pad.

Physical examination

Generally pain is not deep or localized and is present immediately after the sport activity. Pain is elicited by motion of the heel pad.

Biomechanics

The shearing of the fat pad when abnormal motion occurs is most likely the cause of the problem. This is probably inflammatory and not a purely mechanical problem.

Treatment

The use of a well supported shoe with the heel cup and soft heel will generally solve this problem.

Achilles tendinitis

This is a very frequent complaint in all sports, presenting as an overuse type of injury. Often the individual will relate difficulties running up hills or on uneven surfaces. Individuals with a laterally inserted tendon and a valgus heel are often susceptible. Of note is the fact that there does not appear to be a correlation of Achilles tendinitis and Achilles tendon rupture. The corollary is that individuals with Achilles tendon ruptures generally experience this as an acute episode during a sport without antecedent problems.

Physical examination

There may be pain, point tenderness, crepitus, or medial swelling. Pain is generally present anywhere from the insertion to the muscle tendinous junction.

Biomechanics

Of interest in Achilles tendinitis is the fact that there is direct correlation between flexibility, training, and Achilles tendinitis. Individuals with a 'tight' Achilles tendon may develop inflammation as a result of minimal overpull. Individuals who embark on a running type of training programme will develop tendinitis if stretches are not done with increased training. This is presumably due to the lack of flexibility that occurs as the muscle hypertrophies and strengthens.

Treatment

One must be able to perform stretching exercises and if the inflammation is too severe, then it must be reduced by conservative means. Once this is done both the superficial and deep tendon must be stretched. Usually performance of a set of stretches is not enough and the use of a negative heel shoe is recommended for nonplaying times. This works by placing a gentle, prolonged stretch on the heel cord. A small heel lift is used during actual sport to remove stress on the tendon. It must not be used for walking without the sport shoe. The use of an orthosis decreases the valgus component at the subtalar joint.

Surgery is rarely needed, but when a tendon has been inflamed for a prolonged time, the sheath may become constricted and tendinitis occurs each time vigorous activities are begun after rest. A simple division of the tendon sheath is performed, allowing the individual to return to activities soon after skin healing. Occasionally a nodule is found which is a degenerated nodule or an old partial rupture. This needs to be oversewn and occasionally supported with a plantaris graft.

Achilles bursitis

This occurs in much the same sports and with the same mechanism as Achilles tendinitis. It is generally the precalcaneal bursa or retrocalcaneal bursa which becomes inflamed.

Physical examination

Examination is important to differentiate bursitis from tendinitis. Careful palpation of the tendon area can elicit tenderness or peritendon pain separate from bursal pain.

Biomechanics

This is the same as for Achilles tendinitis.

Treatment

Anti-inflammatories, rest and heel lifts generally are used. The sports shoe should be stretched over the area of pain. Occasionally a steroid injection is indicated, but must be done with care, avoiding entry into the Achilles tendon sheath.

Calcaneal apophysitis

Heel pain which is present in the young athlete should be differentiated from Achilles tendinitis. Calcaneal apophyseal pain is obviously self limited when closure of the apophysis occurs. X-rays of the area are not helpful since they often show a sclerotic looking apophysis on the symptomatic contralateral side. This is not an osteochondritis and should not be elevated to the level of diagnosis by the application of an eponym.

Physical examination

There is point tenderness at the calcaneal insertion of the Achilles tendon. Occasionally there may be signs of inflammation.

Treatment

Generally rest, anti-inflammatories and heel elevation are used. In contrast to bursitis, these individuals do not need injection. Apophysitis is generally a self limited process.

BIBLIOGRAPHY

Baker B T 1979 Foot orthotic devices to modify selected aspects of lower extremity mechanics. Am J Sports Med 7(6): 338–341

Blechschmidt 1982 The structure of the calcaneal padding. Foot Ankle 2(5): 260–283

Edwards C A 1981 Orthopedic Shoe Technology for the Orthopedic Shoe Technician, Precision Printing Company, Muncie, Indiana.

Gould N 1983 Hyperpronation and pes planus in the adult. Clin Ortho 181: 37–45

Lutter L 1981 Cavus foot in runners. Foot Ankle 1(4): 225–228

Lutter L 1980 Injuries in runners and joggers. Minn Med 63: 45–51

Mann R, Baxter D, Lutter L 1981 Running Symposium. Foot Ankle 4: 190– 224

Simon L 1979 Le pied du sportif. Masson 1: 135–167

G. James Sammarco

The foot and ankle in dancers

Dance is a predetermined set of steps through space usually accompanied by music. It is an art form which requires the conditioning of a high performance athlete. This special consideration elevates sport to its ultimate level, that of a fine art. There are several types of dance including classical ballet and modern dance as well as folk, jazz and variety dancing of musical shows. Dance may have begun as religious ritual in prehistoric time, but through history it has become an expression of reverence, joy and man's emotion.

The foot and ankle have determined the nature and style of dance. Certain conditions of the foot have caused changes in technique, such as the development of 'ballon' created to hide its inventor's foot deformity. This chapter deals with conditions determining the shape and development of the dancer's foot and ankle, as well as static conditions which affect style and technique throughout his career. Acute conditions including fractures and sprains are included as well as overuse syndromes.

The dancer is a highly motivated, goal-oriented person. To achieve the special body shape required for dance, a diet approaching starvation in calorie content may be chosen (Calabrese & Kirkendall 1983). This unusual behavior may be compounded by an 'artistic personality' which may include an affective disorder (Jamison 1985). The physician must be aware of these special conditions in dealing with these fine artists since rapport is essential in achieving the dancer's compliance to treatment.

TRAINING

Young dancers choose their vocation and hobby for a variety of reasons. The young girl often begins dancing at the age of 5 or 6 years. For the first several years classes are taken once or twice a week. As interest and proficiency develop, she is advanced to more difficult steps. When the child has developed strength, poise, balance and maturity and has mastered the basic steps of ballet, she is permitted to begin dancing 'sur les pointes', that is on her toes. An appropriate toe shoe is chosen (Fig. 49.1). Although there is variation in maturity of young girls, this milestone in her training is seldom reached before the age of 11 or 12 years and requires at least three years of training. With some exceptions, young men begin dancing in their mid-teens. At this point, the foot may be somewhat stiffened and mature. Although dancing en pointe occasionally, male dancers generally stand on half pointe, on the ball of the foot.

The shape of the foot is important because it imparts an aesthetic sense of intent and motion as part of the profile position when the dancer stands in turnout. Artistic directors favour a foot with a high

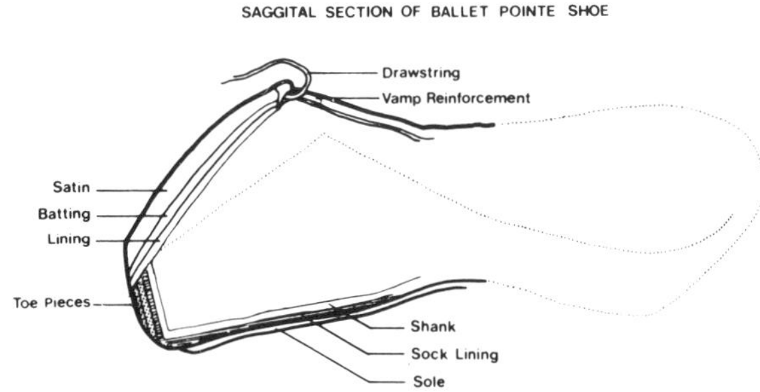

Fig. 49.1 The stiff box of the ballet pointe shoe is constructed of burlap and wheat paste. Layers of cardboard are used in the weight-bearing toe. A dancer may use two or three pairs during a single performance. The shoes are one shape only, not right and left. The foot molds the shoe shape

arch (Fig. 49.2). In fact, such a foot may be graded as a first or second degree cavus deformity by an orthopaedist. While such a high arched foot is often desired, some dancers may begin dancing with a depressed arch, valgus heels, or flexible pes planus. The classical barre is a dance programme designed in part to develop and maintain the dancer's arch. It is rare for the dancer to develop a well formed arch in less than six months. More often, two to three years are required (Nikolic & Zimmerman 1968, Pelipenko 1973).

FAULTS OF THE DANCER'S FOOT

For purposes of reference, certain faults are considered in this chapter. Though not pathological entities in themselves, they are aesthetically unacceptable and may predispose the dancer to injury (Ronconi 1983).

Knuckling down

This occurs when the young dancer has been advanced to pointe dancing before she is ready. The toes collapse inside the shoe and thus the fault may be missed by the teacher (Fig. 49.3). Subsequent strain and predisposition to injury occurs. Rarely, is one able to dance en pointe like this. Treatment includes restricting pointe dancing until the dancer is ready.

Rolling in

Rolling in is a condition whereby the medial longitudinal arch is flattened. Dancers with flexible

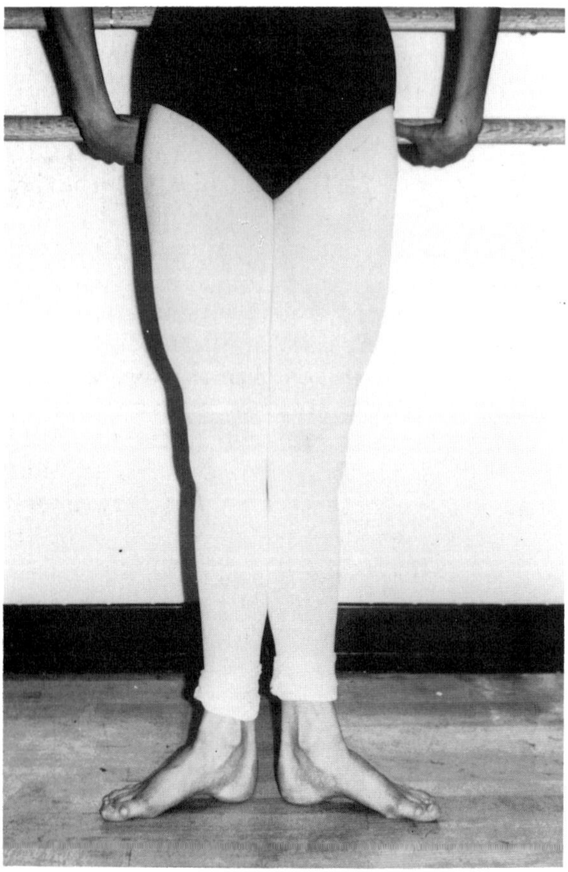

Fig. 49.2 Natural turnout at the hip and a high arch in the foot are desirable physical attributes for the classical ballet dancer

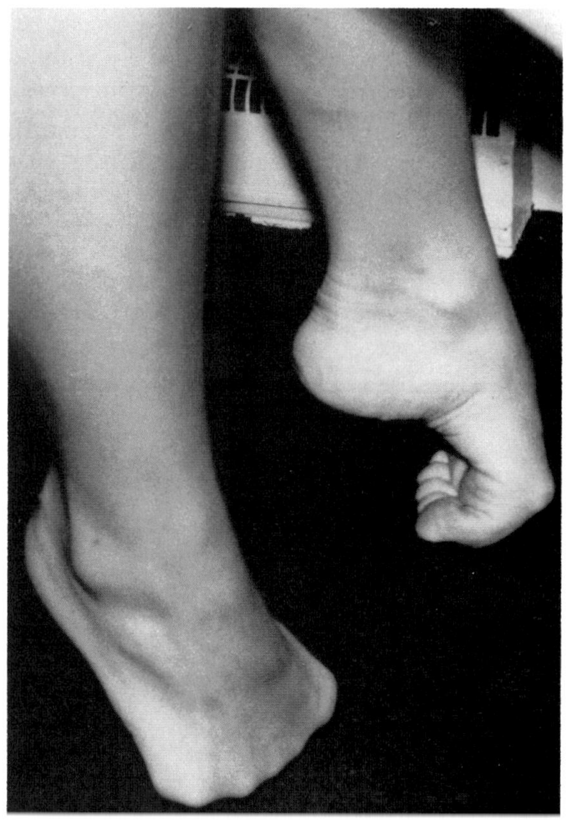

Fig. 49.3 Knuckling down: This dancer is able to demonstrate this 'fault' both in and out of her pointe shoe. If not corrected it usually leads to additional faults and injuries

pes planus unable to develop an arch often have this condition. Attempting to develop a turnout by placing the feet in external rotation rather than externally rotating the hips also strains the medial arch, causing it to flatten. This condition is remedied through correcting turnout technique.

Rolling out

Rolling out is a condition characterized by weight bearing along the lateral border of the foot, rolling the arch upward, sometimes lifting the ball of the foot from the floor. This often occurs as the dancer attempts to increase turnout while performing a grande plié.

Sickling

There are two forms of sickling, sickling in and sickling out. It can be produced with the foot weight bearing or non-weightbearing. Sickling in is an unaesthetic posturing of the foot with the heel pointed inward and the forefoot adducted (Fig. 49.4). It is caused by poor classical technique, a stiff foot or general fatigue, any one of which predispose the lateral foot and ankle to acute injury when the foot is placed in the weight-bearing position. Males who are affected often have begun dancing in late adolescence after the feet have matured and the joints of the midfoot have completed growth. Correction of this fault includes correcting technique which is the responsibility of the dancer and requires the help of a teacher or artistic director.

A foot may sickle out as the heel is brought into valgus and the forefoot is slightly abducted. In some recent classical techniques, it is considered a preferred positioning of the non-weightbearing foot in such dance positions as attitude or arabesque. In the weight-bearing foot, however, it is unaesthetic and can predispose to injury. An attentive teacher recognizes these positions and corrects them.

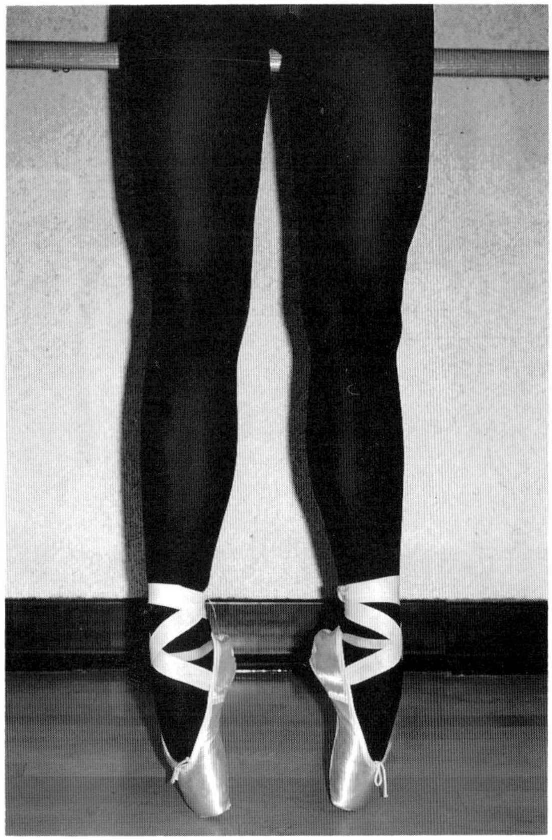

Fig. 49.4 Sickling in: The dancer is standing sur les pointes in first position demonstrating the fault. This can cause lateral ankle ligament strain as well as tendinitis and more severe injuries

ACUTE JOINT CONDITIONS

Ankle ligament injuries

The most common soft tissue injury of the dancer's ankle occurs to the lateral ligaments. As the dancer stands in the half pointe, that is demi pointe, position on the ball of the foot stability is maintained in the ankle (Fig. 49.5) (Hamilton 1982b). If through previous injury the anterior talofibular ligament is lax, it is predisposed to further injury. Acute injury occurs when returning from a leap or jump into the demi pointe position, usually inversion of the foot and ankle (Stojanovie et al 1963). The most common injury occurs at the anterior talofibular ligament. This may be accompanied by a tear of the fibulocalcaneal ligament. Usually such injuries are of grade I or grade II types. Initial treatment includes a compression dressing for 48 hours followed by early motion and a flexibility programme in an air splint. If a complete tear of one or more of the lateral ligaments occurs, a weight-bearing cast is applied and immobilization for three weeks is required. This is followed by an air cast and a power building flexibility programme. The air splint is worn for an

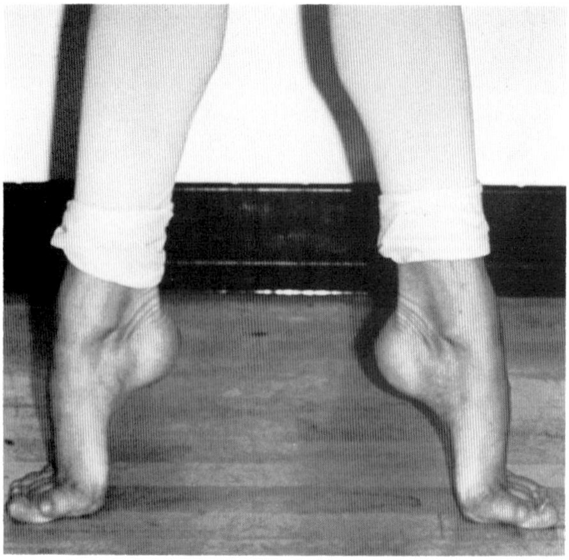

Fig. 49.5 Demi pointe position: The ankle is quite stable in this position (Courtesy: Hamilton W G 1982b)

additional four weeks but is removed at night and for bathing.

Acute third degree ligament injuries to the lateral ankle are uncommon but can be catastrophic. Cast immobilization for six weeks is recommended. Surgical intervention is reserved only for the most severe injuries since the risk of losing motion is high, particularly dorsiflexion, or 'foot flexion' in the dancer's jargon. The patient should be advised that loss of motion follows such a procedure and that a considerable period of time is required to regain complete flexibility.

A foot and ankle flexibility programme following removal of the cast can be performed even with the air splint applied. The dancer is taught to do special foot and ankle exercises at home.

Ligament injuries to the midfoot

These injuries occur at the dorsolateral ligaments of the tarsometatarsal joints by sudden inversion of the foot. They are mild and unless accompanied by avulsion fractures heal within several days. Compression dressing for the first 48 hours is recommended followed by whirlpool, the foot and ankle exerciser board and a flexibility programme. Oral analgesics for the first few days followed by anti-inflammatory medication is also prescribed.

Hyperflexion injury of the hallux

When landing from a leap the tip of the great toe may be caught on the floor, particularly if the toe of the shoe has been rosined (Sammarco & Miller 1979). This, associated with lack of coordination or fatigue, may produce an acute flexion injury of the hallux. Diagnosis includes sudden pain at the metatarsophalangeal joint which may then become red, swollen and tender dorsally and medially. Tenderness is not present at the sesamoids. X-rays fail to reveal fracture, but show soft tissue swelling. Treatment includes compression dressing, elevation and ice for the first 48 hours. The dressing is then removed and buddy taping the hallux to the second toe is performed as active range of motion in a whirlpool is started. A foot and ankle flexibility programme is instituted five days post injury. Limited barre exercises may be resumed as soon as the dancer is able to tolerate motion. The course of convalescence may take as long as three weeks but dancing may only be interrupted by symptoms of pain and stiffness.

ACUTE TENDON INJURIES

Acute injuries to dancers' tendons are related to sudden change of activity. The most common acute tendon condition is Achilles tendinitis. There are three areas where the tendon can be injured, (Sammarco 1982), the most common occurring 3 cm above the insertion of the tendon into the calcaneus. The onset of symptoms occurs after vigorous activity following a period of laying off where the dancer has not been diligent and has not done a flexibility programme on a daily basis. This condition is characterized by tenderness in an area approximately 3 to 4 cm behind and just above the ankle joint. Redness and swelling may be present. Classical ballet dancers secure their toe shoes to the foot with a broad ribbon above the ankle. The ribbon occasionally leaves a mark on the skin and the swelling around these ribbon marks should not be confused with tendinitis. Achilles tendinitis occurs equally in both sexes. Treatment consists of daily supervised physical therapy including ultrasound, whirlpool, a foot and ankle exerciser board, anti-inflammatory medication and decreasing the work schedule until such time as the symptoms subside.

Complete rupture of the tendon carries a guarded prognosis unless the tendon is repaired and its length restored (Lynn 1966, Thomasen 1982).

Partial rupture at the musculotendinous junction of the Achilles tendon is less common. It occurs most often when landing from a leap. The injury occurs at the junction of the gastrocnemius with the thin splayed portion of the Achilles tendon. Tenderness is present in the posterior midcalf over the area of disruption. Swelling and decreased range of motion of the ankle secondary to pain are characteristic. Ecchymosis is rarely seen. No defect is palpable. Treatment includes a posterior plaster splint with compression dressing for a period of 48 hours after which the splint is removed and crutch ambulation is begun. Gentle stretching, ultrasound, whirlpool and anti-inflammatory medication are all important treatment modalities. The dancer may return to dancing within 14 to 21 days depending upon the severity of the tear and the symptoms. Flexibility programmes, such as stretching and conditioning including floor exercises, should not be interrupted since limited use of preconditioning may have been, in part, a cause of the condition. The water barre, ballet barre exercises performed in a pool with the dancer submerged chest deep, is an important adjunct to therapy. The sound leg is used as the 'leg of support' and the injured leg as the non-weight-bearing 'working leg'.

Partial avulsion of the tendo Achillis from the calcaneus occurs in young dancers whose epiphyseal growth plates are still open. Tenderness occurs at the insertion of the Achilles tendon, and is associated with redness and the inability to perform a plié. X-rays may or may not reveal a calcaneal apophysitis. Since these are usually young dancers, dance class may be interrupted until such time as symptoms subside. A ¾ in heel is recommended. The dancer may require crutches if walking is painful. A 'water barre' is also recommended. The entire barre exercise routine is performed without weight bearing on the injured part and with the elimination of gravity so that flexibility and conditioning may be maintained throughout the healing process.

Dancer's tendinitis

Tendinitis of the flexor hallucis longus tendon, called dancer's tendinitis, often occurs after a change in dance technique or following long rehearsals (Hamilton 1977). It is characterized by pain in the posterior ankle and difficulty standing in demi pointe. Symptoms are insidious in onset over several days. The differential diagnosis must include posterior impingement syndrome although such symptoms occur over a longer period of time. The tendon is irritated as it passes posterior to the ankle through its pulley on the posterior and inferior aspect of the talus. There is tenderness in this region and crepitus may be palpable. Pain is elicited by actively flexing and extending the ankle. Treatment includes some restriction of dance activity, anti-inflammatory medication and foot and ankle exerciser board with a flexibility programme until symptoms subside. Dancing may then be increased as tolerated.

Tendinitis of the peroneus longus and brevis tendons occurs at the lateral malleoleus and lateral hindfoot. This, too, occurs as a result of improper conditioning particularly during laying off periods. It is characterized by swelling and tenderness posterior to the lateral malleolus and may be associated with redness. The peroneus longus tendon, in particular, may be tender as it passes from the lateral to the inferior borders of the cuboid toward its insertion at the medial plantar aspect of the foot. The differential diagnosis includes apophysitis of the 5th metatarsal or avulsion of the peroneus brevis tendon from its insertion. Treatment, as with other tendinitides of the ankle, includes anti-inflammatory medication and a light compression dressing, foot and ankle exerciser board and reduction of dance activity until symptoms subside. An elastic adhesive dressing may be worn about the ankle and foot during rehearsal, but not during a performance because it is unaesthetic (Fig. 49.6).

Tendinitis of the extensor tendons of the foot

Tendinitis in the anterior compartment is uncommon. When it does occur it is treated as tendinitis elsewhere.

FRACTURES AND DISLOCATIONS

Fractures of the ankle

Fractures of the ankle in dancers are caused by

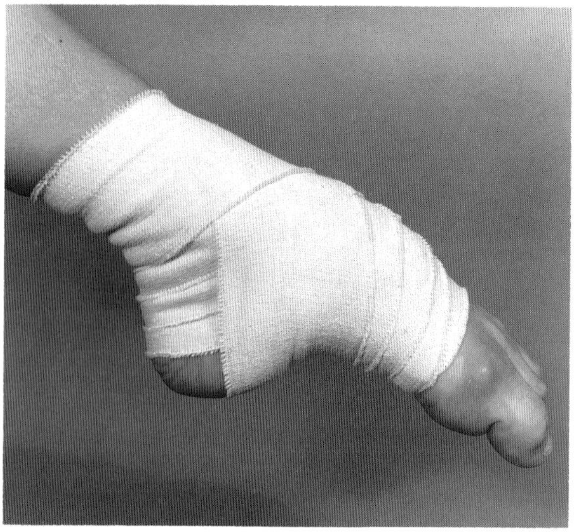

Fig. 49.6 Elastic adhesive strapping of the ankle and hindfoot enables the dancer with tendinitis to attend classes and rehearsals while undergoing treatment

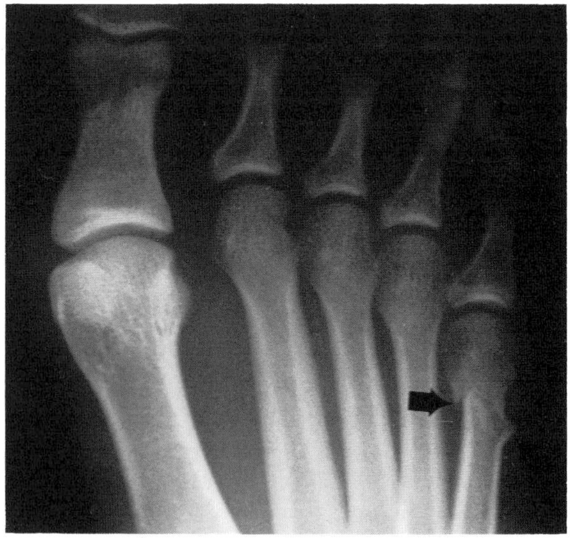

Fig. 49.7 Fracture of the distal 5th metatarsal: This is the most common fracture of the foot in dancers. It may take several months to heal

sudden inversion or eversion of the joint. Fatigue, dancing beyond one's technical ability or unsupervised horseplay can contribute to these injuries. Fractures medially or laterally, as well as fracture dislocations can occur. Immediate anatomic reduction of displaced fractures is an important aspect of treatment. If anatomic reduction cannot be obtained by closed methods, open reduction is recommended. Range of motion of the ankle, particularly in dorsiflexion, 'foot flexion' in dancers' jargon, is decreased with fracture and surgery. The dancer must be advised of this consequence prior to surgery since all forms of dance require full range of motion of the ankle in both dorsiflexion and plantarflexion. Asymmetrical plié due to a stiff ankle is a difficult postoperative sequel to treat. It may affect the dancer's career.

Fractures in the foot

The most common fracture in the dancer's foot occurs in the 5th metatarsal (Fig. 49.7). It is usually caused from an inversion injury, when the dancer is tired or lands improperly from a leap (Sammarco 1984). The fracture occurs at the neck of the metatarsal. Since the foot may be placed in a ballet pointe shoe proper reduction is important. If anatomic reduction cannot be achieved by closed methods open reduction may be indicated. The dancer should be counselled as to the length of time required to heal such fractures; this may be five months. This healing time may be necessary with or without surgery due to the nature of the fracture and stresses in the bone.

Fractures at the base of the 5th metatarsal occur more commonly in nonprofessional dancers (Jones 1902). These are also caused by inversion of the foot. Avulsion of the peroneus brevis tendon from the styloid of the 5th metatarsal also tends to be uncommon in the professional dancer (Fig. 49.8). This may be treated by a compression dressing or cast, depending on the comfort required, and ambulation with crutches. Fractures at the base of the 5th metatarsal may take up to five months to heal and the dancer should be so advised.

FRACTURES AND DISLOCATIONS OF THE TOES

Acute fractures

Acute fractures of the toes are uncommon as are dislocations. The most common dislocation occurs at the metatarsophalangeal joints of the lesser toes, usually the second and third toes. Often the dancer strikes a piece of scenery when leaving a brightly lit stage into the dark wings. Treatment includes a gentle manipulation after infiltration with local

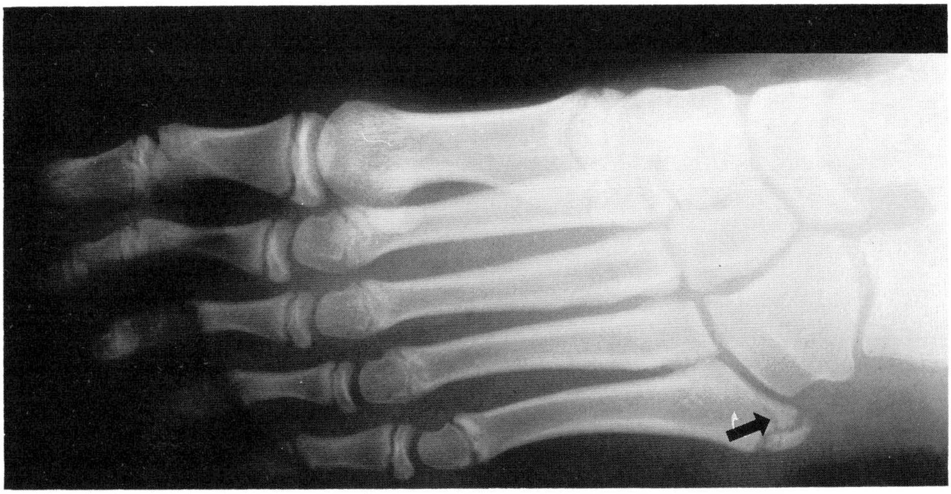

Fig. 49.8 Avulsion fracture of the 5th metatarsal styloid in a dancer whose apophysis has not yet closed. This fracture is uncommon in professional dancers

anaesthetic, a compression dressing and buddy taping. The patient may return to limited dancing shortly after removal of the compression dressing. The post injury programme includes whirlpool, foot and ankle exerciser board and power building of the foot and leg.

Fractures occur when the dancer is barefoot or wearing a soft ballet shoe leaving the toes unprotected. 1% lidocaine anaesthesia is used for reduction. Buddy taping to the adjacent toe or toes is necessary to maintain reduction. A compression dressing is then applied for a period of 10 days after which the dressing is removed, buddy taping applied, and active range of motion is permitted to tolerance.

Patients with fractures of the phalanges should be restricted from dancing for three weeks. However, a flexibility rehabilitation programme and water barre may be continued with the injured part as the working leg, that is the non-weightbearing leg. Floor exercises, that is non-weightbearing dance exercises, are also prescribed.

Fractures of the sesamoid

Acute fractures of the sesamoid bone occur when landing from a leap (Fig. 49.9). As with most acute injuries they are the result of fatigue, poor training or horseplay. They are treated with a ⅜ in horseshoe-shaped felt pad and a compression dressing until symptoms begin to subside, approximately two to three weeks (Sammarco & Miller 1982b). Following this healing period dancing may be permitted using the felt pad around the fracture site to relieve pressure. Fractures occur with equal frequency both in the tibial and fibular sesamoids. They tend to occur more frequently in males.

CONDITIONS OF SOFT TISSUE

Plantar fasciitis

Occasionally after a dancer has neither danced nor performed a flexibility programme during a period of laying off, plantar fasciitis may develop within the first ten days of class. Such symptoms include pain in the plantar aspect of the midfoot which is tender on palpation and increases when the dancer stands in the demi pointe, or half pointe, position. Treatment includes anti-inflammatory medication, elevation, slow stretching exercises and a warm shower prior to dance class. If symptoms persist for more than two to three weeks, a flexible arch support is recommended to be placed in character shoes and ballet shoes. This cannot be used in a ballet pointe shoe.

OVERUSE SYNDROMES

Stress fractures

Stress fractures are common in dancers particularly in the leg and the foot (Burrows 1956, Devas 1975,

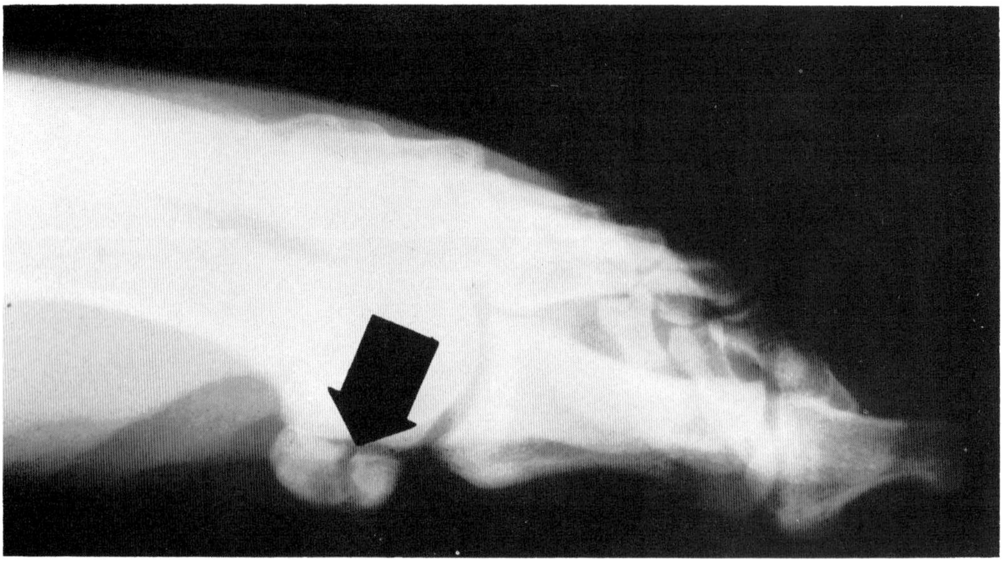

Fig. 49.9 Sesamoid fracture: Caused by landing from a leap on the ball of the foot. This is treated with a felt pad surrounding the sesamoid, relieved in the centre, for a period of three weeks

Howse 1972, Schneider et al 1974, Wilcox et al 1977). They are often multiple and bilateral and may take a considerable period of time to diagnose. Factors contributing to the development of stress fractures include the age and technical proficiency of the dancer, technique, the type of dance shoe worn and the floor of the studio or stage (Mann 1975, Seals 1983). The mechanics of stress fracture development are as well known as the chronicity of symptoms. Stress fractures develop over several weeks or months. Symptoms are subtle in onset and may at first present as diffuse ache or pain. Thereafter, the tenderness localizes over a specific area of the bone. Repeated examinations may be necessary to appreciate these subtle changes over a period of several weeks. Bone scan is important in diagnosis (Wilcox et al 1977). The concentration of the radioactive phosphate activity is often seen within one month of symptom onset. Other diagnostic aids include the use of laminoroentgenograms and axial CT scans. The axial CT scan shows the stress fracture clearly whereas routine X-rays often do not.

Stress fractures of the tibia may take several months and even years to diagnose. They occur most commonly along the anterior border in the region of the tibial midshaft, and are often bilateral and multiple. Although early symptoms may include diffuse pain at the anterior tibia, within a few months tenderness localizes to a specific area. A bone scan confirms the presence of a stress fracture by concentration of radioactive material in the area of tenderness. Many later stress fractures may be visible on standard X-rays.

Treatment includes restriction of dance. Because symptoms have often been present for several months, the dancer must be counselled in the need for this important aspect of treatment. Crutch ambulation is necessary, and a cast may also be required if symptoms warrant. Although dance is restricted, water barre exercises are permitted as well as non-weightbearing floor exercises. The dancer performs the barre exercises submerged to chest level in a pool using the sound leg as the 'leg of support' and the injured leg as the 'working leg'. This modality provides conditioning by maintaining proprioception of the injured leg, coordination of muscles and maintaining strength while eliminating gravity on the injured part. Anti-inflammatory medication is an important therapeutic adjunct. The dancer is permitted to return to partial barre after symptoms have completely subsided. If a dancer resumes dancing too early symptoms will recur.

Stress fractures of the fibula are also common. The most common site of stress fracture is 10 cm above the lateral malleolus. These commonly occur in classical ballet dancers following performances and rehearsals on a hard unyielding floor, such as concrete. Treatment includes reducing activity, particularly weight bearing, while maintaining coordination and flexibility until healing occurs. Since symptoms may have been present for several months, the dancer must be counselled as to the healing time. Anti-inflammatory medication is an important adjunct to therapy. Such medications include Motrin®, Naprosyn®, etc. Dance should be restricted until healing is complete. Treatment also includes use of the water barre. Pain may persist even after healing has occurred and some patients have mild pain on resuming dance. The use of a transcutaneous nerve stimulation unit (TNS) has been suggested and may be effective in decreasing mild pain.

Stress fractures of specific areas

Tibia

Stress fractures of the tibia may be present for up to 18 months and symptoms may be present for up to two years prior to diagnosis (Sammarco 1984, Thomasen 1982). X-rays seldom reveal the presence of fractures early on, they may be visible after a year or more. These fractures occur in the anterior tibial shaft. They are often multiple and bilateral. Treatment may require restriction from dance for as long as six months.

Fibula

Stress fractures of the fibula can occur in two areas. The most common is 10 cm above the lateral malleolus (Fig. 49.10) (Sammarco 1982, 1984). Symptoms are usually present for a shorter period of time, about two months. Bone scan is important in localizing the presence of such a fracture. Treatment includes prohibiting the dancer from bearing full weight on the extremity, and an air cast and crutches are prescribed. Healing occurs approximately eight weeks after initiating therapy, during which time X-ray may reveal the presence of a transverse stress fracture at the area positive on bone scan.

The second common area of occurrence is in the proximal one-third of the fibular shaft. Rehabilitation is an important part of treatment and is discussed below.

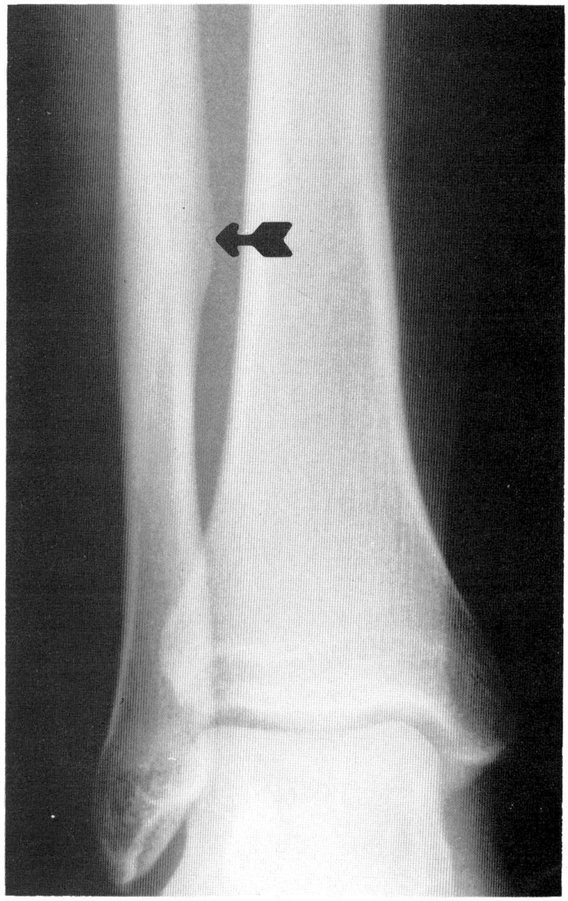

Fig. 49.10 Stress fracture of the fibula: It takes six weeks to become visible 10 cm above the lateral malleolus. A bone scan may be positive within two weeks of symptom onset

Metatarsals

Stress fractures of the foot occur most commonly in the proximal second and third metatarsals at the junction of the shaft and metaphysis (Collis & Jayson 1972, Manter 1946, Sammarco & Miller 1982a, Teitz et al 1985). Fractures of the base of the 5th metatarsal may present as stress fractures. Surgery has been recommended for these as well as for fractures of the tarsal navicular. The author has not found it necessary to perform surgery on stress fracture in the dancer. For persistent symptoms an external electrical bone simulator has been found to be effective but this treatment requires immobilization in a cast and, therefore, prolongs rehabilitation.

Tarsals

Stress fractures can also occur in the tarsal bones, the navicular or cuboid (Figs. 49.11 and 12). Because of the high stresses within the foot and various postures of the foot, symptoms tend to become disabling within a shorter period of time. Thus, a dancer with a stress fracture of the tarsal navicular may present for treatment with vague symptoms of medial foot pain two weeks to a month after symptoms begin. Since standard X-rays usually fail to detect fracture, bone scan is an important diagnostic tool (Figs. 49.13a and b). If the scan is positive, an axial computerized tomogram helps to delineate the actual fracture. Such fractures are incomplete and show fracture lines halfway through the bone. In addition to the treatment outlined above, a compression dressing is recommended for the first 10 days. This is followed by an elastic support stocking with weight bearing limited to toe touch on the affected side. The foot and ankle exerciser board is initiated along with a general rehabilitation programme only after symptoms have become minimal. Time of healing is often in excess of two months and rarely six to eight months.

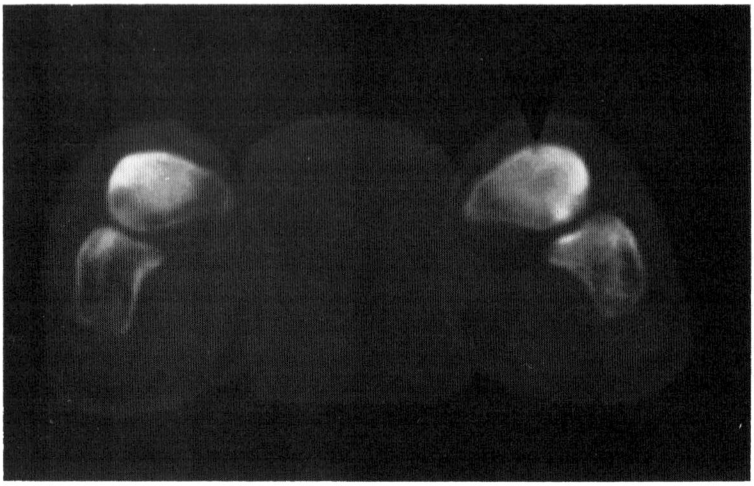

Fig. 49.11 Stress fracture of the navicular: Treated as tendinitis for three months prior to diagnosis. Treatment includes restricting dance for six weeks but permitting a 'water barre' and non-weightbearing floor exercises

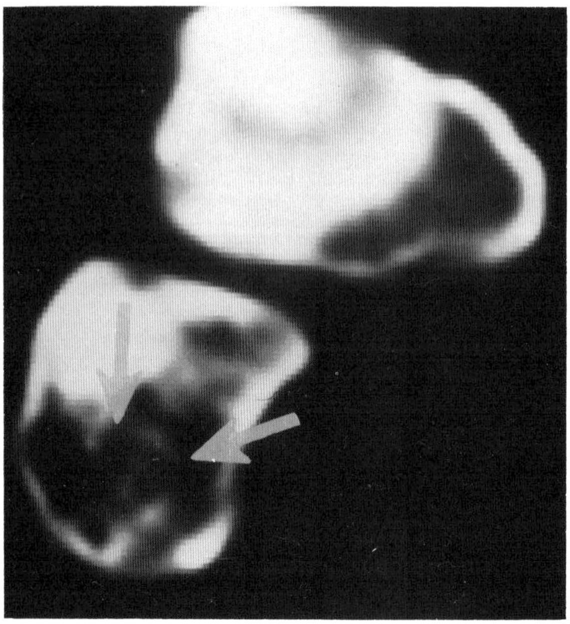

Fig. 49.12 Stress fracture of the cuboid: A rare fracture. Symptoms of lateral foot pain were present for four months prior to diagnosis. Treatment included foot and ankle board, water barre, and floor exercises. The patient remained away from the dance company for eight months

Phalanges

Stress fractures of the toes, although less common, take two to three months to elicit symptoms significant enough to require the dancer to seek medical attention (Fig. 49.14a and b). Specific treatment includes buddy taping and a compression dressing for 10 days to permit early healing prior to initiating the rehabilitation programme.

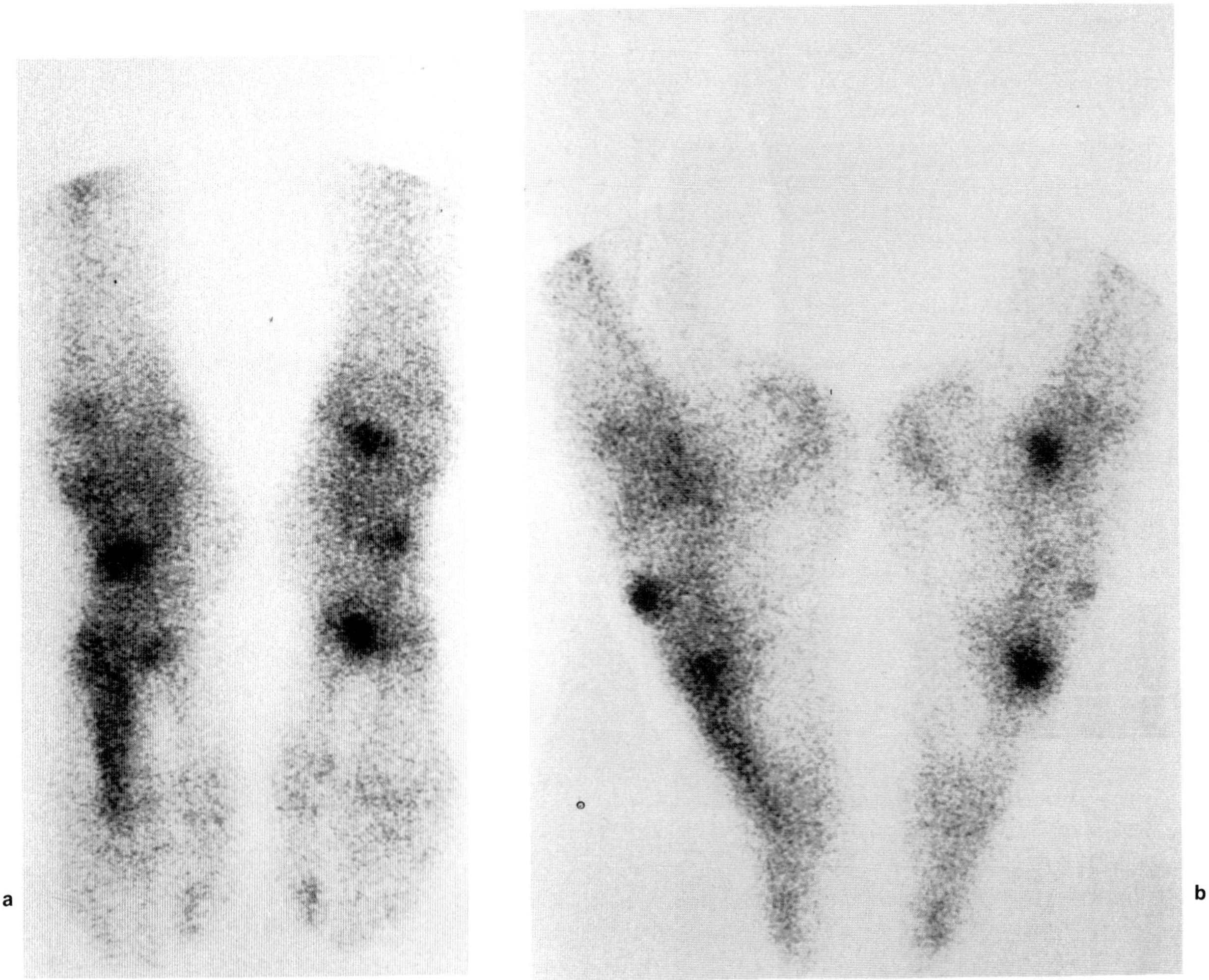

Figs. 49.13a and b Bone scan of feet in anteroposterior and lateral views showing stress fracture of left cuneiform and 'chip' fracture of right talonavicular joint. Decreased activity is seen in the right lateral foot as the dancer inadvertently favours the painful left foot

Sesamoids

Sesamoid fractures, including compression fractures, may have an insidious onset. Symptoms develop over several months or a year. Special X-ray views include lateral and oblique views of the sesamoids as well as tangential views (Fig. 49.15). A manoeuvre helpful in diagnosis is to apply pressure to the sesamoid with the hallux in neutral position, then extend the hallux drawing the sesamoid distally to see if the area of tenderness moves distally. In addition to a flexibility programme, treatment of such chronic compression fractures includes the use of a half inch thick felt pad shaped in a half moon with the central opening large enough to permit the tender area beneath the fracture to sit freely within it. This may be placed into any shoe and allows dancing while, at the same time, relieving pressure beneath the injured part. Symptoms subside within three to six weeks.

Trigger toe

Partial rupture of the flexor hallucis longus tendon occurs in the tendon tunnel as it passes posterior to the ankle joint and beneath the sustentaculum tali (Hamilton 1982a, Sammarco & Miller 1979).

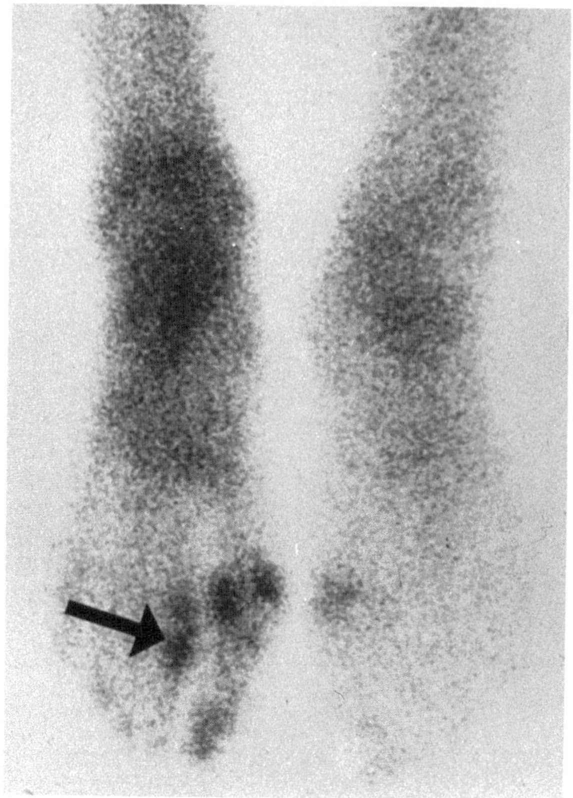

a

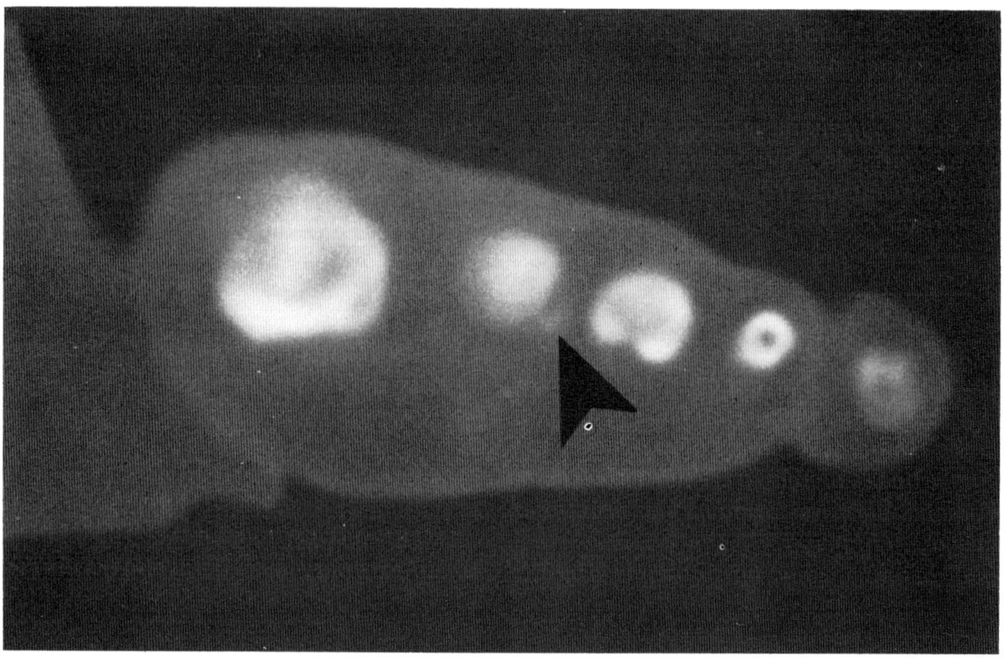

b

Fig. 49.14 a, Bone scan demonstrating stress fracture of the 2nd toe proximal phalanx. Symptoms were present for three months. This dancer had discontinued dancing; b, Same patient. Axial CT scan of left foot demonstrating bone chip at proximal portion of the proximal phalanx

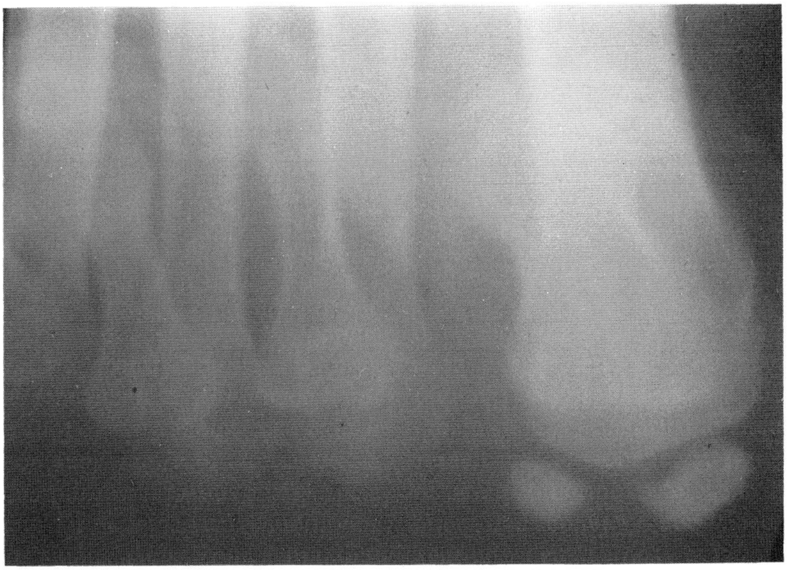

Fig. 49.15 Compression fracture of tibial sesamoid shown in tangential X-ray view of foot. Symptoms were present for 18 months

Symptoms include triggering of the hallux as the dancer rises from half pointe to full pointe position. The dancer feels a loss of strength in the foot. A snap then occurs as the tendon nodule pops into the tunnel and the dancer rises to full pointe (Figs. 49.16a and b). On descending from pointe, the toe remains flexed and pain occurs in the region of the tarsal tunnel until the nodule is snapped distally out of the tunnel. This snapping is palpable over the flexor hallucis longus tendon anterior to the Achilles tendon. It is caused by a chronic partial tear of the flexor hallucis longus (Fig. 49.17). The tendon fibres collapse on themselves in the tendon causing a fusiform thickening to form distally which then hangs up in the tendon tunnel. Treatment includes release of the tendon tunnel through a posteromedial incision at the ankle, shaving the swelling in the tendon and repair of the longitudinal tear in the tendon with 5–0 braided polyester suture. Physical therapy is started within three days, weight bearing at five days, and a full rehabilitation programme within two weeks. It may take several months before the dancer is able to return to a pre-injury level.

CHRONIC JOINT INJURIES

Ankle

The dancer spends a considerable period of time standing on demi pointe, that is, half pointe position on the ball of the foot. In this position, stability of the ankle is achieved through the bony malleoli as well as the posterior deltoid ligaments and laterally through the posterior talofibular ligament and fibulocalcaneal ligament. This unusual posturing for prolonged periods at the limits of the normal range of motion contributes to stretching of the ankle ligaments. This increases joint laxity. In addition, poor technique and fatigue are important factors in lack of control in the foot and ankle.

Laxity of the ankle joint is common in dancers because a complete range of motion is used. The ankle owes its stability both to its shape and to the multiplicity of ligaments attached to the medial and lateral malleoli (Sammarco et al 1973). The most common chronic condition is laxity of the anterior talofibular ligament which may be associated with chronic synovitis. Standard stress X-rays may not reveal such a condition. Performing an anterior drawer manoeuvre, holding the tibia firmly and pulling the heel forward reveals the asymptomatic subluxation of the tibiotalar joint. Such a condition is not treated unless symptomatic (Figs. 49.18a and b). Chronic synovitis on the other hand may be present for periods greater than a year and may be accompanied by chronic pain with motion, particularly with the dancer standing in demi pointe on the ball of the foot. The pain may be disabling; in

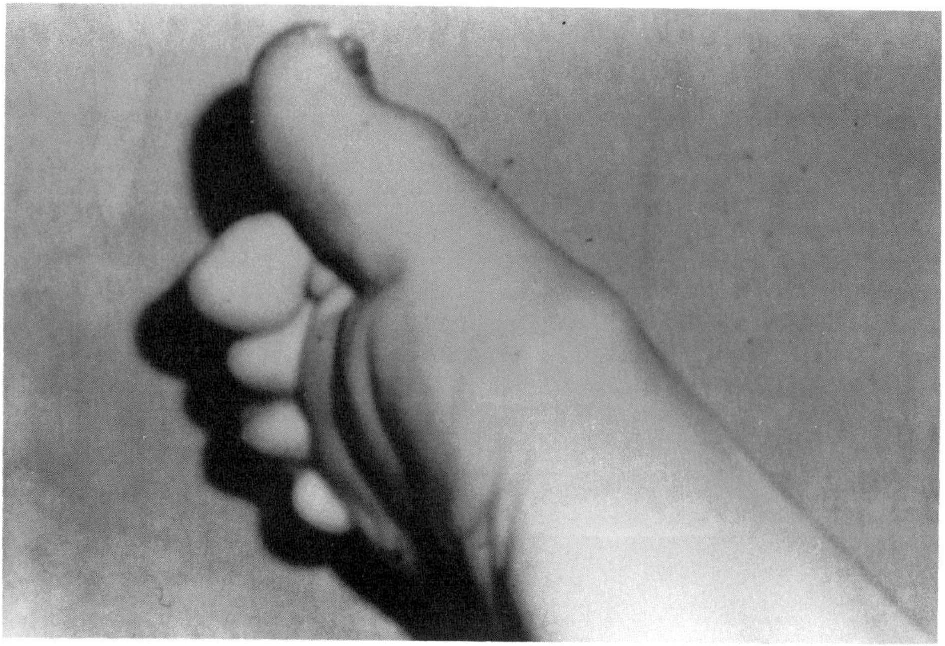

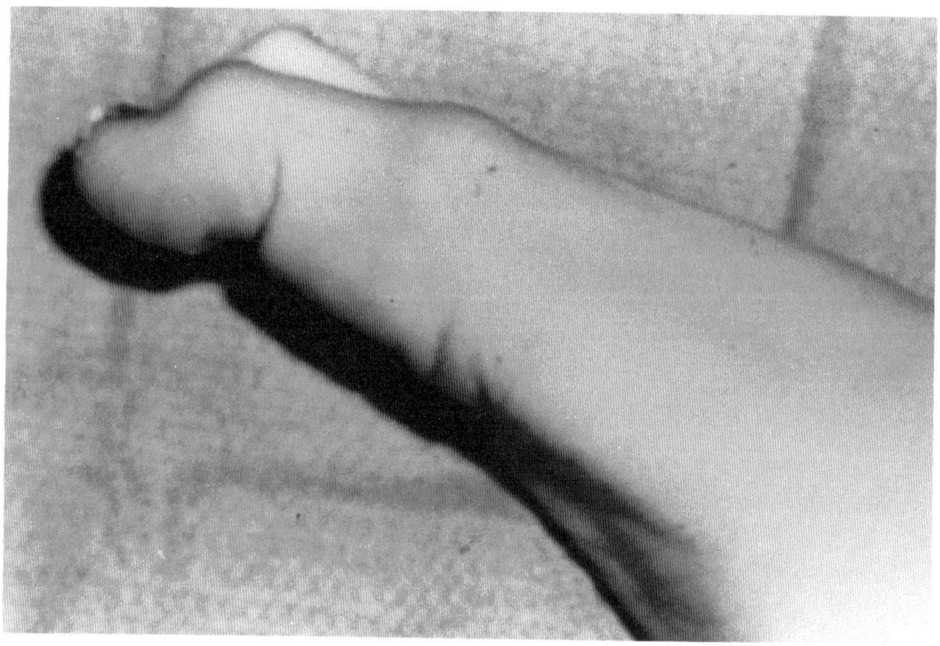

Fig. 49.16 Trigger toe: The toe remains extended as the dancer attempts to pointe the foot. The tendon nodule lies distal to the canal and hangs up giving a feeling of weakness in the foot and pain in the ankle. The tendon then snaps into the canal as the dancer attains pointe position; When the dancer extends the ankle and foot, the distal phalanx flexes because the flexor hallucis longus tendon cannot slide distally. Snapping and pain occur at the ankle as the tendon nodule is passively pulled distal

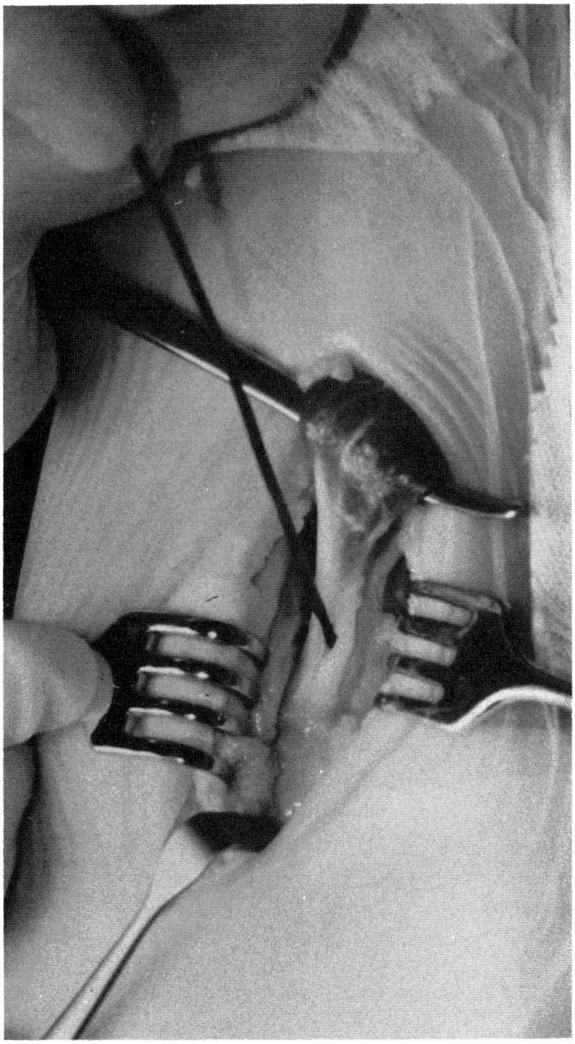

Fig. 49.17 Trigger toe: Operative photograph showing chronic tear in the flexor hallucis longus tendon. A fusiform thickening is present distally

fact painful enough to terminate a young dancer's career (Sammarco 1984).

As with all chronic conditions, the psychological aspect of the dancer is important. The dancer may blame a mild chronic condition for his or her inability to perform sophisticated dance steps required for advancement. Treatment of symptomatic ankle laxity includes a flexibility and power building programme with a foot and ankle exerciser board along with instruction and reinforcement so that the program is continued daily after symptoms subside. Surgical intervention, such as ligament reconstruction and debridement, should be considered only when all other treatment modalities have failed. The dancer must be counselled as to the risks of surgery since reduced motion of the ankle particularly in dorsiflexion may result. The dancer requires full dorsiflexion of the ankle in all forms of dance and ill advised surgery may result in an asymmetrical plié, a step used in all dance. Such a result is unaesthetic and requires a change in the dancer's style and technique.

Anterior and posterior impingement of the ankle

Impingement of the ankle may occur anteriorly or posteriorly. Posterior impingement occurs when the dancer stands on demi pointe, that is half pointe (Howse 1982, Quirk 1982). The tibia impinges against the calcaneus posteriorly as the dancer stands with the ankle positioned at the limits of plantar flexion. Symptoms include stiffness, a feeling of fullness and pain at the posterior ankle deep to the tendo Achillis. A differential diagnosis includes os trigonum syndrome, tendinitis in the flexor hallucis longus tendons, trigger toe and rarely, a synovial cyst. Treatment includes anti-inflammatory medications, a flexibility programme and use of the foot and ankle exerciser board. The symptoms subside in two to three months. Improving technique is an important adjunct to therapy.

Os trigonum syndrome

The os trigonum is present in approximately 8% of the normal population. In the dancer this is of particular significance since impingement of this bone can occur between the tibia and calcaneus. In fact, it may be fractured (Fig. 49.19). Healing of the fracture may cause the bone to enlarge inhibiting the dancer's ability to stand on half pointe. Primary treatment of this condition is similar to that of simple impingement syndrome. However, if asymmetry on half pointe is present with pain resistant to conservative treatment, excision through a small medial incision is recommended (Hamilton 1982a, Quirk 1983, Sammarco 1982, 1984). A compression dressing is applied postoperatively and gentle active stretching is begun within the first 48 hours. A flexibility programme is begun in the immediate postoperative period. The patient is advanced to

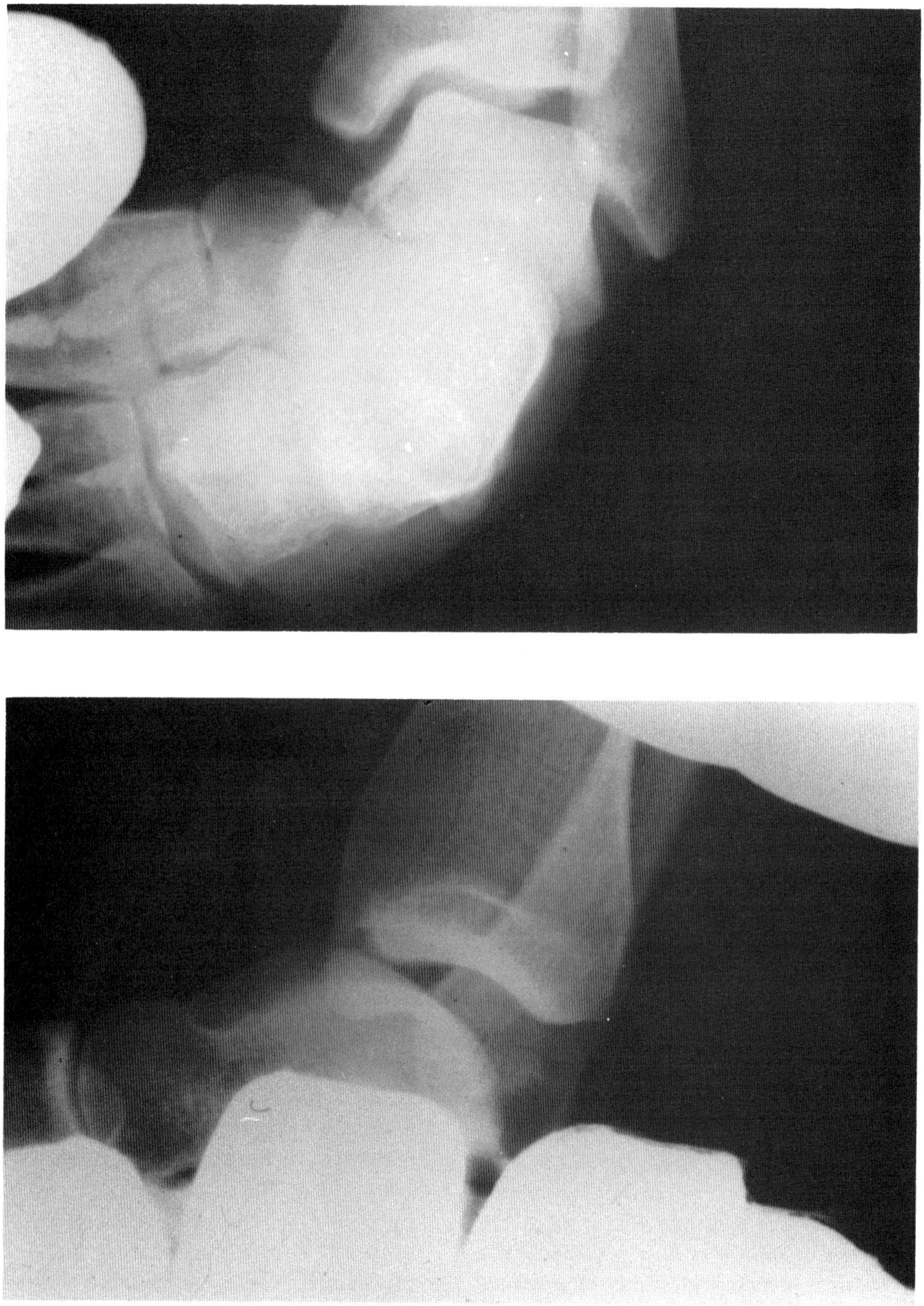

a

b

Fig. 49.18 Ankle ligament laxity: a, Inversion stress in this dancer fails to show instability; b, Same dancer. An anterior drawer sign is easily demonstrable. The dancer is asymptomatic and requires no treatment

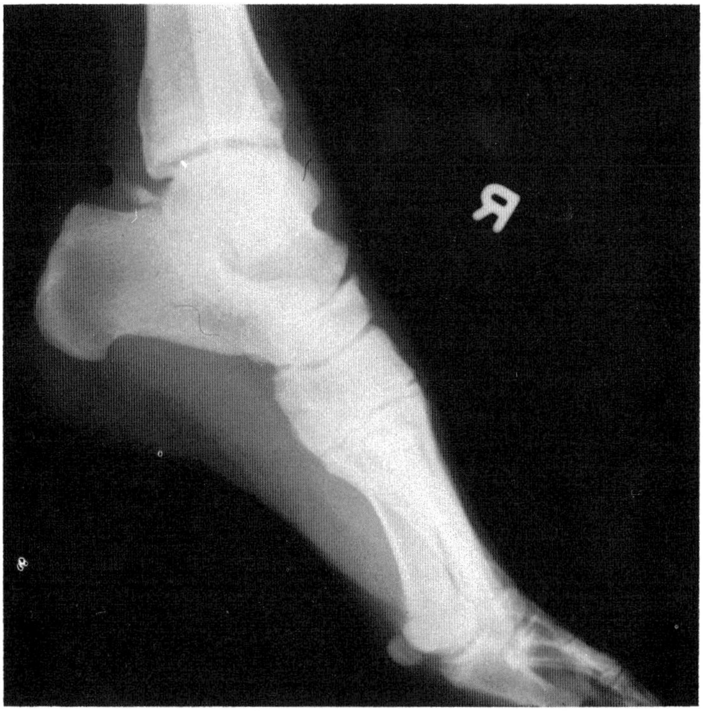

Fig. 49.19 Os trigonum syndrome: The accessory bone is pinched between the tibia and calcaneus when the dancer stands in the half pointe position

barre exercises using the operated leg as the working leg and the sound limb as the leg of support. A full dance schedule may be resumed as symptoms warrant. If stiffness of the ankle persists beyond three weeks, closed manipulation under general anaesthesia should be considered.

Anterior impingement syndrome

Grande plié, that is, bending deeply at the knees while standing at the ballet barre, is used primarily in barre exercises. Demi plié, bending the knee halfway, is common to all forms of dance. In classical ballet symmetry in this position is an important aesthetic quality. Anterior impingement syndrome occurs when the ankle is dorsiflexed as the dancer performs a demi plié forcing the anterior tibia against the neck of the talus (Kleiger 1982). The synovium is pinched between the bones causing symptoms of swelling, tenderness and a decrease in range of motion secondary to pain. Over the years, osteophytes form at the opposing surfaces and are seen best on lateral X-ray of the ankle (Fig. 49.20). Conservative treatment includes the use of anti-inflammatory medication and a flexibility programme along with the foot and ankle exerciser board. Symptoms should subside within six to eight weeks. Surgical excision of the osteophyte can be performed through a small anteromedial incision if necessary.

Uncommon conditions in dancers include the development of cysts. Symptoms may persist for several months prior to diagnosis particularly in the subtalar joint (Fig. 49.21). Treatment for these cysts is surgical excision through a lateral incision. Such problems are rare and the dancer should be counselled as to the prolonged recovery, the possibility of stiffness and also the altering of dance style. Injections of corticosteroid preparations into the dancer's joints and tendons is not recommended. Inadvertent injection into a tendon may simply dissolve it, risking rupture. The formation of sterile abscess of the tendon sheath is also not uncommon after steroid injection.

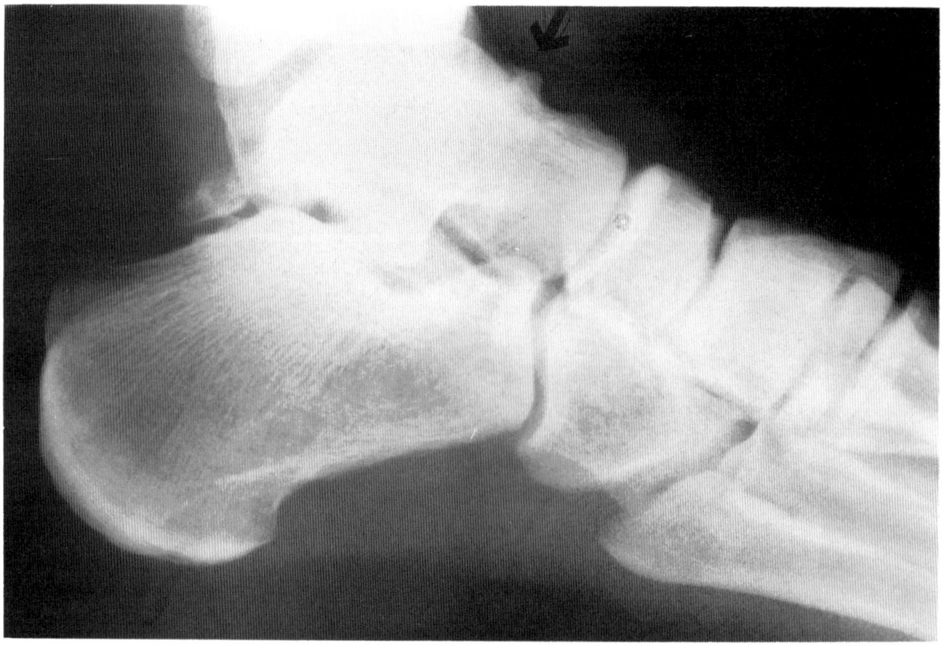

Fig. 49.20 Anterior impingement syndrome: Full dorsiflexion is a necessity in all dance. Painful osteophytes may form resulting in loss of motion and asymmetry on stage. Treatment includes arthroscopic excision of the osteophytes. Note that this dancer has an asymptomatic os trigonum

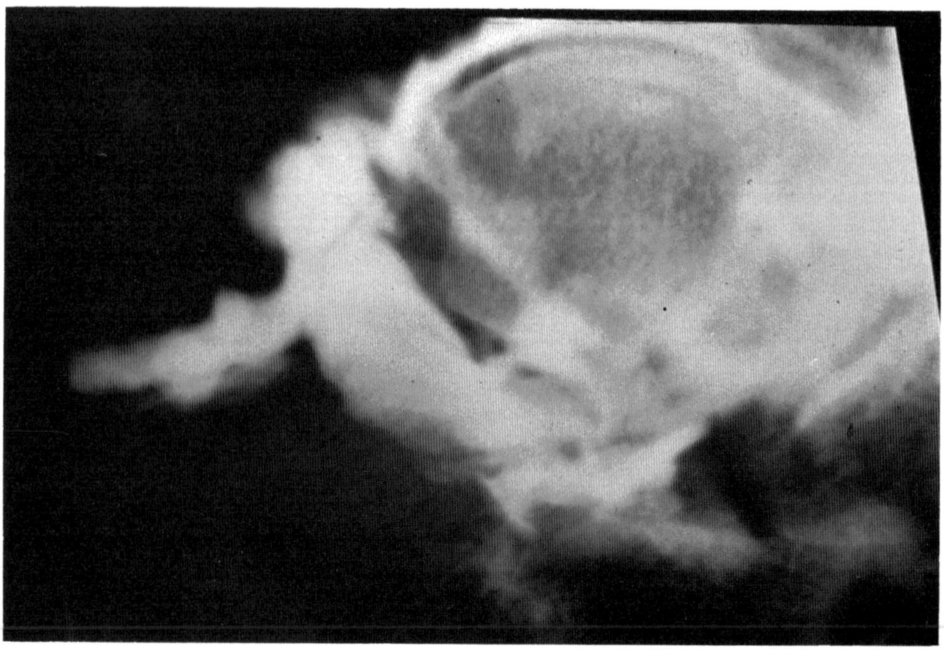

Fig. 49.21 Cyst of the posterior facet of the subtalar joint: A rare condition with symptoms present for four months. Surgical excision relieved symptoms. The dancer returned to a full dance schedule three months post surgery

Chronic midfoot strain

Medial strain of the foot is usually chronic in nature and develops over a period of months. It is characterized by aching along the medial aspect of the longitudinal arch. Physical examination reveals only mild tenderness in the soft tissues and about the first tarsometatarsal joint. X-rays may reveal mild degenerative changes in the midtarsal joints, even in adolescents, but otherwise are unremarkable. Treatment includes the use of anti-inflammatory medication, a foot and ankle flexibility programme and the use of an arch support in the ballet shoe during barre exercises and class. This condition is seldom disabling.

Hallux rigidus

Hallux rigidus in the dancer can be quite disabling. The dancer requires a full range of motion particularly dorsiflexion at the hallux metatarsophalangeal joint. Pain occurs at the metatarsophalangeal joint in the demi pointe position (Ambre 1978, Howse 1983). Mechanical restriction of this motion requires the dancer to invert the foot slightly on rising to the ball of the foot. This altered position predisposes the dancer to inversion injuries. Diagnosis is made by comparing the painful side with the usually asymptomatic opposite foot. Motion is restricted and often osteophytes are palpable. X-rays reveal a decreased joint space with osteophyte formation at the metatarsophalangeal joint of the hallux.

Early treatment includes a flexibility programme designed to increase motion at this joint. Anti-inflammatory medication is also beneficial. By the time the dancer seeks medical attention he may have learned to alter technique enough so that the change in position of the foot while in demi pointe still appears aesthetic. Since the condition usually occurs in the fourth or fifth decade of life, symptoms generally remain mild for years and the dancer may choose to alter his career.

Surgical treatment is recommended only when symptoms are significant enough to warrant termination of a career or severely impair the dancer's style because of pain and stiffness. Cheilectomy of the metatarsophalangeal joint is recommended. Some authors have recommended the use of a Silastic® prosthesis in the proximal phalanx. The results of such surgical treatment have been inconsistent and the dancer should be so advised prior to surgery.

Subluxing toes

Metatarsalgia may be due to several causes. Vague pain occurs in the region of the metatarsophalangeal joints of the lesser toes which may be due to ligament laxity with subluxation of the toe at this joint (Sammarco 1984). The second and third toes are most commonly affected (Ronconi 1983). Symptoms are characterized by metatarsalgia developing over several months while the dancer continues to dance.

On physical examination joint laxity is noted with dorsal-plantar manipulation at the metatarsophalangeal joint. This is usually associated with pain. Direct pressure at the head of the involved metatarsal with the proximal phalanx dorsiflexed also produces pain (Fig. 49.22).

Differential diagnosis should include interdigital neuroma, which is less common in the second web space than in the third. Treatment includes the use of appropriate padding around the metatarsal heads with lamb's wool, anti-inflammatory medication and a flexibility programme for the foot. If these measures fail, excision of the proximal 20% of the proximal phalanx is recommended through a dorsal incision. The capsule should be closed over the metatarsal head and the plantar plate sutured to the surrounding tissues so as to protect the head and prevent the plantar plate from retracting. Postoperatively the toe is held in position with an axial smooth Kirschner wire for three weeks. Following this, active range of motion with physical therapy rehabilitation is begun. The dancer may return to a full schedule as the decrease in symptoms permits.

Traumatic cysts

Traumatic cysts of the second metatarsal joint develop insidiously over several weeks or months. As the cyst forms it may become 'dumb-bell'-shaped as it passes from the plantar to the dorsal aspect of the foot between the metatarsal heads. The web space widens and metatarsalgia develops particularly when the dancer stands in the demi pointe position.

Diagnosis is made on physical examination by

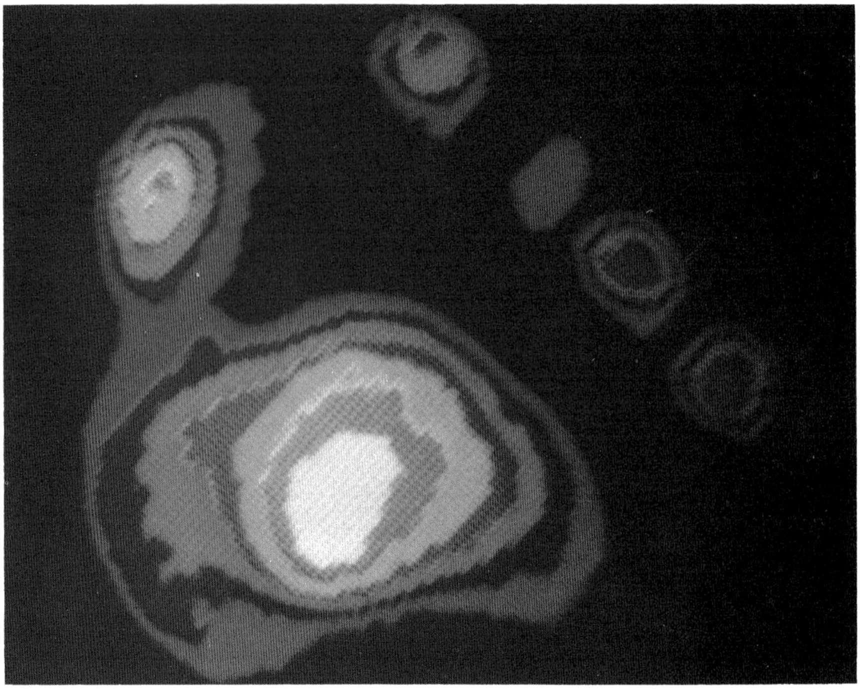

Fig. 49.22 Subluxating 3rd toe: A pressure podogram of a female dancer with metatarsalgia beneath the 3rd metatarsal head for 8 months. Note decreased pressure as indicated by pale gray area beneath 3rd toe

palpating the tender cyst in a widened web space. Differential diagnosis must include chronic abscess due to an unrecognized puncture wound with a foreign body, traumatic aneurysm, and infected soft corn with abscess. A complete blood count with sedimentation rate is performed preoperatively. Standard X-rays may show only soft tissue swelling. An axial CT scan may outline the cyst (Fig. 49.23). Treatment includes surgical excision through a dorsal approach. The dancer should be advised that, although a flexibility programme and limited barre may be permitted early in the recovery period using

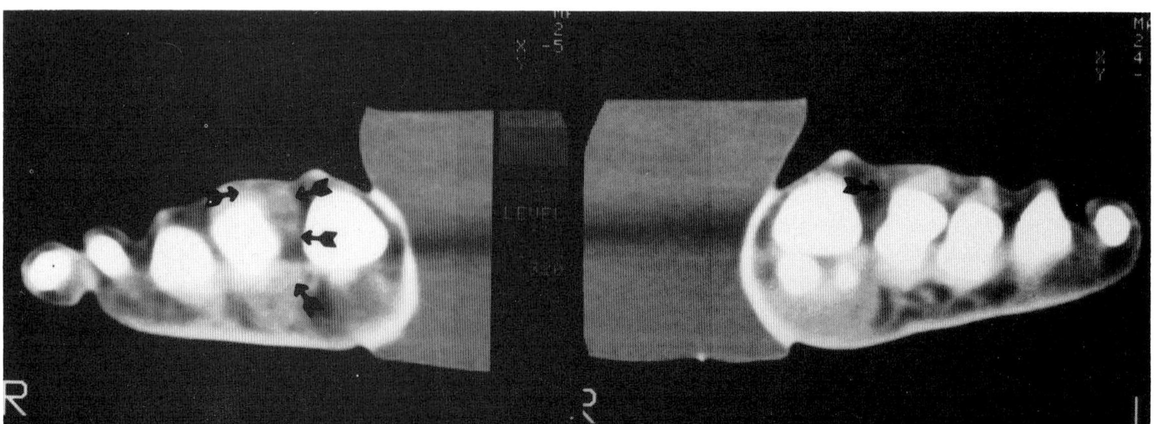

Fig. 49.23 Traumatic cyst of the 2nd metatarsophalangeal joint: CT scan of both feet showing presence of dumbbell shaped cyst on the right (outlined in arrows) and normal soft tissue density on the left (single arrow)

the affected limb as the working leg, a full schedule should be permitted only when pain subsides and full dorsiflexion has returned.

STATIC DEFORMITIES

Acquired flat foot

Dancers who have danced for several decades may develop an acquired flat foot deformity due to the stretching of the ligaments in the foot. This deformity tends to be flexible. When symptomatic a soft leather arch support made of Silastic® is recommended to be placed in a dance or character shoe. A flexibility programme is encouraged.

Splay foot deformity

Splay foot deformity occurs in the fourth and fifth decades. This is thought to be caused by standing for long periods of time in the half pointe position stretching out the intermetatarsal ligaments. Over the years the structures of the forefoot become so lax as to permit the long flexor tendons of the toes to subluxate between the metatarsal heads. Symptoms are characterized by metatarsalgia after class (Sammarco 1982). Treatment includes a flexibility and power building exercise programme for strengthening the foot and ankle musculature, anti-inflammatory medication and a moulded arch support. A metatarsal pad of Silastic® is added to spread out the weight-bearing area behind the metatarsophalangeal joints.

Hallux valgus

Hallux valgus occurs in the dancer at a younger age than in the general population (Hardy & Clapham 1951, Howse 1983). It does not appear related to the adolescent or inherited form of bunion (Fig. 49.24). Symptoms occur following rehearsal with pain medially at the head of the first metatarsal. Over a period of one to two years, a bunion prominence may develop. Resting and elevating the foot following dance relieves the symptoms. There is no loss of flexibility. X-rays reveal no gross osteophyte formation.

Treatment includes examination of the box of the ballet pointe shoe. Since shoes come with different length boxes and with varying stiffness, the dancer

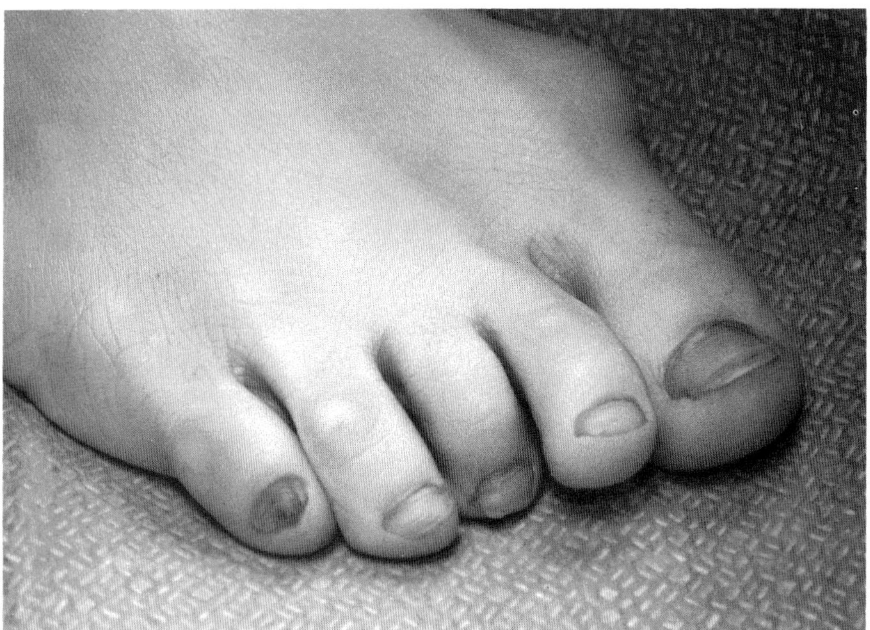

Fig. 49.24 Bunion and hallux valgus: This occurs more commonly in young dancers than in the general population. Since recovery may require one full year, surgery is not recommended unless the dancer has tried all other treatment modalities and is considering terminating her career

should change the shape or style of the pointe shoe. Lamb's wool may be used to pad around the bunion. Surgery is seldom required since it often stiffens the hallux and causes a dramatic change in the dance style.

Dancers who begin to dance late in their second and third decades try to increase their turnout by pressing their knees against a firm surface and anchoring with counter pressure against the ball of the foot. Bunions which occur in later years are often caused by inadvertent rehearsal and dance techniques, such as forcing the hips into a turnout position while doing a grand plié and putting inordinate extra strain on the metatarsophalangeal joints.

Bunion associated with hammertoe deformity occurring in the fifth decade may be symptomatic. If symptoms are mild, however, this may be treated with an arch support or with a bunion flare which can be placed in the ballet shoe. Surgery is not recommended unless pain is severe and disabling even when not dancing. Advanced bunion is often associated with metatarsus primus varus and hallux valgus. Corrective surgery carries with it the possibility of stiffness in the forefoot as well as postoperative pain. Surgical procedures which stiffen or shorten the toes are not recommended since they alter the weight-bearing character of the forefoot. If such surgery is to be undertaken, the dancer must be counselled appropriately as to the possibility of changing dance styles or even her dance profession. Recovery from forefoot reconstruction is often long and although dancing may be resumed when postoperative pain and stiffness allow it, full recovery requiring one year is often the case.

Hammertoe

Hammertoes are common in dancers, are usually flexible in nature and may cause callous formation over the dorsal aspect of the proximal interphalangeal joint. They are usually asymptomatic but may be associated with other static deformities such as hallux valgus, bunion and splay foot. They are caused by placing the foot in a tight toe of a ballet pointe shoe. When pain is present it is usually mild and treated with anti-inflammatory medication and appropriate lamb's wool padding around the toes. Surgery is not recommended since symptoms are usually minimal.

Fixed hammertoe deformity associated with symptomatic hallux valgus, bunion and metatarsus primus varus usually occurs in the fifth and sixth decades. By this time, many dancers have become teachers with reduced schedules and fewer physical demands. A full insole leather arch support with appropriate Silastic® metatarsal pad and proper relief beneath the tips of the toes and metatarsal heads is indicated. If symptoms do not abate a forefoot surgical reconstruction is recommended.

NAIL PROBLEMS

Subungual haematoma

In the ballet pointe dancer, the toenail becomes part of the weight-bearing surface. Several conditions including subungual haematoma can occur. This condition is usually asymptomatic, although unsightly. It is not tender and does not require drainage.

Ingrown toenail

Ingrown toenail is a common malady in dancers. It is treated by partial excision of the affected toenail performed under local anaesthesia. Approximately 20% of the toenail is removed. Removal of the entire nail is not recommended since the great toenail requires more than nine months to regenerate during which time the nail bed is tender and restricts the dancer from dancing sur les pointes.

Onycholysis

This condition occurs as a result of dancing en pointe, permitting the tip of the nail to become a weight-bearing surface. The nail then begins to delaminate. This condition is benign and generally not symptomatic and should not be treated.

Calluses

Corns and calluses are common in dancers. The dancer learns to pad the foot to protect the toes (Fig. 49.25). Often during rehearsal the pads are changed from one toe to another as the dancer's needs change.

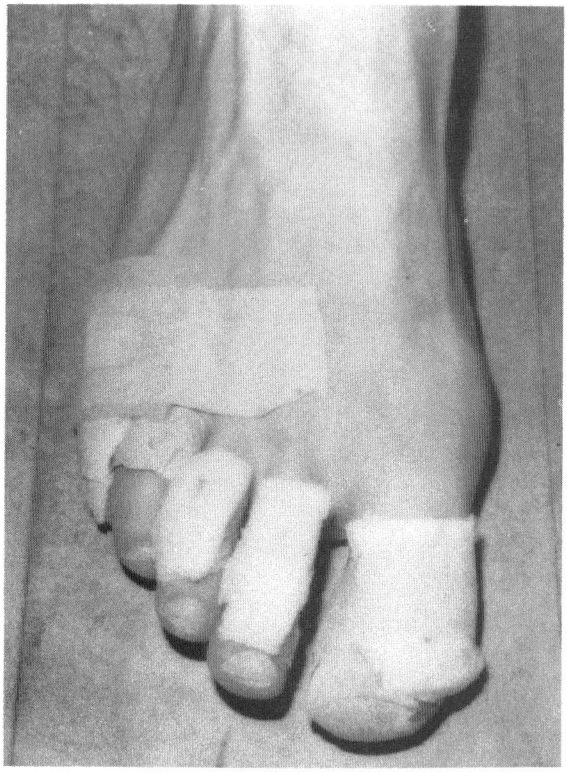

Fig. 49.25 Normal dancer's foot: Pads and tape over corns and calluses protect tender areas during rehearsals and class

Corns

Soft corns between the toes are caused by compression of the adjacent toes and against a prominent condyle of the phalanx. These are usually treated by placing a horseshoe-shaped pad of one-quarter inch felt between the toes, taping the two toes together with the open area of the pad surrounding the corn. The base of the horsehoe pad is placed distally. This permits the foot to be placed in a ballet pointe shoe. Surgical excision of the phalangeal condyle or injection is not recommended since this may destroy collateral ligaments of the small toe joints and permit deformity to occur.

If a dancer delays treatment of such soft corns a dissecting abscess extending into the web space can occur and present as a mass. This requires surgical incision and drainage with appropriate antibiotics. Trimming the corns with a razor is often done by dancers. When corns become infected, the recommended treatment includes appropriate cultures and antibiotics. The most common bacterium isolated is *Staphylococcus aureus* and is treated with cephalexin, 250 mg 6 hourly for 10 days. A pad, in the shape of a doughnut so as to admit the soft corn into the hole, relieves pressure on the centre. The dancer should be counselled as to proper foot hygiene.

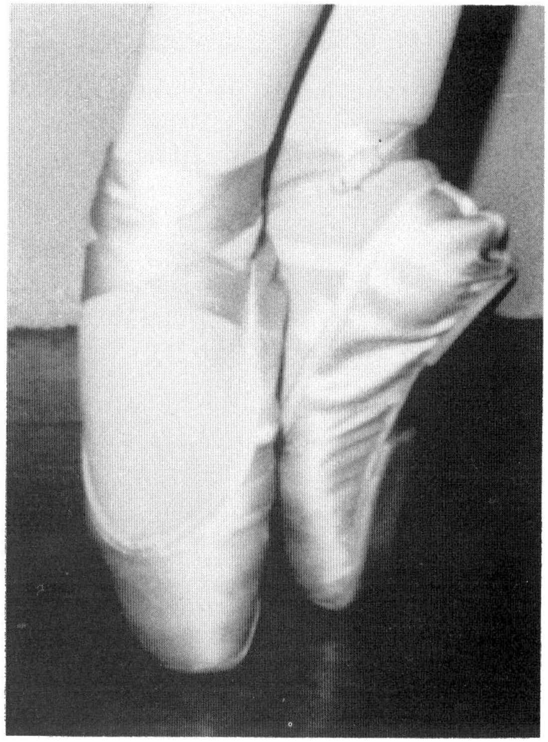

Fig. 49.26 Dancer's feet in full pointe

REHABILITATION

Rehabilitation of the dancer is an important adjunct to therapy. The dancer has the finest body awareness of any athlete and is easily instructed in programmes which are performed at home. The principle of maintaining range of motion, power and co-ordination while protecting an injured part is especially important to the dancer (Cobb & Sammarco 1984). Below are listed the modalities commonly used in helping the dancer recover from injury to the leg, foot and ankle.

Barre exercises

These basic classical ballet exercises are modified to be performed by the dancer so that the injured leg is non-weightbearing and the sound leg is the leg of support.

Water barre

The same exercises are performed with the dancer submerged chest deep in a pool to eliminate gravity. The injured leg is the working leg.

Foot and ankle exerciser board

Exercises are performed using this special board to develop flexibility, coordination and strength about the ankle following injury (Figs. 49.27a and b).

Foot and ankle flexibility programme

See Table 49.1 which is commonly used in the author's rehabilitation programme for injury to the leg, foot and ankle.

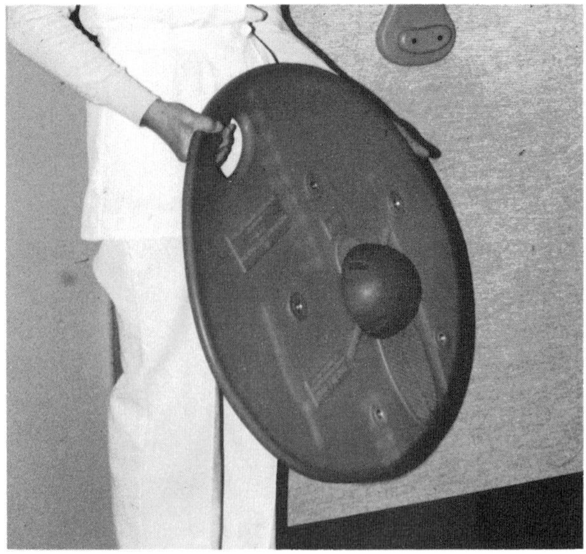

a

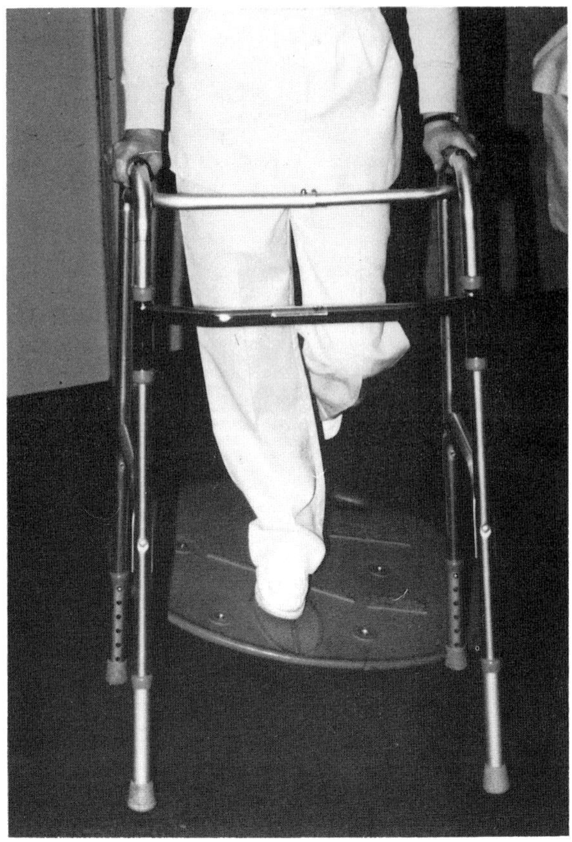

b

Fig. 49.27 (a) The exerciser board ('wobble' board or 'Baps' board). (b) The board in use

Dance medicine — Glossary of terms

Attitude One leg is bent either behind the dancer or in front. The supporting leg is either bent or straight.

Arabesque One leg is extended behind the dancer with straight knee and pointed foot. The supporting leg is either bent or straight.

Ballet pointe shoe A shoe with papier maché at the tip of the toe and batting support around the toes to form a box. This is done for stability when dancing en pointe.

Ballet shoe A slipper which unlike the toe or pointe shoe is very soft.

Ballon A quality of movement by which the impression is given that the dancer, by a reversal of the laws of gravity is continuously thrown off the ground, instead of pushing himself away from it.

Barre A wooden bar, fastened on the walls of a dance studio which helps the dancer to stabilize his balance while going through the initial exercises of the daily practice.

Character shoe A low-heeled leather shoe for character dances such as Folk or National Dances.

Choreography The art of composing a dance or ballet.

Class The place where dancers exercise on the barre, are taught, and practise their ballet.

Table 49.1 Dancer flexibility programme (School for the Performing Arts)

	Joint/muscle group	Objective	Position	Description
1.	Lower Back and Hip	Flexibility	Stand	Stand with feet two feet apart, hands on hips, make a circle with the upper torso, keeping the hips motionless. Repeat with the upper body still making a figure '8' with the hips.
2.	Groin	Stretch	Sit	Sit on the floor with the soles of the feet in contact with each other. Pull the feet towards the buttocks while pressing the outside of the knees to the floor. Relax. Repeat. Then with the legs spread apart as far as possible. Reach with both hands to grasp the right foot while leaning out over the right leg. Hold. Relax. Repeat with the left leg.
3.	Lateral Hip	Flexibility	Sit	Right hip: Sit on the floor, bend the left knee beneath the hip. Put the right foot on the left side of the left knee. Turn the body to the right and pull the right knee to the chest with left arm. Hold. Relax. Repeat for the left hip.
4.	Hamstring and Thigh	Stretch	Stand	Standing with legs straight try to touch the toes with the fingertips; then bend the knees and put palms on the floor. Slowly straighten legs. Hold. Relax. Repeat.
5.	Hamstring	Flexibility	Stand	Cross the right foot over and in front of the left foot. Bend at the waist to touch the toes with the fingertips, keeping legs straight. Hold. Relax. Repeat. Repeat crossing the left foot in front of and over the right foot.
6.	Quadriceps	Stretch	Sit	Sit on the floor with the right leg straight ahead and the toes pointed upward. Bend the left leg and place the left foot behind hip. Lean backwards and hold. Lean forward trying to touch the toes. Relax. Repeat. Repeat with the other leg.
7.	Quadriceps	Stretch	Stand	Bend the left knee and grab the ankle with the left hand, pull the left foot toward the buttocks. Hold. Relax. Repeat. Repeat the exercise with the right leg.
8.	Calf	Flexibility	Stand	With the feet together facing a wall, lean the body at a 45° angle, keep the heels flat on the floor and hold stretch. Relax. Repeat.
9.	Soleus and Achilles	Flexibility	Stand	With the feet together facing a wall, and heels on the floor, lean into the wall bending the knees. Stretching will be felt lower down the leg and in the Achilles tendon area. Hold. Relax. Repeat.
10.	Ankle	Flexibility	Stand	Rotations: Keep the leg straight and make circles with the foot moving first clockwise, then counterclockwise. Repeat. Flex and Point: Keep the leg straight. Bring the foot toward the face. Hold. Next point the toes. Hold. Repeat.

Note: Stretching movements are slow, smooth, and without bouncing. Hold each stretch for 10 seconds, relax and next time stretch further.

Classical ballet The purest stage tradition of gestures and expressions and of steps based on the five absolute positions of the classic dance.

Demi-plié Designates a movement position, or pose, executed in half measure only (or hinted at). Lowering the body by bending the knees half way.

Ethnic dance This was created for worship such as Hindu Natya, the ancient Hawaiian Meles, and highly stylized theatre dances such as the Javanese Wayang-Wang. This form of dance is richest in the Orient.

Fault Incorrect position or movement of the body during a dance step.

Foot flexion Dorsiflexion of the ankle as the foot is brought upward.

Jeté Designates a jump from one leg to the other in which the working leg seems to be thrown forwards, sideways, or backwards.

Kow-tow Kneeling and touching the ground with the forehead.

Leg of support The weight-bearing leg used during a dance step.

Modern dance A form of dance based on dynamism, on the collision of two opposites, such as contraction and release, fall, and recovery formulated from natural rhythms. It is characterized by asymmetry.

Plié In ballet designates the bending of the knees, for instance before commencing or on landing from any jump; also particularly the exercise of the daily class-routine which serves to loosen the muscles and tendons and to strengthen the dancers balance.

Pointe Dancer stretches with pointed foot (Fig. 49.26).

Sur les pointes Standing on the tips of the toes, usually in pointe shoes.

Tendu Stretched or held, as in pointing and stretching the leg in a straight line.

Working leg The nonweight-bearing leg used during a dance step.

REFERENCES

Ambre T 1978 Degenerative changes in the first metatarsophalangeal joint of ballet dancers. Acta Orthop Scand 49: 317–319

Burrows J J 1956 Fatigue infraction (incomplete fracture) of the middle of the tibia in ballet dancers. J Bone Joint Surg (Br) 38B: 83–84

Calabrese L, Kirkendall D G 1983 Nutritional and medical consideration in dancers. Clin Sports Med. W. B. Saunders. 2(3): 539–548

Cobb S, Sammarco G J 1984 Flexibility program for the dancer. Clinic for the Performing Arts. Presented at the Sixth Annual Dance Medicine Symposium. Cincinnati, Ohio

Collis, W J M, Jayson M I V 1972 Measurement of pedal pressures. Ann Rheum Dis 31: 217

Devas M B 1975 Stress Fractures. Churchill Livingstone, Edinburgh

Hamilton W G 1977 Tendinitis about the ankle joint in classical ballet dancers. J Sports Med 5: 84

Hamilton W G 1982a Stenosing tenosynovitis of the flexor hallucis longus tendon and posterior impingement upon the os trigonum in ballet dancers. Foot Ankle 3: 74

Hamilton W G 1982b Sprained ankles in ballet dancers. Foot Ankle 3: 99

Hardy R H, Clapham J D 1951 Observations on hallux valgus. J Bone Joint Surg 33: 376

Howse A J G 1972 Orthopaedists aid ballet. Clin Orthop 89: 52–63

Howse A J G 1982 Posterior block of the ankle joint in dancers. Foot Ankle 3: 8

Howse A J G 1983 Disorders of the great toe in dancers. Clin in Sports Med. W. B. Saunders 2(3): 499–505

Jamison K 1985 Creativity and mood disorders. Harvard Medical School Health Letter. Grinspoon L (ed) 1(12): 4–6

Jones R 1902 Fractures of the fifth metatarsal bone. Liverpool Med Surg J 42: 103–107

Kleiger B 1982 Anterior tibiotalar impingement syndromes in dancers. Foot Ankle 3: 69

Lynn T 1966 Repair of the torn Achilles tendon, using the plantaris tendon as reinforcing membrane. J Bone Joint Surg 48: 268

Mann R A 1975 Biomechanics of the foot. In: Atlas of Orthotics: Biomechanical Principles and Applications. C. V. Mosby Co, St. Louis

Manter J T 1946 Distribution of compression forces in the joints of the human foot. Anat Rec 96: 313

Nikolic V, Zimmerman B 1968 Functional changes of tarsal bones of ballet dancers. Rad Med Fak Zagrebu 16: 131

Pelipenko V I 1973 Specific characteristics of the development of the foot skeleton in pupils of a choreographic school. Arkh Anat Gistol Embriol 64: 46–50

Quirk R 1982 Talar compression syndrome in dancers. Foot Ankle 3: 65

Quirk R 1983 Ballet Injuries: The Australian Experience. Clin in Sports Med 2(3): 507–514

Ronconi P 1983 (Physician to Rome Ballet) Personal communication

Sammarco G J 1982 The foot and ankle in classical ballet and modern dance. In: Jahss M (ed) Disorders of the Foot. W. B. Saunders, Philadelphia, pp 1626–1659

Sammarco G J 1984 Diagnosis and treatment in dancers. Clin Orthop 187: 176–187

Sammarco G J, Miller E H 1979 Partial rupture of the flexor hallucis longus in classical ballet dancers. J Bone Joint Surg 61A: 140

Sammarco G J, Miller E H 1982a Forefoot conditions in dancers. Part 1. Foot Ankle 3(2): 85–92

Sammarco G J, Miller E H 1982b Forefoot conditions in dancers. Part 2. Foot Ankle 3(2): 93–98

Sammarco G J, Burstein A H, Frankel V H 1973 Biomechanics of the ankle; a kinematic study. Orthop Clin North Am 4: 75

Schneider J H et al 1974 Stress injuries and developmental change of lower extremities in ballet dancers. Radiology. 113: 627–632

Seals J 1983 A study of dance surfaces. Clin in Sports Med Presented at the Fifth Annual Dance Medicine Symposium. Cincinnati, Ohio 3(2): 557

Stojanovie S, Marenie S, Ukropina D 1963 Diseases in ballet dancers. Srp Arh Celok Lek 91: 903

Teitz C C, Harrington R M, Wiley H 1985 Pressures on the foot in pointe shoes. Foot Ankle 5(5): 216–221

Thomasen E 1982 Diseases and injuries of ballet dancers. Universitetsforlaget I Arhus. Copenhagen, Denmark

Wilcox J R, Moniot A L, Green J P 1977 Bone scanning in the evaluation of exercise related stress injuries. Radiology 123: 699–703

Militaria

MEDICAL STANDARDS

Prior to entry, all members of the armed services are expected to reach a high standard of fitness, though some reduction in medical standards may be allowed for injury and disability sustained while serving. Should the manpower situation or the need for particular skills demand, certain fitness reductions are made, but this is unusual in peacetime.

It is not infrequent for patients to seek advice on their future acceptability for a service career. All cases should be critically assessed and unless they measure up to an L2 (see below) standard are well advised to consider careers in other walks of life. It is not infrequent for potential recruits to present letters from their medical advisors stating they have had, for example, successfully treated club feet and are now fit for all forms of service life. A career rejection in these formative years can be very disturbing to the young person.

Many of the service trades and branches are predominantly sedentary, but they all have to undergo strenuous recruit or officer initial training which includes the use of arms. It is here that undeclared or misssed physical defects are frequently shown up.

A high degree of physical fitness is maintained in all units. Sport participation is strongly encouraged and periodic fitness and endurance tests are made throughout a service career.

In an emergency or under hostile conditions all may have to engage in combat. Even in normal unit duties guards have to be mounted and parades performed. In hostile conditions the disability of one of a party may prejudice the survival of the others, who are most unlikely to leave the disabled one behind.

Another aspect of physical fitness relates to promotion. Not only do the individual's merits enter into consideration, they must also be physically fit for the promotion. A lowered medical category is a very potent cause of disappointment, premature career arrest and medical discharge.

It is for these reasons that the services maintain their strict criteria on medical standards.

FITNESS ASSESSMENT

The armed services of Great Britain in common with many other countries, use the 'PULHEEMS' system.

PULHEEMS represents: P — Physical capacity; U — Upper limbs; L — Locomotion; H — Hearing; E — Eyesight Right; E — Eyesight Left; M — Mental capacity; S — Emotional stability.

Disabilities of the foot will affect the 'L' assessment. When there is also a constitutional disturbance as in rheumatoid arthritis, this is reflected in the 'P' assessment.

Each lettered assessment is divided into eight degrees as follows:

1. Above average with full combatant capacity and no climatic restriction
2. Average with full combatant capacity and no climatic restriction. It is that normally given to a fit person
3. Below average with restricted combatant capacity without climatic restriction
4. As 1 but restricted to temperate climates only
5. As 2 but restricted to temperate climates only
6. As 3 but restricted to temperate climates only
7. Markedly diminished capacity with restricted combatant ability
8. Unfit for any form of service.

'L' assessment

This includes functional assessment of the lumbar spine, coccyx, pelvis, hip joints, thighs, knees, legs, ankles and feet.

The functional abilities required in each 'L' degree are as follows:

L1 Capable of very severe locomotor activity for five or six days. Able to run, jump, crawl and perform all kinds of manual labour quickly. This assessment is reserved for troops capable of the very severe physical endurance required of a Commando.

L2 Having the same physical capabilities as L1, but performing them at a slower pace. This is the category given to the average fit person.

L3 Able to march five miles or more in an emergency and able to stand for two hours. The grade permits some defects in locomotion

L4, L5 and L6 These grades correspond to the categories L1, L2 and L3 respectively, but with a restriction to temperate climates only. Other climatic restriction, such as exposure to low temperature, is reflected in the individual services' employment gradings.

L7 Able to walk two miles a day at his own pace and able to stand for a moderate though not prolonged period. It restricts the person to duties in the home country or a base area. It is frequently applied as a temporary assessment for a person recovering from a condition such as a fracture.

L8 Unfit for all service.

Assessment of common foot conditions

All assessment is *functional*. For example, a foot may be held in some degree of valgus, but provided it is symptomless it may be given the highest assessment.

Hallux valgus and hallux rigidus when mild and symptomless allow an L2 grading, otherwise L7 or L8 is appropriate.

Single toe deformities, such as a hammer toe, are compatible with L2. Generalized toe clawing is graded L7 or L8.

Rigid and structural flat foot is graded L8.

Pes cavus if slight, symptomless and mobile allows an L3 category, but with symptoms, limited movement or evidence of high pressure areas (callosities), L7 or L8 is indicated. Any persisting talipes deformity normally indicates an L8 grade. Even when symptomless in civilian life, talipes equinovarus after correction has been found to withstand service life and footwear badly.

Conditions of the ankle joint (often due to previous injury) with pain, limited movement or instability are graded L8.

Remediable conditions

These include minor abnormalities such as an exostosis, which would permit the highest assessment following successful treatment.

Normally recruits are not accepted until such conditions have been rectified, full rehabilitation completed and a further medical assessment performed.

TRAINING

On entry primary training has the main objectives of testing the recruit's physical capabilities to prove his fitness for a service career, rendering him fit enough for further training and examining his ability to make decisions or perform skilled tasks when fatigued.

Foot care should be taught, all men should wash their feet at least once a day, after which they should be steeped in cold water for a short time; those with soft feet should use a solution of alum or salt 30 g : 2 l. They should then be carefully dried and dusted with foot powder. A clean pair of socks should always be available. Socks should be washed daily and dried. If this is not possible they should be turned inside out and dried.

Socks, which should be of wool, shrink by 2.5 cm after two washes, so they should at first be a little larger than the foot to allow for this.

If there is any soreness a careful inspection of the footwear should be made for any projections and the fit.

Blisters should be drained, after iodine application, by inserting a sterilized needle and allowing the fluid to drain past it, followed by a small dressing to keep the skin in place. Hyperhidrosis should be managed by bathing in 0.5% formaldehyde solution.

Instruction is given in the care of footwear, boots should be well dubbined to keep them pliant and soft. Recruits must be taught always to have spare dry socks and boots available especially if liable to be wet shod as in beach assaults. They must change into dry socks and boots at the first available opportunity. They are further instructed to dry out the wet wear as a priority task.

The common foot problems include blisters, callosities, foot strain, compartment syndromes, and stress fractures, most of which rapidly resolve with temporary training modification, physiotherapy and chiropody attention. Persisting pain suggests more serious pathology.

Stress fracture, despite negative X-rays primarily, are treated on clinical diagnosis. The verification of stress fracture may take some time, especially when rest treatment is started promptly and callus formation is likely to be minimal. A technetium scan is helpful in the early stages.

The following table gives an indication of when X-ray changes are likely to be seen:

Metatarsals	2 to 3 weeks
Calcaneum	3 to 12 weeks
Fibula (lower $\frac{1}{4}$)	3 to 6 weeks
Tibia (lower $\frac{1}{3}$)	4 to 12 weeks

In the management of stress fracture, cast immobilization is advised as the patient is liable to be disbelieved by his fellows and the NCOs since there are few outward signs. The danger is that he will ignore medical advice and attempt to work it off with prolongation of the process, often a contralateral lesion and a poor result.

Physical defects usually manifest themselves during early training when they have been missed or not declared in the pre-entry screening. Care is required to pick out recruits who are having symptoms but are failing to report them. The instructing staff have this responsibility and rapidly become skilled in detecting it especially if there is an unexplained reduction in a recruit's performance or a limp.

FOOTWEAR

Service footwear is supplied in full length and width fittings, special care is required to see that the recruit and the trained serviceman are correctly fitted. Fitting should be carried out with the recruit standing, carrying a full marching load and wearing regulation socks. This allows for the spread of the feet under these conditions. Should it be impossible to get a correct fit facilities should be available for the footwear to be individually made.

The same care is necessary for special task footwear such as flying boots.

The modern DMS (direct moulded soles) shoes and boots on issue are waterproof up to the tongue attachments. When particularly wet terrain is likely special high waterproof boots are issued. Foot powder containing a fungicide should also be standard issue.

The main task of instruction rests with the serviceman's section commander and especially his noncommissioned officers. The importance attached to foot care, so utterly necessary for the efficient serviceman, is seen in the frequent 'spit and polish' inspections when the state of footwear has special emphasis.

The same care is applied to the footwear needed for sport and physical training.

COLD INJURY

Servicemen, if liable to cold injury, must be given instruction in its prevention, recognition and emergency treatment. This is the responsibility of the section commanders and medical officers. These injuries should be minimal with correct equipment, training and discipline.

Dry cold

This occurs at temperatures below –5°C. Then, snow and frost made worse by wind (the chill factor) and altitude can result in frostbite. It is avoided by suitable clothing with adequate insulation and windproofing, dry underclothes and shelter from wind. Under extreme conditions servicemen should work in pairs, watching for signs of frostbite and treating affected parts by warming, but never rubbing, at once. The foot can be revived on a companion's abdomen or axilla.

A modern form of the Eskimo Muckluk is the footwear of choice though this is not waterproof. It comprises an outer canvas boot with a thick rubber sole, inside which there is a double insole of open nylon mesh which lies on the 1 cm thick solid insole to form an air insulating layer. A felt inner boot and two or three pairs of socks or a pair of sea boot stockings complete the footwear.

Hot food and drink is important and should be taken whenever possible but alcohol is forbidden.

Wet cold

The temperature is between -5C and +5C, not as low as in dry cold, but operating over a longer period. It occurs typically in trenches where the foot is wet shod in cold, muddy conditions, often for days, giving the trench foot syndrome. An aetiologically similar condition of immersion foot occurs when the feet are in sea water frequently dependent and immobile for long periods.

The foot must be kept clean, dry and dusted with foot powder containing a fungicide at all times. Boots must be of correct waterproof height and in good repair.

The ground should be as dry as possible; it should be drained and duck boards used.

Frostbite

Cold injury of the foot must be considered with general hypothermia of which it is often a part.

Battle casualties may also have cold injury when hypovolaemia, resulting from blood loss, will enhance the effect of cold.

In the earliest phase of frostbite the toes are white and numb. This is easily reversed by warming which is accompanied by tingling and redness.

In the next phase the toes are marbled white and insensitive. They are firm but the skin moves over the bony points. On warming they become a mottled blue-red colour. They swell and give a sensation of stinging and burning but no blistering occurs. With more severe damage blisters will form which later dry out forming eschars which are later shed.

Finally, the toes and perhaps other parts of the foot exhibit a frozen, waxy appearance; they feel cold, solid and the skin will not move over bony points. Condensation may form on them in a warm atmosphere. On warming pain occurs with oedema and blisters which turn black and form eschars. Severely involved tissue may not blister but later it will be sloughed.

Assessment of the extent of irreversible damage is difficult and it only becomes clear with time. It takes about 10 weeks for the lines of demarcation to form. Dry gangrene will form unless there is infection, in which case wet gangrene occurs.

Trench and immersion foot

The victim complains that his feet are cold, numb and tingling. In this first or prehyperaemic phase, they appear either white or mottled red-blue and they are stiff, tender and heavy. Sensation may be absent in a stocking distribution but the tissues are resilient. The pulses are usually impalpable.

On warming, the foot passes into the hyperaemic phase, with pain, gross swelling, flushing, blistering and petechia. The pulses return but where irreversible damage has occurred these parts will not become warm. As with frostbite, the differentiation in the early stage is difficult, dry gangrene will appear unless infection supervenes when more extensive wet gangrene will form.

First aid

Heat loss is avoided by adequate covering and warmth, if possible, is given. Where several casualties are carried under adverse conditions, they can be bundled together to provide mutual warmth for the journey. The feet should be exposed to room temperature, if feasible, as in a heated ambulance, otherwise sterile dressing should be applied and the feet covered.

Morphine should be given for pain. Antibiotics should be administered orally as a prophylactic against infection. Smoking is strictly contra-indicated.

Though under emergency conditions it is possible to walk on still frozen feet without greatly increasing the injury, normally cases with cold foot injury must be treated as stretcher cases to prevent more severe foot damage occurring.

On arrival at a treatment centre the feet, after gentle removal of clothing, are rapidly warmed, preferably by immersion in a warm bath. Then following aseptic care to avoid infection and usually conservative management. Hyperbaric oxygen has a place in the treatment.

MISSILE INJURY

As with all surgery, correct management depends on an understanding of the pathology of the lesion. For this it is necessary to have some knowledge of ballistics and the mode of tissue damage.

It is a sad observation that in all wars to date ignorance of this has resulted in incorrect wound management with consequent increased morbidity and loss of limb and life.

Missiles

Taking the speed of sound in air as 350 m/sec, missiles travelling at a faster rate are classified as 'high velocity' and slower, as 'low velocity'. The significance is in the kinetic energy they possess and hence their destructive power.

Tissue damage is caused by the energy imparted to the tissues by the missile. The kinetic energy of a missile is given by the formula K.E. = $\frac{1}{2}mv^2$ where m = mass and v = velocity.

If the missile passes through the part then the energy transfer is $E = \frac{1}{2}m(v_1-v_2)^2$ where v_1 is the velocity on entry and v_2 the velocity on exit.

The importance of the velocity of the missile is clear, and it is helpful in management to know this. It is frequently not apparent from an inspection of the wound.

Ballistics

On leaving a gun a bullet is seldom stable since the resistance to its flight is about its point and tapered end while its centre of gravity is behind this. Due to centrifugal effects the spin imparted by the rifling of the barrel will tend to correct the instability.

When it enters tissue, the density of which is more than 800 times that of air, the instability is increased and becomes more so with passage through the tissues. This greatly increases the energy transfer to the tissues by the mechanism to be described.

Figure 50.1 shows three typical rounds and data on the energy of each.

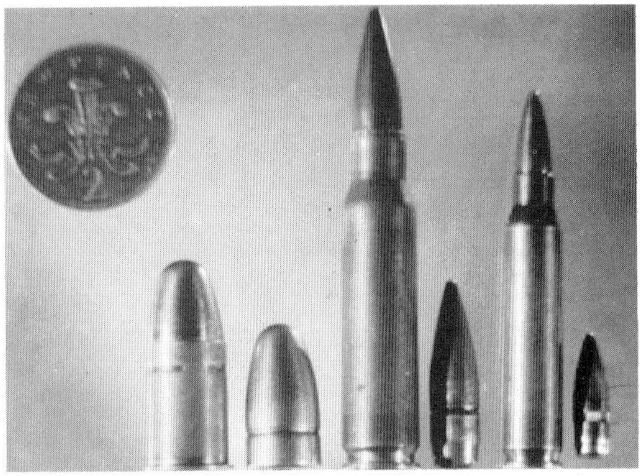

Fig. 50.1 Typical rounds:

	Round	Weight	Muzzle velocity	Energy
		g	m/s	J
a.	Hand gun	17.2	200	344
b.	NATO rifle	9.4	800	3008
c.	Armalite rifle	3.6	1000	1800

Fragments

Following the explosion of bomb, shell or grenade, irregular metal fragments fly out in all directions initially at high velocity and with gross instability. The velocity decreases with distance travelled until they fall to the ground (Fig. 50.2).

Casualties near to the explosion will have high velocity missile injuries. Further away low velocity missiles will be encountered. Secondary missiles, due to the explosive effect on surrounding material or lifted by the impact of the primary missiles, include stones, rock chips and splinters. Secondary missiles are a common finding in injury from antipersonnel mines.

MECHANISM OF INJURY

Laceration and crushing

This happens ahead of the missile, is local and with smooth stable missiles can be slight. With irregular unstable ones, like grenade fragments, it can be extensive.

Missiles are not sterilized by the heat generated in their passage through the air. They may acquire

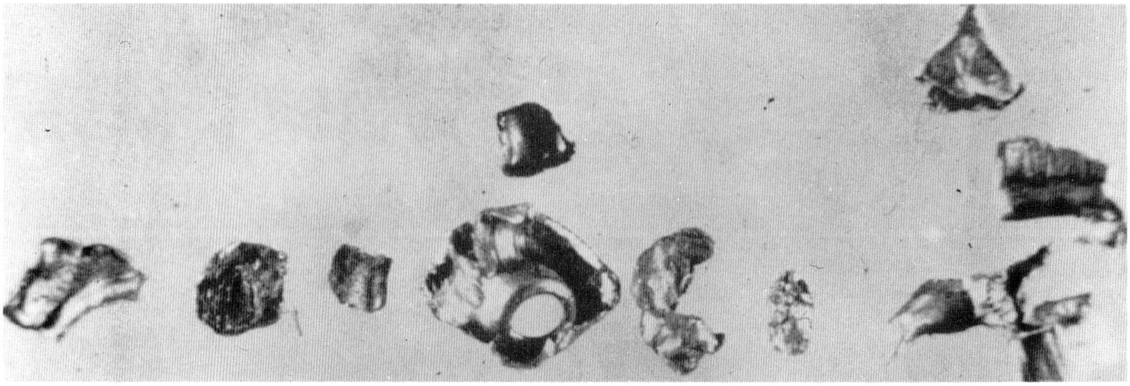

Fig. 50.2 Metal fragments of shrapnel removed from a victim

bacteria on passage through the clothing and may indeed carry pieces of it into the wound. All wounds therefore should be regarded as contaminated.

This tissue damage occurs in all missile wounds and is the chief factor in injuries from low velocity projectiles.

Shock wave

This and cavitation, discussed below, occur only in high velocity wounding.

The shock wave travels ahead of the missile, spreading out as a wave of high pressure of up to 100 atmospheres, moving at the speed of sound in water. It lasts about one millionth of a second and can travel along blood vessels damaging the intima and also may shatter bone.

Cavitation

When the tissues receive the energy from the missile they fly apart forming a vacuum cavity, the size of which is proportional to the energy imparted. It is in communication with the outside at both the entrance and exit wounds.

The lining of the cavity consists of severely crushed and devitalized tissue and torn blood vessels. If bone is included, it may be shattered. The susceptibility to damage of the tissue varies; those containing elastic and fibrous tissue are resistant, including skin, lung, tendon and ligament. Tissues having high water content are very susceptible and include muscle, liver and brain.

The cavity oscillates for a short while and is grossly contaminated by the vacuum effect which sucks in anything in the vicinity of the entrance and exit wounds. It will then fill with blood and exudate.

When a missile is fired through blocks of 20% gelatin and certain soap preparations, their behaviour simulates that of muscle. They are used to study cavitation (Fig. 50.3).

The flask shape is due to the increasing instability of the missile, with greater release of energy to the tissues and hence increasing cavitation, as it passes through the tissues. The lesion illustrated would be found typically in the thigh or calf, but in the foot, where the missile tract is often short, a high velocity missile could pass through causing relatively little damage. However, the reverse would occur if the missile was unstable on entry.

MANAGEMENT OF MISSILE WOUNDS

First aid

Lifesaving takes priority. This will concern chiefly establishing and maintaining an airway, care of the unconscious patient, closure of sucking chest wounds and the control of accessible haemorrhage.

Little further damage is likely to ensue from missile wounds of the foot. Emergency field dressings may be used on large wounds, but inflatable splints are strongly advised since they are quick to apply, help control bleeding, give adequate immobilization and allow X-rays to be taken through them. The opposite limb can be used to help immobilization when practicable.

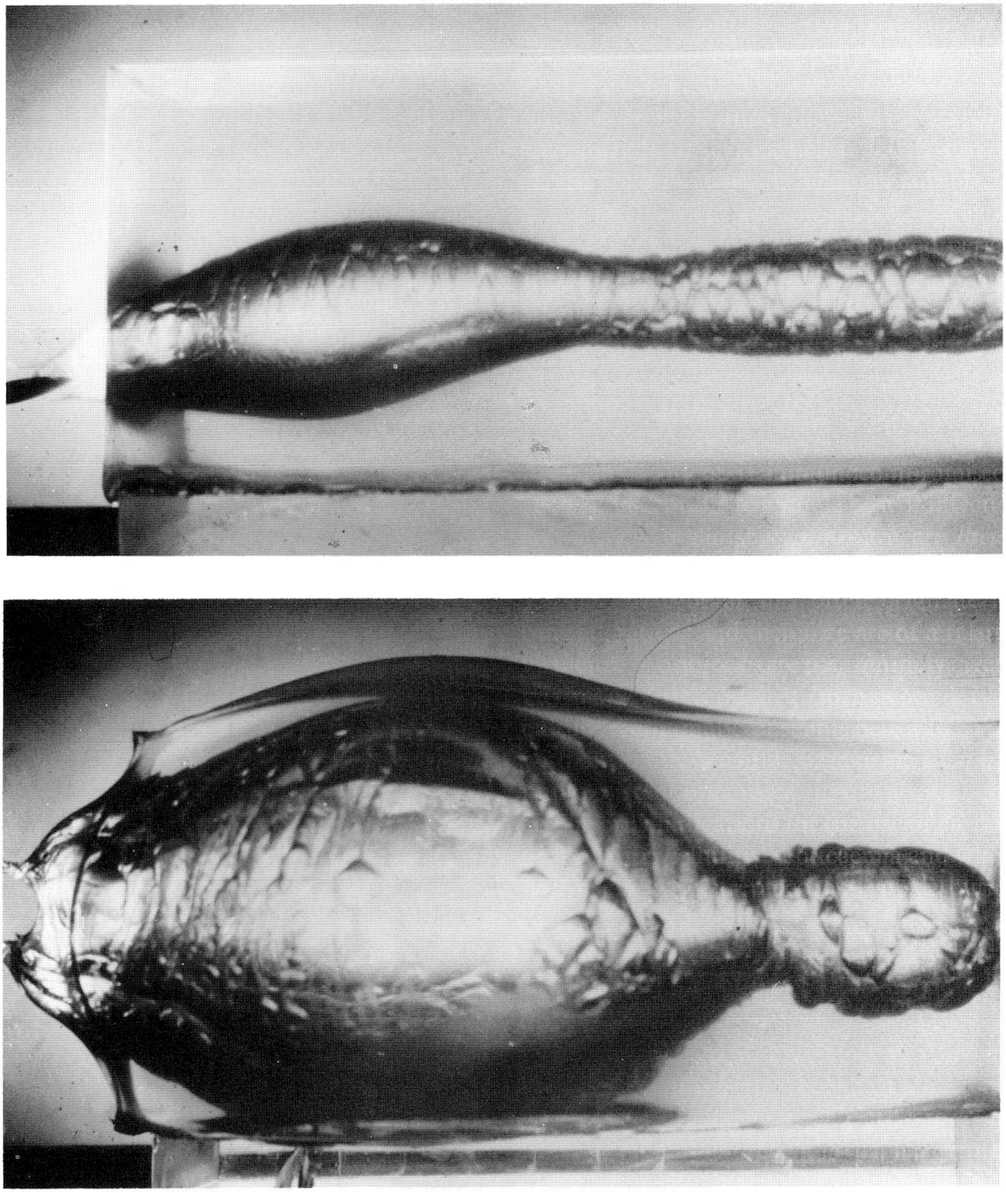

Fig. 50.3 Simulated cavitation. A 7.62 mm rifle bullet, weight 9.4 g, fired through a block of 20% gelatine at a muzzle velocity of 800 m/sec. (a) taken at the moment of strike plus 572 μs, shows the bullet leaving. The point has turned through 180° due to instability exaggerated by its passage through the block. The cavitation process has commenced. (b) is taken at strike plus 1632 μs. The cavitation is now well developed with the entrance and exit holes wide open. The cavity is larger near the exit due to the turning bullet transferring more energy to the gelatine (Photos by C.D.E.)

Rapid transfer to a surgical facility is the ideal, but if delay is likely and certainly if more than six hours will elapse before surgical toilet is performed, then a wide spectrum antibiotic in large dosage should be given. This reduces morbidity and approximately doubles the allowable time to surgery.

Triage

This is the sorting of casualties into treatment groups. It is an essential procedure to get the minimum mortality and morbidity from an incident by the most effective use of the staff and facilities available. It requires a continually updated knowledge of the theatre workload and delay, expected further casualties, transport availability, and the state of more distant surgical facilities to where the less urgent cases may be transferred.

Four categories are recognized:

A. Relative minor cases who, with simple treatment, can walk and manage themselves.

B. Those who, following simple treatment, can be safely left to await transport to a less busy unit for definitive management.

C. Those requiring immediate surgery and who would then have a reasonable chance of survival.

D. Those with mortal injury requiring medical comforts.

The category criteria must be variable, they will depend on the prevailing conditions, available staff and facilities. It is a highly responsible position and, wisely, should be given to the most experienced clinician available who must be realistic throughout the incident.

Practice in mass casualty management is of great value and the desirability of regular exercises by all hospital groups cannot be overemphasized.

WOUND TOILET

This should be done within six hours of wounding. If antibiotics have been given more time is available but should not exceed 12 hours.

The principles are those of any compound wound, bearing in mind the pathology of missile wounds. Unless the weapon used is known all should be considered as caused by high velocity missiles. This is often not clear from external inspection.

Under anaesthesia a sterile dressing is applied and the surrounding skin generously shaved and prepared. An inflatable tourniquet should be used on the limbs where practicable; it allows better inspection and reduces blood loss, but should be released as soon as possible.

The wound edge is excised, but since skin has high resistance to missile injury, not more than 2 mm need be taken. Subcutaneous tissue is examined; if it is pulped or grossly contaminated, it must be meticulously excised. The missile track is then thoroughly explored and the skin will need to be incised to allow this without heavy retraction occurring. The deep fascia is then widely opened in all the compartments involved. Further skin incision may be required for a thorough exploration, it should be planned bearing in mind the blood supply and will usually be along the length of the limb.

Finger examination of the tract and cavity is helpful — foreign matter, shrapnel, grit and pieces of fabric can be felt. The full extent of the track and cavity is ascertained and is laid open.

Now follows the meticulous removal of all blood clot, exudate, foreign matter and all dead and devitalized tissue. Dead muscle is identified by the four 'C's': Colour, Consistency, Contractility, Capillary bleeding.

The tourniquet should have been released by this stage, copious irrigation is required, and the procedure methodically performed. Devitalized muscle is 'mushy', coming away readily with the forceps in clumps, its colour varying from maroon, purple or green to black. It should be excised until it contracts on gentle pinching with forceps, and capillary bleeding is seen.

Large bone fragments with periosteal attachment should be cleaned and preserved. They are scrubbed if necessary, and returned to act as a spacer; frequently they will form a graft. If possible, blood vessels, nerves and tendons should be covered with fascia or muscle.

Joints need thorough irrigation and exploration. Besides the removal of all contaminating matter, care is required especially to remove any lead fragments which could later set up a lead arthrosis. The synovium should be closed if possible, but failing that the joint should be closed using the capsule or some fascia.

The wound is dusted with antibiotic powder and a loose fluffed gauze and cotton wool dressing applied. This ensures free drainage and aeration. The wound must never be packed.

If suitable, external fixation of a fracture is excellent management. Otherwise conventional immobilization is applied. Plaster casts must be well padded and either completely split or bivalved.

Delayed primary closure

Delayed primary closure is performed on day 3, 4 or 5 following wound toilet. Not only has this worked well in practice, but it has also been shown experimentally to be biologically sound. At this stage swelling has settled, any remaining particulate matter has been carried off in the exudute and the vascular response prior to granulation has commenced.

On removing the dressing under anaesthesia, the whole wound should be covered in clear serum, provided the toilet procedure was correctly performed. It should now be completely closed. The healing by this procedure compares most favourably with that obtained by primary closure. Following dressing the wound should be left for 10 to 14 days.

If nonviable tissue is still present, it must now be removed and the initial procedure repeated. Reinspection is done 3 to 5 days later when the wound, if satisfactory, should be closed. However, healing is now of the secondary type.

It should be noted that by this system the patient may be evacuated, after wound toilet, from the forward areas to a safe, less busy base area.

This system provides the optimum management of all missile wounding and has much to commend it in grossly contaminated and high velocity injuries so common in modern road traffic accidents. It is being used increasingly for such cases.

BLAST INJURY

Explosive blast is a frequent cause of injury in war. The sudden conversion of the charge into gas gives rise to a blast wave, a mass movement of air and heat. When the charge is contained, as in a grenade, bomb or shell the casing is shattered producing multiple missiles in addition.

The interval between peace and war is blunted and getting more so. Urban terrorism is now widespread throughout the world. The bomb, often home made, is usually placed in a public place where it can cause a large number of casualties.

For the correct management of these injuries a knowledge of the wounding mechanism is necessary.

Blast wave

This is a wave of high pressure spreading out from the explosion and lasting a few milliseconds, followed by a negative phase of not greater than one atmosphere lasting a little longer. It gets rapidly less with distance. It can travel at 90° to the main wave as an 'incident pressure', as over a blast wall, and it can rebound from a wall or building as the 'reflected pressure'.

The main damaging effect is on the gas-containing organs, the lungs, bowel and middle ear.

The blast effect on the lungs is to break the aveolar vascular barrier allowing air into the pulmonary arteries. It is the main cause of sudden death by coronary air embolism. In cases of lesser injury with survival, cerebral air embolism may occur and this is a cause of a shocked state often incorrectly diagnosed as 'battle neurosis'.

The less severe blast lung syndrome may become manifest later, sometimes 12 to 36 hours after the incident. This possibility must be kept in mind when managing and resuscitating a patient with a peripheral injury, which often appears as the more obvious and florid lesion.

The shock wave is propagated more rapidly and much further in water. The effects are much more serious when the victims are immersed and are produced at a greater distance from the explosion.

Mass movement of air

The rapidly expanding gas from the explosion displaces air which travels outward following the shock wave and is known as 'windage'. At first it is at very high pressure, but this rapidly falls with distance.

At close range it can cause complete disintegration of the body. Further away large portions of the victim may be separated and traumatic amputation of varying extent may occur. Still further away the person may be thrown into the air suffering then conventional injury. At yet greater distance, he may be blown over.

The other effect is on surrounding structures; injury may then be caused by falling masonry and secondary missiles. Injury is more severe in enclosed spaces and traumatic amputation is then frequent (Fig. 50.4).

Amputation. In the emergency situations discussed, amputation should be performed through, or just above, the level of trauma. The site should be concerned more with the level of bone injury than the soft tissue damage.

Viable skin should be preserved. If there is a

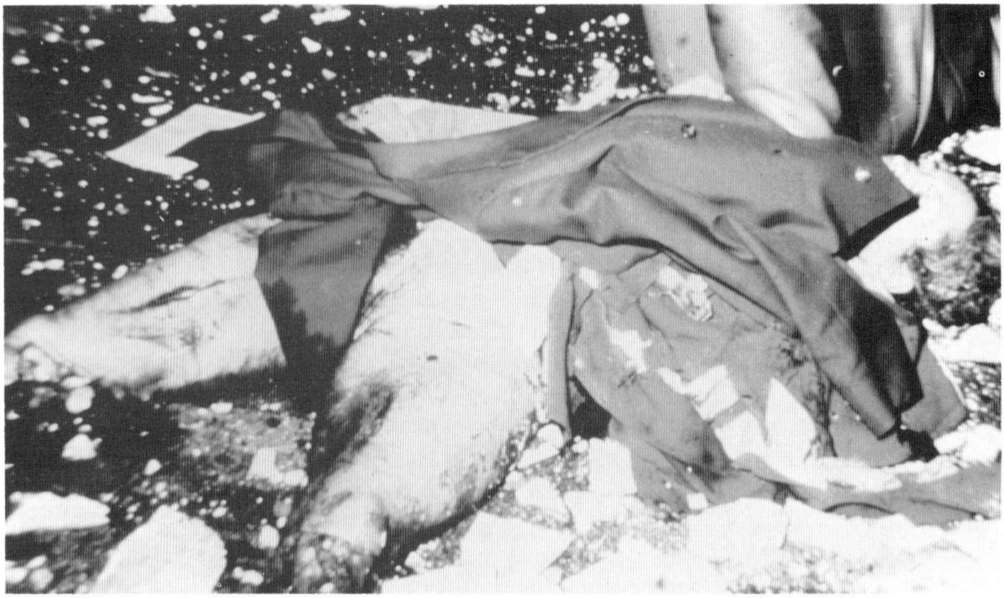

Fig. 50.4 Traumatic amputation caused by a bomb explosion in a confined space. The dead victim was quite near the bomb which had been placed in a hotel foyer

tendency for it to retract a few sutures over the stump dressing should be inserted.

The management of the wound should be that of a missile wound, aiming to avoid infection and to permit closure at delayed primary suture between 3 and 5 days later. Primary closure should not be attempted as the risk of infection, especially anaerobic, is high.

Amputation is required after blast amputation and where the damage to the foot is very severe, especially with neurovascular injury.

Late amputation may be required for a complication such as gangrene or to provide a better stump for prosthetic fitting. Experience has shown that amputations at sites other than those of election can be fitted with good serviceable protheses in the majority of cases.

SHOTGUN WOUNDS

These are found more in civil insurrection, criminal activity or accidents.

At close range, under 5 m, the immense tissue damage is caused by the shot, which moves at high velocity, the charge and the wadding (which is placed between the charge and the shot in the cartridge). The wounds should be managed as for high velocity missile injuries.

Intermediate range injury produces multiple penetrating wounds to below the level of the deep fascia. They are of low velocity type and should be treated by exploration, toilet and delayed primary suture.

At a distance there is peppering of the skin. This should be treated by skin cleansing, removal of the pellets and dressing.

REHABILITATION

This important aspect of the final management of military injury is commenced as soon as possible in hospital to keep optimum function in all uninvolved parts. It is supported by occupational therapy and welfare attention.

As soon as his condition allows, often when the injured part is still under treatment, in a cast or awaiting further reconstructive procedures such as tendon grafting or nerve surgery, the victim is transferred to a rehabilitation unit. These units are sited in pleasant, country areas and are run as a service mess with the usual facilities for sport and recreation. They have a full staff of physiotherapists, remedial gymnasts, occupational therapists and welfare workers. They are commanded by a medical officer with a staff of remedial consultants, specialists and administrative staff and are supported by visiting consultants.

Treatment is arranged individually, but classwork is done by all to maintain and improve general fitness. Suitable games are an important aspect of this and competition is encouraged.

Centres are planned to have good residential accommodation with the usual unit freedom and weekend leave completely to wean the patients from the hospital atmosphere, where they have frequently spent a long time. A spirit of optimism is fostered; much of the encouragement comes from others who have overcome disabilities sometimes more severe.

These rehabilitation centres have proved highly cost-effective and they are much preferred by the patients to hospitals. They release urgently required acute hospital beds and they ensure the maximum and most rapid recovery of injured servicemen before return to useful duty or to civilian life. They are of particular value in foot and lower limb disorders. Unless fully recovered servicemen are of little use in a fighting service. All these considerations are of greater significance in time of war.

BIBLIOGRAPHY

Berlin R 1976 Local effects of assault rifle bullets in live tissues. Acta Chir Scand: Suppl 477

Berlin R 1977 Local effects of assault rifle bullets in live tissues. Acta Chir Scand: Suppl 459

Candole C A 1967 Blast injury. Can Med Assoc J 96: 207–214

Clevland M, Manning J G, Stewart W J 1951 Care of battle casualties and injuries involving bones and joints. J Bone Joint Surg 33A: 517–521

Coates J B, Beyers J C 1962 Wound Ballistics. Medical Department United States Army: Washington DC

Coppell D L 1976 Blast injury of the lung. Br J Surg 63: 735–737

De Muth W E 1969 Bullet velocity as applied to military rifle wounding capacity. J Trauma 9: 27–38

Devas M 1975 Stress Fractures. Churchill Livingstone, Edinburgh

Furlong R, Clark J M P 1947 Missile wounds involving bone. Br J Surg, War Surgery Supplement 2: 291–310

Hadfield J, Hobsley M 1978 Current Surgical Practice. Edward Arnold, London. pp 204–229

Hampton O P 1951 Wounds of Extremities in Military Surgery. Henry Kimpton, London

Howland W S, Ritchey J S 1971 Gun shot fractures in civilian practice. J Bone Joint Surg 53A: 47–55

Kirby N G, Blackburn G (eds) 1981 A Field Surgery Pocket Book. HMSO, London

Livingstone R H, Wilson R I 1975 Gunshot wounds of the limbs. Br Med J 1: 667–669

Lowry K F, Curtis G M 1950 Delayed suture in the management of wounds. Am J Surg 80: 280–287

Moore F D 1969 Post Traumatic Pulmonary Insufficiency. W B Saunders Co, Philadelphia

Owen Smith M S 1979 Explosive blast injury. J R Army Med Corps 125: 4–16

Owen Smith M S 1981 High Velocity Missile Wounds. Edward Arnold, London

Rawlins J S P 1978 Physical and pathophysiological effects of blast. Injury 9: 313–320

Sellier K 1979 Effectiveness of small caliber ammunition. Acta Chir Scand, Suppl 489: 71–80

Skepanovic D 1979 The effect of shooting steel spheres at blocks of soap. Acta Chir Scand, Suppl 489: 71–80

Whelan T J, Burkhalter W E, Gomez A 1968 Management of war wounds. Advances in Surgery, vol 3, Year Book, Medical Publishers Inc., Chicago. pp 227–349

Industrial and occupational disorders

INDUSTRIAL INJURY OVERVIEW

In 1984 the National Safety Council reported that foot injuries represented 4% of all work-related injuries in the United States. This claim followed only 13 years after the same Council's figures had led Kleiger (1976) to estimate that foot and ankle injury accounted for 16.5% of all work injuries.

In terms of compensation costs, the National Safety Council estimated that almost $600 million was paid out for injuries to the foot and ankle in 1971. In 1978 that Council recorded 130 000 cases of compensable foot injuries. By 1984 the number of foot injuries had dropped to 80 000, at an estimated cost of $2104 per case.

This radical change in the picture for industry in general is poorly documented. However, the trend is reflected in the records of the Construction Safety Association of Ontario, which represents the industry most affected by foot and ankle injury, according to a survey submitted by the CSAO to the American National Standards Institute in 1975. In that document it was stated that 48.6% of all industrial foot and ankle injuries occurred to construction workers. The next largest single group similarly affected constituted only 9.6% of the total. Hence it seems justifiable to review the consistently maintained figures of the construction industry to gain a perspective on the current foot and ankle injury situation in the workplace.

Litster stated in 1984 (1984a) that there had been a greater than 60% reduction of foot injuries amongst construction workers in Ontario since 1969. That statistic represented more than 18 000 fewer foot injuries for that period of time, and a saving in direct compensation costs of over $47 million.

The 1975 survey of the CSAO found that 30% of injuries to the foot had occurred on the sole, 23% involved the midfoot, and 22% affected the toes. Punctures were the most common type of injury, accounting for 31% of the total. About 25% of the injuries involved fractures. 1984 estimates of that association demonstrated a vastly different situation. Only 5.1% of injuries occurred on the sole, 3.8% involved the metatarsal region, 8.8% affected the toes and 7.1% were related to the heel, while 48.6% of all foot injuries involved the ankle. Punctures accounted for only 6.3%, and fractures 19.6% of the foot and ankle injuries. The dominant type of injury identified was sprains and strains, which defined 34.3% of all injuries to the foot and ankle. This corroborated the finding of the high incidence of ankle as opposed to foot injuries, which has created a new priority of concern.

INDUSTRIAL INJURY TO THE ANKLE

Ankle injury was found to have a 32% incidence in a comprehensive overview of the North American industrial accident pattern conducted in 1975. CSAO 1984 estimates present an even greater percentage (48.6%) of ankle relative to foot injuries. The last figure reflects both a dramatic reduction of foot injuries in recent years, and the fact that ankle injury has not been proportionately reduced, although actual occurrences are fewer.

The major ankle injuries seen are sprains and strains caused by slipping or tripping accidents. Most soft tissue ankle injuries are the result of tears to either the anterior talofibular ligament, the calcaneofibular ligament, or both. In marked equinus the anterior talofibular ligament is taut, and functions as the primary static, soft tissue stabilizer on the lateral side of the ankle. The typical trip over a low step or runner forces the ankle into equinus, rendering the anterior talofibular ligament vulnerable. Acute ligamentous tears are the most common form of injury, but in some occupations chronic injuries predominate. As will be elaborated later in this chapter, a theatrical dancer who needs absolute stability in plantar flexion, lacks the support necessary to maintain this position if ankle ligaments are stretched or scarred.

Treatment of single ligament injuries is generally conservative. A pressure dressing employing a contoured pad around the lateral malleolus may be applied at the worksite. When combined with ice and elevation, this significantly retards oedema formation and accelerates recovery. An adhesive strapping may allow isolated anterior talofibular ligament tears to be managed in an ambulatory fashion. The use of a firm high-cut boot can facilitate the worker's return to regular employment with little or no delay.

Lateral ligament injuries involving both the calcaneofibular and anterior talofibular ligaments can produce gross instability, combining both talar tilt and anterior drawer movement. These injuries require, at least, a below-knee walking cast. In selected cases strong consideration should be given to primary surgical repair.

The prognosis in most ligamentous ankle injuries is good, although residual discomfort may persist for several months. Adequate ankle support during the rehabilitation period, and a programme of regular exercise to recover strength and proprioception, should be initiated in all cases where the residual symptoms interfere with the return to work.

While it is impossible to protect against all hazards, slipping exemplifies the usually avoidable accident. Slipping occurs when there is insufficient friction between the soles or heels of the worker's shoes and the floor surface. Frequently poor housekeeping, such as failure to clean or dry surfaces following a spill, is responsible for a dangerously slippery surface. The obvious management for this problem is better housekeeping. However, a more reliable solution is the application of abrasive or non-slip materials to the floor surface. Industrial carpeting virtually eliminates slipping.

Another approach to the prevention of this major cause of ankle injury is the wearing of slip-resistant safety shoes. These rely upon abrasive material and specific tread design. Until recently no satisfactory slip-resistant sole had been designed. However, with refinements of non-slip rubber and non-slip neoprene, and in the past year the introduction of polyurethane as the primary material used for the manufacture of safety shoes, a significant reduction is expected in slip-accident statistics.

Hitherto, high-cut boots have had little impact on ankle injury caused by slipping and tripping, since workers tend not to lace them properly. Apparently the current procedure for securing ankle support is too time-consuming or cumbersome for most workmen. In order for the ankle covering to become an effective ankle support, greater refinement of the usage mechanism will have to be built into that feature of safety boots.

Another common source of ankle injury in industry is blunt trauma to the soft tissue from a moving object. The result of blunt ankle trauma is often superficial abrasion of the skin overlying the malleoli. The impact may be from the moving wheel of a truck or dolly, or from the foot being wedged between moving boxes. Because of their inaccessibility, tendon injury around the ankle is rare from this mechanism. Unless fracture occurs, the trauma is usually minor and can be dealt with by simple first aid measures.

High-cut boots and leather or canvas gaiters provided protection to the ankle against blunt trauma, and may guard against lacerations and burns. However, misused boots can increase the severity of chemical and thermal burns to the ankle or foot, and of injury from metal or glass fragments which enter the unlaced boot and are difficult to remove. Second degree burns have resulted from hot water being accidentally hosed inside a worker's boot. The depth of the burn is increased by the hot water being held in contact with the skin by the sock and boot. Not all burns are as obvious. Chemical burns can occur gradually, if the heavy socks usually worn with work boots absorb toxic materials and hold them in close proximity to the skin of the ankle and foot. Because of the insidious onset, the worker may not be aware of the severity of the resulting injury.

INDUSTRIAL INJURY TO THE TOE

Toe injuries in the industrial setting have become

considerably less frequent in recent years. Between 1975 and 1984 the incidence of toe injuries dropped from 25% to 8.8% of all foot injuries according to CSAO estimates. Most of these injuries are caused by a striking object, which is second only to slipping in the overall causes of foot and ankle injury.

Contusions and minor soft tissue injuries to the toes are rare in the properly protected foot. However they may occur as the only sequelae of severe crush injuries to the toe cap of a well-constructed work boot. Hall (1982) points out that only minor contusions were noted in the toes of a worker who had an eight-ton cylinder of steel plating roll across the front of his safety boot.

Fractures and crush injuries to the toes are far less common in protected work situations than in most leisure-time activities. These injuries generally occur as the result of direct impact, or from the foot being trapped under a wheel or in the moving parts of a machine. Crush injuries to the great toe are usually associated with fractures of the phalanges. These can be severely disabling, and may lead to prolonged discomfort and difficulty with shoe fitting. In cases of significant angular deformity of the great toe, operative intervention is usually required. Fractures of the remaining four digits are of less clinical significance, and except for symptomatic treatment can frequently be ignored. Treatment of an accompanying subungual haematoma by drainage through a hole burned in the toenail should be carried out immediately, even in the suspected presence of a distal phalangeal fracture.

Lacerations to the toes are uncommon with proper protection. When injuries do occur they are generally the result of contact with cutting devices, the most common of which is the power lawnmower. More than 10 000 lawnmower injuries to the foot are recorded annually in North America. Most of these occur away from the workplace. A worker who might refuse to remain on the job without proper foot protection, often ignores comparable safety procedures at home.

Between 1969 and 1984 industrial toe injury had been significantly reduced, largely due to the increased effectiveness of the steel toe cap in safety shoes. However, Litster (1984b) claimed that the maximum energy protection level had not yet been achieved. He advocated that the 100 joules standard operative in the United States, and the Canadian standard of 125 joules should be upgraded to 150 joules to meet the real need for adequate toe protection.

Clearly the decrease in toe injuries is a direct result of the widespread use of safety shoes that has evolved during the past few years. In the 1977 Canadian Injury Survey, only 57% of construction workers were reported to be wearing safety shoes. By 1984, 95% of these workers were wearing protective footwear. In 1977 safety shoes were heavy and box-like, and therefore failed to gain consumer acceptance. Today safety shoes are available in styles ranging from dress shoes to sneakers. They are attractive, comfortable and convenient, and to some people with heightened safety-awareness they have become the shoe of choice, even off the job. With the recent introduction of polyurethane as the major material in the manufacture of safety shoes, even the highest grade, heavy-duty work boots are light-weight. This innovation should further reduce injury as workmen performing heavy labour, who have hitherto opted for lower-grade protective footwear because of its lighter weight, switch to the more appropriate type of boot.

INDUSTRIAL INJURY TO THE HEEL

Trauma to the heel represented 7.1% of all foot and ankle injury in 1984, a percentage only slightly smaller than toe injury estimates. Loss of footing was found to have caused the greatest number of injuries to the foot and ankle overall, and is generally the source of injury to the heel. Construction workers and firefighters who frequently work at a height are particularly susceptible to this type of injury. Heel damage may also result from repetitive minor trauma, such as prolonged walking on hard surfaces.

Trauma to the heel pad, while not a serious structural injury, may produce considerable functional limitation. The injury results from forceful or repetitive impacts to the cushioning fat-containing elastic cells between the tuberosity of the os calcis and the plantar skin. Pain on walking may be sufficient to curtail normal work activity. Treatment generally consists of a cushioned insole and adequate rest. Modifications of the standard safety shoe to treat this condition are difficult, and a change in the floor surface is seldom possible.

Plantar fasciitis occurs along the anterior margin of the tuberosity in front of the heel pad. Again, the pain may limit the worker's ability to walk. Cushioned insoles or arch supports are the usual treatment, but resistant cases may necessitate anti-inflammatory medication, local cortisone injections and, rarely, surgical division of the fascia. It is important to bear in mind that this is generally a self-limiting condition. Workers should be encouraged to continue their regular activities in spite of low levels of discomfort, and should be reassured that continued activity does not cause further damage.

Fractures of the os calcis may result from a fall even from a low height, and are by far the most serious of the heel injuries. 75% of these fractures involve the subtalar joint and most have a degree of displacement causing loss of the longitudinal arch of the foot, widening of the heel, and a reduction in heel height. Failure to restore the normal contour to the hindfoot leads to serious long-term problems with shoe fitting, and may preclude the use of safety boots. This injury can significantly limit the worker's possibility of further employment. Early treatment should include some attempt at restoration of normal hindfoot anatomy. The period of non-weightbearing may be prolonged, but early movement is recommended. The worker who fractures his os calcis is unlikely to return to anything more than a sedentary job in less than six months.

INDUSTRIAL INJURY TO THE SOLE

The incidence of sole injuries relative to injuries to other parts of the foot and to the ankle was 30% in 1975. By 1977, statistics showed a 6% incidence. According to 1984 estimates the incidence of sole injury had fallen yet further to 5.1%.

This dramatic change was largely due to the inclusion of steel insoles in safety shoes. These rapidly became mandatory in the construction industry where workers were most vulnerable to puncture wounds in the sole of the foot, which had been the most common industrial injury prior to this safety innovation. Another factor which contributed to the reduction of sole punctures was replacement of the wooden formwork and shoring used to pour concrete, with prefabricated metal ones.

Notwithstanding the decrease in incidence, puncture wounds do still occur through the side of the shoe beside the insole, or in association with crush injuries to the rest of the foot. Although they generally involve only fat and subcutaneous tissue, on rare occasions punctures may damage a joint or disrupt a tendon. With the exception of lacerations of the flexor hallucis which are generally repaired surgically, treatment of isolated tendon lacerations is conservative and the functional result usually surprisingly good. However, the incidence of established infections following untreated punctures is high, and the subsequent chronic drainage and continuing pain can become a serious complication. Appropriate treatment for deep plantar lacerations should include thorough debridement, full exploration to determine the extent of the injury, and restoration of normal anatomy wherever possible.

While not specifically injurious to the sole, electrical current may be conducted to ground through the feet. Therefore nonconductive soles, composed of outsoles and heels of high electrical resistance, should be worn by workers in industries where high-voltage electrical equipment is an occupational hazard.

INDUSTRIAL INJURY TO THE METATARSALS

The frequency of metatarsal injury was estimated to have decreased from 23% in 1975 to 3.8% in 1984. This decrease in incidence is yet further evidence of the remarkably effective foot safety programme that evolved in the industrial workplace during this period of time.

Most fractures of the metatarsals occur as a result of a direct impact on the top of the foot. Fractures of the first metatarsal can substantially alter the contour of the longitudinal arch of the foot, and make it difficult for the worker to wear the standard safety boot. Restoration of normal bony alignment is desirable. Fractures to the remaining metatarsals can generally be treated symptomatically, and may often be managed in an ambulatory fashion with adequate protection within an oversized shoe. An early weight bearing programme helps to prevent post-traumatic oedema and to maintain normal joint mobility in the ankle and hindfoot.

Flexion or severe pronation or supination injuries can occur when the forefoot is caught in a moving belt or roller. Severe rotational injuries may lead to disruption of the tarsometatarsal junction, as well as to fractures of the metatarsals themselves. Operative reduction and internal fixation are generally required in cases of severe displacement. Long-term complications may include post-traumatic osteophyte formation on the dorsum of the foot, with chronic pain and sufficient bony enlargement to make shoe fitting difficult.

Protection for the metatarsals is achieved by inclusion of a metatarsal shield in safety shoes. An effective shield completely covers the dorsum of the foot, is built into the shoe, and overlaps or rests upon the toe cap.

INJURY VICTIMS

Younger age and inexperience continue to correlate highly with susceptibility to industrial accidents. The 1977 Canadian Injury Survey reported that 55% of industrial accidents involved workers under 30 years of age, and 65% affected those with less than five years experience. 1976 Statistics Canada data found 65% of workers under age 24 to be at risk of injury, while those over 24 years had only a 35% probability of injury. Similar percentages were confirmed by the CSAO for foot and ankle injury. The higher percentage of incidence amongst younger workers is disproportionate to their numbers; hence inexperience rather than greater numbers accurately explains this phenomenon.

PREVENTION

The vastly reduced incidence of industrial foot and ankle injury in recent years seems to be largely due to the growing contemporary concern with safety and accident prevention. Safety education and regulations, together with increasingly refined safety equipment, have imposed a high degree of awareness and practical application of safety measures among workers and management in industry.

As far back as the early 1940s some companies made safety equipment mandatory. Subsequently industrial associations began to research and develop standards for the quality control of safety equipment, and to recommend safety regulations. Governmental legislation obligating companies to provide for the safety of workers, and more recently recognition of the right of workers to refuse to perform unsafe tasks, have given safety issues a high priority in industrial settings. In Canada, the original governmental position was so general as to have been little more than an acknowledgement of the need for safety measures. The virtual impossibility of enforcement may explain the government's evasion of confining legislation. However, their relationship of safety conditions in industry to the issue of human rights, has forced industries to invest substantially in safety measures and research, increasingly to reduce industrial injuries.

DANCE INJURIES

Dance injury to the ankle

As in the industrial setting, sprains and strains are the most common acute injury sustained by dancers. In this occupation these injuries tend to be caused by incorrect landing while the foot is in the plantarflexed position. Anterior talofibular ligament strain resulting from forced inversion of the ankle is seen most often.

Mild sprains involve a stretch or partial tear of the talofibular ligament, or combined injury to the anterior talofibular and calcaneofibular ligaments. Pain occurs in the area anterior to the fibular, and there may be tenderness over the calcaneofibular ligament behind and below the lateal malleolus. Generally these types of sprains do not produce instability. Treatment involves elevation, analgesics and immobilization of the specific area by serial taping or a plaster cast, depending on the degree of sprain. In order to maintain flexibility, strapping should be removed and the ankle re-examined frequently, and exercise should be continued.

When instability is demonstrated either clinically under local anaesthetic block or radiologically with anterior drawer or inversion talar tilt, both the anterior talofibular and the calcaneofibular ligaments should be considered completely torn. Treatment includes a below-knee walking cast or surgical repair or both. A rehabilitation programme should be prescribed to restore range of motion to the ankle and contiguous joints initially, and subsequently to strengthen all muscle groups crossing the ankle, particularly the peroneals. After six months the dancer should be able to return to a normal routine.

Gross instability of the ankle subsequent to major ligament disruption requires surgical repair. Traditional lateral ankle reconstitution with complete transfer of the peroneus brevis is not recommended, since this muscle is the primary dynamic stabilizer of the lateral side of the joint. For dancers who require absolute stability in plantarflexion, primary ligament repair with retinacular plication can improve stability without sacrificing peroneal motor function. Alternatively, a longitudinal division of the peroneus brevis may provide material for repair while maintaining the muscle's normal activity.

Ankle strain resulting from eversion causes injury to the anterior portion of the deltoid ligament, and may involve the anterior tibiofibular ligament. Most dancers are able to continue to dance despite the pain which persists for several months. Treatment stresses adequate warm-up exercise, avoidance of fatigue, strapping of the ankle while dancing, and periodic elevation. Analgesics and anti-inflammatory medication are prescribed where indicated. An isolated complete tear of the deltoid ligament is rare. With or without surgical intervention, this condition requires cast immobilization for six weeks.

The anterior and posterior aspects of the ankle joint are commonly involved in talar impingement syndromes. Extreme plantarflexion, as occurs with dancing 'en pointe', forces the posterior tibial lip against the posterior facet of the talus. The intervening soft tissue, including the synovium and joint capsule or the os trigonum if present, are trapped between the border of the tibia and the calcaneus. If the activity is repeated without modification, inflammation may develop in the posterior joint, with secondary osteophyte formation at the posterior tubercle of the talus or enlargement of the os trigonum. Pain is experienced above the calcaneus at the posterior joint line, as well as medially and laterally deep to the peroneal tendons.

Radiographic finding of a large posterior tubercle or enlarged os trigonum is, however, not necessarily evidence of painful posterior impingement. Similar posterior ankle pain is produced by Achilles tendinitis, tendinitis of the flexor hallucis longus, peroneal tendinitis at the lateral malleolus, and nonspecific synovitis of the ankle. To establish a diagnosis of posterior impingement the symptoms must be reproduced by plantarflexion of the ankle, to which the other conditions do not react. Traction on the heel relieves the symptoms.

Treatment of this condition consists of elastic adhesive dressings and anti-inflammatory medication. Prolonged warm-up exercises are also advocated prior to dancing. In cases where pain persists and there is X-ray evidence of ectopic bone or osteophyte formation, posterior arthrotomy of the ankle with excision of the bone may be necessary. Return to 'en pointe' dancing may not be possible for up to a year subsequent to surgery.

Impingement of the anterior margin of the tibia on the talar neck can be caused by extreme dorsiflexion, as occurs with the demi plié dance position. Initial symptoms are poorly localized. However, on examination tenderness is present between the medial malleolus and the tibialis anterior tendon, and between the lateral malleolus and the extensor digitorum communis. In advanced cases, exostoses may be present on the anterior talar neck and the anterior lip of the tibia. If the trauma is repeated, these may become increasingly prominent and eventually fill the normal sulcus on the superior surface of the talar neck.

Treatment of mild anterior impingement syndrome consists of a half-inch heel lift in street shoes, and nonsteroidal anti-inflammatory medication. Advanced cases may require surgical excision of the exostoses in order to extend the dancer's career, but recurrence of exostoses must be expected after several years.

Ankle fractures tend to occur when the dancer is tired, balance is poor and timing is off. The fracture pattern is not unique. Eversion fractures are more common, and usually occur in the supporting ankle during an incorrectly executed turn. Inversion fractures occur through the same mechanism, and more commonly produce lateral ligament tear. Following treatment of the acute injury, rehabilitation must include range of movement and stretching exercises, with particular emphasis on passive dorsiflexion. The passive range of movement is generally greater than the active range, so the deficit may not be recognized in a routine ankle examination. With the patient seated, pull the foot backwards until the heel leaves the floor. Comparing the normal and injured sides may demonstrate a variation in passive range of up to 20°. Loss of this movement is a significant disability to the performer in both modern dance and classical ballet. Even with aggressive post-fracture management, a return to full, painfree ankle function may take up to two years.

Inflammation of the tendons or tendon sheaths occurs frequently. Most common is Achilles tendinitis or peritendinitis, which seems to be related to the performance of unusual dance movements and to unyielding floor surfaces. This condition generally involves inflammation of the unsheathed region a few centimetres above the insertion of the Achilles tendon into the os calcis. However symptoms may be localized to the area proximal to the calcalneal bursa. Tenderness over an area of the tendon may be accompanied by swelling, erythema or crepitus. Pain is experienced on landing after a jump, as deceleration is produced by the triceps surae. Treatment for this condition includes refraining from jumping until pain has subsided, rest, elevation, the application of local heat, and nonsteroidal anti-inflammatory medication. A heel lift can be used in street shoes. Stretching and strengthening exercises should be performed.

Tendinitis of the flexor hallucis longus tendons at the medial aspect of the ankle is also common. With the repeated stress of extreme plantarflexion when standing 'en pointe', inflammation may occur where the tendon enters its fibro-osseous canal. When the muscle belly of flexor hallucis longus extends too far distally, positions of extreme dorsiflexion wedge the muscle fibres into the entrance of the fibro-osseous tunnel behind the talus, causing pain. Treatment is symptomatic, and includes rest, local heat, elevation and anti-inflammatory drugs.

Dance injury to the midfoot

Improper technique causes many acute and chronic injuries to the midfoot. For example, fundamental to all dance is the ability to externally rotate the lower extremity. Ideally this facility, termed 'turn out', depends upon an almost 90° external rotation at the hip, a small degree of knee rotation, and the 20 to 30° of natural outward inclination of the foot and ankle. Dancers with increased femoral anteversion, an anterior-oriented acetabulum, or tight anterior hip capsule and ligaments, are not able to achieve the required rotation at the hip. They often try to compensate by increasing rotation at the knee, foot and ankle, causing undue stress to the medial ligaments of the knee and foot. The increased laxity in the midtarsal joints results in abduction of the weight-bearing part of the foot, and flattening or pronation of the medial longitudinal arch. Inflammation of the plantar fascia and abductor hallucis may be associated conditions. Repeated excessive pronation causes pain at the medial aspect of the first metatarsophalangeal joint, and may eventually result in severe hallux valgus.

Conditions rising from abnormal positions such as 'rolling in', 'rolling out' and sickling, which involves faulty instep positioning while 'en pointe', should be treated by balancing the foot and ankle complex to correct movement technique, anti-inflammatory medication, elastic taping and specific orthotics.

Dance injury to the forefoot

Acute hyperflexion injury of the metatarsophalangeal joint of the hallux is common among dancers. Tearing of the dorsal portion of the capsule occurs when tripping causes the entire body weight to bear upon the forcibly flexed digit. Reaction to the event is immediate pain and loss of movement. Treatment involves elastic adhesive strapping of the great toe and forefoot, and the use of crutches for 10 days, followed by graduated active and passive exercise until return to full motion is achieved in about six weeks.

Hyperextension of the interphalangeal joint of the great toe is also a common injury. However it is seldom symptomatic, and treatment is usually limited to padding the toe to prevent recurrent excessive movement. Less common injuries to the hallux include fractures of the proximal phalanx and sesamoiditis. Interphalangeal joint strain is sometimes caused if pointe dance shoes lack adequate stiffness in the toe box.

Minor capsular tears and even frank dislocation of the metatarsophalangeal joints of the lateral toes are also frequently seen in dancers. The complete dislocation is immediately incapacitating. Reduction is achieved by hyperextension of the toe while applying sustained traction. Following reduction, the injured digit is taped to an adjacent toe for three to four weeks.

DANCE INJURY MANAGEMENT — AN OVERVIEW

Disorders of the foot and ankle in dancers are generally managed conservatively. Even in more severe cases operative intervention must be approached with caution. The dancer places extraordinary demands on the foot and relies upon a perfect response. Surgery rarely returns the injured structures to the required level of function. Even in successful cases the postoperative rehabilitation is lengthy and often frustrating. The scar will remain painful for a year or more, and if it is positioned in an area of pressure, may create a new problem.

ACKNOWLEDGEMENT

I gratefully acknowledge the assistance of Ms. Chartrand of the Construction Safety Association of Ontario, and Mr. Munnings and Mr. Norman of ISECO Safety Shoes Ltd. I would particularly like to acknowledge the help of Adrianne Cohen. Without her literary skill I could not have completed this chapter.

BIBLIOGRAPHY

Anderson L D 1977 Injuries of the forefoot. Clin Orthop 122: 18–27

Beals R K, Hickman N W 1972 Industrial Injuries of the Back and Extremities. J Bone Joint Surg 54A: 1593–1611

Beaumont C W, Idzikowski S 1970 A Manual of the Theory and Practice of Classical Theatrical Dancing. Dover, New York

Burrows H J 1956 Fatigue Infraction of the Middle of the Tibia in Ballet Dancers. J Bone Joint Surg 38B: 83–94

Collis W J M, Jayson M I V 1972 Measurement of Pedal Pressures. Ann Rheum Dis 31: 215–217

Coltart W D 1952 Aviator's Astragalus. J Bone Joint Surg 34B: 545–566

Construction Safety Association of Ontario 1975 Summary of a Foot Injury Study. CSAO, Toronto

Construction Safety Association of Ontario 1984 Lost Time Injury Summary. CSAO, Toronto

Construction Safety Association of Ontario 1986 Ontario Construction Industry: Lost Time Foot Injuries, 1980–1986. CSAO, Toronto

Ecker M L, Ritter M A, Jacobs B S 1967 The Symptomatic Os-Trigonum. JAMA 201: 882–884

Fitzgerald R H, Cowan J D E 1975 Puncture Wounds of the Foot. Orthop Clin North Am 6: 965–972

Giannestras N J, Sammarco G J 1975 Fractures and Dislocations in the Foot: In: Rockwood C A, Green D P (eds) Fractures. J B Lippincott, Philadelphia

Gould N 1976 Safety Shoes for Industry. In: Bateman J E (ed) Foot Science, W B Saunders, Philadelphia

Grahame R, Saunders A S, Maisey N 1979 The Use of Scintigraphy in the Diagnosis and Management of Traumatic Foot Lesions in Ballet Dancers. Rheumatol Rehabil 18: 235–238

Hall H 1982 Industrial Injuries to the Foot and Ankle and Their Prevention. In: Jahss M H (ed) Disorders of the Foot. W B Saunders, Philadelphia

Hamilton W G 1977 Tendinitis About the Ankle Joint in Classical Ballet Dancers. J Sports Med 5: 84–88

Hamilton W G 1982 Sprained Ankles in Ballet Dancers. Foot Ankle 3: 99–102

Hamilton W G 1982 Stenosing Tensynovitis of the Flexor Hallucis Longus Tendon and Posterior Impingement upon the Os-Trigonum in Ballet Dancers. Foot Ankle 3: 74–80

Hardaker W T, Margello S, Goldner J L 1985 Foot and Ankle Injuries in Theatrical Dancers. Foot Ankle 6(2): 59–69

Hardy R H, Clapham J C 1951 Observations on Hallux Valgus. J Bone Joint Surg 33B: 376–391

Hillegass R C 1976 Injuries to the Midfoot: A Major Cause of Industrial Morbidity. In: Bateman J E (ed) Foot Science. W B Saunders, Philadelphia

Howse A J G 1982 Posterior Block of the Ankle Joint in Dancers. Foot Ankle 3: 81–84

Howse A J G 1983 Disorders of the Great Toe in Dancers. Clin Sports Med 2: 499–505

Inman V 1976 The Joints of the Ankle. Williams & Wilkins, Baltimore

Kay D B 1985 Sprained Ankle: Current Therapies. Foot Ankle 6(1): 22–27

Kleiger B 1976 Work-Related Injuries of the Foot and Ankle. In: Bateman J E (ed) Foot Science. W B Saunders, Philadelphia. pp 254–256

Kleiger B 1982 Anterior Tibial Talar Impingement Syndromes in Dancers. Foot Ankle 3: 69–73

Litster R 1978 Review of 1977 Canadian Injury Survey. Proceedings Paper, Conference on Protective Equipment, Toronto

Litster R 1984a Foot Injuries in North America. Proceedings Paper, Conference on Protective Equipment, Toronto

Litster R 1984b Applied Personal Protection Technology. Proceedings Paper, Conference on Protective Equipment, Toronto

McDougall A 1955 The Os-Trigonum. J Bone Joint Surg 37B: 257–265

Miller E H, Schneider H J, Bronson J L, McLain D 1975 A New Consideration of Athletic Injuries — The Classical Ballet Dancer. Clin Orthop Rel Res 111: 181–191

National Safety Council 1972–1985 Accident Facts. National Safety Council of America. pp 23–39

Rovere G D 1983 Musculoskeletal Injuries in Theatrical Dance Students. Am J Sports Med 11: 195–198

Sammarco G J 1982 The Foot and Ankle in Classical Ballet and Modern Dance. In: Jahss M H (ed) Disorders of the Foot. W B Saunders, Philadelphia. 2: 1627–1659

Sammarco G J 1984 Diagnosis and Treatment of Dancers. Clin Orthop 187: 176–187

Sammarco G J, Miller E H 1979 Partial Rupture of the Flexor Hallus Longus Tendon in Classica! Ballet Daners. J Bone Joint Surg 61: 149–150

Sammarco G J, Burstein A H, Frankel V H 1973 Biomechanics of the Ankle: A Kinematic Study. Orthop Clin North Am 4: 75–96

Seligson D, Gassman J, Pope M 1980 Ankle Instability: Evaluation of the Lateral Ligaments. Am J Sports Med 8: 39–42

Cold injury

POPULATIONS AT RISK

Populations of 100 million or more may be at risk from cold injury yet it is relatively uncommon in civilian life and associated with illness, injury or unusually harsh climatic conditions. In wartime, the position is different as large numbers may be exposed to climatic extremes against which they cannot take normal precautions. Cold injury was of considerable significance in Napoleon's Russian campaign and in many previous wars. In World War II in the US Army there were 90 000 casualties due to cold, 87% from rifle companies, and in the winter of 1943 frostbite injuries among US heavy bomber crews were greater than all other casualties put together. In the British Army because of vigorously enforced foot hygiene — a legacy from World War I when there were 115 000 cold injuries — cases were minimal. In the Korean Campaign, 1950–1952, 25% of all casualties were due to cold and in the Falklands in 1982, 15% were due to cold injury of the lower limbs. A small number of cases occur in polar travellers and mountaineers despite improvements in equipment, technique and knowledge (Schechter & Sarot 1968, Hanson & Goldman 1969, Washburn 1962, Ward 1974, Marsh 1983).

Acclimatization

Convincing evidence for general acclimatization to cold is difficult to obtain though cold habituation occurs. Local acclimatization has an essentially vascular basis. Newcomers cannot work as long with bare hands as those who have spent long periods in cold conditions and indigenous Central Asian highlanders can walk comfortably in bare feet on snow for long periods without cold injury.

Studies on a Nepalese pilgrim in the Everest region who walked with bare feet in snow at -5°C and who slept in the open wearing light clothing at temperatures of −13°C at night showed that he maintained a metabolic rate 50% above normal by light shivering. He complained neither of numbness nor tingling in either hands or feet and the skin temperature of his toes dropped only to 8°C so that frostbite did not occur (Pugh 1963). Meditation, hypnosis and biofeedback training may increase peripheral blood flow through vasodilatation. Toe temperatures may rise as much as 8.3°C through G Tum-mo yoga (Benson et al 1982).

TEMPERATURE REGULATION

A useful but oversimplified concept is to imagine the body as consisting of a central core with a relatively uniform temperature of 37°C and an insulating shell with a temperature of 33°C. Heat transfer within the body occurs by convection through the circulation and conduction through peripheral tissue to skin surface.

As the maintenance of the central core temperature is essential to life this may occur at the expense of the peripheral 'expendable' structures such as toes and fingers. The control of body temperature depends on interaction between heat production and heat loss. The former depends on normal body metabolism which at rest corresponds to an oxygen consumption of the order of 5 ml/kg/min. During heavy exercise and shivering, heat output may rise considerably; maximal oxygen consumption in athletes may be as high as 85 ml/kg/min though this level cannot be maintained.

Heat loss in dry cold conditions is mainly by convection or transfer of heat by bulk movement when air adjacent to the body is heated. If air so heated remains trapped it will serve as insulation. If it is disturbed by external wind, considerable heat loss can occur and this is prevented by windproof clothing. Loss of heat by conduction occurs when clothes become wet due either to rain, sweat or melted snow. As water is a good conductor of heat, heat loss is increased.

Heat loss by radiation is independent of air movement. If the body heat is greater than the surroundings heat is lost, if less the body gains heat. In polar and high mountain environments heat gain by both direct and indirect radiation (the albedo) from snow may be of prime importance in survival (Chrenko & Pugh 1961). Heat gain at high altitude (5800 m) can be three times that occurring at sea-level in desert regions (Pugh 1962).

Heat loss by evaporation may occur through perspiration or in expired air and at the high ventilation rates of altitude the latter may be most important. Disordered lung function or 'Eskimo-lung' due to exposure for long periods at subzero temperatures has been reported, and this will depress oxygen uptake and, therefore, heat production (Schaeffer et al 1980). Exhaustion may lead to reduced stroke volume, a falling peripheral resistance and shift in the distribution of blood to capacitance vessels. This failure of vasomotor regulation with pooling of peripheral venous blood, in cold conditions will accelerate heat loss (Ekelund 1967) and low blood pressure states have been described following ascent to extreme altitude (Pugh & Ward 1956).

Perspiration occurs as a result of exercise and emotional stimulus and the soles of the feet, palms of hands and axillae are particularly affected. On military operations emotional sweating may be increased when periods of great activity followed by immobility are common. Neglect in the designs of footwear can lead to serious cold injury. Varicose veins of the lower limbs may increase heat loss by convection and cold phlebitis has been reported. Heat loss from the body is prevented by the insulation of tissues, air and clothes, and that provided by clothes is the most important. Insulation of the feet is by means of boots which should be designed to keep the feet both dry and warm. Though less subject to cooling, the foot is less easy to rewarm than the hand as local metabolism and heat store are both poor. The part played by blood flow in heat input is relatively larger in the foot than in the hand.

Footwear in cold, underdeveloped countries often consists of animal skin packed with grass or leaves, and Eskimos use the mukluk which operates on the same principle.

Normally a leather boot with a firm sole is worn with one or more pairs of socks and with an insole. Double leather boots with a detachable inner have been developed but are very heavy and clumsy. Vapour barrier boots suffer from the defect that feet remain constantly wet and liable to skin disorders.

Modern ski-boots with a plastic outer and moulded foam inners are remarkably warm and this same principle is now used in the manufacture of mountaineering boots which have a plastic outer shell and detachable inner boot of manmade fibre. This is much lighter and less clumsy than the double leather boot. Over all, a gaiter should be fixed to the boot and this should extend to the *knee*. Snow may easily enter the boot if only an ankle gaiter is used and this will melt and cause cold injury.

For permanent shelter, huts, tents, snow-caves or individual snow slots should be used. In snow conditions, particularly if there is danger of avalanche, a snow hole or individual snow slot may be preferable to a tent. One accommodating four people takes about three to four hours to dig. It has the advantage of permanence, safety, warmth and relative exclusion from wind noise. The entrance should be clearly marked.

HIGH ALTITUDE AND COLD INJURY

Oxygen uptake falls with altitude. At extreme altitudes the margin between maximum oxygen consumption and that necessary for adequate heat production and work narrows and cases of frostbite of the feet have been recorded in fully clad mountaineers. Both cold and high altitude raise the packed cell volume and viscosity and slow peripheral blood flow. Cold injury to capillary walls leads to plasma leakage and intravascular sludging. This local haemoconcentration will be increased at altitude and impaired tissue nutrition and necrosis may occur more rapidly.

Dehydration, the result of abnormal water loss from the lungs due to increased respiration will also increase blood viscosity and thrombosis may be encouraged by relative inactivity. Even at normal temperatures the blood flow in the skin is reduced at high altitude, the result of arteriolar vasoconstriction. Cardiac output is also decreased as may be basal metabolic rate and the ability to shiver. Hypoxia and cold blunt mental function and precautions taken against cold injury may be inadequate. Deterioration at altitude leading to poor appetite, with decreased calorie intake, results in diminution of the insulating layer of subcutaneous fat.

Cold injury to the feet often occurs during forced bivouacs. A snowcave must be dug, both crampons and boots removed and feet warmed in the companion's armpit or abdomen. Both fluid and food should be taken if available. With these precautions it has been possible to survive at night at 28 700 ft at −35°C without supplementary oxygen and without frostbite (Ward 1975, Clarke 1976, Heath & Williams 1981).

COLD INJURY COMPLICATING TRAUMA

The risk of frostbite in exposed subdermal tissue is considerable. Devitalized tissue freezes in 1 minute at 0°C if wind speeds rise above 2 metres per second.

If hypotension or haemorrhagic hypovolaemia are present the normal signs of hypothermia may be masked. The risk of hypothermia is also increased in victims with partially perfused exposed tissue at subzero temperatures. When warmed, these hypothermic patients may start to bleed profusely from injured tissue. In addition, the analgesic protection afforded by cold will be lost on rewarming. Wounds should be thermally protected as soon as possible and a balance struck between thermal protection and necessity for close observation (Pearn 1982).

Cold injury and renal failure

Incipient renal failure associated with rhabdomyolysis has been recorded following severe frostbite of both lower limbs and in nonfreezing cold injury of the feet in children. Severe exercise may also be a factor (Raifman et al 1978, Rosenthall et al 1981).

COLD INJURY AND THE ELDERLY

The elderly are less active, may have an inadequate diet and a sluggish metabolic and vasomotor response with progressive impairment of thermoregulatory mechanisms. The long-term conservative management particularly of freezing cold injury with the possible complications of hypostatic pneumonia, bedsores and urinary infection has to be balanced against amputation and early mobility. Much will depend on the mental age and physical activity of the patient (Emslie-Smith 1981, Ramstead et al 1980).

PHYSIOPATHOLOGY

Nonfreezing cold injury may progress to freezing cold injury and both may occur in the same lower limb and be associated with hypothermia. Nonfreezing cold injury usually occurs in wet/cold conditions between 0°–15°C though the upper limits are not precisely known as feet exposed in water at 21°C for hours may become swollen, hyperaemic and painful. Frostbite occurs at temperatures of 0°C and below in dry/cold conditions.

In nonfreezing cold injury the skin is less affected than deeper structures and probably the major damage is to the nerves due to the direct action of cold and indirectly to hypoxia, the result of vasospasm and haemagglutination. Nerve conduction may cease after 1–3 hours of prolonged cooling. Muscle is very sensitive to local cooling and the temperature of deep muscle after two hours immersion may be only 1°–2°C above the fluid surrounding it. After eight hours of such exposure the speed of muscle movement is greatly decreased. Cold-induced vasodilatation with hyperaemia follows the ischaemic phase. General body cooling can affect both the degree of vasodilatation and hyperaemia, which if suppressed results in the temperature of the affected part falling to that of the air or water surrounding it (Fig. 52.1).

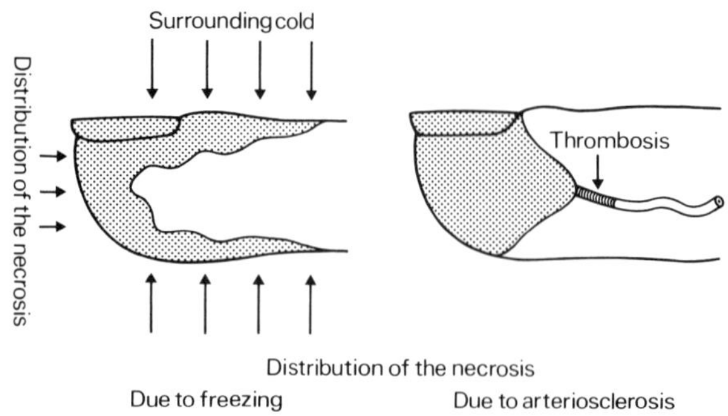

Fig. 52.1 Physiopathology of frostbite and arteriosclerosis

Tissues vary in their resistance to freezing cold injury; skin appears to freeze at -0.53°C whilst muscle, blood vessels and nerves are highly susceptible. Connective tissue, tendons and bone are relatively resistant. Fat necrosis and atrophy occur.

Nerves

Decreasing temperature increases proportionally the clinical severity which is matched in peripheral nerves by an increasingly severe morphological change. The main findings are an immediate increase in the mean diameter of myelinated and nonmyelinated fibres, marked oedema, a delayed and selective axon degeneration, and infrequent, segmented and paranodal demyelinization. There is a selective vulnerability to cold based on nerve fibre diameter with myelinated fibres more susceptible than nonmyelinated. Degeneration of nerve fibres is probably due to increased permeability of endoneurial vessels which leads to diffuse oedema, the production of toxins, changes in osmolarity and increase in endoneural pressure. Whilst there is clear clinical and pathological evidence of ischaemia in freezing cold injury this is less clear in nonfreezing cold injury though some change in vascular endothelium occurs.

Once the temperature falls below freezing for more than a few seconds, nerve degeneration occurs affecting all nerve fibres equally. There is complete necrosis of all structures within the perineurium except the endothelial lining of blood vessels (Peyronnard et al 1977, Nukada et al 1981).

Skin

The freezing of skin at temperatures of -1.9°C for seven minutes caused no lasting injury, whereas after 11½ minutes the skin was red and tender for several days. Repeated exposure for 20 minutes or more caused blistering.

Blood vessels

Damage to blood vessel walls depends on the period of contact and degree of cold, and plasma leaks into the tissues forming blisters. These contain tissue breakdown products associated with vasoconstriction, increased leucocyte sticking and platelet aggregation occur.

Intravascular blood becomes more viscous and haemagglutination with blood vessel blockage and gangrene occurs. Due to the actions of precapillary sphincters, arteriovenous shunts open and close in cycles and blood bypasses the frozen part. Complete closure of the A-V shunts renders the part avascular and this mechanism protects the hypothalamic temperature-regulating centre from cooled blood and the patient from hypothermia.

Ice crystal formation in environmental freezing cold injury

Interstitial ice-crystals form which enlarge at the expense of intracellular water, osmotic pressure rises and enzyme mechanisms are disturbed with subsequent cell death.

Muscle

In freezing cold injury to muscles, the degree of injury depends on the degree of exposure. The superficial coldest layer shows coagulation necrosis, followed by slow necrosis with muscle atrophy alone in the deepest layer. Repair is by fibrous tissue.

Neither ice-crystal formation nor ischaemia are necessary to produce these changes which are due to cold alone (Lewis & Moen 1952).

Bone and joints

Bone cells are more sensitive than overlying skin and epiphyseal cartilage is more sensitive than bone. The direct action of cold on chondrocytosis or microvascular changes with end artery thrombosis or both may be the cause (McKendry 1981).

Oedema

Primary

Normally cold is associated with tissue dehydration, however the longer the limbs take to cool the more likely is oedema to occur, possibly the result of changes in tissue pH.

Secondary

This is the result of rewarming and vasodilatation and forms within 12–24 hours. Plasma passes through the cold damaged capillaries into the interstitial tissue.

Exercise

Continuous submaximal exercise over several days produces an expansion of the extracellular compartment with either subclinical or overt (pitting) oedema of the ankles and feet, partly due to fluid retention and partly to shift from the intracellular compartment. This is independent of fluid balance and is affected by altitude. Compression of the tissues of the feet may occur as a result with increased susceptibility to cold injury (Williams et al 1979, Milledge et al 1982, Ross and Attwood 1984).

CLINICAL FEATURES

Nonfreezing cold injury

Paraesthesia, numbness leading to loss of sensation and a feeling of 'walking on cotton wool' are usual. At night pain like an electric shock, together with swollen feet, makes sleep difficult. In the morning, weight bearing becomes almost unbearable for the first 10–15 minutes and this is then replaced by numbness. The affected area spreads proximally. Following the 'ischaemic' phase and after 2–5 hours in a warm environment, a high blood flow with full arterial pulses and hot, swollen and painful feet follows. Blistering may occur with partial return of sensation and power. Patchy gangrene with loss of tissue may be present. Sensory loss can persist and profuse sweating may be present. Loss of muscle power with resulting contraction can be serious. Freezing cold injury may intervene if the temperature falls further (Ungley et al 1946).

Freezing cold injury

Superficial (Figs. 52.2–4)

Only the skin and subcutaneous tissue are involved and the tissue though white is soft and pliable.

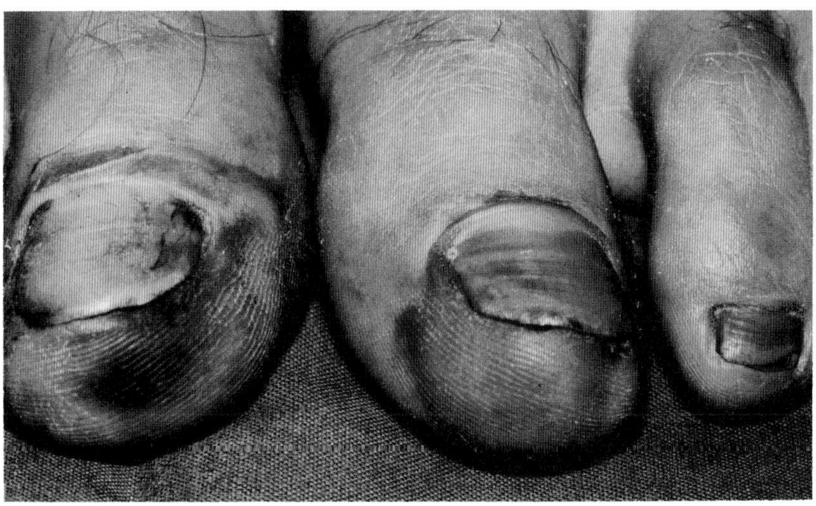

Fig. 52.2 Superficial frostbite: initial discolouration

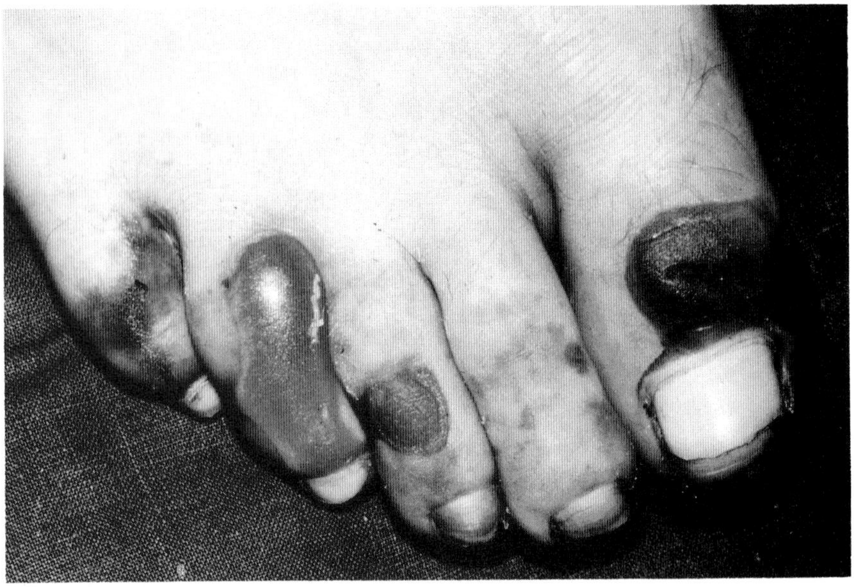

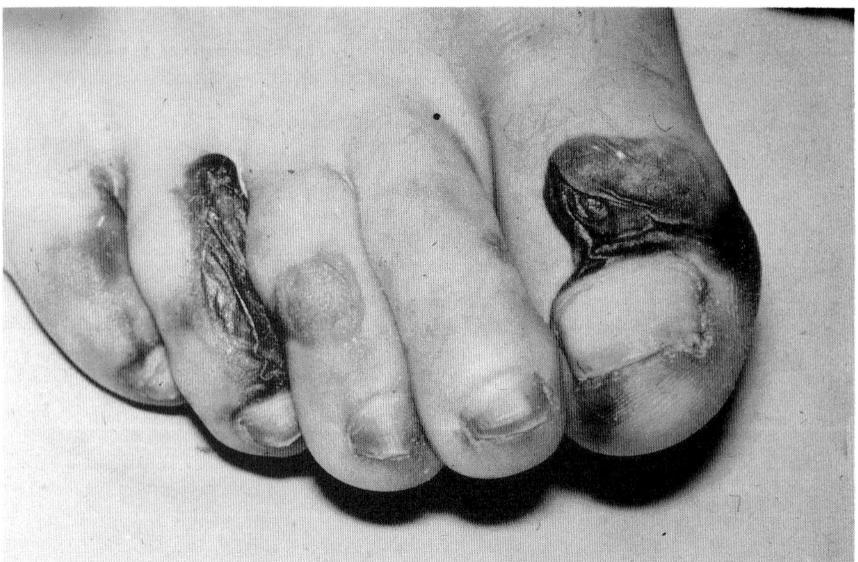

Fig. 52.3 Superficial frostbite: a, blistering on dorsum of toes with some blackening of tissue; b, some weeks later. Superficial carapace formation with crinkling of dead skin which is finally discarded spontaneously. There is no loss of outline or mummification

Blisters may occur within 24–48 hours — they are more common on the dorsum of the foot and toes, where tissue is lax, than on the plantar surface. The blister fluid absorbs leaving a black insensitive carapace. There is associated oedema and within days a very definite line of demarcation occurs. If the contour of the black carapace corresponds to that of the original part, loss of tissue is unlikely, but if mummification and loss of contour occurs, tissue loss is likely. The gangrene is essentially superficial, only a few millimetres thick and peeling off like a glove over the months leaving shining red baby-skin which is abnormally sensitive to temperature and touch. Abnormal sweating may occur. In two to three months it will take on the general appearance of normal skin. The nail may be lost but is likely to grow again normally or slightly deformed.

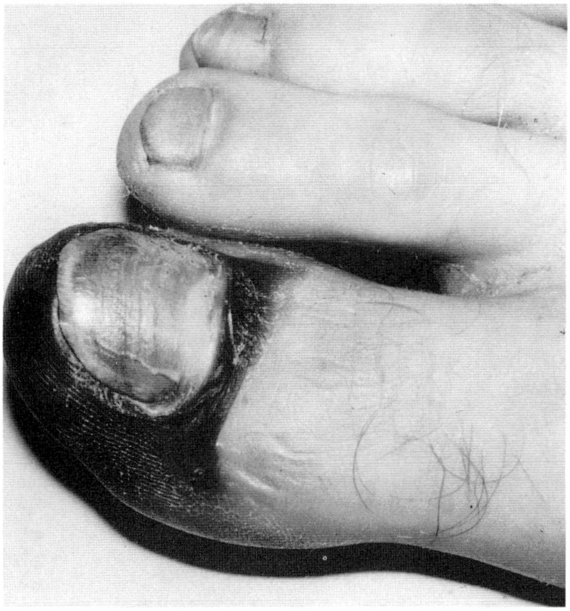

Fig. 52.4 Superficial frostbite: later black carapace which separated spontaneously with no tissue loss (right big toe)

Deep (Figs. 52.5–7)

This involves the skin and subcutaneous tissue as well as muscle, tendons and bones. The affected part is cold, mottled, blue or grey and may remain swollen for months. Blistering, if it occurs, may take weeks to develop. Initially painless, shooting and throbbing pain may develop. Permanent tissue loss is almost inevitable and the loss of contour and form with a mummified appearance develops. Eventually a complete cast of toe or part of the foot separates.

As the muscles are at a distance from the most affected part and as tendons are resistant to cold it will be possible to move the toes or the foot at the ankle.

TREATMENT

Prevention

It is extremely important to dress for the temperature with which the part will be in contact. The feet can be below freezing in deep powder snow or in near freezing water while the environmental temperatures may be many degrees above freezing. Feet must be kept as dry as possible.

Principle

No form of violent therapy should ever be used. In a

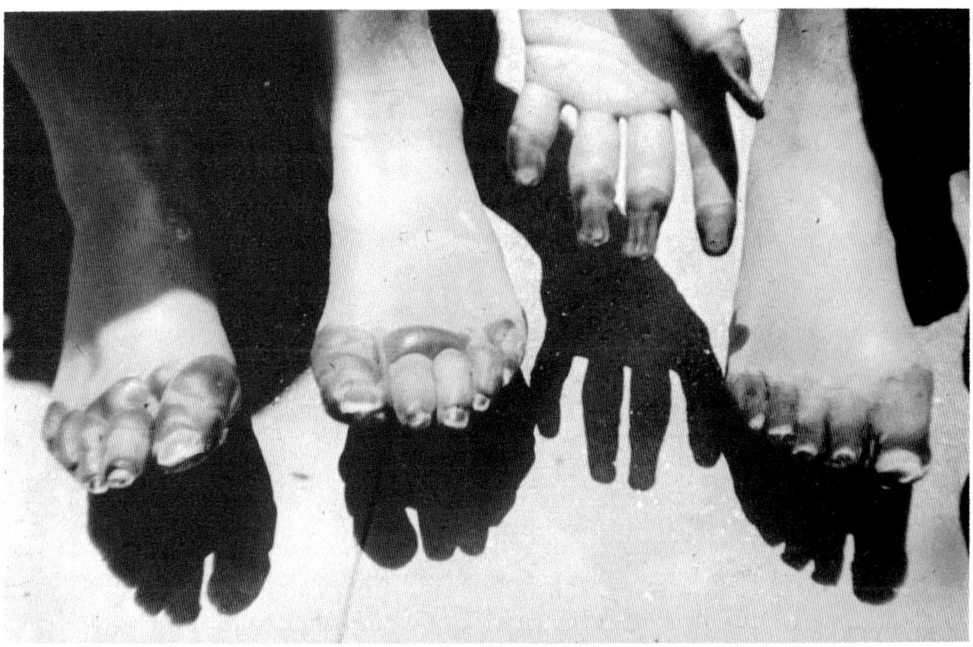

Fig. 52.5 Deep frostbite: loss of outline of fingers is obvious here. Blistering of toes with some loss of outline and mummification has occurred

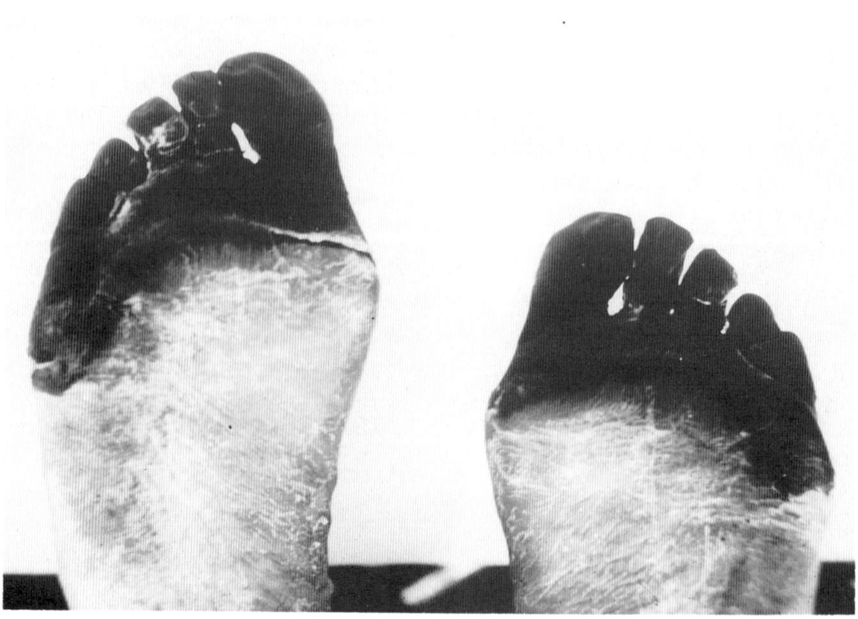

Fig. 52.6 Deep frostbite: obvious line of demarcation in region of metatarsophalangeal joints. Mummification and loss of outline can be seen. This is a later stage of Figure 5. Courtesy Mr. C J C Renton, Hereford County Hospital

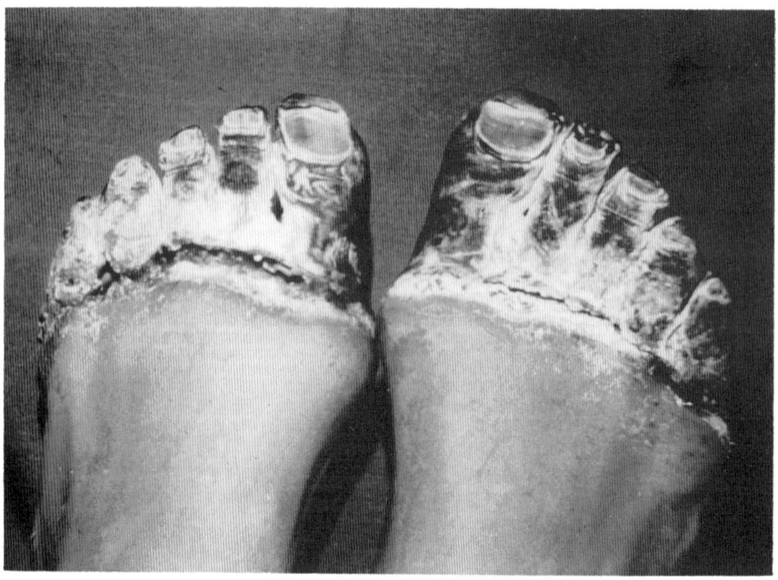

Fig. 52.7 Deep frostbite: a later stage of Figure 6. Dorsum of the foot shows the line of demarcation (covered in antibiotic powder). Courtesy Mr. C J C Renton, Hereford County Hospital

bivouac boots should if possible be removed and feet warmed in the axillae, groin or on the abdomen of a companion. Crampons must be removed and extra clothing put on. At high altitude if supplementary oxygen is available its use will cause peripheral vasodilatation. Protection from the wind is essential. A snow hole should be dug if possible as within it the environmental temperature will be higher than outside.

Nonfreezing cold injury responds to conservative measures such as local and general warming, food and shelter. If frostbite supervenes rapid rewarming should be started, preferably using a water container, to 44°C using a thermometer to check water temperature. Vasodilator drugs do not appear to improve tissue survival nor are the results of sympathectomy striking. Low molecular weight dextran, immediate sympathectomy using intra-arterial reserpine and intravenous blockade with guanethidine using the Bier technique have also been used but with limited success. Hyperbaric oxygen seems to have been discarded. Dissolution of a blood clot by intra-arterial streptokinase has been used. Raised tissue compartment pressures may interfere with venous return and relief incisions may be considered. Rewarming in a pHisohex® whirlpool bath should last for 20 minutes at a time and a thermometer used to check water temperature.

The extent of tissue loss is hard to estimate. Radioactive technetium seems to act as a prognostic indicator only some time after initial exposure. Doppler examination will indicate the degree of arterial flow. Blisters should not be removed. Active movements must be encouraged using whirlpool baths and silicone oil. Unless infection has occurred antibiotics should not be given and the patient should be nursed in as sterile conditions as possible. Thrombolytic enzymes are being evaluated (Flora 1985) but there is a risk especially if intracranial injuries are present. Fractures should be treated conservatively by closed rather than open methods; and dislocation reduced immediately to prevent tissue pressure.

Patients should be kept in pleasant surroundings, given a high calorie and high protein diet and antitetanus serum. Premature surgery is the most potent cause of morbidity, though relief of pressure by escharotomy may be beneficial. Surgical intervention should be minimal. If amputation is necessary, as little tissue as possible should be removed, and it should be delayed for several weeks (Figs. 52.8 and 9). Closure with viable skin is preferable to a skin graft. Further reconstruction can be considered in appropriate cases. Mental preparation is important for patients who may be emotionally labile (Ward 1983).

AFTER EFFECTS

Both short and long-term effects of freezing and nonfreezing cold injury have been reported.

Skin may crack even at normal temperatures and cause painful fissures. Fungating and ulcerating squamous cell carcinoma of the heel have been reported in individuals frostbitten 40 years previously. The lesions were well differentiated, of low malignancy and with no evidence of spread. Treatment was by local excision and skin-grafting. Block dissection of regional lymph glands was not carried out. Unstable scar tissue, chronic irritation and pressure were factors in aetiology (Rossis et al 1982).

Muscle may be replaced by fibrous tissue. Cold

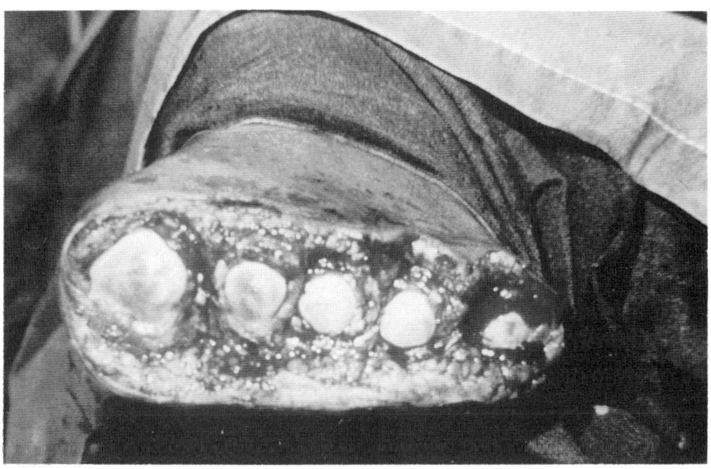

Fig. 52.8 Deep frostbite: Metatarsophalangeal disarticulation. Courtesy Mr. C J C Renton, Hereford County Hospital

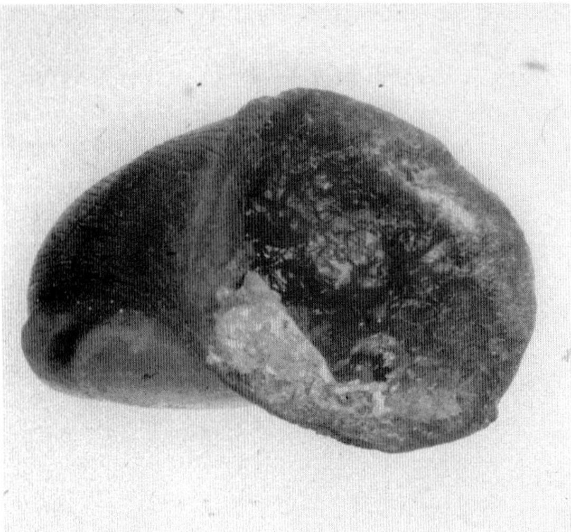

Fig. 52.9 Cast of frostbitten toe which separated spontaneously

sensitization with an unusual degree of vasospastic response to cold and relative resistance to rewarming is well known. A high incidence of nonfreezing cold injury occurs in those with a history of local cold injury and this raises the question particularly in the Armed Forces of whether cold injured troops should be used again in a cold environment. Problems with rigidity of the feet and fallen arches have been reported as has osteoporosis (Francis & Golden 1985).

There is histological evidence of axon regeneration in both myelinated and nonmyelinated fibres together with a gradual return of nerve function. Full return of function after nonfreezing cold injury may take nine months or longer. A burning sensation in the feet has been noted in 61% after apparent full recovery and intractable pain may occur for periods of up to 35 years. Other late sequelae include disturbance of autonomic function — both hyperhidrosis and anhidrosis have been reported (Suri et al 1978, Kumar 1982).

Changes in the epiphysis may occur in frostbitten children and cartilage and bone abnormalities with deformity have been reported. Either the direct actions of cold on chondrocytes or microvascular change with end artery thrombosis or both may be implicated (McKendry 1981).

REFERENCES

Benson H, Lehmann J W, Malhotra M S, Goldman R F, Hopkins J, Epstein M D 1982 Body temperature changes during the activity of G Tum-mo Yoga. Nature 295: 234–236

Chrenko F A, Pugh L G C E 1961 The contribution of solar radiation to the thermal environment of man in Antarctica. Proc R Soc Lond, Series B 155: 243–265

Clarke C R A 1976 On surviving a bivouac at high altitude. Letter Br Med J 1: 92

Ekelund L G 1967 Circulatory and respiratory adaptation during prolonged exercise. Acta Physiol Scand 70 (Suppl) 292

Emslie-Smith D 1981 Hypothermia in the elderly. Br J Hosp Med 26: 442–453

Flora G 1985 Secondary treatment of frost bite. In: Rivolier J, Cerretelli P, Foray F, Segantini (eds) High Altitude Deterioration. Karger, Basel. pp 159–169

Francis T J R, Golden F St C 1985 Non-freezing cold injury. The pathogenesis. J Roy Navy Med Serv 71: 31–38

Hanson H E, Goldman R F 1969 Cold injury in man. A review of its aetiology and discussion of its prediction. Milit Med 134: 1307–1316

Heath D A, Williams D R 1981 Man at high altitude. The pathophysiology of acclimatisation and adaption. Churchill Livingstone, Edinburgh

Kumar V N 1982 Intractable foot pain following frostbite. Arch Phys Med Rehabil 63: 284–285

Lewis R B, Moen P W 1952 Further studies on the pathogenesis of cold induced muscle necrosis. Surg Gynecol Obstet 95: 543–551

McKendry R J R 1981 Frostbite arthritis. Can Med Assoc J 125: 1128–1132

Marsh A R 1983 A short but distant war — The Falklands Campaign. J R Soc Med 76: 972–982

Milledge J S, Bryson E I, Catley D M et al 1982 Sodium balance, fluid homeostasis and the renin-aldosterone system during the prolonged exercise of hill walking. Clin Sci 62: 595–604

Nukada H, Pollock M, Allpress S 1981 Experimental cold injury in peripheral nerves. Brain 104: 779–813

Pearn J H 1982 Cold injury complicating trauma in sub-zero environments. Med J Aust 1: 505–507

Peyronnard J M, Pedneault M, Aguayo A J 1977 Neuropathies due to cold — quantitative studies of structural changes in human and animal nerves. Proceedings of 11th World Congress of Neurology, Amsterdam 303–329

Pugh L G C E 1962 Solar heat gain by man in the high Himalaya. UNESCO Symposium on Environmental Physiology and Psychology in Arid Conditions. Luck-Now pp 325–329

Pugh L G C E 1963 Tolerance to extreme cold at altitude in a Nepalese pilgrim. J Appl Physiol 18: 1234–1238

Pugh L G C E, Ward M P 1956 Some effects of high altitude on man. Lancet 2: 1115–1121

Raifman M A, Berant M, Lenarsky C 1978 Cold weather and rhabdomyolysis. J Paediatrics 93: 970–971

Ramstead K D, Hughes R G, Webb A J 1980 Recent cases of trench foot. Postgrad Med J 56: 879–883

Rosenthall L, Kloiber R, Gagnon R, Damtew B, Lough J 1981

Frostbite with Rhabdomyolysis and renal failure. Am J Roentgenol 137: 387–390
Ross J H, Attwood E C 1984 Severe Repetitive Exercise and haematological status. Postgrad Med J 60: 454–457 454–457
Rossis C G, Yiacoumettis A M, Elemenoglou J 1982 Squamous cell carcinoma of the heel developing at site of previous frostbite. J R Soc Med 75: 715–720
Schaeffer O, Eaton R D P, Timmermans J, Hildes J A 1980 Respiratory function impairment and cardio-pulmonary consequences in long term residents of the Canadian Arctic. Can Med Assoc J 123: 997–1007
Schechter D C, Sarot I A 1968 Historical accounts of injuries due to cold. Surgery 63: 527–535
Suri M L, Vizayan G P, Puri H C, Barat A K, Singh N 1978 Neurological manifestations of frostbite. Indian J Med Res 67: 292–299
Ungley C C, Channell G D, Richards R 1946 The immersion foot syndrome. Br J Surg 33: 17–31
Ward M P 1974 Frostbite. Br Med J 1: 67–70
Ward M P 1975 Mountain medicine. A clinical study of cold and high altitude. Crosby Lockwood Staples, London
Ward M P 1983 Thrombosis and frostbite. 'Man at altitude'. Seminars in Respiratory Medicine 5: 202–206
Washburn B 1962 Frostbite. What it is — how to prevent it — emergency treatment. N Eng J Med 266: 974–989
Williams E S, Ward M P, Milledge J S, Withey W R, Older M W J, Forsling M L 1979 Effect of the exercise of seven consecutive days hill-walking on fluid homeostasis. Clin Sci 56: 305–316

Burns

INTRODUCTION

The burned foot offers an important but often relatively neglected aspect of management in the burned patient. It is a measure of this 'relative unimportance' that there are few publications on the management of the burned foot in the medical literature. A burn of the foot is not commonly seen in isolation and it is usually part of a more extensive thermal injury. The plantar surface of the foot in particular is rarely accidentally burned in a western civilization. This is presumably because of the remoteness from the hands which often cause the injury, the upright stance with plantar contact, the wearing of adequate protective footwear and the brisk flexor withdrawal response of the foot to painful stimuli. Clearly unconscious patients and those suffering from a neuropathic disorder do not possess this protective sensory mechanism and the burns tend to be deep. In countries with warmer climates footwear is often not worn and there is thus little protection to thermal injury. In some third world countries burning of the feet is practised as a supposed therapeutic measure in some medical conditions (Ofodile & Oluwasanmi 1978).

Each foot comprises approximately 2.5% of the total body surface area in adults and the tissues respond to thermal injury as elsewhere in the body. The management, however, must be adapted to each individual case.

CAUSES OF BURN IN GENERAL

The types of thermal injury and their relative incidences are approximately as follows:

75%	Flame or flash burns	
12%	Scalds	
	Direct contact burns	i.e. Molten metal, bitumen, radiator
13%	Chemical burns	i.e. Concentrated acids and alkalis, phosphorus, hydrofluoric acid, cement
	Electrical burns	inc. Flash injury, arc injury, high voltage entry and exit injury

It has been shown that approximately 50% of burns occur in the home and that two-thirds of these are preventable (Lynch 1979). This is obviously alarming as the aesthetic, social and functional disabilities can remain for the lifespan of the patient. The aetiology of the foot burn will indicate the depth of tissue damage. For example, scalds are associated with superficial burns of the skin. Flame contact and chemical burns are associated with full thickness injury; and electrical exit injuries, burns in epileptics, paralysed or unconscious patients are associated with deep structural damage. The burns with massive tissue destruction involving skin and deep structures are associated with prolonged thermal contact, especially flame injury, and high voltage electrical conduction injury.

The cause of thermal injury tends to vary with the age of the individual. From birth to six months of age burn injury is rare and nonaccidental injury (NAI) must be excluded. As a baby starts to crawl and walk then scalds are a frequent mode of injury. Climbing or being put into a bath of hot water can be a more serious injury in children than in adults because the skin on a child's foot is thinner and consequently will burn to a greater depth. With the onset of adolescence thermal injury appears to be more commonly associated with experimenting or 'playing' with such dangerous materials as matches, petrol and electricity. Into adulthood occupational burns of the foot are common and include electrical burns (often complicated by spontaneous ignition of clothing), chemical burns and the many varieties of contact burn that form a part of the hazard of everyday life. Attempted suicide by burning is not uncommon in this age group.

A sudden episode of deep unconsciousness in the proximity of a fire may lead to a foot being engulfed in the flames for a prolonged period and sustaining charring and very deep burns commonly involving bone.

NORMAL SKIN ANATOMY

The anatomical basis of the foot has already been described in Chapters 3 and 4. Each individual structure burned is a potential reconstructive problem. The skin itself has considerable powers of regeneration after thermal injury provided that some epithelial elements survive in the wound. Figure 53.1 shows the important structures and their position within the skin layers. The cutaneous blood supply is through axial pattern vessels that feed a

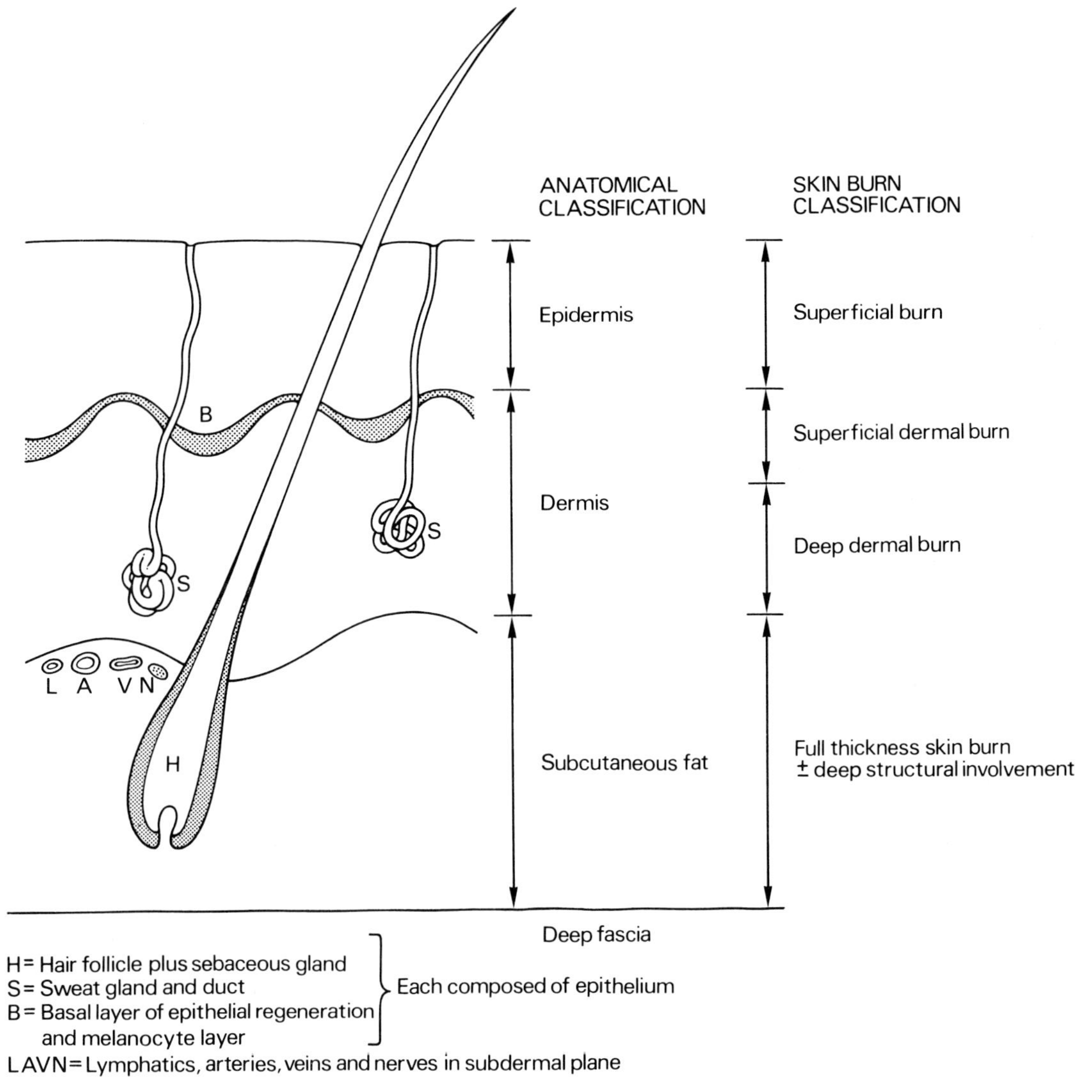

Fig. 53.1 Positions of important structures within skin layers

rich subdermal plexus and these are obviously important in the healing process. It should be noted that the sole skin is different to the other areas of skin in the foot because it has:

1. A thicker keratin layer
2. No hair follicles
3. Sweat glands deeper in the dermis and often adjacent to superficial fascia.

In addition the sole is highly adapted for its role in weight bearing and thus after a full thickness burn it is often difficult adequately to replace and provide good function.

PATHOLOGY

The old classification of first degree, second degree and third degree burns has been superceded. Excluding simple erythema, skin burns are classified as superficial, dermal (superficial or deep), or full thickness. A combination of all these types is usually present in a significant thermal injury and it is well known that burn depth can progress over the first 8 to 12 hours post-burn (Lawrence 1974, deCamara et al 1982). Figure 53.2 shows that if the intermediate zone of stasis is at the dermosubcutaneous junction and the deep hair follicle epithelium has been included in this zone, then an initially deep dermal burn may progress to a full thickness burn. It is by maintaining adequate hydration, preventing oedema and controlling sepsis that burn depth progression is limited.

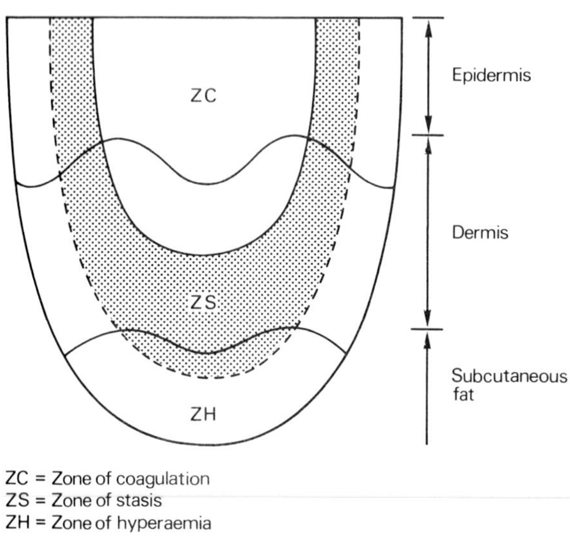

Fig. 53.2 Burn depth progression

A burn injury will heal by a process of epithelial regeneration based on intact basal epithelium and the epithelium related to the skin adnexae. The greater the density of viable epithelium at the base of the burn wound the faster the burn will heal. Thus superficial burns heal very quickly, i.e. within 10 days, superficial dermal burns will heal within three weeks, deep dermal burns will heal between three and six weeks and full thickness burns with no residual epithelial remnants may never heal. A full thickness burn can only heal by epithelial ingrowth from the healthy nonburned skin edges and there appears to be a finite gap over which epithelium can bridge. Clearly therefore a narrow band of full thickness burn may eventually heal but large areas will not heal without surgical intervention. A sterile moist environment enhances epithelialization but there must be a concomitant adequate nutritional intake. The thicker keratin layer on the sole helps to protect the area from thermal injury and the more deeply positioned sweat glands compensate for the lack of hair follicles with regard to available epithelium for healing purposes.

Deep structural burns essentially contain necrotic tissue which can be life-threatening if left. Acute renal failure, disseminated intravascular coagulation, and deep seated sepsis (including clostridial) are all causes of burn mortality associated with deep burns.

Extensive damage from a high voltage electrical injury is a possible cause of such an injury where an early amputation may save the patient's life but a heroic attempt at salvage may cause the patient's demise.

The physiological swelling in and around the burned area is produced in accordance with the rules of inflammation by a wide range of locally and systemically acting vasoactive substances, including fibronectin. Their combined effects can last for about three days and thereafter, especially with the larger burns, a diuresis will herald a reduction in the swelling. The degree of swelling can be controlled to some extent by leg elevation, bed rest and a pressure dressing. It is important to control spreading cellulitis within the oedematous layer of the burned lower leg and foot and of particular importance is careful daily toilet between the toes.

CLINICAL FEATURES

An adequate history will indicate burn depth even before viewing the injury. It is important to know the cause of burn, the duration of contact of the burning substance on the foot, the type of clothing and footwear worn at the time of burn and the immediate local management of the burned area. The exact time of injury, the percentage body surface area burned and the weight of the patient (kg) must be known to calculate an intravenous fluid resuscitation programme if appropriate.

A superficial burn will present rather similarly to simple erythema and the skin often appears intact but if the burned area is gently rubbed with a gloved finger the superficial epidermis will 'peel' off to leave a raw, red, moist, tender bed. Blisters tend to develop some hours after the burn. The amount of burn oedema lost from such an injury is small and the area heals rapidly to leave a minimal scar. This type of thermal injury of the foot can often be managed on an out-patient basis.

A superficial dermal burn will present with a very painful area of early blistering (Fig. 53.3). The blisters are typically more thick walled than the superficial burns and are often burst by the time of presentation. The bed of the deroofed blister is very tender, red/pink in colour and is rather moist in the acute phase. The area that is deroofed will blanche significantly if pressed with a gloved finger and rapidly return to its original colour on release.

A deep dermal burn may be blistered and the roof is composed of a relatively thick dead skin layer (Fig. 53.4). When deroofed the bed is white, but still sensitive to pin prick. The healing time is rather prolonged in a deep dermal burn and the scars tend to become hypertrophic if allowed to heal without surgical intervention.

A full thickness skin burn often does not blister but appears as an area of thick leathery eschar (Figs. 53.5–7). If it includes the adjacent subcutaneous tissue thrombosed vessels may be visible confirming the diagnosis. As the cutaneous nerve ends have been destroyed the burned area is insensitive except at the junction between the burned and nonburned skin. In practice it is often difficult accurately to distinguish between a deep dermal and a just full thickness burn but in theory pin prick sensation is present in the former. This investigation in an acutely burned and distressed patient is commonly inaccurate and may be superfluous as the clinical management does not alter. Perhaps the only indication is in the patient with a circumferential burn where an escharotomy is being considered.

In electrical burns where the foot is an exit point then the heart should be checked for conduction defects. Surgery is deferred for five days to allow tissue necrosis to be completed. Excision and cover

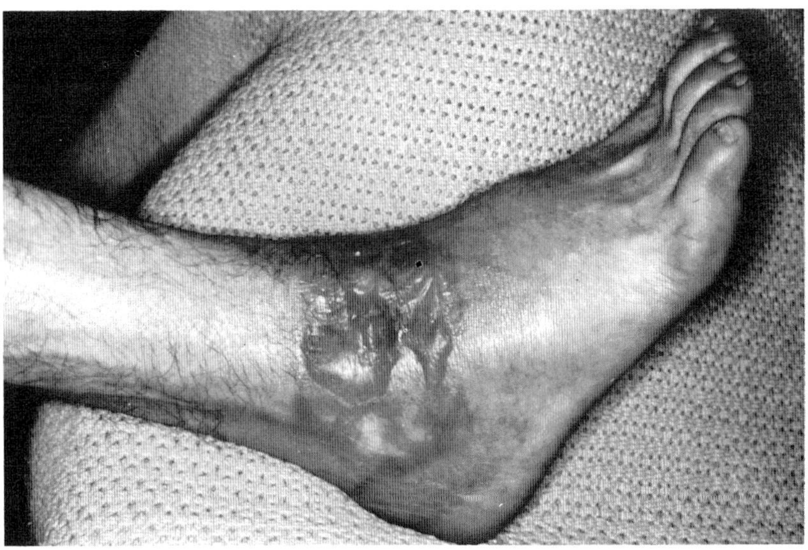

Fig. 53.3 Superficial dermal burn caused by brief contact between skin and a chemical. Note that the blisters are thin walled

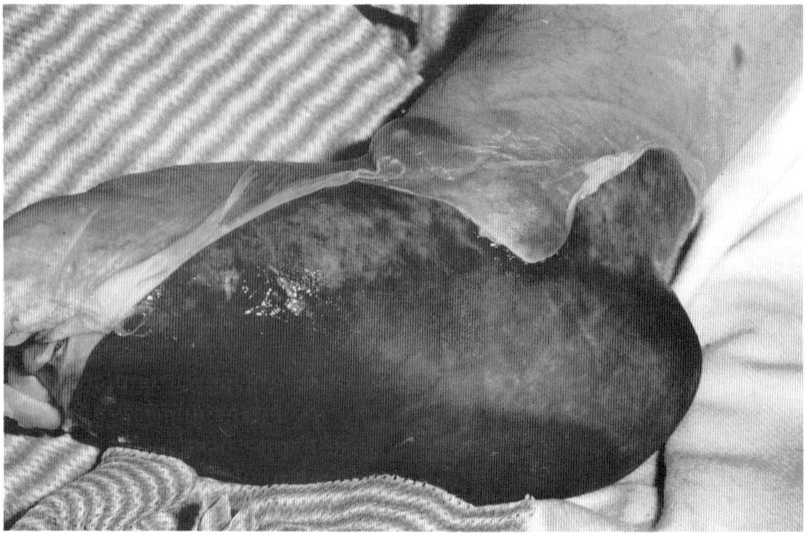

Fig. 53.4 Contrast the injury in Figure 3 with this deep dermal and full thickness injury on the plantar and dorsal surfaces of the foot which was caused by prolonged immersion in very hot bath water. In this particular case a non-accident injury was identified. The blister roof is thick and the moist red base contains a few thrombosed veins. A child will tend to suffer a deeper burn than an adult in similar circumstances because a child's skin is thinner

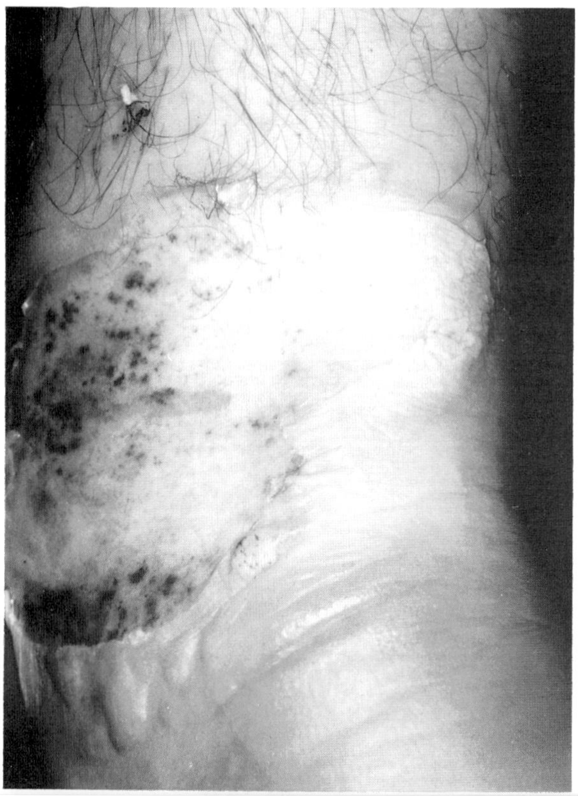

Fig. 53.5 Full thickness skin burn caused by direct contact with molten metal. The white base contains numerous small thrombosed vessels within the eschar

with a flap or skin graft if appropriate is then carried out. In high voltage electrical burns joints may be rigid due to severe muscle damage which may lead to myoglobinuria and renal failure if not ruthlessly debrided. Venous and arterial thrombosis will intensify the volume of tissue damage. Amputation early in this process should be seriously considered to preserve life (Figs. 53.8 and 9).

TREATMENT

The primary aim of treating foot burns is to achieve healing in as short a time as possible. The secondary aim is to achieve a functional, cosmetically acceptable foot. In some respects the management to achieve these aims overlaps in that correct early treatment may prevent the need for further procedures.

Superficial burns of the feet should be managed conservatively with infrequent dressings as described later. They should heal within 10 days. Superficial dermal burns should be managed conservatively as above and they should heal within three weeks.

Deep dermal and full thickness skin burns should be treated surgically to obtain early skin cover and a better quality scar. The surgical management

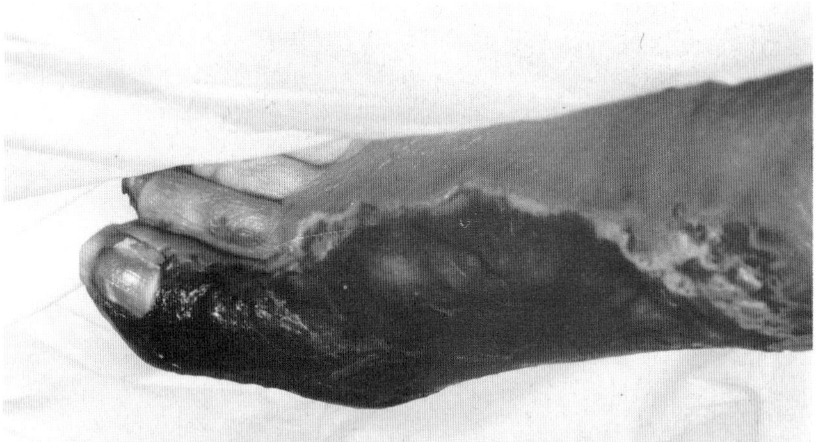

Fig. 53.6 Full thickness skin burn with deep adjacent structural damage in an epileptic patient whose foot was in contact with a burning surface for a prolonged period. The injury is one week old and the thick discoloured eschar contains a thrombosed vein

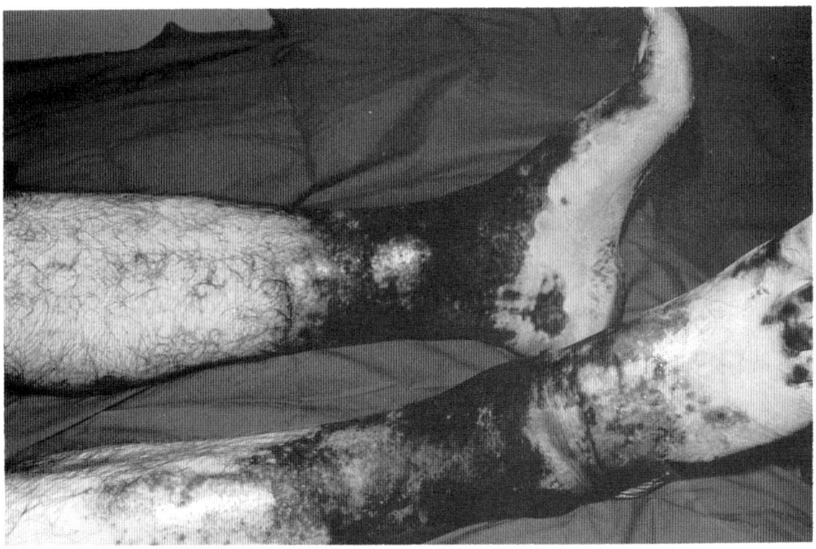

Fig. 53.7 A case of severe cement burn affecting both ankles and feet. The cement tends to collect inside footwear and when the skin perspiration activates the cement dust a burn will develop quite insidiously. Despite the appearance these burns were only just full thickness

consists of tangential serial excision of the burn down to healthy tissue and covering the area with skin graft (either as a sheet, fenestrated, or meshed). It is sometimes difficult to identify burned tissue under a tourniquet and in this situation the clue to viability is bleeding of the tissues after release of the tourniquet. Under an exsanguinating tourniquet the phrase 'red is dead' is appropriate and excision down to a 'white is right' plane ensures a healthy base. Excision and grafting should be performed either before the fifth day post burn or after the third week. Intermediate grafting, i.e. between five days and three weeks, is not generally practised because of difficulty in assessing the depth of the tissue damage with no satisfactory plane of demarcation. Septicaemia due to bacterial spillage from the excised burn wound cannot be met by an adequate host immune response at this stage as this has not had time to develop. A circumferential full thickness skin burn of the leg or foot should have an escharotomy done as soon as diagnosed and similarly a deep structural burn should have a fasciotomy.

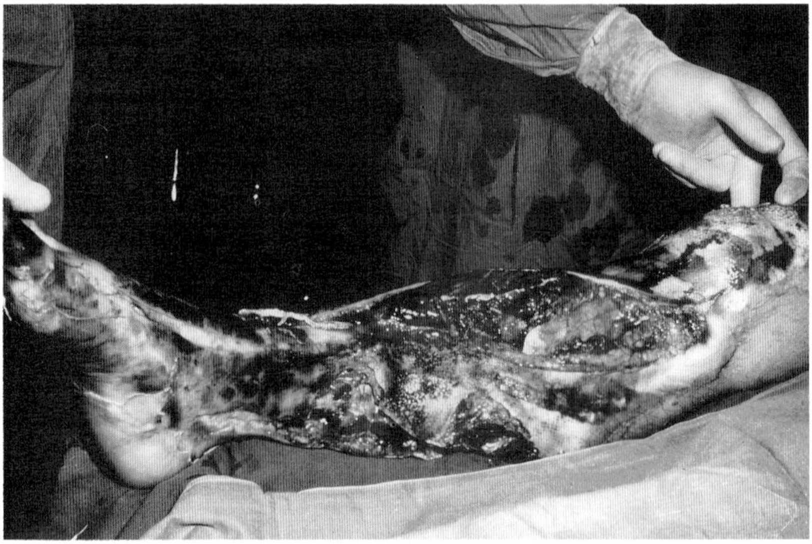

Fig. 53.8 An extensive burn with considerable tissue destruction caused by high voltage electrical contact. Despite early amputation this patient died

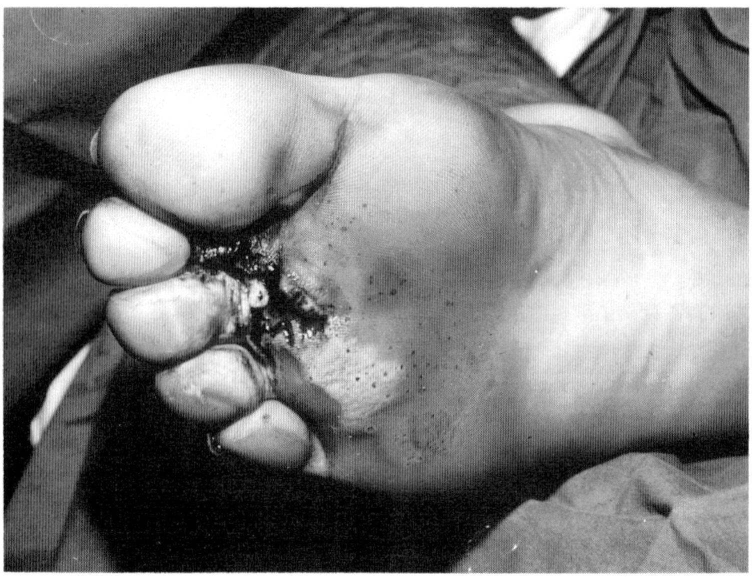

Fig. 53.9 Electrical exit point on the sole of the foot. This contrasts with the patient in Figure 8, with a large electrical entry point, in that there is little destruction of the deeper structures. In this case the burned area is left for five days and, after demarcation, the dead tissue removed and the defect covered

By three weeks post-burn the eschar of a full thickness skin burn will have separated to leave a granulation tissue-based defect. A skin graft will take on such a surface but it is usual to rub the area with a gauze swab or even to shave the granulations down first. Recently dermabrasion has been used effectively in deep dermal burns at three weeks to create a good bed on which to lay a skin graft and to produce cosmetically acceptable scars.

Full thickness skin burns with deeper structural damage should be excised before five days post-burn when the necrotic zone may be easily assessed. In the

admission and from the burn at each change of dressing. The surface colony counts on burned surfaces can be reduced by bathing or soaking the foot in a chlorhexidine bath regularly. It is very important to clean meticulously between the toes in a burned foot as it is often the harbouring site of bacteria.

BURN DRESSINGS

There are many types of commercial dressings available on the market often with antibacterial action, but the usual dressings are:

1. For superficial and superficial dermal burns vaseline impregnated gauze (tulle gras) is the cheapest and most commonly used contact dressing. A foot with this type of burn can also be treated in a plain freezer bag or a freezer bag containing chlorhexidine or silversulphadiazine (Flamazine®). The foot could also be equally well managed by the exposure method where the elevated limb is allowed to produce a dry eschar by exposing it to the air and perhaps even using a commercial hairdryer for assistance. The eschar falls off at about three weeks.
2. For deep dermal and full thickness burns the decision must be made whether there will be an early or a late grafting technique employed. For early grafting the burn need only be dressed with tulle gras as previously described. In late grafting cases frequent Flamazine® bags or dressings should be used. The Flamazine® is particularly effective in controlling *Pseudomonas* on the burn and also provides some pain relief to the patient.
3. The deep structural burns should be dressed with tulle gras as they will all be operated upon within five days.

SKIN REPLACEMENT

The ultimate aim in the management of the burned foot must be to obtain a cosmetically acceptable, functioning foot that will fit comfortably into a shoe and cause no long-term problems. In the first instance the priority is to gain complete wound healing and in the vast majority of cases the most superficial burns will heal on their own. The deep dermal and full thickness burns, however, are best treated by the early tangential excision and skin graft technique. This applies to both burns on the dorsum and the sole of the foot. Obviously a skin graft on the weight-bearing area of the sole is not ideal but once the skin graft has matured it can be replaced by a flap. Flaps carried out early are often inset into an infected environment and are more likely to fail. A thin skin graft will take better than a thick skin graft but will also contract more. Thus a thicker skin graft should be preferred around a joint but a thinner graft should be preferred elsewhere. A thin skin graft donor site will also heal faster and be available for reharvest earlier.

Skin grafts can be lost for a variety of reasons including an unhealthy bed, colonization with group A β-haemolytic streptococcus, an unsupported graft with leg dependency at an early stage and haematoma under the graft. It is to minimize the latter cause that a sheet of skin graft is often fenestrated or meshed. For a combination of an excellent chance of skin 'take' and good cosmesis a mesh of 1.5 : 1 is recommended (Fig. 53.11). The most recent advance in skin graft technique is in the use of cultured autograft and homograft. At present though this method is not suitable in the coverage of the burned foot because not only is the 'take' poor but also the skin that does take contracts by over 50% of its original surface area.

A skin graft will not take on exposed tendon or bare cortical bone and if these structures are to survive then they must be covered with a vascularized flap. After debriding the burned foot a local, regional, distal or free flap can be used. These have been discussed in Chapter 62. To enable the foot to fit into a shoe a flap often needs to be thinned and this is done when the flap and scars have matured. An example of a full thickness skin burn with deep structural involvement is shown in Figure 53.12. A latissimus dorsi myocutaneous free flap has been used to cover the defect on the dorsum of the foot and ankle. Note that the flap is still bulky and will need thinning and the toes are also in an unsatisfactory position. To preserve movement in exposed joints flap cover is essential at an early stage and a vascularized tendon graft can be included in the free flap if indicated. Relatively early arthrodesis is recommended by some authors to obtain a stable pain-free limb if joint destruction is inevitable (Jackson 1976).

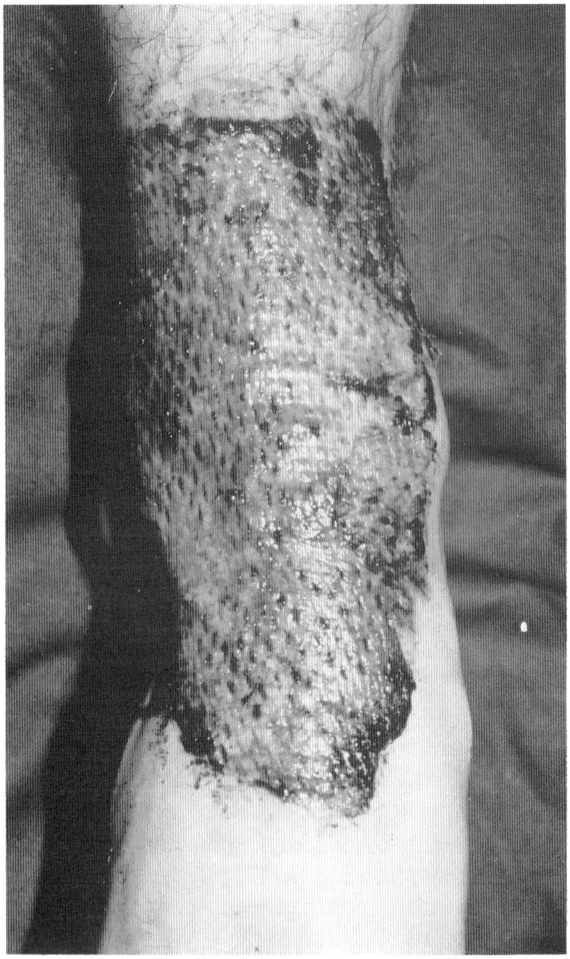

Fig. 53.11 Fully taken 1.5 : 1 mesh graft on the dorsum of the foot and anterior aspect of the ankle

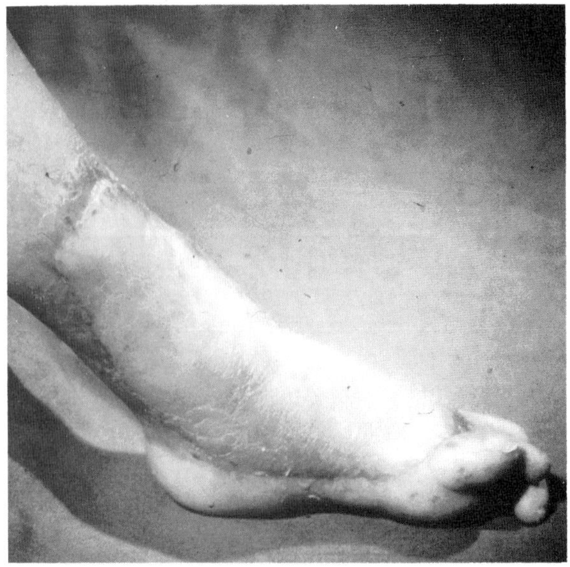

Fig. 53.12 Latissimus dorsi myocutaneous flap inset into a large area on the dorsum of the foot and ankle that had been deeply burned, causing exposure of deep structures

SCAR AND CONTRACTURE CONTROL

In general the longer a burn takes to heal the deeper the burn and the greater the chance of developing an unsightly scar and problems with joint contractures. The superficial burn will heal rapidly with minimal scar formation but the deep dermal burn can take three weeks to heal and then form an unsightly scar with progressive contracture formation. A skin grafted or a flap covered burn tends not to become hypertrophic except at the margins. A normal scar can be expected to mature within one year, but a hypertrophic scar may take as long as five years to mature and a keloid scar can be present for decades. It is during the active phase that a scar is red, firm to hard, raised, unsightly and itchy, but the scar will then become pale, soft, flat and non-itchy. During the active phase the scar length tends to contract and if this is not countered then deformity will result. Thus at the earliest possible time, i.e. just before complete healing, patients with deep dermal and full thickness burns should be considered for pressure garment scar and contracture control. Custom measured garments as provided by Pan Med Ltd. (Fig. 53.13) are extremely useful in enhancing burn

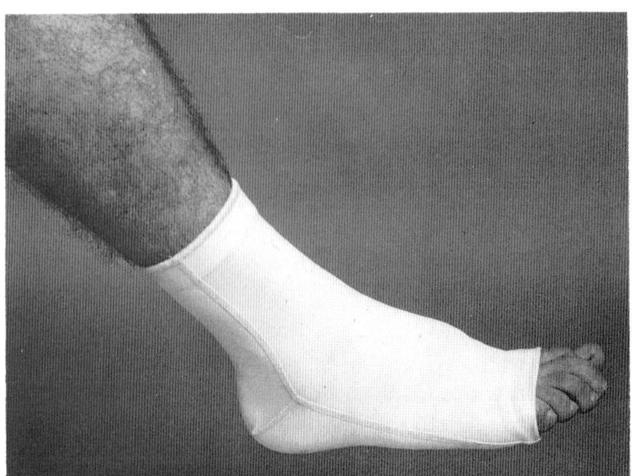

Fig. 53.13 Use of a custom made pressure garment on the foot and ankle

scar maturation and preventing contractures. In suitable cases spacers can be fitted to prevent burn syndactyly. These garments can be used alone or in combination with silicone gel which has recently been shown to have scar maturation properties of its own (Perkins et al 1982). The burn scar should be regularly massaged with oily cream during the infrequent times that the pressure garment is not being worn.

For established hypertrophy pressure therapy is still of use, but in addition triamcinolone injections, intralesional scar excision, or tangential shave and overgraft are useful alternatives.

Burn scar contractures will cause anatomical distortion of joints which could lead to secondary irreversible joint changes. The deformity will vary with the site of the burn contracture:

1. *The dorsum of the foot*

Hyperextension of the metatarsophalangeal and ankle joints with impaired or abnormal growth pattern in children is not uncommon. Joint contractures such as these can sometimes be prevented by using pressure garments, oyster splints (Fig. 53.14), or custom-made moulded silicone shoes (Feldman et al 1974). Once established, however, a surgical release and skin graft or, in the case of a narrow linear contracture, a Z-plasty will correct the contracture. This is provided that the joints are not themselves irreversibly damaged. Occasionally, such as when tendons are exposed during the release of contracture, a skin graft will not take and flap cover is necessary. To assist in obtaining a good graft take, the joint over which the contracture was acting should be immobilized until the graft has consolidated, i.e. about 10 days. Figure 53.15 shows a burn scar on the dorsum of the foot which is extending the metatarsophalangeal joints and preventing the wearing of reasonable footwear. The contracture was released and skin grafted, and the metatarsophalangeal joints were immobilized by using Kirschner wires. The early result is shown in Figure 53.16. In such cases a flexor to extensor transfer may also be of use.

2. *The sole of the foot*

Flexion deformity of the toes can cause problems with footwear. These contractures can be released

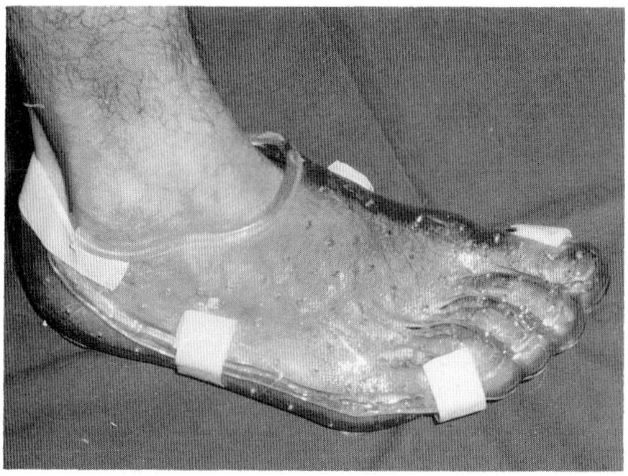

Fig. 53.14 Use of a moulded oyster splint in the prevention of post burn contractures. Spacers can be fitted to prevent post burn syndactyly

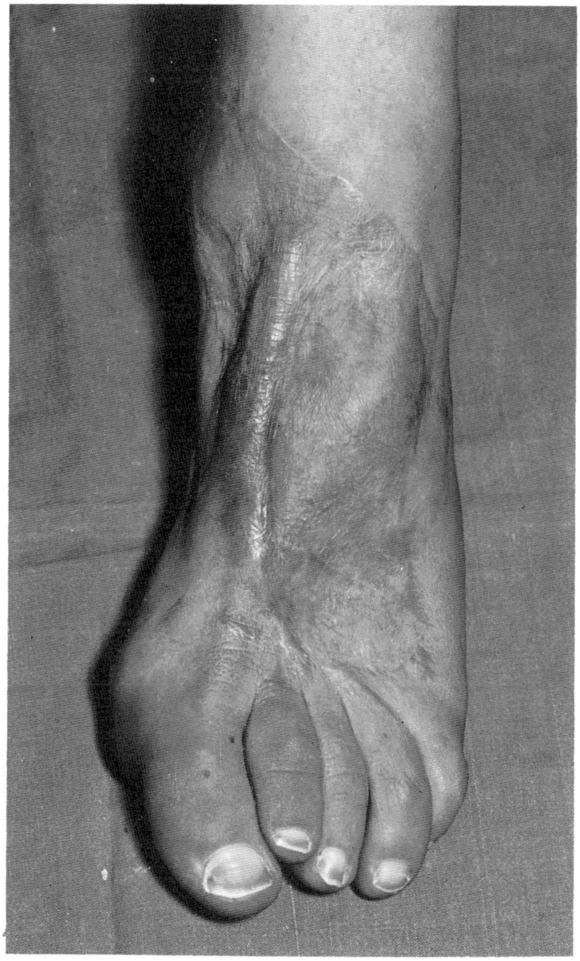

Fig. 53.15 Post burn contracture on the dorsum of the foot which is pulling the toes into a dorsal position and causing discomfort on wearing normal footwear

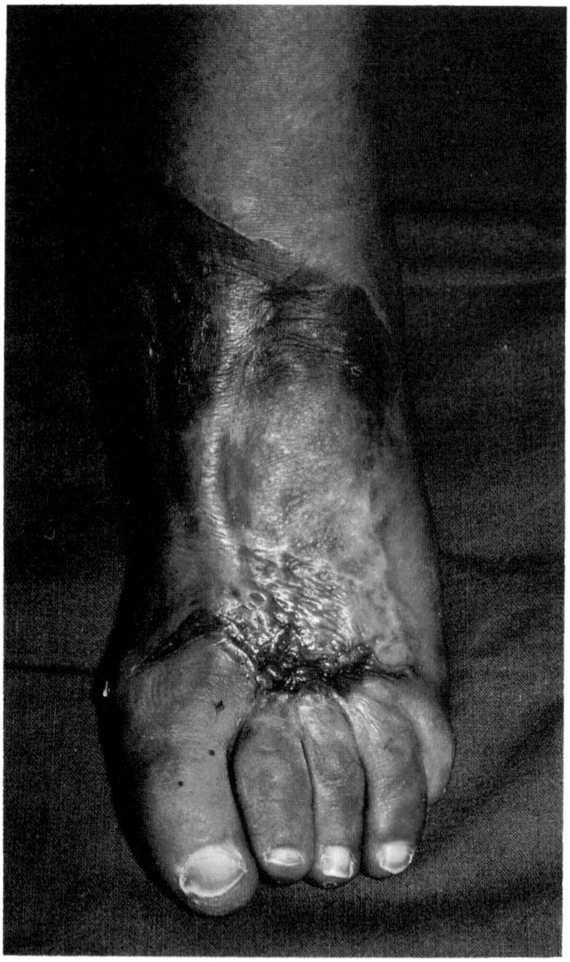

Fig. 53.16 Result of transverse release of the contracture in Figure 15 and skin grafting of the defect. The metatarsophalangeal joints were immobilized by using Kirschner wires until the graft had stabilized

and grafted as above but flap cover is more appropriate over the weight-bearing areas.

3. *Lateral and medial contractures around the ankle joint*

Burn scar contractures at these sites will tend to pull the forefoot into valgus and varus respectively. Although the deformity may be immediately correctable it will often recur if the release and skin graft technique alone is used. It is better to release the contracture and provide flap cover if possible.

4. *The heel and tendo Achillis region*

A contracture in this region will produce an equinus deformity which is often difficult to correct. It is far better to avoid this problem by splinting and providing early flap cover if appropriate.

The problem with thick hypertrophic scars, areas of skin graft and noninnervated flaps are that they remain relatively insensitive and consequently trophic ulcers are not uncommon, especially on the sole. In these cases careful attention to foot hygiene and adequate protection are needed for the rest of the patient's life.

Other complications

Unstable scarring without contracture of any significance is a difficult problem. In the first instance the scar should be managed conservatively with avoidance of pressure in the form of footwear over the unstable area, keeping the area clean and then massaging the area with oily creams when healed. Adjacent hyperkeratotic areas should be pared down preferably by a chiropodist. If these methods fail then the unstable scar will need reinforcing either by a shave and overgraft technique or by excising the area and introducing new tissue in the form of a flap. The overgraft method involves shaving the unstable epidermis and then covering the exposed dermis with a thick skin graft, thus providing a more stable base.

Syndactyly of the toes is not a functional problem unless there is a deformity due to differential growth patterns of the toes or due to concomitant dorsal or plantar contractures. In most instances therefore toe syndactyly is not operated upon. Toe nail dystrophy is commonly associated with forefoot burns and can usually be managed satisfactorily by a chiropodist (Fig. 53.17).

Acquired vertical talus deformity can follow some severe burns of the foot and leg in infancy (Jackson 1980). This is due to a shortening of the calf muscles which pulls the talus and calcaneus into equinus, a scar contracture which pulls the forefoot into eversion, valgus and dorsiflexion, and an underdeveloped sustentaculum tali which is a feature of the first year or two of life. It is the sustentaculum tali which normally prevents the downward dislocation of the head of the talus.

Septic arthritis has rarely been reported in burned patients and often the cause is iatrogenic (Jackson 1980).

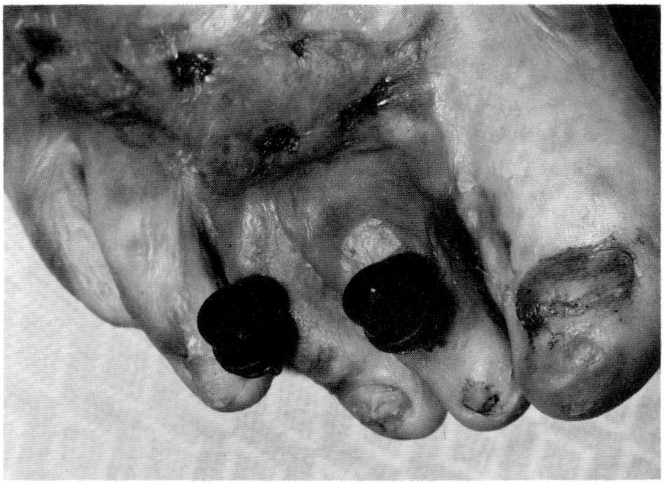

Fig. 53.17 Toe nail dystrophy in a well healed burned foot

ACKNOWLEDGEMENTS

We would like to thank Elsa Gordon for typing the script; Pan Med Limited, Imperial Chemical Industries and Mr. G. Wilson FRCS for providing some of the photographs, and the staff at Mount Vernon Hospital who successfully manage such patients.

REFERENCES

de Camara D L, Raine T J, London M D, Robson M C, Heggars J P 1982 Progression of thermal injury: A morphologic study. Plast Reconstr Surg 69: 491–499

Feldman A E, Thompson J T, MacMillan B G 1974 The moulded silicone shoe in the prevention of contractures involving the burn-injured foot. Burns Inc Therm Inj 1: 83–95

Jackson D MacG 1976 Burns into joints. Burns Inc Therm Inj 2: 90–106

Jackson D MacG 1980 Destructive burns: Some orthopaedic complications. Burns Inc Therm Inj 7: 105–122

Lawrence J C 1974 The perinecrotic zone in burns and its influence on healing. Burns Inc Therm Inj 1: 197–206

Lowbury E J L 1979 Wits versus genes: The continuing battle against infection. J Trauma 19: 33–45

Lynch J B 1979 Thermal burns. In: Grabb W C, Smith J W (eds) Plastic surgery. 3rd edn. Little, Brown and Company, Boston pp 453–483

Ofodile F A, Oluwasanmi J O 1978 Burning the feet to treat convulsions. Br J Plast Surg 31: 356–357

Perkins K, Davey R B, Wallis K A 1982 Silicone gel: a new treatment for burn scars and contractures. Burns Inc Therm Inj 9: 201–204

Algodystrophy

Loss of function associated with seemingly inappropriate pain, circulatory changes and tenderness, occasionally developing some time after injury when improvement would be expected, has been recognized for many years but the condition is still poorly understood.

Mitchell and his coauthors (1864) described excessively painful injuries incurred in the American Civil War and introduced the term 'causalgia.' They emphasized the peculiar burning pain and recorded the associated damage to nerves.

In 1937, de Takats took the description a stage further and introduced the name 'reflex dystrophy.' Later, in 1965, to emphasize that it was the sympathetic nervous system that was mainly concerned, he changed it to 'sympathetic reflex dystrophy.'

Meanwhile, others had used various names to identify different aspects of the disorder. Sudeck, in 1900, making use of the recent discovery of X-rays, described the osteoporosis that occurs and was rewarded by the syndrome being termed 'Sudeck's atrophy.' Leriche and Fontaine (1930) thought 'painful post-traumatic osteoporosis' a better name and Steinbrocker (1968) drew attention to the 'shoulder-hand syndrome.'

Because of shortcomings in all these names, the term 'algodystrophy,' which was introduced by de Sèze & Ryckwaert in 1951, seems the best for general usage.

A UNIFYING CONCEPT

In addition to the florid forms described and documented by authors, there are probably many other cases of pain, with or without circulatory changes or where changes are missed because more sophisticated investigations such as technetium bone-scanning are not used. These too should be diagnosed as algodystrophy. Perhaps the so-called 'transient osteoporosis of the hip' (Valenzuela et al 1977, Langloh et al 1973) is another clinical form. Could 'migratory osteoporosis' be yet another (O'Mara & Pinal 1970)? Perhaps many of the stiff, painful hands seen after fractures of the radius are really mild forms of algodystrophy. Likewise, might not many of those cases which are slow and difficult to rehabilitate after lower limb injuries be suffering from an incomplete form of algodystrophy?

CLINICAL COURSE

The typical presentation when the foot is affected is limping on a painful swollen foot without an obvious, adequate cause. There may have been previous trauma but this was either too long ago or too minor to explain satisfactorily the present condition. Alternatively, the previous trauma seems to have been properly treated and there is no reason for new pain and swelling. If surgery was the precipitating factor, the new symptoms are usually attributed to infection, but tests fail to confirm this and antibiotics are ineffective.

When it follows a fracture of the ankle, the patient complains of increasing pain and the toes protruding from the immobilizing plaster cast are discoloured. Causalgia cases following nerve injury have constant, intense, burning, distressing pain aggravated by touch or movement. All sensory stimulation tends to cause a highly unpleasant burning sensation. The foot is usually red, but not necessarily warm.

About 50% of cases are associated with trauma and

may occur a few days after. The onset may be delayed for several weeks or months but an average interval is one month (Portias 1977, Renier et al 1973, Serre et al 1967).

The onset is usually fairly rapid. Over a period of one to two weeks increasing pain in the foot leads to the use of one or possibly two crutches. Normal walking is impossible. Onset may occasionally be very acute and the degree of pain frequently seems inappropriate from the appearance of the foot. In about 10% of cases the pain has a peculiar distressing burning character.

In approximately one-third of cases, swelling is also present at the onset. It is a pitting oedema which may affect only part of the foot but usually involves the whole foot and possibly the ankle and the lower leg. If not present initially, swelling develops later in most, but not all cases. There is usually marked hypersensitivity of the foot so that footwear and even bedclothes cause discomfort.

Initially, in about half of reported cases, there is erythema and increased temperature of the foot, changing after a period of days or weeks, to a cold cyanosis. Sweating is increased during both phases and movements of the foot are restricted because of pain and tenderness.

Gradually, with or without treatment, the pain and swelling subside but the foot tends to remain cold and perhaps blue. In less severe cases and with active movements and use, improvement tends to occur at this stage. Movements increase, the circulation improves and normal walking gradually resumes. Resolution usually takes several months and commonly a year.

In a small proportion of cases resolution does not take place. In these more severe cases or where active therapy or patient effort have been insufficient, the foot remains cold and perhaps cyanosed. Movements do not return to normal but pain and tenderness clear gradually. The skin becomes light, thin and shiny. The foot remains stiff and weak.

AETIOLOGY

The aetiology is unknown but there are certainly two factors which commonly seem to initiate the disorder, namely, trauma and pain. A third factor, emotional stress, is frequently associated. A basic question, yet to be answered, is whether certain people are inherently prone or at risk to develop algodystrophy by virtue of some constitutional, perhaps hereditary, diathesis, should they be subjected to precipitating factors such as trauma or acute pain, or could anyone develop algodystrophy in certain circumstances.

Familial and hereditary factors

There are no reported family studies, but recently the occurrence of algodystrophy in three members of one family has been reported.

Genetic predisposition could be shown by HLA phenotyping. Reports have not yet shown any convincing association, but these studies are still in their early stages.

Is there an algodystrophic diathesis?

If a person was constitutionally prone to algodystrophy, he could be expected to suffer several episodes during a lifetime. Although cases of multiple attacks of algodystrophy have been reported (Langloh et al 1973), this is an infrequent occurrence and most people have one attack only.

There is evidence of sympathetic nervous system overactivity in the syndrome, but no definite evidence of a primary abnormality of other autonomic function has yet been shown to be present in a majority of cases. Some writers have mentioned as examples of predisposing sympathetic hyperactivity, pre-existing hyperhidrosis and tendency to cold hands and feet.

Similarly, it has not been shown that sufferers from algodystrophy have a lower tolerance of pain than normal or an increased responsiveness to painful stimuli.

Trauma

Injuries, fractures and surgical procedures are by far the most common precipitating factors of algodystrophy. Both minor and major trauma may be responsible.

Painful conditions

Many different and diverse causes of pain have been

reported as initiating factors. Root pain from lumbar disc disorders is one of the commonest in the case of foot involvement (Carlson et al 1977).

Systemic diseases and drug therapy

Upper limb algodystrophy is certainly related to cardiac disease and neurological syndromes such as hemiplegia. It is uncertain whether a suspected relationship with epilepsy is due to the disease, trauma or barbiturate therapy. Isoniazid therapy has been implicated (Good 1970) and diabetes mellitus is suspected of predisposing to the syndrome (Lequesne et al 1977).

Psychological factors

Anxiety and overprotection of the affected part are common features of the syndrome, but these could well be secondary to the pain and loss of function and not causative features. Indeed, many typical cases are seen in patients with a normal positive attitude. As the condition frequently develops at a time when improvement following injury is expected, the patient often has a sense of grievance. Some authorities consider the grievance a contributory aetiological factor in the development of the condition whereas others consider it a natural reaction to the nonimprovement. This feeling is certainly not always present and while it cannot be dismissed as a possible factor in some cases, it is not possible to give it a definite role.

However, when present, both anxiety and grievance act as negative factors against resolution of the disorder.

Much has been written on the mechanism of this disorder but no satisfactory and generally accepted explanation has emerged. It is suggested that in peripheral trauma, injury to nerves causes abnormal excitation of nonmedullated or finely medullated 'C' afferent fibres (Granit et al 1944, Seltzer & Devor 1979), or 'cross-circuiting' to these fibres from efferent fibres (Doupe et al 1944), such that in the spinal cord, abnormal sympathetic reflexes are stimulated and the 'gate mechanism' controlling pain sensation (Melzack & Wall 1965) is disturbed.

A similar hypothesis is that whereas a normal nerve only conducts one impulse when stimulated and then has a refractory period, in algodystrophy this dampening down effect is lost and the small C fibres keep firing sensory impulses after the stimulus has ceased.

Another idea is that the C fibres become hypersensitive to noradrenaline and are activated by the minute amounts normally present in the tissues (Korenman & Devor 1981). Increased sympathetic efferent activity releases more noradrenaline and produces a vicious circle.

PATHOLOGY

There is no clearly defined picture. In the early stages, the skin and subcutaneous tissue show oedema and in the later stages, atrophy. The synovium tends to be hypervascular, but only slightly, if at all infiltrated with inflammatory cells. Bone is soft with loss of trabeculae. Osteoclasts and bone resorption are increased, but osteoblasts are plentiful.

PHYSICAL EXAMINATION

The appearance of the foot in the early stages varies greatly between cases. It may look quite normal, it may be pink, oedematous and warm or it may be just a little puffy (Fig. 54.1).

The foot is usually tender to touch and painful to move. The patient frequently objects to the foot being examined and seeks to protect it with his hands. Sweating is usually increased.

After days or perhaps weeks the pink erythema disappears and the temperature drops so that the foot becomes blue, cold and sweaty. This is frequently the stage at which it is seen for a 'second opinion'.

Except in minor cases, the patient walks with a limp and usually uses a stick or crutch in one or both hands.

Sometimes only part of the foot is affected. Skin sensation is normal in most cases but in a small number, any stimulation produces a distressing burning sensation (hyperpathia). As the condition slowly resolves, the tenderness and hypersensitivity disappear.

Many patients display a very anxious concern about their algodystrophic foot but occasionally the

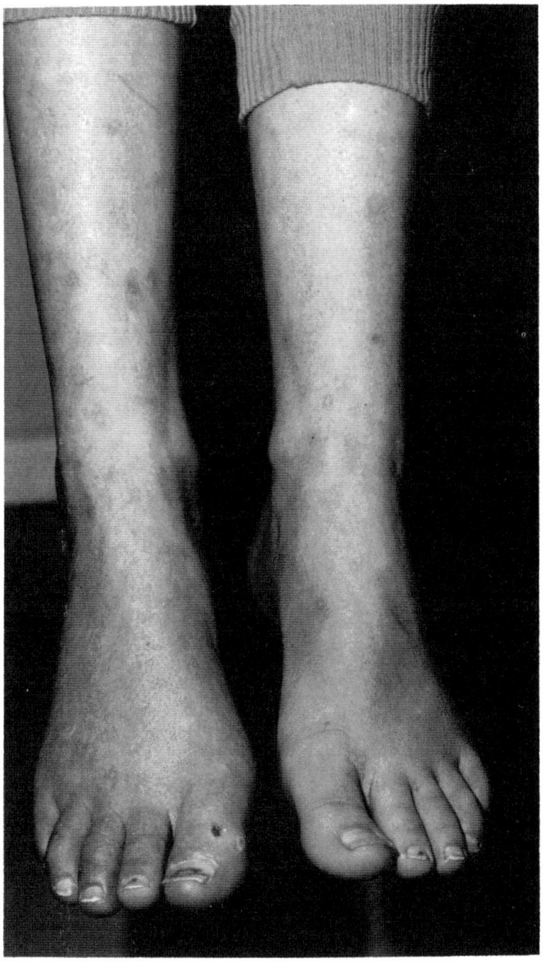

Fig. 54.1 Appearance in early stage

patient may appear more or less unconcerned about it.

There are no associated abnormalities on examination of the rest of the patient.

INVESTIGATIONS

Clinical pathology

The white cell count and erythrocyte sedimentation rate remain normal. Serum biochemistry estimations are all within normal limits. There have been reports of increased urinary excretion of calcium and hydroxyproline. Hypercalcinuria seems to be a less common and variable feature, but increased hydroxyprolinuria appears to occur fairly often and may parallel the course of the disease.

X-rays

The earliest sign is subchondral bone resorption with disappearance of trabeculae. This may occur in discrete lacunae giving a very typical honeycomb or 'spotty' osteoporosis. There is also general osteoporosis of the foot. Subchondral bone laminae and cortical bone may also be resorbed to the extent of giving the appearance of 'disappearing bone.' The changes are quite different from the osteoporosis and erosions of rheumatoid arthritis or the tophaceous deposits of gout (Fig. 54.2).

X-ray changes are usually not visible for at least two to four weeks after the start of symptoms and may not develop for two to three months. Therefore, if changes are not present on initial radiographs, further films should be taken after an interval.

Although osteoporosis may be confined to one or two metatarsals and phalanges (partial algodystrophy), it usually affects the whole foot and ankle and may be very severe. When established, X-ray changes are frequently more severe than would be expected from physical examination and may take years to return to normal (Genant et al 1975).

Bone scan (scintillography)

Uptake of radioactive technetium 99m isotope-labelled pyrophosphate is a most valuable investigation in suspected algodystrophy (Doury et al 1979, Greyson & Tepperman 1984, Kozin et al 1981). Recordings taken two to five hours after injection almost always show increased isotope uptake in the affected part and a normal finding probably negates the diagnosis. The bone scan changes occur very early and may show increased uptake when other features are indefinite or absent. Increased isotope uptake may persist for several months. The changes, however, are not specific and the main value in differential diagnosis is to show the presence of a unilateral pathology (Fig. 54.3).

Thermography

It is possible to record circulatory changes by

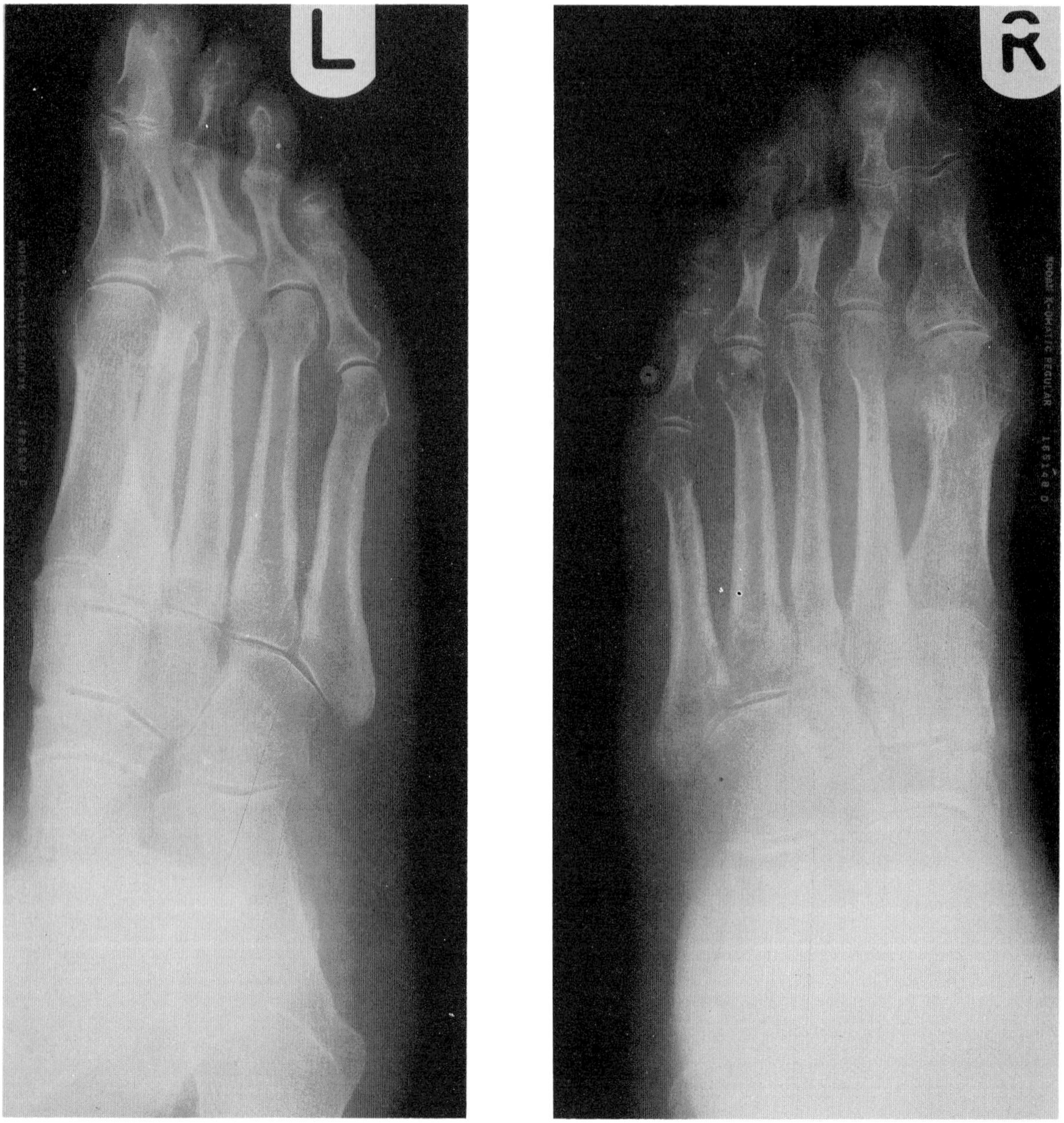

Fig. 54.2 X-ray views of both feet show widespread osteoporosis on the right

measuring surface temperature using an infrared camera. In this way, differences in circulation between the feet can be demonstrated even when it is not obvious visually or palpably. The response of one foot to cooling of the opposite limb or even of the hand gives valuable information regarding blood flow and its responsiveness. Different patterns have been recognized. Two typical variations have been seen in algodystrophy. In the early stages, the response to contralateral cooling is hyperdynamic with quick and strong vasoconstriction followed (after the cooling) by rapid vasodilatation. During the later cold cyanotic stage the resting circulation is reduced and further slow vasoconstriction occurs with contralateral cooling. Relaxation of the vasoconstriction afterwards is slow and poor.

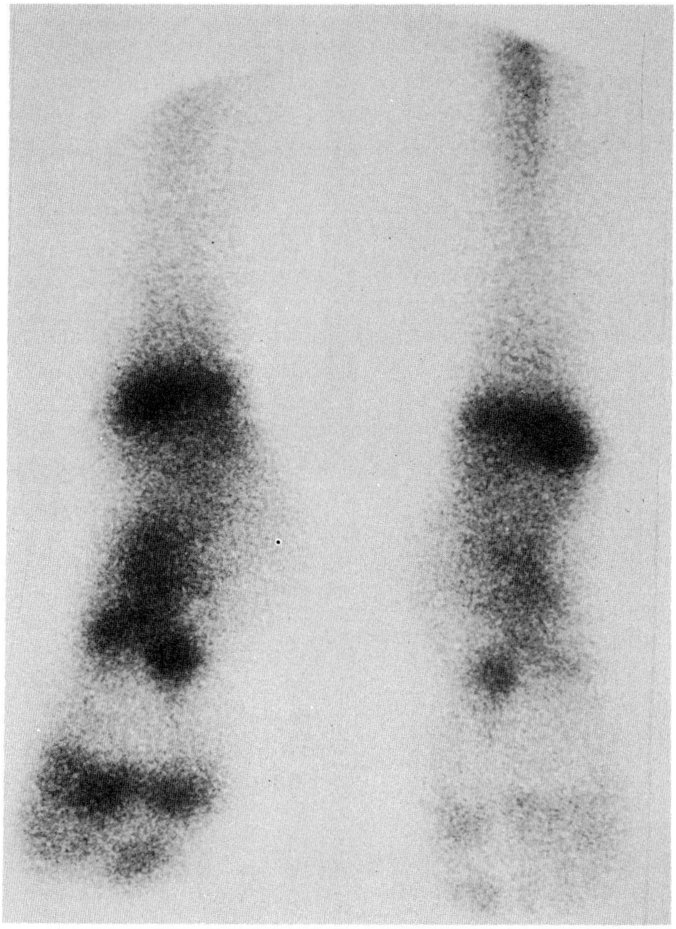

Fig. 54.3 Bone scan changes

DIFFERENTIAL DIAGNOSIS

The cardinal features of algodystrophy are pain, hypersensitivity, circulatory changes, increased sweating and osteoporosis. Swelling, loss of function and a history of recent surgery or trauma are additional pointers to the diagnosis. However the condition started, if a foot demonstrates these features, algodystrophy can be regarded as having developed and having become the main problem.

Infection is always suspected if the foot is red, warm, swollen and painful but if there is no obvious source of infection and the foot is sweating as opposed to hot and dry, algodystrophy should be considered. To allay doubt, a short sharp course of an appropriate antibiotic can be given, but failure to improve should strengthen suspicion of algodystrophy.

Gout has several similar features but rarely constitutes a diagnostic problem. The foot is dry instead of sweaty, the serum urate level is raised and there may be a history of previous attacks.

The pain of rheumatoid arthritis is rarely as severe as in algodystrophy and circulatory changes are minor. Osteoporosis is usually relatively mild and not of the spotty type.

Some patients with algodystrophy demonstrate hysterical unconcern as a feature of their pre-existing personality, but whilst a 'hysterical foot' may be swollen, cold, blue and slightly osteoporotic, it does not show the sequence and intensity of circulation changes of algodystrophy nor the severe osteoporosis and increased sweating. Bone scan and thermography are normal.

Similarly, although the malingerer may complain of intense pain and tenderness and produce some oedema and cyanosis as a result of disuse, X-rays, bone scan and thermography are normal as is sweating.

A good response to sympathetic blockade, even if temporary, can be taken as confirmatory proof of the diagnosis of algodystrophy and this can be particularly helpful in litigation cases when further investigations prove inconclusive.

TREATMENT

Of primary importance is the early establishment of a positive diagnosis so that intensive therapy can be started. The longer diagnosis and treatment are delayed the more difficult and protracted does therapy become (Wynn Parry 1980, Schutzer & Gossling 1984). Having made the diagnosis it is vital to reassure the patient that the condition is recognized and that it is curable although it will take time and much effort. This reassurance needs giving repeatedly during the prolonged period of treatment and especially if there has been preceding doubt and anxiety regarding the diagnosis, suspicion of infection or of surgical error.

With reassurance and establishment of patient confidence must go exhortation and encouragement of effort and exercise.

Some authors are convinced that early muscle contractions and mobilization after fractures and surgery reduce the incidence of algodystrophy but there are no controlled studies reported.

Physical treatment

Physiotherapy

The essence is to encourage voluntary movements. Ultrasound, whirlpool baths, electrotherapy and other techniques have been suggested. These are all adjuncts to soothe and gain patient cooperation in the vital part of the treatment, active exercises. These can be performed on apparatus such as a cycle or treadle, in water, or working with the therapist in assistance/resistance, or movement pattern techniques. It is the reestablishment of normal reflexes and circulation by normal active movements that will restore normal function.

Certainly in the early stages and frequently even in the recovery phase, it is not possible for the ordinary patient to perform adequate exercises without the aid of a remedial therapist and it is important to stress to the therapist the necessity for frequent therapy sessions, preferably daily or twice daily.

In cases of minor severity, physical treatment alone will suffice but in more severe and established cases the foot is too painful or too unresponsive for physiotherapy. Medical therapy is needed in order to make active exercise possible.

Transcutaneous electrical nerve stimulation (TENS)

As disturbance of the normal balance of sensory nerve impulses arriving in the substantia gelatinosa of the spinal cord is considered to be a main cause of the pain, electrical stimulation of myelinated sensory fibres should theoretically be very effective. Results are best in treatment of causalgia due to nerve injury and less satisfactory, although frequently useful, in algodystrophy due to other causes (Wynn Parry 1980, Richlin et al 1978) (see Fig. 54.4).

Acupuncture and electroacupuncture

Good results have been reports for these forms of therapy. It is suggested that they release endorphins and thus relieve the pain but they may act on the 'gate mechanism' similarly to TENS (Chan & Chow 1981).

Drug therapy

Oral medication using analgesics, nonsteroidal anti-inflammatory drugs, or antidepressants, is on the whole disappointing. These preparations may be given in addition to other measures, but seldom seem to play a significant part in therapy.

Beta-blocking agents given orally may occasionally be effective (May & Glowinski 1979).

Calcitonin

Calcitonin injections have been strongly advocated by French workers (Acquaviva et al 1976, Doury et

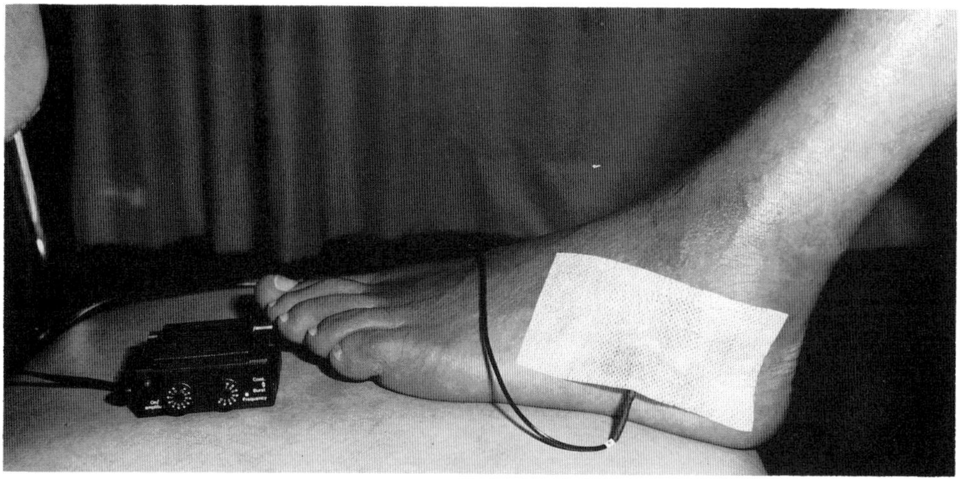

Fig. 54.4 Patient undergoing TNS treatment

al 1981, Fournié et al 1979) and seem very effective when given within the first few months (or preferably weeks) of the disorder. After six months, the response is less satisfactory. Dosage can be varied but a suggested regime would be 50 to 150 IU of salmon calcitonin given intramuscularly daily for 10 days and then three times a week for three weeks. As nausea is fairly common after injections, the dose should start at 50 IU and be increased in stages. If the patient experiences nausea, he should rest for a while after the injection. If necessary 10 mg of metoclopramide can be given intramuscularly at the same time to reduce the nausea.

Sometimes the response is dramatic; at other times slower. If there has been no improvement after the 10 days of daily treatment it is probably useless to continue. If the injections are effective but improvement is slow, there is no danger in continuing calcitonin for two or three weeks longer. It is, however, very expensive.

Corticosteroids

These drugs have been used both systemically and locally with reported good results (Christensen et al 1982). Where there is local joint swelling, tenosynovitis or a tender ligament attachment which seems to be serving as a 'focus' for the syndrome, most authorities would agree to local steroid infiltration. Systemic administration is more controversial because of its possible side effects and because doses of the order of 40–60 mg prednisolone daily may be needed initially. However, in an otherwise fit person careful steroid dosage should be quite safe for a few weeks (Glick 1973, Kozin et al 1981). Corticosteroids are particularly useful in longstanding cases where sympathetic overactivity has diminished and fibrosis or contractures appear to have started. Other forms of therapy are ineffective in such cases, but under the influence of steroids, intensive physiotherapy may become feasible and worthwhile.

Sympathetic blockade

The sympathetic nerve supply to the foot can be blocked by the paravertebral injection of bupivacaine. If the response is good, improvement in colour of the foot and relief of pain should be obvious within a few minutes. Function should also improve. The improvement should last for at least a day but as the anaesthetic wears off the full syndrome may recur. With injections repeated every second or third day, progressive and more lasting improvement may be achieved. If the response is good but relapse repeatedly occurs, permanent sympathetic blockade should be carried out by either phenol injection or surgical sympathectomy.

An alternative technique is to block the sympathetic receptors in the foot by intravenous administration of guanethidine to the leg after a tourniquet is applied according to the technique of

Biers, as described by Hannington-Kiff (1974, 1977). 1000 IU of heparin and 20 mg of guanethidine sulphate made up to 50 ml with saline, are injected slowly with the tourniquet round the thigh at 50 mmHg above the patient's systolic blood pressure. After five to ten minutes the tourniquet is released intermittently whilst the blood pressure is monitored. As the procedure is painful it needs to be carried out under a general anaesthetic and with resuscitation equipment at hand in case the guanethidine causes a severe fall in blood pressure when the tourniquet is released. Here also, the benefit should be immediate but may only last 24 hours. This procedure can be repeated several times (Loh et al 1980).

Psychotherapy

Some form is necessary in all cases but this can usually be given in the form of sympathetic reassurance by the doctor and remedial therapists during regular visits. There are cases where more specialized psychiatric assessment and management can be necessary and helpful.

Surgery

It is sometimes necessary to consider a surgical operation on a patient who has had algodystrophy, perhaps as a result of surgery, and perhaps to remedy contractures resulting from the dystrophy. Any limb surgery is best avoided, but two precautions can be advised if surgery is essential. It should not be attempted on an algodystrophic foot without a preceding sympathectomy. Immediately following surgery, prednisolone therapy should be started. The initial dose should be 20 mg daily and this can be reduced gradually over the next few weeks.

PROGNOSIS

The earlier the condition is recognized, the better the prognosis. If diagnosis and treatment are delayed until after contractures and trophic changes have begun, the chances of full recovery of function are reduced. The pain will eventually diminish or disappear but normal movements may not return. The patient may be left with a cold, stiff, cyanosed foot.

On the other hand, if active intensive therapy is commenced in the first few weeks, even though a great deal of prolonged effort may be required, full recovery is usually achieved.

Poor prognostic factors are late recognition, low pain tolerance by the patient, litigation and adverse psychological features.

MEDICOLEGAL ASPECTS

As previously mentioned under 'Aetiology' there is not infrequently a suspicion that the syndrome of pain and dysfunction has been aggravated if not initiated by the desire for compensation. Whereas in some instances, such suspicions are definitely incorrect, there remain other cases where, despite doubt, the possibility remains. In such patients, it is important to confirm the diagnosis by positive findings on X-ray, bone-scanning and thermography. If these are abnormal, a firm diagnosis of a somatic disorder can be made.

The occurrence of algodystrophy after surgery or after treatment of a simple injury, may lead to a claim of negligent or incorrect therapy. This is more likely if the onset of algodystrophy is not recognized and provokes noticeable doubts and anxiety on the part of the surgeon. Early recognition of the typical features and confirmation by tests allows a firm diagnosis and explanation to be given to the patient.

No prophylactic measures have been shown to be effective in preventing the onset of postoperative or postfracture algodystrophy.

REFERENCES

Acquaviva P, Eisinger J B, Schiano A, Recordier A M 1976 Traitement des algodystrophies par la calcitonin. Mediterr Med 4. 33–44

Bonica J J 1973 Causalgia and other reflex sympathetic dystrophies. Postgrad Med 53: 143–148

Carlson D H, Simon H, Wegner W 1977 Bone scanning and diagnosis of reflex sympathetic dystrophy secondary to herniated lumbar disc. Neurology 27: 791–793

Chan C S, Chow S P 1981 Electroacupuncture in the treatment of post-traumatic sympathetic dystrophy (Sudeck's atrophy). Br J Anaesth 53: 899–901

Christensen K, Jensen E M, Noer I 1982 The reflex dystrophy

syndrome. Response to treatment with systemic corticosteroids. Acta Chir Scand 148: 653–655
Churcher M D 1984 Algodystrophy after aortic bifurcation surgery. Lancet 2: 131–133
De Seze S, Ryckewaert A 1951 Algodystrophies sympathiques du membre supérieur. Maladies des os et des articulation. Flammarion, Paris
De Takats G 1937 Reflex dystrophy of extremities. Arch Surg 34: 939–956
De Takats G 1965 Sympathetic reflex dystrophy. Med Clin North Am 49: 117–129
Doupe J, Cullen C H, Chance G Q 1944 Postraumatic pain and causalgia syndrome. J Neurol Neurosurg Psychiatry 7: 33–48
Doury P, Dirheimer Y, Pattin S 1981 Algodystrophy. Springer Verlag, Berlin. p 123
Doury P, Granier R, Pattin S 1979 La place de la scintigraphie osseuse aux pyrophosphates de technetium 99m dans le diagnostic des algodystrophies. A propos de 74 observations. Ann Intern Med 130: 553–557
Fournié A, Ayrolles C, Guyard C 1979 Résultats de l'épreuve d'hypolcalcémie aiguë a la calcitonine dans les algodystrophies décalcifiantes. Rev Rhum 46: 55–56
Genant H K, Kozin F, Bekerman C, McCarty D J, Sims J 1975 The reflex sympathetic dystrophy syndrome. A comprehensive analysis & using fine detail radiography, photon absorptiometry and bone and joint scintigraphy. Radiology 117: 21–32
Glick E N 1973 Reflex dystrophy (Algoneurodystrophy): Results of treatment by corticosteroids. Rheumatol Rehabil 12: 84–88
Glynn C J, Basedow R W, Walsh J A 1981 Pain relief following post-ganglionic sympathetic blockade with I.V. guanethidine. Br J Anaesth 53: 1297–1301
Good A E 1970 Rheumatism and chemotherapy of tuberculosis. Ann Intern Med 72: 752–753
Granit R, Leskell L, Skaglund C R 1944 Fibre interaction in injured or compressed region of nerve. Brain 67: 125
Greyson N D, Tepperman P S 1984 Three phase bone studies in hemiplegia with reflex sympathetic dystrophy and the effect of disuse. J Nucl Med 25: 423–429
Hannington-Kiff J G 1974 Intravenous regional sympathetic block with guanethidine. Lancet 1: 1019–1020
Hannington-Kiff J G 1977 Relief of Sudeck's atrophy by regional intravenous guanethidine. Lancet 1: 1132–1133
Korenman E M D, Devor M 1981 Ectopic adrenergic sensitivity in damaged nerve axons in the rat. Exp Neurol 72: 63–81
Kozin F, Ryan L M, Carerra G F, Soin J S, Wortmann R L 1981 The reflex sympathetic dystrophy syndrome (RSDS). III. Scintigraphic studies, further evidence of the therapeutic efficacy of systemic corticosteroids and proposed diagnostic criteria. Am J Med 70: 23–30
Langloh N D, Hunder G G, Riggs B L, Kelly P J 1973 Transient painful osteoporosis of the lower extremities. J Bone Joint Surg 55A: 1188–1196
Lankford L L 1980 Reflex sympathetic dystrophy. In: Omer G E Jr, Spinner M (eds) Management of peripheral nerve problems. W B Saunders, Philadelphia
Lequesne M, Dang N, Bensasson M, Mery C 1977 Increased association of diabetes mellitus with capsulitis of the shoulder and shoulder hand syndrome. Scand J Rheumatol 6: 53–56
Leriche R, Fontaine R 1930 Des ostéoporoses douloureuses post-traumatiques. Presse Med 30: 617–621
Loh L, Nathan P W, Schott G D, Wilson P G 1980 Effects of regional guanethidine infusion in certain painful states. J Neurol Neurosurg Psychiatry 43: 446–451
May V, Glowinski J 1979 Algoneurodystrophie traitement par les bétabloquants. Nouv Presse Med 13: 1095
Melzack R, Wall P D 1965 Pain mechanisms: A new theory. Science 150: 971–979
Mitchell S W, Morehouse G R, Keen W W 1864 Gunshot wounds and other injuries of nerves. J B Lippincott, Philadelphia
O'Mara A E, Pinal R S 1970 Bone scanning in regional migratory osteoporosis. Case Report. Radiology 97: 579–581
Portias L H 1977 Les algo-neuro-dystrophies réflexes des membres inférieurs. Resultats d'une étude basée sur l'observation de 78 cas de 1969 à 1975. Sem Hop Paris 53(2): 133–138
Renier J C, Bregeon C, Boasson M, Billabert C 1973 Les algodystrophies du membre inférieur. Arch Med Ouest 5: 107–118
Richlin D M, Carson H, Rowlingson J C, Sussman M D, Baugher W H, Goldner R D 1978 Reflex sympathetic dystrophy: Successful treatment by transcutaneous nerve stimulation. J Pediatr 93: 84–86
Schutzer S F, Gossling H R 1984 The treatment of reflex sympathetic dystrophy syndrome. J Bone Joint Surg 66A: 625–629
Seltzer Z, Devor M 1979 Ephaptic transmission in chronically damaged peripheral nerves. Neurology 29: 1061–1064
Serre H, Simon L, Claustre J 1967 Algodystrophie réflexe du pied (A propos de 45 observations). Rev Rhum Mal Osteoartic 34: 722–732
Simson G 1974 Propranolol for causalgia and Sudeck atrophy. (Letter) JAMA 227: 327
Steinbrocker O 1968 The Shoulder-hand syndrome: present perspective. Arch Phys Med Rehabil 49: 388–395
Sudeck P H M 1900 Uber die akute entzundliche knockenatrophie. Arch Klin Chir 62: 149
Valenzuela F, Aris H, Jacobelli S 1977 Transient osteoporosis of the hip. J Rheumatol 4: 59–64
Wyn Parry C B 1980 Painful conditions of peripheral nerves. Aust NZ J Surg 50: 233–236

Chiropody

INTRODUCTION

Chiropody, traditionally the care and removal of superficial lesions of the feet has undergone drastic changes within the last 15 years and is currently defined as 'Chiropody comprises the maintenance of the feet in a healthy condition and the treatment of their disabilities by recognized chiropodial methods in which the practitioner has been trained'. The recognition of the profession by a State Register in 1960 was followed by the introduction of the use of local anaesthesia.

This innovation allowed chiropodists to develop and use a range of minor surgical techniques mainly in the treatment of toenail disorders and removal of verrucae. More recently the introduction of biomechanics into the diagnosis and treatment of foot disorders has allowed management to go beyond the treatment of symptoms. The fact that science has taken the place of art in no way diminishes the very real importance of traditional techniques. The need still remains for pain-free removal of corns and callosities, and the skilful use of padding and taping.

During their three year course the students will fabricate a wide range of devices, insoles and orthoses which later they will prescribe in practice. Training stresses the need to differentiate between local and systemic disorders, particularly important as practitioners receive patients direct, making their own diagnosis and treatment regime.

Within the hospital environment the chiropodist will work closely with other medical disciplines, particularly endocrinology, rheumatology, orthopaedics and dermatology. Post-registration degree courses have now been introduced and the profession looks forward to the Diploma course being replaced by a Degree course in the near future.

HISTORICAL PERSPECTIVE

The earliest British text dealing with the treatment of corns, callosities and other minor foot disorders was written by Heyman Lion in 1802. The emphasis of this book was on the painless and long-term removal of corns and the treatment of painful nails. The dressings described in the text are mainly of the strapping variety and are medicated in various ways. No protective or corrective paddings are mentioned. 'An experienced Chiropodist in 1878' describes how plantar corns may be removed and the areas protected by thick hat felt with holes cut into it. It is suggested that the pad be glued into the shoe. Early chiropodists certainly used a variety of materials in order to protect parts of the foot following treatment, felt being most commonly used. This was often applied to the foot with zinc oxide adhesive. Chiropodists themselves frequently prepared these adhesive pads spreading zinc oxide on the felt and finishing them with an iron.

Dagnall (1985) maintained that Lewis Durlacher (1792–1864), in writing his book *A treatise on corns, bunions, and diseases of nails, and the general management of the feet* established Chiropody as a branch of medicine and surgery. Durlacher was surgeon chiropodist to several British sovereigns, including Queen Victoria, and first described plantar digital neuritis. The *Lancet* in 1827 describes his treatment for onychocryptosis as a 'most important improvement in this Department of operative surgery'. Runting, a founder of the first British Chiropodial Society in 1912, describes not only a range of adhesive pads, but also various remedial straps. He also emphasized the importance of adequate footwear — a point which still presents the modern chiropodist with many difficulties in the course of treatment.

An attempt has been made in this chapter briefly to describe the specialist approach of Chiropody and to illustrate the clinical application of these principals in outlining the management of a range of conditions.

FUNCTION OF THE FOOT

1. The foot must be capable of acting as an adaptor to uneven surfaces and as a shock absorber.
2. It must become a rigid lever in propulsion.

Gait

These requirements are met in the normal foot by a cycle of pronation and supination.

Pronation of the rear foot allows an unlocking of the subtalar joint and then the midtarsal joint. As the foot moves into supination at midstance with the foot in the neutral position the subtalar and midtarsal joints are locked. The foot can then act as a rigid lever.

The stable supinated foot goes into the propulsive phase and toe-off. In order to establish a point of reference it is helpful to define a position of the foot in which it is most efficient. This position will be determined by a range of individual joint variations and angular relationship. When the rear foot is neither pronated nor supinated and the forefoot is locked against it then the foot is in the *neutral* position.

BIOMECHANICAL FOOT ABNORMALITIES

Langer & Wernick (1978) clarify the five most common biomechanical foot abnormalities as:

1. Subtalar varus (calcaneal varus): an inversion deformity of the calcaneus when the subtalar joint is in the neutral position.
2. Forefoot varus: a fixed osseous inversion deformity as related to a bisection of the calcaneus when the subtalar joint is in the neutral position. This condition must be distinguished from the nonfixed positional forefoot deformity of supinatus.
3. Equinus: a foot in which there is a marked lack of dorsiflexion of the subtalar joint in the neutral position with the knee extended (Fig. 55.1).
4. Forefoot varus: a constant structural eversion of the forefoot.
5. Plantarflexed first ray.

Table 55.1 indicates the management of these disorders.

The normal foot

The requirements for a foot to function normally are shown in Fig. 55.1. Function of the foot is, of course,

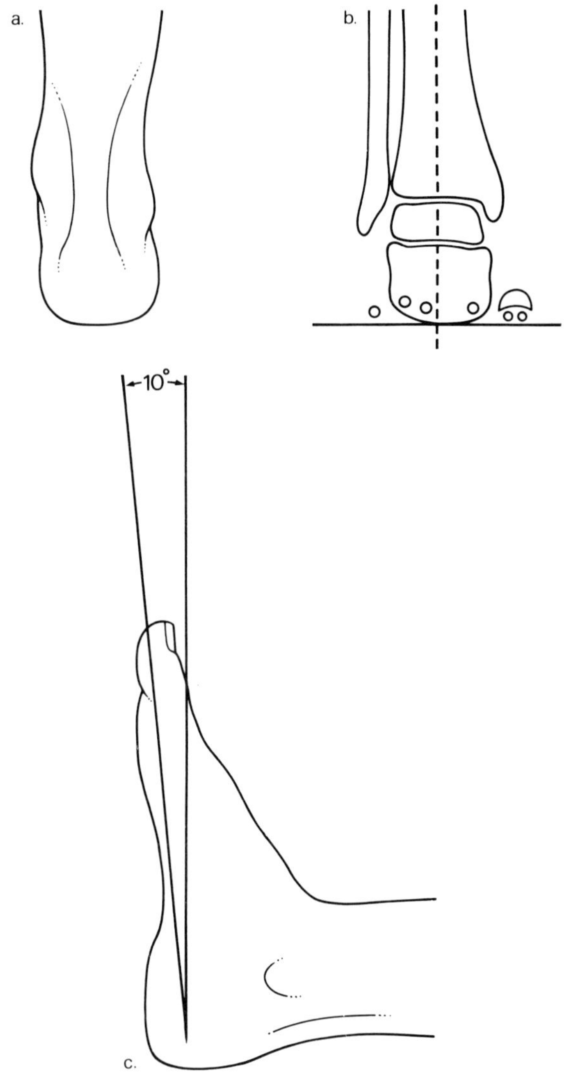

Fig. 55.1 a: The calcaneum is vertical and parallel to the lower ⅓ of the leg; b: The rear foot and forefoot should be parallel to each other; c: There should be a minimum of 10° of dorsiflexion with the knee extended and the foot in neutral

Table 55.1 Management of biomechanical foot abnormalities

Foot type	Lesions	Symptoms	Treatment
Subtalar varus (Rearfoot varus)	Bunion Corn on 5th toe Hammer toes Talar bunion Deep plantar lesions 2:3:4 Haglund's deformity	Leg fatigue Low back pain Neck spasm	Treatment of lesions Heel to be maintained in neutral by using a rearfoot medial (varus) post. Allowance must be made for normal pronation to occur
Forefoot varus	Hallux abductovalgus deformity Corn on 5th toes Overlapping toes Plantar lesions particularly affecting metatarsal heads 2:3:4 Calcaneal spur on X-ray	Bunions Plantarfasciitis Inferior calcaneal bursitis Foot strain Chronic low backpain Anterior shin splints	Treatment of lesions Rigid or semirigid orthosis with forefoot medial (varus) post
Equinus (must be differentiated from dynamic muscle imbalance (Runner's equinus))	Subluxation of hallux Corns on toes 2:3:4:5 Toe deformity Deep plantar callus Genu valgum and recurvatum	Sciatica Intermetatarsal neuromas Fatigue	Palliative treatment of lesions Attempts to correct a compensated equinus may make matters worse although a *pronated* device may help Heel lifts Surgery Stretching
Plantarflexed first ray	2 types: 1. Pronation originates from rearfoot varus 2. As in forefoot varus		As subtalar varus As forefoot varus
Forefoot valgus (rigid plantar flexed first ray)	Metatarsus adductus Pes cavus foot type Claw toes Elevated 1st toe Deep corn under 1st and 5th metatarsal heads	Pain in tissues around sesamoid Chronic ankle sprain Haglund's deformity (Heel bump) Morton's toe Leg and back pain.	Semirigid or accommodative Reinforced cork is useful Give rigid foot 'soft' support

subject to abnormality in the structures above it (see below).

The abnormal foot

Changes in position may occur in an attempt to balance or neutralize positional or structural deviations elsewhere. This mechanism is called *compensation*.

MECHANICAL STRESSES OPERATING ON THE TISSUES OF THE FOOT AND THEIR EFFECT ON THE SKIN

Stress, the force that is applied over the area of the object, can be divided into three groups:

1. Compressional — as in tissue beneath the calcaneum
2. Tensile — an extension of tissue
3. Shearing — as between the foot and the shoe.

Blakeman (1985) reviews the various mechanical forces and suggests that padding and shock absorption materials should also be identified by their ability to resist these forces.

The forces listed are normally combined and when abnormally high, result in corns, callosities, bursae and blisters. Intermittent pressure on the stratum corneum produces overactivity and results in hyperkeratosis. The effect of excessive hyperkeratosis is to reduce the elasticity of the skin and, through its bulk, cause pain and discomfort. Callus is a diffuse hyperkeratosis whilst corns are more localized areas of impacted hyperkeratosis with central nuclei.

CLASSIFICATION OF CORNS

Corns can be classified as follows:

Hard (Heloma durum)
Soft (Heloma molle)
Vascular (Heloma vasculare)
Neurovascular (Heloma neurovasculare)
Seed corns (Helomatu miliare) — plugs of cholesterol

Removal of hyperkeratotic lesions by nonincisional scalpel technique

Whilst treatment is aimed at the prevention of lesions a most important part of the chiropodist's work remains the removal of callosities and corns and reduction of nails (see clinical applications — nails). Charlesworth (1947) describes the methods of removal.

Whole section

This technique involves undermining the overgrowth with a sharp scalpel and picking the complete lesion free using a chisel-type instrument. It is not normal practice in the UK.

Part section

This method involves removing hyperkeratosis in small sections or flakes with a lateral slightly scooping motion. Any nuclei are then removed as one piece. This is the preferred method.

Minute section

As above but the nucleus of any corn is removed in section with the skin held taut to avoid drag on nerve filaments. This is a method particularly used in vascular and neurovascular lesions. Scullion (1984) lists the criteria for good chiropodial scalpel technique as:

1. Firm skin tension
2. Light, easy balancing of the instrument
3. Flexibility of the wrist
4. Sideward movement of the blade
5. Debriding in an ordered fashion — starting at the softer outer edge of the lesion.

Instruments

The advent of replaceable blades has largely made setting and stropping a thing of the past although some specialized fixed blade knives such as those used to reduce and treat nails are still popular. Modern instruments are now made from stainless steel to facilitate autoclaving.

PADDING, TAPING AND STRAPPING

Modern methods of measuring dynamic and static

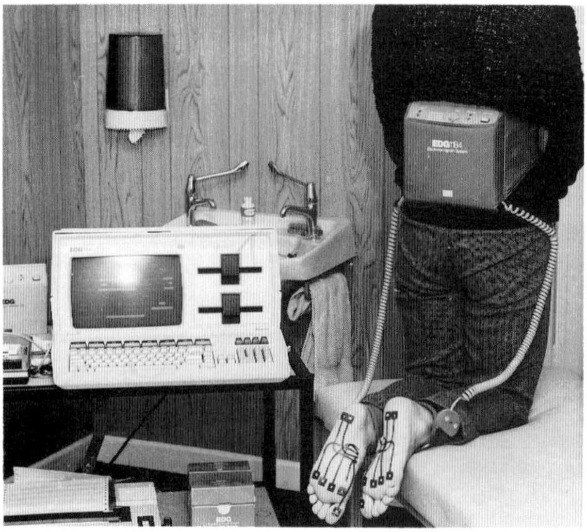

Fig. 55.2 The electrodynagram. The relationship between the foot and leg must be determined in all three planes

foot pressures ranging from Harris and Beaths inked ridged pressure pads to the pedobarograph and dynamic gait analyser (Fig. 55.2) have challenged the traditional theories of chiropody padding.

Dhanedran et al (1980) showed that pressure on the lesser metatarsal heads is not significantly reduced by applying a felt metatarsal pad. Dalton (1982) challenges the concept of pressure being responsible for corns and callouses, and argues that friction is the most important dynamic component. These observations follow the work of Root et al (1977) and Scarlatto (1971) whose books largely introduced systemic biomechanics of the foot and lower limb to UK chiropody.

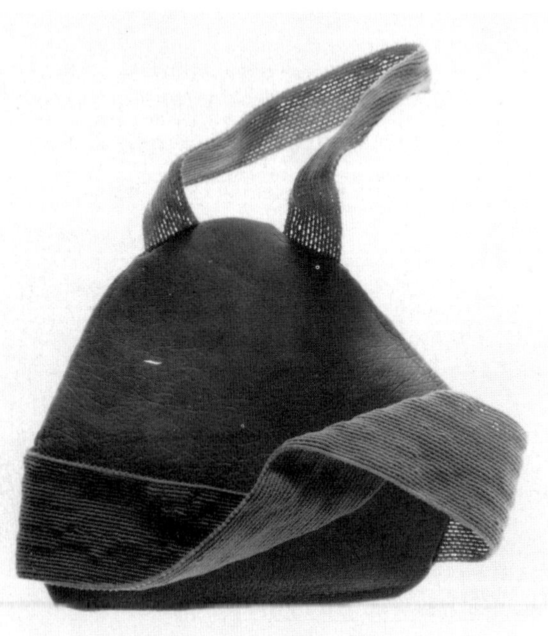

Fig. 55.3 A replaceable plantar pad

Hanby & Walker (1960) extended the work of Charlesworth (1947) in presenting a concise theory of padding starting with the precept that the function of the chiropodist was to combat the effects of overwork on the foot. They stated that padding should aim to:

1. Provide cushioned protection
2. Give rest to particular tissues of the foot generally
3. Redirect or combat undesirable stresses
4. Correct malposition of the foot and parts of it.

Neale & Walker (1984) reviewed various paddings and usefully describe a range of shoe modifications using felt and other adhesive materials.

Materials and techniques

Adhesive dressings, in spite of the difficulties of sensitivity, good hygiene and resilience, remain the favourite material of the chiropodist. In spite of the many technological advances in orthoses and shoe gear there remain a group of patients for whom padding and strapping uniquely seem to offer comfort and pain relief. Most padding and tape is now available in hypoallergic grades in addition to the traditional zinc oxide spread. Padding is available as felt, compressed or semicompressed, to protect or redirect stresses, and foams in various densities to provide shock absorption and to cushion debilitated tissues. Thinner materials such as fleecy web or stockinette are used to reduce skin friction. Foam is also available in tubular form and can be used to protect lesions over phalangeal joints. These are easily replaced by the patient.

Padding materials may be applied to the feet, stuck into the shoes, made into replaceable pads (Fig. 55.3) or used in an appliance. Where weight transfer is required the material is applied proximal to the articulation of the joint. Where the head of a joint is subluxed then this should be accommodated within a 'U' (Fig. 55.4d) and cushioned with a light density foam. Similarly a cavus type foot with a

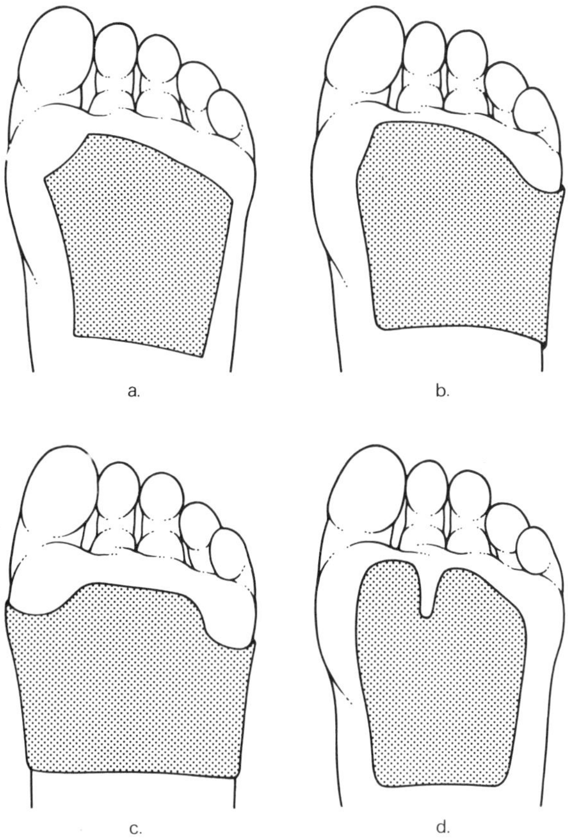

Fig. 55.4 a: Plantar metatarsal pad; b: Single wing plantar metatarsal pad; c: Double wing plantar metatarsal pad; d: "U" plantar metatarsal pad

painful plantar corn can be treated with a firm double wing felt pad (Fig. 55.4c) to transfer pressure and a foam cushion above it. Pads intended as cushions or shock absorbers are placed over the lesion or painful area.

Silicone rubber devices

Silicone rubber offers the chiropodist the opportunity to construct easily and at the chairside, a wide range of devices which are durable and hygienic. Coates (1977) discusses the advantages of silicones and details a wide range of devices.

However, many of the products available today are difficult to use and unstable. Considerable practice is required to gain expertise and the products' shelf-life and storage conditions require monitoring. One of the simpler compounds is a putty-like silicone which can be premoulded to the foot to assess the quantity required and shaping requirements. It is then fixed with a tinted hardener, spatulated well and moulded on the foot. Although the device can be used immediately, a total setting time of 24 hours is preferred. The device can be washed and, although torn easily, can be very durable. A combined interdigital wedge and toeprop is illustrated (Fig. 55.5).

Digital casting

This technique produces protective devices used to protect lesions on toes and bunions. Plaster of Paris bandage or dental alginate are used to make a mould and the positive plaster cast is made from this. The cast is dipped in liquid latex and successive layers added until a resilient skin has formed. The protective padding is then applied and further layers of latex added. The resulting device is easily removable and simple to keep clean (Fig. 55.6).

Common uses of taping

1. After mobilization of a sprained ankle
2. In plantar fasciitis and painful heels (Fig. 55.7)
3. Tendo Achillis problems

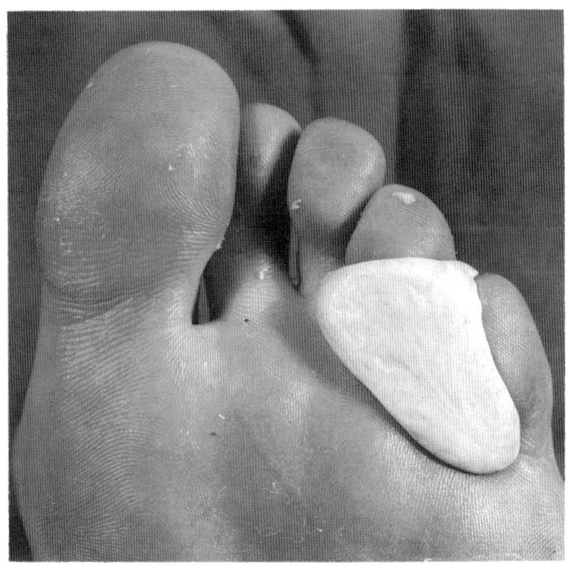

Fig. 55.5 A combined interdigital wedge and toe prop made of silicone rubber

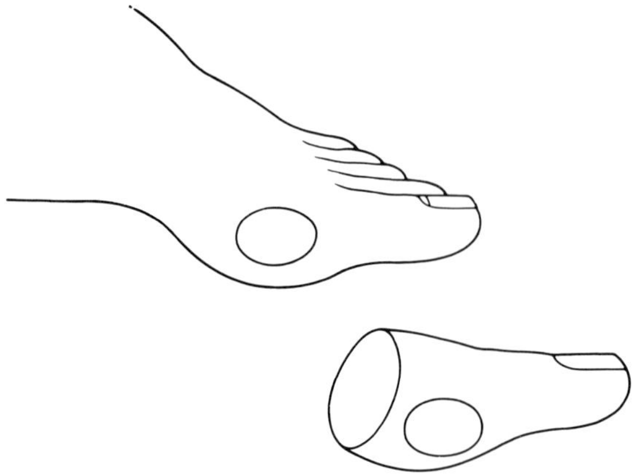

Fig. 55.6 The cast is dipped in liquid latex and successive layers added until a resilient skin has formed

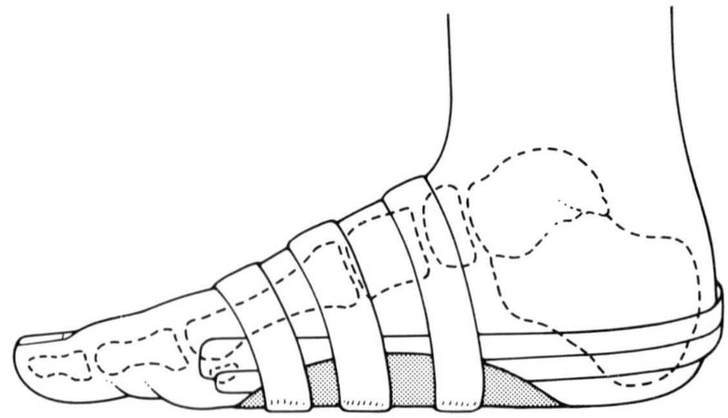

Fig. 55.7 Low dye strapping combined with an arch pad

4. Maltracking of the patella and other knee injuries
5. To limit inversion and eversion of the heel.

The rigid tape is applied over a thin protective foam layer. Anchor straps are applied distally and proximally and further tape applied to limit movement as required. Modified figure-of-eight strapping may also be used to achieve a similar result.

Thermoplastic foams

Nonadhesive foams of varying density can also be used to construct moulded insoles incorporating pads. This foam (Plastazote) can also be used to construct light seamless boots and shoes (Drushoes) for feet that are not accommodated in normal footwear. These materials can be moulded directly to the foot after heating to 140°C and can be reinforced in layers to improve their function.

Nonthermoplastic shock absorbing materials

1. PPT, a poromeric rubber material
2. Sorbothane, a recently developed viscoelastic polymer material which is available with two recovery rates (30 and 50 durometer)
3. Spenco, a material made from neoprene with nitrogen bubbles in it. This material absorbs friction and vertical forces.

These three materials, which are available in sheet and shaped form, are suitable for the construction of simple devices or for incorporating into orthoses and padding. All three materials have relatively fast recovery rates and keep their shape over long periods. Sorbothane, which is very useful in cases where high levels of shock absorption are required, does have the disadvantage of being rather heavy. The material, which mimics the properties of connective tissue (Niehans 1985), can be applied to itself without the use of adhesives.

PPT is available in a wide range of thicknesses and is very light and easily machined.

Spenco is available in thin sheet form and is more suitable for covering.

All these materials make excellent base materials in the treatment of rheumatoid, diabetic and other feet where there may be loss of fibrofatty tissue, poor shock absorption or debilitated tissues.

Effect on the knee of overpronation

Subotnick (1975a), Steadman (1979) and Landry & Zebas (1985) all describe the effects of overpronation on patellofemoral problems (Fig. 55.8) especially on the sports participant and the young. Abnormal pronation in the foot can give rise to rotation of the knee altering the Q angle and the pull of the quadriceps. Orthotic therapy to hold the foot in the neutral position is indicated.

BIOMECHANICAL AND ORTHOTIC THERAPY

Biomechanical therapy works at its simplest through reducing movement and bringing the ground up to

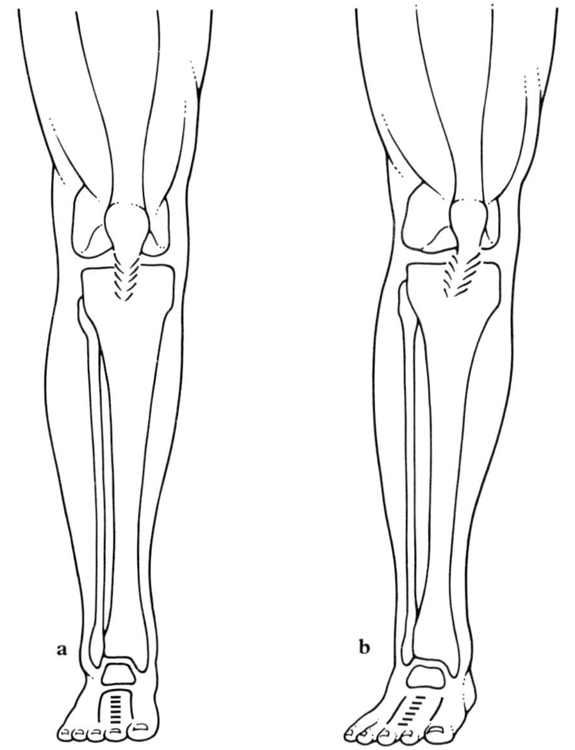

Fig. 55.8 a, Normal neutral foot; b, Pronated foot

the foot. Long term, it is hoped that orthotic therapy combined with physical therapy and perhaps surgery will rehabilitate muscle imbalances. In some conditions functional devices are not effective and simpler accommodative devices may give better relief from symptoms (Gibbard 1968). Improvements in shoes, especially sports shoes, have reduced injury and these, combined with temporary orthoses, may be sufficient. The use of orthoses in the management of foot problems connected with cerebral palsy especially when a foot orthosis is combined with an ankle orthosis is fully discussed by Rosenthal (1984). Conditions treated included balancing, stance phase and swing difficulties as well as dynamic muscle imbalances.

Orthoses

Are constructed from a variety of materials including rigid Rohadur (Fig. 55.9) and semirigid Vitrathene (Fig. 55.10). A rule of thumb is that rigid orthoses are prescribed for a soft foot and vice versa. Shells are constructed from these thermoplastic materials on

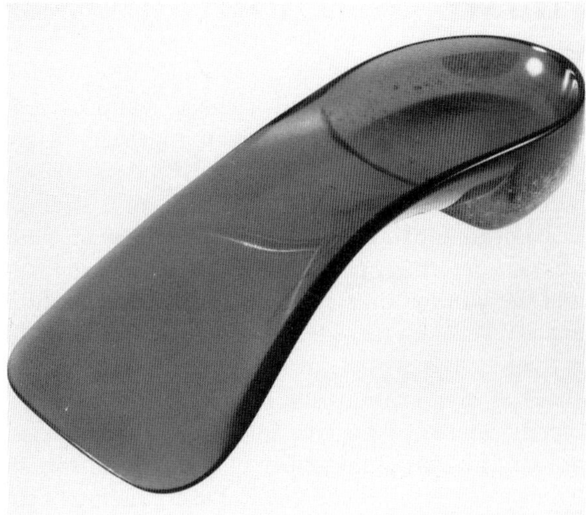

Fig. 55.9 A rigid orthosis showing rear foot posting

neutral position casts of the foot. Wedges or posts are applied to the rear or forefoot either in rigid acrylic materials or high impact rubber. It is important to allow for normal pronation when posting.

In addition to casted devices, heel lifts to compensate for leg length irregularities and shoe modification may be necessary. Wernick (1978) and Subotnick (1975b) discuss the biomechanical problems associated with skiing. Where the problem is intrinsic to the foot it is suggested that an orthosis be worn. Where it is extrinsic then the boot should be canted (tilted). It is also speculated by this writer and Bell (1985) that angling the bindings on the ski where restrictions exist in the hip or knee might enable the skis to be brought parallel with less difficulty.

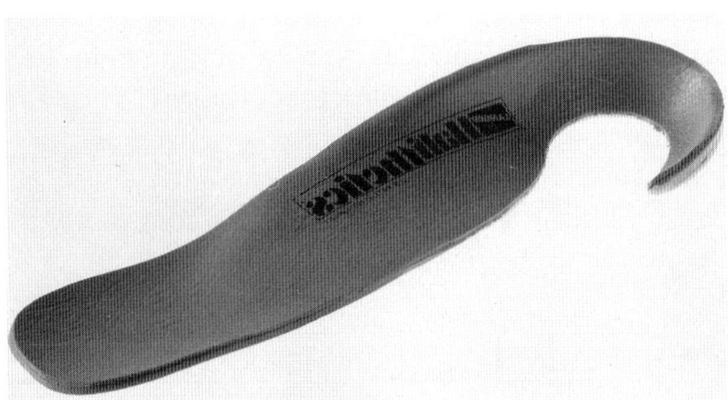

Fig. 55.10 A semi-rigid device cut away for easier shoe accommodation

CLINICAL APPLICATION

Examination

The patient is examined sitting, standing and walking. A full history is taken together with a general medical history. The nature and position of superficial lesions, the presence of swelling, discolouration and change in temperature and any obvious deformity noted. The foot pulses are taken and the skin colour and texture recorded. The shoes are checked both for size wear patterns, and flare (the medial, central, or lateral bias of the forepart of the shoe). A brief examination of the patient walking is carried out and any gait or anatomical abnormalities noted. If a gait abnormality is seen or the history warrants it, a full biomechanical examination of the lower limbs is carried out with note being taken of any problems in the upper body. Radiological examination may also be necessary.

THE NAILS

The chief purpose of the nail is to protect and assist the sensory functions of the distal phalanges of the fingers and toes. However, because of this protective role the nails are often damaged themselves, and being the most peripheral tissues are sensitive to changes and interruption in vascularity. The need for regular cutting also puts the nail at risk from selfinflicted injury.

The nails arise from the matrix within an invagination of the skin immediately superior to the base of the distal phalanx. The nail plate is composed of densely packed keratin cells ridged on the inferior surface to conform with a similarly ridged underlying nail bed. Lewis (1954) argued that part of the bed also contributes to nail growth, although Samman (1965) qualifies this by stating that this only occurs under pathological conditions. The nails are affected by trauma, infection, ischaemia and a wide spectrum of systemic disease. As well as acquired disorders, the nail may less commonly be affected by congenital factors.

The painful nail

Aetiology

Pain may arise from the nail grooves or bed and may be due to one or a combination of the following:

1. Corns or calluses in the nail sulci — onychophosis
2. Infection of the sulci or toe pulp caused by a spike of ingrowing toenail — onychocryptosis
3. Involuted nail pressure from an excessively curved nail
4. A gross thickening of the nail with or without distortion — onychauxis, onychogryphosis
5. Subungual haematoma
6. Irritation of the sulci arising from a rotational deformity of the phalanx, often the hallux, and usually associated with overpronation
7. A relaxed nail sulcus in conjunction with hyperhidrosis.

Treatment

Corns and callosities in the sulcus. Friction between the nail and sulcus may result in the formation of corns or calluses. These must be differentiated from verrucae or, in rare cases, glomus tumour.

The fitting of footwear, including socks, should be checked and any gait abnormality compensated for where possible.

The nail plate often requires thinning down and this is done by using a chiropody drill. The nail groove is gently cleared using a fine scalpel such as a Beaver handle fitted with a No. 67 blade. It may be necessary to soften the tissue in the sulcus by using hydrogen peroxide or applying a weak paste of salicylic acid. Wherever possible removal of nail sections should be avoided as regrowth of these may produce further irritation. When any corns have been enucleated and the groove irrigated then the sulci should be packed with one of the following:

1. A light foam
2. Copalene — a woven cotton fabric
3. Amadou — a bark treated with sodium nitrite which acts as a slight astringent
4. Silicone rubber

The packing may be secured using collodion or cement such as acrytensil.

Where hyperextension of the toe exists and the footwear is tight a corn may form on the nail bed beneath the distal edge of the nail. In order to remove this it is normally necessary to cut the nail back although occasionally the lesion can be removed without this if access permits. Following removal, advice should be given regarding footwear and adhesive padding or a removable device issued to protect the lesion.

Involuted nails

In this case the nail is excessively curved across the plate and may result in a pinching of the soft tissue of the toe pulp.

Aetiology

1. The distortion may be associated with a rotational deformity of the toe
2. The shape of the nail may be inherited
3. A subungual exostosis — a bony overgrowth — may develop on the tip of the distal phalanx and push up against the nail distorting the lateral borders (Fig. 55.11).

Treatment

Back (1970) describes a technique of 'unrolling' the nail plate with heated pliers.

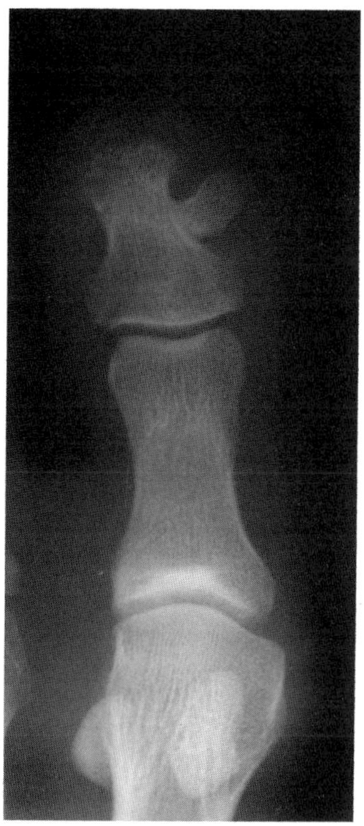

Fig. 55.11 Subungual exostosis

Corrective bracing is a useful method of treating the involuted nail, although it may require long-term application. The braces may be constructed from stainless steel wire (Fig. 55.12) or a rubber band secured to small plastic hooks which are glued to the edges of the nail plate (Fig. 55.13). Severe cases may require surgery.

Clinically the presence of a subungual exostosis may be demonstrated by a cherry red appearance beneath the distal edge of the nail plate. Lateral X-rays will confirm the diagnosis.

Onychauxis — hypertrophied nail

In this condition the nail plate is thickened and discoloured.

Aetiology

1. Trauma
2. Onychomycosis
3. Psoriasis and other skin disorders
4. Systemic factors

Treatment

This condition is normally irreversible and may affect one or all of the toenails. The patient will

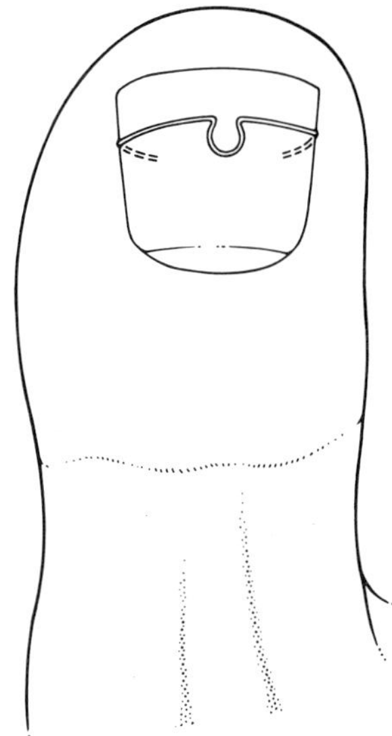

Fig. 55.12 Stainless steel wire nail brace

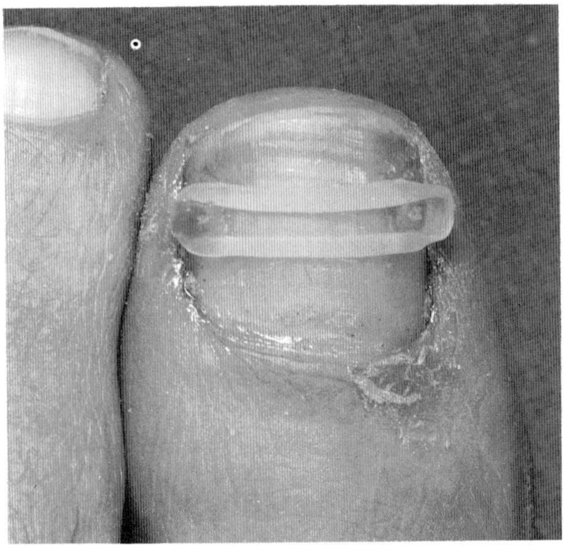

Fig. 55.13 Nail brace with rubber band secured with plastic hooks

require regular chiropody treatment to have the nail reduced.

Where only a single nail is affected it may be worthwhile considering a total nail ablation with phenolization of the nail matrix.

Onychogryphosis — ramshorn (Fig. 55.14)

In this condition the nail plate is not only grossly thickened, but is deformed so that the nail frequently has a spiral-like appearance resembling a ram's horn. The nail may also grow over the distal edge of the toe and penetrate the plantar surface of the toe in severe cases.

Aetiology

1. Trauma
2. Neglect

Treatment

As with onychauxis the nail may be thinned down using an electric drill. Occasionally vascular tufts are situated within the nail and care must be taken to avoid cutting these.

Onychocryptosis — ingrowing toenail

Poor cutting of the nail in attempting to shape it may

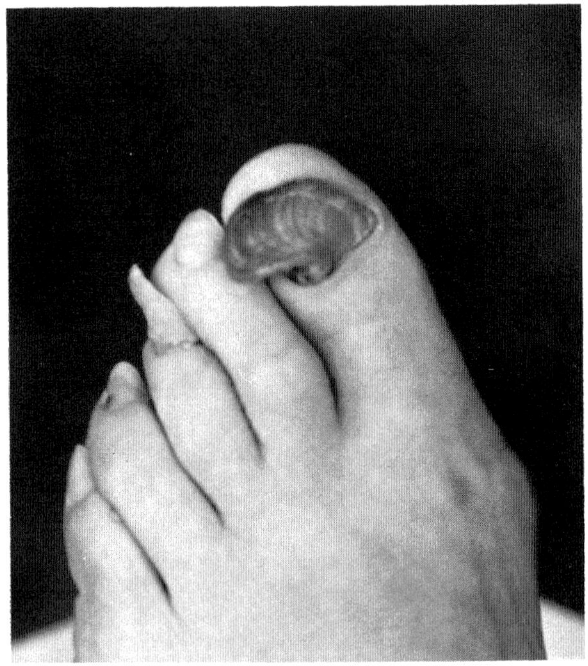

Fig. 55.14 A ramshorn nail

result in a spike of nail being left. This grows forward into the pulp of the toe causing infection and hypergranulation along the lip of the nail sulcus (Fig. 55.15). This infection will not resolve until the nail spicule is removed and any antibiotic therapy should normally only accompany such treatment. Local

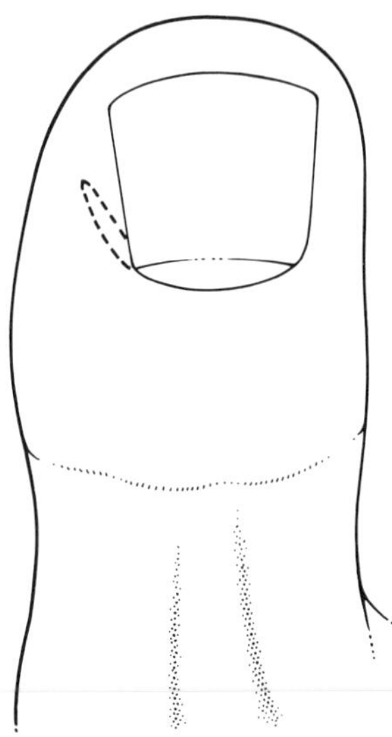

Fig. 55.15 An onychocryptosis showing a typical nail spike

anaesthesia may be used to ensure pain-free removal, but the injections should be made as proximal as possible to the area.

The spicule of nail may be freed using Thwaites nippers and a Francis chisel or Beaver knife. Once loosened the section of nail can be extracted with fine mosquito forceps. The edge of the remaining nail plate should be carefully smoothed using a Blacks file. The wound should be irrigated with hydrogen peroxide solution and flushed with 0.5% Hibitane® in spirit. A dry iodine powder spray makes a satisfactory postoperative dressing, although it may be necessary to recommend postoperative saline foot baths in order to promote drainage. An interdigital wedge constructed of silicone rubber or felt and a shoe with the toe area removed will assist in removing pressure from the area during healing. Hypergranulation may be reduced by applying a 70% stick of silver nitrate. It is of course mandatory that advice should be given on the correct cutting of the nail. The nail generally should be cut so that the distal edge follows the contour of the toe and no attempt should be made to shape the nail. The edges must be free of the sulci. A recurrence or delayed healing may indicate the need for more radical nail surgery or bracing.

Subungual haematoma

Bruising beneath the nail plate is usually associated with a blow or trauma from a shoe. The condition is often known as runners nail. In the over pronating foot the length of the foot increases and impaction of the tips of the toes against the shoe causes bruising beneath the nail. A semicircular felt pad beneath the tongue of the shoe will enable tighter lacing to secure the foot. The depth of the toe puff must be adequate and toe props to assist extension where appropriate are helpful. A group of sportsmen particularly affected are footballers. Modern football boots are soft topped and injury to the toe and nails is not uncommon.

Early decompression is important to prevent deformity. This can be carried out using a heated needle or, alternatively, the plate can be drilled with a fine burr.

Irritation of the sulci arising from conjunction with hyperhidrosis

This condition usually occurs in boys aged between 12 and 17. Often the nails are cut badly. Dagnall (1983) surmises that this is analogous to fingernail biting from tension. He reports Englands' (1909–1980) theory that hormonal levels play an important part in the condition. Advice and encouragement regarding correct cutting should be the first step in management and the prescription of mild astringents such as 3% salicylic acid in surgical spirit can be effective.

Nonsurgical removal of dystrophic nails

Port & Sanicola (1980) review the work of Farber & South (1978) and report their own findings using a combination of 40% urea and occlusion to remove nails. An average occlusion period of 12 days was reported. For those cases where surgery or local anaesthetic is not indicated this is a useful alternative treatment.

NAIL SURGERY

Where conservative methods are not successful in resolving the nail problem then total or partial ablative surgery may be considered. As in all surgery the procedure should be carried out only where the patient's general status permits and where there is a reasonable peripheral circulation. High risk patients such as diabetics must be carefully evaluated preoperatively.

As surgery of the toenail is covered elsewhere in this book, here only an outline is presented of nail procedures carried out by chiropodists.

In all cases the surgery is carried out under aseptic conditions and local anaesthesia. A list of instruments suitable for nail surgery is illustrated (Fig. 55.16).

Partial or total nail ablation with sterilization of the matrix using phenol

This technique was first described by Boll (1945) and Wee (1972) in the US and later in the UK by Francis & Furness (1974), Dagnell (1974) and Bell (1977). Its relative simplicity and reliable results as reported by Ashcroft et al (1979) make it the treatment of choice.

The toe is first exsanguinated and a tourniquet

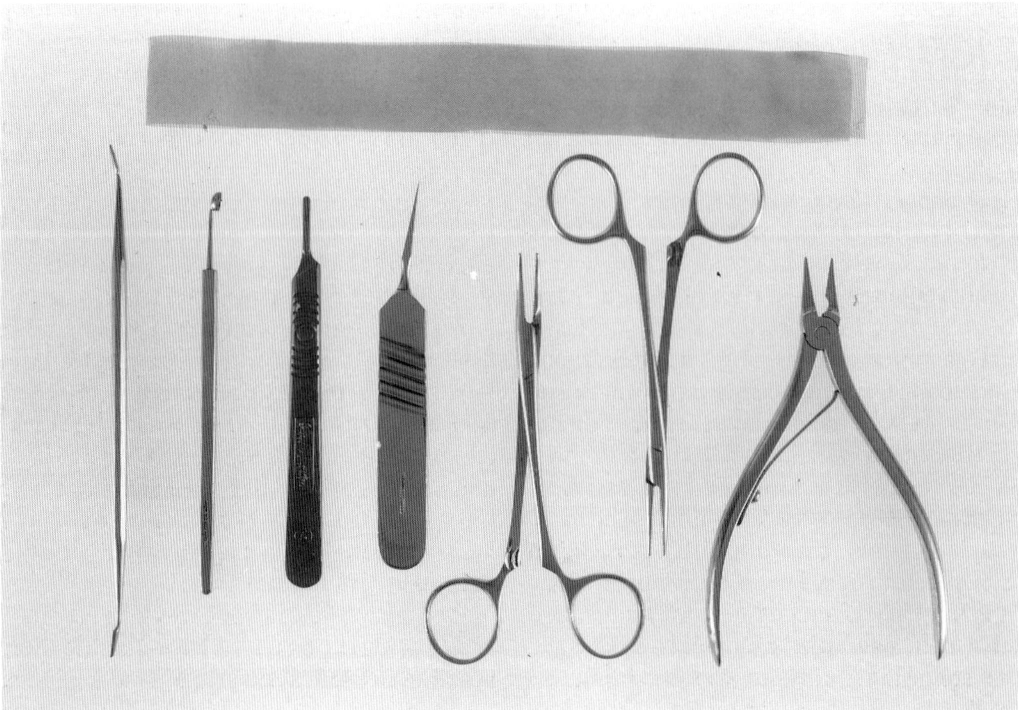

Fig. 55.16 A nail instrument kit. From left to right: Black's file, curette, scalpel handle, Francis chisel, Halstead forceps (straight and curved), Thwaite's nippers. Top: latex Esmarch bandage

applied. This is important as the phenol will be ineffective in the presence of bleeding. The nail is partially or totally ablated and the matrical area treated with a saturated solution of phenol applied with a wooden applicator. When the area is blanched, normally around two minutes, the tourniquet is released and the area irrigated with sterile saline or 5% hibitane in spirit. The toe is dressed once haemorrhage ceases. Hawes (1975) discusses postoperative care following this procedure and there is wide agreement that Ponoxylan Gel® or Betadine® ointment are satisfactory medications. The action of the latter is said to be enhanced in the presence of pus and serum.

Steindler technique

This approach is indicated where narrowing of the nail plate is required without any loss of ungualabial tissue. It has the advantage over the phenol method of rapid healing. The method is described by Francis (1981).

A single incision through the nail plate is made which is split and extended to the eponychium and into a hockey stick shape over the matrical area. A second incision within the ungualabia completes a wedge distally. The nail tissue and matrix are dissected out.

Winograd technique

This involves the removal of a wedge of nail and tissue and is indicated where hypertrophy of the ungualabia is present.

Subungual exotosis

This bony overgrowth or 'tufting' of the dorsodistal surface of the terminal phalanx is associated with a tubular deformity of the nail. It is reported that this is connected with a 'wedging' effect caused by an associated ossicle or sesamoid on the plantar articulation of the distal interphalangeal joint. The overgrowth can be removed through a fishmouth incision at the distal aspect of the toe removing the distal one-third of the nail plate. A double elliptical wedge of skin is removed to close the dead space left following removal of the exostosis.

Where surgery is contraindicated because of the patient's general condition an open-toed or deep shoe is recommended.

DEFORMITIES OF THE LESSER TOES

The toes are important during the propulsive phase of gait. Ground force results in dorsiflexion, whilst the toe flexors increase plantar flexion. At the same time the phalangeal joint is extended by toe extension in order that the toe can act as a stabilizer. While functional orthoses and insoles may be able to control rear and forefoot abnormalities they are often not able to improve toe function significantly without the use of separate bolsters or toe props.

Deformities of the toes can arise as a result of intrinsic or extrinsic factors and may result in painful corns, callosities and nails. When primary biomechanical abnormalities are present, badly fitting shoes and hosiery can initiate or exacerbate toe deformity. Toes are often affected by systemic factors.

Hammer toes

The commonest deformity of digits is the hammer toe. Klenerman et al (1976) suggested that the term should be limited to flexion deformities that cannot be overcome by stretching. Higgs (1931) postulated that stretching was prevented by contraction of the skin and soft tissue beneath the flexed joint. However, in many cases of fixed hammer toe deformity bony changes can be observed on X-Ray, demonstrating that ankylosis and subluxation have occurred. The hammer toe presents as a flexion of the proximal interphalangeal joint. The term mallet toe is used when only the distal joint is involved.

Retracted toes

Where limitation of dorsiflexion at the ankle exists, together with a tight tendo Achillis, weak tibialis anterior and substitution of the digital extensors then the toes may be retracted into a dorsiflexed position. Stretching exercises may increase ankle dorsiflexion where there is no bony abnormality; heel lifts can assist. Digital splinting will improve alignment. Shoes should have deep toe puffs to remove pressure from the dorsum of the toes.

Claw toes

Flexion of the interphalangeal joints with extension at the metatarsophalangeal joints directs the toes up into a claw toe deformity. In common with all toe deformities, badly fitting shoes may be responsible, although neurological involvement as in Charcot–Marie–Tooth disease is more usual. Intrinsic muscle imbalance and inflammatory disease of the joints can also bring about this deformity. Conservative management is directed at protecting painful lesions. Further details of treatment are given under 'Conservative Treatment'.

Corns may also occur between the toes as a result of intermittent stress. These lesions are often macerated and the area requires the application of astringents such as a weak solution of silver nitrate, following removal. An interdigital wedge may then be constructed to protect the bony prominences.

Less common deformities of the toes include syndactylism, overriding and underriding fifth toes and juvenile curly toe.

Factors affecting toe function

1. Neurological impairment
2. Biomechanical abnormalities
   a. Increased knee flextion may cause internal tibial rotation, subtalar and prolonged midstance pronation. This may result in clawing of the toes
   b. Equinus. Lack of 10° dorsiflexion with knee extended
   c. Hammer toe deformity as a result of partial compensation of subtalar pronation and poor compensation by the first ray
   d. Short first metatarsal or big toe
3. Trauma
   a. Toe amputation
4. Systemic
   b. Bone changes, especially hypertrophy and subluxation
5. Congenital

a. Short metatarsal or big toe
b. Unusual metatarsal and toe lengths
6. Specialist sports activities including fencing and raquet sports where clawing occurs during stabilization
7. Effect of unsuitable footwear.

Conservative treatment

As a result of the various soft tissue and bony deformities corns and callosities may form on weight or pressure areas and bursae may develop over the phalangeal joints. These may occur either dorsally or over the medial or lateral aspects of the toes.

Infection may be introduced into these deeper structures along sinuses linking the bursa with the epidermis. Particularly in the case of patients with poor peripheral circulation the consequence of such infection may be cellulitis. Careful removal of keratin plugs from these sinuses is required and, where necessary, drainage.

Lesions on the dorsum of the toes can be protected by shaped felt pads. These pads — crescent shaped around the lesion — should extend to the base of the toe (Fig. 55.17) whilst the horns of the crescent should extend along each side of the lesion to protect it. Lesions on the fifth toe particularly may need to be protected from all directions and a cavitied felt cover may be used (Fig. 55.18). It is also a useful method of holding a medicament in place. Where the toe is flexible a pad may be placed beneath it to extend it. This pad may also be shaped to protect any lesions on the apices of the toes. A single interdigital pad incorporating plantar and dorsal elements is illustrated (Fig. 55.19). The wing of this pad extending to the dorsum and the whole pad is secured with extension or elastic strapping.

Where more than one toe is affected or where correction of one toe may cause tendon overloading of adjacent toes, then orthodigital splinting is indicated. This may be:

1. Stuck to the foot
2. Made as a replaceable pad with elastic rubber (Fig. 55.20)
3. Constructed from silicone rubber.

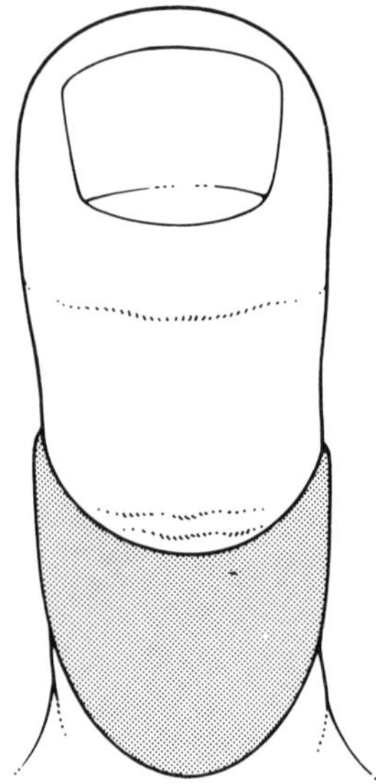

Fig. 55.17 Felt digital crescent

The prop should extend from the base of the toe or toes to a point around the distal interphalangeal joint. It is essential that it should, however, conform to the individual contours of the toes. The dorsal pad should be used as described.

Digital pads and splints may also be constructed in

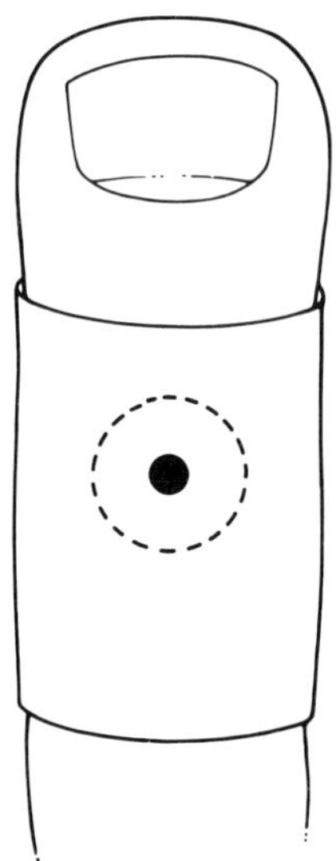

Fig. 55.18 Felt digital cover

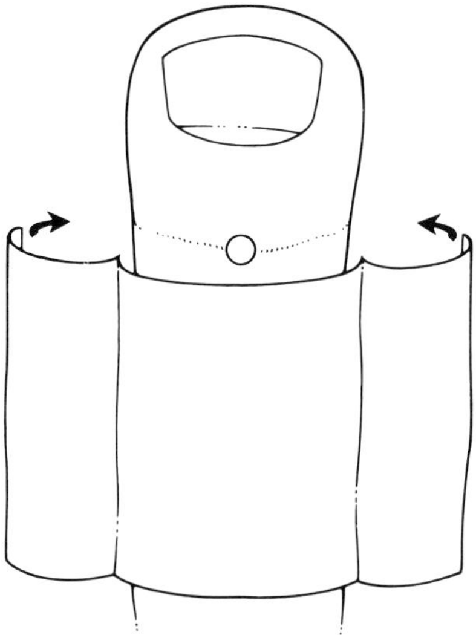

Fig. 55.19 Digital cover with wings extending around the toe

latex using the technique described earlier. Disposable tubular foam (Tubefoam®) can also be reinforced to provide effective toe devices. This foam can also be cut to provide protection for the plantar surface, and bony enlargements of the great toe joint. Simple interdigital wedges are helpful in reducing shearing stress between the toes and are best constructed from silicone rubber. They may be combined with toe props or orthodigital splints.

Prostheses where amputation or injury has resulted in a loss of digits are easily constructed using silicone rubber materials. The device is moulded directly onto the foot and is held in place by the sock or stocking. Where there is a contraction of the digital extensor tendon with consequent hyper-extension of a toe, up and over elastic splinting (Fig. 55.21) can be used to hold the toe temporarily in the corrected position.

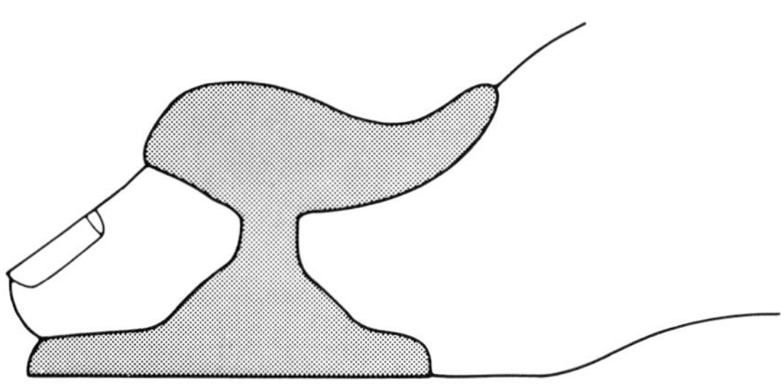

Fig. 55.20 Replaceable pad with elastic rubber

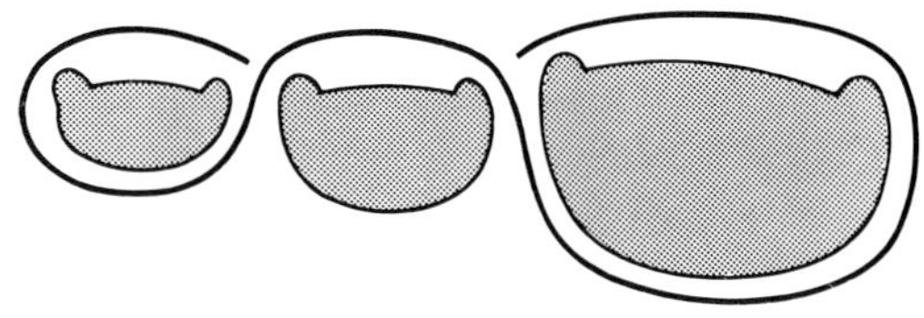

Fig. 55.21 Elastic splint

FIRST RAY DEFORMITIES

Hallux valgus

Lateral deviation of the great toe with medial deviation of the head of the first metatarsal. A similar problem may arise on the fifth toe giving rise to a bunionette or tailor's bunion.

Aetiology. Root et al (1977) and Gerbert & Sokoloff (1981) both agree that the commonest cause of first ray deformity leading to bunion formation and other degenerative diseases of the first metatarso-phalangeal joint is pronatory abnormality producing hypermobility of the first ray. Other causes including metabolic (Fig. 55.22) disease and congenital abnormalities are much less common. Hypermobility is due to an inability of the peroneus longus tendon to stabilize the first metatarsal. As a result of the fulcrum of the peroneus longus being rendered ineffective the first ray is not stabilized by it. The hypermobility helps the first metatarsal to adduct, the intermetatarsal angle increases and the intrinsic muscles operating on the base of the proximal phalanx are put to a mechanical disadvantage. Deformity then increases. In the presence of these primary biomechanical ab-normalities poor footwear can increase both the deformity and painful lesions associated with it.

Treatment. Early stabilization of the pronated foot may allow the deformity to be arrested although some changes are irreversible. There are many factors responsible for overpronation and in some cases orthotic therapy can control the deforming force.

Well established joint disease causing discomfort and malfunction can be treated by surgery or conservatively to relieve the symptoms. The prominent joint may develop overlying corns, and the bursae which frequently form between the skin and the joint may become inflamed with the formation of tracking sinuses. The risk of infection, especially in debilitated tissues is substantial.

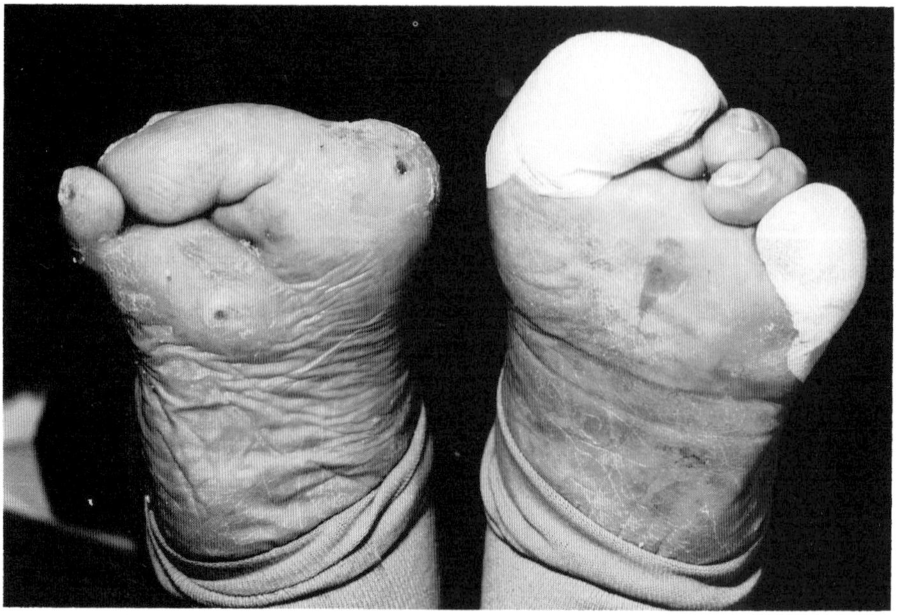

Fig. 55.22 Diabetic feet illustrating changes in neurotrophic joints

Because of the bony deformity, footwear may exert pressure and friction and therefore great care must be taken in its selection and modification to accommodate lesions.

It may be necessary to provide surgical footwear or modify existing shoes with balloon patches to accommodate the enlarged joint. The short-term treatment should aim at removing pressure and reducing any inflammation or infection that may be present. Felt padding, together with corrective strapping, is helpful. Flask strapping (Fig. 55.23) is a convenient method of holding the joint in the corrected position. Medication may be applied through the cavity of the padding without removing this. Physical therapy, such as heat to reduce inflammation, also has a place in the treatment.

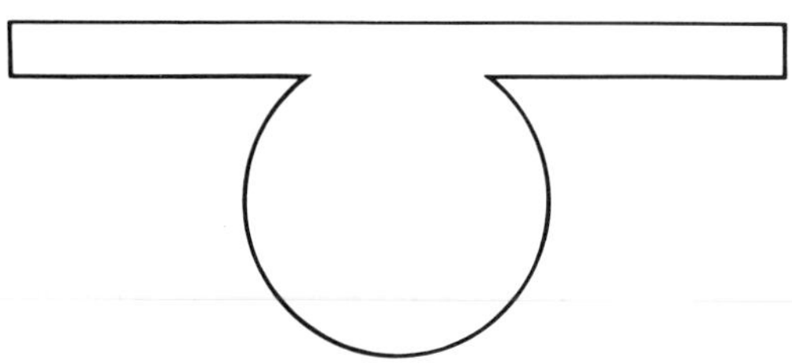

Fig. 55.23 Flask strapping

More durable protection can be provided by taking a cast of the joint and producing a dipped latex device incorporating protective padding. This device can be removed at will and is of low bulk. Wedges inserted between the first and second toes are helpful when strapping the toe into the corrected position, but have little long-term value. Any protective padding should be supplemented with valgus or arch pads and, in the presence of plantar lesions, wing pads should be used. Where functional orthoses are not indicated, then an accommodative device designed to support the foot and protect any plantar lesions should be provided.

Hallux limitus and hallux rigidus

In these conditions there is a limitation of movement at the first metatarsophalangeal joint varying in severity.

Aetiology

As in the case of hallux valgus, over pronation, together with secondary biomechanical factors is the most important cause. However, trauma, particularly in the active sportsperson, can also contribute. Systemic factors must also be considered.

Pathology

Degenerative changes in the joint with or without hypertrophy of the head of the first metatarsal.

Treatment

In the early stages heat or other physical modalities are used to reduce pain and inflammation. Treatment must be aimed at removing pressure from the affected joint and reducing movement. Single wing pads with metatarsal strapping may be used initially or, alternatively, posted or wedged insoles. Figure-of-eight strapping is helpful in stabilizing the joint. Orthoses or insoles with a shaft over the stiffened joint are of value. Shoes should be stiff soled with rigid shanks and a metatarsal bar can be of value. In severe cases, surgery to fuse the joint or replace it with a Silastic® implant will be required.

PLANTAR PROBLEMS

Most metatarsophalangeal joint deformities arise from frontal and transverse plane variations of the foot, but sagittal plane deformities of elevatus should also be considered.

Aetiology

Pressure deviations caused by biomechanical abnormalities, the loss of fibrofatty padding caused by disease, and subluxation of the metatarsal head may all result in pain and deformity. The presence of underlying disease such as diabetes or the collagen diseases presents special problems. Loss of sensation may occur in the diabetic with a greater tendency for lesions to become infected (Fig. 55.24). In the rheumatoid patient atrophy and joint derangement in the foot may result in very real disabilities. Certain skin diseases, such as psoriasis, also result in a marked overgrowth of epidermis on the plantar surface of the foot. Superficial lesions may be aggravated by the presence of bursae and cysts. Problems not related to pressure and friction, such as verrucae and porokeratoma (a blocked sweat gland) may also occur and problems such as plantar interdigital neuritis or Morton's toe are generally considered to have plantar origins.

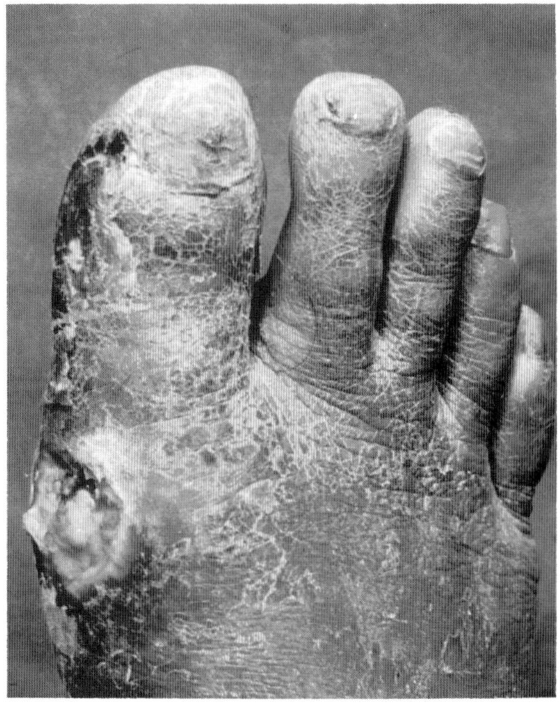

Fig. 55.24 A diabetic foot showing the effects of a hot water bottle

Treatment

Hyperkeratotic lesions

Commonly the lesions present are corns and hyperkeratosis. Corns and callosities must be carefully removed and, where necessary, the application of medication to act as a kerolytic or caustic agent should be used. Useful agents are a 60% paste of salicylic acid and wheat germ and pyrogallol which is particularly useful on hard fibrous lesions. Lesions containing nerve fibres, such as neuro-vascular corns, can be treated with 20% pyrogallol paste.

Local anaesthesia is rarely necessary for the painless removal of these lesions. In debilitated tissue as in the presence of collagen or metabolic disease, it may be advisable to underoperate, but to treat more frequently due to the increased risk of infection.

Various pads as already described can be adapted to protect and improve plantar lesions. By placing a pad behind the lesser metatarsal heads regrowth of callus can be reduced and the pain from strained ligaments and other soft tissue structures alleviated.

These various causes are sometimes unhelpfully if conveniently labelled metatarsalgia.

Seed corns (heloma milaire) are small multiple lesions, often found on the plantar surface where the skin is anhydrotic. After removal the area should be covered initially with a thin dressing such as fleecy web. A friction-reducing insole made from material such as Spenco will give relief.

Verruca pedis

Verrucae, the result of papovavirus infection of the skin, are widespread in the population particularly affecting the young. The infection causes a papilloma in the skin of man and electromicroscopic studies demonstrate the presence of the virus throughout the prickle cell layer in infected tissue. The verruca frequently presents as a well defined, space-occupying tumour, overlaid with hyperkeratosis. There are changes in the cellular activity leading to elongation and hypertrophy of the rete pegs. The skin lines are sharply interrupted. Red and black points within the lesion representing intravascular thrombosis can be seen. The tumour is benign, although Neufeld et al (1985) reports a rare case of verrucous squamous cell carcinoma of the foot stressing the need for accurate differential diagnosis. Verrucae can occur anywhere on the feet although they are commonest on the plantar surface, presumably associated with the surface from which the infection is transferred. The lesions may be confused with hyperkeratotic lesions although diagnosis is easier once overlying callus has been removed.

Differential diagnosis

1. Unlike the majority of corns and callosities the lesions are very painful on lateral pressure
2. Neurovascular and other corns occur only on pressure-bearing areas
3. Age — verrucae are more common in the young
4. Skin lines are broken rather than realigned.

The verruca lesion may occur singly or in groups (multiloculated) and sometimes as a shallow mosaic pattern.

The condition is contagious and it is speculated that transmission takes place during barefoot activities such as swimming or showering after sport. Prohibition of such activities when infected is socially impossible and unacceptable.

Regression does take place when there is a good immunological response so treatment should be delayed unless there is pain. A period of six months is sufficient and treatment should take place after this. Spontaneous resolution is often preceded by pain and inflammation.

Treatment

Topical agents. There is a range of topical agents available none of which appear to be very effective on plantar warts. Neale (1984) reports disappointing results with iodoxuridine in dimethyl-sulphoxide (DMSO). Dinitrochlorobenzene has also been used (Carrel & Davidson 1973). The initial sensitizing dose is applied to the skin and this is followed by the application of the agent to the lesions. There is an allergic response and, as a result of this immune reaction, resolution. Because of the possibility of a systemic reaction to the drug it may only be used under close supervision.

Chemical cautery. The destruction of the lesion is achieved using one or a combination of acids; those commonly used are:

1. Salicylic acid paste 60%
2. Monochloracetic acid in saturated solution. The lesion should be masked before application to protect surrounding tissue and the medicament applied at intervals of about one week. Tissue is debrided at each visit.

Cryotherapy

Destruction by freezing. The commonest methods are:

1. Using nitrous oxide (−88.5° centigrade)
2. Liquid nitrogen (−196.0° centigrade)

The methods of application are discussed by Barrett (1976), Rottschafer & Weil (1977) and Luciano (1977) who emphasizes the three principles when employing cryotherapy:

1. There must be a phase of rapid cooling and slow thawing
2. The lowest temperature for that agent should be reached
3. The lowest temperature should be maintained for a predetermined therapeutic time.

Both methods produce varying degrees of pain and discomfort both during and after treatment and in many cases the use of local anaesthesia is worthwhile. The treatment often results in painful blisters which may require early drainage. The advantages of this approach are early healing, reliability and lack of scarring. The equipment, however, can be expensive and bulky although liquid nitrogen can be applied with a cotton wool bud. More usually a probe or spray is used attached to an insulated flask. Nitrous oxide is stored as a gas in a cylinder and is used via regulated probes. A treatment time of 2–3 minutes is usual.

ELECTROTHERAPY

This must be carried out using a local anaesthetic.

Dessication or fulguration

This technique is not new and was described by Francis (1970). The electrode is either inserted into the tissue (Dessication-drying) or close to it (Fulguration-lightening) until the area blanches. The whole of the lesion must be treated. Healing may be delayed due to the profound tissue destruction and good drainage is important to avoid discomfort. Scarring may result so that this method must be avoided in those individuals with a history of keloid or hypertrophic scarring. Where the lesions are situated on weight-bearing areas other methods should be considered.

Electrosurgery

A pure high frequency current is utilized to obtain a fast cutting speed. Thin wire electrodes are preferred.

Curettage

McGlamary (1980) considered that stubborn lesions which are painful are candidates for excision. The area is infiltrated with local anaesthetic and the margins of the lesions lightly demarcated with a scalpel. The edges of the verruca are sharply undermined and the lesion 'teased' out using blunt dissection. Laceration of the germinal layer should be avoided. After removal of the mass the cavity may be touched with a saturated phenol solution to reduce postoperative pain, or lightly fulgurated (McLaughlin 1948) and dressed with nonadhesive gauze. A haemostatic dressing may be required. The foot should be elevated for 12 hours and kept dry for three or four days. Healing is normally rapid but there may be scarring.

PLANTAR DIGITAL NEURITIS

This condition, first described by Durlacher (1845) and later by Morton arises from a lesion on the plantar digital nerve at its point of bifurcation to supply the digits. The third interdigital space is normally affected but the second interdigital space may also be involved. The condition commonly affects women in the second to fourth decades.

The pain arises proximal to the base of the toes and frequently radiates into the middle three digits and occasionally into the leg. Classically, Morton's toe only describes the pain in the fourth toe. Pins and needles and tingling may also be experienced. Pain is not normally felt on rising, but develops through the day, especially when tight fitting or unsuitable footwear is worn. Removing the footwear and massaging the area often relieves the pain.

The main diagnostic feature is pain when the forefoot is compressed laterally and the metatarsal interspace is deeply palpated. A painful click (Mulder's click) is often elicited through this and must be distinguished from the painless click produced by the displacement of a fatty lobule. Mulder's click is probably due to the lesion being squeezed in and out of the intermetatarsophalangeal bursa.

Klenerman et al (1976) stress that the lesion around the nerve is degenerative and that the term neuroma is a misnomer. The lesion is probably ischaemic (Nissen 1948) and is connected with a traction on the plantar digital artery from the intermetatarsophalangeal bursa.

Treatment

It is vital that any biomechanical abnormality should be treated either by plantar and digital padding or orthoses to reduce stress. Footwear must be examined and, if constricting, discarded. Injections of local anaesthetic and hydrocortisone are also helpful in reducing discomfort possibly by breaking up fibrosis. Conservative treatment as described can be most effective in the early stages and may obviate the need for surgical excision.

Stress fracture (march fracture)

Stress fractures may occur in the shaft of the middle three metatarsals. The fractures arise from repetitive abnormal stress (unaccustomed walking or marching). The area above the fracture is swollen and tender and the pain is relieved by rest. X-Rays are not conclusive until callus formation is observed.

Treatment

Strapping with or without metatarsal padding will splint the bone. A wooden-soled shoe is helpful in reducing movement. Casting is rarely necessary.

Osteochondritis (Freiberg's infraction)

This condition is thought to be an aseptic necrosis of the second or third metatarsal head and usually occurs in childhood. The child may complain of pain and frequently limps. The result is a flattened metatarsal head with arthritic changes. X-Ray may demonstrate the presence of joint mice.

Treatment

Protective insoles are helpful to deviate pressure from the affected metatarsal head. In the adult, surgery may be indicated.

Plantar fasciitis

This is frequently the cause of pain under the heel although it must be differentiated from pain arising from bursae or nerve entrapments and neuromas. It may well be that pain in the central portion of the plantar fascia is also neural in origin.

Fasciitis may be present in association with systemic disease such as ankylosing spondylitis, Reiter's syndrome (of venereal or enteric origin) or less commonly a gut disorder such as Crohn's disease. 'Functional' fasciitis can be brought about by excessive pronation, obesity or trauma.

A calcaneal spur may form as a result of inflammatory changes at the junction of the bone and plantar fascia (enthesopathy). It is unlikely, however, that the spur is often responsible for pain and discomfort and indeed it is frequently found radiologically without any clinical signs or symptoms.

Treatment

In the acute stage rest and ultrasound are useful together with the use of insoles to relax the plantar fascia and to take pressure from the painful area (Freiberg 1957). More effective insoles can be constructed from cork and covered with foam to hold the foot in the neutral position. In true plantar fasciitis horseshoe-shaped pads in the heel have little effect. Low dye and figure-of-eight strapping are helpful. Accurately placed injections of hydrocortisone and local anaesthetic will reduce pain although they may exacerbate the condition initially. Injections or physical therapy should only be used in conjunction with padding or orthotic therapy. Extending the ideas of Hicks, who propounded the windlass effect in which there is an overpull on the plantar fascia, it is important that there is a good range of dorsiflexion at the ankle joint by stretching the calf muscles in the acute phase. Surgery to release the plantar fascia and/or remove the heel spur is seldom indicated.

Calcaneal apophysitis (Sever's disease)

This condition occurs in children between the ages of 7 and 12 years and is more common in girls than boys. It presents as a pain in the rear part of the heel which is made worse by exercise. The condition is frequently found in children who are keen gymnasts, dancers or runners.

Lateral pressure over the area will elicit pain. Fixen (1976) describes the condition as chronic strain at the attachment of the tendo Achillis to the apophysis, similar to Osgood–Schlatters' disease of the tibia tubercle. The use of cushioning heel pads or neutral position orthoses will relieve pain whilst the condition resolves.

CONCLUSION

Space has only permitted the description of management and treatment of a limited range of conditions. The chiropodist is increasingly involved in treatment of the injured athlete and of children both within the Health Service and private practice. Chiropody is an evolving profession and the changes that we have seen within the last few years will no doubt be followed by very many more within the near future, so that the practitioner will become an integrated member of the Health Team.

REFERENCES

American College of Foot, Surgeons Complications in Foot Surgery. Williams & Wilkins, Philadelphia. pp 41–42

Ashcroft D, Lavis G, Russell L 1979 Retrospective analysis of partial Nail Avulsions. The Chiropodist 34(4): 100–103

Back A C 1970 Thermal Correction of Involuted Nails. The Chiropodist 25: 11

Barrett C E 1976 Verruca Treatment Using Cryotherapy. The Chiropodist 31(10): 276–277

Beck J 1977 Chiropodist 32(11): 380–383

Becke, Rosenthal R K 1984 Foot Ankle 4;4 174–201

Bell D R C 1977 Advanced Techniques. The Chiropodist 32(7): 238–245

Bell D R C 1985 Personal Communication

Blakeman P 1985 Forces, Stress and Appliance Materials; A Discussion. The Chiropodist 40(5): 132–135

Boll O F 1945 Nail Phenolisation. J of the Nat Assn of Chiropodists 35: 8–7

Bremner D N, McCormack J, St Price M H, Hunter E 1976 The Chiropodist 31: 320–325

Carrel J, Davidson D 1973 Topical Immunotherapy of Recalcitrant Verrucae. J Am Pod Assoc 63: 293

Charlesworth F 1947 Chiropody Theory and Practice. Actinic Press, London

Coates I S 1977 Silicone Orthodigita and Shielding. Private Publication

Costain D S 1978 Chairside Silicone Devices. The Chiropodist 33(4): 105

Dagnall C J 1974 Nail Phenolisation. Br J Chiropody 39(6): 133

Dagnall C J 1983 Onychocryptosis in Boys. The Chiropodist 38(5): 191–192

Dagnall C J 1985 The Formation of the Society of Chiropodists in 1945. Its Significance in Chiropodial History. The Chiropodist 40(11): 355–361

Dalton B 1982 Friction, Intermittent or Otherwise. The Exciting Cause of Corns and Callous. The Chiropodist 37(11): 372–379

Dhanedran M, Robertson K, Hutton W C The Effects of Metatarsal Padding on the Load Distribution under the forefoot. The Chiropodist 35: 43–52

Durlacher V 1845 A Treatise on Corns, Bunions and Diseases of Nails, and the General Management of the Feet. Simpkin, Marshall & Co, London

Edgar M A 1976 Hallux Valgus and Associated Conditions, Blackwell. The Foot and its Disorders. Klenerman Scientific Publications, Oxford 118–119

Farber E M, South D A 1978 Urea Ointment in the Nonsurgical Avulsion of Nail Dystrophies. CUTIS 22: 689

Francis B E 1970 The use of high frequency current in the treatment of Verrucae. The Chiropodist 25(8): 295–298

Francis B E 1981 Steindler technique for nail correction. J Pod Assoc March 44–45

Francis B E, Furness W 1974 Nail Correction using Phenolisation. Skin Surgery for Chiropodists, North London Post-Graduate Group, London pp 37–45

Frazer E R 1967 Orthonyx Theory and Practice, Br Chiropody J 32: 229, 277, 33: 53, 105, 129, 249, 34: 5, 55, 125, 177, 221, 246, 35: 26; 9 37: 29, 79, 269

Freiberg J A 1957 The Diagnosis and Treatment of Common Painful Conditions of the Foot. Amer Ac Orth Surgeons 14: 238

Fixen J A 1976 The Foot and Its Disorders. Klenerman Blackwell Scientific Publications, Oxford. p 74

Gerbert J, Sokoloff J H 1981 Text Book of Bunion Surgery. Futura Publications Co, N.Y. p 46–50

Gibbard L C 1968 Charlesworths Chiropodial Orthopaedics, 2nd Edn. Baillière Tindall and Cassel, London

Hanby 5th, Walker F E 1960 Principles and Practice of Chiropody 2nd Edn. Baillière-Tindall, London

Hawes K D 1975 Experience with a Standardised Postoperative Procedure following Nail Resection with Matrix Sterilisation. The Chiropodist 30(10): 291

Higgs S S L 1931 Hammer Toe. Postgrad Med J 6: 131–133

Klenerman L, Nissan K, Baker H 1976 The Foot and its Disorders. Blackwell, Oxford. pp 147–150

Landry M E, Zebas C 1985 Analysis of 100 Knees in High School Runners. J Am Pod Assoc 75(7): 382–384

Langer S A, Wernick J 1978 A practical Manual for a basic approach to Biomechanics. Langer Acrylic Lab. Inc. New York

Lewis B L 1954 Microscopic Studies of Foetal and Mature Nail and Surrounding Soft Tissue. Arch Derm Syph (Chic) 79: 732

Lord M 1981 Foot Pressure Measurements; A Review of Methodology. J Biomed Eng 3: April

Luciano C S 1977 Verruca Plantaris. J Am Pod Assoc 67(12): 858–869

Maddocks M 1985 Winograd Technique. J Am Pod Assoc 14–15

Marr S J 1984 Toe Buttressing for Forefoot Problems. J Am Pod Assoc 74(3): 136–140

McGlammary E D 1980 Nail Correction in the Presence of Infection. A Monograph on Foot Surgery. Penn College of Podiatric Medicine. p 12

McLaughlin C R 1948 Plantar Warts — a Plea for Rational Treatments. Lancet 1: 69

Neale, Walker, 1984 Common Foot Disorders Diagnosis and Management. Churchill Livingstone, Edinburgh pp 185–208

Neufeld R I, Kurtzer C M, Estersohn H S, Napoli J D 1985 Verrucous Squamous Cell Carcinoma of the foot. J Am Pod Assoc 75(6): 300–305

Niehans L P 1985 Sorbothotics (R) Soft Tissue Supplement Orthoses. J Am Pod Assoc 75(1)

Nissen K I 1948 Plantar Digital Neuritis; Morton's Metatarsalgia. J Bone Joint Surg 30B: 84–94

Port M, Sanicola K F 1980 Nonsurgical removal of dystrophic nails utilising Urea ointment occlusion. J Am Pod Assoc 70(10): 521–423
Robertson K, Crawford S 1976 Nail Wedge Resection. A Retrospective Analysis. The Chiropodist 31: 225
Root M L, Orien W P, Weed J H 1977 Normal and Abnormal Functions of the Foot Vol. II. Clinical Biomechanics Corporation, Los Angeles
Rosenthal R K 1984 The Use of Orthotics in Foot and Ankle Problems in Cerebral Palsy. Foot Ankle 4(4): 195–200
Rottschafer W C, Weil L S 1977 Cryosurgery and its Utilisation in Podiatry. J Am Pod Assoc 67(9): 603–608
Runting E G V 1933 Practical Chiropody 4th Edn. Faber and Faber, London. pp 103–125
Samman P D 1965 The Nails in Disease. Heinemann Medical Books, London. pp 2–3
Scarlato T E 1971 A Compendium of Podiatric Biomechanics. Californian College of Podiatric Medicine
Scullion P G 1984 Scalpel Technique in removing heloma and Hyperkeretosis. J Foot Surg 23(4): 344–349
South D A, Faber E M 1980 Urea ointment and the nonsurgical avulsion of nail atrophies; a reappraisal. Cutis 25: 609
Sperryn P N, Restan L 1983 Orthoses and the Painful Foot. Br J Sports Med 17(4): 129–134
Steadman J R 1979 Nonoperative Measures for Patellofemoral Problems. Am J Sports Med 7(6): 374–375
Subotnick S 1975a Orthotic Foot Control and the Overuse Syndrome. The Physician and Sports Med Jan. 75–79
Subotnick S 1975b Podiatric Sports Medicine. Futura Publishing Co, New York. pp 117–221
Wee G C 1972 Atlas of Improved Surgical Procedures for Common Foot Disorders. Springfield
Wernick J 1978 Orthotics: New relief for skiers feet. Ski Dec. 78: 60–62

FURTHER READING

Charlesworth F 1961 Chiropody Theory and Practice. 5th Edn. Actinic Press, London
Klenerman L et al 1984 The Foot and Its Disorders. Blackwell Scientific Publications, Oxford
Read P J 1978 An Introduction to Therapeutics for Chiropodists 2nd Edn. Actinic Press, London
Rossignol L E 1980 Encyclopaedia of Material Media and Therapeutics for Chiropodists. Faber, London
Spencer A M 1978 Practical Podiatric Orthopaedic Procedures (revised Edition). Ohio College of Podiatric Medicine
Sammans P D 1978 The Nails in Disease. 3rd Edn. Heinemann, London
Subotnick S I 1975 Podiatric Sports Medicine. Futura Publishing Co, New York

Rehabilitation

PRINCIPLES

Restoration of function in the foot following injury or surgery should take account of the patient's general health, local pathology and future potential abilities or requirements.

The foot not only transmits body load to the ground when standing but achieves deceleration and propulsion by a complex balance of muscular and articular forces. Disruption of these forces for whatever reason may result in loss of function.

Because the leg is dependent for most of the waking day, pathology in the arteries, veins or lymphatics of the leg or foot will result in persistent swelling. This may lead to pain, stiffness and loss of function.

Many general conditions, either directly or indirectly, produce problems in the foot. Not only may they initiate local pathology but also they may compromise recovery from an unrelated injury or operation.

LOCAL PHYSIOLOGY

The development of the human foot as a load-bearing and propulsion system has been achieved by a balance of forces between articular surfaces, soft tissues and both intrinsic and extrinsic muscle power.

The microclimate of the foot in a shoe is markedly variable between different footwear materials, different environments, and different activities. Most general purpose shoes achieve a balance of factors to permit foot function within a limited budget. However, in the presence of local pathology the balance may be unsatisfactory either by virtue of shape, texture, vapour permeability, or load distribution. Good bare-foot function may not extend to good shod function, particularly with women's fashion shoes.

Viability, healing and performance of the tissues of the foot are determined by sensibility, vascularity and muscle function interacting with structural stability. Abnormalities of any of these factors can derange overall foot function.

Proprioception

Proprioception from the foot and ankle is an essential component of normal gait; any neural pathology locally or more proximally which detracts from the basic sensory input will modify gait, muscle forces or balance. Where it is completely lost, as in some sensory neuropathies, central awareness of foot-strike may be achieved by increasing the mechanical transmission of the compression wave of heel strike, by a stamping type of gait.

Conversely where there is a central disturbance of coordination such as Parkinson's disease, the raising of the heel and accentuation of heel strike may improve gait (Knutsson 1972).

In children with marginal spasticity or habitual toe-walking, acoustic enhancement of heel strike can also be shown to improve gait. This is achieved by a mechanical heel-clicker or a load sensitive electrical transducer in the heel of the shoe which signals a correct heel strike (Conrad & Black 1980).

INNERVATION

Sensibility

Sensibility in the foot protects the skin from damage

due to external forces. Obviously it is helpful to feel a stone in a shoe since if undetected it will rapidly cause skin damage and ulceration. In many peripheral neuropathies, such as leprosy or diabetes, or central dysfunction such as meningomyelocele or spinal cord injury, this ability is lost and ulcers develop. Thus the sufferer should examine the skin of the foot and the inside of the shoe every day (Shipley 1979).

Peripheral nerve lesions may lead to loss of sudomotor function. This leads to dry skin which easily breaks down and heals slowly. The choice of footwear materials may be of great importance in this situation.

Sympathetic innervation of the foot controls the microvascular circulation. Disturbances of autonomic function may lead to vasospasm in conditions such as Raynaud's phenomenon, or arteriovenous shunting as in some cases of diabetes mellitus (Ward et al 1983).

In peripheral vascular disease sympathectomy may maintain skin viability in the marginal case, but at the expense of muscle function if the majority of limited limb flow goes to the foot.

VASCULARITY

Arterial flow

Arterial pathology to the leg commonly results in poor foot function. Arteriosclerosis can reduce flow sufficiently to cause muscle claudication and a cold foot. If more severe the foot may become ischaemic or gangrenous. Chronic arterial insufficiency may allow good skin viability with a resting temperature of 20° or less but a sudden exposure to cold, dropping the temperature a few degrees more, will result in gangrene.

Arteriovenous shunting is a normal mechanism of controlling the microcirculation. However, in autonomic dysfunction it may be excessive due to changes in precapillary sphincter tone and result in diminished skin flow but high limb flow. It is demonstrated by elevating the leg and demonstrating full veins at heights up to more than 30 cm.

Venous return

Venous drainage of the foot is both active and passive. Directional flow is maintained by the valves described by Harvey (1628). Damage to the valves results in increased venous pressure in the dependent foot; oedema results.

Active venous flow is produced as a result of both arterial pressure and the 'muscle pump' effect of activity. It is also influenced by the diameter of the veins — larger veins having slower flow. Thus to maximize flow the veins should not be permitted to dilate. Where the valves are incompetent this may have to be achieved with elastic stockings (Scurr et al 1977). Passive venous flow is increased by elevation of the leg. Femoral vein flow is maximal with 15° of head down tilt.

Normal venous flow is from deep towards superficial. Following episodes of phlebothrombosis the valves of the deep veins may become incompetent and allow reflux from superficial to deeper layers. With increasing intraosseous pressure the lower leg and foot may start to ache. The symptoms are often reduced by ligation of the major perforating vessels. However, it is important to evaluate dilated veins to be clear whether they are the source of pathology or major collateral vessels assisting venous return (Thulesius et al 1973).

To assess the adequacy of the venous pump a direct measurement of venous pressure in the foot or of foot volume is made (Partsch 1982). During knee bending exercise the pressure record from the foot vein will oscillate around the baseline. The varicosities are now occluded by digital pressure together with the saphenous trunk. The exercise is repeated. If the muscle pump is working effectively the baseline pressure in the foot veins will fall and the foot volume diminish. If the pump is incompetent the pressure will oscillate around the same baseline; these cases are unlikely to benefit from surgical ligation of perforators (Fig. 56.1).

Lymphatic drainage

Lymphatic problems in the foot are less common than venous. However, chronic venous disease can lead to chronic lymphatic obstruction. Lymphatic flow is influenced by the same factors as venous flow but with the important difference that where channels are obstructed, few effectively dilate to restore efficient flow.

Chronic lymphatic oedema is difficult to disperse.

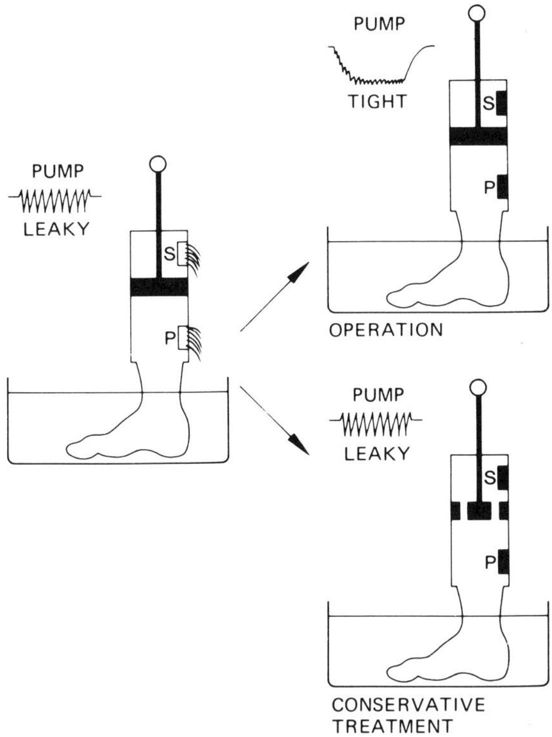

Fig. 56.1 Functional assessment of venous pump function. If there is no adequate volume and/or pressure reduction in the foot with exercise, the measurement is repeated with a digital compression of the saphenous trunk *(S)* and of incompetent perforators *(P)*. An improvement of the curve is an indication for operation. If the curve stays unchanged the main cause for the pumping deficiency is assumed to be localized in the deep veins. Such cases are treated conservatively. (From Partsch 1982; reproduced with permission from the editor of Year Book Medical Publishers, Inc.)

It may be necessary to elevate the leg for several days (Bourne 1975). The process is accelerated by intermittent compression and graded elastic pressure stockings.

Oedema

Oedema of the leg and foot may have many causes, the commonest local factors are venous or lymphatic insufficiency. General disorders include cardiac, hepatic or renal failure. In diabetes mellitus and leprosy the mechanism may be neuropathic involvement of the sympathetic innervation of the arteriovenous sphincter mechanism resulting in venous hypertension.

Benign conditions causing leg oedema include rheumatoid arthritis, myxoedema, pregnancy, and lipoedema. Occasionally malignancy, drug reactions and nutritional deficiencies may be responsible.

Compartment syndromes

These may be acute, intermittent or chronic.

Following an acute injury in the leg blood loss from the soft tissues or bone may result in a rise of pressure in the tight fascial compartments of the leg or foot. The effect is minimized by early immobilization, elevation and cold packs. Differentiation must be made early from arterial occlusion or rupture, which require surgical management.

Wick catheter studies have shown a correlation between compartment pressures in the leg in excess of 40 mmHg and subsequent muscle and nerve fibrosis (Mubarak et al 1976). Fasciotomy is the only acceptable treatment (Mubarak & Owen 1977). Failure to intervene within 12 hours may result in chronic irreversible fibrosis of muscles in the deep compartments of the leg and consequent fixed deformities of the ankle or foot as the result of Volkmann's ischaemic contracture. The chronic effects of a compartment syndrome may include joint stiffness and deformity, loss of muscle power, reduced walking or running tolerance, pain and loss of normal sensibility. Occasionally these problems are insoluble in the lower leg and foot and require surgical soft tissue release, joint stabilization or even amputation.

Intermittent compartment syndromes may develop in athletes in endurance events. The thigh, leg or foot may be the site of pain which may mimic a stress fracture. The commonest site is the anterolateral compartment of the leg resulting in reduced power in tibialis anterior. This leads to high foot strike force and sometimes stress fractures in the forefoot, Achilles tendinopathy due to excessive heel strike or low back pain from gait imbalance. Surgical decompression is a simple, safe and effective remedy.

Bone strength

This is the result of local and general factors. It is gained in response to the loads applied to the bone according to Wolff's law (1892). The process takes time and thus excessive loads over short periods may result in stress fractures — an example being a ballet dancer working or rehearsing on a concrete as opposed to a sprung floor.

Prolonged load relief will result in rapid loss of bone strength, particularly after major injury or surgery. The catabolic effect of such events leads to an overall loss of protein, including bone matrix and articular cartilage.

Nutritional deficiencies may lead to significant osteopoenia. Marginal deficiencies, particularly of vitamin C, may result in delayed restoration of bone strength after mobilization and probably delayed healing of fractures. Malabsorption syndromes may result in deficiency of vitamin D. While this is less common as a nutritional deficiency with the fortification of milk, bread or cereals, it is still a feature of gastric, biliary, pancreatic or small bowel disease. It may be a feature both of jejunoileal bypass surgery for obesity and of anorexia nervosa (Hey et al 1982).

Local bone resorption may be the result of specific pathology such as Paget's disease or bony metastasis. It is seen as a complication of arteriovenous shunting and may be responsible for the high incidence of stress fractures in diabetes mellitus (Heath et al 1980, El-Khoury & Kathol 1980).

Hyperparathyroidism may result in a loss of bone strength as the result of calcium deficiency. Renal dialysis has also been associated with brittle bones where deionized water has not been used (Leather et al 1981).

Well-known causes of reduced bone strength such as senile osteoporosis, osteomalacia, rheumatoid disease, thyroid dysfunction and osteogenesis imperfecta should not be forgotten. These and many other conditions may present with a fracture around the foot or ankle.

Soft tissue healing

This is a function of collagen maturation. Experimental wounds have shown that in health full collagen strength is not achieved for six months. After injury or in disease this time may be greatly prolonged. Local ischaemia results in production of relatively weak collagen.

With a normal blood supply in a previously healthy patient soft tissue strength is gained slowly if immobilized, but more rapidly with normal anatomical and physiological function. Hence active rehabilitation following soft tissue injury yields better results than complete immobilization.

The soft tissue response to trauma includes microvascular thrombosis and capillary leakage. The resultant oedema reduces oxygen and nutrient perfusion to the healing cells.

Healing is optimal where oedema and microvascular occlusion is prevented. This may be achieved with prompt use of ice, compression and elevation, supported by local application of thrombolytic heparinoid medications (Lester 1981). The pain-reducing effect of an ice pack allows earlier mobilization. Where pain is excessive a two week period of rest in a plaster cast is justified followed by mobilization with supportive strapping.

Articular cartilage

The quality of articular cartilage is maintained by movement. It has been shown that rigid immobilization of a joint for as little as 14 days results in significant loss of articular cartilage thickness and mechanical resilience (Puhl & Iyer 1973). Direct crush injuries are often sustained by articular cartilage in the absence of radiologically evident bone injuries, particularly on the talus at the time of ankle fractures or dislocations. Such injuries must be protected from significant loads during healing, but will be helped by motion. In the knee joint injuries to articular cartilage have been shown to heal most rapidly under passive motion with protected load bearing (Salter 1981).

The precise amount of joint movement needed adequately to nourish articular cartilage is not known. The desire for at least a modest amount of movement may be a major factor in electing for internal fixation of fractures around the foot and ankle. Particularly in the case of os calcis fractures resulting in disruption of the subtalar joint complex some form of early reduction and fixation may result in greatly improved long-term results (Shannon & Murray 1978). If there is no gross displacement early mobilization gives the best results.

Thus there are three hidden enemies for the three basic structures: load relief of bone, swelling of soft tissues and immobilization of articular cartilage. Furthermore subchondral bone remodelling does not occur without motion, articular cartilage needs a degree of loading for adequate nutrition and soft tissue oedema can reduce motion. Where there has been an injury to a joint all these factors are involved. Slow rehabilitation may be the consequence of failure to identify these features upon initiation of treatment.

BIOMECHANICAL FACTORS

Biomechanical factors influencing foot function are described elsewhere. In the rehabilitation of the painful or deformed foot they may play a critical role. Forces are applied to the foot in varying magnitude and direction both in health and disease. Disturbance of joint function by either stiffness or hypermobility may result in pathology either locally or at a distance.

Furthermore the rate at which the forces are applied is also significant. Thus on heel strike the subtalar joint moves from a position of inversion to one of eversion, absorbing force as it does so. By preventing this rotation, foot strike compression forces to the more proximal parts of the skeleton may be increased. However, should it be too rapid, the resultant excessive torsional force to the tibia may result in knee pain.

Under the influence of a hard heel strike the subcalcaneal soft tissues are subjected to massive distortions or even disruptions; further proximally the soft tissues of the leg suffer a substantial distortion as the shock wave is transmitted to them and the same effect probably occurs in the spine all the way to the brain (Hawes et al 1979, Light et al 1979).

Thus walking or running in hard-heeled shoes on hard surfaces may aggravate conditions such as subcalcaneal pain, Achilles tendonitis (MacLellan & Vyvyan 1981), anterolateral shin soreness, knee pain, hip pain, low back pain (Voloshin & Wosk 1981, Voloshin et al 1981) migraine and Menieres disease. Compliant footwear can help to minimize these diverse complaints in conjunction with appropriate local therapy.

Forces acting locally in the foot may cause problems both by vertical loading and horizontal shear. High shear forces may result in forefoot ulceration but generally only occur at points of high vertical loading. Thus by minimizing vertical load transients shear is reduced. This permits healing of ulcers and, if continued, prevents their recurrence (Pollard & Le Quesne 1983).

Shear forces may be aggravated by the materials with which the foot is in contact when under load (Hertzman 1973). Adhesion to an insole material made moist by perspiration may predispose to skin blistering. With other materials the hard dry skin of the leprotic or diabetic foot may increase shear.

In athletic shoe design account must be taken of the purpose for which the shoe is to be used. Thus while some sole constructions result in excellent grip, with prolonged use they may result in pushing the toes hard into the toe-box, resulting in subungual haematoma of the hallux or abrasion of the lesser toes (Sperryn 1980).

Endurance running on hard surfaces requires a very stable rear foot with good cushioning of heel strike forces — the former to minimize torsional phenomena and the latter to compensate for the consequent loss of subtalar shock absorption which would otherwise deliver a large shock wave to the skeleton.

These biomechanical principles can well be employed when considering rehabilitation of the injured foot in nonathletes. Thus if extremes of motion of the subtalar joint cause pain the limitation of motion resulting from the stable heel cup and firm arch support of a running shoe may be the only treatment needed to restore normal activity (Sneppen et al 1977).

Where hard heel strike produces subcalcaneal pain a compliant material beneath the heel and the soft tissue control resulting from a well contoured heel cup generally permit healing and prevent recurrence.

Biomechanical data

This may conveniently be obtained from force platforms or pedobarographs. The sophisticated system of Cavanagh & Michiyoshi (1979) has allowed objective measurement of forces beneath different areas of the foot. However, simpler systems such as the optical pedobarograph with intermittent stance phase imaging (Betts & Duckworth 1978, Minns & Craxford 1984) or the Electrodynogram worn within the shoe (Polchaninoff 1983) may give valuable at a glance information upon which surgical or orthotic measures may be based (Hennig et al 1980).

The optical pedobarograph

This records forces beneath the foot on a plane surface during a single stance phase. It will reveal high-spots of pressure on a 'contour map' principle and suggest bony or soft tissue procedures which may correct painful pressure symptoms (Fig. 56.2).

It is of particular value on the neuropathic foot in identifying points of high pressure which may predispose to ulcer formation. Thus in the insensitive foot of meningomyelocele or spinal cord injury or the impaired foot of diabetes or leprosy it could play an important role in preventing foot ulcers (Pollard & Le Quesne 1983, Shipley 1979).

The socioeconomic significance of prevention of foot ulceration in these conditions cannot be stressed too strongly. In the diabetic foot the time from first ulcer to amputation is on average five years.

The Electrodynogram (EDG)

EDG has been found to be of value in assessing foot forces in running or walking. Where problems have arisen suggesting the need for an orthotic device in this specialized area the machine can record forces within the shoe over a number of strides before and after the fitting of an orthosis.

This system is available in some centres for use in general orthopaedic problems of the foot where modular off-the-shelf orthotics are available and gives immediate evidence of adequate mechanical effect.

DIAGNOSIS

In the assessment of a patient with a foot or ankle problem it is essential to take a clear history. This must include details of occupational activities, sport, any pending litigation, secondary gain factors and alcohol abuse.

General physical examination should include observation of the hands for evidence of osteoarthritis or rheumatoid arthritis. The forces developed during normal gait are sufficient to deform a marginally involved toe joint afflicted with rheumatoid arthritis producing subluxation or dislocation at the metatarsophalangeal joints. The changes of rheumatoid arthritis may be more subtle in the hands but early involvement of these equivalent joints in the hands should alert one to the possibility of this underlying cause for foot pain. Staining of the fingers in a smoker may suggest

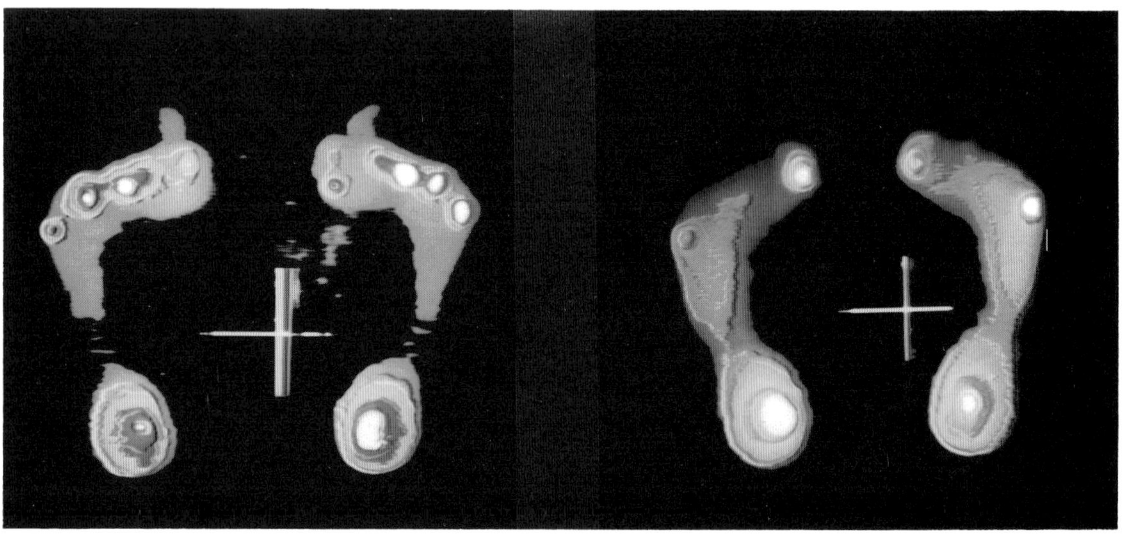

Fig. 56.2 Optical pedobarograph display of pressures beneath the foot. Points of peak pressure are shown at the centre of the 'contour map' (courtesy of Mr. L. Klenerman)

peripheral vascular disease as a contributory factor in the slow healing of wounds or injuries to the foot. Cardiovascular examination should exclude cardiac failure, chronic pulmonary disease or peripheral vascular disease. Any of these may result in persistent oedema in the foot and slow healing of wounds and the deeper tissues.

Any history of associated inflammatory conditions such as conjunctivitis or urethritis should be elicited and sought out. Reiter's syndrome is a potent cause of foot pain, particularly in the heel, and the inflammatory softening of the plantar ligaments in gonorrhoea may be the cause of an acute flat foot (Huskisson & Hart 1975).

Some cases of toxic arthritis may produce spasmodic flat foot or foot pain. A large number of drugs have been incriminated in causing joint pains. For example acute gout may be precipitated by oral diuretics, some antihypertensive drugs, cytotoxic therapy etc. Rheumatoid arthritis may be exacerbated by iron dextran when given by total dose method and arthralgia may be experienced by patients who do not have rheumatoid disease. Systemic lupus erythematosus may be exacerbated or precipitated by a large number of drugs, the commonest being penicillin or sulphonamides but oral contraceptives may rarely be responsible (Adverse Drug Reaction Bulletin 1971).

Fixed deformities of the joints proximal to the foot should be recorded. Examine the skin for abnormal pigmentation or dermatosis and the spine for evidence of dysraphism. Other abnormalities such as scoliosis, winged scapulae, tight hamstrings, or hand intrinsic weakness may suggest an underlying dystrophy.

The normal limb should be examined to give a reasonable assessment of goals that may be achieved. Neuromuscular assessment should be detailed and recorded including power testing of individual muscles or groups using the MRC grade or, where available, mechanical devices such as spring balances or strain gauges.

Areas of sensory disturbance should be drawn and labelled, including proprioception. Note should be taken of foot hygiene, nail care, socks worn and shoe condition; wear patterns on the shoe may indicate significant gait abnormalities.

Examination of the urine should be undertaken routinely. In particular a routine test for sugar should be made. Presence of excess amounts of protein in the urine may indicate underlying amyloid disease, systemic lupus erythematosus, myeloma, Henoch–Schönlein purpura, polyarteritis nodosa and many other inflammatory arthropathies. In addition patients who are on haemodialysis or who have had renal transplantation from time to time develop arthralgia which may be manifest in the foot.

SPECIAL INVESTIGATIONS

Electrodiagnostic techniques

Electrodiagnostic techniques are valuable in detecting denervation, when there is doubt clinically of neurological involvement, in assessing the site of lesion in the lower motor neurone (i.e. anterior horn cell, nerve or muscles) and in establishing the level of the lesion in a suspected entrapment neuropathy (Nakano 1975). The detection of a widespread disorder of sensory and motor conduction will point to a generalized neuropathy. The presence of normal sural/vertebral transmission or normal conduction in the lateral popliteal nerve, then slowing across the medial tibial nerve at the ankle will suggest the diagnosis of the rare tarsal tunnel syndrome. The inability to detect denervation in a wasted muscle will suggest disuse atrophy and not neurological disorder. Finally root pain may be a symptom of spinal nerve root compression. The detection of denervation in appropriate muscles supplied by the suspect root and the presence of normal sensory motor conduction will confirm the suspicion.

Electromyogram (EMG)

Where there is evidence of muscle weakness, EMG can differentiate between upper and lower motor neurone disorders and myopathies. Substantial degrees of muscle wasting in the calf can result from years of abnormal gait with a painful foot.

Nerve conduction studies

Should be requested when suspecting a peripheral neural dysfunction in neuropathy or compartment syndrome. An occasional cause of foot pain is the tarsal tunnel syndrome. Peripheral neuropathies such as diabetes mellitus, alcoholic neuritis and leprosy may be demonstrated. Where there has been a previous history of nerve injury causalgia should be considered.

Transcutaneous Po_2 measurement

Where skin viability is in doubt this method is safe and reliable as an indicator of perfusion and response to treatment.

Compartment pressure measurement by wick catheter

Recent work in fracture management in the leg has evolved a system of percutaneous measurement of deep compartment pressure. A needle containing a wick is introduced into the selected compartment(s) and a reading of pressure is obtained in thigh, calf or foot. The technique can be applied to both trauma and exercise-induced compartment syndromes (Mubarak et al 1976).

PAIN MEASUREMENT

There is no objective way to assess pain. The patient's subjective assessment is influenced by factors like time of day, hunger, thirst, demands of work or money, family pressures and many other things. Because of observer variability consecutive assessments should be made by the same examiner.

The visual analogue scale of pain is sometimes of value in assessing change in pain experienced. The patient is shown a horizontal line with 'no pain' at one end and 'extreme and intolerable pain' at the other and asked to indicate on that line where his or her pain may be. Different qualities or locations of pain should be assessed on a fresh scale each time. Each must be clearly labelled with date, time and observer and retained in the patient's clinical record (Fig. 56.3).

Name

NO PAIN X————————————X MOST PAIN

Observer

Date: Time:

Fig. 56.3 Visual analogue scale for pain

AIDS TO REHABILITATION OF THE FOOT

Exercises

Joint mobilization

Active exercises to increase the range of motion of ankle and foot joints can be undertaken without load or pain (Shannon & Murray 1978). Dorsiflexion, plantar flexion, circumduction, inversion and eversion should be achieved separately at least three times in every 24 hours to the maximum degree within the limits of comfort. In the healthy foot with good intrinsic muscles, shortening of the longitudinal arch, flexion, extension and abduction of the toes can be separately achieved.

With improving function and healing these exercises can be enhanced initially by therapist-assisted active movements and then further by passive stretching by the therapist or the patient using a sling around the foot. Where there is fixed deformity proximally correction may be essential to allow normal foot function.

Muscle strengthening

Very weak muscles can initially be assisted to act by faradic stimulation.

Having initiated effective muscle activity exercise can continue actively, initially without and later with resistance. Particular attention should be directed to the intrinsic muscles of the foot, particularly with forefoot problems.

Resisted exercises can initially be against the physiotherapist or isokinetic exerciser, and subsequently against gravity (Fugl-Meyer et al 1979). If the changeover is hampered by pain normal gait may be initiated by weight-relief in the hydrotherapy pool or suspension harness.

Proprioceptive neuromuscular facilitation. Movements tend to occur as part of a mass spectrum of movement any component of which, when resisted, may enhance others (Knott & Vors 1968).

Thus toe flexion is the first phase of the sequence, toe flexion → forefoot adduction → foot and ankle plantar flexion → knee flexion with external tibial rotation → hip extension, adduction and external rotation. Toe extension is the first phase of the sequence progressing with foot abduction → foot and ankle dorsiflexion with eversion → knee extension with internal tibial rotation → hip flexion, abduction and internal rotation.

These patterns are used to enhance the action of a weak member of the sequence. By resisting the normally powered functions and preventing the movement complex from occurring the weaker muscles are enhanced; to achieve toe flexion, movements at the hip, knee and ankle are prevented until toe flexion is achieved. The normal progression of the patterns if from distal to proximal.

Weak muscles may also be enhanced by activation of the antagonist. For example to activate a profoundly weak dorsiflexor of the ankle the patient is instructed to plantarflex the ankle as strongly as possible and then quickly 'pull up'. This sometimes promotes dorsiflexor activity.

When there is full tolerance to gravity-resisted exercise further improvement can be obtained by running or wobble board training. Wobble board work should start with a low amplitude over one axis and progress to a longer amplitude. It is very effective in both intrinsic and extrinsic muscle exercise and if well tolerated also rapidly increases the range of joint motion.

Muscle endurance is best improved by sustained submaximal muscle contraction. The contraction should be maintained for six seconds, then relaxed for six seconds. This cycle should be repeated six times followed by a two minute rest. During this rest time another muscle group can be worked. Six repetitions of the sets should be completed in each session and at least three sessions be completed each 24 hours. Thus for a single group such as intrinsic foot exercises the daily minimum time is 12 minutes. At least one hour should elapse before repeating each set.

Recent studies with isokinetic measurement of muscle power shows that a single muscle may have normal power in part of its range of action but be weak in another part. The value of isokinetic exercisers in recognition and management of these patients is well established following surgery on the tendo Achillis and is now becoming evident in neurogenic abnormalities.

Balance training

Following a period of immobility in bed or persisting foot pain one of the major disabilities resulting in inefficient locomotion may be lack of proper balance and coordination.

In order to restore this balance all joints must first be adequately mobilized to operate at least within their minimal range of motion. Thus, although in normal gait the hip and knee rarely flex beyond 40°, a greater arc than this is required in order to produce a normal cadence. Likewise muscle power in the lumbar region, pelvis, hamstrings, quadriceps and calf must be restored to at least MRC grade 3, i.e. the power to resist the pull of gravity, and to MRC grade 4 in order to achieve anything approaching normal ambulation. In order to achieve these grades of power initial walking may have to be in the hydrotherapy pool or within parallel bars. Subsequently progress may be made to a walking frame, crutches or sticks.

Balance training in hemiplegia may be assisted by use of the noninvolved limb to carry weight with the involved limb being accustomed to load bearing gradually (Bobart 1978).

Cross-legged standing is a technique sometimes used in adult hemiplegia. With the therapist in attendance the patient stands on the good leg and gradually transfers weight cross-legged to the involved limb until confidence is obtained.

Using a wheeled trolley beneath the foot the involved leg is moved backwards and forwards under control to develop proprioceptive and balance skills. Progression to increased load bearing on the trolley can be made safely with support from the therapist or wall bars.

After graduating to full load bearing without external support it is then appropriate to progress to standing on a wobble board, mini-trampoline or spring board, either with a harness or the physiotherapist's support. At each stage it is valuable to progress to doing the same activity with the eyes closed.

Relief of spasm

Regular passive stretching of all involved joints is essential to prevent the development of fixed deformity. Having overcome any such deformities either by stretching or even on occasions by surgery it is possible to progress to active exercises in the expectation that goals will be achieved. Weak muscles initially may develop more rapidly with eccentric exercise than concentric exercise. Particular attention should be paid to the more proximal muscles, since commonly spasm is generated by a number of different components, one of which may be failure through weakness of one particular muscle group; this may set off generalized or localized limb spasm.

When any specific muscle or muscle group appears to initiate a general spasm it is valuable to concentrate on stretching this muscle and its associated group and to exercise it in its normal function. Spasm may sometimes be broken by use of resisted work on an antagonist group. For example where calf muscle spasm generates an equinus gait it may be of value for the physiotherapist to resist the patient's active attempts to dorsiflex the ankle. This may result in a degree of relaxation of the calf muscles as well as improving the power of the ankle dorsiflexors. An alternative approach may be to use an exercise cycle with a low saddle thereby driving the ankle into dorsiflexion passively using the quadriceps. A few minutes cycling each morning is frequently sufficient to break up the pool of spasm in the calf muscles for many hours.

Where external splints are required in order to use normal footwear they should not be spring-loaded since this often appears to aggravate spasm.

In all patients with focal limb spasm local pathology in the foot or leg may increase the overall pool of spasm. Therefore careful search for aggravating factors such as foot ulcers or infected toe nails should be made on a regular basis.

Prevention of fixed deformity

Put all joints through the maximum possible active and passive range *at least* twice in every 24 hour period.

In the absence of muscle spasticity, resting splints are of great value particularly at night. Not only may they prevent contracture of scar tissue but they reset the point of resting muscle tone. They should be adjusted regularly to keep up with gains in joint position until the required position is reached and a little overcorrected.

Fibrous tissue contracture may still be initiated as much as six months after healing has commenced. Scar tissue may achieve 80% of its ultimate strength in only six weeks so follow-up intervals should be no longer than this in healthy adults.

Dynamic splinting

Early mobilization of joints involved in soft tissue injury with ligament disruption may be assisted by supportive strapping. Nonextensible strapping should be used in the line of action of the injured ligament and applied to overcorrect the joint. When applied to the lateral ligament of the ankle it may also raise the resting tone of the underlying peroneal muscles and further assist stability. Care should be taken to avoid circumferential taping in a manner that could compromise venous return and cause swelling. Elasticated support may be applied over the strapping.

If the skin condition is poor a pneumatic brace may be used to assist in the dispersal of oedema in addition to providing stability. In severe injuries a hinged cast-brace may be preferred.

Persistent equinus may be controlled with an in-shoe ankle–foot orthosis. This simple device will allow a normal swing-through phase of gait and achieve a firm heel-strike and good stability when the foot bears weight. Alternative methods are a spring-loaded toe strap or a lateral caliper with heel block.

Subtalar movement may be limited by a rearfoot orthosis, built up laterally or medially if necessary to correct excessive valgus or varus tilt. This will allow normal ankle movement. Greater deformities or instabilities can be controlled with a lateral caliper, boots and a T-strap to control ankle joint movement.

Metatarsophalangeal joint pain or subluxation may be controlled by a bar proximal to the heads of the second, third and fourth metatarsals. Where the medial ray is not fully loaded during walking or standing as in hallux valgus or following excision arthroplasty (Keller's operation) a medial arch support may also be needed.

Footwear

When functional deformities have been corrected by strapping, splintage or support, residual vertical or horizontal stresses should be controlled with a compliant insole material.

Insole materials should be vapour permeable or

have a high surface capillarity to prevent skin maceration from perspiration. Shoe uppers should be vapour permeable. For problem feet most of these conditions are met by well fitted jogging shoes. Insoles are also available made in Plastazote, Poron, neoprene foam and other materials which meet these criteria.

Where excessive foot moisture is a problem the feet should be washed and dried regularly. Synthetic socks should not be used except as the minority reinforcing component of a natural fibre. This is particularly important in adolescents suffering from fungal infections of the forefoot (athlete's foot) or ingrowing toenails with paronychia.

Long toenails may abut in the toe-box of a shoe and result in a painful subungual haematoma or a paronychia. However, it is often difficult to distinguish between a haematoma and a subungual melanoma.

Shape

The optimal shoe is of a shape that allows normal passive forefoot function and good rearfoot stability. Fashion shoes rarely achieve either of these criteria, particularly for women.

There should be sufficient room in the shoe for the foot, sock and orthosis if needed. Motion should not be excessive in order to limit friction and blister formation.

Materials

The upper should be of a material with vapour permeability appropriate to the amount of sweat formation in the foot. Most is secreted on the dorsum and can be vapourized from the upper. In sport shoes many modern fabrics can release larger volumes than leather, allowing more choice of midsole materials.

In diabetic feet sweat production is reduced or absent. The skin tends to be dry and crack easily, even with moderate forces. Thus a degree of fluid retention may be helpful.

The texture should be sufficiently compliant to yield to moderate pressure and prevent shear. Where a manmade fabric is used it should not have a directional flock on the surface as this may generate friction during activity.

The insole material should normally have a degree of capillarity which can transmit excessive fluid from beneath the forefoot to the side of the shoe. It should be sufficiently compliant to allow deformation under load. It should not have a directional flock.

The midsole should have a degree of compliance which will minimize the larger force peaks generated at heel strike and toe-off.

Some of the modern viscoelastic materials can absorb these peaks in vertical or horizontal directions, so minimizing the problems associated with structural deformities.

Load distribution

General purpose footwear with low heel heights and adequate, forefoot space generally require only a moderate degree of arch support.

In the presence of structural or functional abnormalities orthotic devices may be required to modify gait-related loads. If these are to be used shoes must be fitted with the device inserted. If the fit is good the patient should be prepared to use the device for up to six weeks before expecting symptomatic relief. Commonly the foot is initially less comfortable and the patient should be warned of this.

SPECIAL TREATMENTS AND EQUIPMENT

Ice

Ice broken up to small fragments should be mixed with cold tap water in a plastic bag and sealed. This is at 0°C. Solid ice must *never* be used since its temperature is not known and it may cause skin necrosis. Wrap the ice pack in a towel and apply to the affected part for up to 20 minutes to reduce pain and swelling. Repeat after 30 minutes if necessary.

Heat

Topical heat in the form of warm water, wax or infrared radiation may be used to increase circulation. On its own it is not of a great benefit in the foot. However, in combination with cold water as contrast bathing it assists in the dispersal of oedema or haematomata when used in alternating two-minute cycles for 10 to 20 minutes. Patients may be taught to do this at home.

Cold bathing

Reduced venous tone is made worse by hot baths. Patients with incompetent veins and foot oedema should be advised against taking hot baths and encouraged to shower; regular cold bathing of the feet and legs helps to increase venous tone.

Compression

This may be static or dynamic. Static compression should be applied with graduated pressures from toe to knee or above (Holford 1976, Scurr et al 1977). Stockings above the knee have a tendency to roll down and form a tight constriction ring; if so they must be supported to a waist-belt. They may be removed at night if the foot of the bed is elevated. Tubular compression bandages of uniform diameter should not be used since they may concentrate pressure in the calf and minimize it at the knee, thereby increasing the tendency to distal venous pooling, oedema or deep venous thrombosis. Custom-made pressure garments can be made to control swelling of flaps or grafts after plastic surgery and may need to be used for up to six months.

Intermittent compression may be produced in a single cavity envelope or by a series of separate cavities filling and emptying in sequence. Some systems can be fitted on the operating table to prevent venous stasis during proximal surgery and should always be considered when there is a past history of venous thrombosis.

At moderate pressures (35–40 mmHg) the compression may be used for up to 20 minutes in comfort and safety. It is suitable for use in acute injuries to reduce swelling and haematoma formation in conjunction with a heparinoid cream. For chronic resistant oedema higher pressures (up to 60 mmHg) can be used in the presence of a normal arterial blood supply.

Intermittent compression around the ankle can be achieved with the Aircast brace in which pressure rises and falls while walking or running. It is comfortable as well as effective in stabilizing the ankle and can be used immediately after a soft tissue injury.

Friction

Some soft tissue injuries respond well in the early stages of treatment to friction therapy. It is of particular value in the foot and ankle for treatment of Achilles tendon pain (Smart et al 1980).

The mechanism of action may be either by prevention of adhesion formation or dispersal of oedema and enhancement of blood supply. Where there are small haematomata it will help to keep them soft and easy to resorb. Deep friction can be instituted early in treatment after local pain relief with ice.

Ultrasound

After the cessation of bleeding from a soft tissue injury and in the presence of stable vascular plugs (four to seven days), ultrasound may be used to reduce haematomata by liquefaction and to stimulate fibroblast proliferation and alignment.

Treatments can be given up to twice daily in a dose that is not painful to the area involved. Penetration should be adjusted to the depth of the involved tissue. It is effective for capsular and ligamentous injuries. Where early adhesions are forming, as around tendon repairs or transfers, treatment with ultrasound may assist mobilization. Treatment should not be given earlier than four weeks and is probably not beneficial after three months when the scar tissue is largely mature.

Controlled studies of ultrasound on stress fractures have not shown convincing evidence of therapeutic benefit but on occasions it causes pain over the lesion and may aid diagnosis.

Interferential therapy

Low voltage interferential therapy is effective in relieving pain and enhancing the blood supply of deep tissues when used in an alternating mode of frequency cycles from 10–80 per second. It may be of value in bursitis and small joint arthritis. The electrodes are applied to give a net interferential current at the point to be treated. Using a probe it is sometimes possible to provoke pain in a deeply situated lesion and thereby confirm that treatment is applied to the correct area.

If it is effective in relieving pain it may be used prior to assisted active or passive joint mobilization. Alternatively it may be of value in selection of sites for transcutaneous nerve stimulation (TNS) treatment as well as the optimum frequency for the stimulator. The optimum analgesic frequency tends to lie in the 5–15 Hz range and maximum hyperaemia in the 70–90 Hz range.

Application of the electrodes to produce an interferential current over the lumbar sympathetic chain has been used temporarily to block sympathetic activity and produce a transient 'sympathectomy' in the leg and foot for assessment purposes.

Pulsed magnetic fields

There is increasing evidence that this form of treatment assists in the healing of soft tissue as well as bone (Wilson 1972, Fenn 1969).

It may be of value in assisting or enhancing nerve growth after injury or repair and particularly in inhibiting perineural fibrosis. Thus in the long term it may prevent some of the painful sequelae of nerve repair. Studies continue on its use in promoting healing of skin ulcers in the foot.

Transcutaneous nerve stimulation (TNS)

The place of TNS is firmly established in the management of chronic pain. Its correct use requires great attention to detail both from patient and therapist. A diagram should be made of the siting of the electrodes; the optimum current may only be found after many days of trial and error. This should be done under in-patient supervision.

The stimulator should be used early in the treatment of pain. Delay to the chronic painful state may result in reduced efficiency. Chronic pain from the periphery will establish biochemical changes in the spinal cord which may be permanent within six months and it is important to minimize this risk.

Acupuncture

This ancient form of pain relief is being found to be of increasing value in the management of chronic conditions where muscle spasm is a major feature. Variations include acupressure and electro-acupuncture.

In addition to its effect in reducing pain, electroacupuncture may be used to induce skin blood flow changes in sympathectomized limbs, probably by release of vasoactive peptides from the brain (Ballard et al 1970, Owen et al 1979).

In Raynaud's disease and diabetes mellitus skin temperature in a sympathectomized limb may rise by as much as 8–10° within 40 minutes of stimulation in the hand (Abram et al 1980). Low frequency (2–5 Hz) impulses applied to the first web space of the normally innervated hand at an amplitude below that which induces muscle contraction or pain is a suitable method (Kaada 1982). The resultant increase in blood flow may substantially speed the healing of ulcers of the foot. The temperature rise may persist for several hours after discontinuing stimulation. Some TNS machines are suitable for this treatment.

Some observers using TNS for pain relief in the back have observed a significant temperature rise in the periphery. In one series only one patient did not experience a temperature increase.

Biofeedback

Biofeedback is a system in which biological activity such as muscle power, skin temperature, and pressure distribution is converted electronically into an audible or visible signal. The patients can learn to modify relevant parameters with this information in order to work towards a more normal gait pattern.

EMG feedback

EMG feedback uses skin mounted electrodes which indicate the extent of muscle activity beneath them. By placing the electrodes over agonist and antagonist groups audible or visible signals are generated either on an analogue scale or at a preset threshold. Thus antagonists can be trained to relax while agonists achieve the desired level of activity. By modifying the selected thresholds gradual learning patterns can be established.

Treatment should be undertaken initially as an in-patient until good dissociation is learned. This may take 2–3 weeks. Thereafter self-training can be continued as an out-patient with review by the therapist at weekly intervals which may be extended as progress is achieved. When the learned pattern is established the biofeedback may be discontinued. This may be in six weeks or more depending on associated pathology or motivation.

Skin temperature feedback

This can be used for management of Raynaud's phenomenon, chilblains and other related circulatory problems.

A skin thermocouple is applied to the area of abnormal perfusion. An audible or visible signal is generated at the desired temperature threshold. The patient is then asked to attempt to influence the skin temperature. This alone may achieve a result which the patient can then appreciate and monitor. Additional enhancement may be by the patient imagining the foot in a warm bath, on the beach, in front of the fire or any environment in which the phenomenon does not occur or to which it usually responds.

The signal may be set to emit at intervals of 0.1 °C, these being extended as learning progresses. After the first success has been experienced the patient can continue at home with therapist supervision on alternate weeks. This may be discontinued after an at-risk period during which the patient has been able to remain symptom-free.

Pressure related feedback

Pressure related feedback is used to retrain foot loading patterns. In habitual equinus gait in children where there is good or normal ankle mobility and muscle power, but inappropriate toe-walking, an audible signal can be transmitted from the heel of the shoe on achieving a correct pattern of heel strike; if the shoe heel touches the ground without an adequate load the signal is not generated. With regular threshold achievement additional rewards may be given in a progressive pattern if necessary. In general, the achievement of the sound in itself may be an adequate reward.

Pharmacotherapy

Diuretics

Chronic venous insufficiency commonly responds to a course of diuretics in reducing the volume and discomfort of oedema. However, they should not be used if there are hazards of electrolyte imbalance; they demand regular biochemical review. The potential alteration of renin-angiotensin regulation which may result in resistant oedema is sometimes the result of prolonged diuretic therapy.

Venotonic drugs

Selective constriction of peripheral veins can be achieved experimentally by intravenous injection of 1 mg dihydroergotamine. This results in a significant decrease in blood volume in the legs but the side effects of such doses, including headaches and vertigo, render this method unsuitable. However, early results of a trial of an oral dose of 10 mg dihydroergotamine suggest that this may be of benefit without substantial disadvantages (Partsch 1982).

Arteriovenous shunting as seen in the high-flow oedematous diabetic foot can be reduced with ephedrine up to 60 mg orally three times daily (Edmonds et al 1983). As the oedema recedes the dose may be reduced. The arterial blood pressure should be carefully monitored with the patient being treated as an in-patient on initiating this form of treatment.

Sympathectomy

As discussed above there are cases where sympathectomy would seem appropriate, particularly in Raynaud's disease. A transient chemical block can be produced by injection of lignocaine around the lumbar sympathetic chain. If this produces the desired effect a more permanent block with phenol can be performed. This must be done under X-ray control since injection into the major vessels or peritoneum would be catastrophic.

Local injection therapy

Despite extensive animal experimental evidence that intra-articular steroid injections may damage a joint there is considerable clinical evidence of benefit from its use in the foot. A combination of 25 mg hydrocortisone acetate with 1 ml 1% lignocaine is frequently helpful when given after manipulation of a joint under anaesthetic. Other preparations such as prednisolone sodium phosphate (Codelsol®) methylprednisolone acetate (Depo-Medrone®) and triamcinolone (Ledercort®, Kenalog®) are also widely used.

Injections should not be given into tendons or into the substance of a ligament for fear of rupture. Thus tendon sheath injection must be given with care.

Confirmation of accurate location of the needle can be gained by injecting a small volume of contrast medium under X-ray control to perform a tenogram prior to injection of the steroid. Then if the therapy is ineffective it is reasonable to review the diagnosis prior to further therapy.

Steroid injections into the painful heel 'spur' area are frequently very painful for two or three days. Thereafter symptoms may subside for a few weeks. Review in less than six weeks will miss the late recurrence. Injections should not be given unless a trial of an effective viscoelastic compliant heel cushion has failed. More than three injections should not be given in view of the degree of collagen liquefaction that may occur, particularly in very active people. If more are required the diagnosis is probably wrong.

Anti-inflammatory agents

Pain relief in the inflamed foot can often be aided by nonsteroidal anti-inflammatory drugs. They are of particular benefit in the acute management of crystal arthropathy. In this situation prompt administration of indomethacin 50 mg eight hourly may rapidly abort an attack.

Long-term use of these agents is probably best avoided. There is evidence in the hip joint that high or long-term dosage may aggravate destructive changes in bone. In the foot it is usually possible to modify painful forces either by orthotics or by surgery and provide adequate relief of symptoms without serious hazard. If the expected improvement does not materialize within the expected time span the diagnosis should be questioned.

Systemic steroid medication in severe cases of rheumatoid arthritis may result in more rapid thinning of the skin and subcutaneous tissues of the sole of the foot than that caused by the disease itself. Thus where metatarsal heads are prolapsed or the subcalcaneal pad is thinned care should be taken to prescribe compliant insole materials in adequately fitting shoes for the foot to prevent the risk of skin ulceration.

SAMPLE REHABILITATION PROGRAMMES

Rehabilitation of the foot following injury or surgery varies according to the nature of the injury and the treatment already undertaken. Whilst it is not possible to itemize a programme for every conceivable pathology an outline of the philosophy of rehabilitation for some common injuries follows. However, we emphasize that these should be varied appropriately according to local and general factors.

Fractured calcaneus

Undisplaced

Exclude vertebral crush fracture
Ice
Compression until oedema dispersed
Elevation

Mobilize the ankle and subtalar joints as soon as pain permits. Allow non-weightbearing with crutches for six weeks, when bone union is becoming 'sticky', and protected weight bearing until full body weight can be accepted without pain, remembering that equinus load is all taken by the tendo Achillis. Compliant footwear with a stable heel counter to limit excessive passive subtalar motion should be worn.

Displaced

1. Reduce by preferred method and fix by percutaneous pinning
2. Ice
3. Compression
4. Elevation

Mobilize non-weightbearing for six weeks (to bone union) with efforts to restore subtalar motion. If subtalar joint stiffness persists, manipulate under an anaesthetic at 8–10 weeks and continue exercises.

Swelling may persist for up to six months, therefore use elasticated support for foot and ankle. Stable compliant heeled shoes should be worn.

The patient should avoid jobs such as roofing which require good subtalar mobility.

Ankle fracture

Aetiology: Rotation force to the loaded ankle

Pathology: Fractures of lateral, medial or posterior malleoli with or without collateral ligament injury

Aim: Achieve stable reduction until adequate union in order to restore full function.

Nonoperative treatment

This consists of above knee cast to control rotation, with foot in neutral, non-weightbearing, and change to below knee cast at three to four weeks.

Progress to full weight bearing, then remove cast at six weeks and X-ray.

If union is satisfactory, then:

1. apply elasticated support
2. mobilize ankle by walking or cycling
3. at two weeks progress to wobble board or mini-trampoline
4. at six weeks gentle running in a stable training shoe and normal running after three months (if full function), but sometimes as much as six months, depending on the injury
5. if there was a ligament injury use support strapping for at least three months of sport and no sport without compliant footwear for at least two years.

Operative treatment

Indication: Stable reduction not achieved by closed methods.

Principle: Stable internal fixation of anatomically reduced fracture(s).

Post-operation regime:

1. Elevate foot at least 40 cm above hips for 48 hours, in a
2. Padded bandage or a bivalved below knee cast.
3. At 48 hours start active ankle motion — strictly non-weightbearing.
4. Discharge home, when wounds permit, provided there is minimal oedema and ankle motion of 10° dorsiflexion to plantar flexion 30°, in a below-knee weight-bearing cast, usually 5–10 days after operation.
5. Remove the cast at six weeks and X-ray. If union looks satisfactory mobilize to full weight bearing as for closed fracture.
6. Remove implants at two years, although diastasis screws must be removed at six weeks, as ankle dorsiflexion beyond neutral cannot occur freely without tibiofibular mobility.

Problems

Persistent deformity. If union has occurred with more than 10° of valgus or 5° of varus a correcting heel wedge should be used.

Persistent instability. Support strapping with low heeled shoes, an out-flared heel and a stable heel counter.

Persistent stiffness. Manipulation under anaesthetic of ankle and subtalar joints at four to six weeks after union.

Persistent swelling. See section on oedema on page 1113.

Persistent pain. Exclude nonunion, instability, loose body, compression neuropathy of lateral popliteal, sural, posterior tibial or saphenous nerves, ischaemic contracture of long flexor or intrinsic muscles, Sudeck's atrophy, secondary gain and low grade infection of the implant.

If all the above are excluded and the pain is considered due to gross joint destruction and persists despite full mobilization consider arthrodesis (Mazur et al 1979, Harrington 1979). Arthroplasty of the ankle for post-fracture pain is not recommended.

Forefoot arthroplasty

Elevate well for 2–3 weeks. Maintain mobility and strength of arms to allow effective use of walking aids (especially shoulders with rotator cuff defects) during bed rest period.

When wounds are fully healed, mobilize in deep shoes with a double thickness of Plastazote or similar compliant material and with protected weight bearing on crutches. Progress to two walking sticks at six weeks when wound healing is secure.

Change the insole material as soon as it has 'bottomed out', often every two weeks and no later than six weeks.

Diabetic forefoot ulcers (Figs. 56.4a and b)

Treatment

1. Clean the ulcer
2. Bed rest
3. Pare down edge of ulcer
4. Debridement
5. Occasional antibiotics

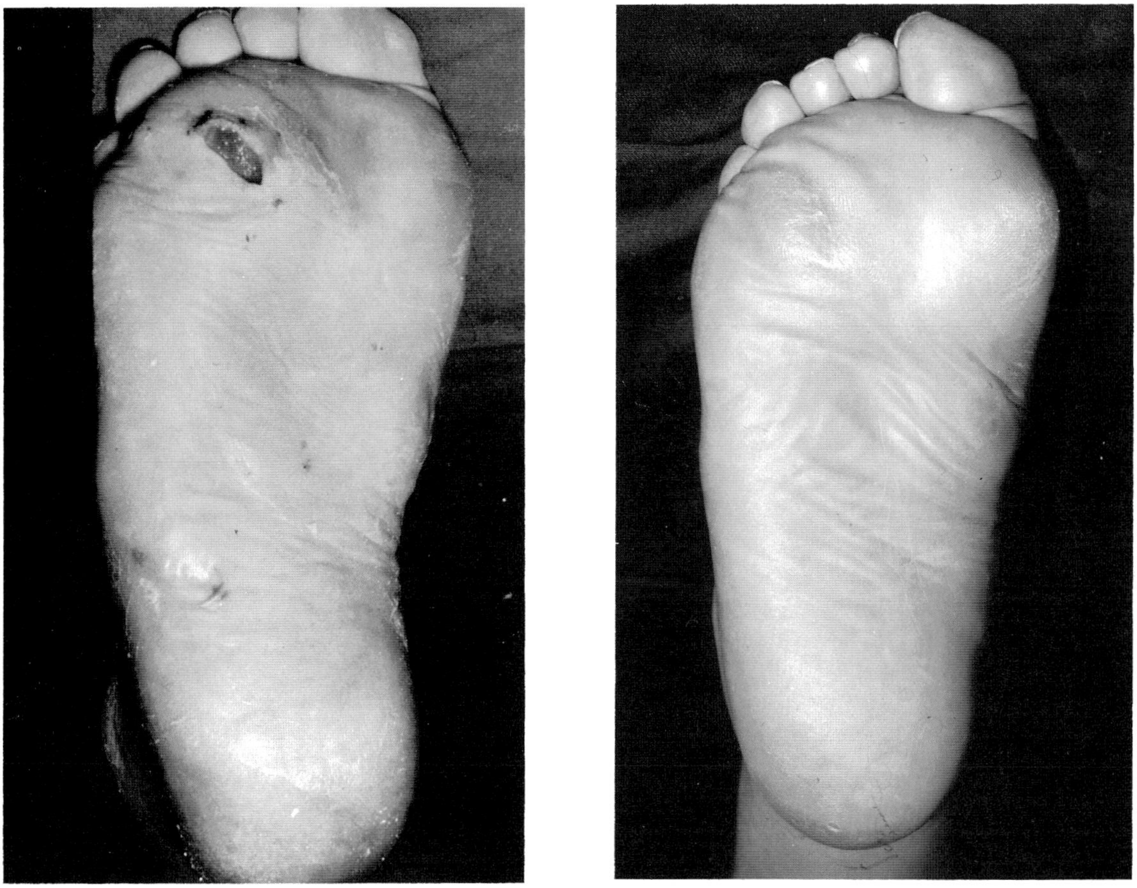

a b

Fig. 56.4 Diabetic forefoot ulcer before (a) and after (b) six weeks in plaster cast (reproduced by permission of Mr. John Pollard FRCS)

6. Sterile dressing to forefoot ulcer
7. Well padded below knee cast with self-adhesive foam around the malleoli, trimmed to the level of the mid-point of proximal phalanges of the toes to allow changes of dressings and with a walking rubber rocker. If the cast is soiled by discharge, water etc., change it.

Redress daily until healed and remove the cast two weeks after healing is complete.

After healing of the ulcer the foot is protected in deep shoes with a double Plastazote insole, one layer medium density and upper layer low density (Pollard & Le Quesne 1983, Wood et al 1977). Change low density Plastazote when it bottoms out — often every week.

N.B. This method is not suitable for cases with osteomyelitis. In this situation ray excision may be required before healing is obtained. Undiagnosed osteomyelitis may lead to amputation.

The forces which caused the ulcer still operate after healing; unless footwear is carefully controlled they will recur. If load relief by surgery is not possible the choice of insole material is critical to limb survival.

Sports injuries

Foot and ankle pain in sport are commonly the result of overuse or concentration of stress (Bertram 1970). In managing the injury it is essential to identify the causative factors and eliminate them as far as possible. Poor posture, bad balance, weak upper limbs, leg length discrepancy or limb rotational deformities may all be manifest as foot problems in sport.

Whenever possible observe the action which may be causing the problem. Treadmill running may give some clues, but does not approach the forces generated on the road or track either in magnitude or direction and is therefore not a diagnostic substitute. Laboratory based gait assessment is often unrepresentative and misleading in difficult cases.

Many sports injury remedies can usefully be applied to the nonathlete.

Subcalcaneal pain

Aetiology

Hard heel strike in hard shoes on hard ground. Radiological spurs are probably irrelevant (Ali 1980). Soft tissue arthropathy such as Reiter's syndrome, rheumatoid arthritis, ankylosing spondylitis etc. should be excluded.

Treatment

Treatment consists of rest for three days with local ice and elevation. A heel pad support bandage to prevent fat pad shear and a transcutaneous or systemic anti-inflammatory agent should be used. Correct footwear with a shock-absorbing heel pad and radius to heel cup to constrain the soft tissue heel pad under load must be worn (MacLellan & Vyvyan 1981).

If pain persists excavate the heel pad beneath the area of maximal tenderness and build up to full activity over 2–3 weeks within limits of pain. Maintain cardiovascular and muscle fitness on an exercise cycle or with weights etc. Use local injection with steroid only as a last resort.

Achilles tendon pain

Aetiology

Hard heel strike in hard shoes on hard ground, often with an excessive exercise rate or degree of pronation. Sometimes there is heel tab friction, metaphyseal spur, partial subcutaneous rupture, ankylosing spondylitis etc.

Treatment

This consists of walking only in soft shoes for two weeks. Ice can be used. Gradually increase activities and running, minimizing pain with good shock-absorbing shoes with a stable heel counter and an adequate arch support.

Then, implement regular passive stretching of hamstrings and Achilles tendons, but no running with leg or body weights. In chronic cases, use local ultrasound or interferential therapy and deep frictional massage. Maintain upper limb and cardiovascular fitness with use of weights and bicycle. Avoid local steroid injection, not only may they mask important signs in recovery, but also if injected into the tendon may predispose to rupture.

Stress fracture

Aetiology

Excessive activity with excessive load, usually on a hard surface or in military footwear. Sometimes there is underlying bone pathology (Heath et al 1980).

Treatment

Withdraw the precipitating activity at once. If the fracture is incomplete walk with protected weight bearing for two weeks, but if complete, immobilize if indicated by location of fracture (e.g. tibia, but not metacarpal neck 'march' fractures).

Return gradually to function within the limits of comfort, but stop before pain begins — pain indicates progression of the fracture and activity must be discontinued. Keep to compliant shoes and minimum loads for six weeks, then gradually increase tolerance to greater loads or harder footwear if demanded.

Identify the causative factor in order to prevent recurrence. Bone can usually respond to a major load increase if phased in over a six week period.

PAINFUL PERIPHERAL NERVE DISORDERS OF THE FOOT

The term causalgia was first used by Weir Mitchell (1872) in his account of the results of damage to peripheral nerves in the American Civil War. The word means 'burning pain' and is the characteristic feature of a small but significant number of patients with partial lesions of peripheral nerves, in particular the median and sciatic nerves. Classically the condition follows partial lesions of nerves due to gunshot wounds, but in civilian life, the condition can follow stretching injuries of nerves after severe sprains and fractures of the ankle joint, following accidental division of sensory nerves, such as in operations on varicose veins and following excision of traumatic neuromas.

The clinical features of causalgia have never been better described than by Weir Mitchell in his book of 1872. He described the severe spontaneous burning pain in the hand or foot, the marked hyperaesthesia which we now call hyperpathia, in which the slightest touch causes severe pain, indicating a profound disturbance of the peripheral and central nervous system. He noted that there was little or no sensory loss, marked colour changes with cyanosis and swelling, occasional skin eruptions, joint swelling, marked changes in the nails with overgrowth, pitting and roughening, loss of hair, the gradual spread of pain and the hyperaesthesiae to adjacent nerves outside those of the autonomous distribution of the original nerve damaged, then finally, the appearance in a small number of cases of bizarre involuntary movements which could persist for many years. This severe burning pain would demoralize even the most hardy soldier and one of the characteristic features was the way it was aggravated by physical and emotional stimuli. Weir Mitchell described the case of Private Corliss, who lay in his bed in the military hospital writhing in pain exacerbated by the footsteps of visitors nearby and the sound and vibration of a military band in the square outside.

In the Second World War, the commanding officer of a large United States Airforce base hospital had to persuade the commanding officer of an airbase a mile away to divert the aircraft from flying over his hospital, for the vibration and noise severely affected his patients with causalgia from gunshot wounds of the nerves.

In 1900 Sudeck described a curious osteoporosis of the bones of the foot, following a trivial injury to the ankle. Sudeck's atrophy or reflex sympathetic dystrophy, as it is often known, usually follows mild trauma. Two distinct stages are recognized: in the acute stage, when the part is swollen, there is a marked spontaneous pain and hyperpathia with cyanosis. Some months later, the part becomes cold, and the joints very stiff with skin atrophy and nail changes. Clinically, the condition of causalgia and Sudeck's atrophy are virtually indistinguishable and it is now believed that both these conditions have the same pathological mechanism in common, which is damage to peripheral nerves. Loh & Nathan (1978) argue that the two conditions are at either end of the same spectrum, in which causalgia involves damage to major nerve trunks, while in Sudeck's atrophy there is damage to the very fine axons. Not only are the clinical features similar in both conditions, but the response to treatment also is similar.

Until recently, Sudeck's atrophy was believed to be due to a disorder of the sympathetic nervous system. It is now realized that the sympathetic nervous system is, in fact, behaving normally, but there is hypersensitivity to circulating noradrenalin of the large diameter afferent fibres subserving touch, position sense and vibration.

Wallin et al (1976) recorded the ongoing sympathetic activity with microelectrodes in the sympathetic nerve fibres in patients with severe spontaneous pain from causalgia. The sympathetic activity persisted unchanged despite the complete abolition of pain by the application of TNS. Wall & Devor (1978) have cogently summarized the effects of damage to peripheral nerves. The neuroma at the site of damage is the seat of ongoing spontaneous discharges of varying frequency. Demyelination can cause ectopic foci of spontaneous discharges to develop and there can be crosstalk between myelinated and unmyelinated fibres, so that spontaneous reverberating discharges are set up. Furthermore, there are profound central changes following peripheral damage, including spontaneous firing, abnormal sprouting, abnormal discharging circuits, and the uncovering of normally quiescent neural circuits. In addition there is the marked hypersensitivity to noradrenalin already mentioned, which explains the exacerbation of pain to emotional and environmental stimuli.

The diagnosis presents no problem. Following damage to a peripheral nerve, the patient will complain of severe spontaneous burning pain, first in the distribution of the damaged nerve and then gradually spreading to the territory of adjacent nerves. The patient will be unable to bear the touch of bedclothes or light clothing, but will often be able to tolerate firm pressure. This suggests that the large diameter afferents are being stimulated and activity in these fibres helps to damp down the nociceptive traffic centrally (Wall & Gutnik 1974). Colour changes in the skin follow rapidly and the patient may be quite unable to bear weight on the leg.

In Sudeck's atrophy, classically following a trivial injury such as a slight sprain or strain, the patient develops acute swelling of the foot, with severe spontaneous burning pain and marked hyperpathia. If the condition does not rapidly settle spontaneously, chronic changes ensue, with stiffness of joints, atrophy of skin and the classical nail changes already described. The natural history of both these conditions is poor.

Weir Mitchell's son, who was also a neurologist, followed up 22 of his father's patients with causalgia 27 years after injury and found that over half of them were still having very severe pain.

Subbarao & Stillwell (1981) described a long-term follow-up of 125 patients with Sudeck's atrophy and showed that a significant proportion (35%) were unable to work and 70% were having persistent pain and disability.

All authors, and we can confirm this in our work, have shown that early treatment is essential if the condition is not to become chronic. Once the condition is set, it is extremely difficult to correct the joint deformities and reverse the circulatory and skin changes.

Management

It has seemed logical, when confronted with a painful nerve lesion following trauma, to resect the neuroma and to repair the nerve by suture or graft. However, the results have been extremely disappointing and over and over again in the literature one finds the recurrence rate of pain after such procedures distressingly high. Repeated surgical procedures are often applied, leading to more and more pain, often spreading far beyond the original territory of the damaged nerve. It is only recently, with the explosion of neurophysiological research in this field, that we now realise why this is so. Further damage to the peripheral nerves leads to more neuroma formation, more ectopic foci, more cross talk, more sensitivity to noradrenalin and even greater central changes of deafferentation. It is not surprising, therefore, that repeated surgery often leads to an exacerbation of the symptoms.

The basic pathophysiological disorder that we now recognize has given us the clue to the management of these patients. Because there are many different results of damage, a variety of treatments must be applied. Since the work of Wall & Sweet (1967) it is known that transcutaneous nerve stimulation is effective in reducing or abolishing pain after nerve damage. This is presumed to be due to its effect on inhibiting the spontaneous firing of the neuroma. More recently it has been suggested that there is a central effect also. Stimulation of the large diameter fibres encourages the secretion of encephalins or endorphins in the spinal cord, which in turn have the effect of damping down spontaneous firing or inhibiting the transmission of the nociceptive stimuli further centrally.

Sympathetic block was first used by Barnes in 1948 in patients with causalgia following nerve injuries in the Second World War with spectacular success and stellate block for Sudeck's atrophy or causalgia in the hand, or lumbar sympathetic block or sympathectomy for the condition in the foot have long been practised with success. Although we now know that the sympathetic nervous system is not at fault, reducing the sensitivity of the large diameter afferents to circulating noradrenalin will prevent the triggering of spontaneous discharges.

Hannington Kiff (1974) introduced the technique of guanethidine block. We have found this the most valuable treatment of all techniques for sympathetic block. It is considerably easier than stellate blocks, it can be carried out by the house officer (whereas stellate blocks require a highly experienced anaesthetist), the effect lasts longer and it can be repeated frequently.

We have learned that in our early work, we were too timid in our approach to this technique, giving the patient one or two blocks and if these were unsuccessful, abandoning the procedure. We have now learned that at least six blocks on alternate days should be given. If the patient shows even the slightest sign of responding to treatment, with relief of pain for an hour or two after the injection, then it is well worth continuing.

Furthermore, it is important that the patient should not be sedated, but that as soon as he is clear of the intensive treatment area (usually one hour after the injection) he should be encouraged to undergo desensitizing procedures and to use the affected limb as much as possible, attempting to restore more normal movement patterns in the spinal cord and to break up the abnormal circuits caused by the distorted profile reaching the spinal cord.

The best results in these difficult patients are obtained by admission to an inpatient intensive rehabilitation programme. We have a minicare ward where patients are admitted on a five-day basis, where they are accommodated in hostel-type accommodation and have intensive treatment throughout the day. Thus, serial guanethidine blocks can be given over a two or three week period and the correct site for application of the electrodes for TNS and the selection of the particular parameters for that particular patient can be studied at leisure by the physiotherapist (Frampton 1982).

TNS is a widely abused treatment, many patients being insufficiently instructed in the application of the stimulator and the treatment being given for far too short a time. It is far too common in our experience to find that patients are being given a stimulator without adequate instructions and told to wear it for half an hour or an hour at a time. Many of our patients wear our stimulator 8 or 12 hours a day for many months on end (Frampton 1982). During their stay, patients are exposed to the full rehabilitation regime of active exercises, games, workshop activities and desensitization techniques. The therapists and the patients themselves are encouraged to stroke and rub and handle the painful skin when they are under the influence of the guanethidine block or the TNS.

In 1984, Withrington & Wynn Parry reported on 86 patients with severe painful peripheral nerve disorders, including partial peripheral nerve injury, Sudeck's atrophy, phantom pain and postherpetic neuralgia. 71% of these patients who had had pain for an average of 3.4 years before admission, obtained complete or substantial relief of pain. Follow-up must be indefinite. In some patients, the pain gradually returns some months after discharge and it is important to readmit them for a top-up with a few more guanethidine blocks and a further intensive rehabilitation programme. Some of our patients are readmitted every year or 18 months, often in the winter when symptoms tend to return with the cold weather.

One of the most disturbing results of our study was the effect of surgery. 50 of our patients had had 71 operations specifically to relieve pain before being referred to our service and in only one of them had this operation been successful. It must be emphasized that further attempts to cure pain by surgery are almost invariably doomed to failure. Rolfe Birch, the Surgical Director of the Peripheral Nerve Unit of the Royal Orthopaedic Hospital, Stanmore, Middlesex, has established with our rehabilitation team a number of maxims for guidance in this field. They are:

1. Continuity should always be restored if possible, burying nerve ends in bone, or leaving a nerve unsatisfied, is liable to lead to more neuroma formation with further sprouting and ectopic foci of discharges.

2. Peripheral nerve surgery demands the highest quality technique, and particularly where painful nerves are concerned, must not be left to the inexperienced surgeon.

3. Internal neurolysis should never be carried out — this does further damage with all the effects already described. Sympathectomy also demands the highest technique.

4. Finally, one surgical attempt only should be allowed to relieve pain. The temptation to continue excising neuromata or painful segments of nerves and replacing with grafts should be resisted at all costs.

5. Long-term follow-up is essential and intensive rehabilitation is a vital part of the total management.

REFERENCES

Abram S E, Asiddao G B, Reynolds A C 1980 Increased skin temperature during transcutaneous electrical stimulation. Anesth Analg 59(1): 22–25

Adverse Drug Reaction Bulletin 1971 Drug Induced Arthralgia and Arthritis 30: 88

Ali E 1980 Calcaneal spur in Guyana W I Med J XXIX: 175–183

Ballard D R, Abboud F M, Mayer H E 1970 Release of a humoral vasodilator substance during neurogenic vasodilatation Am J Physiol 219(5): 1451–1457

Barnes R 1954 Causalgia. A review of 48 cases in 'Peripheral nerve injuries'. Report of the Medical Research Council, 156
Bertram J 1970 Stress fractures in Royal Marine recruits. J Roy Nav Med Serv 56: 78–91
Betts R P, Duckworth T 1978 A device for measuring pressures under the sole of the foot. Eng Med 7: 223–228
Bobart B 1978 Adult Hemiplegia: Evaluation and Treatment. William Heinemann, London
Bourne I J H 1975 Results of treatment of swollen legs by vertical leg drainage. Folia Angiologica XXIII: 288–297
Cavanagh P R, Michiyoshi A 1980 A technique for the display of pressure distributions beneath the foot. J Biomech 13: 69–79
Conrad L, Black E E 1980 Augmented auditory feedback in the treatment of equinus gait in children. Dev Med Child Neurol 22: 713–718
Edmonds M E, Anker A G, Watkins P J 1983 Ephedrine: A New Treatment for Diabetic Neuropathic Oedema. Lancet 8324: 548–551
El-Khoury G Y, Kathol M H 1980 Neuropathic fractures in patients with diabetes mellitus. Radiology 134: 313–316
Fenn J E 1969 Effect of pulsed electromagnetic energy (diapulse) on experimental haematomas. Can Med Assoc J 100: 251–254
Frampton V 1982 Pain control with the aid of transcutaneous nerve stimulation. Physiotherapy 68: 77
Fugl-Meyer A R, Nordin G, Sjöström M, Wählby L 1979 Achilles tendon injury: A model for isokinetic strength training using bio-feedback. Scand J Rehabil Med 11: 37–44
Hanington-Kiff J 1974 Intravenous regional sympathetic block with guanethidine. Lancet i: 1019
Harrington K D 1979 Degenerative arthritis of the ankle secondary to long standing lateral ligament instability. J Bone Joint Surg 61A: 354–361
Harvey W 1628 Exercitatio Anatomica de Motu Cordis et Sanguinis in Animalibus. Translated by K J Franklin 1957. Blackwell, Oxford
Hawes D, Light L H, Repond E 1979 Modelling the distortion produced by heel strike transients in soft tissue. J Physiol 296: 10–11 P
Heath H, Melton L J, Chu C-P 1980 Diabetes mellitus and the risk of skeletal fracture. N Engl J Med 303(10): 567–570
Hennig E M, Cavanagh P R, MacMillan N H 1980 High Resolution In-Shoe Pressure Distribution Measurements by Piezoelectric Transducers. Proc. of Special Conference of the Canadian Soc. for Biomechanics. London, Ontario
Hertzman C A 1973 Use of Plastazote (TM) in foot disabilities. Am J Phys Med 52: 289–303
Hey H, Lund B, Sorenson O H 1982 Delayed fracture healing following jejunoileal bypass surgery for obesity. Calcif Tissue Int 34(1): 13–15
Holford C P 1976 Graded compression for preventing deep venous thrombosis. Br Med J 2: 969–970
Huskisson E C, Hart F D 1975 Joint Disease: all the Arthropathies. 2nd edn. John Wright & Sons, Bristol
Kaada B 1982 Vasodilatation induced by transcutaneous nerve stimulation in peripheral ischaemia (Raynaud's phenomenon and diabetic polyneuropathy). Eur Heart J 3: 303–314
Knott M, Vors D 1968 Proprioceptive Neuromuscular Facilitation. Harper & Row, New York
Knutsson E 1972 An analysis of Parkinsonian gait. Brain 95: 475–486
Leather H M, Lewin I G, Calder E, Braybrooke J, Cox R R 1981 Effect of water de-ionisers on 'fracturing osteodystrophy' and dialysis encephalopathy in Plymouth. Nephron 29: 80–84
Lester A A 1981 Management of sprained ankles. A double blind study. Practitioner 225: 935–936
Light L H, MacLellan G E, Klenerman L 1979 Skeletal transients on heel strike in normal walking with different footwear. J Biomech 13: 477–480
Loh L, Nathan P W 1978 Painful peripheral states and sympathetic blocks. J Neurol Neurosurg Psychiatry 41: 664
MacLellan G E, Helal B, Vyvyan B, Light L H 1982 Achilles Paratenonitis — Prevention by control of passive Microtrauma. Current Topics in Sports Medicine p 867
MacLellan G E, Vyvyan B 1981 Management of pain beneath the heel and Achilles tendonitis with visco-elastic heel inserts. Br J Sports Med 15: 117–121
Mazur J M, Schwartz E, Simon S-R 1979 Ankle arthrodesis. Long term follow up with gait analysis. J Bone Joint Surg 61A: 964–975
Minns R J, Craxford A D 1984 Pressure under the forefoot in rheumatoid arthritis. Clin Orthop 187: 235–242
Mubarak S J, Owen C A 1977 Double incision fasciotomy of the leg for decompression in compartment syndromes. J Bone Joint Surg 59A(2): 184–187
Mubarak S J, Hargens A R, Owen C A et al 1976 The wick catheter technique for measurement of intramuscular pressure. J Bone Joint Surg 58A(7): 1016–1020
Nakano K K 1975 The entrapment neuropathies of rheumatoid arthritis. Orthop Clin North Am 6(3): 837–860
Owen S, Atkinson E R, Lees D E 1979 Thermographic evidence of reduced sympathetic tone with transcutaneous nerve stimulation. Anesthesiology 50: 62–65
Partsch H 1982 Treatment of chronic venous insufficiency. Year Book Medical Publishers, Inc., New York
Polchaninoff M 1983 Gait analysis using a portable Microprocessor-based segmental foot force measuring system. Proceedings of the Seventh Annual Symposium on Computer Applications in Medical Care. IEEE Computer Society Press, Maryland
Pollard J P, Le Quesne L P 1983 Method of healing diabetic forefoot ulcers. Br Med J 286: 436–437
Puhl W, Iyer V 1973 S.E.M. Observations on the structure of the articular cartilage surface in normal and pathological condition. Proc. Workshop S.E.M. in Pathology 1.1.F Research Inst., Chicago, Ill.
Salter R B 1981 Presidential Address to Canadian Orthopaedic Association (June 1981)
Scurr J H, Ibrahim S Z, Faber R G, Le Quesne L P 1977 The efficacy of graduated compression stockings in the prevention of deep vein thrombosis. Br J Surg 64: 371–373
Shannon F T, Murray A M, 1978 Os calcis fractures treated by non-weight bearing exercises. J R Coll Surg Edinb 23(6): 355–361
Shipley D E 1979 Clinical evaluation and care of the insensitive foot. Phys Ther 59(a): 13–18
Smart G W, Taunton J E, Clement D B 1980 Achilles tendon disorders in runners — a review. Med Sci Sports Exerc 12(4): 231–243
Smith C L 1980 Physical therapy management of patients with total ankle replacement. Phys Ther 60: 303–306
Sneppen O, Christenson S B, Kvogsol O, Lorentzen J 1977 Fracture of the body of the talus. Acta Orthop Scand 48(3): 317–324

Sperryn P N 1980 Running and training shoes. Medisport 2: 42–46

Subbarao J, Stillwell G K 1981 Reflex sympathetic dystrophy syndrome of the upper extremity. Analysis of total outcome of management of 125 cases. Arch Phys Med Rehabil 62: 549

Sudek P 1900 Uber die akute eutzu nahiche knockens thopi. Archiv für klinische chirurgie 62: 147

Thulesius O, Norgren L, Gjores J E 1973 Foot volumetry — a new method for objective assessment of oedema and venous function. Vasa 2: 325

Voloshin A, Wosk J 1981 The influence of artificial shock absorbers on human gait. Clin Orthop 160: 52–56

Voloshin A, Wosk, Brull M 1981 Force wave transmission through the human locomotor system. J Biomech Eng 103: 48–50

Wall P D, Devor M 1978 Physiology of sensation after peripheral nerve injury, regeneration and neuroma formation. In: Waxman S G (ed) Physiology and Pathobiology of Axons. Raven Press, New York

Wall P D, Gutnik M 1974 Properties of afferent nerve impulses originating from a neuroma. Nature 248: 740

Wall P D, Sweet W H 1967 Temporary abolition of pain in man. Science 155: 108

Wallin G, Torebjork E, Hallin R 1976 Preliminary observations on the pathophysiology of hyperalgesia in the causalgic pain syndrome. In: Zotterman Y (ed) Sensory Function of the Skin in Primates. Pergamon Press, Oxford. p 489

Ward J D, Symms J M, Knight G, Boulton A J M, Sandler D A 1983 Venous distension in the diabetic neuropathic foot. J Roy Soc Med 76: 1011–1014

Weir-Mitchell S 1872 Injuries of nerves and their consequences. (Reprinted 1965), Dover Publications, New York

Wilson D H 1972 Treatment of soft-tissue injuries by pulsed electrical energy. Br Med J 2: 269–270

Withrington R H, Wynn Parry C B 1984 Management of painful peripheral nerve disorder. J Hand Surg 9: 24

Wolff 1892 Das Gesetz der Transformation der Knochen. A Hirshwald, Berlin

Wood R A B, Williams R H P, Hughes L E 1977 Foam elastomer dressing in the management of open granulating Wounds. Br J Surg 554–557

George Murdoch

Orthotics

THE FOOT AND NORMAL HUMAN LOCOMOTION

It is sufficient for our purpose to consider the part played by the foot in normal gait. The start of a gait cycle is when the heel of the swinging leg strikes the ground — 'heel strike' or 'heel contact'. Thereafter the foot goes through a period of rapid plantar flexion to the position when the foot is in contact with the ground throughout its length — 'foot flat'. At the end of this period of mid stance the heel leaves the ground — 'heel off' until the stance phase is completed by the lifting of the toe from the ground at 'toe off'. The stance phase from heel contact to toe off occupies some 60% of the gait cycle. The limb then enters the swing phase initially accelerating and towards the end of this phase decelerating just before the next cycle begins at heel contact (Fig. 57.1).

It is evident that there is a period of double support beginning when one foot is in its most stable mode, foot flat, and the other foot is toward the end of its swing, and striking the ground before heel off on the original foot occurs. The length of this period of double support varies with many factors and is of greatest duration when walking slowly. It ends with toe off on the original foot; if the foot of the swinging leg fails to make contact before toe off then the subject is no longer walking but is trotting or running.

The muscles acting on the foot clearly play a distinct role in the gait cycle; the dorsiflexors dampen the rapid plantar flexion at the ankle at heel contact produced by the lever arm of the calcaneum; the calf muscles maintain foot flat and produce an extension moment about the knee and later plantarflex the foot at heel and toe off; and finally,

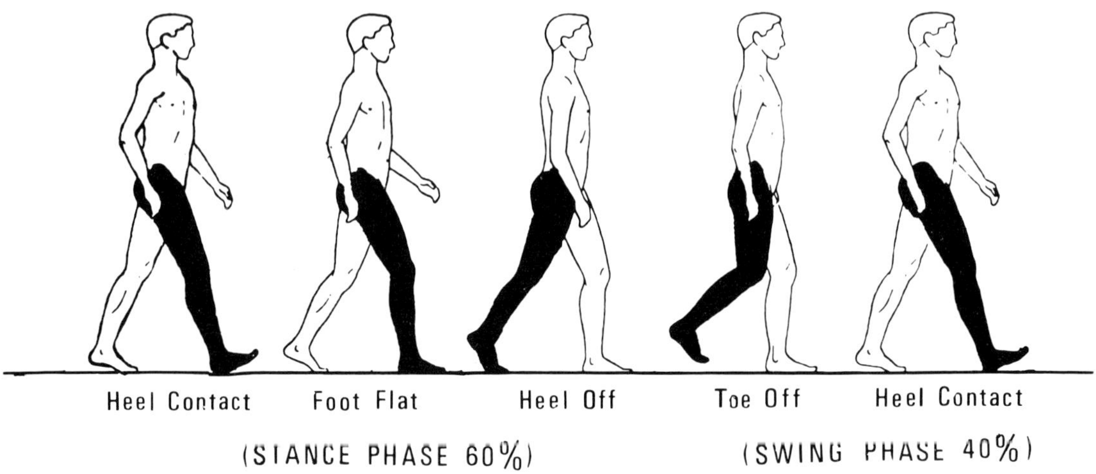

Fig. 57.1 The gait cycle

the dorsiflexors ensure toe clearance during swing (Fig. 57.2).

This interplay of function and foot position is a small but vital element of the gait cycle which is a vastly complicated system of harnessing the large forces generated to produce a very efficient and smooth locomotion (Fig. 57.3). These forces are compounded of gravity effects, muscle action and inertial effects and finally have to be absorbed by the foot in contact with the ground. We know from force plate studies the magnitude and direction of these forces. The resultant forces can be broken down into forces acting along three axes, vertical to the ground, in the line of progression and from side to side and the torque forces around the axes. Vertical force can be shown to increase steadily from heel strike to foot flat, momentarily exceeding body weight as the body mass acting through its centre of gravity loads the new stance foot. At mid stance the vertical force drops below body weight as the centre of gravity rises again.

A forward shear force occurs at heel contact and is reversed as the foot thrusts backwards; again after heel off a further force to the rear is generated.

A medial shear force can be seen as the foot comes to mid stance at which point, with the centre of gravity directly above the foot, equilibrium is established. As the cycle proceeds and the heel comes off the ground, lateral shear force becomes evident.

The convention employed above in using terms such as heel contact, foot flat and heel off etc. is hardly applicable when we consider some abnormal gaits, e.g. in the hemiplegic there may be no heel contact or toe off. In these instances 'foot presentation' and 'lift off' may be more useful terms. In abnormal gait the presentation of the foot to the ground may be due to abnormalities unconnected with the foot or directly resulting from an abnormality of the foot. This occurs in the case of a victim of division of the peroneal nerve when the foot may present the head of the fifth metatarsal and

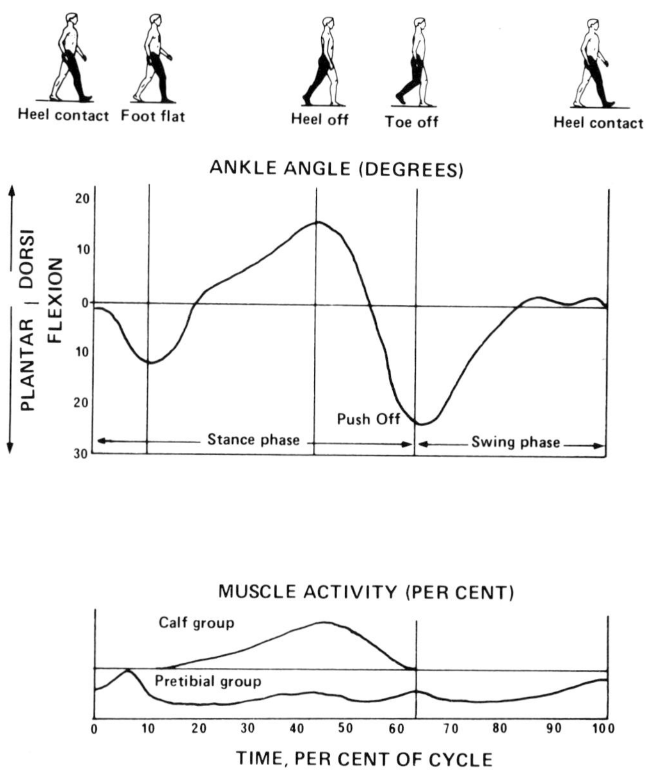

Fig. 57.2 The role of the ankle/foot muscle in the gait cycle

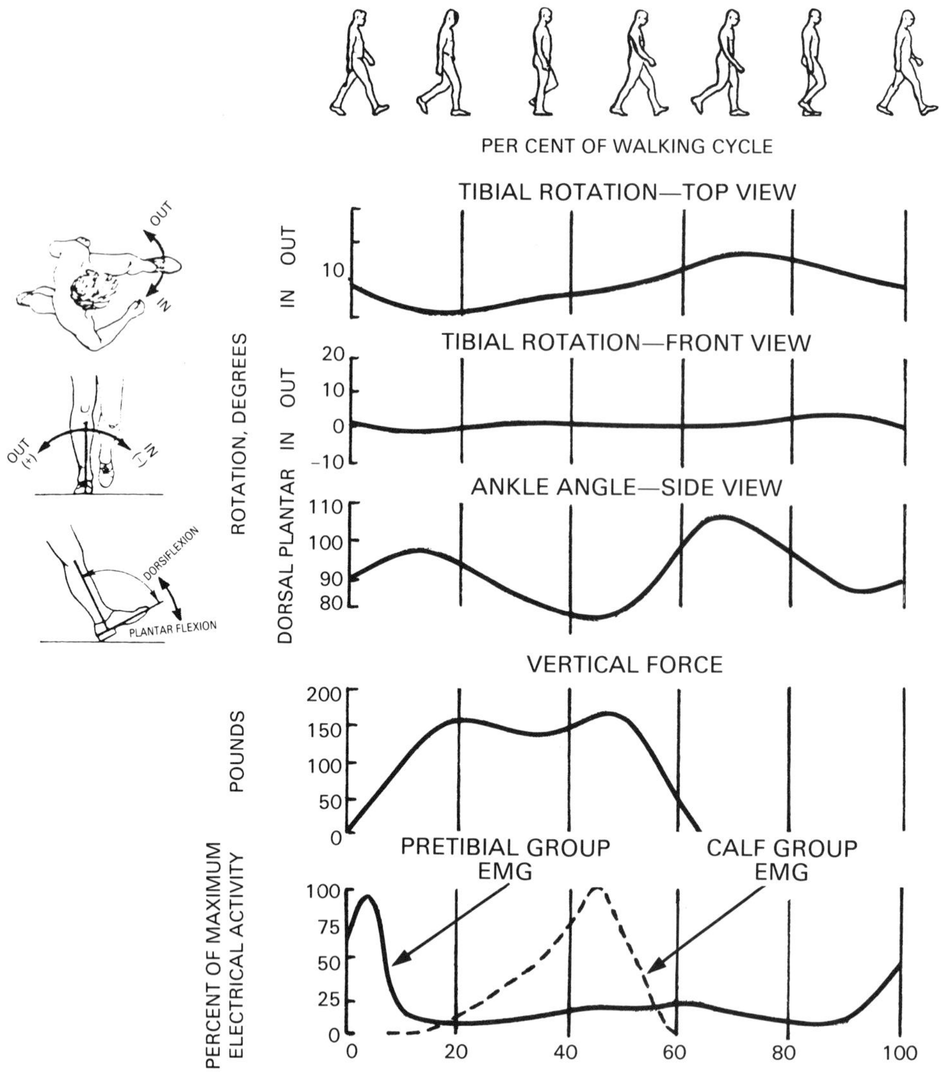

Fig. 57.3 Forces and displacements during gait

lateral border of the foot to the ground followed by the foot falling backwards into the foot flat position. Similarly, there may be no heel off phenomenon but rather a situation wherein the entire foot is lifted off at the beginning of the swing. Where there is a fixed deformity of the foot, e.g. in severe relapsed talipes equinovarus, heel contact may never be made. In all of these situations, at least in the industrial world, the boot or shoe modifies foot presentation, stance and lift off to some extent.

Foot biomechanics

It is necessary therefore to turn to the biomechanics of the foot in more detail. As noted above the role of the foot is an integral part of the biomechanics of the leg. During gait the pelvis, femur, tibia and fibula rotate around the vertical axis (Levens et al 1948); during swing and at the start of stance the leg internally rotates and thereafter reverses direction, reaching maximum external rotation just after toe off. The capacity of the foot to accommodate these movements and to fulfill its role as a stable support in one phase and as a forward propellant in another is a function of the anatomy of the ankle joint and the foot itself. The structure is such that its flexibility permits the foot to adapt to different surfaces and to accommodate to the rotational demands in swing and early stance. Equally the anatomy permits its conversion to a rigid lever arm at toe off.

The axis of the ankle joint (Fig. 57.4) subtends an angle of some 80° with the long axis of the tibia and is externally rotated by some 20–30° in relation to the knee axis. The longitudinal axis of the foot, notionally between the second and third toes, is internally rotated 6° to the axis of the ankle joint with a range of 2° internal rotation and some 7–8° external rotation (Fig. 57.5) (Hicks 1953).

Movement at the subtaloid joint is complex but at its simplest provides 'inversion' when the calcaneum is tilted towards the midline and 'eversion' when tilted away from the midline (Fig. 57.6a and b). The axis of rotation is oblique, passing as it does some 23° to the midline of the foot in the transverse plane, providing motion from 4–47°, and in the horizontal plane passing at an angle of some 41° with a range of 21–69° (Manter 1941). The effect of this disposition is that when the leg is externally rotated the calcaneus is inverted and conversely when the leg is internally rotated the calcaneus is everted.

The conjunction of joint axes of the subtaloid and midtarsal 'joints' is equally contrary and produces important effects. The so-called 'midtarsal' joint composed of the talonavicular and calcaneocuboid joints is directly affected by the attitude of the hindfoot. When everted the axes of the two joints are parallel and movement is relatively free but when the hindfoot is inverted the axes are incongruous and movement is restricted.

The net effect of those joint dispositions can be seen in the gait cycle. At foot presentation (heel contact) the leg is in internal rotation, thus the hindfoot is everted permitting movement in the longitudinal arch of the foot. As external rotation takes over in stance, the hindfoot inverts reducing movement and stabilizing the longitudinal arch. It should be noted that a coincident effect is that external rotation of the leg produces elevation of the longitudinal arch and internal rotation, a flattening.

A composite movement occurs along the line of the metatarsophalangeal joints. This 'metatarsal break' has its axis from the most distal, the second, to its most proximal, the fifth and lies somewhere

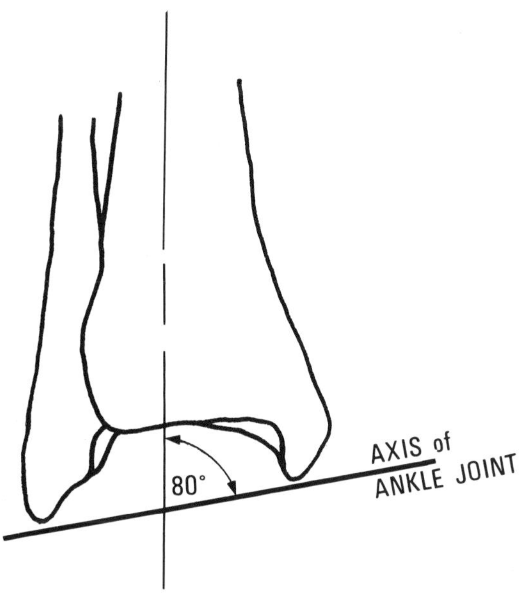

Fig. 57.4 The axis of the ankle joint

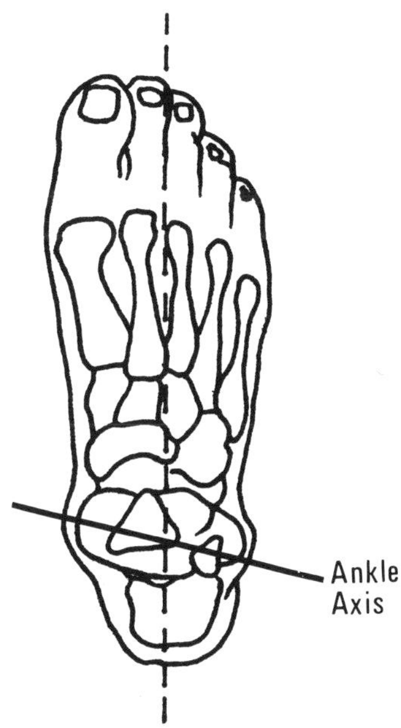

Fig. 57.5 The longitudinal axis of the foot, rotated 6° to the axis of the ankle (range 2° internal rotation, 7–8° external rotation)

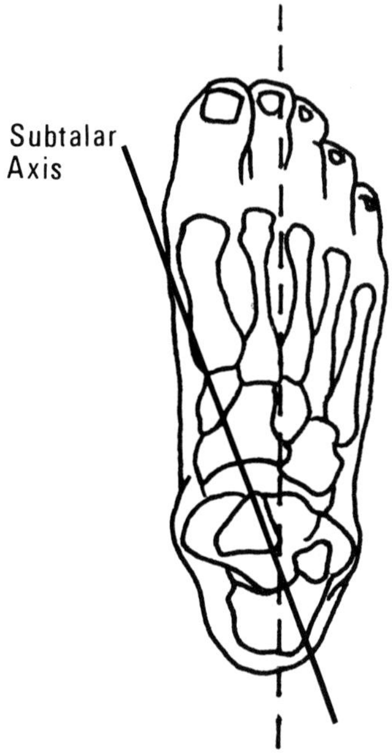

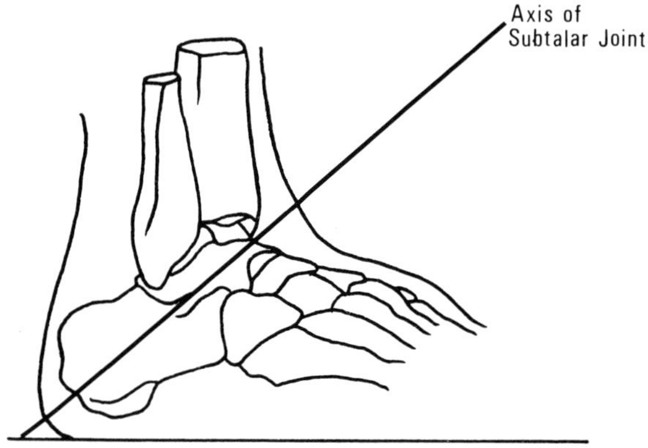

Figs. 57.6a and b The subtalar axis (a) subtends angle of 23° to the midline of the foot in the transverse plane (range of motion 4°–47°); (b) in the horizontal plane subtends angle of 41° (range of motion 21°–69°)

between 50° and 70° to the long axis of the foot (Fig. 57.7). Thus provision is made for further fine tuning in the attitude of the foot as it presents to the ground.

It will be apparent that any factor limiting or otherwise interfering with the movement of these interrelated joints may produce marked alterations to the gait.

The role of the muscles

The actions of the muscles working around the ankle joint and into the foot play an important part in foot function. The dispositions of the muscles in relation to the joints determine their function; accordingly it is obvious which muscles are involved in dorsiflexion or plantar flexion of the ankle joint. Their function in relation to eversion and inversion can be deduced by their relationship to the axis of the subtaloid joint. Similarly their distance from the axis in question will determine the efficiency of their leverage in motion about that axis.

The muscles with origins and insertions within the foot itself stiffen and stabilize the foot during the second half of the stance phase prior to heel off and toe off (Smith 1954, Inman & Mann 1964). When weakened or paralysed, clawing of the toes occurs with reduction of the 'toe lever arm'.

One other structure, the plantar aponeurosis, requires mention (Fig. 57.8) (Hicks 1954). Passing

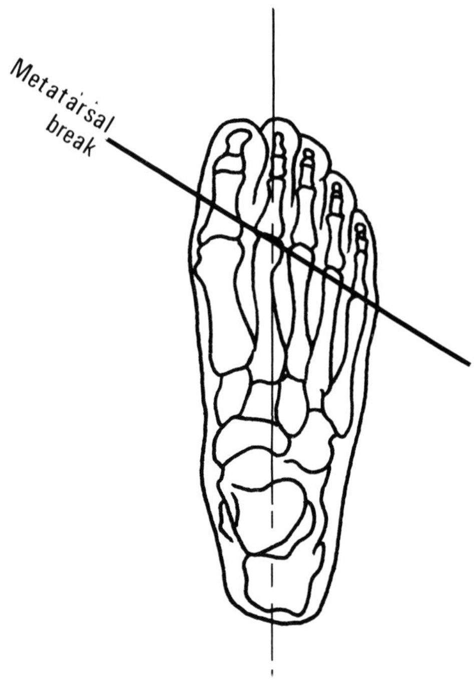

Fig. 57.7 Metatarsal break runs from the second to the 5th metatarsal, lies between 50°–70° to the long axis of the foot

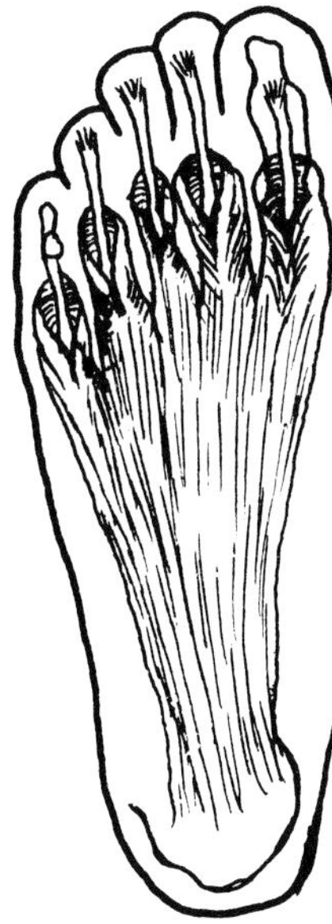

Fig. 57.8 The plantar aponeurosis

forward from the calcaneus and terminating in its extensions as they embrace the flexor tendons and help to form the plantar pads, the aponeuroses stabilize the metatarsal heads. In this way, without any muscle action as such, the arch is raised from heel off to toe off.

It will be apparent that in prescribing, designing and constructing an orthosis to influence the function, presentation or stability of the foot due recognition must be paid to the several joint axes and their interrelationship. The best example relates to any orthosis traversing the ankle joint and seeking to control it: it must be based on the best compromise for the ankle axis, i.e. a line joining the tip of the medial to the tip of the lateral malleolus. It should also reflect the relationship between the longitudinal axis of the foot and the ankle axis.

THE SHOE

In an industrial society the boot or shoe is an integral part of any orthotic system or device seeking to correct or otherwise affect the function of the foot. Shop shoes vary considerably in design, especially since the advent of a range of manmade materials. However, it is perhaps still useful to describe the component parts of the traditional shoe, although in some modern versions some of these components may be combined or even absent (Fig. 57.9a and b).

The upper includes the toe box, vamp, lace-up and tongue and heel counter. The sole consists of an insole with lining, usually a filler between the insole and the sole itself. The sole is joined to the insole by the welt, a strip of leather which ensures a smooth seamless inside to the shoe. The heel of the shoe should be broad enough to give adequate stability and be 2–3 cm in height. The shank, that part of the sole running from the heel to the ball of the shoe, should be stiff.

Where a foot problem consists of no more than unwelcome bony protruberances, a shop shoe with a decent toe box and soft upper such as suede may be sufficient especially as the accommodation necessary can be enhanced by mechanical stretching. A paralysed foot will function more effectively with a light soft shoe for easier forefoot lift off.

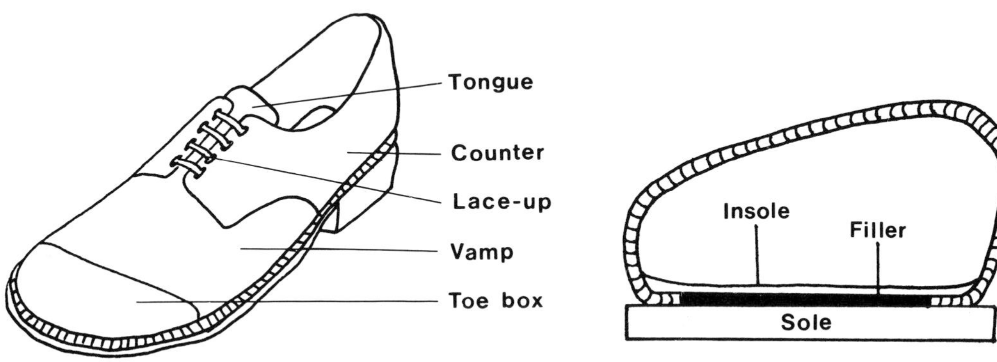

Fig. 57.9 The shoe: a, upper; b, sole

Shoe adaptations

Internal adaptations

These are easier to accommodate if the shoes are one-half to one size larger than the patient's normal footwear. They are usually fixed to the insole or to a separate and additional insole. When an additional insole is prescribed the space in the contralateral shoe should be satisfied by the provision of an additional insole without alteration. The commonly prescribed adaptations are metatarsal domes or pads and arch supports.

Metatarsal support. The metatarsal dome or support made of firm rubber or plastic material is placed just proximal to the metatarsal heads protecting principally the second, third and fourth metatarsal heads (Fig. 57.10). They also have another important effect in increasing the efficiency of the intrinsic muscles of the foot and/or the efficacy of the toe grip by inducing plantar flexion at the metatarsophalangeal joints and extension at the interphalangeal joints.

Arch supports. Arch supports are usually constructed of half domes fixed to the medial border of the insole and constructed of cork or rubber (Fig. 57.11). To be effective they must control the attitude of the heel and ensure a median position or even slight inversion. This sometimes requires a supplement in the form of an internal medial heel wedge of 2–3 mm in height.

Excavations of the heel, the insertion of soft foamed rubber and a low medial support can be effective in relieving symptoms of plantar spur.

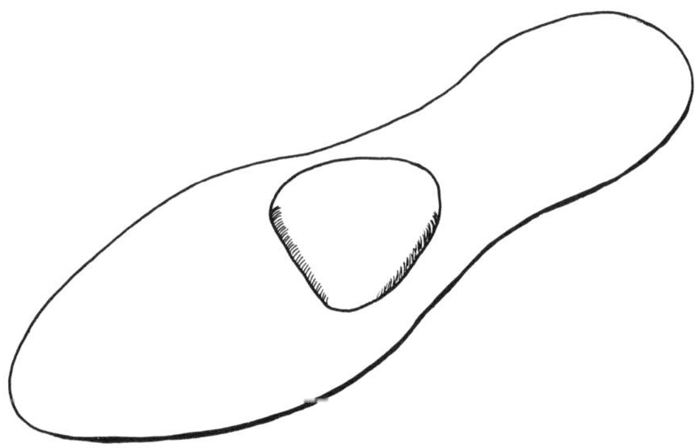

Fig. 57.10 Metatarsal dome or support

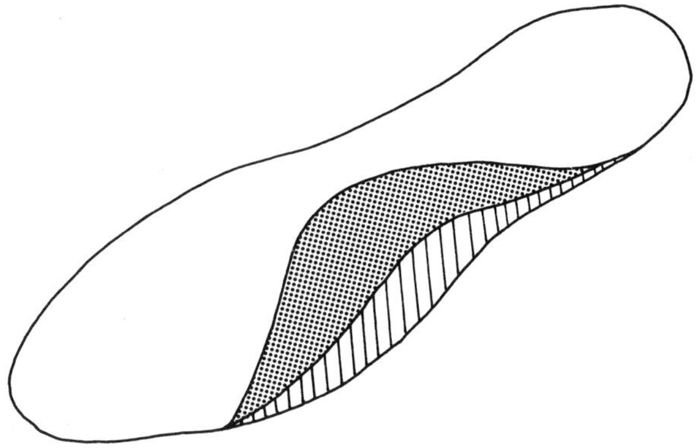

Fig. 57.11 Valgus support

External adaptations

Wedges. These adaptations typically include a variety of heel and sole wedges. External wedges by themselves are unlikely to exert any corrective force even in children but may supplement other corrective measures (Fig. 57.12). Certainly the wedge must be modest, from 3–5 mm, as otherwise the foot will slide laterally within the shoe negating any inversion effect and possibly exaggerating eversion of the heel and flattening of the foot. What they do achieve is to provide a plantigrade position for the shoe.

Floating out. The sole, heel, or both may be 'floated' out on the medial or more commonly lateral aspect to increase stability (Fig. 57.13).

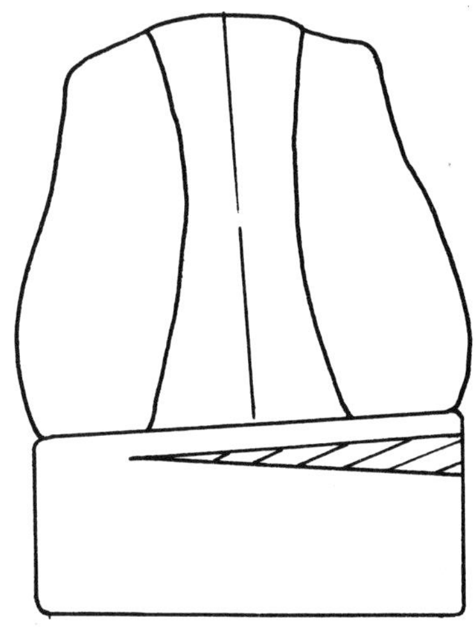

Fig. 57.12 Medial heel wedge on left shoe

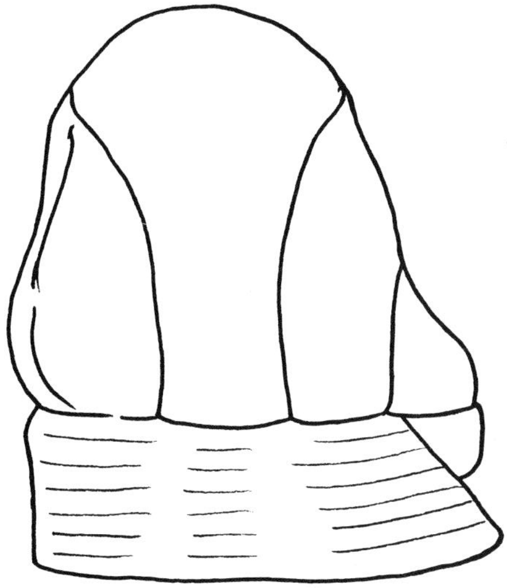

Fig. 57.13 Heel floated out on lateral aspect

Metatarsal bar. Metatarsal bars, usually of leather, are commonly prescribed to relieve pressure on the metatarsal heads; this is effected by placing them proximal to the metatarsal heads, thus producing earlier force transfer (Fig. 57.14).

Stiffeners. The sole of the shoe may be stiffened by the insertion of steel into the shank or simply by an additional sole, usually in conditions such as hallux rigidus.

Thomas heel. An anteromedial extension of the heel, the Thomas heel is commonly prescribed to provide additional support for the shank of the shoe and thus the longitudinal arch of the foot (Fig. 57.15). In the heavy patient already provided with an arch support a Thomas extension is a sensible adaptation. Floating out of the Thomas heel is sometimes prescribed to increase heel stability but the common combination of a painful valgus foot

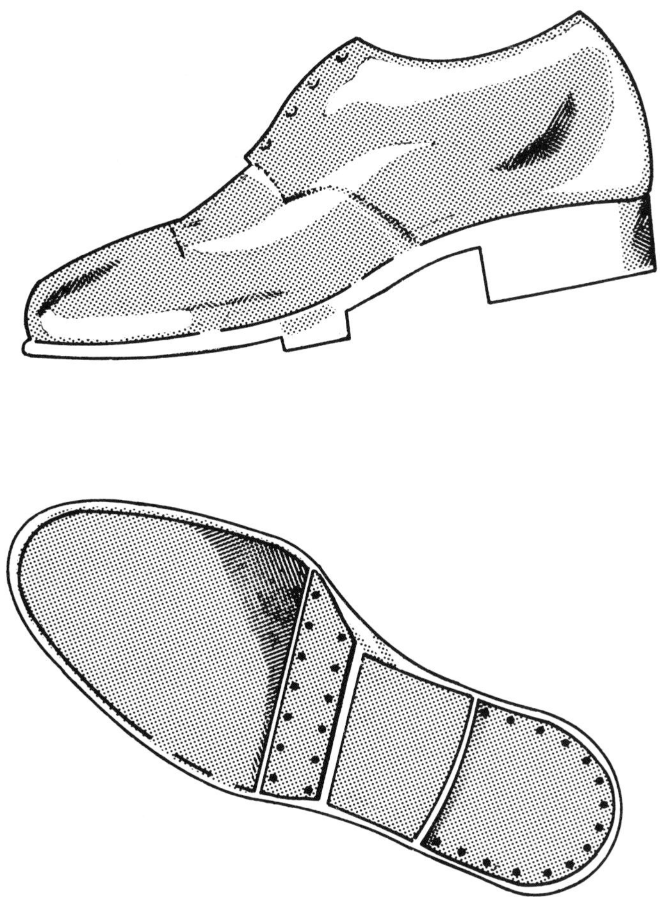

Fig. 57.14 Metatarsal bar

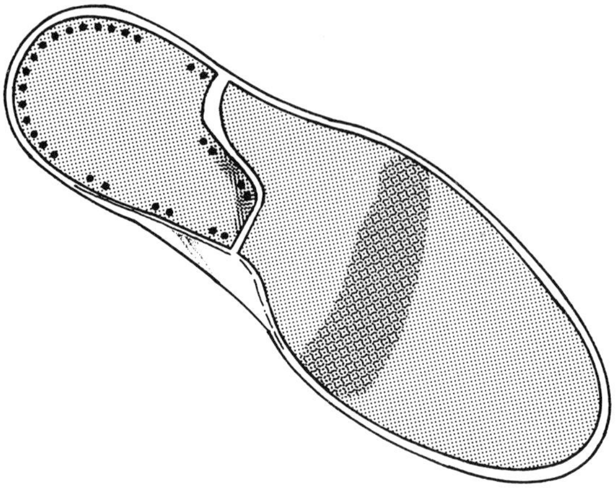

Fig. 57.15 Thomas heel

and a chronic strain of the lateral ligament of the ankle (produced by repeated involuntary heel inversion in an attempt to alleviate *medial* pain) may require floating out of the heel on the lateral aspect in addition to the Thomas heel.

Elevation of the heel in conditions affecting the Achilles tendon can be effected by a raise of 4 or 5 mm tapering forwards.

Limb discrepancy. Shortening can be compensated for by raises of heel or sole or both. Large discrepancies if fully compensated produce an ugly shoe which may be unacceptably heavy even with the judicious use of cork. In addition the sole is quite rigid thus requiring a 'rocker' surface to present to the ground (Fig. 57.16). Height compensation of the order of 15–17 mm can be achieved and for the most part be disguised by a careful sharing of adaptation — a minor reduction of the heel on the long leg, combined with a minimal raise inside the shoe and a small exterior raise of the heel on the short side.

Care should be taken when attempting to reduce the pitch of the heel by raising the sole of the shoe. If the heel counter is closely fitting as in the moccasin or non-lacing type of shoe, the change in position of the centre of gravity forces the back of the heel of the foot against the edge of the counter with consequent extreme discomfort and even blistering.

Orthopaedic shoes

A limited range of orthopaedic shoes or deep footwear is available. They are produced on a commercial basis and usually incorporate the following features (Fig. 57.17):

1. A straight inner border to the shoe
2. The forefoot is relatively broader in relation to the heel than in the normal commercial shoe
3. There is extra depth not only in the toe box, but throughout the length of the shoes to accommodate deep insoles and arch supports of up to 10 mm in depth.

The introduction of this range of shoes has materially reduced the need for individually made surgical shoes as the orthopaedic shoe with a suitable insole can usually accommodate a range of minor deformities such as hallux valgus, claw toes, etc.

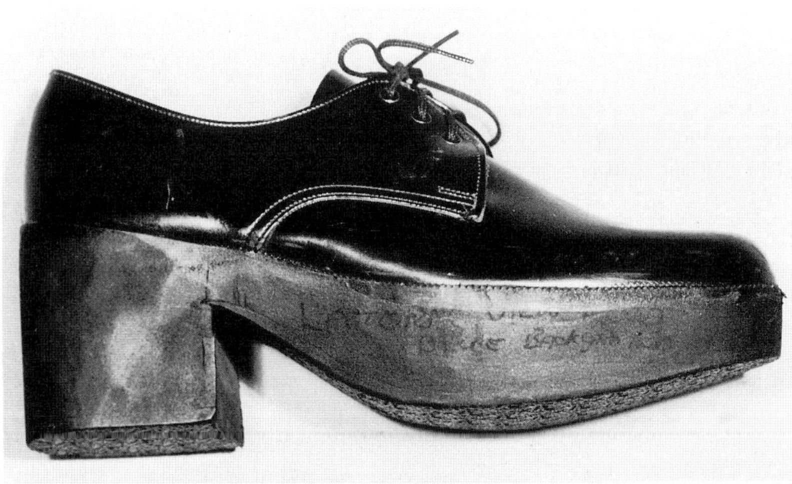

Fig. 57.16 Sole and heel raise on shop shoe — note rocker sole

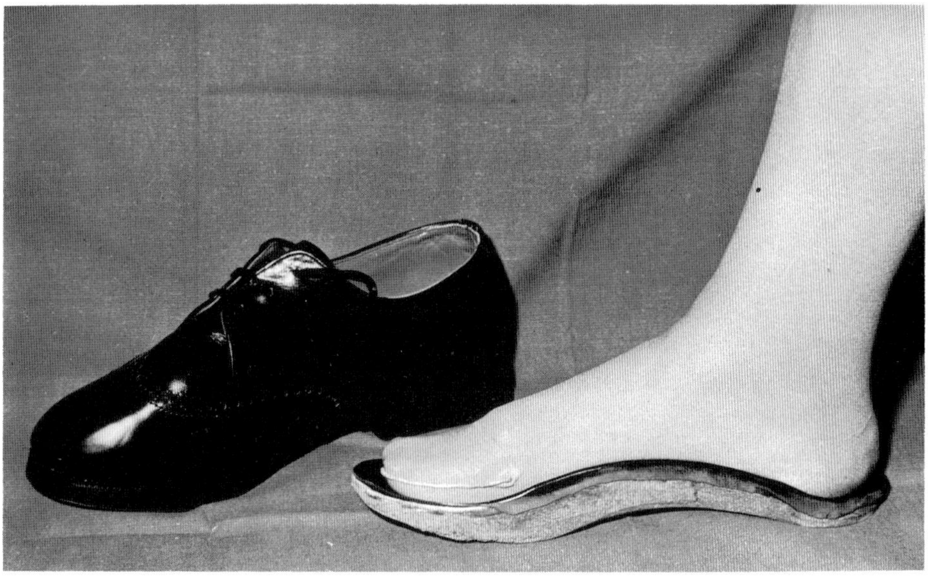

Fig. 57.17 Orthopaedic shoe with insert

Space shoes

This range of footwear, again produced on a commercial scale, is designed to accommodate feet with marked and usually rigid deformities. They usually are combined with a very thick, say 25 mm sole of resilient material — usually a rubber or polymer (Fig. 57.18a and b). The sole and other alterations within the space shoes may well be specially designed and constructed for the individual patient. Velcro fastenings readily attached and disconnected by the disabled hand are now commonly supplied rather than a lace-up fastening. Where space shoes are required for indoor use only they can be made very simply directly onto a plaster of Paris cast of the foot without any rectification. The construction is based on a moulded combined sole and heel unit, an upper of stretch material, a sponge sock and cement.

The surgical shoe and boot

This type of bespoke footwear is made for the individual patient with the objective of correcting or accommodating a foot deformity.

There are four essential elements in surgical footwear: a) the last, b) the cradle or insole, c) the upper, d) the sole — the surface presented to the ground (Fig. 57.19).

The last is the insole which determines the shape of the shoe or boot. It must ensure that the final footwear will accommodate the foot at rest, under load and in walking. It must allow for the actual height of heel required and provide as far as possible, an acceptable appearance. Whatever else it must transfer the force actions efficiently and provide comfort for the patient whether it is intended to correct or simply accommodate the foot. Lasts may be made of wood, plaster of Paris, plastic compounds or a combination of materials. They may be derived from a series of measurements and drawings or a plaster of Paris model of the foot. Whatever the method, modification of the model is required to ensure a good fit and so some dimensions are increased and others reduced to effect the best compromise to accept the changes in shape that occur in motion.

The upper may be made of a variety of materials but leather remains the material of choice because of its plasticity, elasticity and permeability. It can thus be moulded to shape, retain that shape and conversely can accommodate to the changes that take place on walking. With improved cements and cementing techniques the welt is used less and by far the majority of shoes today are made by direct attachment of the upper between the insole and sole of the shoe, and are lighter in weight and appearance.

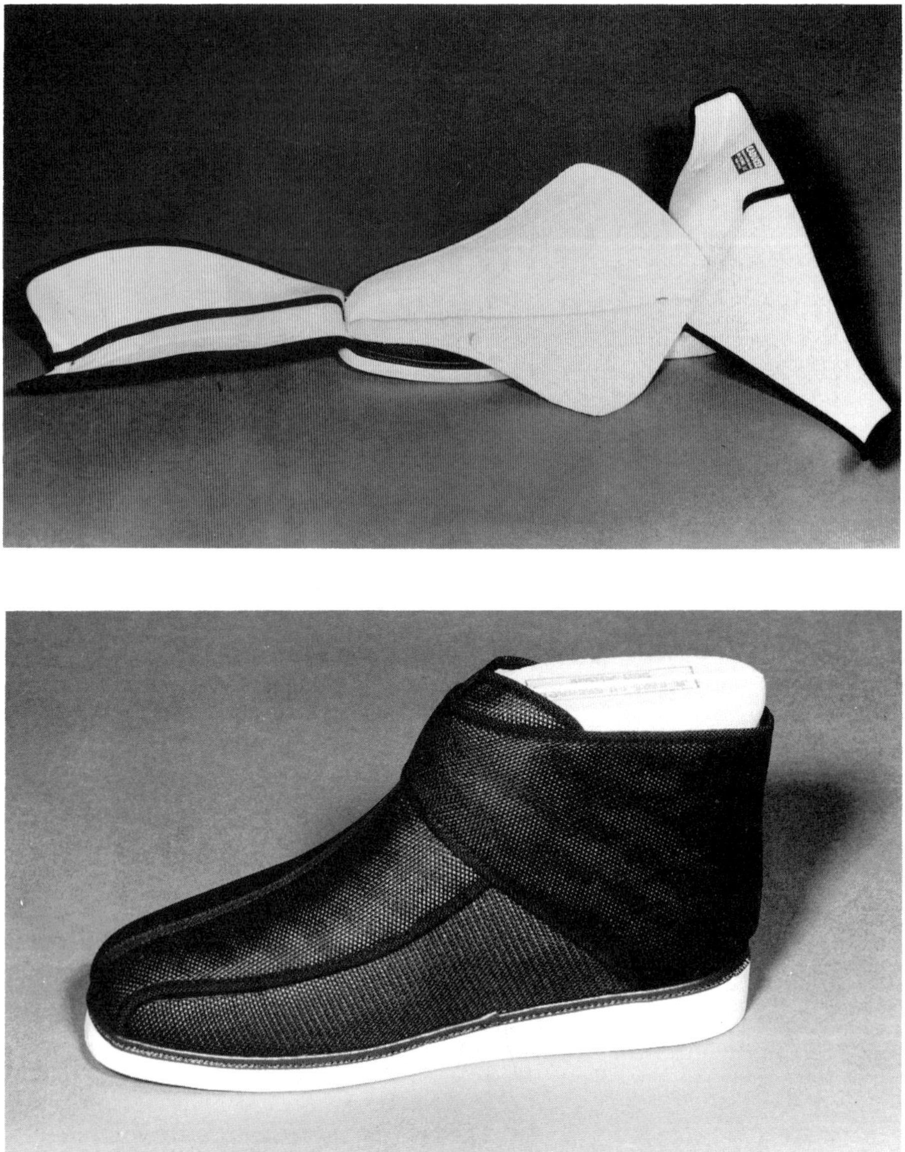

Fig. 57.18 Example of a Space shoe. a: full provision for access of foot; b: as worn

The cradle is the key to comfortable surgical footwear (Fig. 57.20a and b). The body weight is transferred to the sole and thence to the ground via the insole. It must therefore not only reflect the shape of the foot at rest but also accommodate for the changes in contour which take place under load as in standing and in the cyclic changes occurring in walking.

The sole or bottom of surgical footwear has traditionally been made of leather but many alternatives are now available. They may offer advantages in terms of lightness, wear properties, antislip characteristics or much appreciated cushioning. Nowadays the sole is fixed to the upper and insole by direct attachment using one or other of the modern cements.

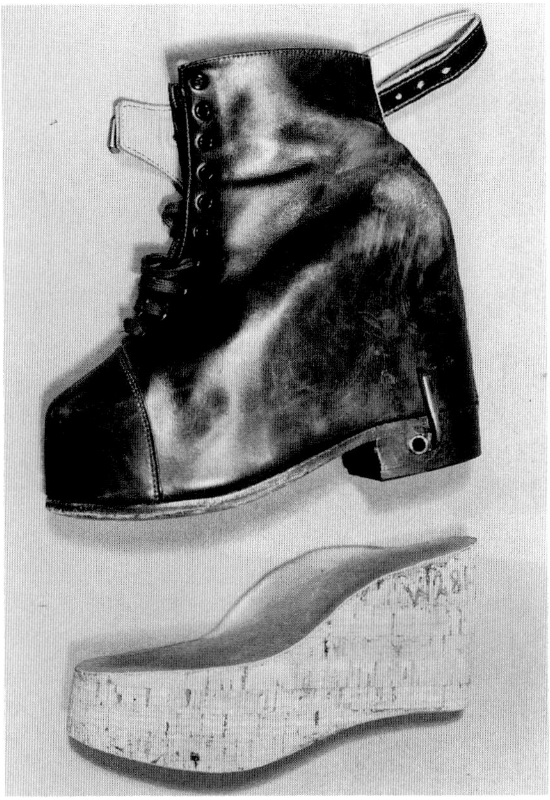

Fig. 57.19 Surgical boot demonstrating cradle and height compensation

Shop shoes with adaptations, so-called orthopaedic shoes with insoles or surgical shoes built individually may be prescribed with the objectives of either correcting deformity, preventing its deterioration or simply accommodating.

Correction can be obtained by the shaping of the last of the footwear either by itself or in combination with an ankle foot orthosis (AFO) or an even longer device. A nicely balanced prescription and design is often required as forces have to be transferred without discomfort to the patient and yet high forces may have to be employed to effect correction. It may be that full correction can be produced, for example by the examining hands, but the forces exerted are so high that surgical footwear alone cannot succeed. In these situations orthotic devices extending above the ankle may be needed or correction achieved in stages.

When the deformity is fixed and cannot be corrected except by operation then the design of the surgical footwear must be based on accommodating the deformed foot. In these circumstances the cradle conforms very closely to the contours of the foot and transfers the body weight to the sole of the shoe in a plantigrade mode thus distributing the forces as widely as possible. Because of the rigidity of the footwear cushion heels and rocker soles may be required to dampen heel contact and ensure a smooth transfer through mid stance to roll over and lift off.

Children's shoes

Generally speaking a shoe for a child should encompass a straight last and a wide toe box. The next important point is that children outgrow their shoes very rapidly, often in a matter of months. Accordingly the shoe must allow for this growth in terms of length and a generous toe box; most importantly it should have a snug fit at the heel. Lacing shoes are preferable as retention of the foot in the shoe is more readily obtained. For children with 'normal' feet a large range of entirely acceptable shoe designs are available including 'trainers' and sports shoes. The notion of the need for a firm child shoe embodying so-called orthopaedic principles remains popular but has not been proven. Equally the influence of shoe corrections on the child's foot remains clouded by myth, fashion and the concern of parents for the apparent deformities of their children's feet. Few, if any, long-term studies of the effect of these corrections exist and none provide scientific proof. Nonetheless, some shoe designs, adaptations and corrective devices require comment.

Shoe wedges usually located between sole and insole may be employed in the sole or heel or both. Maximum height should be no more than 5 mm and should be used with care — a lateral sole wedge may well tend to correct a metatarsus varus but will accentuate the commonly associated heel valgus. Again, an inner heel wedge used for arch support may do no more than aggravate a tibial torsion deformity. The Thomas extension to the heel is commonly prescribed, sometimes associated with a 5 mm medial heel wedge.

Inserted supports are available, from individually constructed valgus supports or insoles made of cork or rubber to shelf items like the heel cup (Fig. 57.21) (Helfet 1957) which seeks to control the attitude of the calcaneum.

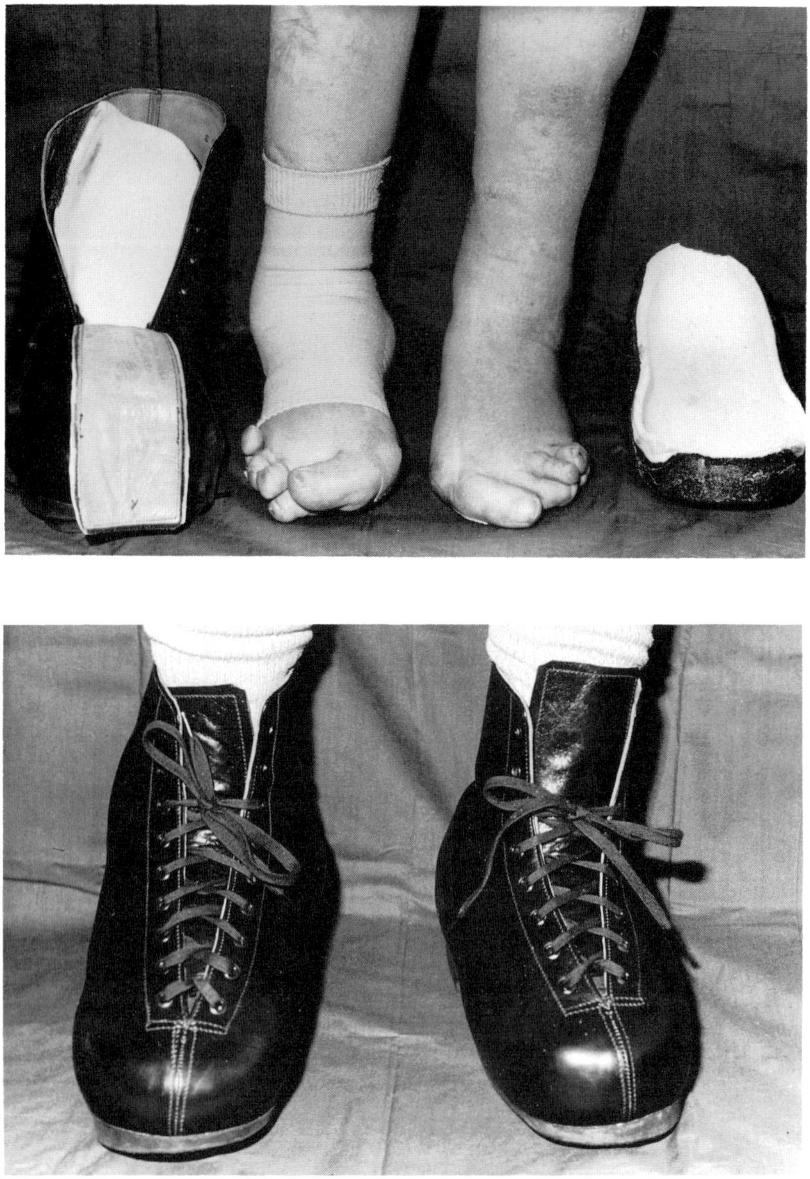

Fig. 57.20 Rheumatoid arthritis with fixed deformities. a: demonstrating cradles; b: fitted boots

ORTHOTIC COMPONENTS

Ankle joints

A free movement ankle joint consists of a side bar and joint made of aluminium or a variety of steels. It provides the basis for controlling varus or valgus by an anchoring strap.

Other ankle joints are available which permit ankle movement in one direction but limit it in the other. A solid ankle joint preventing all ankle movement would normally require the addition of soft heel to dampen heel contact and a rocker sole to aid roll over and toe off.

T and Y ankle straps

Usually made of leather, these adaptations are sewn onto the medial or lateral aspect of shoe at the level of

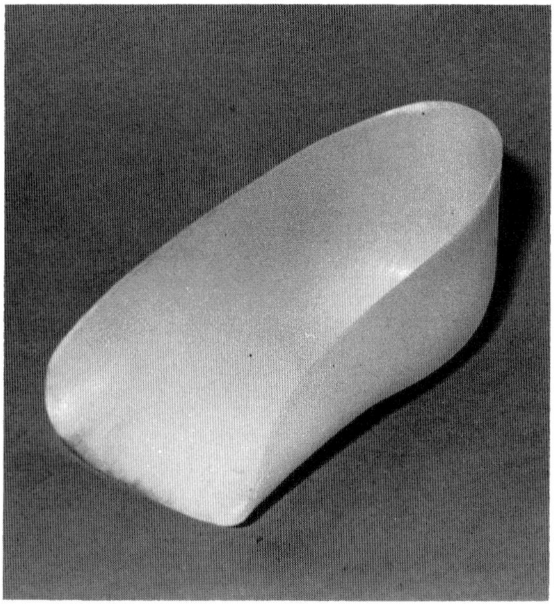

Fig. 57.21 Heel cup

the shank and encircle the ankle to be fastened around a rigid bar on the opposite side thus exerting an inversion or eversion force on the shoe for transmission to the foot (Fig. 57.22).

Moulded inserts

These are usually based on a plaster of Paris model of the foot and are made of thermoplastic material such as polypropylene (Fig. 57.23). They control the posture of the foot and can be used on their own or in conjunction with a bar orthosis (Inman 1969).

An increasing number of these inserts are prefabricated; in these instances they must be selected with care.

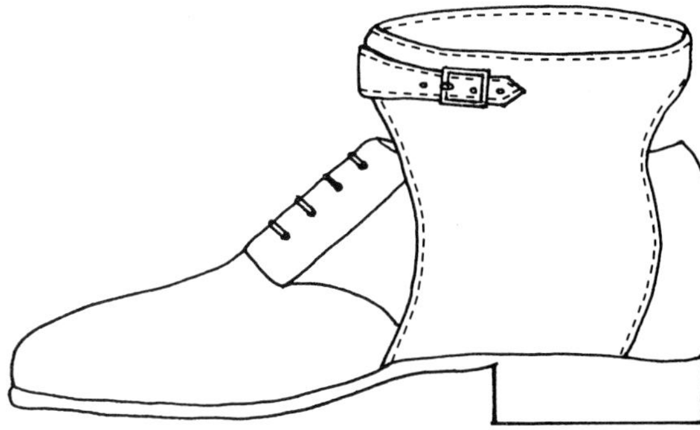

Fig. 57.22 Medial T-strap

Double-bar AFO

This device can be used to prevent foot drop or to limit or stop plantar flexion (Fig. 57.24). T-straps are commonly added to control varus or valgus.

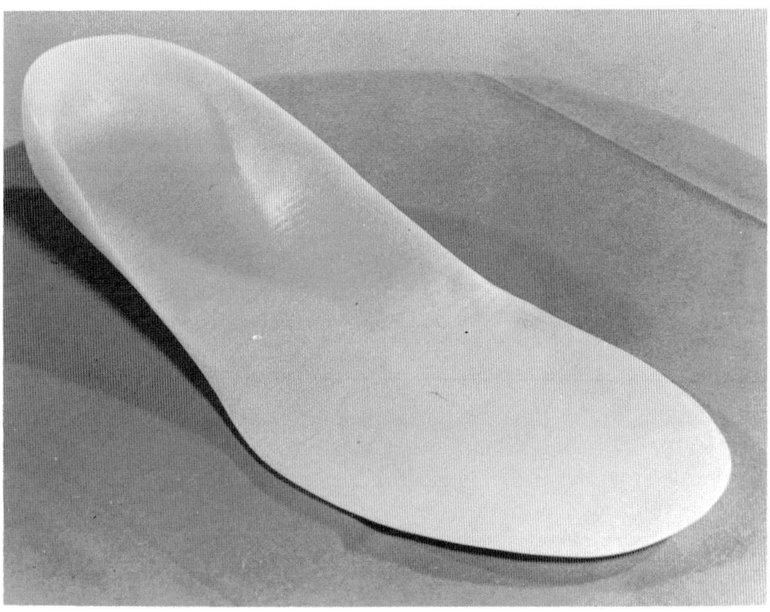

Fig. 57.23 Moulded insert

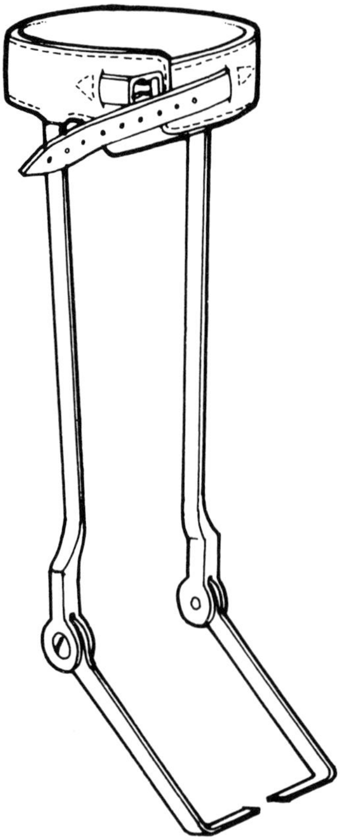

Fig. 57.24 Double bar AFO with ankle joints. This design is preferable to side irons tubed into the heel of the shoe

A variety of the double bar AFO still prescribed has the side irons tubed into the heel of the shoe with or without anterior and/or posterior stops to control the degree of plantar or dorsiflexion. This device should not be prescribed as the axis of movement is not consonant with the axis of the ankle. Furthermore, the stops need repeated adjustment to maintain the required functional control.

Single-bar AFO

This may be prescribed for a similar purpose as a double-iron AFO. It is clearly lighter and when used on the lateral aspect damage to the contralateral ankle is avoided. There is little control of movement of the foot inside the shoe if used without a moulded insert.

All bar AFOs require care in aligning the joints to accommodate tibial torsion.

Plastic shell AFO

By employing the appropriate material and matching the design to the requirements it is possible to produce whatever function is desired. All are constructed over a plaster of Paris model of the lower leg and foot. All are worn inside the shoe or boot.

Rigid AFO

This device blocks all movement at ankle and subtaloid joints and markedly restricts movement in the remainder of the foot (Fig. 57.25). It may be laminated using polyester, fibreglass and nylon stockinette or made out of a sheet plastic such as polypropylene. The movement blocking effect is achieved by choosing thicker material and by the trim line. Strapping with Velcro closure completes the orthosis. As with more conventional braces which block ankle movement a cushion heel and rocker sole on the shoe is required.

Flexible AFO

A very light weight unobtrusive AFO to maintain dorsiflexion of the foot in swing but otherwise permit movement can be constructed using another plastic, Ortholen (Fig. 57.26). It is available as a preformed leaf spring which can then be heat moulded over the cast and trimmed as required. Minor adjustments can be made by a heat gun or by cold forming.

Where more control of the foot is required in addition to maintaining dorsiflexion, polypropylene, pioneered by Gordon Yates (1968), is the material of choice. It can be obtained in a variety of thicknesses and thus, along with precise trimming the exact amount of movement required can be achieved. The material is so resistant to fatigue that flexion at ankle level can be provided sufficient to give a smooth roll over in stance and yet rupture of the material may not occur for years. Yet another version, the TIRR (Texas Institute for Rehabilitation and Research) (Engen 1971) device uses polypropylene with reinforcing corrugations posteriorly making for a light but durable orthosis (Fig. 57.27). This AFO has been well received but it does require more time to fabricate and for many patients offers no more

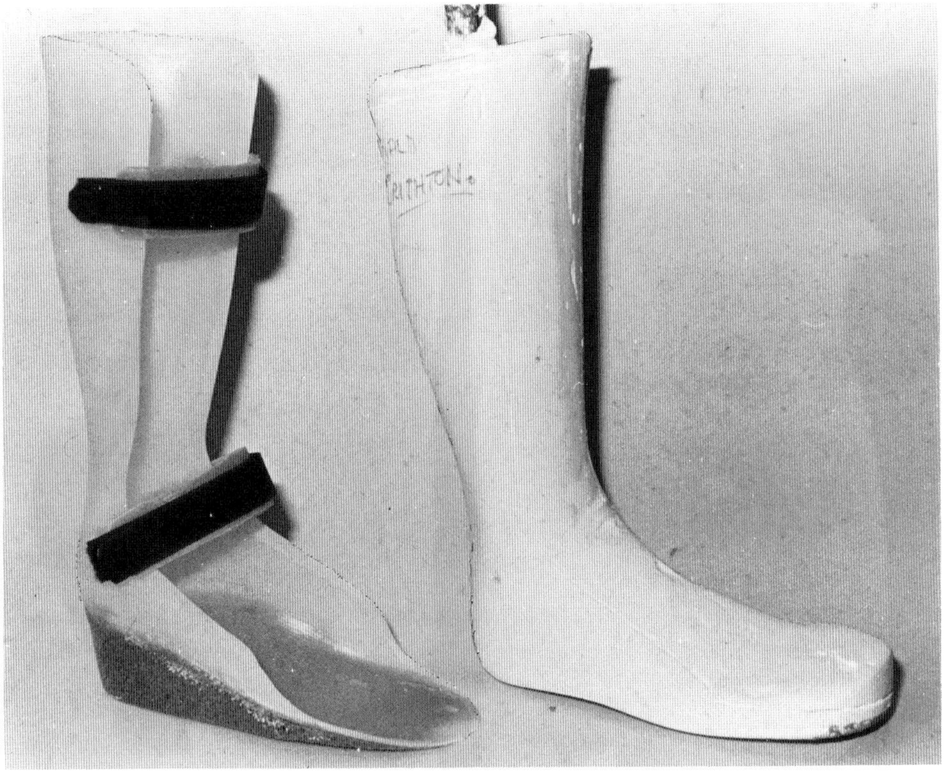

Fig. 57.25 Rigid AFO made of polypropylene. In this instance there is an additional heel wedge to accommodate an equinus deformity

advantages than a polypropylene AFO without corrugation but with carefully chosen thickness and precise trimming.

The plastic Hemispiral Below Knee Orthosis designed at the Institute of Rehabilitation Medicine, New York University Medical Center (Lehneis 1972), provides for transverse rotation as well as movement in the frontal and sagittal planes (Fig. 57.28). The material is transparent and springy and composed of an acrylic nylon. The spiral configuration permits controlled plantar flexion and dorsiflexion. At heel contact the spiral unwinds allowing plantar flexion and from foot flat onwards the forward movement of the leg over the foot is assisted by the spiral as it returns to its unstressed position and then as dorsiflexion takes place energy is stored and then released from heel off to toe off. In swing the stiffness of the device prevents plantar flexion and ensures toe clearance.

The device is indicated for patients who lack overall muscle power in the ankle/foot complex. It is lightweight and the shoe insert portion provides a built in foot support with moderate mediolateral stability. Patients find it aesthetically pleasing. It has to be said that it is a difficult brace to fabricate, trim and fit and requires experience to avoid stress concentration at the point where the brace turns from the leg into the foot. Its virtues are perhaps best seen in the case of the hemiplegic patient.

Finally the Patellar Tendon Bearing AFO (McIlmurray & Greenbaum 1958) (Fig. 57.29a and b) offers a method of partially unloading the foot and ankle while retaining, if required, some plantar and dorsiflexion. It derives its name from the below-knee prosthesis described by Radcliffe & Foort (1961) and its design is based on similar principles. Anteroposterior forces are transferred through the patellar tendon in front and the flattened, broad calf at the back. Mediolaterally, forces are transferred through the flare of the medial tibial condyle and the anterolateral muscle mass and fibula. The design has developed considerably since first described and in

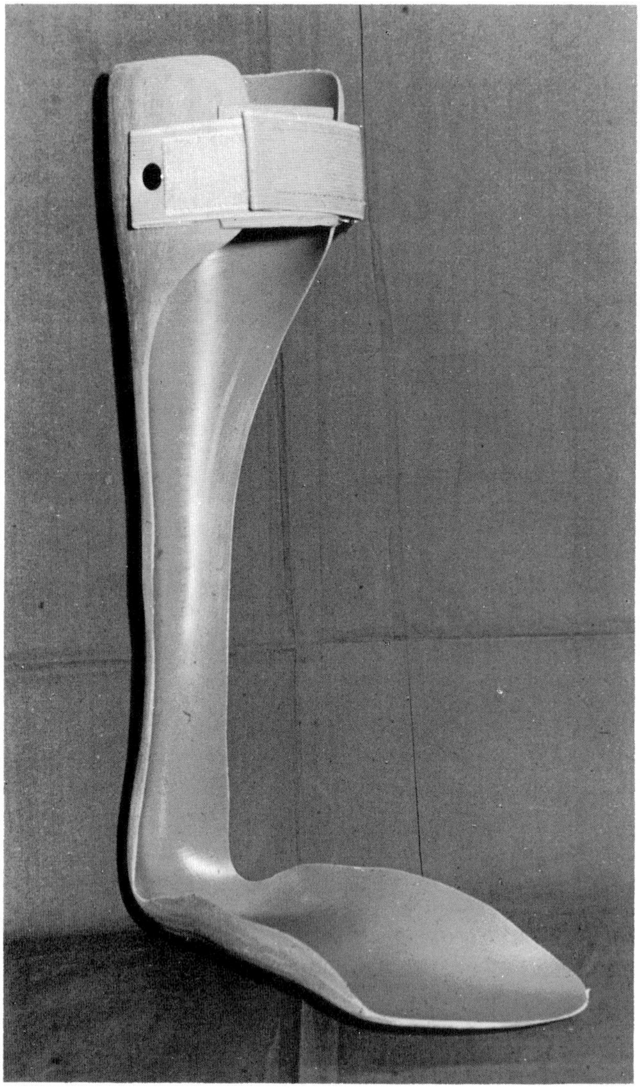

Fig. 57.26 Flexible AFO using Ortholen®

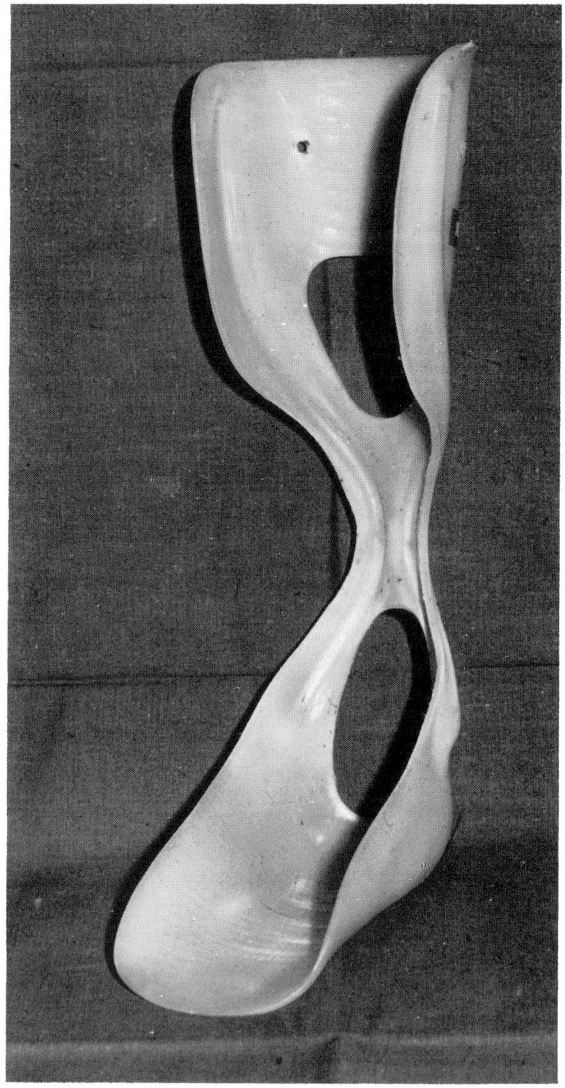

Fig. 57.27 TIRR AFO

our hands is made entirely of polypropylene. Only a proportion of the ground reaction forces can be transferred through the brace and to do so requires considerable skill. The degree of unloading also depends on the tolerance of the tissues and the amount of movement permitted at the ankle. Short of a long leg brace with tuber bearing, it is virtually the only alternative to surgery for some patients with painful arthritis of the ankle and hindfoot joints or full thickness skin loss of the heel pad.

The importance of an accurate fit of any orthosis with the leg and foot is clear. Platts et al (1979) point out that it is equally important to so shape the device externally that it fits the shoe as well. They describe their method of construction and underline that the orthotist should have access to the intended footwear before making the orthosis.

Conditions amenable to orthotic management

Genu valgum

Shoe alterations have no place in the management of

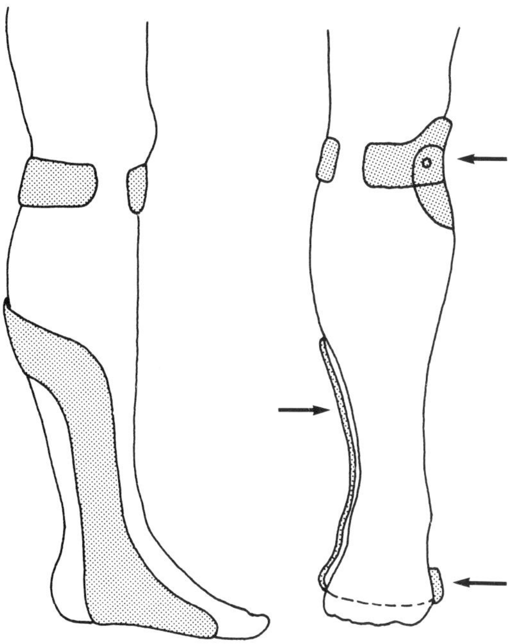

Fig. 57.28 Hemispiral brace. Note 3 point pressure system as embodied in design

infantile knock knee. If there is a coincident flat foot, a 3 or 4 mm medial wedge on a Thomas heel may improve the gait. In older age groups a knock knee deformity of substance requires a long leg brace or surgery. The alterations will exert no corrective influence although a coincident pes plano valgus may merit alterations.

Genu varum

The bow legs of infancy correct spontaneously and no shoe alterations are required.

Tibial torsion

There is no evidence that a shoe alteration or insole influences this deformity or its possible spontaneous recovery. When persistent in the older child valgus of the foot may appear and be sufficient to merit a Thomas heel and, if the child is heavy, an arch support.

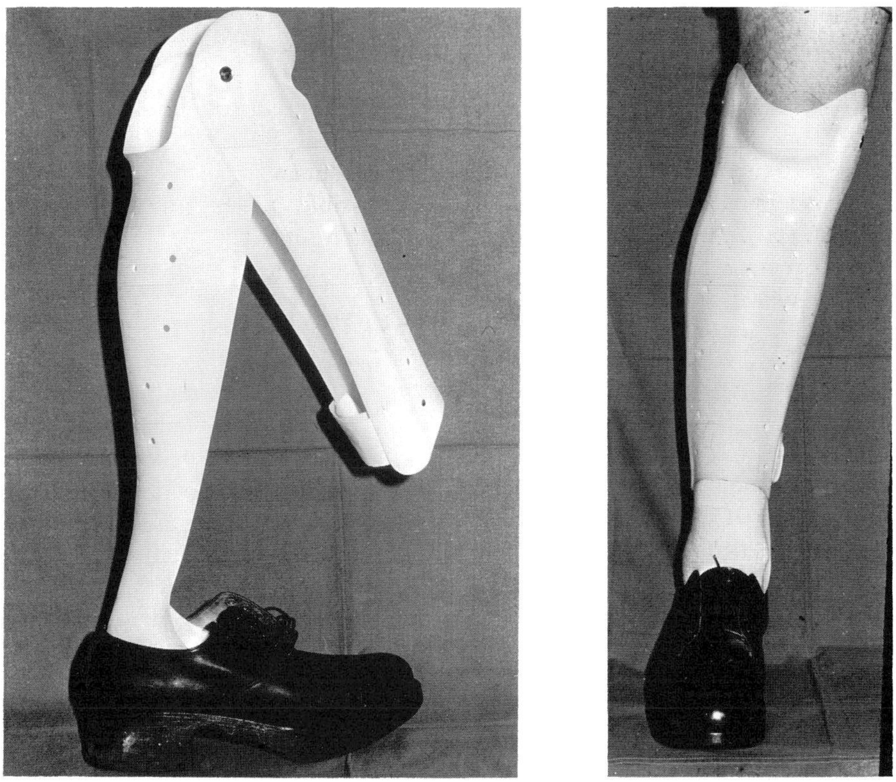

Fig. 57.29 PTB AFO demonstrating (a) method of access and (b) the close fitting nature of the brace

Congenital talipes calcaneovalgus

Where all muscles are active and the foot fully mobile albeit with increased plantar flexion spontaneous correction is the rule. The child should be examined some 6–12 months after weight bearing has started and, if any calcaneovalgus remains, a 5 mm inside raise to the heel can be prescribed.

Pes plano valgus

This is perhaps the commonest foot 'condition' seen in children. In fact some foot valgus is a normal finding. Morley (1957) found that 97% of children under 18 months old were flatfooted while only 4% of 10-year-old children were flatfooted. This strong tendency to spontaneous correction as part of normal development points to the primary requirement of reassuring the parents and advising them on the choice of footwear with particular reference to a snug heel grip, a firm shank and sufficient room in the toe box. Examination of the child sometimes aided by radiographs of the foot should exclude abnormalities such as a short Achilles tendon or a varus or cavus forefoot, where the heel valgus is secondary. Examination of the shoe may reveal undue wear on the medial side, or a broken medial counter at the heel.

Sharrard (1958) lists four circumstances in which he will recommend shoe alterations, including pain, a deformed shoe counter, failure to restore the longitudinal arch on tiptoe, and undue wear of the heel of the shoe on the inner side. The author's own inclination in these circumstances is not to prescribe wedges affixed to a normal shoe although they are acceptable as an integral part of the shoe design. The shank of the shoe needs to be stiff to control the foot attitude and depending on the age and/or weight of the patient this can be achieved by a steel insert, additional leather stiffening or simply a Thomas heel extension. Where there is a gross valgus of the hindfoot with a break at the talonavicular, or the naviculocuneiform joint even these supports may not be sufficient and virtual destruction of the shoe is inevitable. In these circumstances, short of surgery, an outside bar with inside T-strap or preferably a moulded AFO or insert will offer the only control.

Congenital tarsal coalition

Whether talocalcaneal or, more commonly, calcaneonavicular the condition usually presents as the so-called 'spastic flat foot' in the early teens. A lateral iron and inside T-strap is commonly needed after immobilization or as part of the management following excision of the cartilaginous or bony bar. Thomas heels with or without valgus supports may be employed later on a permanent basis.

Talipes equinovarus

This developmental abnormality has been known since the beginning of medical history. The management of the deformity consisting of equinus, adduction and inversion of the hindfoot and adduction and inversion of the forefoot has over the years developed on the basis of manipulation and splintage. Setting aside the question of operative treatment and its timing, once manipulation has achieved its objectives the position is maintained by adhesive strapping. With the advent of modern plastics the strapping can be replaced by a device located over the flexed knee and retaining the foot in valgus (Fig. 57.30a and b) (Lyquist 1976). Being thermoplastic the splint can be adjusted to take advantage of improvements obtained by manipulation.

The choice of techniques, strapping or splintage, will depend on how often manipulation is to be carried out and available orthotic expertise. As soon as possible, usually 2 or 3 months from birth, Reimann & Lyquist (1970) recommend that a dynamic splint be employed. Their design is based on Manter's (1941) observation on the precise axis about which pronation and supination take place — the axis deviates independently in relation to the longitudinal axis of the foot and forms an angle of 42° with the horizontal plane (see Fig. 57.6). The joint arrangements follow this compromise and permit adjustment about 'ankle' and 'subtalar' joints. Because of the modular form of the design and the range of sizes available, Lyquist maintains that some 90% of children in the age group 3–60 months can be fitted satisfactorily (Fig. 57.31).

For the older child Denis Browne boots to maintain forefoot abduction with variable degrees of abduction determined by an adjustable bar joining the boots, can be used (Fig. 57.32). When ambulant these same boots may be used or alternatively boots may be worn on the opposite feet with wedges on sole

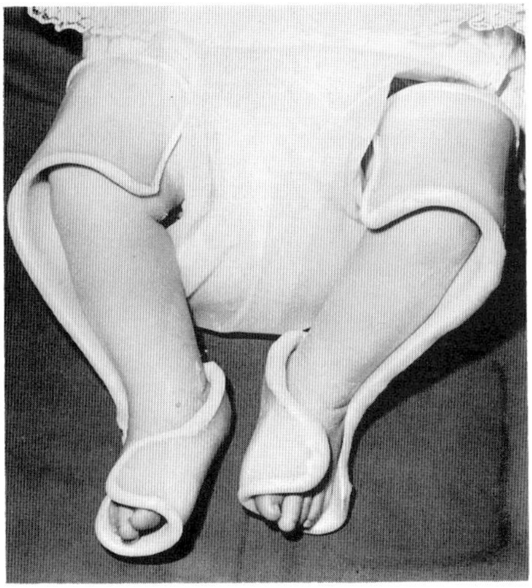

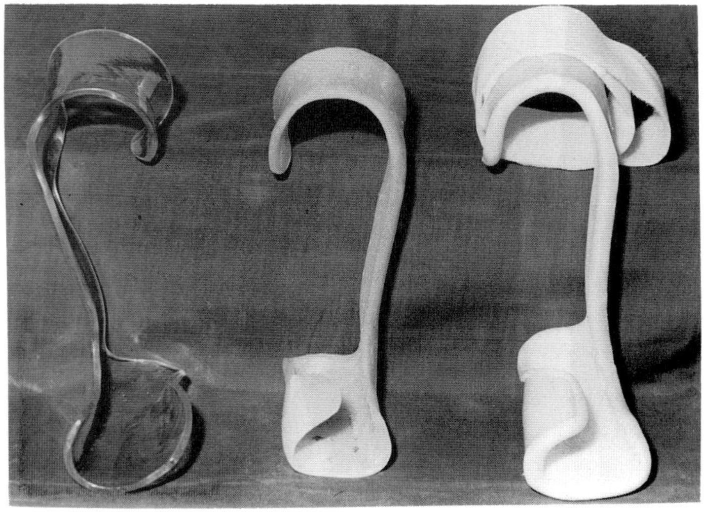

Fig. 57.30 a: Plastic devices holding feet in the corrected position b: alternatives

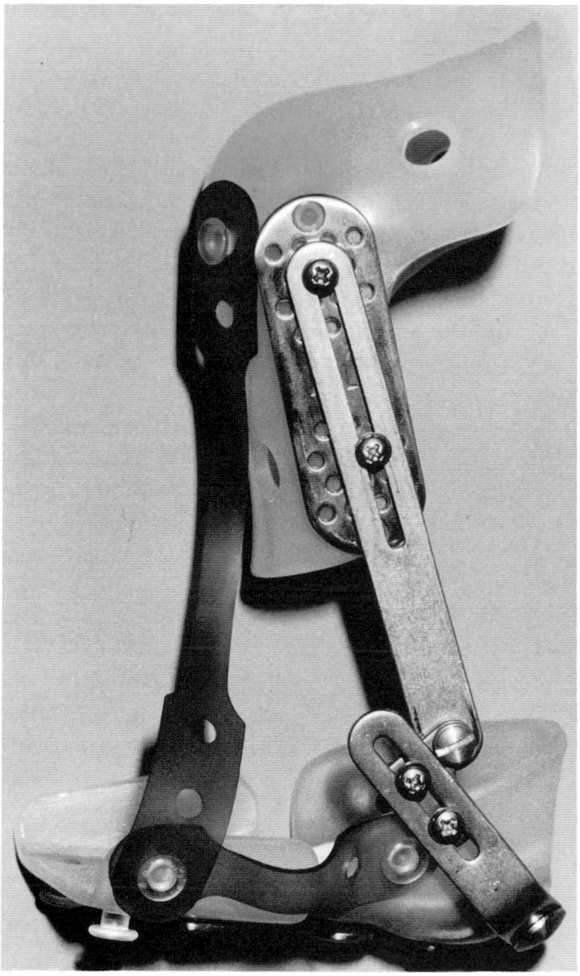

Fig. 57.31 Lyquist dynamic splint

and heel initially medial, working on the lateral side of the foot.

As with all orthoses an accurate fit is essential for control. It is difficult to ensure such control with Denis Browne boots and splints. It is also doubtful if any orthosis is really effective in correcting the deformity. However, Reimann & Lyquist (1970) believe that the dynamic club foot splint influences the tension in the tissues, the muscles and the ligaments in such a way that the foot becomes 'softer' at a much greater rate.

Finally, with the thermoplastic materials now available it seems sensible to use individually designed polypropylene AFOs controlling with accuracy the correction obtained by manipulation with strapping or following operative correction. It is appreciated that it is not always possible to implement this regime — there must be competent orthotists available.

Cerebral palsy

The hypotonic child. In myotonia, joint laxity may occur resulting in valgus feet on standing. AFOs will prevent feet going into valgus and may aid knee stability; a standing frame or baby walker will further extend the child's environment.

The dystonic child. The persistent tendency to equinus foot attitude may prevent rising to stand, standing balance and controlled walking and, of course, if persistent and untreated, result in fixed

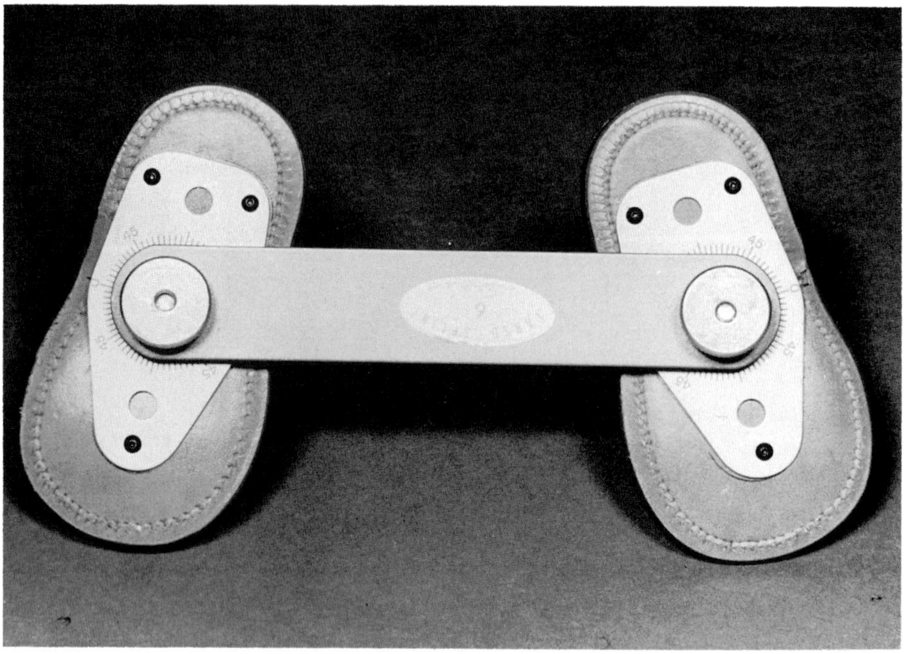

Fig. 57.32 Dennis Browne boots

equinus at the ankle, dorsiflexion at midfoot and a fully developed rocker-bottom foot. Furthermore, the equinus deformity will ensure an extension moment about the knee producing repeated sudden forced extension in walking and ultimately joint laxity and hyperextension.

The use of an AFO to prevent equinus, indeed to maintain a slightly dorsiflexed attitude, induce knee flexion, establish balance and smooth out gait should be considered seriously irrespective of any other treatment regime (Fig. 57.33a and b). At the least the AFO can alter materially the biomechanical environment to the child's benefit without causing any harm. This view had developed after an extended clinical experience by the Dundee Clinic Team as outlined by Meadows et al (1980). It is also the basis of a number of opinions and recommendations expressed in this section on cerebral palsy.

The spastic child. It is in this stage that contractures are most likely to occur due to muscle imbalance and hypertonicity. Accordingly the wearing of AFOs even when the child is at rest should be encouraged. AFOs may be used to reduce contractures by use during both day and night. It is not necessary to attempt to overcorrect but simply to ensure that the child's foot is held in maximum dorsiflexion. Serial AFOs over some months may be required.

Where surgery to lengthen the Achilles tendon is deemed necessary the use of AFOs postoperatively in maximum dorsiflexion and inversion is desirable after removal of plaster both during the night and at rest periods.

Care is required in the use of AFOs in dealing with contractures. A mild contracture of the soleus can be overcome by serial AFOs with increasing dorsiflexion but a contracture of gastrocnemius requires special care. If a cast is taken with the knee flexed and thereby some dorsiflexion gained, subsequent extension of the knee will generate large forces possibly resulting in plantarflexion of the hindfoot and the production of a rocker-bottom foot.

When a valgus deformity appears it cannot be solved by the inclusion of a valgus support in the AFO; rather, better results are obtained by ensuring some inversion in the foot piece of the AFO (Fig. 57.34a, b and c). In casting the AFO the foot should first be fully plantarflexed, then fully inverted and only then, dorsiflexed. With younger children it is usually better to cast when lying down. In those patients who still exhibit primitive neurological reactions the prone position is preferable.

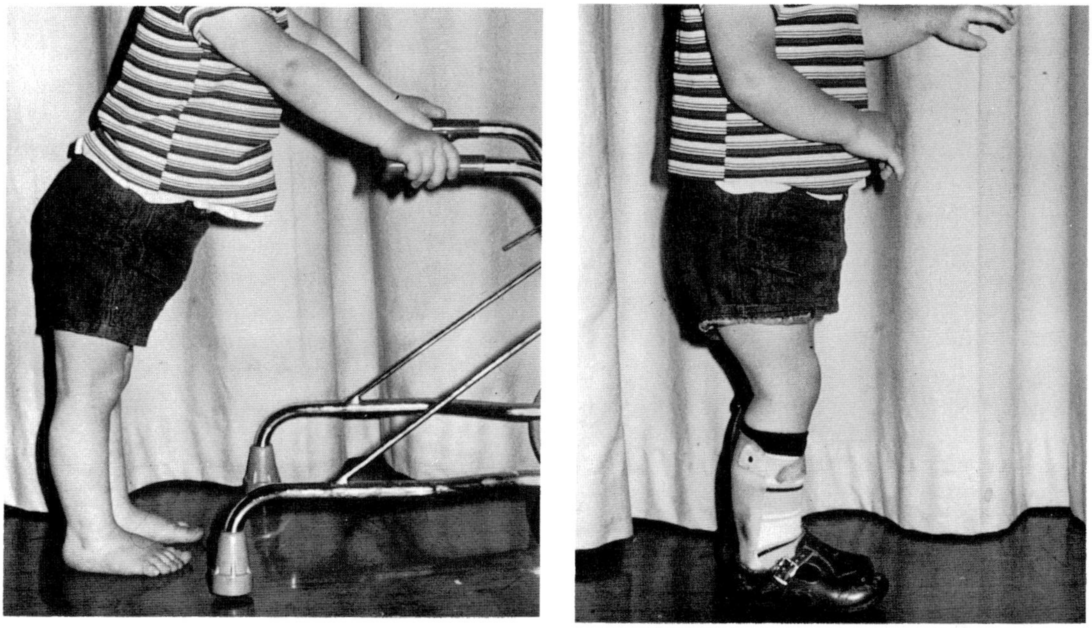

Fig. 57.33 Cerebral palsy. a: typical standing posture with hyperextended knees and inability to balance; b: fitting of AFOs prevents equinus, induces knee flexion and establishes good standing balance

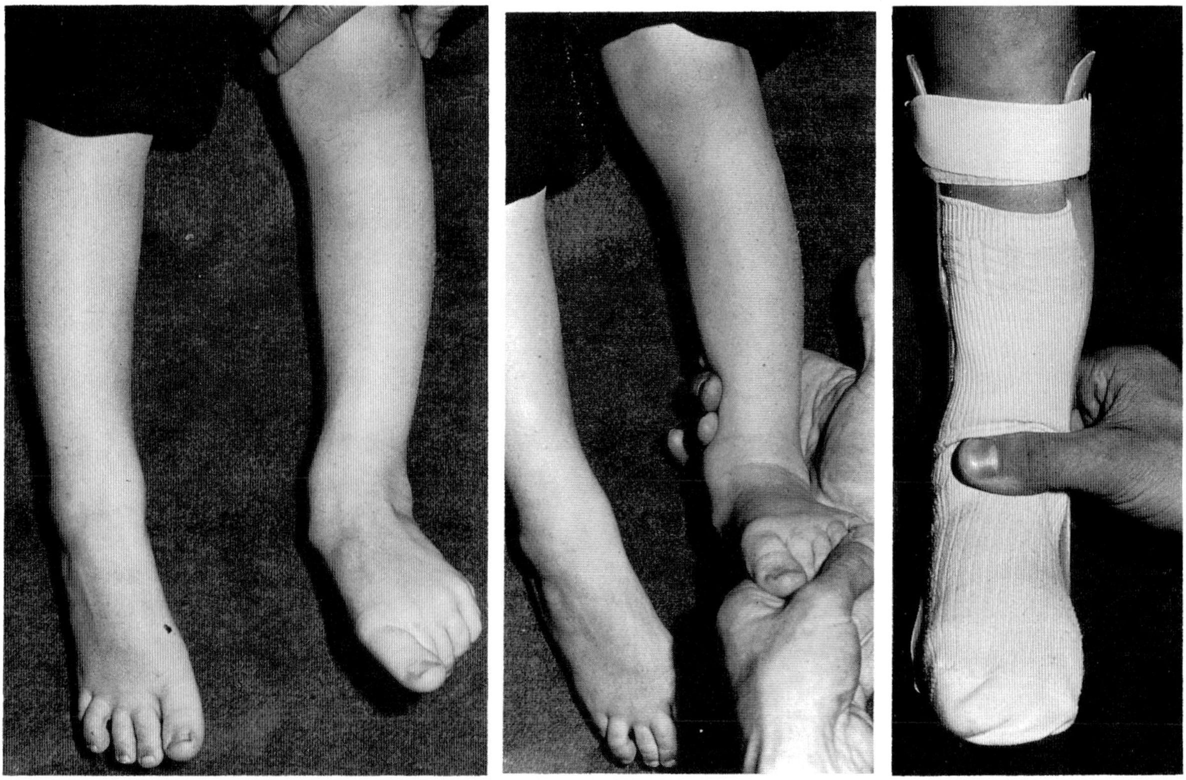

Fig. 57.34 a: Gross valgus; b: illustrating 3 point pressure required to invert the hindfoot; c: foot encased in polypropylene AFO embodying this principle

Care must be exercised in preparing the positive model to ensure that the trim line of the plastic AFO is rolled out and the forefoot part extended beyond the toes. Finally the ankle strap should be at 45° and pointing towards the heel so that it will resist any tendency to plantarflex. The foot should be placed in the fully corrected position before donning the device. A 'peep hole' in the plastic AFO enables a check to be made that the heel is properly positioned and full correction obtained.

Attention must be paid throughout for signs of pressure whether it be due to increased tone, increase in size with growth or unusual activities; normally, these circumstances require renewal of the AFOs. Several modern styles of footwear are satisfactory as they permit easy access of a foot fitted with an AFO. It is important that the shoes worn, both for indoor and outdoor should have effectively the same heel height.

In the hemiplegic child where the leg and/or foot may be smaller, height compensation is provided, but normally partial compensation is sufficient. High density Plastazote® moulded to the sole of the AFO may be enough and may even be accommodated within the shoe. Where build-ups are required on both the inside and outside of the AFO orthopaedic footwear may be required to accommodate them.

In the case of deformed feet which are smaller than normal or the contralateral foot, the opportunity may present to use shop shoes of the appropriate size or standard 'deep shoes' and occupy the unsatisfied space with a self-generating polyurethane foam as described by Platts et al (1982). They point out that the overlarge shoe may require stiffening, e.g. using an insole of high molecular weight polyethylene shaped to the last of the shoe. Wedge shoes may need no additional stiffening. Their criteria for patient selection are the wish to wear normal looking footwear, foot dimensions within those of the proposed footwear and finally, sufficient forefoot and near normal heel to ensure that the foot stays in the shoe.

Once AFOs have been completed and fitted, the ability to stand and walk may be determined by the amount of dorsiflexion provided. Initially the degree of dorsiflexion should provide forward leaning of the lower leg. If sufficient dorsiflexion is not possible heel wedges may be added to the orthoses. Walking can be improved by providing a shoe with a cushion heel to improve knee stability and with a rocker sole to ensure a smooth transition into knee flexion at the end of the stance phase.

The striking phenomenon in observing the cerebral palsied child walking after a switch from a plantigrade AFO to a dorsiflexed one is the extraordinary change in gait: the effect is virtually instantaneous with a much smoother and much better controlled gait and the difference in ankle attitude may be no more than 10°. Meadows (1984), a rehabilitation engineer who has a long, closely observed experience in a clinic team involved in the management of the cerebral palsied child, postulates that the phenomenon is due first to the alteration of the biomechanical environment and second to the interaction of biomechanical and neurological factors.

Noting that when the ankle is in some 10–20° of dorsiflexion the spasm in the plantarflexors is markedly reduced — the so-called quiet zone — Meadows believes that by restraining the ankle within that quiet zone with the AFO the threshold is maintained and spasm does not occur so readily (Fig. 57.35). The set of the AFO/shoe configuration in relation to the ground also conditions the position of the joints above and brings the knee joint closer to the ground-to-foot force vector. This in turn reduces the moment about the knee and thus the amount of force required to be produced by the quadriceps to balance. By maintaining the force vector close to the knee throughout the gait cycle, reducing impact forces by a cushion heel and ensuring a centre of pressure (the origin of the ground-to-foot force vector) that moves smoothly with the changing kinetic picture, a notably smoother gait is produced. It would seem that this can only occur if the altered biomechanical environment influences the underlying level of muscle tone and the functional demand made upon the neuromuscular system.

Rheumatoid arthritis. This inflammatory disease has direct effects on joint function. The inflammation of the tissues results in synovial overgrowth and distension of the joint which in turn restrains joint motion. Muscle function is also distorted by changes in joint capsules and weakened fascial planes. In the most acute phase the muscles splint the joint to avoid all motion to reduce pain. Later there is reflex immobilization of all but the

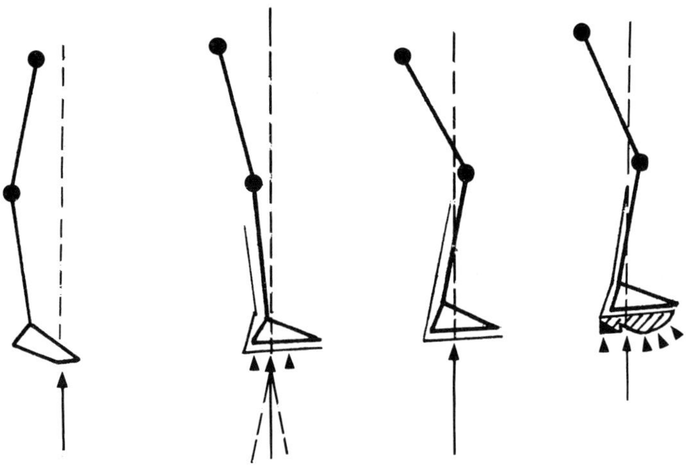

Fig. 57.35 a: Foot in equinus, ground to foot force vector is well in front of knee joint generating high moment about the knee; b: alterations in AFO characteristics influence the direction of the force vector and its point of origin; c: alteration to the shank attitude moves the knee nearer the force vector; d: the cushion heel and rocker sole ensures that the centre of pressure moves smoothly with the changing kinetic picture

mildest muscular action which inhibits exercise programmes. The use of orthotics is limited by the chronic nature of the disease. Splinting by one orthotic device or another is clearly useful in this acute phase. However, if splintage is prolonged the orthoses will inhibit function. Thus the main requirement is to make judgements regarding rest and activity and make judicious use of orthoses intermittently.

The patient suffering from rheumatoid arthritis may well require special footwear; indeed, feet are more commonly affected than hands. Park & Craxford (1981) reviewed 100 patients suffering from rheumatoid arthritis and wearing surgical shoes, and noted that the common deformities were splayed forefoot (87%), clawed toes (82%), and hallux valgus (57%). Flat foot was observed in 40%. They further point out that amelioration of symptoms normally required insoles usually constructed of sponge, rubber or Plastazote®. The deformities that present are in infinite variety but the metatarso-phalangeal joints are often the first to be involved. The subsequent clawing of the toes and an increase in the circumference from the fifth to first metatarsal usually prevent the wearing of most shop shoes. An increase in the toe box is usually the least that is required. Typically a gross hallux valgus, claw toes and a large callosity over the second metatarsal head require a shoe with a deeply cushioned insole and it may have to be bespoke. If the ankle has been affected the patient may not be able to point the toes into the shoe and an opening extending forward to the toes may be necessary.

Prosthetic requirements

Syme's amputation

The stump that results from the Syme's amputation possesses the full length of the leg except the heel. The stump end is bulbous thus permitting a self suspending design of the prosthesis which in turn must also provide access for the stump end. Its nature is such that it may be end-bearing to a varying degree (Murdoch 1976).

While there are biomechanical factors to consider, the functional loss is not great (McLaurin 1970). The prosthesis can be seen as a passive extension of the stump and at heel contact there is a force commensurate with normal on the end of the stump and smaller but significant forces tending to rotate the prosthesis clockwise on the stump producing forces acting on the stump on the posterior aspect proximally and on the anterior aspect distally (Fig. 57.36a and b). Conversely, at push-off the prosthesis is tending to rotate anticlockwise and the forces on the stump act anteriorly on the proximal end and posteriorly at the distal end. Because the stump is

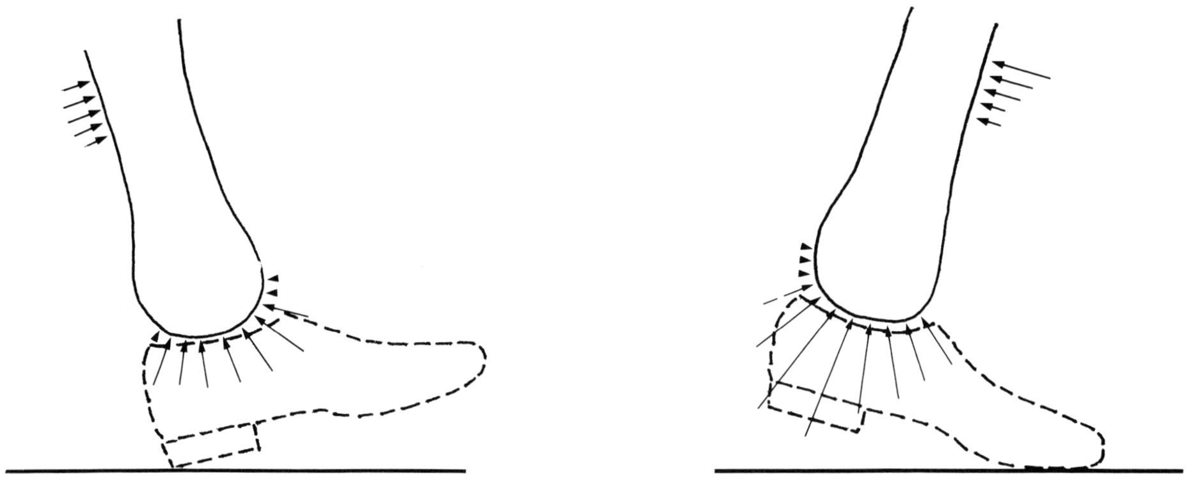

Fig. 57.36 Syme's amputation. a: application of force at heel contact; b: force pattern at push-off

long it is not difficult to stabilize the socket. However, as the stump, at least in its distal half, is nearly round, stabilization against rotation of the socket can be more difficult. If the foot is aligned with some toe-out a force couple tends to rotate the prosthetic toe inwards. This couple is linked between the ground reaction force's horizontal component and the horizontal component of the stump forces (Fig. 57.37). At mid stance the stump rotates clockwise as the patient moves forward causing further inward rotation of the prosthesis. At push off inward rotation occurs yet again as the force couple again takes effect. The most effective way to counter this tendency is to ensure accurate keying of the proximal part of the stump into the prosthesis by fitting in a similar way to the Patellar Tendon Bearing Prosthesis.

Thus the socket design should encompass weight

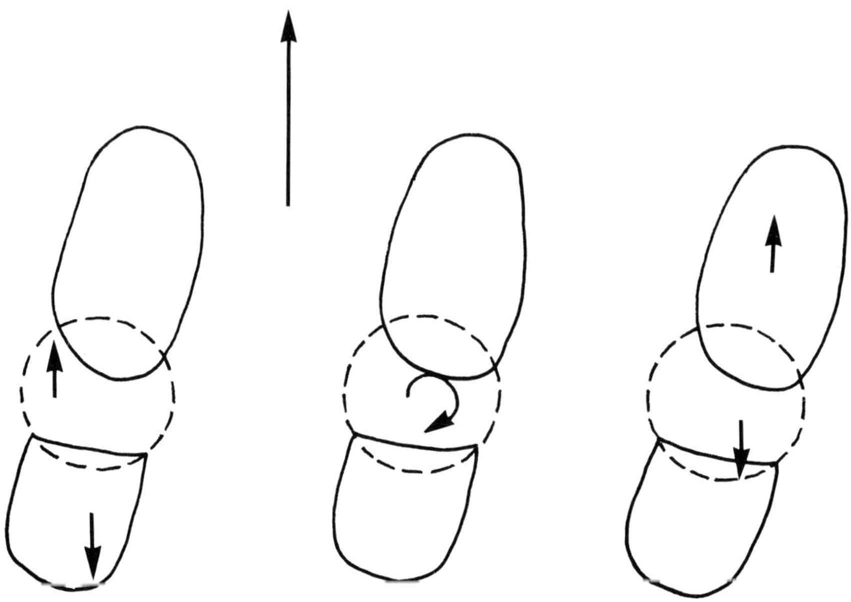

Fig. 57.37 Syme's amputation. a: forces acting to rotate the prosthesis inward to the stump at heel contact; b: mid stance arrow shows the direction the stump tends to take); c: just prior to toe-off

bearing, suspension, resistance to rotation and control of anteroposterior and anterolateral forces to ensure stability.

A variety of prostheses are available and some examples are illustrated in Figures 57.38 and 39. Types (b) and (d) made of plastic material are those most commonly prescribed. The provision of a window to provide access of the bulbous end to the distal part of the socket provides the main fabrication problem as there is clearly a stress concentration problem just above the ankle. This difficulty has usually been overcome by the inclusion of judiciously placed glass fibres, nylon stockinette, carbon fibre, etc.

A typical alignment requires a few degrees of dorsiflexion to provide roll over prior to toe-off. In standing the knee should be centred on a vertical line passing midway between the back of the heel and the ball of the foot. Toe-out should be provided for cosmetic reasons, but may be difficult to maintain.

In congenital absence of the fibula and some other conditions the stump is short enough to permit a PTB type of prosthesis with a measure of end-bearing. In these circumstances a standard SACH foot can be prescribed.

With a full length stump an artificial foot with a lower profile may be required. One drawback with a foot of this kind is that it may preclude the use of an adequate heel cushion, especially as a softer heel may go some way to reduce rotation within the socket.

Chopart amputation

The Chopart amputation produces a stump which is the full length of the leg as it retains the whole of the os calcis and talus (Fig. 57.40). The stump, such as it is, tends to be in equinus and varus. Insertion of the tibialis anterior and the other extensors into the talus can overcome the equinus problem, but the shape of the bones gives the shape and appearance of a varus disposition. If the stump cannot be stabilized except by a prosthesis encompassing a part or the whole of the lower leg then the whole 'leg' will be longer than the contralateral leg, and it is very unlikely that normal footwear can be employed: the resultant 'high' boot may be very heavy, bulky and ugly. The prosthesis described by MacDonald (1955) (Fig. 57.41) can be worn inside a normal shoe. This type of fitting requires considerable expertise as the device must grip the concavities on each side of the os calcis in a precise and comfortable manner. When successful the patient can use the full range of dorsiflexion if required. With the development of modern plastic technology a number of analogues are being produced. The amputation itself remains very uncommon.

Modern plastics such as high molecular weight polyethylene (Ortholen) have been deployed widely in orthotics and an adaptation of a widely used AFO can be used for the Chopart amputation stump.

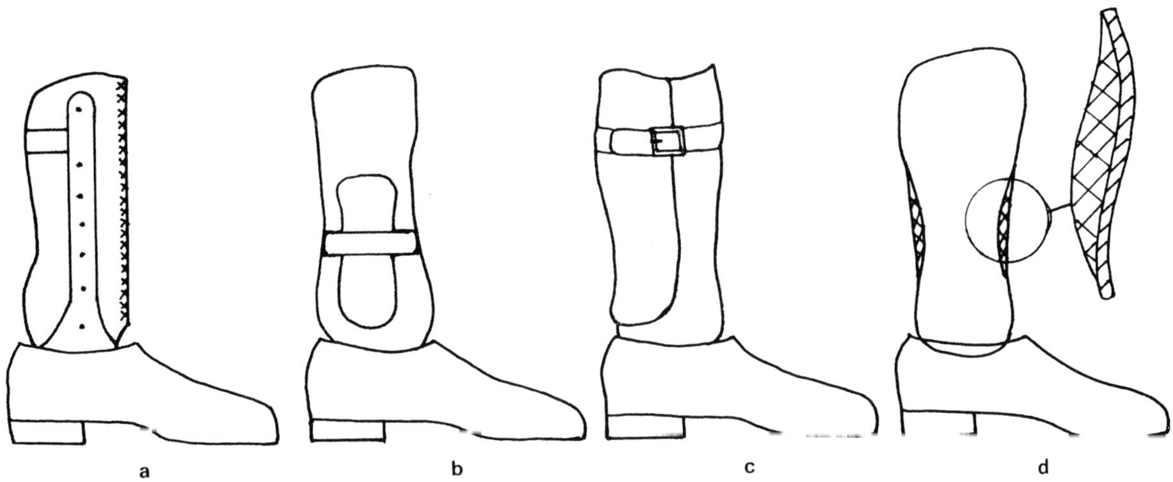

Fig. 57.38 Various types of Syme's prostheses

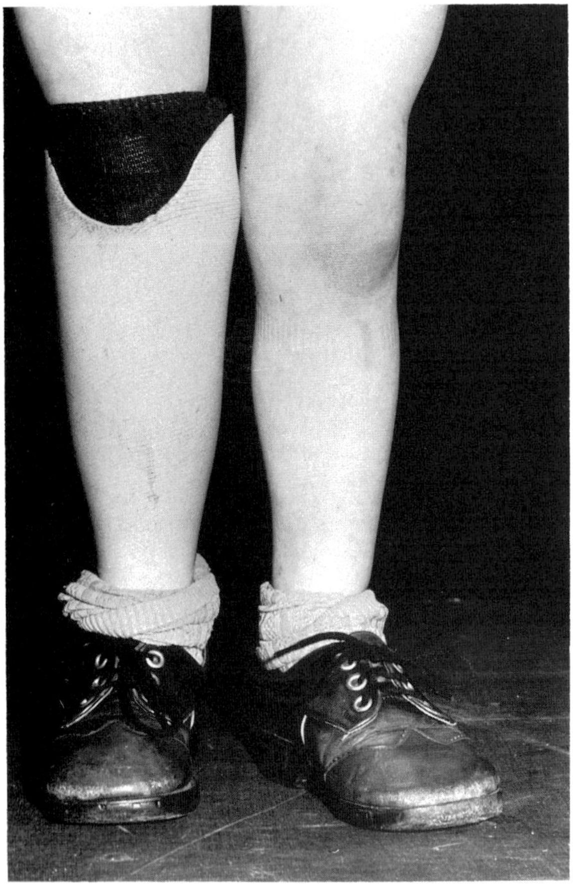

Fig. 57.39 Child wearing type (d) prosthesis (see Fig. 38). Amputation was at 10 months for congenital absence of fibula. State of shoes testify to level of activity achieved

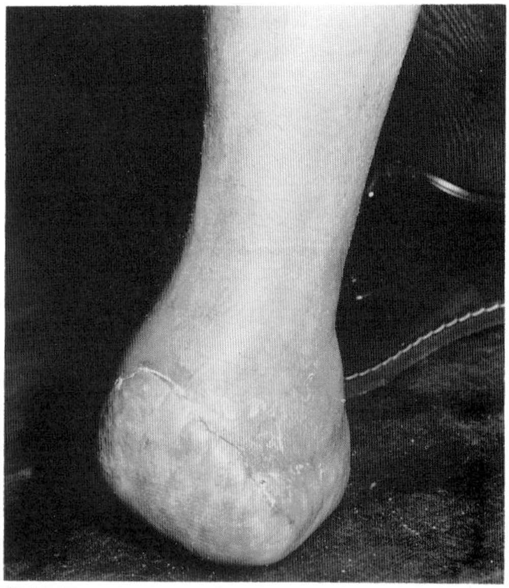

Fig. 57.40 Chopart amputation stump

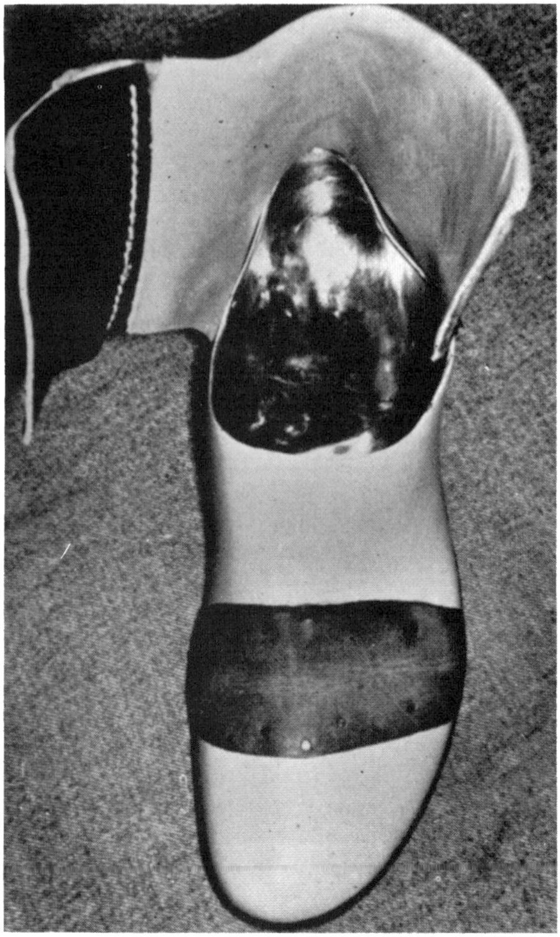

Fig. 57.41 MacDonald type prosthesis

Rubin & Danisi (1971) describe a design employing a commercial version of the Ortholen drop foot AFO where the sole of the device is extended to the end of the shoe, incorporating a filler for the missing part of the foot and Velcro straps to retain the stump in the orthoprosthesis. The sole has to be thinned to provide 'toe-break' but such spring resistance as there is should be retained to provide assistance at push-off.

Lisfranc amputation

This procedure consisting of disarticulation along the tarsometatarsal line, with either division of base of the second metatarsal or reduction of the medial cuneiform, provides a stump just long enough to be fitted with a device which can be worn inside a normal shoe. Clearly it must encompass the whole of the remaining part of the foot and be fitted with precision to the hollows on both sides of the calcaneum and ensuring that the whole of the dorsum of the foot is employed in force transference; if pressures remain unacceptably high then the 'socket' will have to be extended proximally with consequent loss of dorsiflexion.

Transmetatarsal amputation

This procedure leaves a significantly large part of the foot to permit the use of a normal shoe. An insert used simply as a filler may be sufficient in some cases or require a device to encompass the remaining part of the foot and properly to locate it within the shoe (Fig. 57.42). Standard materials such as leathers or any of a combination of modern plastics may be used, e.g. expanded polyethylene, polypropylene or polyurethane. All of these types are based on a positive model of the foot stump duly modified to ensure force transference to resistant tissues and to decrease pressure on the more sensitive parts. Some use laminated plastic with a foam lining, but more recently more flexible designs have been developed to reduce the tendency to skin breakdown and to improve the foot profile built onto the socket (Childs & Staats 1983). Designs using RTV elastomers (Wilson 1979) and reinforced silicone are examples of these types. However, the construction of these orthoses can be quite complex and demanding and the reader is referred to the relevant publications.

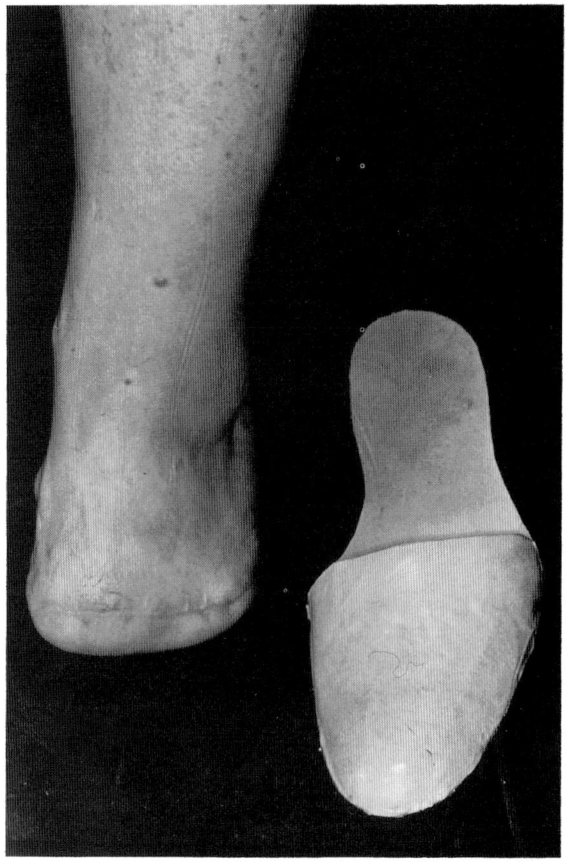

Fig. 57.42 Transmetatarsal amputation with shoe filler

REFERENCES

Childs C, Staats T 1983 The slipper type partial foot prosthesis, Advanced below-knee, prosthetic seminar. UCLA Prosthetic and Orthotic Education Program, Fabrication Manual

Engen T J 1971 Instructional manual for fabrication and fitting of a below knee corrugated polypropylene orthosis. Texas Institute for Rehabilitation and Research, Houston

Helfet A J 1957 Treatment of flat feet in children. (Proceedings of the 5th Congress — South African Orthopaedic Association) Abstract. J Bone Joint Surg 39B(1): 160

Hicks J H 1953 The mechanics of the foot. I The Joints. J Anat 87: 345–357

Hicks J H 1954 The mechanics of the foot. II The Plantar Aponeurosis. J Anat 88: 25–30

Inman V T 1969 UC-BL dual-axis ankle-control system and UC-BL shoe insert. Biomechanical considerations. Bull Prosthet Res Spring: 130–145

Inman V T, Mann R A 1964 Phasic activity of intrinsic muscles of foot. J Bone Joint Surg 46A: 469

Lehneis H R 1972 New developments in lower limb orthotics through bioengineering. Arch Phys Med Rehabil 53 (7): 303–310

Levens A S, Inman V T, Blosser J A 1948 Transverse rotation of the segments of the lower extremity in locomotion. J Bone Joint Surg 30A(4): 859–872

Lyquist E 1976 The dynamic club foot splint as a modular system. In: Murdoch G (ed) The Advance in Orthotics, Arnold, London. pp 433–439

MacDonald A 1955 Chopart's amputation. The advantages of a modified prosthesis. J Bone Joint Surg 37B: 468–470

McIlmurray W J, Greenbaum W 1958 A below-knee weight-bearing brace. Orthop Pros App J 12 (2): 81–82

McLaurin C A 1970 The Syme type prosthesis. In: Murdoch G (ed) Prosthetic Orthotics Practice. Arnold, London. pp 125–137

Manter J T 1941 Movement of the subtalar and transverse tarsal joints. Anat Rec 80: 397–410

Meadows C B 1984 The influence of a polypropylene ankle-foot

orthosis on the gait of cerebral palsied children. Ph.D Thesis University of Strathclyde
Meadows C B, Anderson D M, Duncan L M, Sturrock M P T 1980 The use of polypropylene ankle foot orthoses in the management of the young cerebral palsied child. Tayside Rehabilitation Engineering Services
Morley A J M 1957 Knock knee in children. Br Med J ii: 976–979
Murdoch G 1976 Syme's amputation. J R Coll Surg 21(1): 15–30
Park C, Craxford A D 1981 Surgical footwear in rheumatoid arthritis — a patient acceptability study. Prosthet Orthot Int 5: 33–36
Platts R G S, Field A, Knight S 1979 Orthoses to fit shoes. Prosthet Orthot Int 3: 89–90
Platts R G S, Knight S, Jakins I 1982 Shoe inserts for small deformed feet. Prosthet Orthot Int 6: 108–110
Radcliffe C W, Foort J 1961 The Patellar Tendon Bearing Prosthesis. Biomechanics Laboratory, University of California, Berkeley and San Francisco
Reimann I, Lyquist E 1970 Dynamic splint used in the treatment of club foot. Acta Orthop Scand 40: 817–824
Rubin G, Danisi M 1971 Functional partial-foot prosthesis. Bull Pros Res Fall: 149–152
Sharrard W J W 1958 Minor orthopaedic disability in childhood. Practitioner 180: 415
Smith J W 1954 Muscular control of the arches of the foot on standing; electromyographic assessment J Anat 88: 1952
University of California 1957 Installation of the Solid Ankle Cushion Heel (SACH) foot for adult male amputees
Wilson M T 1979 Clinical application of RTV elastomers. Orthotics and Prosthetics 34(4): 23–29
Yates A 1968 A method for the provision of light weight aesthetic orthopaedic appliances. Orthopaedics I (2): 153–162

Surgical approaches

INTRODUCTION

The purpose of foot surgery is to rectify a symptomatic abnormality. The final result should be a pain-free functioning foot, without any complications resulting from the surgery. In order to achieve this the surgeon should thoroughly familiarize himself with a detailed anatomy and physiology of the foot. A correct surgical technique plays a very large part in obtaining a successful result.

GENERAL PRINCIPLES

Adequate blood supply

The foot must be assessed with regard to an adequate blood supply. Peripheral pulses should be easily palpable. The texture of the skin and nails should be normal. In doubtful cases, the patient should be referred to a vascular surgeon for further investigation. Diabetic patients and patients on steroids should be carefully assessed before surgery is advised. The presence of vasculitis in rheumatoid patients is a contraindication to surgery, so is an obviously ischaemic foot. In borderline cases, where surgery has to be carried out, the limb should not be exsanguinated or a tourniquet applied, as the use of these techniques will jeopardize an already precarious blood supply.

Haemostasis

A tourniquet should always be used unless there are contraindications. A clear surgical field makes an operation that much easier and quicker as important structures such as nerves can be identified and preserved. The use of an exsanguinating Esmarch bandage is not necessary and may even be dangerous as it has been shown that rough application may result in damage to nerves and other tissues. Of course, its use in tumour surgery is absolutely contraindicated as tumour cells may be squeezed into the general circulation. Elevation of the limb for a few minutes, usually the length of time taken to apply a pneumatic tourniquet, will suffice for adequate exsanguination of the limb. The torus sausage exsanguinator does not have the damaging effects of a badly applied Esmarch bandage and can be used if a completely bloodless field is required.

During surgery, meticulous haemostasis should be carried out, as a bleeding wound will result in delayed healing and, worse still, may favour a wound infection. A bipolar diathermy unit is preferable as there is less tissue damage. Blood vessels, especially veins, should not be ligated unnecessarily as an inadequate venous drainage will predispose to swelling of the extremity. Removing the tourniquet at the end of the operation and controlling any bleeding points should be practised. A compression bandage, using plenty of cotton wool, and a crepe bandage with or without suction drainage can eliminate haematoma formation if extensive dissection of soft tissues has been carried out. Postoperative elevation of the foot of the bed as well as resting the operated foot on two pillows, will avoid any postoperative oedema.

Early mobilization

Following surgery, early mobilization should be encouraged to ensure an adequate circulation to the extremity with efficient functioning of the 'peripheral heart', i.e. the contractions of the muscles of the lower limb, in particular, the calf muscles. This in turn will minimize deep venous thrombosis and swelling of the extremity. When seated, the patient should elevate his or her feet to avoid dependent oedema. It must be emphasized that prevention of swelling is more rewarding than reducing a swelling once it has formed. Early weight bearing, when the sole of the foot has been operated upon, minimizes neuroma formation and the patient should be encouraged to get onto his or her feet as soon as possible, usually 48–72 hours after surgery.

Surgical incision

A surgical approach should allow for easy access to all the necessary structures in the operation. The incision should be long enough to carry out the operation, but not too long as the resulting scar will not only be bigger and more disfiguring, but important structures may be unnecessarily disturbed or even damaged. If an old surgical scar is present, it should be made use of, by making the skin incision through it. An incision parallel to it is not only more disfiguring but the skin between the present incision and the old surgical scar may undergo ischaemic necrosis.

As far as possible, incisions should not be made over bony prominences as these may be subjected to pressure which may be painful. Also, incisions should follow Langer's lines or natural cleavage lines as they result in fine scars. Incisions should not be made across normal skin creases or Langer's lines as the subsequent scar is not only unsightly but may contract and restrict joint motion. On the dorsomedial side and on the plantar surface of the foot, Langer's lines are longitudinal in direction (Fig. 58.1), but on the dorsolateral side of the foot these lines run distally and laterally (Fig. 58.2).

Incisions should be straight wherever possible. If an incision has to be curved, it should not be too curved otherwise the skin flap may be devitalized. It is better to have a longer straight incision along a skin crease than a shorter curved one, as not only will the wound heal better, but will be less disfiguring. Undermining of the skin must be avoided. Any incision should, as far as possible, be carried down to bone or deeper tissues and dissection carried out deep to the deep fascia. Muscles must be separated rather than cut through. Important nerves and blood vessels must be left intact. They should be identified and protected if they are in danger of being injured. On the other hand, if they can be avoided completely they should be left alone and not searched for by dissection.

If previous surgery has been carried out on the foot, incision through the old scar has to be considered even though the scar may not be ideally situated. However, forceful retraction must be avoided at all costs for the skin edges may necrose.

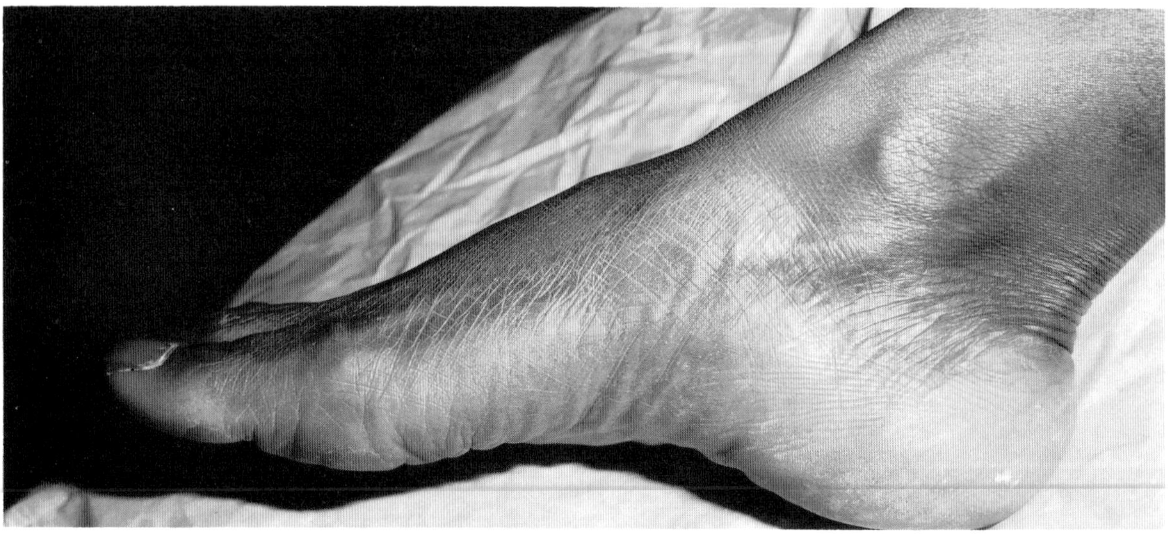

Fig. 58.1 Langer's lines on dorsomedial and plantar surface of the foot

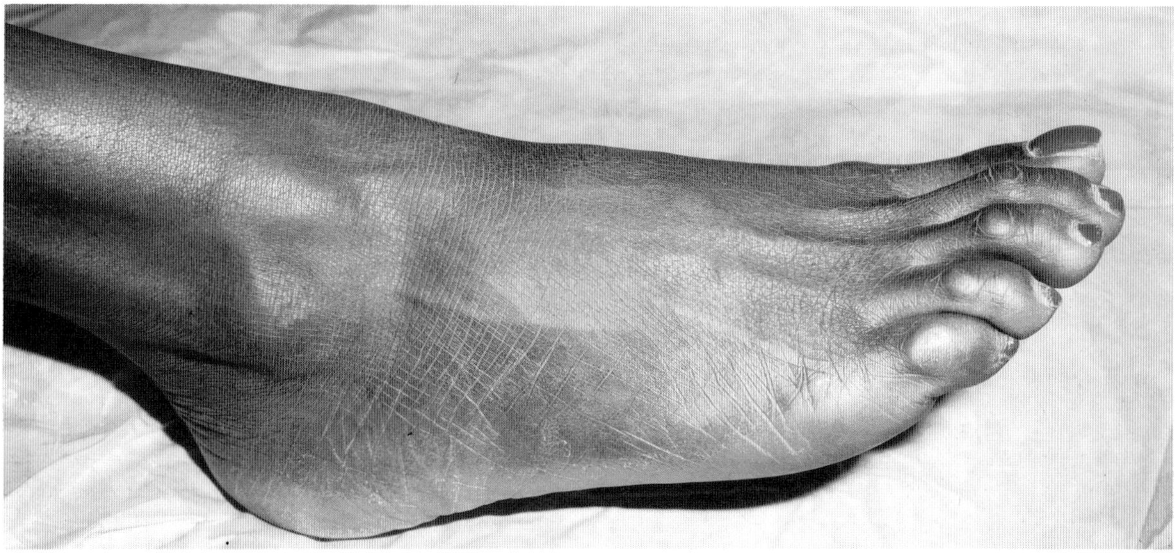

Fig. 58.2 Langer's lines on dorsolateral side of the foot

Tissue retraction

Retraction of skin should be gentle and be for short periods only to prevent necrosis of the skin edges. The skin on the dorsum of the foot is thin and devoid of any rich vascular plexus, and heals poorly if subjected to unnecessary abuse (Fig. 58.3). The skin on the sole of the foot, on the other hand, is very thick and vascular like the palm of the hand, and heals quickly, (Fig. 58.4). The subsequent scar is not tender when subjected to weight bearing. Therefore the surgeon should not hesitate to incise the plantar skin if this will provide him with the necessary access to the structures in which he is interested.

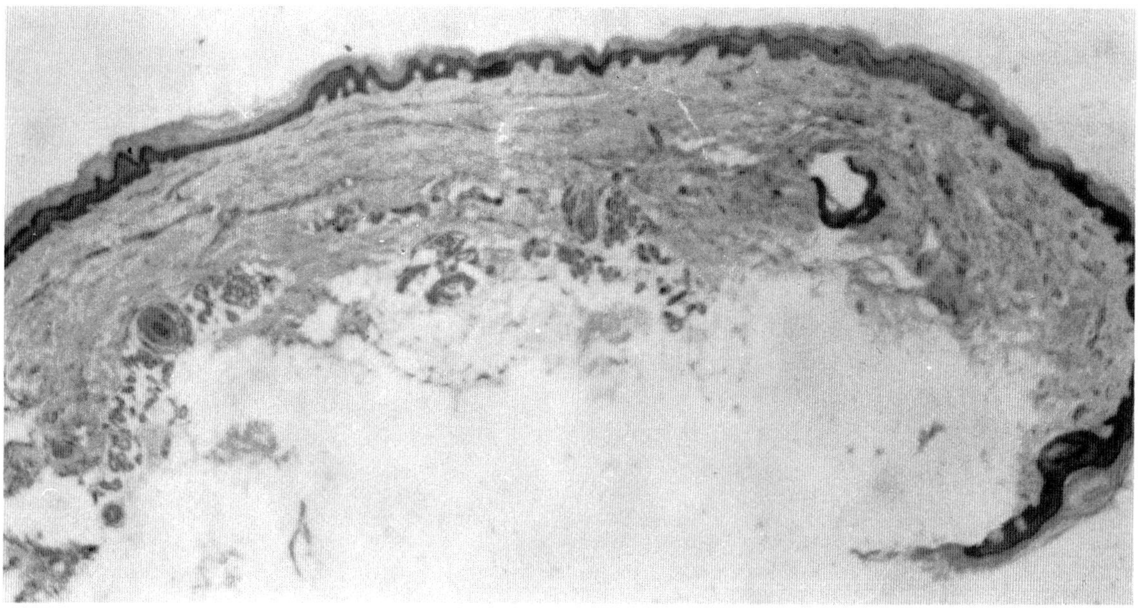

Fig. 58.3 Skin on dorsum of the foot showing the thin layers of cells (×25). (Courtesy of Dr. Harold Caplan, Consultant Pathologist, Enfield District Hospitals)

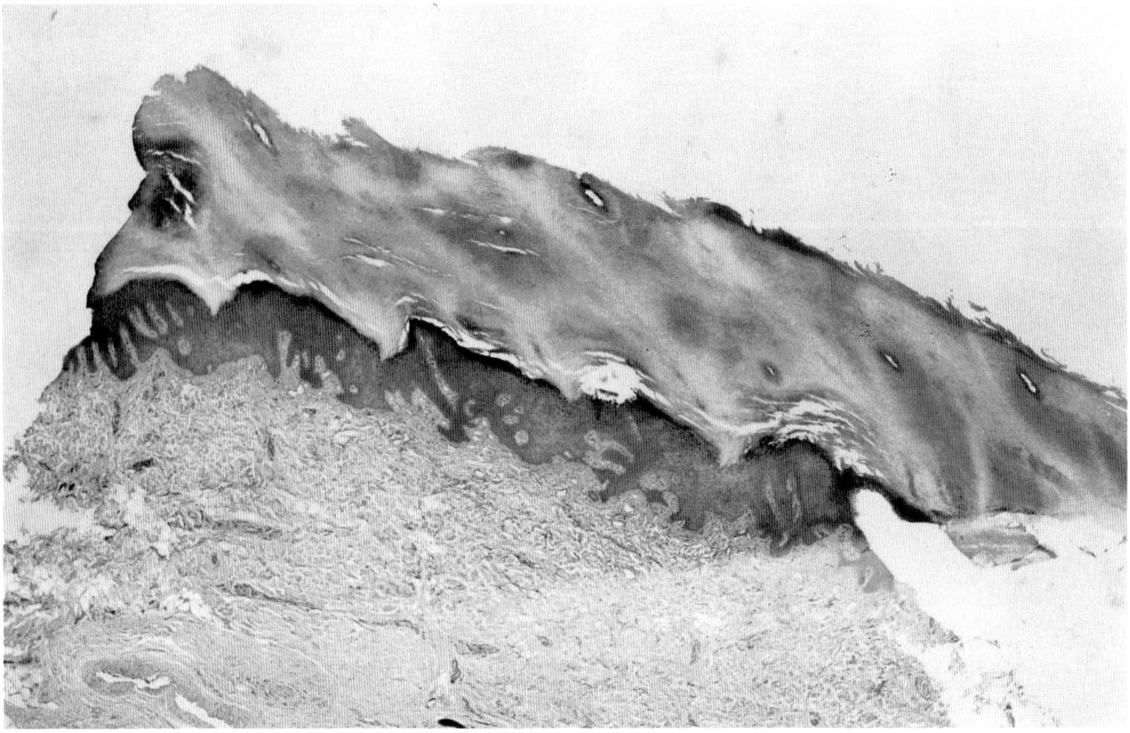

Fig. 58.4 Skin on sole of the foot, showing the thick layers of cells (×25). (Courtesy of Dr. Harold Caplan, Consultant Pathologist, Enfield District Hosptials)

Cutaneous nerves

Cutaneous nerves should be respected, as unwitting damage to even a small nerve could give rise to a painful neuroma, (Figs. 58.5 to 9). This is especially distressing to the patient if the scar is subjected to constant pressure or frequent distortions. These nerves usually accompany blood vessels and when the latter are clamped, care must be taken to ensure that the accompanying nerves are not damaged. Complete division of these cutaneous nerves results in loss of sensation, and numbness especially around the heel and on the plantar surface will not only be annoying, but also dangerous, as penetrating injuries can occur without the patient being aware of such occurrences, and foreign material can be left in the foot unknowingly.

Position of patient on the operating table

Depending on the various surgical approaches and the preference of the surgeon, the patient can lie either supine or prone, or with a sandbag under either buttock, or in the lateral position. However, the position should be decided beforehand, and the anaesthetist notified so that he may pass an endotracheal tube, if necessary, and arrange for sufficient pillows to be placed under the patient, e.g. if the patient is to be in the prone position. Nothing is worse than for the surgeon to find that he is not able to obtain an adequate exposure because the patient happens to be in the wrong position.

Operations on the dorsum of the foot can be done with a sandbag under the ipsilateral buttock for a dorsolateral approach, or under the contralateral buttock for a dorsomedial approach. Operations on the sole of the foot can be done by the surgeon sitting at the foot of the operating table and tilting the head of the table downward. The posterior parts of the sole including the Achilles tendon, the calcaneum, the posterior structures of the ankle and subtalar joints can be approached by lying the patient prone on the table.

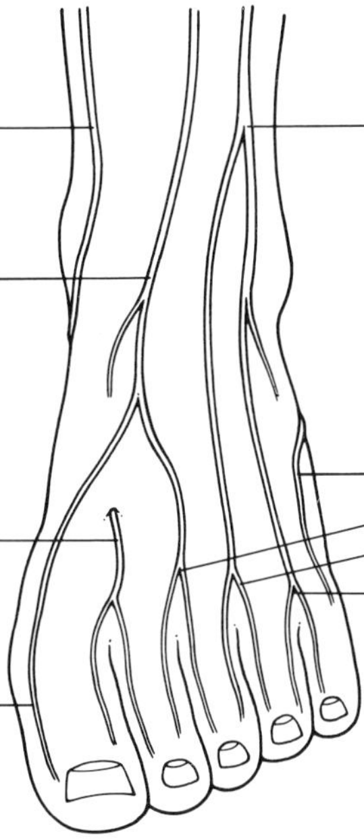

Fig. 58.5 Cutaneous nerves on dorsum of the foot

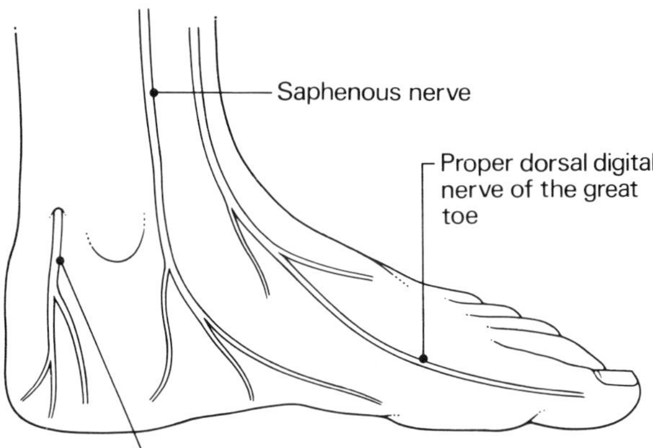

Fig. 58.6 Cutaneous nerves on dorsomedial side of the foot

In certain surgical procedures, such as subtalar or ankle arthrodeses and ankle joint replacements, it is necessary to correct or maintain a plantargrade position of the foot in relation to the rest of the lower limb. This is easily achieved by hanging the leg to be operated upon over the end of the operating table, which is raised high enough to allow the foot to rest on a flat wheeled trolley which can be moved about or locked in position. By moving the trolley about, ankle movements can be reproduced. Also, by applying pressure on the knee the weight-bearing foot can be simulated.

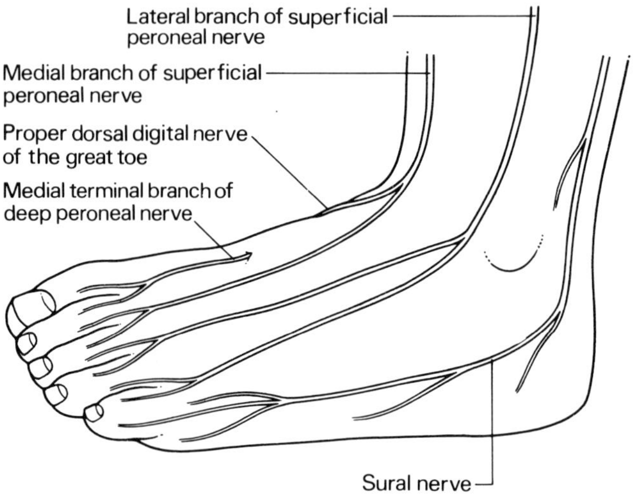

Fig. 58.7 Cutaneous nerves on dorsolateral side of the foot

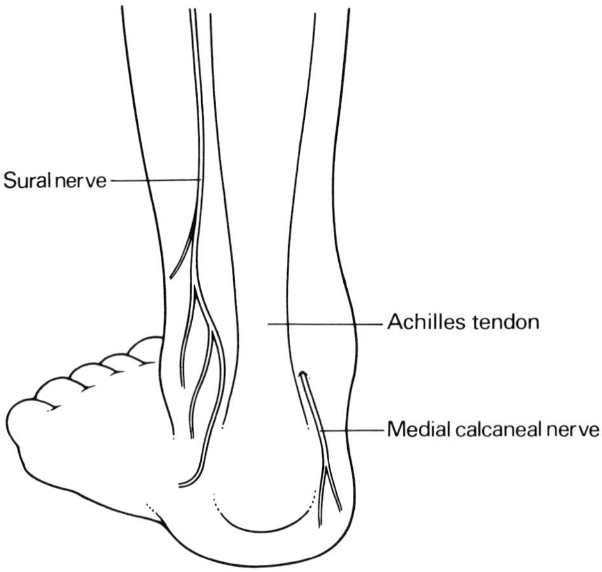

Fig. 58.8 Cutaneous nerves on back of the ankle

SURGICAL APPROACHES TO THE FOOT

The great toe

Access to the terminal phalanx (Fig. 58.10)

Access to a subungual exostosis of the terminal phalanx can be achieved by removing the nail and incising through the sterile matrix of the nail bed.

The patient lies supine on the operating table. A fish mouth or transverse incision at the tip of the great toe can be made to expose the tuft and distal part of the terminal phalanx. In screw arthrodesis of the interphalangeal joint, because the tuft of the terminal phalanx has a thin edge, the drill hole is made in a retrograde fashion from the base of the terminal phalanx after exposing the interphalangeal

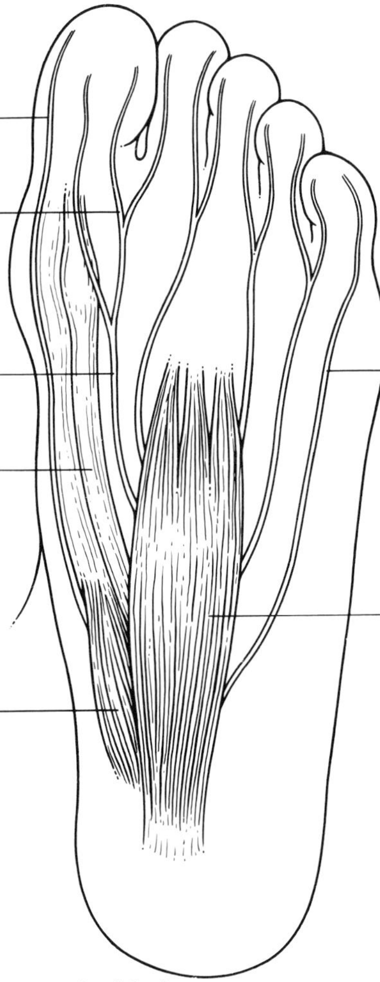

Fig. 58.9 Cutaneous nerves on sole of the foot

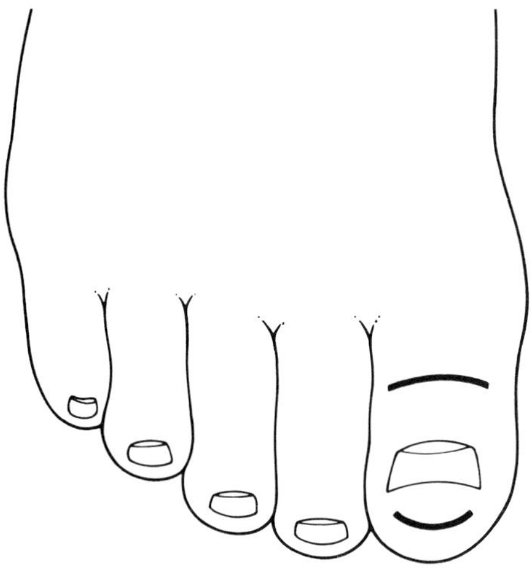

Fig. 58.10 Fish mouth incision to terminal phalanx of the great toe and transverse incision to interphalangeal joint

joint, care being taken not to damage the nail bed. The screw is then introduced distally through the fish mouth incision, withdrawing the drill bit with the screw in contact in order to locate the drill hole.

Access to the interphalangeal joint

The patient lies supine on the operating table. A transverse incision is made across the dorsum of the joint. The incision should not extend beyond the midlateral line on either side of the great toe so as to avoid the digital nerves and vessels. This midlateral line is demarcated by a change in the texture of the skin from the relatively thin dorsal skin to the thick and coarse plantar skin.

The head of the proximal phalanx is rounded and in order not to make the incision too proximal, the interphalangeal joint should be flexed and the incision made across the apex of the head. If an arthrodesis of the joint is carried out the extensor tendon can be incised across with the skin incision, but if the mobility of the joint is to be retained, e.g. in operations on intra-articular fractures involving the head of the proximal phalanx, the extensor tendon must be incised more proximally in order to leave sufficient tendon attached to the terminal phalanx to be sutured back to the proximal end.

The interphalangeal joint can also be approached by a dorsomedial longitudinal incision, but this gives a limited exposure and should be used only if the extensor tendon has to be kept intact for early mobilization of the joint, such as in intra-articular fractures which have been internally fixed. The transverse or longitudinal incisions could be extended into an 'L' or 'Z'-shaped incision if more exposure is required, taking care not to transgress the midlateral line on either side.

Access to the metatarsophalangeal joint

Dorsomedial approach (Fig. 58.11) The patient lies supine on the operating table. A dorsomedial straight longitudinal incision across the metatarsophalangeal joint, medial to the extensor hallucis longus tendon, is the usual approach for exposing this joint in procedures such as the Keller's or Mayo's operations, or when replacing the joint with a Helal silicone ball or Swanson prosthesis. It is medial to the proper dorsal digital nerve of the great toe, which must be identified and protected. Thereafter the incision should be carried straight down to bone and the capsule dissected off the exostosis of the first metatarsal, which is usually present. It is important not to undermine the skin unless absolutely necessary as healing in this region is usually slow and any damage to the vascular supply of the skin, such as rough handling and hard retraction will result in skin necrosis.

Look out for the large medial branch of the superficial peroneal nerve. This runs parallel and lateral to the extensor hallucis longus tendon on the dorsum of the foot, and it in turn gives off three branches: the medial branch, which is the proper dorsal digital nerve of the great toe and which crosses the extensor hallucis longus tendon running distally on its medial side and anastomosing with the terminal branches of the saphenous nerve to supply the dorsomedial side of the big toe; the central branch which is the dorsal digital nerve to the second cleft supplying the adjacent halves of the second and third toes; and the lateral branch which divides into the dorsal digital nerve to the third cleft and the dorsal digital nerve to the fourth cleft. The terminal

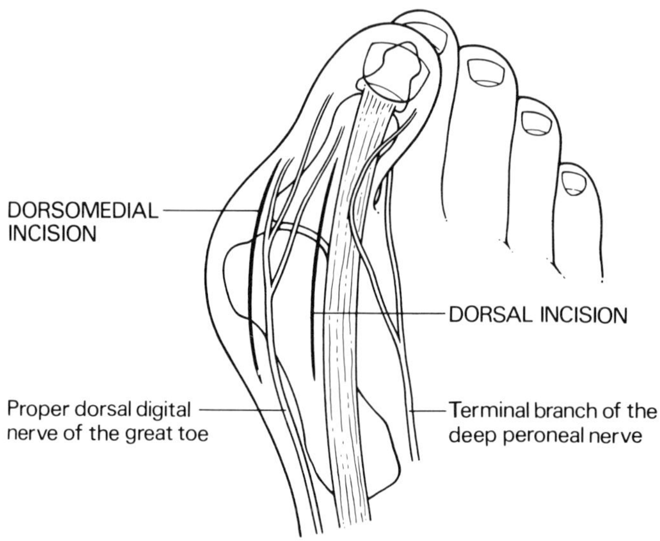

Fig. 58.11 Dorsomedial approach to the metatarsophalangeal joint of the great toe

branch of the *deep* peroneal nerve supplies the adjacent halves of the great and second toes.

To summarize, the skin of the first cleft is supplied by the deep peroneal nerve whereas the skin of the other clefts is supplied by the superficial peroneal nerve (McMinn et al 1982).

Dorsal approach (see Fig. 58.11). A dorsal approach is made between the proper dorsal digital nerve of the great toe and the extensor hallucis longus tendon.

Medial approach (Fig. 58.12) A more medial incision is used to expose the attachment of the abductor hallucis. A curved incision with its convexity upwards, starting from the middle of the shaft of the proximal phalanx and ending at the neck of the first metatarsal is used if a capsular reefing is part of the surgical procedure. The incision should not be too curved as skin healing may be slow.

Dorsolateral approach (Fig. 58.13). A 3 cm incision, lateral to the extensor hallucis longus tendon, centred on the metatarsophalangeal joint can be used

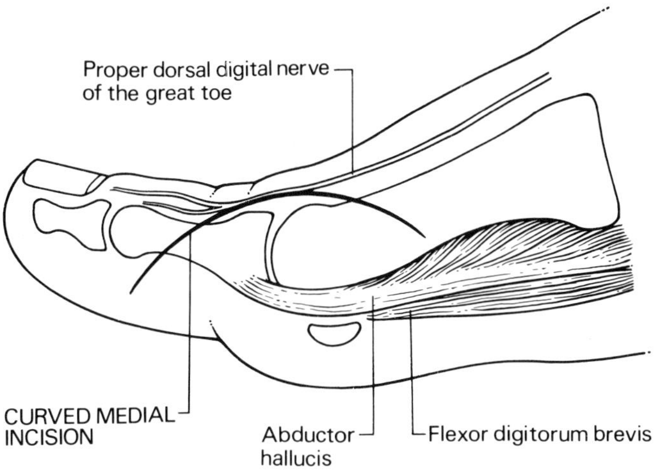

Fig. 58.12 Medial approach to the metatarsophalangeal joint of the great toe

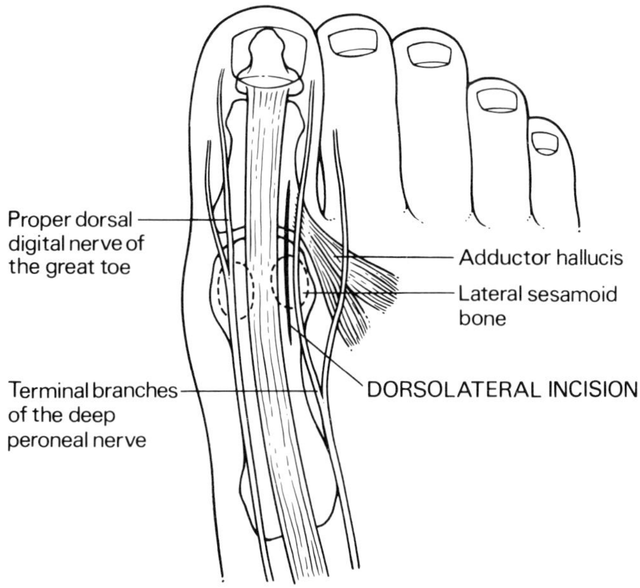

Fig. 58.13 Dorsolateral approach to the metatarsophalangeal joint of the great toe

to expose the lateral sesamoid from above. The attachment of the adductor hallucis can also be exposed by this approach. Care should be taken of the terminal branch of the deep peroneal nerve to the lateral side of the great toe, which lies lateral to the skin incision.

Access to the nail bed (Fig. 58.14)

1 cm incisions are made from the two proximal corners of the nail and extending proximally and outwards. The skin flap so formed is dissected back proximally to expose the nail bed and insertion of the extensor tendon. This is used in radical ablation of the nail bed (Zadik 1950).

Plantar approach (Fig. 58.15). A longitudinal incision directly under the head of the first metatarsal, usually 3 cm in length, will provide sufficient access to the medial or lateral sesamoid bone, the flexor sheath and the flexor hallucis longus tendon.

If a sesamoid bone is to be removed, the flexor sheath is incised and the tendon of the flexor hallucis longus retracted away. Take care to protect the first common plantar digital nerve which lies very close to the lateral sesamoid bone. This nerve supplies the plantar surfaces of the adjacent halves of the great and second toes. Its damage leads to anaesthesia of this area of which the patient is constantly aware. On the medial side the proper plantar digital nerve of the great toe does not lie as close to the medial sesamoid bone, but being a thin delicate nerve can also be easily damaged unless it is carefully looked for and protected.

The lateral four toes

The approaches to the lateral four toes are essentially the same as for the great toe, namely (a) a transverse fish mouth incision to expose the terminal phalanges; (b) a transverse incision across the dorsum of the distal or proximal interphalangeal joint. The extensor tendon and the dorsal capsule are divided, and the joint is exposed by flexion and division of the collateral ligaments. This approach is useful for arthrodesis of the interphalangeal joints. Remember to make the skin incision across the apex of the metatarsal head so as not to be too proximal to

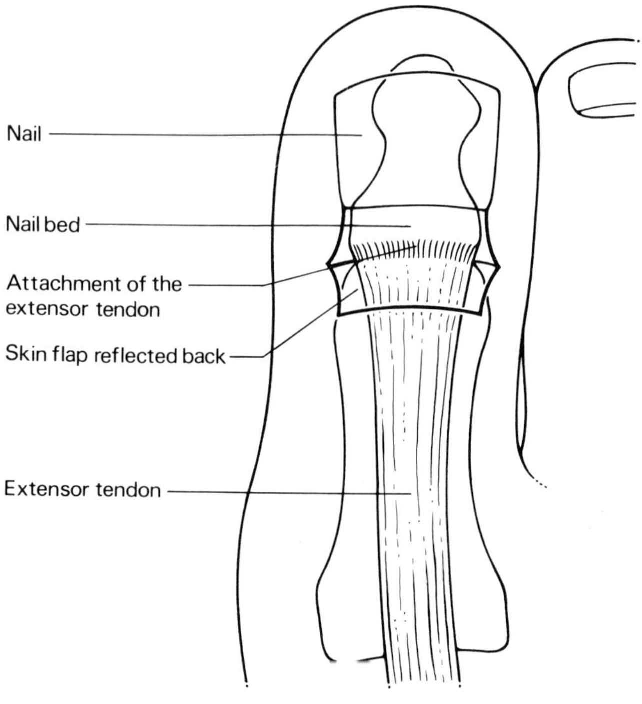

Fig. 58.14 Access to the nail bed

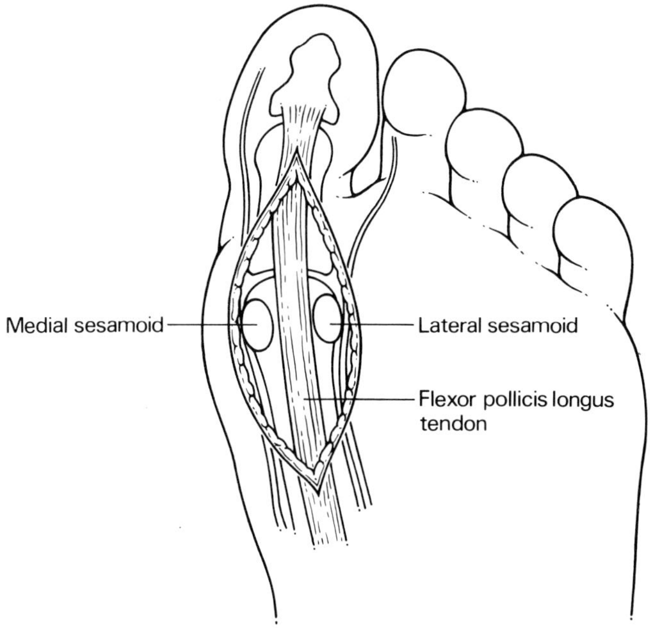

Fig. 58.15 Plantar approach to the metatarsophalangeal joint of the great toe

the joint; and (c) a midlateral incision to expose the extensor tendon in certain procedures, such as the Girdlestone procedure of flexor to extensor tendon transfers (Taylor 1951).

A longitudinal incision on the dorsum of the metatarsophalangeal joint can lead to a contracted scar resulting in a cocked-up toe. If a dorsal incision is necessary to expose the metatarsophalangeal joint, as in open reduction of a dislocation or an osteotomy of the metatarsal neck in osteochondritis of the second metatarsal head, an S-shaped incision is preferred.

If several metatarsal heads have to be exposed, a transverse elliptical incision on the plantar surface is the best surgical approach (Fig. 58.16). The lymphatic and venous drainage of the foot are on the dorsum and a transverse incision on this surface would predispose to delayed skin healing and postoperative oedema due to disruption of these vessels. The transverse elliptical plantar incision is very useful in the multiple excisions of the metatarsal heads, as in the Hoffman's operation, or in the Kates–Kessel operation. The advantage of this incision is that the metatarsal heads are prominent on the plantar surface and are, therefore, easily accessible in the sole of the foot due to the dislocation of the metatarsophalangeal joints in late claw toes. Furthermore, excess tissue, including the skin callosities, can be excised in an elliptical incision and the toes and distally displaced metatarsal fat pads can be brought down when the skin edges are stitched together. The metatarsophalangeal joints are exposed by longitudinal incision of the plantar capsule. In claw toes, the metatarsal heads displace the vessels, nerves and flexor tendons to one side and care must be taken to protect these structures.

Weight bearing can be carried out very early — in a few days following the operation, and even before the skin sutures are removed at two weeks. Skin healing is very good due to the rich vascularity of the plantar skin.

The metatarsal shafts

If an incision has to be made on the dorsum of the forefoot, it should be longitudinal in order to minimize damage to the lymphatic and venous drainage. Fortunately the skin creases or Langer's lines are in almost the same direction, and the cutaneous nerves lie parallel to a longitudinal incision and therefore escape damage.

If a particular metatarsal shaft is to be exposed a

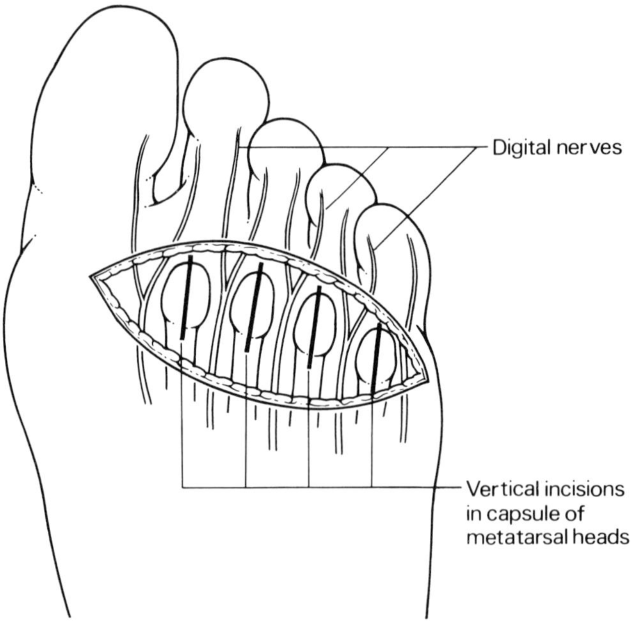

Fig. 58.16 Transverse elliptical plantar incision to the lateral four toes

longitudinal incision is made directly over it. If several metatarsal shafts have to be exposed, as in the Helal metatarsal osteotomy, the longitudinal skin incision should be of adequate length, about 3 cm along the distal shaft of the third metatarsal bone (Fig. 58.17). By gently retracting the skin, the periosteum of the second metatarsal bone is incised longitudinally and the shaft exposed. Similarly the fourth metatarsal shaft is exposed by retracting the other side of the skin incision. To ensure that the first and the fifth metatarsal bones are not accidentally osteotomized, these two bones should be palpated along their whole length after the bone retractors are in place to check that the retractors are not exposing these two bones. Also it is advisable to keep dissection of soft tissues down to a minimum to prevent cross union of the osteotomized bones.

The digital nerves

Like the dorsum of the foot, the plantar surface should be incised in a longitudinal direction in order to avoid damage to any of the nerves, vessels and tendons. This is the best approach to the digital nerves (Betts 1940). In conditions such as Morton's metatarsalgia, a long straight incision is made in the sole of the foot overlying the affected digital nerve and between the metatarsal heads (Fig. 58.18). The thick subcutaneous fat is incised and gently retracted. The deep fascia is incised to expose the digital nerve and vessels to the cleft. The skin incision should extend from the cleft distally to the hollow of the medial longitudinal plantar arch proximally, and the affected digital nerve is excised sufficiently proximally in order to site the cut nerve end in a non-weightbearing part of the foot, so that if an end-neuroma forms it will be out of the way when weight bearing (Nissen 1951). This incision exposes not only the digital nerve very well, but also allows easy access to the interdigital bursa, which not infrequently accompanies a Morton's 'neuroma'.

In the rare instance where several digital nerves are affected, and to prevent multiple incisions in the sole of the foot, a transverse incision across the sole of the foot, distal to the metatarsal heads, can be made (Kaplan 1950). The subcutaneous tissue is incised across in line with the skin incision, taking special care not to cut any digital vessels or nerves. The digital extensions of the plantar aponeurosis, the flexor tendon sheaths, the tendons of the lumbrical muscles and transverse metatarsal ligaments are exposed. The affected digital nerves are dissected

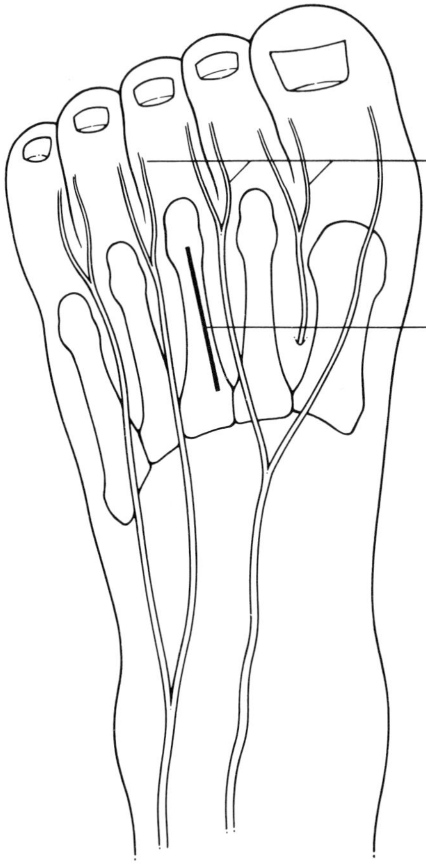

Fig. 58.17 Common incision on dorsum of the foot for metatarsal osteotomies

free and sectioned as proximally as possible. Unfortunately this exposure does not allow for adequate proximal sectioning of the affected nerves. Fortunately not more than two digital nerves are usually involved, and therefore a longitudinal incision can frequently be employed.

If two adjacent nerves are affected, a longitudinal plantar incision can be made between the two nerves, and both nerves exposed simultaneously and sectioned proximally in the hollow of the medial longitudinal plantar arch.

A longitudinal dorsal incision between the metatarsal heads to expose the digital nerve has been described (McKeever 1952). However, in such an exposure the transverse metatarsal ligament is divided, which may lead to splaying of the forefoot (Fig. 58.19). Also the digital nerve is difficult to expose as it lies more on the plantar side of the foot.

The plantar structures of the foot

Medial exposure (Henry 1957) (Fig. 58.20)

In a full exposure of all the plantar structures, the skin incision is made from the first metatarso-phalangeal joint to a point 3 cm above the medial malleolus between the Achilles tendon and the posteromedial border of the tibia. The incision is slightly curved with its convexity downwards and lies just below the navicular bone between the medial calcaneal nerve and the saphenous nerve. Care is taken to avoid damage to these nerves. The incision is deepened through the deep fascia and flexor retinaculum of the tarsal tunnel to expose the posterior tibial tendon, flexor digitorum longus tendon, posterior tibial artery and venae comitantes, tibial nerve and flexor hallucis longus tendon. Below the medial malleolus and lying on the medial side of

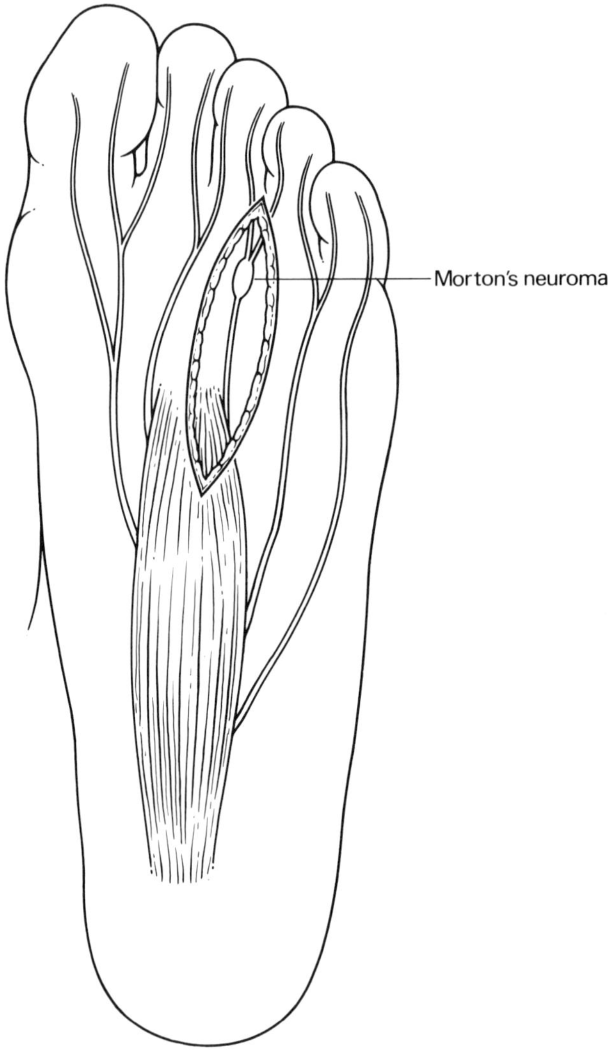

Fig. 58.18 Plantar approach to Morton's neuroma

the calcaneum is the muscle belly of the abductor hallucis with its distal tendon lying on the belly of the flexor hallucis brevis.

About 2 cm proximal to the tubercle of the navicular bone, the flexor digitorum longus tendon crosses medial to the flexor hallucis longus tendon. The tibial nerve divides 2 cm below the medial malleolus into lateral and medial plantar nerves. The lateral plantar nerve passes along the lateral border of the flexor digitorum brevis muscle.

The abductor hallucis is identified and its tendon is detached distally. The muscle belly is dissected off the navicular bone and medial tuberosity of the calcaneum, taking care to preserve its nerve supply which enters its deep side. By retracting this downwards the plantar structures are exposed.

This medial approach gives access to all the plantar structures, including the calcaneum, navicular, medial cuneiform and first metatarsal bones.

Depending on which structures are to be exposed, the incision can be limited either to the posterior half or the anterior half. On the other hand, if a more extensive approach is required, the medial approach can be combined with a posteromedial approach to expose the ankle and subtalar joints. The incision is

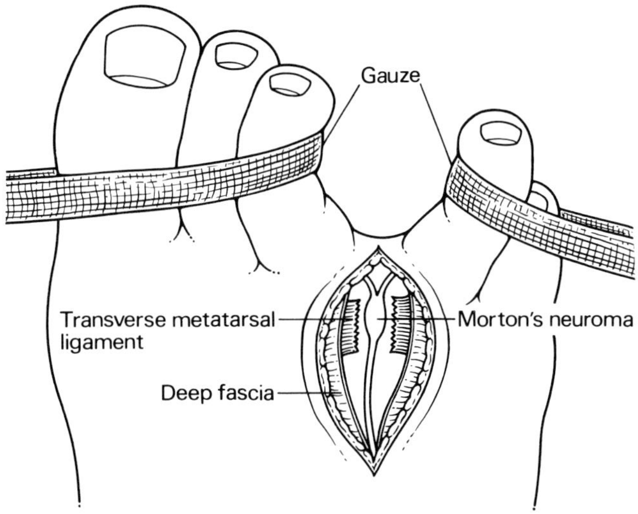

Fig. 58.19 Dorsal approach to Morton's neuroma

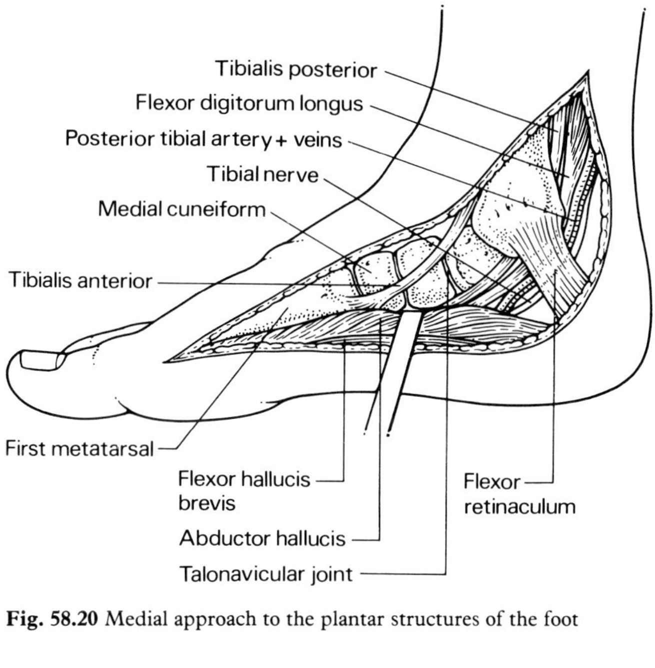

Fig. 58.20 Medial approach to the plantar structures of the foot

extended proximally upwards between the Achilles tendon and the tibia. This extended incision is useful in conditions like congenital talipes equinovarus where the ankle, subtalar and talonavicular joints are exposed. In the operation described by Brockman (1930) the incision extends vertically between the tibia and Achilles tendon, downwards behind and below the medial malleolus, and curves forwards to end at the medial cuneiform.

Structures at the back of the heel

Achilles tendon

The Achilles tendon, its superficial and its deep bursae can be exposed by vertical incisions placed medially, laterally or posteriorly to the tendon. Of these three positions, the medial incision is favoured because it gives rise to a less obvious scar, which is not irritated by the back of a shoe, and it heals well. A transverse incision extending from the medial to the lateral sides of the tendon along the skin creases can be made, but the exposure is not as good. It is not advisable to split the Achilles tendon in order to gain access to structures deep to the tendon as it is important not to damage any fibres. The fibres of the tendon spiral clockwise in a superior direction on the right and anticlockwise in a superior direction on the left, (Fig. 58.21), and even if some fibres are cut exposure is still inadequate. Furthermore, even separating the fibres of the Achilles tendon may damage the proprioceptive nerve fibres which are present within the tendon.

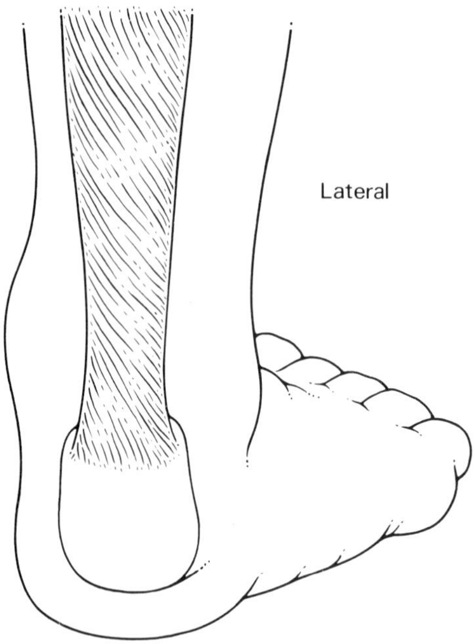

Fig. 58.21 Direction of fibres in the Achilles tendon in the right foot

Calcaneum

The calcaneum can be exposed medially, laterally, inferiorly or posteriorly. It can also be split posteroinferiorly.

Medial approach (Fig. 58.22). A medial exposure is used for an open wedge type of oblique osteotomy of the calcaneum for residual congenital talipes equinovarus (Dwyer 1963), Steindler release of the plantar aponeurosis, and exploration of the structures posterior to the medial malleolus, such as in tarsal tunnel syndrome. An incision is made between the Achilles tendon and the tibia 3 cm above the tip of the medial malleolus. It is curved downwards behind and below the medial malleolus to the tuberosity of the navicular bone parallel with the inferior border of the calcaneum. The saphenous nerve and vein lie in front of this incision.

Lateral approach (Fig. 58.23). The patient lies supine with a sandbag under the ipsilateral buttock. Lateral exposure of the calcaneum is made by a vertical incision starting 3 cm above the tip of the lateral malleolus between the fibula and Achilles tendon. It curves downwards behind and below the tip of the lateral malleolus, passing across the peroneal trochlea of the calcaneum to the base of the fifth metatarsal bone. The sural nerve and its

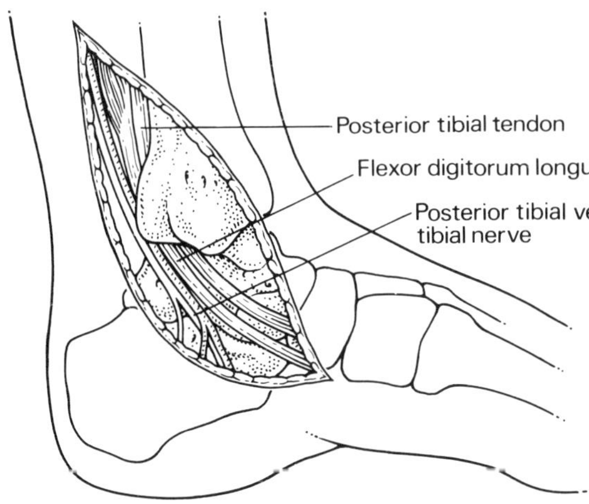

Fig. 58.22 Medial approach to the calcaneum

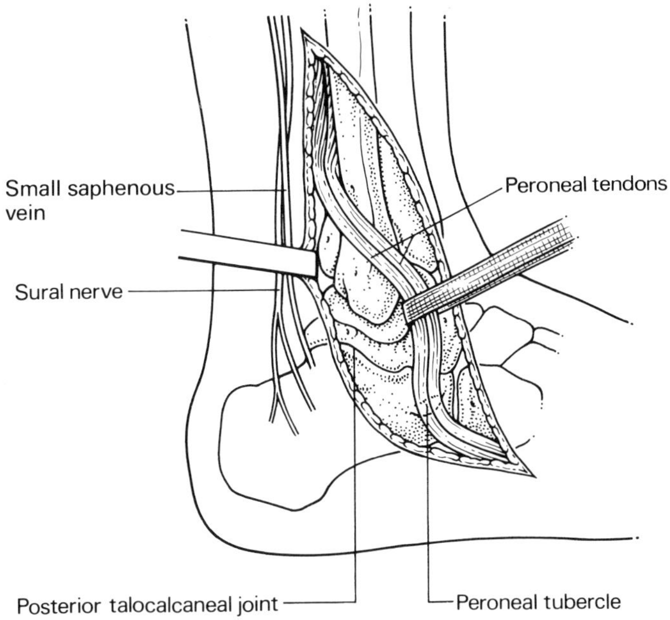

Fig. 58.23 Lateral approach to the calcaneum

branches are identified and retracted anteriorly, and the soft tissues incised down to bone. If the peroneal tendons have to be retracted anteriorly the peroneal sheath is incised. If the tendon sheath is incised it has to be repaired at the end of the surgical procedure. If the peroneal sheath is not incised, the incision lies behind and below these tendons. This approach gives access to the calcaneum in bone grafting for crush fractures, in reconstruction of the lateral ligament, and to the posterior facet of the talocalcaneal joint.

Inferior approach (Fig. 58.24). The patient lies

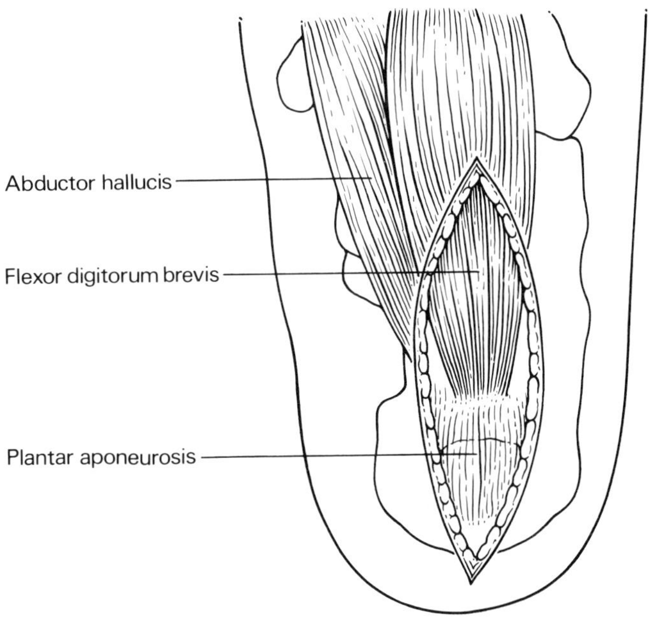

Fig. 58.24 Inferior approach to the calcaneum

supine on the operating table. An inferior approach to the calcaneum is made by a midline incision along the longitudinal axis of the foot in the heel pad, and through the plantar aponeurosis. This approach is useful to excise a troublesome calcaneal spur and to insert an intramedullary nail for a plantar arthrodesis. As long as the incision is kept to the midline, there is no danger to the important nerves of the sole, which are on the medial side.

Posterior approach (Fig. 58.25). The patient lies prone on the table. A posterior exposure of the calcaneum is made by a transverse incision along the skin crease centred on the back of the heel. The skin is undermined and retracted above and below to expose the posterior part of the calcaneum.

Posteroinferior approach (Fig. 58.26). The patient lies prone on the table. The posteroinferior split heel exposure of the calcaneum (Gaenslen 1931) is rarely carried out nowadays. It was used in complete or partial excision of the calcaneum for infection and in comminuted fractures. The incision extends from just above the insertion of the Achilles tendon, splitting the tendon and the bone anteriorly to the calcaneocuboid joint in the sole of the foot. The bone is split longitudinally using an osteotome or saw.

The subtalar and midtarsal joints

Anterolateral approach (Campbell 1956) (Fig. 58.27)

This approach is the most versatile of the dorsal approaches to the foot, and gives the best exposure to the tarsal joints. Being in the line of a vascular watershed it heals well.

The patient lies supine with a sandbag under the ipsilateral buttock. An anterolateral exposure of the subtalar and midtarsal joints, as well as the ankle joint can be made by an incision starting from 4–5 cm above the ankle joint in front of the fibula to 1 cm below the tip of the lateral malleolus. It curves gently to end at the base of the fourth metatarsal bone and passes above the peroneal tendons and between the sural nerve and the lateral branch of the

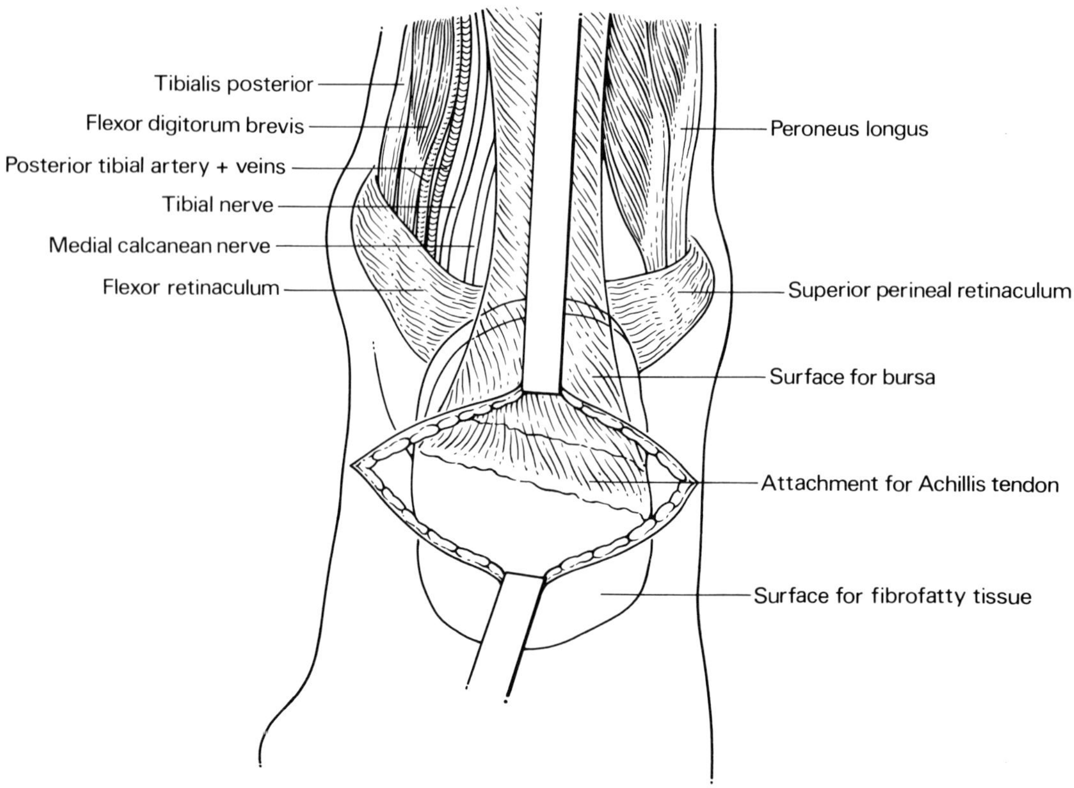

Fig. 58.25 Posterior approach to the calcaneum

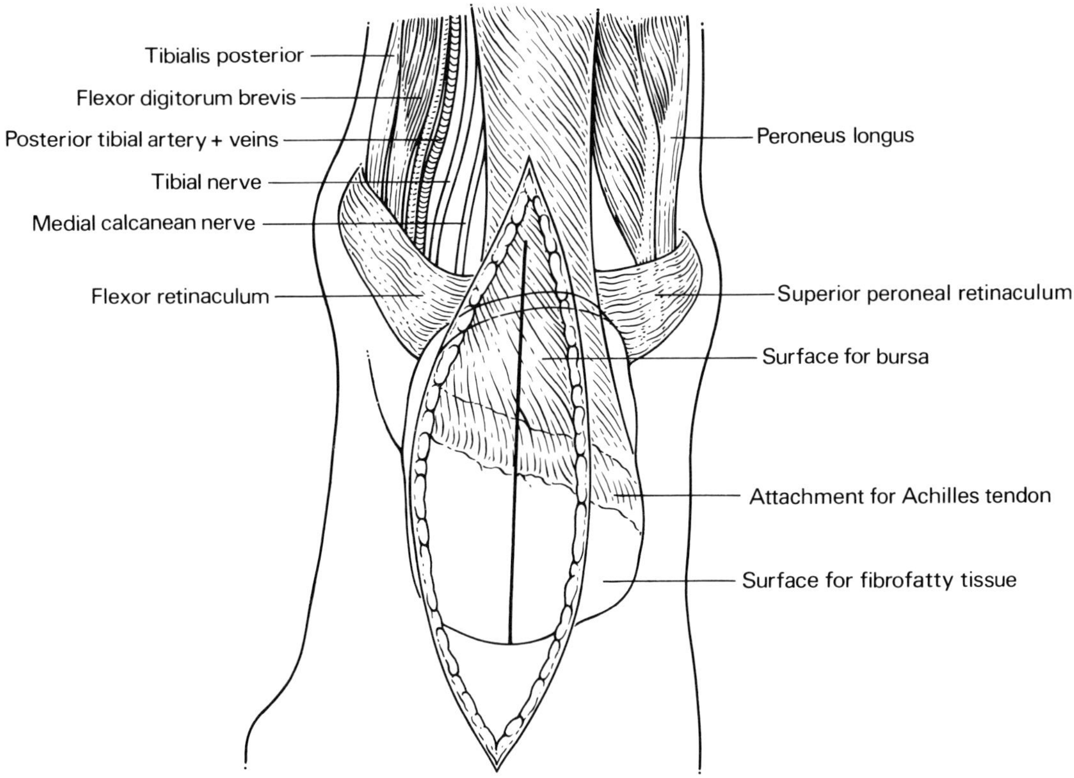

Fig. 58.26 Posterior-inferior approach to the calcaneum

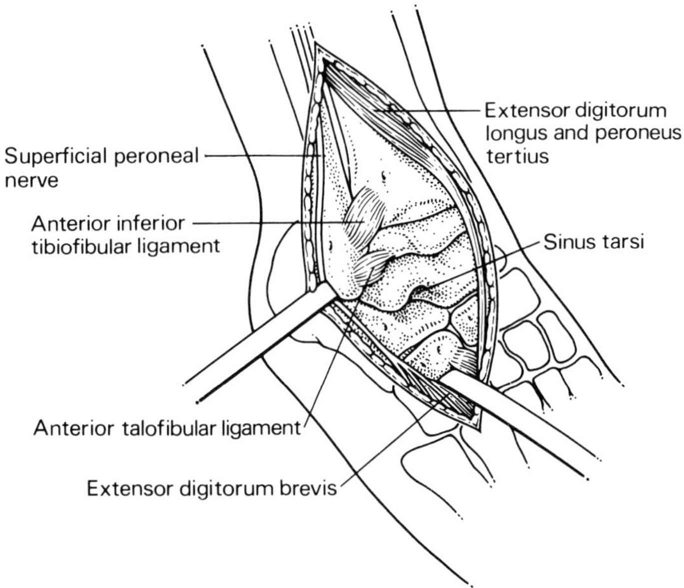

Fig. 58.27 Anterolateral approach to the ankle (Campbell)

superficial peroneal nerve. The peroneal tendons are identified and protected. The deep fascia and inferior extensor retinaculum are divided just lateral to the peroneus tertius, and the muscle belly of the extensor digitorum brevis is partially dissected upwards from its attachment to expose the anterior part of the ankle, the talonavicular joint, the calcaneocuboid joint and the lateral part of the subtalar joint and sinus tarsi. It is not always necessary to use the full extent of the approach.

This approach is used for artificial replacement or arthrodesis of the ankle joint, repair of the anterior tibiofibular ligament, arthrodesis of the talonavicular, calcaneocuboid or subtalar joints either separately or in combination as in a triple arthrodesis or a pantalar arthrodesis.

Lateral approach (Ollier 1891) (Fig. 58.28)

The subtalar joint can also be exposed by a lateral incision from below the tip of the lateral malleolus, curving across to the talonavicular joint. The sural nerve, the lateral branch of the superficial peroneal nerve, the terminal branches of the deep peroneal nerve and the dorsalis pedis artery cross the incision and should be protected. The tendons of the extensor digitorum longus and peroneus tertius are retracted medially, the peroneal tendons retracted downwards and the extensor digitorum brevis partially dissected upwards to expose the subtalar and midtarsal joints. This is a limited approach to the subtalar and midtarsal joints, and is useful for a triple or a subtalar arthrodesis. A more limited exposure of the sinus tarsi can be made, as in the extra-articular arthrodesis of the subtalar joint in severe pes planovalgus (Grice 1952) by an incision extending from 1 cm below the tip of the lateral malleolus upwards and forwards across the sinus tarsi. The lateral branch of the superficial peroneal nerve, which lies at the anterior part of the incision, must be preserved. The fat and deep fascia are dissected away to expose the sinus tarsi.

SURGICAL APPROACHES TO THE ANKLE JOINT

The ankle joint can be exposed from many approaches, medial, lateral, anterior, posterior and a combination of the above.

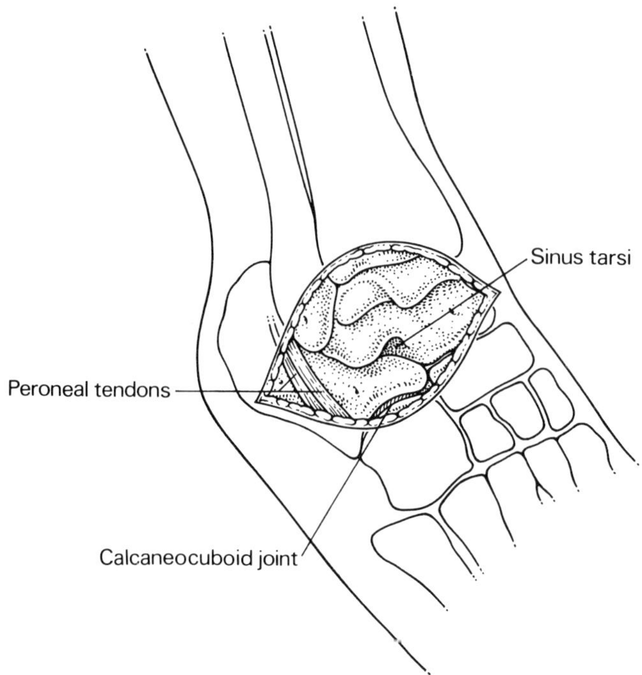

Fig. 58.28 Lateral approach (Ollier) to the ankle

The simplest are the short medial and lateral approaches. A vertical incision is made over the medial or lateral malleolus down to its tip, the length of the incision varying according to the purpose of the exposure. These incisions are frequently used to reduce and internally fix fractured malleoli. If a more extensive approach is necessary this vertical incision can be curved forwards or backwards below the tips of the malleoli, and in such instances the vertical limb of the incision can be placed anterior or posterior to the malleolus, depending on whether the incision is to be curved backwards (in the former) or forwards (in the latter). The important structures to be looked for on the medial side of the ankle are the deltoid ligament, the tibialis posterior tendon, flexor digitorum longus, tibial nerve, posterior tibial vessels, the saphenous nerve and great saphenous vein, and on the lateral side, the peroneal tendons, the calcaneofibular ligament, the lateral branch of the superficial peroneal nerve, the sural nerve and the small saphenous vein.

Short medial approach (Fig. 58.29)

The patient lies supine with a sandbag under the opposite buttock. A vertical incision 4–5 cm is made over the medial malleolus down to its tip. Take care of the saphenous nerve and the great saphenous vein, which lie along the anterior border of the medial malleolus, and the tibialis posterior, flexor digitorum longus, the posterior tibial artery and vein, the tibial nerve and flexor hallucis longus, behind the medial malleolus. The periosteum is incised and stripped off the bone to expose the medial malleolus. Subperiosteal stripping anteriorly will expose the ankle joint and this manoeuvre is useful in obtaining a perfect reduction of a medial malleolar fracture.

Transmalleolar approach (Koenig & Schaefer 1929) (Fig. 58.30)

The ankle joint can also be more fully exposed by osteotomizing the medial malleolus transversely, just below the level of the roof of the ankle. By everting the foot the superior surface of the talus and the ankle joint can be exposed.

The patient lies in the lateral position. The affected leg is below the normal one, which is flexed at the knee to expose the ankle of the leg affected.

A curved transverse incision is made just proximal to the medial malleolus. The medial malleolus is exposed, taking care not to damage the medial

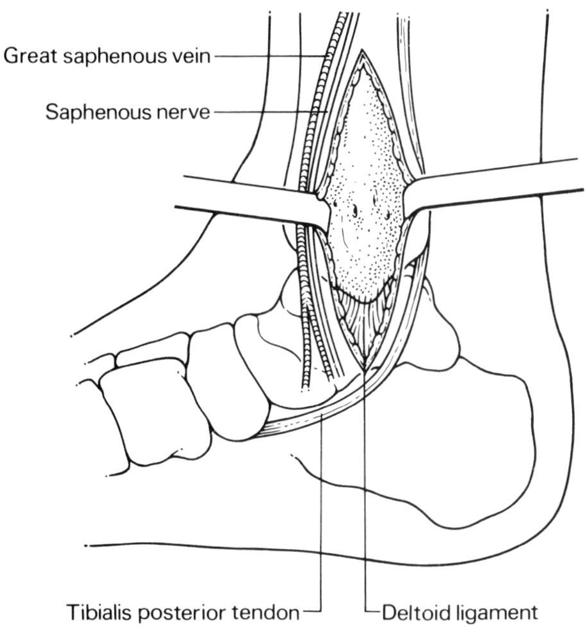

Fig. 58.29 Short medial approach to the ankle

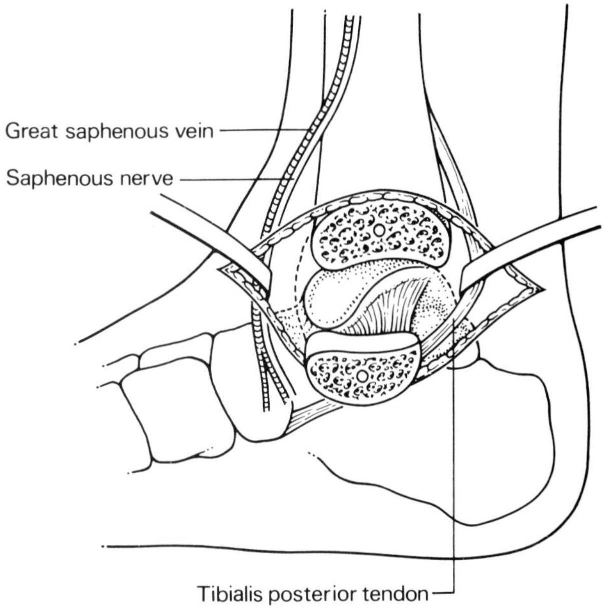

Fig. 58.30 Transmalleolar approach to the ankle

ligament. A drill hole is made into the medial malleolus in an oblique direction to a depth of about 6 cm and the track tapped. The medial malleolus is osteotomized in an oblique direction, so that the plane of osteotomy is at right angles to the screw track. By everting the foot, the talus is dislocated laterally and the ankle joint exposed. The wound is closed by screwing back the medial malleolus.

This approach is not commonly used as, in a sense, osteotomizing the medial malleolus is creating an intra-articular fracture and reduction and re-positioning of the medial malleolus must be perfect to avoid secondary osteoarthritis. In addition the anterior tibial artery and deep peroneal nerve can be easily damaged unless great care is taken. However, it is useful in fracture-dislocations, intra-articular fractures and osteochondritis dissecans of the talus.

Short lateral approach (Fig. 58.31)

The patient lies supine with a sandbag under the ipsilateral buttock. A vertical incision 4–5 cm is made over the lateral malleolus down to its tip. Care is taken of the lateral branch of the superficial peroneal and the sural nerves. The periosteum is incised and stripped off the bone to expose the lateral malleolus. Further stripping of the periosteum anteriorly will expose the anterior part of the inferior tibiofibular joint.

Lateral approach (Kocher 1911) (Fig. 58.32)

The patient lies supine with a sandbag under the ipsilateral buttock. A 5–6 cm vertical incision is made between the Achilles tendon and the posterior border of the fibula and curved down 2 cm below the tip of the lateral malleolus and across to the talonavicular joint. The deep fascia is incised after identifying and protecting the sural nerve, the small saphenous vein and the peroneal tendons. These structures are retracted backwards. The anterior talofibular and calcaneofibular ligaments are divided to expose the subtalar and calcaneocuboid joints. By inverting the foot, the ankle joint is subluxated and exposed to view.

This approach gives a very good view of the ankle, subtalar and midtarsal joints, but there may be slow healing of the skin wound due to the wide retraction and if the incision is made too curved.

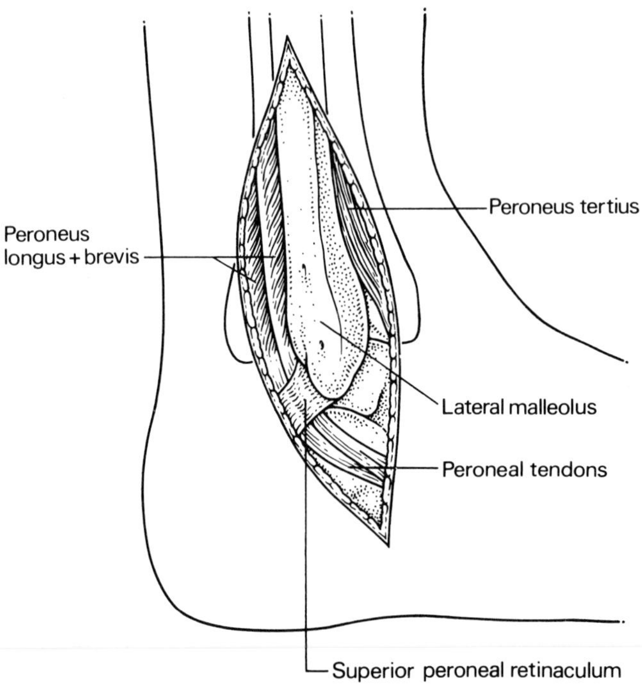

Fig. 58.31 Short lateral approach to the ankle

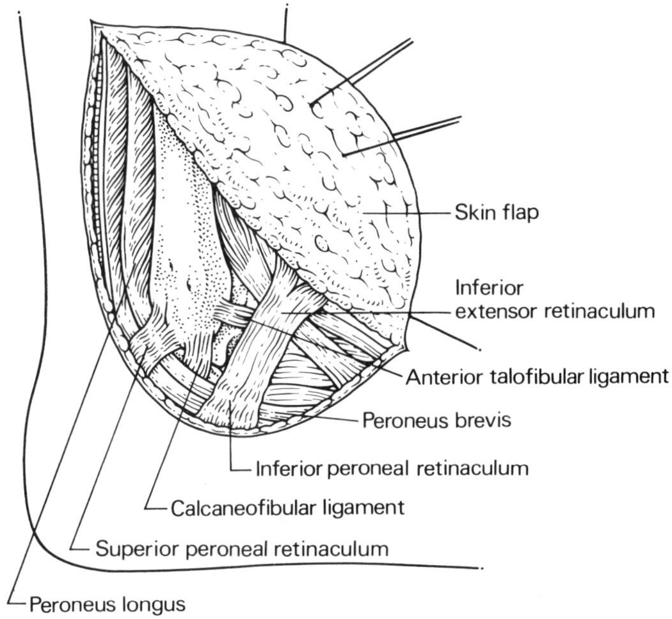

Fig. 58.32 Lateral approach (Kocher) to the ankle

Anterolateral approach (Campbell 1956) (see Fig. 58.27)

This gives an excellent approach to the ankle, subtalar and midtarsal joints as well as the talus and other tarsal bones, except the navicular, medial and intermediate cuneiform bones.

The patient lies supine with a sandbag under the ipsilateral buttock. An incision about 4–5 cm proximal to the ankle is made along the anterior border of the fibula, to 1 cm below the tip of the lateral malleolus, across the calcaneocuboid joint to the base of the fourth metatarsal. The deep fascia and the inferior extensor retinaculum are incised. The extensor digitorum brevis muscle is dissected off its attachment to the underlying bone and retracted distally. The lateral malleolar and lateral tarsal vessels may have to be sacrificed but identify and protect the lateral branch of the superficial peroneal and sural nerves. The blood vessels have to be carefully diathermized to prevent a postoperative haematoma. The long extensor tendons, the anterior tibial artery and deep peroneal nerve are retracted medially and the ankle, subtalar, talonavicular and calcaneocuboid joints are exposed by incising the joint capsules. It is not always necessary to use the full extent of the approach.

Posterolateral approach (Gatelier & Chastang 1924) (Fig. 58.33)

The lateral part of the ankle joint, including the talus, and the posterior and anterior parts of the lower end of the tibia can be exposed by hinging the fibula outwards on the lateral ligament.

The patient lies in a lateral position with the affected leg uppermost. A 10–12 cm vertical incision is made on the lateral side of the fibula down to just below the tip of the lateral malleolus, and carried anteriorly for 3–4 cm in the line of the peroneal tendons. The fibula is osteotomized about 7–10 cm from its tip and stripped subperiosteally. The peroneal sheath is incised and the peroneal tendons retracted forwards. The interosseous membrane and the inferior tibiofibular ligament are divided and the fibula turned outwards on the talofibular and calcaneofibular parts of the lateral ligament to expose the lateral part of the ankle and the posterolateral part of the tibia.

If the fibula is fractured, the interosseous membrane and inferior tibiofibular ligaments may be already damaged and it is not necessary either to osteotomize the fibula or divide these ligaments. However, it is important to make sure that the talofibular and calcaneofibular ligaments are preserved.

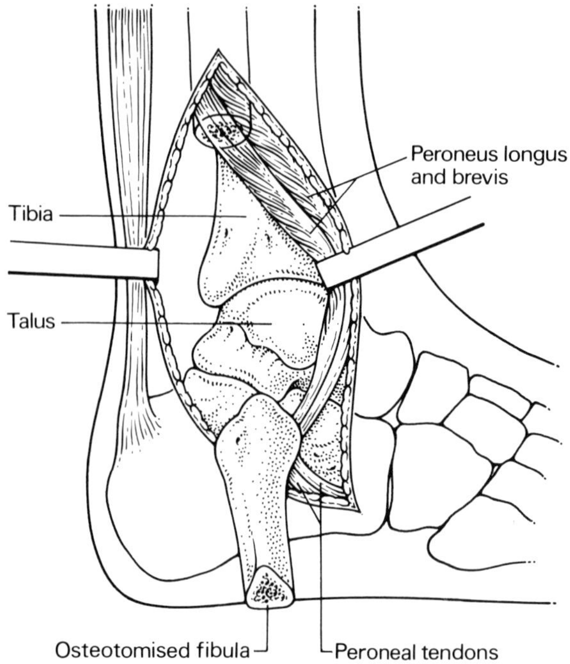

Fig. 58.33 Posterolateral approach to the ankle

During closure, the inferior tibiofibular joint is stabilized by a transfixing screw directed 10° upwards and laterally across this joint and above the ankle joint, taking care not to damage the ankle by drilling too low. It is important to ensure that the fibular osteotomy or fracture is reduced well so that shortening of this bone does not occur. If necessary a short plate may be used internally to fix the fibula. The tendons are replaced and the tendon sheaths repaired.

This approach is useful for intra-articular fractures and osteochondritis dissecans of the talus, and when a wide exposure of the ankle joint is necessary as in pigmented villonodular synovitis and multiple chondromatosis.

Access to the posterior malleolus

The posterior malleolus of the tibia can be exposed either by a posteromedial approach or a posterolateral approach, depending on which part is to be exposed.

Posteromedial approach (Broomhead 1932) (Fig. 58.34)

The patient lies supine with the foot over the end of the table to allow the ankle to be dorsiflexed easily. A vertical incision is made between the Achilles tendon and the posterior border of the tibia and curved downwards and forwards below the tip of the medial malleolus to end at the talonavicular joint. The posterior malleolus of the tibia is exposed by retracting posteromedially the tendons of the tibialis

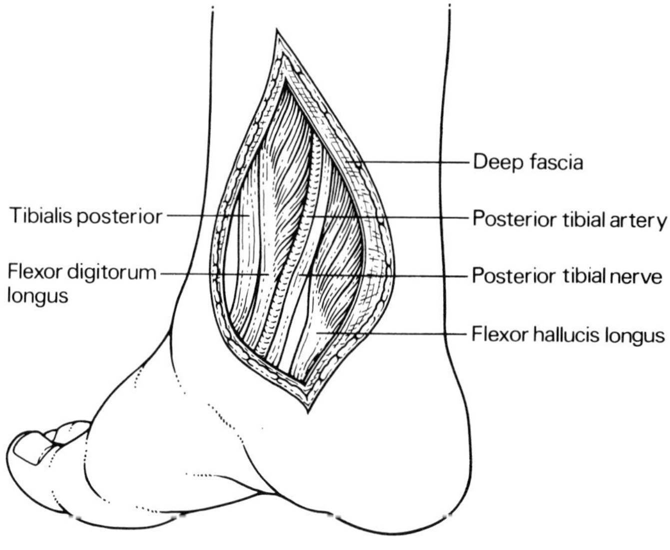

Fig. 58.34 Posteromedial approach to the ankle

posterior, flexor digitorum longus and flexor hallucis longus, the tibial nerve and posterior tibial vessels. It is useful to remember that the flexor hallucis longus has muscle fibres down to the level of the ankle joint, and that the tibial nerve is quite a large structure even in children.

This approach is useful for exposing both medial and posterior malleoli, in cases of trauma, and in the posteromedial release operation for congenital talipes equinovarus.

Posterolateral approach (Fig. 58.35)

The patient lies prone with the foot over the end of the table to allow for adequate dorsiflexion of the ankle. This approach consists of a 10–12 cm vertical incision along the lateral border of the Achilles tendon and curving downwards and forwards below the tip of the lateral malleolus. The tendons of the flexor hallucis longus and peroneus brevis are identified and retracted away from each other, to expose the posterior parts of the tibia, ankle and subtalar joints. The flexor hallucis longus may have to be stripped off the posterior surface of the tibia to obtain an adequate view of the ankle joint.

Anterior approach (Fig. 58.36)

The patient lies supine on the operating table. A vertical incision starts from the anterior border of the tibia 8–10 cm proximally down across the ankle joint (midway between the lateral and medial malleoli) to the base of the second metatarsal. The superficial peroneal nerve lies very close to this incision. This nerve is identified and protected. The plane between the extensor hallucis longus and the extensor digitorum longus tendons is identified. The extensor retinaculum is incised. The anterior tibial artery and deep peroneal nerve are also identified and protected, and with the tendons of the extensor

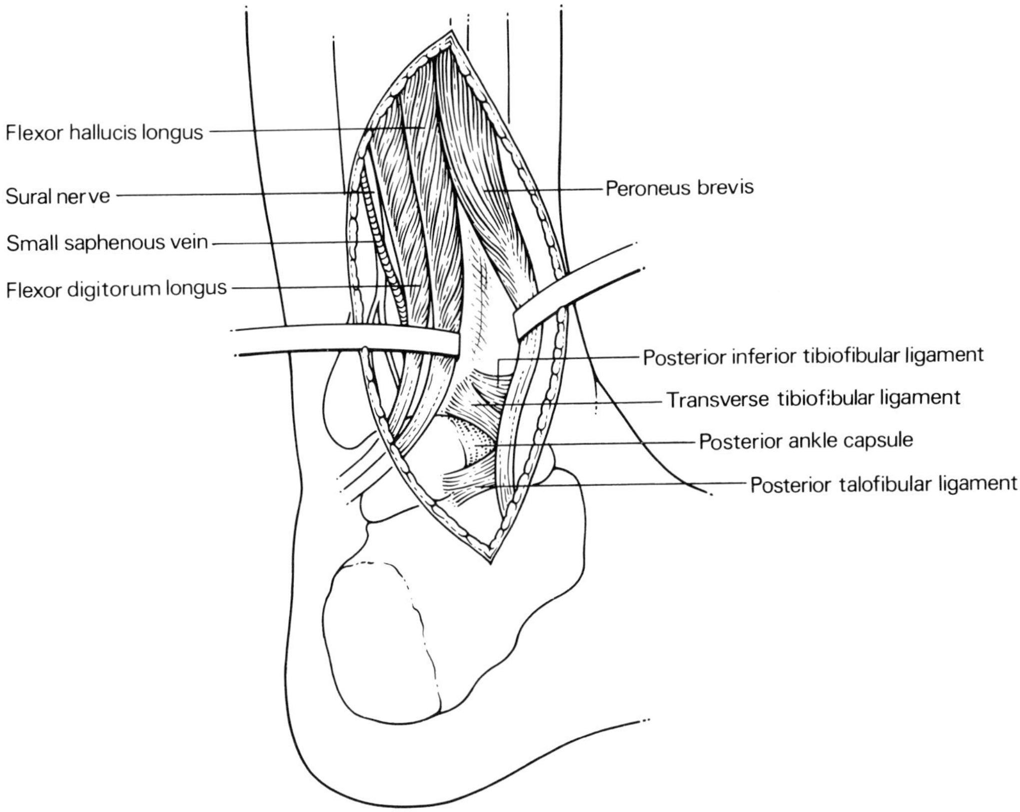

Fig. 58.35 Posterolateral approach to the ankle

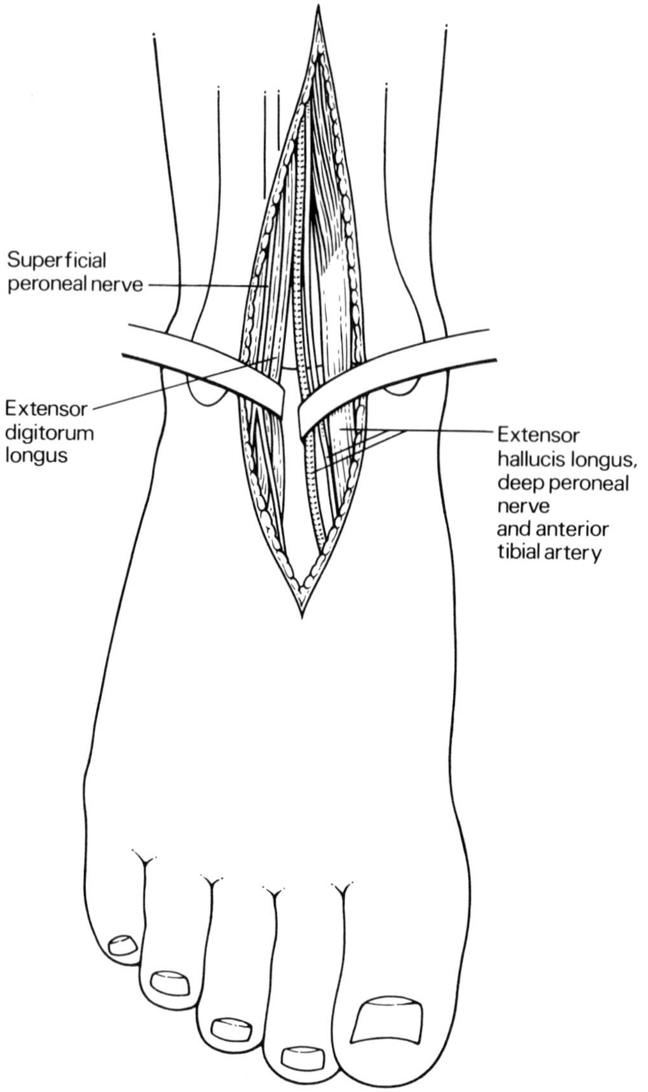

Fig. 58.36 Anterior approach to the ankle

hallucis longus and tibialis anterior are retracted medially, while the tendon of the extensor digitorum longus is retracted laterally to expose the ankle joint. The capsule of the ankle joint is incised in the line of the skin incision. It can be stripped off the tibia and talus for a wide exposure. This exposure can be further extended to include the tibia by retracting the tibialis anterior laterally.

The anterior approach to the ankle joint is useful in arthrodesis procedures, not only of the ankle joint but also of the subtalar joint (Brown's (1968) modification of the Grice operation).

Posterior approach (Fig. 58.37)

The patient lies prone on the operating table. The posterior approach to the ankle joint consists of a 10–12 cm vertical incision along the posterior border of the Achilles tendon. The Achilles tendon is divided by a Z-shaped incision and retracted. The flexor hallucis longus and peroneus brevis tendons are separated to expose the posterior part of the ankle joint. The tibial nerve and posterior tibial vessels are protected by the tendon of the flexor hallucis longus, but care should be taken not to damage them.

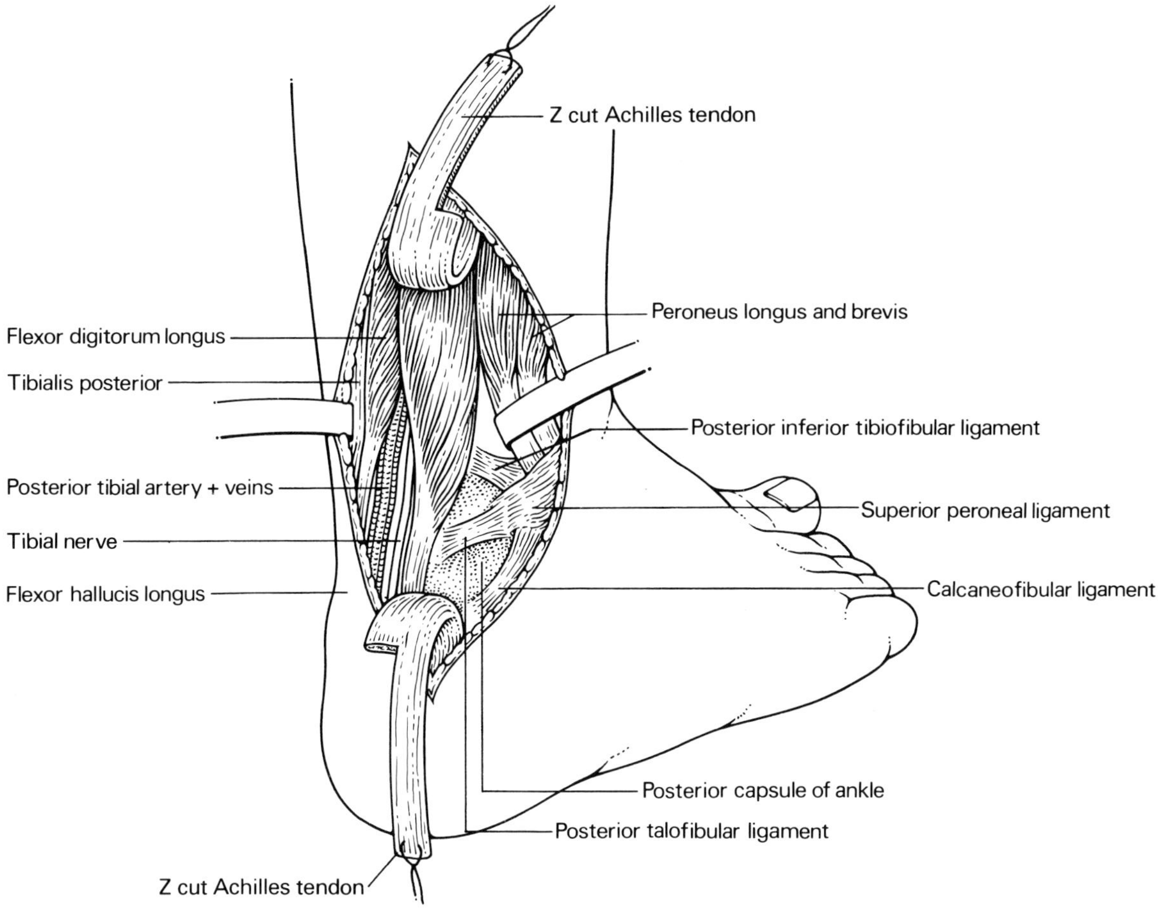

Fig. 58.37 Posterior approach to the ankle

This approach is usually not carried out unless absolutely necessary because of damage to the Achilles tendon by the Z-incision.

REFERENCES

Betts L O 1940 Morton's metatarsalgia: Neuritis of the fourth digital nerve. Med J Aust 1: 514

Brockman E P 1930 Congenital Club Foot (talipes equinovarus). J Wright & Sons Ltd, Bristol

Broomhead R 1932 Discussions on fractures in the region of the ankle joint. Proc R Soc Med 25: 1082

Brown A 1968 A simple method of fusion of the subtalar joint in children. J Bone Joint Surg 50B: 369

Campbell W C 1956 Operative Orthopaedics, 3rd edn. C V Mosby Co, St Louis. p 195

Dwyer F C 1963 The treatment of relapsed club foot by the insertion of a wedge into the calcaneum. J Bone Joint Surg 45B: 67

Gaenslen F J 1931 Split-heel approach in osteomyelitis of os calcis. J Bone Joint Surg 13: 759

Gatelier J, Chastang 1924 Access to fractured malleolus with piece chipped off at back. J Chir 24: 513

Grice D S 1952 An extra-articular arthrodesis of the subastragalar joint for correction of paralytic flat feet in children. J Bone Joint Surg 34A: 927

Helal B 1975 Metatarsal osteotomy for metatarsalgia. J Bone Joint Surg 57B: 187

Helal B, Chen S C 1982 Arthroplastik des Grosszehengrundgelenks mit einer neuen Silastik-Endoprosthese. Orthopäde 11: 200–206

Henry A K 1957 Extensile Exposure, 2nd edn. The Williams & Wilkins Co, Baltimore
Hoffmann P 1911 An operation for severe grades of contracted or claw toes. Am J Orthop Surg 9: 441
Kaplan E B 1950 Surgical Approach to the plantar digital nerves. Bull Hosp Joint Dis 11: 96
Kates A, Kessel L, Kay A 1967 Arthroplasty of the forefoot. J Bone Joint Surg 49B: 552
Keller W L 1904 Surgical treatment of bunions and hallux valgus. N Y Med J 80: 741
Kocher T 1911 Textbook on Operative Surgery, 3rd edn. (Translated by H J Stiles & C B Paul). A & C Black, London
Koenig F, Schaefer P 1929 Osteoplastic surgical exposure of the ankle joint. Z Chir 215: 196
Langer Carl von (1819–1887) Professor of Anatomy, University of Vienna
Mayo C H 1908 Surgical treatment of bunion. Ann Surg 48: 300
McKeever D C 1952 Surgical approach for neuroma of plantar digital nerve (Morton's metatarsalgia). J Bone Joint Surg 34A: 490
McMinn R M H, Hutchings R T, Logan B M 1982 A Colour Atlas of Foot and Ankle Anatomy. Wolfe Medical Publications Ltd. p 50
Morton T A 1876 A peculiar and painful affection of the fourth metatarso-phalangeal articulation. Am J Med Sci New series 71: 37
Nissen K I 1951 The etiology of Morton's metatarsalgia. J Bone Joint Surg 33B: 293
Ollier P 1891 Traité des Résections et des Opérations Conservatrices qu'on Peut Practiquer sur le Systeme Osseux, Vol 3. G Masson, Paris
Steindler A 1920 Stripping of the os calcis. J Orthop Surg 2: 8
Swanson A B 1975 Silicone implant resection arthroplasty of the great toe. J Bone Joint Surg 57A: 1173
Taylor R G 1951 The treatment of claw toes by multiple transfers of flexor into extensor tendons. J Bone Joint Surg 33B: 539
Zadik F R 1950 Obliteration of the nail bed of the great toe without shortening the terminal phalanx. J Bone Joint Surg 32B: 66

Principles of fracture treatment

INTRODUCTION

Fractures involving the foot and ankle joint account for a significant proportion of all injuries. In the young these fractures may lead to permanent deformities, particularly if the growth plate is damaged and unequal growth occurs. In adult life the fracture may result in disability from degenerative changes following damage to the joint, which in turn can lead to long periods off work. In the elderly, fractures of the foot and ankle may result in loss of independence and may indeed confine the patient to bed.

The foot may be involved in a patient who has sustained multiple injuries, in which case the basic priorities are to resuscitate the patient, paying particular attention to the airway, the degree of head injury and the circulating volume of the patient. Once these parameters have been managed, full attention can be directed to the foot and other musculoskeletal injuries.

PRINCIPLES OF TREATMENT APPLIED TO THE FOOT

The principles of fracture treatment applied to the foot can be considered under the following headings:

1. Care of the wound
2. Attention to the vascular status
3. Attention to the neurological status
4. Damage to muscles and tendons
5. Treatment of the fracture

Whilst each of these sections will be dealt with in detail it is obvious that priorities must be given to immediate relief from vascular compression such as occurs following a fracture-dislocation of the ankle (Fig. 59.1). If this fracture is left, the compression of the distal vascular supply can be so severe as to jeopardize the viability of the foot and early reduction is imperative. Equally so, in line with any other form of first line management, if there is skin loss, the wound needs to be covered prior to dealing with the tissues under sterile conditions.

CARE OF THE WOUND

The prevention of infection in open fractures

Open fractures left untreated have in the past led to amputation or death (Billroth 1886). Today, although death from a compound fracture may be rare, amputation may still be necessary. However the

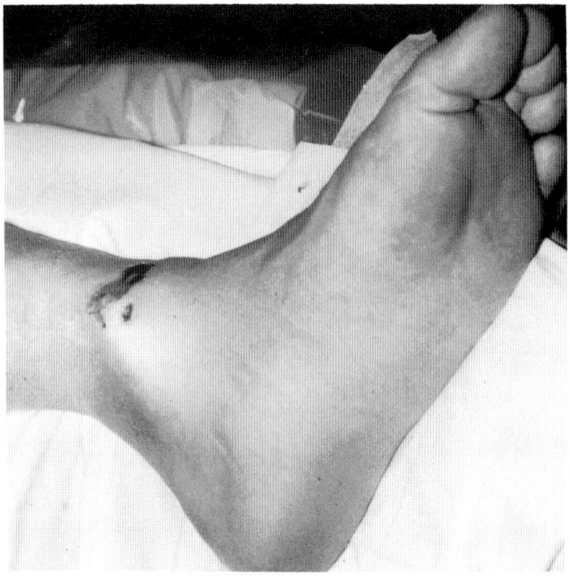

Fig. 59.1 Fracture-dislocation of the ankle

establishment of a chronic osteomyelitis is a persistent problem (Fig. 59.2). Eradication of this infection once it has occurred may be hard to achieve and can lead to significant loss of function.

The wound

The immediate treatment of the patient with a compound fracture is the removal of obvious dirt and debris from the wound. This can be done immediately in the Accident Unit, at which time the wound can be washed and covered with a sterile cloth in order to prevent subsequent infection from further pathogenic organisms. It is important that the patient is transferred to the operating suite as soon as possible for definitive treatment of the wound.

After scrubbing the surrounding skin and wound, a tourniquet can be applied without exsanguination and the patient transferred to the operating theatre. Thorough excision of all dead and devitalized tissue is mandatory. Clearly at this time the wound is further inspected for any foreign material which must be removed. The wound itself can then be washed out with 0.9% saline or other suitable solution such as chlorhexidine or povidone iodine and up to 14 l of saline can be used thoroughly to cleanse a grossly damaged structure (Gustillo & Anderson 1976).

ANTIBIOTICS

The use of 'prophylactic' antibiotics in the management of compound fractures is still contentious. However if the wound is considered to be already infected or at least colonized by pathogenic organisms due to the nature of the injury, it is not unreasonable to consider the use of antibiotics as 'therapeutic'.

The choice of antibiotics

The selection of an antibiotic for treatment should depend on the pathogenic organisms that are encountered. Patzakis et al (1974) isolated a wide variety of organisms from compound fractures, including gram-positive and gram-negative organisms, even though only a small proportion became frankly infected.

Clearly the distribution of pathogenic organisms may vary from area to area, some rural communities having a higher incidence of clostridial organisms than others.

However since most wounds are initially contaminated with pathogenic organisms it is rational to give an antibiotic on admission to hospital. Patzakis and his colleagues, in a prospective trial on a large group of patients, reported an infection rate of 14% in those patients who received

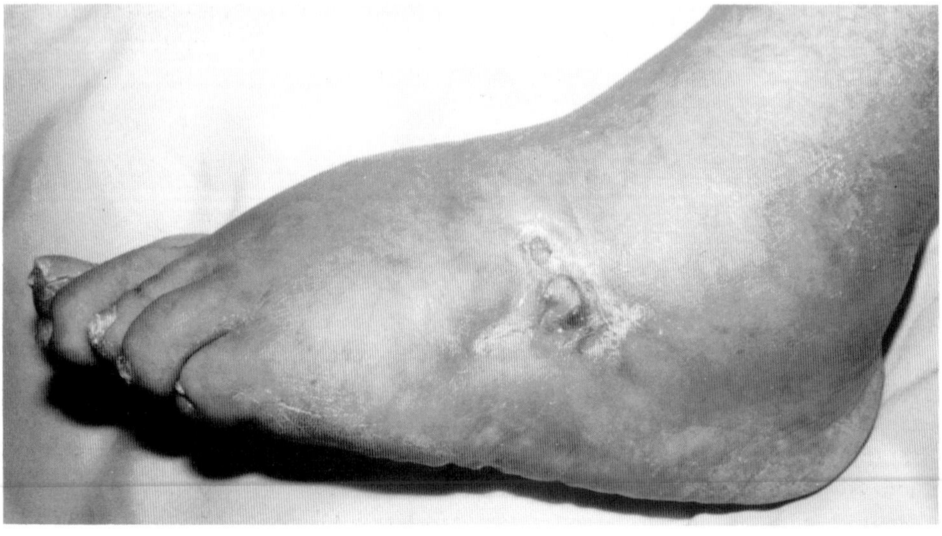

Fig. 59.2 Chronic osteomyelitis involving the foot following a previous fracture

no treatment, 10% in a group receiving penicillin and streptomycin and 2% in patients who had a cephalosporin injected for four days. The difference between cephalosporin and the untreated group and the penicillin with streptomycin group is statistically significant.

On the basis of this study, it is our practice to use a cephalosporin (cefuroxime) as a therapeutic agent in all compound fractures.

Route of administration

Following any fracture, no matter how severe, there is a reduction in the blood flow to the bone. In a compound fracture which by its nature is of high velocity type and therefore severe, the blood supply to the bone will be reduced. In this case, the antibiotics delivered systemically will be reduced particularly if they are administered intravenously. Pollard et al (1979a) showed that following an intramuscular injection of flucloxacillin in a group of patients undergoing total hip replacement, the amount of flucloxacillin assayed in the femoral head removed at surgery was at or below the mean inhibitory concentration (MIC) for most pathogenic organisms. Hence it is rational, particularly in the period immediately after the fracture to give the antibiotic systemically in large doses, at least to allow a reasonable concentration to reach the area of damage, whilst the bone blood flow is reduced (Hughes & Anderson 1985).

Length of administration of antibiotic

Patzakis et al (1974) advocated four days of intramuscular injection. This is clearly an arbitrary time and must be related to the extent of the skin damage, associated with the fracture and degree of potential area of injection.

For some time fractures have been considered to be compound from within or from without, depending upon whether the bone pierced the skin due to angulation, or whether the skin was damaged from the original fracture. To some extent this approach has been superseded by the numerical classification of Gustillo & Anderson (1976). They divided compound fractures into:

Type I which are comparable to the original compound from within

Type II in which there is skin damage

Type III in which there is extensive damage.

Types II and III are degrees of compound fractures from without. As the classification seems to be accepted widely and has clear merits, it is rational to link the length of antibiotic administration to the type of fracture.

The high-dose short course of antibiotics has been shown to be effective in prophylaxis against infection following total joint replacement (Pollard et al 1979b) and therefore it is our practice to give:

Group I cefuroxime 1.5 g intravenously once

Group II cefuroxime 1.5 g i.v. and i.m. for 48 hours

Group III cefuroxime 1.5 g i.v. and i.m. for five days

In this way we hope to rationalize the antibiotic treatment of compound fractures.

ANTITETANUS PROGRAMME

As a general principle, measures to treat tetanus must be taken in all patients brought to hospital with open wounds. In superficial wounds potentially contaminated, tetanus toxoid 0.5 ml is given, to produce an active immunity. In larger, deeper wounds tetanus toxoid is given in combination with an antibiotic, whilst in heavily contaminated wounds with a great deal of devitalized tissue it is reasonable to give human antitetanus serum along with tetanus toxoid and antibiotics.

Clearly it is of importance to know if the patient has had tetanus toxoid before and requires a boost to his immunity.

TREATMENT OF THE SKIN

In any compound fracture, the skin is damaged. In severe injuries the amount of skin loss may be extensive, as a result of which the wound may not heal and the bone will be exposed, thus leading to chronic bone infection. Skin necrosis may occur from pressure within the foot from swelling (Fig. 59.3).

There are two basic methods for replacing skin loss in the foot, free grafts or flaps. With free grafts the skin is taken directly from the donor site and applied to the recipient area, the graft being

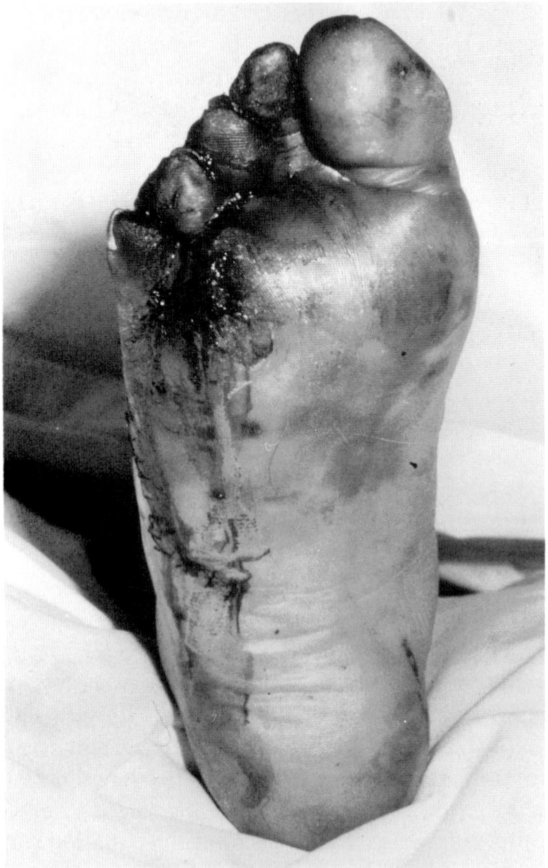

Fig. 59.3 Severe skin necrosis of the foot following a fracture of the 3rd and 4th metatarsals caused by crushing

dependent for survival upon revascularization from its new bed. If a flap is used the skin for grafting remains attached to the area from which it has been raised by its base and therefore retains its blood supply. When new vessels have grown into the flap from the recipient site it is detached from the donor area.

Free grafts

These may be either split skin or full thickness skin.

Split skin

In these, strips of partial thickness skin, consisting of epidermis and part of the dermal layer, but not extending down to the subcutaneous fatty tissue, are cut with a Humby knife. The donor site, depending on the area to be covered, is usually taken from the buttocks or upper thighs. The skin graft is then spread on to a sheet of vaseline gauze which can be cut into smaller squares before being applied to the wound. This allows blood and exudate to drain between rather than collect beneath the grafts. The graft is kept in place by an overlap of sheets of vaseline gauze followed by dry dressings which can be changed after 48 hours or left for up to 10 days. Because part of the dermis remains, full regeneration of skin follows in the donor area.

Split skin provides a very satisfactory immediate treatment for areas of skin loss, but in the foot on the dorsal surface there is no subcutaneous fat and there the graft is adherent to deeper structures and is liable to injury (Fig. 59.4).

Full thickness (Wolfe) grafts

These grafts, in which the whole thickness of the dermis is included, produce a firmer cover and can be of use in the heel or sole of the foot.

Flap grafts

A flap may be raised from one site and the foot brought to it, as in a cross-leg flap. Alternatively a flap could be raised from the abdominal wall and a tube formed which is then detached on one end and transferred to the recipient area, where it is opened out to form a tube pedicle flap.

Vascularized graft

A third type of skin graft is the vascularized graft, in which a full thickness graft is raised on its blood supply and then transferred to the recipient site, say the dorsum of the foot, and the blood vessels reconstituted with the help of an operating microscope.

ATTENTION TO THE VASCULAR STATUS

Early treatment to relieve pressure on the blood supply to the foot is one of the main priorities of management. Fracture-dislocations of the ankle are frequently associated with distortion of the arterial supply which needs to be relieved by prompt reduction.

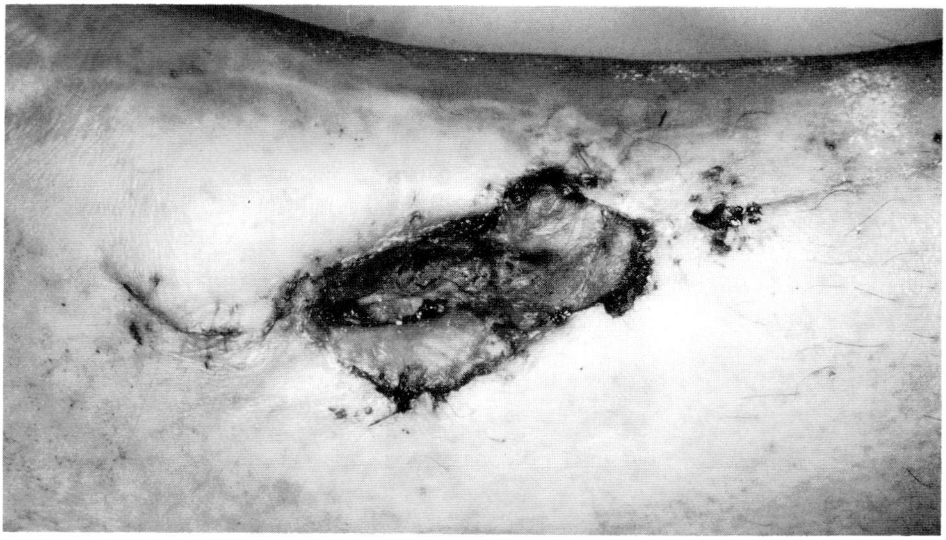

Fig. 59.4 A split skin graft has been applied to the foot to cover a defect caused by a shot gun injury

Clearly if there has been damage to a major vessel proximal to the foot, possibly at the knee joint, this will take priority in treatment as it is imperative to restore normal circulation as soon as possible. After six hours muscle changes become permanent and nerve degeneration occurs. Clinically the important signs to look for are loss of sensation, reduction in capillary return, loss of movement and the presence of pain. A pulse in fact may not be detectable. Also, toe gangrene can occur due to direct tissue damage in crushing injuries.

ATTENTION TO THE MUSCLES AND TENDONS

In most fractures a degree of damage must occur to the muscles and tendons in close proximity. As the haemorrhage resolves, fibrous tissue will form, so that the initial trauma will be the prime cause of some of the stiffness which follows removal of a plaster for a foot and ankle injury. Hence in order to overcome this problem there is every reason for advocating early mobilization after a fracture.

ATTENTION TO THE NERVES

It is relatively infrequent that the nerves to the foot appear to be damaged, following a fracture-dislocation although it is conceivable that a neuropraxia or axonotmesis could affect the posterior tibial nerve. This in itself may lead to involvement of the medial or lateral plantar nerves, the latter supplying the intrinsics to the foot, which in turn may be a cause for intrinsic contracture and stiffness.

However there is no evidence to support this except that stiffness and clawing, the cause of which is not clear, does occur following a fracture.

TREATMENT OF THE BONE

From the point of management, fractures in general fall into three groups:

1. Fractures of flat bones
2. Fractures of long bones
3. Fractures involving joints

Fractures of flat bones

In these fractures treatment is directed primarily towards dealing with the soft tissue lesions, the bone injury being to a large extent ignored. An example of this in the foot is the calcaneum. Where the subtalar or calcaneocuboid joint is not involved, attention is directed towards the soft tissues and early mobilization of the ankle and foot.

Fractures of long bones

In this group the main considerations are towards rotational deformities, producing malunion, and to the establishment of nonunion. Malunion is clearly a problem in injuries of the tibia which implicate the ankle joint, but unless the joint is involved in this region, malunion is not a major complication.

Malunion of fractures of the neck of the talus can limit foot dorsiflexion and union in misalignment of metatarsal fractures can affect adversely weight bearing under the forefoot.

Equally so, nonunion is not a major problem except for fractures of the talus. Nonunion is a complication of impaired bone blood supply and the talus is at risk because of its distally based blood supply (Kelly & Sullivan 1963) which may be severed in a fracture of the neck of the talus. This leads to the notorious complication of avascular necrosis of the talus and to ankle joint degeneration. However, the rest of the bones to the foot have a good blood supply due to the plentiful muscle attachments in this area.

Fractures involving a joint

This is by far the most important factor to be considered following an injury to the foot. It has been generally accepted that a partial or full thickness defect in cartilage cannot be repaired by the surviving chondrocytes (Mankin 1963, Meachin 1963). However, Salter et al (1980) have suggested that cartilage can be reformed by the technique of continuous passive motion. Using the rabbit as the experimental model, Salter produced varying types of full thickness cartilage defects and then maintained the animal's leg in a machine which continuously moved the joints. Salter and his colleagues suggested that this continuous movement was a stimulus to repair of the cartilage defect.

This is an extremely important concept and is very relevant to the foot. The normal function of the hyaline cartilage which covers the ends of all bones in synovial joints is to act as a shock absorber, to bear load and to reduce friction. If these properties are lost following injury then pain and disability will ensue. It is becoming increasingly evident that cartilage does have some capacity to repair; not only from Salter's important work, but also from Mitchell & Shepard's (1980) experiment on the effect of compression to promote healing of intra-articular fractures.

PRINCIPLES OF TREATMENT OF FRACTURES

This can be considered under the following headings:

1. *Reduction of the fracture*. This is not always necessary, but will depend on the degree of displacement, the site and type of bone involved and the age and ambitions of the patient.
2. *Reduction and maintenance of the fracture*.
   1. external means
   2. internal means
3. *Rehabilitation*. Local to the foot and ankle, of the patient as a whole.

Reduction of the fracture

Reduction of fractures of the foot is not always necessary. In these instances early movement should be encouraged and soft tissue swelling controlled either by initial elevation, perhaps with a compression bandage and ice packs or by early exercise. Pain from fractures of the foot will be alleviated in certain circumstances, by the application of a below knee plaster.

Shape. It is important to restore the shape of the foot and the relative lengths of the medial and lateral columns of the foot to as near normal as possible.

However in those fractures of the foot and ankle which involve a joint, manipulative reduction may need to be performed and can be closed or open. Closed reduction prior to internal fixation may be appropriate in certain circumstances, such as fractures and dislocations of the midtarsus, but invariably *open* reduction is required in order to prevent the interposition of soft parts and an inadequate reduction. There are certain well established principles which need to be followed when reducing a fracture by closed means:

1. Adequate X-rays of the fracture in at least two planes are required
2. Complete analgesia of the fractured limb with adequate muscle relaxation
3. The fracture is manipulated by increasing the

deformity in order to disengage the fracture and to try to exclude soft tissues

4. The deformity is reversed to reduce the fracture

5. Check X-rays in two planes need to be taken. (Macnicol 1983).

If this fails it is important to proceed to open reduction, although the decision to expose the fracture surgically should never be taken lightly.

Dewar & Evans (1968) drew attention to missed fracture-dislocations of the midtarsal joint when the displacement had reduced spontaneously. However the whole midtarsus can remain unstable to abduction strain and this can be demonstrated on X-rays taken during examination under anaesthesia.

As a rule, in children open reduction is avoided. However it may be necessary in displaced malleolar fractures and talar fractures. In epiphyseal injuries using the Salter & Harris classification (1963), reduction and fixation of the fracture are necessary in the type IV and in certain type III injuries, because if the displacement is not corrected serious growth disturbances will occur producing deformity in the limb (Fig. 59.5).

Maintainance of reduction of the fracture

Fractures can be held by external or internal means.

External

This may be by some form of external splintage, which can be plaster of Paris or any of the more modern plastics. As a general principle, immobilization of the joint above and the joint below is needed (Fig. 59.6) and three-point fixation is usually essential (Charnley 1970). The time for which the external splintage needs to be maintained varies with the site of the fracture and the age of the patient. On the whole children require plaster casts for about three to four weeks, whilst in adults most fracture-dislocations of the foot and ankle require about six weeks. However, as it is imperative to encourage mobility in the foot, internal fixation may have been practised and the need for plaster immobilization may be shortened, if required at all.

It is clearly important when applying a plaster cast to the lower limb, because of an injury to the foot and ankle, that the ankle joint is placed at 90° to the tibia so that contractures involving this joint do not occur. Equally so, after an injury to the foot and ankle, soft tissue swelling may be enormous and hence a complete plaster need not be applied and a back slab should be used. Without doubt the plaster must be split down to the skin after any surgery to the foot and ankle in order that the vascular supply is not placed in jeopardy. At the same time a careful watch is kept on the circulation and sensory supply to the toes.

Another form of external fixation is traction. This can be applied to control the limb in alignment and hold the fracture. There is little need for this form of traction in foot injuries, although the foot may well be elevated on a Braun's frame in its plaster cast.

Cast-bracing introduced by Sarmiento (1972) has been particularly effective for the treatment of patients with long bone fractures. This system encouraged mobility and loading of the fracture. However it has little role to play in fractures of the

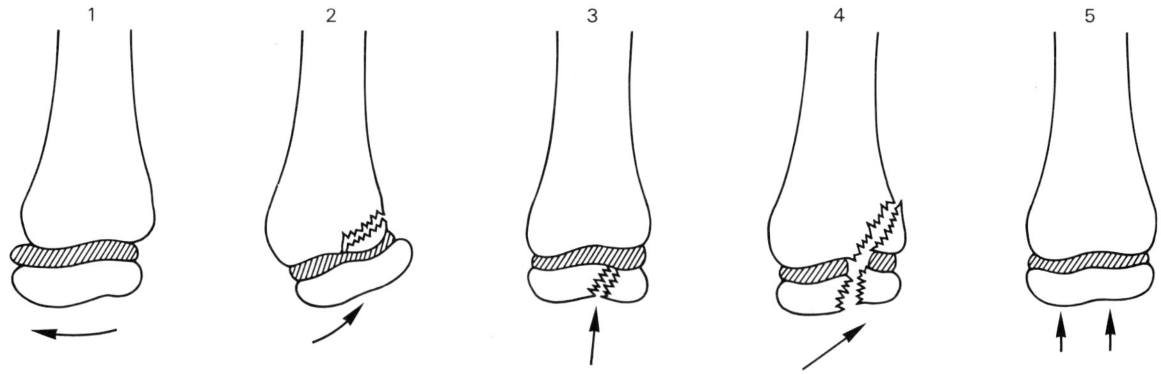

Fig. 59.5 Salter–Harris classification of epiphyseal injuries

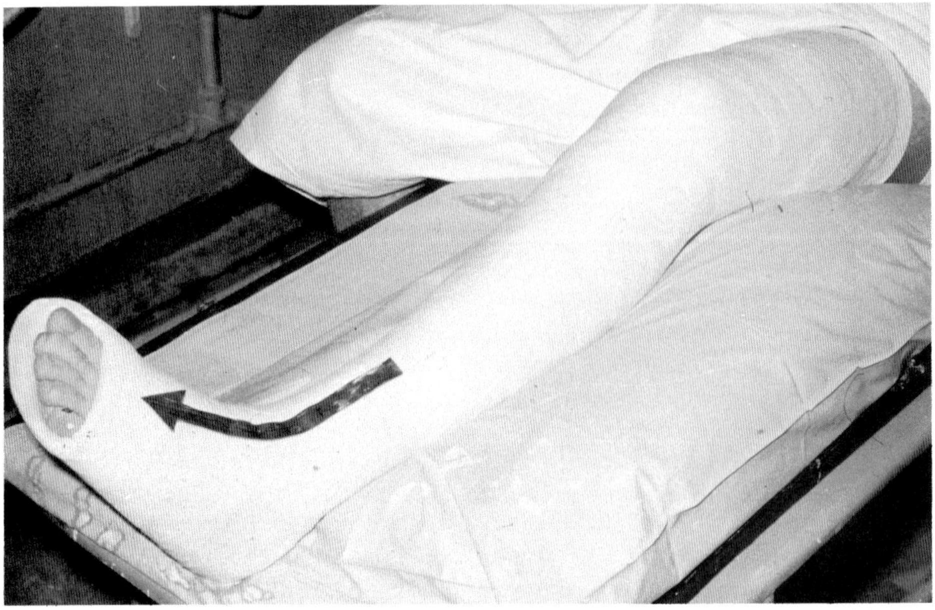

Fig. 59.6 An above knee plaster with the ankle internally rotated and the foot inverted, applied to a patient with an external rotation injury to the ankle. There has been a rupture of the deltoid ligament and a fracture of the fibula at the level of the syndesmosis

ankle and foot. Equally so, whilst external fixation of fractures has provided a useful means of treating many fractures around the skeleton, as yet it does not appear to have an application in fractures of the foot and ankle.

Internal

Internal fixation lends itself to the treatment of certain fractures involving the foot and ankle, particularly when joint surfaces are involved. If the joint surface is to be restored to as near normal as possible, effective internal fixation is required.

Ankle joint injuries are one of the prime examples where accurate reduction is required to ensure the joint surface is realigned and this is complemented by internal fixation using the techniques advocated by the AO group (Müller et al 1979). Once adequate reduction has been achieved (Fig. 59.7) and the swelling of the soft tissues has subsided, the final phase of fracture treatment, rehabilitation of the soft parts, can begin.

In the foot, in order to restore joint alignment, fractures of calcaneum involving the subtalar joint can be treated by bone grafting and elevation of the depression. This technique is particularly applicable to those fractures classified as Type 4A, 4B, 5A and

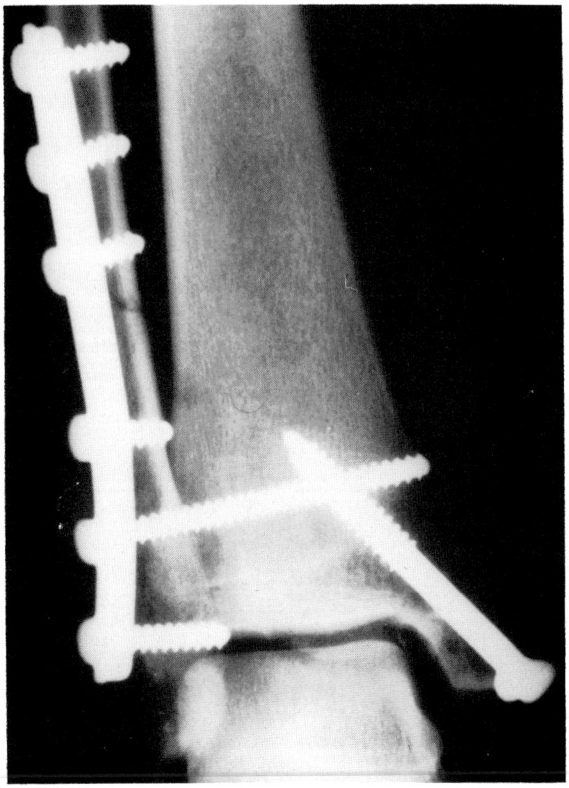

Fig. 59.7 Internal fixation for a fracture-dislocation of the ankle in which there has been disruption of the inferior tibiofibular joint and diastasis

5B by Rowe et al (1963), (Fig. 59.8). Fractures of the talus, navicular and metatarsus with which there is an associated dislocation are best treated, after reduction, with internal fixation using a Kirschner wire. The equipment that is essential for K wire fixation is the availability of an image intensifier, or adequate X-rays and a slow speed hand drill for inserting the wire. The Lisfranc injury in particular needs to be held by internal fixation in order to prevent redislocation (Figs. 59.9a and b).

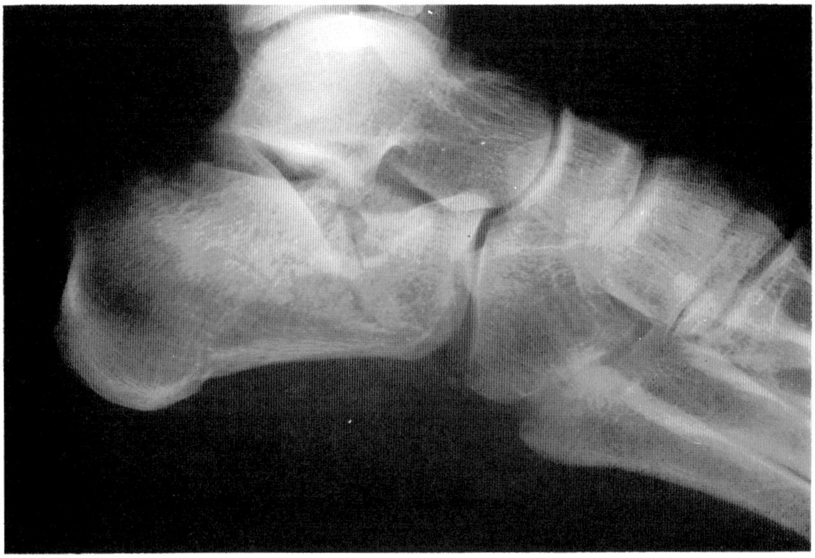

Fig. 59.8 A calcaneal fracture in which the subtalar joint is damaged

a

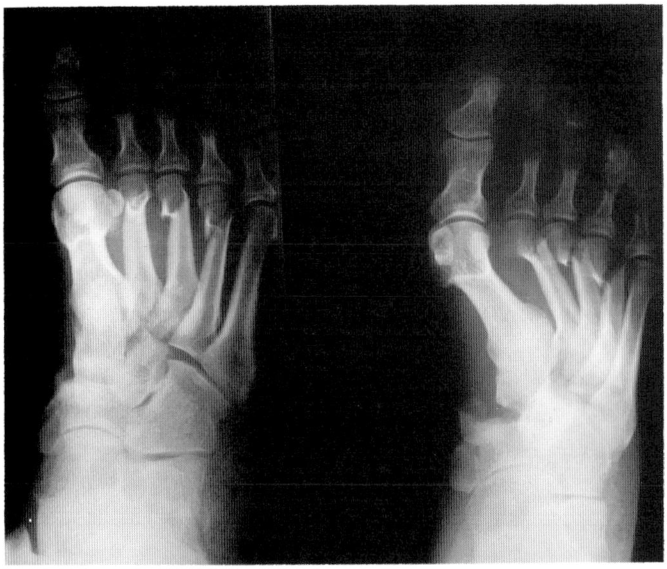

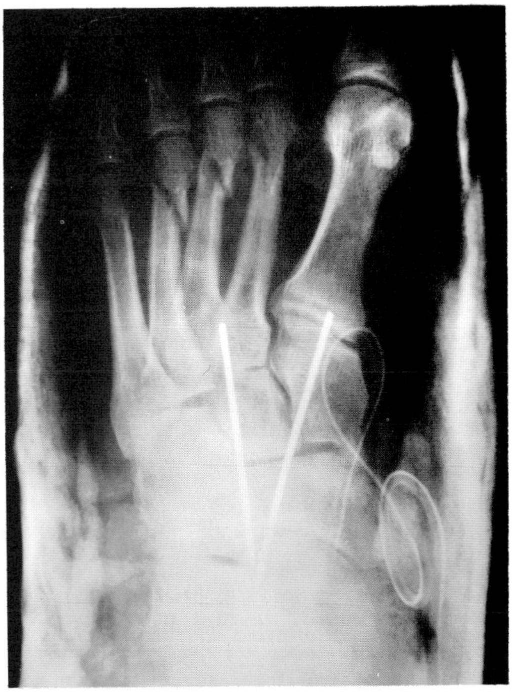

b

Fig. 59.9 a: A Lisfranc fracture-dislocation; b: The same after open reduction and internal fixation

Rehabilitation

Rehabilitation of the foot and ankle following a fracture can be considered under the headings:

1. Local
2. General

Local — the skin

If the skin has not been damaged, early movement is encouraged to prevent adhesions from forming and subsequent stiffness. The following methods are available for this.

Cold therapy such as ice at a temperature of −12°C, can be used in the treatment of recent injuries, particularly when there is an acute swelling. Lee et al (1978) have shown that there is a slowing of conduction in the motor and sensory nerves under this treatment and hence ice therapy not only relieves swelling, but may alleviate pain and muscle spasm.

Ultrasound is available at frequencies of 1–3 Hz and can be used to assist the absorption of tissue fluid, to reduce pain and to stimulate cell activity in the area (Hyde 1980).

Active and passive exercises are commenced as early as possible and should begin with passive or static exercises. These can be followed by free active exercises, which are performed by the patient, and finally by restricted exercises in which the muscles and the joints are encouraged to move against the resistance of springs, pulleys, weights or manual resistance (Hyde 1980).

Local — bones and joints

The essential complications that follow fractures to the foot and ankle are damage to the joint surface leading to osteoarthritis, damage to the growth plate in children, particularly of the distal tibia and leading to a varus or valgus deformity of the ankle joint, nonunion, particularly of the talus and leading to avascular necrosis of the talus in the ankle joint and chronic osteomyelitis.

Damage to the cartilage surface is a risk with all fractures involving the hindfoot and midfoot. The ankle joint surface may be damaged leading to osteoarthritis which in turn may require ankle arthrodesis.

Subtalar joint damage may lead to osteoarthritis and Noble & McQuillan (1979) advocate subtalar fusion within three months of the injury to treat this problem. Occasionally with a severe fracture-dislocation of the mid and hindfoot as a result of vertical compression, triple arthrodesis perhaps accompanied by ankle fusion may be required (Fig. 59.10).

Damage to the growth plate may result in epiphyseal arrest and can lead to varying degrees of deformity, depending on the age of the child at the time of injury. Various treatments have been advocated including the use of fat grafts after removing the fused area of the plate.

Nonunion of the talus is a major complication which invariably results in surgical fusion of the subtalar and ankle joints.

Chronic osteomyelitis may become established in the foot or ankle joint following an injury. The principles of treatment are:

1. Removal of dead tissue
2. Control of the infection
3. Encouraging new bone formation.

Removal of dead tissue

All dead and necrotic tissue needs to be removed. A sequestrum may be identified by means of tomography (Fig. 59.11). The amount of dead tissue that requires removal is not easy to define and one of the techniques available is the injection of disulphylene blue into the patient, in order to demonstrate those areas which are viable and take up the dye and those areas that are nonviable and do not take up the dye.

Control of the infection

Currently the most popular method is to place antibiotic impregnated cement beads into the defect. These beads contain gentamicin which is inserted into Palacos® cement (Klemm 1976). The beads have been shown to be as effective as suction irrigation methods in controlling infection in patients with deep bone infections (Hedstrom et al 1980). This technique for delivering the antibiotic has been studied by Wahlig et al (1978); high doses were found to be delivered to the bone and to persist for several weeks. The beads are inserted usually in a chain of 30 into the already cleaned area, but diffuse

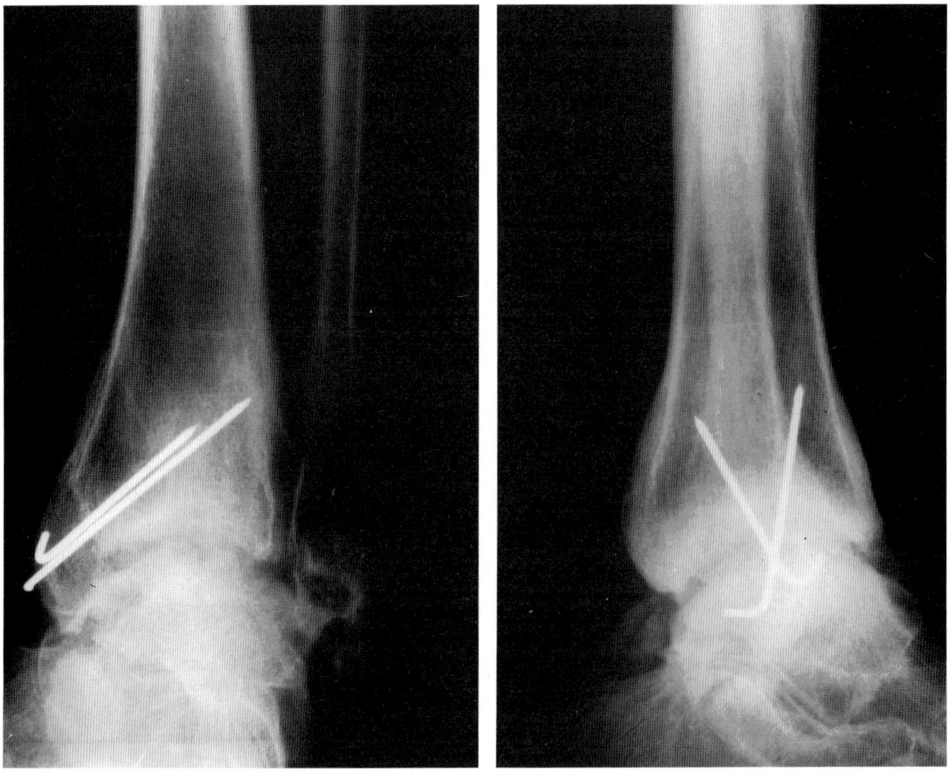

Fig. 59.10 A patient with a grossly destroyed ankle following a severe injury and which will require a pantalar fusion

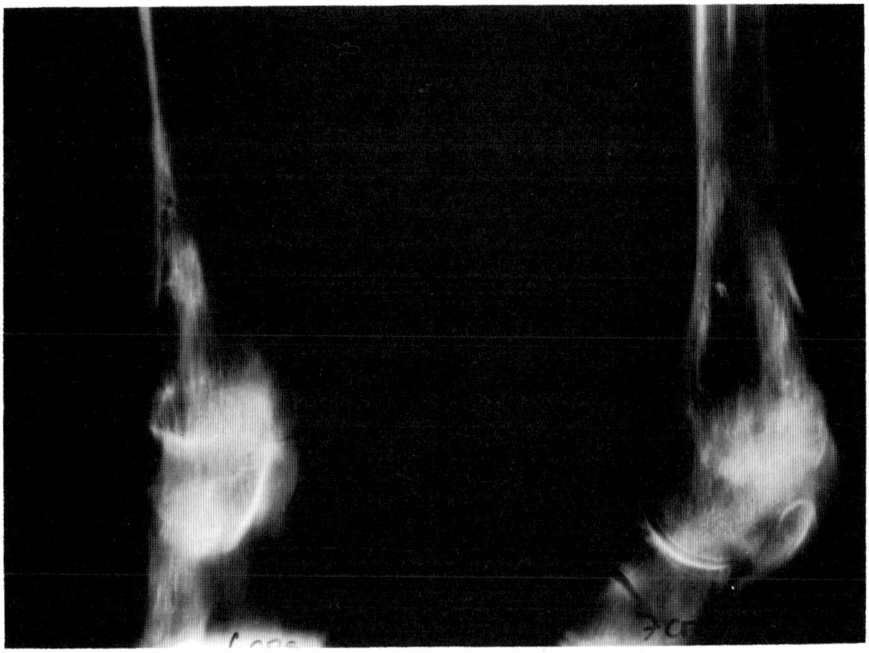

Fig. 59.11 A tomogram showing a sequestrum in the distal tibia

out rapidly and therefore they should be removed by about two weeks. It is advisable to leave one or two of the beads protruding through the surface so that the whole chain can be removed.

Occasionally infection can be managed by complete ostectomy (e.g. astragalectomy) but it will lead to significant disability of the foot which will invariably need to be supported by an orthosis.

Finally if all else fails amputation may need to be considered. Patients for this are particularly those following trauma in which there is gross tissue destruction and loss of blood supply to the foot. It is not unreasonable to leave the distal end of the amputation open. Late causes for removal of the foot would include uncontrolled chronic infection, or indeed intractable pain following previous injury or damage to the foot itself. The level of amputation and the approach to treatment is discussed in Chapter 61 but in principle it would seem reasonable to maintain as much of the foot as is possible bearing in mind that Syme's amputation is a satisfactory procedure for an active adult or child. Older people may not tolerate such a procedure but it should always be considered.

Sudeck's osteodystrophy is a form of post-traumatic dystrophy in which significant osteoporosis occurs. It is a late complication of an injury to the foot and there is an exaggerated stiffness and swelling of the foot which in turn may be warm. This temperature change is associated with a vasodilation and the patient may indeed complain of pain along with the stiffness and swelling. Treatment in the initial stages is by rest and splintage to prevent contractures of the ankle joint from occurring, which is followed by physiotherapy and it may take several months for function to be restored. Guanethidine has been used in the treatment of the resistant case, acting as a preganglionic blocker, to restore the circulation to near normal.

General

After the treatment of his fracture the patient may need advice and help in restoring him to his social situation. This involves adjusting his work pattern as required and adapting the patient to the disability. For this programme the help and advice of the rehabilitation team, the Medical Social worker and the Rehabilitation Officer may be required.

Encouraging bone formation

If a defect has been created by removing dead bone, it needs to be filled. This can be done by bone chips taken from the iliac crest using Papineau's technique (Fig. 59.12) in which all the dead and devitalized

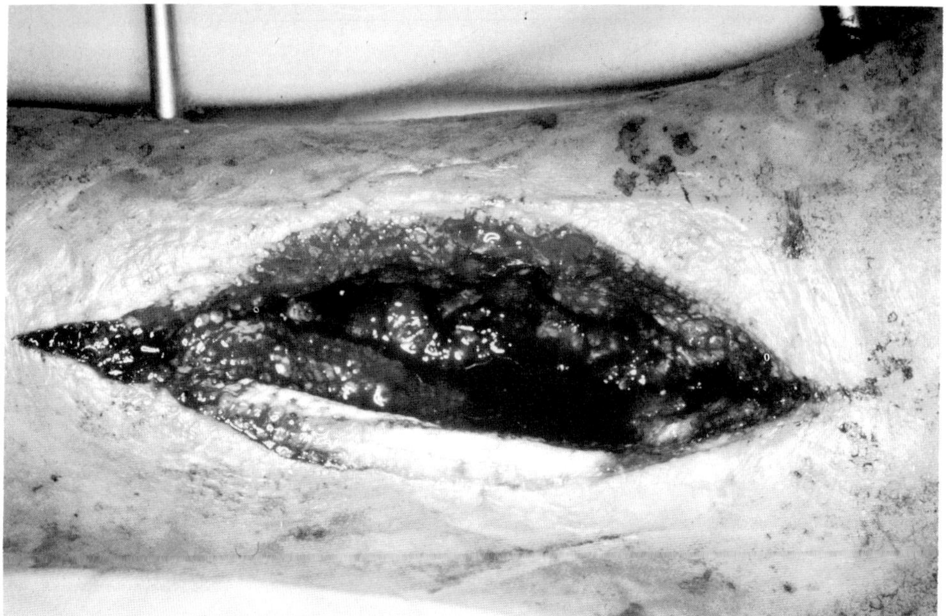

Fig. 59.12 Bone chips filling a defect in the foot, which was produced when all dead tissue was removed

tissues are removed radically. The whole area is cleaned out thoroughly. After a period of usually about one week fresh cancellous bone graft taken from the iliac crest and if need be the greater trochanter and distal femur, are placed into the hole that has been created. Regularly the wound is washed out with normal saline and granulation tissue starts to appear over the cancellous graft. It is possible to apply split skin or indeed a full thickness or myocutaneous flap over this defect at a later stage (Fig. 59.13).

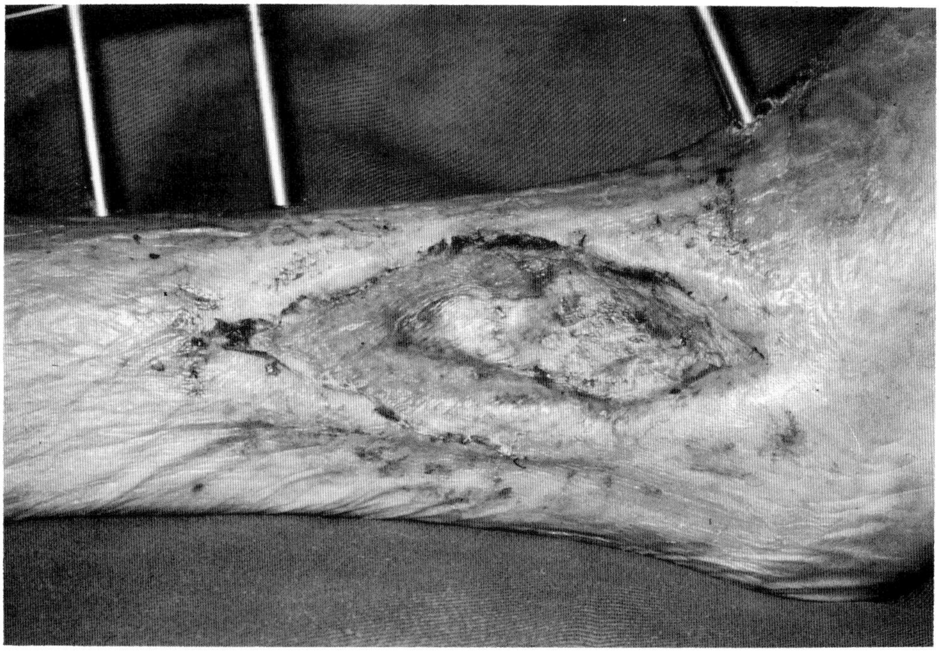

Fig. 59.13 When granulation tissue appeared the defect was covered with a split skin graft

REFERENCES

Billroth T 1886 Die Allgemeine Chirurgische Pathological und Therapic 50 Vorlesungen. Georg Reimer, Berlin

Charnley J 1970 The Closed Treatment of Common Fractures. 3rd edn. E & S Livingstone, London

Dewar F P, Evans D C 1968 Occult fracture-subluxation of the mid-tarsal joint. J Bone Joint Surg 50B: 368–388

Gustillo R B, Anderson J T 1976 Prevention of infection in the treatment of one thousand and twenty five fractures of long bones. J Bone Joint Surg 58A: 453–458

Hedstrom J A, Lidgrew L, Totholm C, Oññerfalt R 1980 Antibiotic containing bone cement beads in the treatment of deep muscle and skeletal infections. Acta Orthop Scand 51: 863–869

Hughes S P F, Anderson F M 1985 Penetration of antibiotics into bone. Leader, J Antimicrob Chemother

Hyde S 1980 In: Hughes S P F, Sweetnam D R (eds) Physiotherapy C.21 Basis and Practice of Orthopaedics. Heinemann, London

Kelly P J, Sullivan C R 1963 Blood supply of talus. Clin Orthop 30: 37–44

Klemm K 1976 Die behandhung Chronischer knockenin fekhonen mit Gentamycin — PMMA — Kelten und — Kugeln in Gentamycin — Kele Symposium Munchen contzen 4 Erlangen ed Verlag für Lenrmille Wissenschaft and Forschung, Germany. pp 20–25

Lee J M, Warren M P, Mason S M 1978 Effects of ice on nerve conduction velocity. Physiotherapy 64: 1

Macnicol M F 1983 Principles of fracture management. In: Hughes S P F (ed) Basis and Practice of Traumatology. Heinemann, London

Mankin H J 1963 Localisation of treated thymidine in articular cartilage of rabbits III Mature articular cartilage. J Bone Joint Surg 45A: 529

Meachin G 1963 The effect of scarification on articular cartilage in the rabbit. J Bone Joint Surg 45B: 150

Mitchell N S, Shepard N 1980 Healing of articular cartilage in intra-articular fractures in rabbits. J Bone Joint Surg 62A: 628

Müller M E, Allgower M, Schneider R, Willenger H 1979 Manual of Internal Fixation. Springer-Verlag, Berlin

Noble J, McQuillan W M 1979 Early posterior subtalar fusion in the treatment of fractures of the os calcis. J Bone Joint Surg 61B: 90–93

Patzakis M J, Harvey J P, Ivler D 1974 The role of antibiotics in the management of open fractures. J Bone Joint Surg 56A: 329

Pollard J P, Hughes S P F, Scott J E, Evans M J, Benson M K D 1979a Antibiotic prophylaxis in total hip replacement, a prospective trial. Br Med J 1: 707–709

Pollard J P, Hughes S P F, Evans M J, Scott J E, Benson M K D 1979b Concentration of flucloxacillin in femoral head and joint capsule in total hip replacement. J Antimicrob Chemother 5: 721–726

Rowe C R, Shellarides H T, Freeman P A, Sorbie C 1963 Fractures of the os calcis, a long term follow up study of 146 patients. JAMA 184: 920–923

Salter R B, Harris W R 1963 Injuries involving the epiphyseal plate. J Bone Joint Surg 45A: 587–622

Salter R B, Simmonds D F, Malcolm D W, Rumble R J, Macmichael D, Clements N D 1980 The biological effect of continuous passive motion in the healing of full thickness defect in articular cartilage — An experimental investigation in the rabbit. J Bone Joint Surg 62A: 1232

Sarmiento A 1972 Functional bracing of tibial and femoral shaft fractures. Clin Orthop 82: 2–13

Wahlig H, Dingelden E, Bergmann R, Reuss K 1978 The release of gentamicin from polymethyl methacrylate beads, an experimental and pharmacokinetic study. J Bone Joint Surg 60B: 270–275

Operative technique of the ankle and hindfoot

INTRODUCTION

The foot and ankle is a unique part of the lower extremity. It contains numerous articulations, is crossed by several tendons and has extensive ligamentous support. Most of the time the ankle and foot, especially the hindfoot, work in concert providing normal stance and gait. This is the first area of the body which is subjected to the stresses of weight bearing. Patients may present with a wide variety of pathology some of which is highly complicated. The area is frequently the site of pathology caused by either trauma, some type of congenital or developmental deformity, or an arthritic disease. Due to the complex nature of the anatomy and the need to provide pain relief and stability, arthrodesis operations are frequently necessary. Osteotomy is probably the second most commonly performed operation in this area, while arthroplasty is rarely considered.

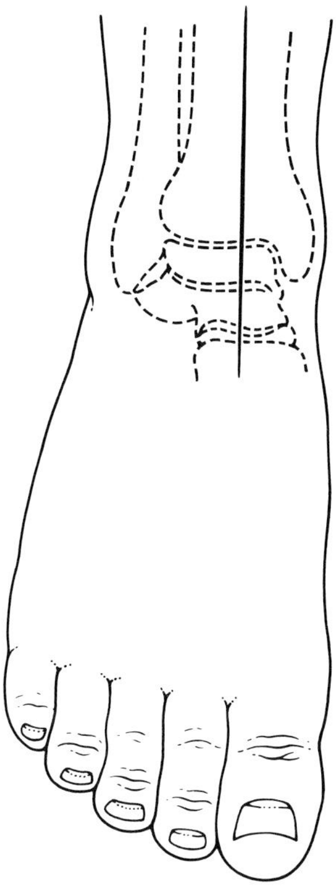

Fig. 60.1a The skin incision for an anterior approach to the ankle joint

SURGICAL APPROACHES

Anterior approach to the ankle

Incision

Centre the skin incision over the anterior ankle joint and extend it about 5–8 cm proximally and distally (Fig. 60.1a). Care must be taken not to place too much tension on the cut skin edges. The incision can always be lengthened. The extensor retinaculum is divided between the extensor digitorum longus and the extensor hallucis longus. The deep peroneal nerve and anterior tibial artery are in this interval and must be carefully retracted. The bundle can be moved medially or laterally depending on the exposure desired. Dissection can also proceed between the anterior tibialis and the extensor hallucis longus (Fig. 60.1b). This protects the neurovascular bundle, but may limit the lateral exposure of the ankle joint. The anterior approach can also proceed through the tendon sheath of the tibialis tendon (Gould 1982).

The next deep structure is the anterior joint capsule which can be opened vertically or horizontally. The periosteum can be elevated from

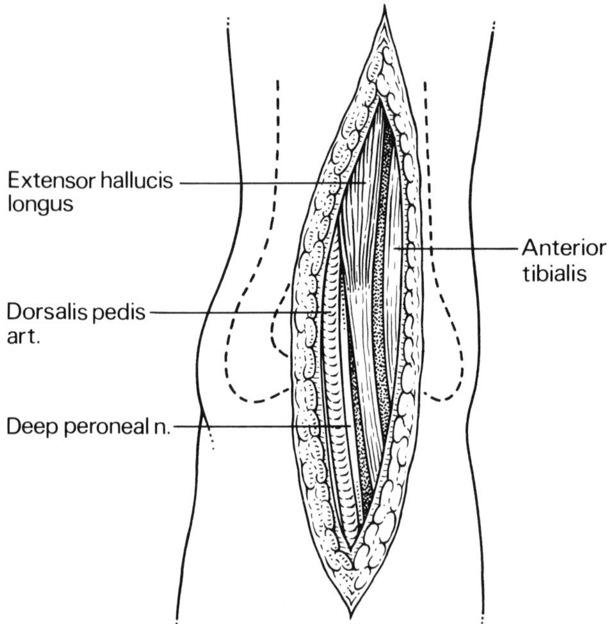

Fig. 60.1b The deep approach to the anterior ankle between the anterior tibialis tendon and the tendon of the extensor hallucis longus. This gives the most protection to the anterior neurovascular bundle and gives good exposure to the ankle

the distal tibia beginning at the joint line. It is possible and quite easy to expose the entire ankle through the incision (Fig. 60.1c). Medially the malleolus and tibial plafond are clearly seen when the capsule is opened. The lateral dissection is a bit more difficult, but the lateral malleolus can be exposed. Depending on the operation to be performed, during exposure of the lateral malleolus, it may be necessary to identify and preserve the anterior talofibular ligament.

Anterolateral approach to the ankle and hindfoot

Patient position

All lateral approaches to the ankle and foot need internal rotation of the hip joint. This can be easily accomplished by placing a sandbag or towel roll under the ipsilateral buttock.

Incision

The incision should begin about 4–6 cm proximal to the anterolateral side of the ankle 2 cm anterior to the anterior edge of the fibula. It curves distally toward the base of the fourth and fifth metatarsals (Fig. 60.2a).

The deeper dissection follows the skin incision cutting through the retinacula. The superficial peroneal nerve should be identified and protected in the posterior part of the wound. The ankle and hindfoot joints are exposed by retracting the peroneus tertius and extensor tendons medially (Fig. 60.2b). The anterior capsule is opened to expose the ankle joint. Excision of the fat pad of the sinus tarsi and distal retraction of the extensor digitorum brevis allow exposure of all three hindfoot joints (Fig. 60.2c).

Posterior approach to the ankle and subtalar joint

Patient position

The prone position is preferred with the distal leg supported on a sterile elevated support.

Incision

A straight incision is made beginning at the distal end of the lateral malleolus and extending

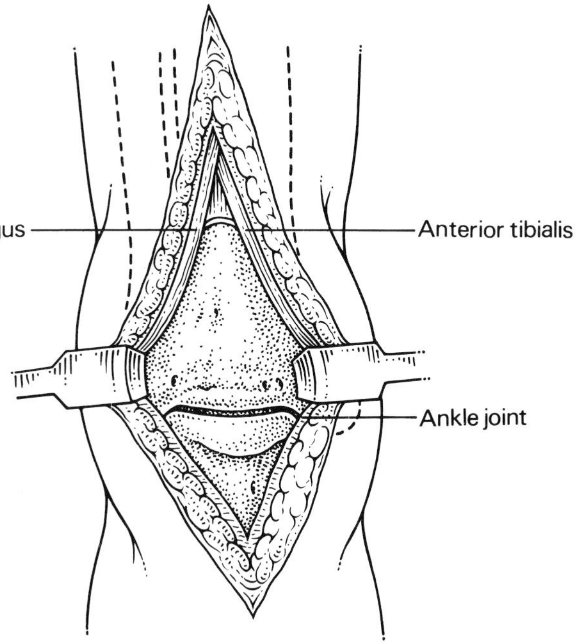

Fig. 60.1c The distal tibia and proximal talus are well exposed through this anterior approach to the ankle

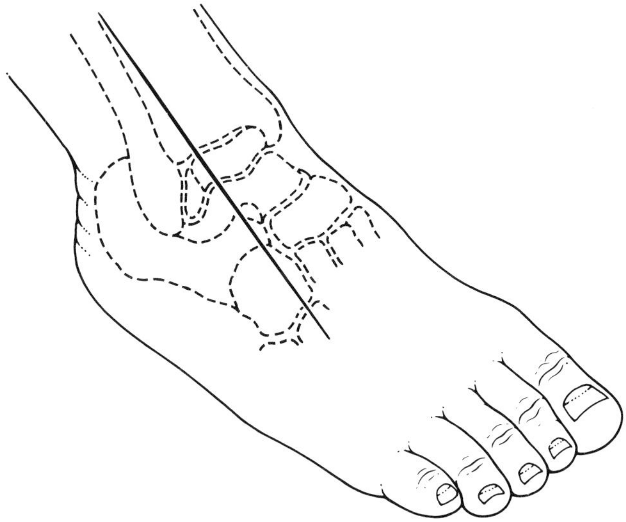

Fig. 60.2a The anterolateral approach to the ankle joint with possible extension to the hindfoot. The skin incision begins just anterior to the distal fibula and courses distally across the sinus tarsi

proximally about 10–12 cm just lateral to the Achilles tendon.

The short saphenous vein and sural nerve should be protected within the anterior flap of the incision. The deep fascia is incised and a plane developed between the peroneal tendons laterally and the flexor hallucis longus on the medial side. It may be necessary to release some of the origin of the flexor hallucis longus from the posterior ridge of the fibula to gain wider exposure. Dissection or retractors should never proceed medial to this muscle to avoid injury to the posterior tibial neurovascular bundle.

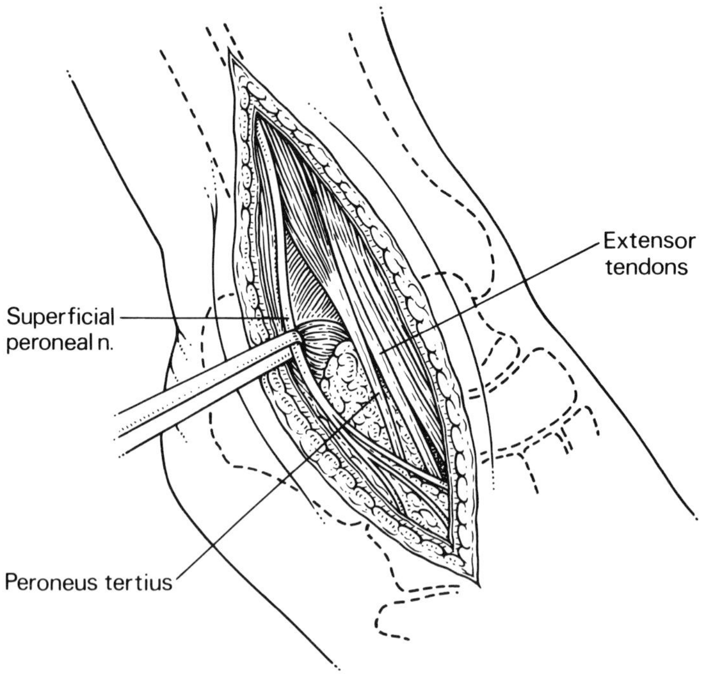

Fig. 60.2b Exposure is carried deep between the superficial peroneal nerve, peroneal tendons and the extensor tendons and peroneus tertius

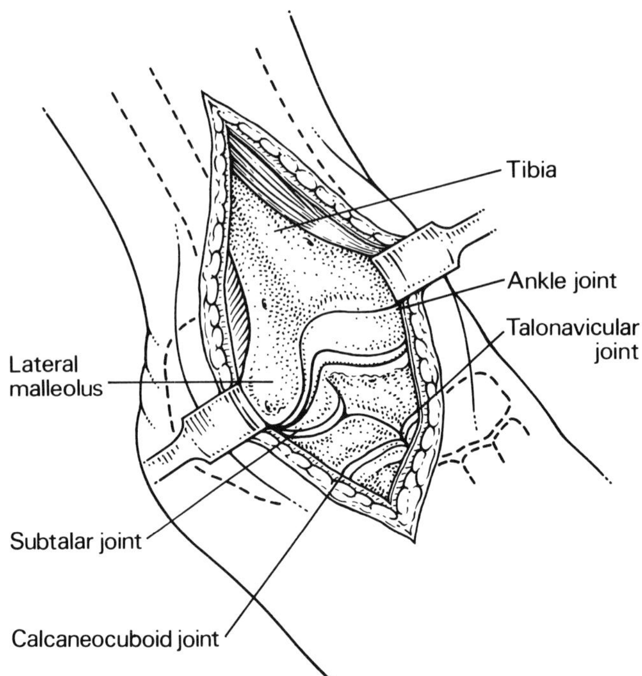

Fig. 60.2c An excellent view is accorded through this exposure of the distal tibiotalar joint as well as the lateral malleolus, the talonavicular, calcaneocuboid joints and subtalar joint

Depending on the pathology, the posterior capsule of the subtalar joint may be the first joint exposed in the deep dissection. However, the ankle joint can be easily recognized. Should an ankle arthrodesis be planned, the tendo Achillis can be transected.

Posterolateral approach to the ankle

(transfibular approach — method of Gatellier & Chastane)

This approach was initially designed to permit fixation of a large posterior tibial fracture at the ankle. In such conditions the fibula is usually fractured, but can be osteotomized about 10 cm proximal to tip of the lateral malleolus for reconstructive or arthrodesis procedures. The incision is along the posterior border of the fibula, approximately 12–15 cm long and curved parallel to the peroneal tendons distally. The peroneal tendons are displaced anteriorly, the fibula osteotomized and freed by dividing the interosseus ligament. The fibula is hinged laterally on the calcaneofibular and talofibular ligaments which are preserved to maintain ankle stability postoperatively during reconstructive operations. A wide exposure is provided to the lateral and posterior ankle, and by subluxating the talus laterally, most of the dome of the talus and distal tibia can be exposed. Should ankle arthrodesis be performed, the fibula can be used as a bone graft.

Medial approach to the ankle

A medial approach to the ankle also offers excellent exposure, especially for an ankle arthrodesis (Thomas 1969, Scranton 1985). The medial approach actually includes a short vertical lateral approach to the distal fibula. The fibula is first osteotomized through a 5 cm longitudinal incision across its lower end centred on the ankle joint. Approximately 10 to 12 mm of distal fibula is resected, usually above the level of the ankle joint either with a rongeur (Thomas 1969) or an oscillating saw (Scranton 1985). The medial incision is a vertical incision exposing the lower 10–12 cm of tibia ending about 4 cm distal to the medial malleolus. Thomas (1969) exposes the distal tibia extraperiosteally and cautions that the posterior retractor should not compress the posterior tibial nerve. He then incises the periosteum about 4 cm proximal to the tip of the medial malleolus and creates an osteoperiosteal flap with a broad osteotome. The medial malleolus is divided at its junction with the lower tibia. Downward traction distracts the ankle and valgus angulation should be avoided so that the posterior tibial nerve is not stretched.

Another medial exposure has been described by Scranton (1985). After making a fibular osteotomy, he proceeds with a 12 cm long incision centred over the medial malleolus taking care to preserve the long saphenous vein. The periosteum and deltoid ligaments are stripped off the medial aspect of the tibia. This allows exposure of the ankle joint. The anterior two-thirds of the medial malleolus is removed with an oscillating saw. The posterior one-third is preserved to protect the neurovascular bundle and the tendons. Obviously these two medial approaches are not entirely suitable for reconstructive procedures about the ankle but are ideally suited for arthrodesis techniques.

Approach to the valgus hindfoot deformity

A severe valgus hindfoot deformity can be seen in patients with rheumatoid arthritis or severe pes planus and requires special consideration as to the proper skin incision. The valgus deformity must be corrected and usually a bone graft or an osteotomy is necessary. It may be impossible to close an improperly placed incision following correction of the deformity.

Patient position

The patient is supine with some type of a lift under the buttock to keep the extremity internally rotated (Fig. 60.3).

Incision

A straight incision, beginning approximately 5 cm above the top of the lateral malleolus and 1 cm anterior to the fibula, extends distally, curving slightly anteriorly toward the calcaneocuboid joint (Fig. 60.4a).

The peroneal tendons and sural nerve remain on the fibular side of the incision and are usually not

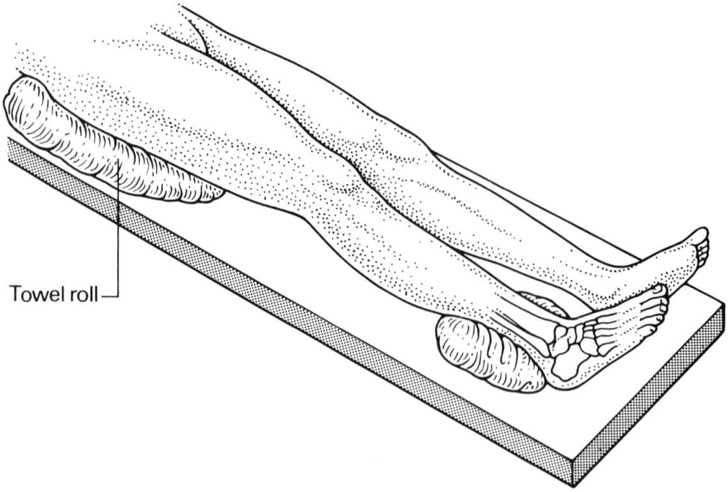

Fig. 60.3 For a patient requiring any operative procedure on the lateral aspect of the ankle, the hindfoot should have a towel roll placed under the ipsilateral buttock to maintain the extremity in some internal rotation

disturbed. In severe deformity it may be necessary to release the peroneus brevis tendon. The sinus tarsi is cleared of soft tissues exposing the posterior facet of the subtalar joint. The origin of the extensor digitorium brevis is elevated from the anterior process of the calcaneus exposing the calcaneocuboid joint (Fig. 60.4b). Dissection is carried more medial

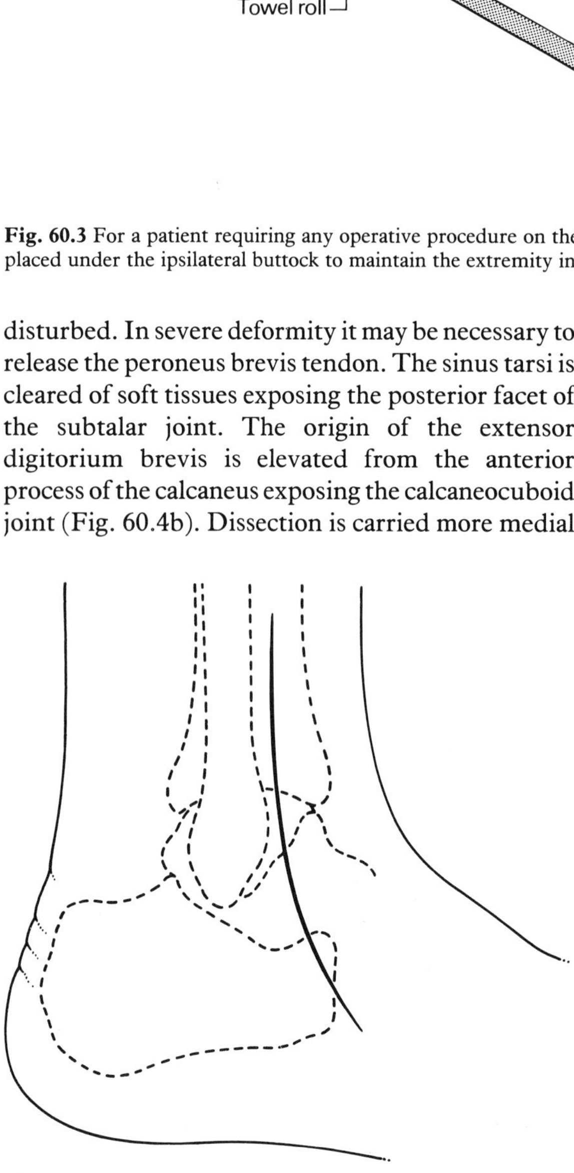

Fig. 60.4a The skin incision for a lateral approach to the ankle joint in the hindfoot. The incision is placed about 1 to 2 cm anterior to the distal fibula and extends distally along the line of the peroneal tendons

at that level to expose the lateral side of the talonavicular joint.

The talonavicular joint is more fully exposed through a separate dorsomedial longitudinal incision just medial to the insertion of the anterior tibial tendon. Through the lateral and medial incisions, a subluxation of this joint can easily be reduced. The valgus deformity of the subtalar joint can then be corrected. Any abutment between the calcaneus and lateral malleolus must be removed. It may be necessary to release the calcaneofibular ligament to achieve correction. This incision must be drained postoperatively especially in the dead space created by clearing the sinus tarsi. Interrupted sutures must be placed carefully, closing the skin without tension.

Approach to the varus hindfoot deformity or a nondeformed hindfoot (Hoppenfeld & de Boer 1984)

Patient position

Similar to other lateral approaches.

Incision

A curved incision is made within the skin lines beginning below the distal posterior end of the fibula. It curves distally and medially over the sinus tarsi, ending at the lateral side of the talonavicular joint.

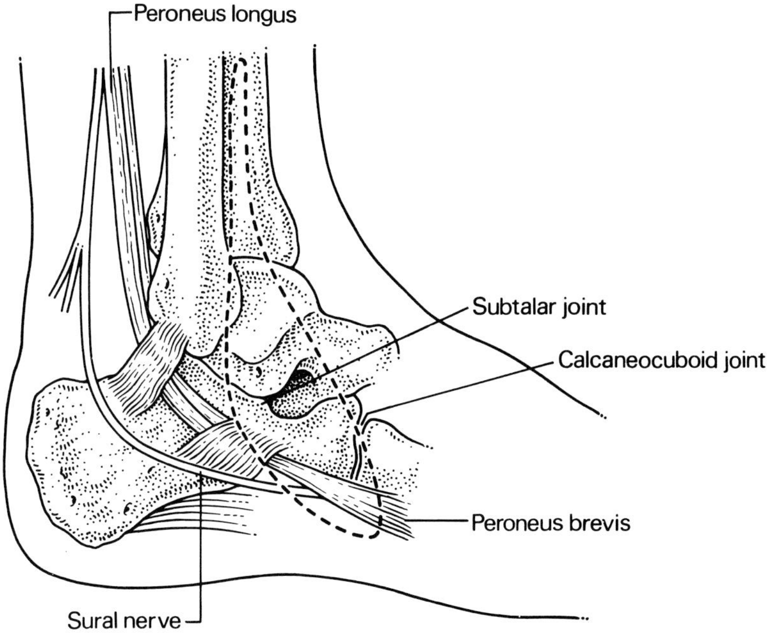

Fig. 60.4b This lateral approach to the ankle and hindfoot exposes the distal fibula and the subtalar joint as well as the calcaneocuboid joint. The peroneal tendons and sural nerve can also be seen in the wound and these must be protected

Large skin flaps should not be mobilized as they frequently heal poorly. The fat pad within the sinus tarsi should be detached and allowed to remain with the proximal skin incision. The fascia over the extensor tendons is also opened in line with the skin incision. Retract these tendons medially exposing the origin of the extensor digitorium brevis which is reflected distally. This exposes the calcaneocuboid joint, and the lateral side of the talonavicular joint. Dissection along the posterior wall of the sinus tarsi exposes the posterior facet of the subtalar joint.

RADIOGRAPHIC ASSESSMENT OF THE MIDFOOT AND HINDFOOT

Penneau et al (1982) evaluated children with bilateral pes planus using a standardized set of anteroposterior radiographs to assess the arch by measuring the talocalcaneal angle. An angle of 25° or greater was noted in patients with a pronated foot. On the lateral weight-bearing radiographs an arch ratio was developed using the length from the weight-bearing surface of the os calcis to the head of the first metatarsal and dividing this by the height of the hindfoot or a perpendicular line drawn to the talonavicular joint (Fig. 60.5). When the ratio was high, it correlated with a normal foot, when low it correlated with pes planus. Anteroposterior radiographs were taken from 100 cm away at a 20° angle from the vertical. The lateral radiograph was taken at 100 cm and was horizontally centred on the calcaneocuboid joint.

Bordelon (1980) also utilized a special weight-bearing lateral radiograph to assess idiopathic hypermobile flat feet in children. The radiograph was made with the foot relaxed and in a normal angle of gait. The lateral talometatarsal angle was measured and classified as: 1. neutral if a 0° measurement was made, that is a line drawn through the talus continued uninterrupted through the first metatarsal (Fig. 60.6). 2. A mild flat foot showed up to a 15° plantar angulation of the talus in relation to the first metatarsal. 3. Severe flat foot was measured as greater than 15° plantar flexion angle of the talus in relation to the first metatarsal.

An extensive radiographic measurement of the normal adult foot was performed by Steel et al (1980). They evaluated 41 pairs of feet from female volunteers between the ages of 40 and 60 years. The normal foot was defined as one which was painless and had no history of significant pain or disability. In

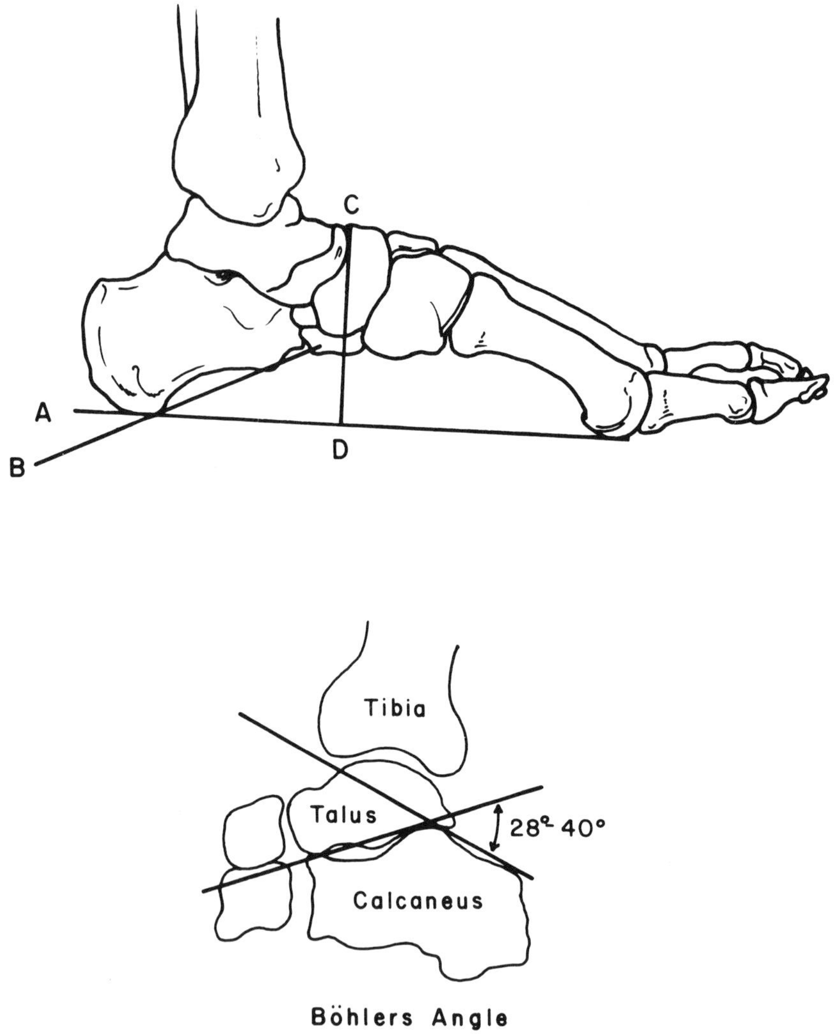

Fig. 60.5 The top diagram shows one method of determining an arch ratio. A ratio is developed by measuring a line on a weight-bearing lateral radiograph of the foot from the weight-bearing surface of the os calcis to the weight-bearing surface of the first metatarsal head. The vertical measurement is perpendicular drawn to the most superior portion of the talonavicular joint. The latter is represented by line C–D. The calcaneal pitch angle is the angle formed by the intersection of line A and line B. Line A traverses the weight-bearing tips of the calcaneus and the first metatarsal head and line B runs across the plantar surface of the calcaneus. The lower diagram depicts the measurement of Böhler's angle. This angle assesses the integrity of the subtalar joint on a lateral weight-bearing radiograph

addition the feet had no history of musculoskeletal disease, had not been operated upon and were without skin or soft tissue lesions. Standardized anteroposterior and lateral weight-bearing radiographs were taken of each foot. The film cassette of the lateral radiograph was in contact with the medial aspect of the foot and the X-ray source was perpendicular to the cassette, 120 cm away. The anteroposterior radiograph was weight-bearing and taken with the subject standing on the film cassette. The X-ray source was 3 m above the cassette and tilted 15° from the vertical anteroposterior plane. Magnification was only 0.5% on the anteroposterior view and only 1.5% on the lateral view.

28 measurements were recorded from the anteroposterior film and 31 measurements from the lateral radiograph. The study showed that there was a range of normality for almost each measurement rather than a single fixed figure. They describe a distribution curve of normality for the measure-

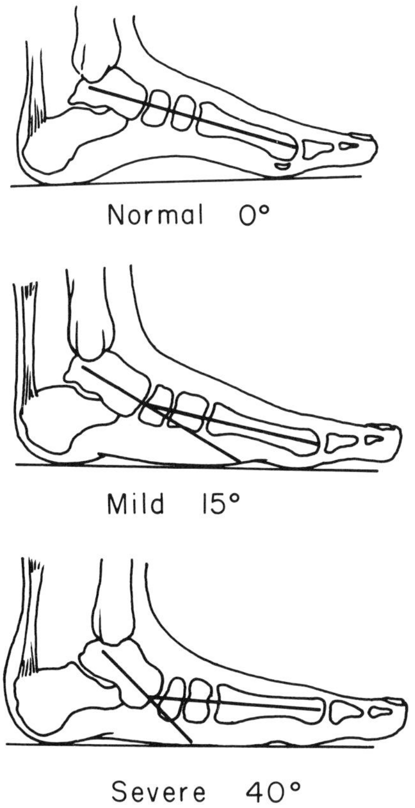

Fig. 60.6 The lateral talometatarsal angle measured to assess idiopathic hypermobile flat feet in children (Bordelon 1980)

ments. For example, Böhler's critical angle was measured between 22° and 48°. However, in 21% of the feet the angle was greater than the upper reported value of 40° (Gamble & Yale 1966). In 9% of the feet, the angle was less than the lower reported value of 20° (Gamble & Yale 1966). Thus almost one-third of the feet they studied were outside of the range reported to be 'normal'.

Although they found a significant positive correlation between the first metatarsophalangeal angle and other forefoot measurements, there was no significant correlation found between that angle and any midfoot or hindfoot measurement. Most importantly they noted that there was little difference between the measurements of the left and the right feet of their subjects. Thus feet were found to be symmetric in their group. This gives credence to the usual clinical practice of using the contralateral foot for comparison particularly if it is normal. On the anteroposterior radiograph the talocalcaneal or hindfoot angle showed a great spread from 15–63°. Half of the subjects had an angle measured from 20–37° while the upper range of normal was between 37° and 54° for the remaining 50%. Other interesting hindfoot measurements were the talometatarsal-two shaft angle and the calcaneus metatarsal-two shaft angle. In addition, the hindfoot width was measured by a line from the most medial aspect of the talus to the most lateral aspect of the calcaneus. A length/height ratio was also developed. However they measured the total length of the foot from the most posterior aspect of the calcaneus to the tip of the long toe in contrast to Penneau et al (1982). The height was measured from the most superior portion of the talonavicular joint on a line perpendicular with the length of the foot. However a length measurement of the calcaneus to the distal first metatarsal was also made.

The calcaneal pitch angle has been described as a true measurement of the longitudinal arch of the foot (see Fig. 60.5) (Drobocky 1986). It is drawn by a line which traverses the weight-bearing tips of the calcaneus and first metatarsal head with another line that runs across the plantar limits of the calcaneus. If above 30° a high arch is noted and if below 20°, a low arch (Gamble & Yale 1966). Böhler's angle is formed by drawing a line from the posterosuperior tip of the tuberosity of the os calcis through the highest point of the os calcis at the posterosuperior margin of the posterior articular facet. A second line is drawn from the highest point of the os calcis anteriorly through the same point at the posterior superior margin of the posterior facet (Gamble & Yale 1966). A normal range from 20–40° is reported.

ARTHRODESIS

Types of arthrodesis techniques

Many different techniques are available to fuse joints.

Excision of the joint surfaces

Excision of the joint surfaces through the subchondral plate can be accomplished by using curettes, an osteotome, a power saw or a power burr. The bony surfaces available for fusion can then be increased by using a gouge to raise small bits of cancellous bone which remain attached to the underlying bed. At this point, a gap exists between the bony surfaces. Soft tissue release is then necessary so that the bone ends fit together. Then these surfaces must be held together until fusion occurs. Traditionally this has been accomplished by a cast.

Grafting techniques

These are usually combined with excising the joint surfaces or can be utilized as the primary method of arthrodesis. Autogenous grafts are the best and occasionally sufficient bone can be obtained from local sites such as the calcaneus and the tibia. However, most often grafts are taken from the iliac crest. Bone grafts can be inlayed across the joint, inlayed into the joint (Campbell et al 1974) or slotted across or into the joint (Figs. 60.7a and b). Rotating a dowel, half of which is composed of adjacent joint surfaces, 90° to the normal axis of the joint usually leads to solid fusion (Fig. 60.8).

Two special circumstances require the addition of significant amounts of bone to obtain arthrodesis.

1. In children with open epiphyseal plates, Chuinard & Peterson (1963) described a method of impacting a full thickness iliac crest graft into a denuded ankle joint. The graft is held in place by the normal compression forces across the ankle. Epiphyseal growth continues and several millimetres of length are added to the lower leg.

2. Patients with failed prosthetic ankle replacement also have significant bone loss and it may be virtually impossible to achieve good bony opposition between the distal tibia and whatever remains of the talus (Fig. 60.9a). Campbell et al (1974) reported an excellent method of placing two or three full thickness iliac crest grafts across the ankle joint for fusion. The technique was designed as a primary arthrodesis, and excised a block containing the articular surfaces of the joint. The posterior cortex of the tibia should remain intact if possible, better to contain the grafts. The grafts are then cut several millimetres wider than the space created between the distal tibia and the calcaneus and are wedged between the malleoli and the bone ends (Fig. 60.9b). Whenever possible the cancellous bone of the graft is made to coapt with whatever cancellous bone remains on the prepared bed. Although they used threaded pins or screws across the fusion site if there was instability, an external fixator would also provide the necessary rigidity and compression. The method used by White (1974) is similar in utilizing a precision preparation of the bed for arthrodesis and in obtaining iliac grafts. However, he used a

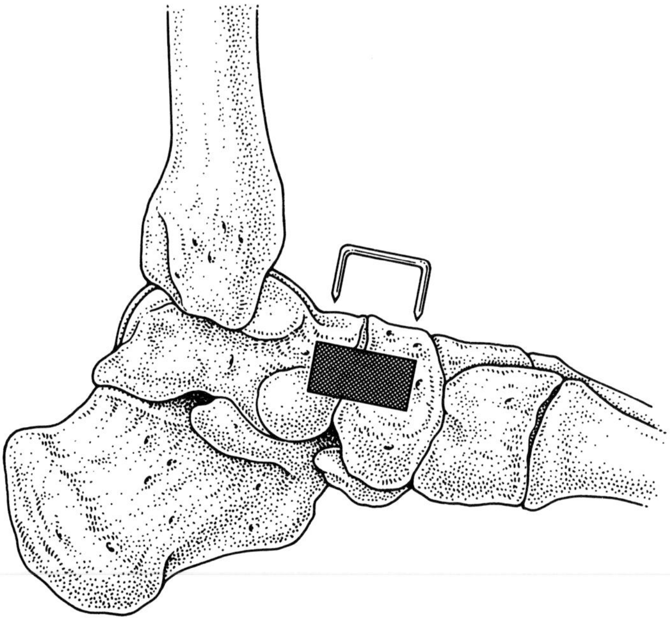

Fig. 60.7a An arthrodesis technique with a slot graft placed into the talonavicular joint and being held in place with a staple

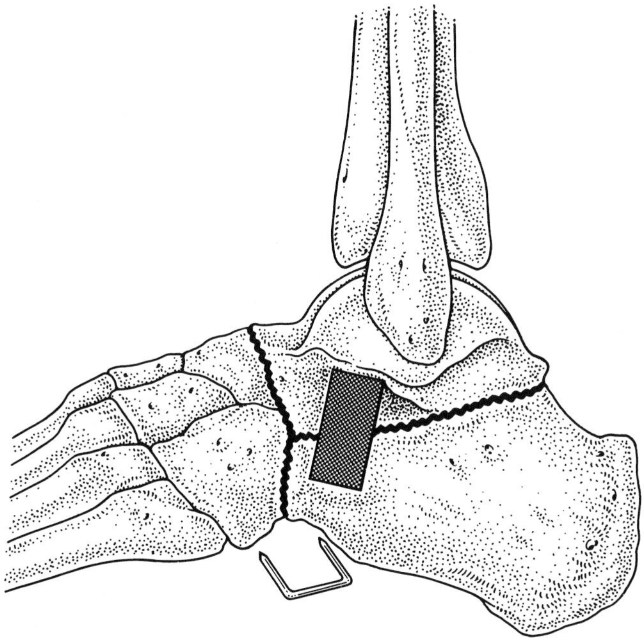

Fig. 60.7b An arthrodesis technique using an inlay graft as well as excision of the surfaces of the hindfoot joints

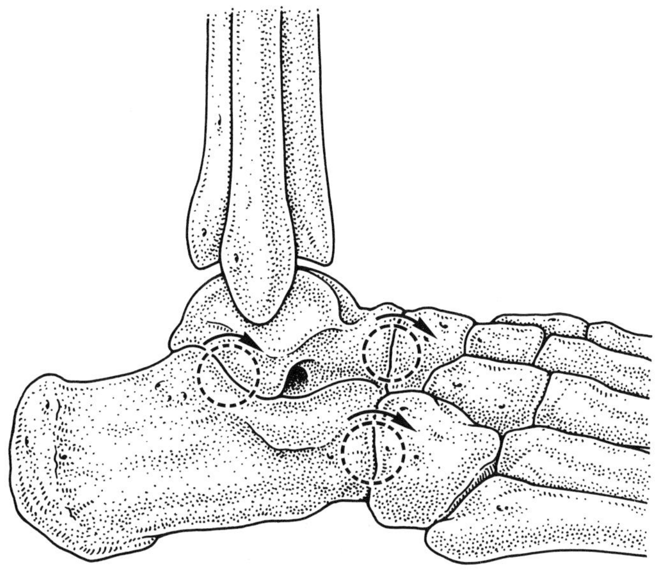

Fig. 60.8 A schematic drawing of the rotation of the dowels across the hindfoot joints. These dowels are composed of one half of each joint surface and are rotated 90° to ensure solid arthrodesis

posterior approach and repaired the posterior capsule. The Achilles tendon was also repaired under enough tension to approximate its initial resting length and to maintain the function provided by the gastrocnemius across the knee joint.

Internal fixation

Once the above steps have been performed, some means is usually necessary to hold the surfaces and grafts stable until fusion occurs. This can be

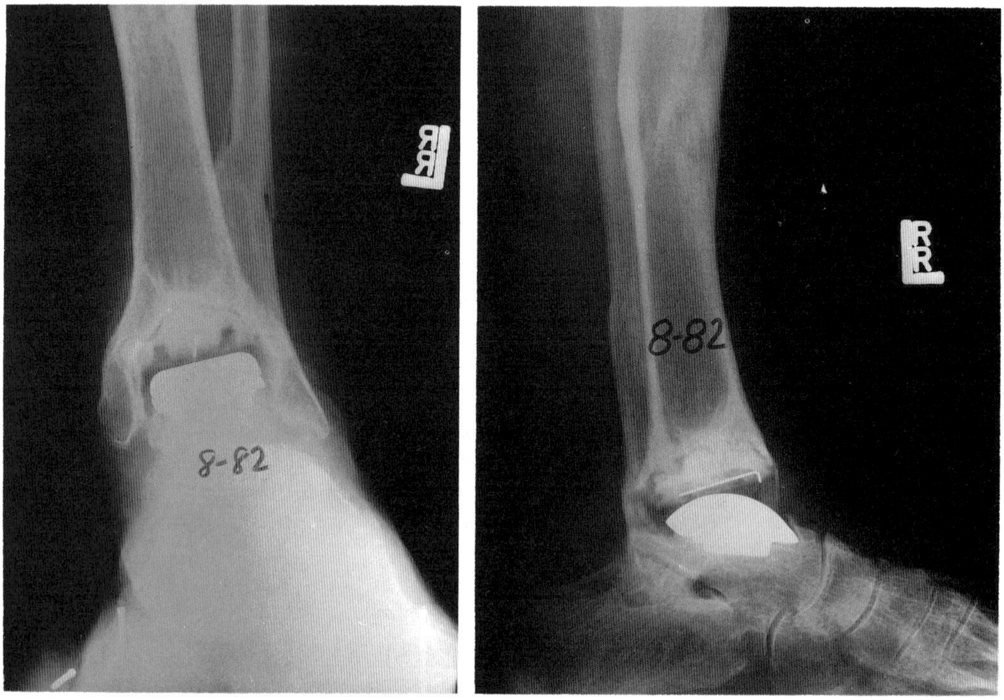

Fig. 60.9a A male patient presented with a loose total ankle prosthesis which was painful. The prosthesis was used to treat a traumatic arthritis from a severe fracture of the lower leg and ankle

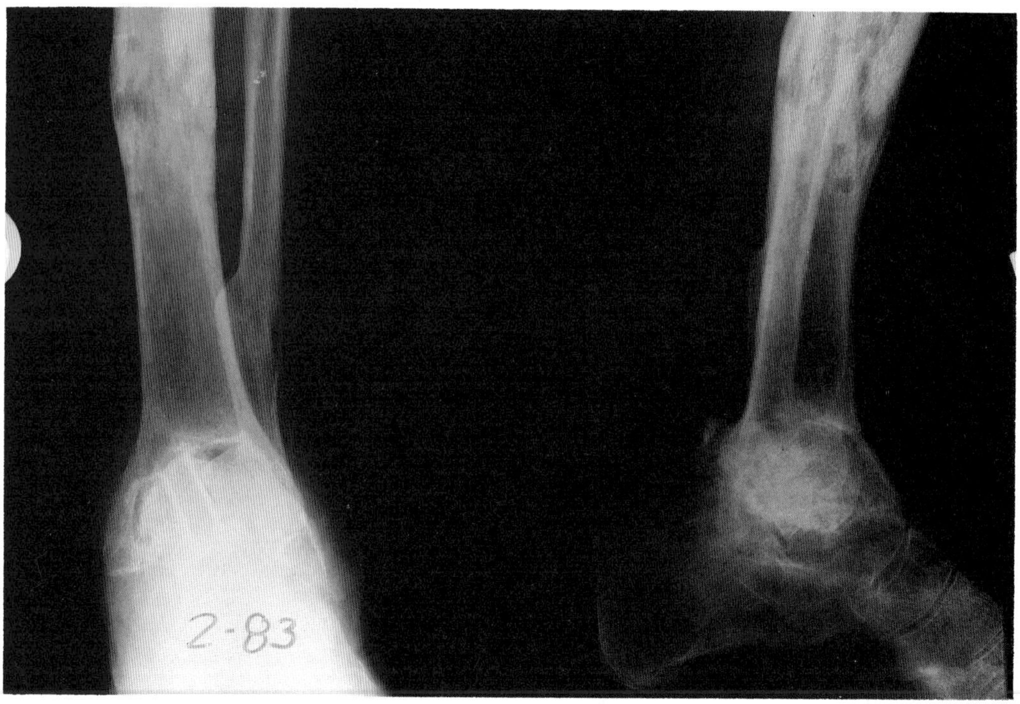

Fig. 60.9b Note the large bone grafts taken from the patient's iliac crest and placed in the ankle mortise. This area was immobilized by an external fixator for 10 weeks. The patient has a solid painless ankle arthrodesis, and only a 1 cm leg length inequality

accomplished with staples, although it is difficult to get compression with a staple and the larger ones require predrilling to allow smooth insertion. Kirschner wires and Steinman pins are also used to transfix smaller joints. However, compression screw techniques probably offer the best fixation, and can be utilized in arthrodesis techniques for the hindfoot joints or the ankle joint. In addition it is possible to utilize a compression plate to achieve ankle arthrodesis (Scranton 1985).

A special technique using a hip compression screw and a modified Stone staple has been reported for the Blair fusion (Lionberger et al 1982). This operation is an accepted method of achieving ankle arthrodesis in the absence of the dome of the talus or when it is necrotic. This modified procedure is a tibiotalar fusion between the anterior tibia and the neck of the talus. A paediatric hip compression screw is passed from the posterior tibia superiorly and directed anteriorly and inferiorly to within 5 mm of the talonavicular joint.

External fixation with compression fixators

Compression arthrodesis techniques using an external fixator are now frequently employed in ankle arthrodesis. Of course, these depend on proper preparation of the bony surfaces and at times bone grafting is also necessary. One should not rely only on the external fixator to provide a successful arthrodesis. External fixation only provides rigid fixation and maintains the proper alignment.

Ankle arthrodesis

Arthrodesis of the ankle has been widely discussed in the literature for many years. Over 10 years ago White (1974) reviewed the French and English literature and documented at least 22 distinctly different techniques for arthrodesis reported since 1900. Although the operations are different, several have common features and can be placed into groups:

1. Compression clamps are currently utilized as an adjunct to many arthrodesis techniques
2. Some operations use the fibula as strut or spike graft
3. Procedures are described where the tibia is used as a donor site, as a strut graft, a sliding graft or a transposed graft through the joint
4. There are other operations which include use of the dowel technique and epiphysis-preserving arthrodesis.

In addition to individual preference by the surgeon, several reasons may exist for the many diverse techniques.

1. The type of pathology for which the arthrodesis is indicated. Frequently fusions are required for an arthritic ankle secondary to trauma where there may have been bone loss or perhaps, osteonecrosis.
2. During the past few decades ankle trauma has frequently resulted in at least one previous primary operation so that internal fixation devices may be present as well as previous incisions all requiring the surgeon to select the most appropriate incision and technique to gain fusion.
3. The anatomy requires that one rather small bone, the talus, be fused to another much longer, bone, the tibia. Hopefully this will occur while the adjacent joints, especially those of the hindfoot as well as the knee remain unimpaired. The indications for ankle fusion are well defined and the most common are pain, stiffness and deformity due to an arthritic joint. Other indications include infection, instability and poor function as a result of paralysis and, recently, failed total ankle arthroplasty (Stazzeri et al 1984, Rothacker & Cabanella 1983).

Probably two of the most important factors in ankle arthrodesis are the final position of the foot to the leg and the final status of the subtalar joint and the transverse tarsal joints (talonavicular and calcaneocuboid joints). Recent studies have shown that the neutral position gives the best overall results (Buck et al 1982, King et al 1980, Ratliff 1959, Mazur et al 1979). King's studies gave the neutral position as a 90° angle between the tibia and the plantar surface of the foot. This position permits some transverse tarsal motion. They measured midfoot motion of 5–20° of plantar flexion with an average of 11°. An ankle fused in equinus of any more than 5°, would not be able to utilize this movement while walking. Morrey & Wiedeman (1980) examined 30 patients an average of seven years after solid ankle fusion. They measured an average range of motion of Chopart's joint of 13°, 2° dorsiflexion and 11° plantar flexion. Dorsiflexion ranged from –5 to +5 degrees and plantar flexion from 0–20°. Almost all subtalar joints were stiff. These findings have been confirmed by Buck et al (1982), who found that fusion in the neutral position provided greater total motion in the sagittal plane. They noted that posterior displacement of the talus resulted in less knee recurvatum. Also, a valgus position of the ankle improved side-slope walking. Jackson & Glasgow (1979) studied a group of patients with a solidly fused ankle whose opposite ankle was normal. Although they did find midtarsal stiffness in 33% of feet after solid arthrodesis, there was also significant dorsiflexion and plantar flexion in 27% of patients on the side with the ankle arthrodesis. In 40% there was no change in midtarsal motion as compared to the opposite normal foot. Stewart et al (1983) reports that 53% of their patients with ankle arthrodesis had a minimum loss of midtarsal motion, 17% had a significant increase in motion and 30% were unchanged. This is also significant because all of the subtalar joints on the side of the ankle arthrodesis were stiff. It is common that the subtalar joint is abnormal in patients requiring ankle arthrodesis as it is frequently involved in the pathology, either trauma or arthritis, which involves the ankle. However, as long as there is eversion of the heel, with the talonavicular and calcaneocuboid joints parallel, transverse tarsal motion is possible. Thus it appears that a better functional result following ankle arthrodesis will be obtained if: (1) The final position is a 90° angle between the tibia and the foot, (2) The talus is posteriorly placed under the tibia, (3) The transverse tarsal motion is maintained (Mazur et al 1979) and (4) Motion of the subtalar joint is maintained if it is present preoperatively or if stiff, so that the calcaneus remains in or is placed into eversion.

Arthrodesis using an external fixator

External fixators were used prior to 1951 in conjunction with ankle arthrodesis to hold the tibiotalar joint in the desired position (Anderson 1945). However, the concept of compression arthrodesis was introduced and popularized by Charnley (1951) when he gained consistent success with arthrodesis of the knee by compression. An external fixator properly applied in compression offers good immobilization of the ankle joint and facilitates fusion. Several external fixation devices have now become available for use. Charnley (1951) gave several criteria that need to be satisfied in the design of an ideal compression arthrodesis: (1) the compression pins must avoid neurovascular structures; (2) normal joints must be excluded from the compressive force; (3) the line connecting the two points at which pressure is applied should pass through, or very near the axis of the joints to be arthrodesed and (4) the cut surfaces of the bone being compressed must have a good blood supply and be free from active disease.

An external fixator should be selected which:

1. Provides compression in more than one plane. The original Charnley device provided adequate medial-lateral rigidity, but allowed some antero-posterior motion especially if the surfaces to be fused were not flat and parallel. The opposite extreme may be the double upright frame of the modified Hoffman external fixator. This device provides excellent rigidity to such a degree that the weakest link of the entire system is at the pin to bone junction.

2. The fixator should be of a reasonable size and permit ambulation with the patient being able to use crutches or a walker. It should also permit access to the incision and, most importantly, the skin about the pins.

3. The device should allow some adjustments to be made so that the compression forces can vary and the alignment be adjusted.

A triangular compression device (Calandruccio 1984) has been used which is relatively simple to apply and adjust and which provides sufficient compression and rigidity to ensure fusion.

Operative technique

Utilizing an external fixator

Anterior approach. An anterior or anterolateral incision is used to expose the ankle for a primary arthrodesis. The talus and tibia are freed of any adhesions, fibrous tissue or debris preventing proper alignment. The talar dome and then the distal tibial surface should be flattened with an oscillating saw to form a 90° angle between the leg and foot. Usually very little bone needs to be excised and removing first the articular surface of the talus facilitates removing the concave surface of the distal tibia.

The surfaces are then prepared as described under the arthrodesis techniques. The first fixation pin is inserted medially into the talus just posterior to the medial malleolus. A small transverse medial skin incision is made in this area, and if necessary the neurovascular bundle can be identified and retracted. Very often a centimetre of the posterior aspect of the medial malleolus is removed so that the pin will not impinge on the bone. The talus is held to the tibia in the proper 90° angle for fusion, and using a hand or power drill a 4 mm or 5 mm diameter centrally threaded pin is inserted at a right angle to the tibia from medially to lateral, carefully protecting the neurovascular bundle and tendons (Fig. 60.10a). The pin should be about 1.5 cm distal to the resected articular surface of the talus. As the pin emerges laterally, expose the fibula and remove sufficient bone to prevent impingement which would prevent compression (Fig. 60.10b). A drill guide and the distal transverse bar of the compression device aid in positioning the second and, if necessary, a third pin in the talus parallel to the first pin. All three pins can usually be placed in the talus. This is most important if the subtalar joint is not involved. However, if the hindfoot is stiff either from a fibrous or bone ankylosis then the pins can be placed either through the joint or in the calcaneus. Should the calcaneus be in varus, this can be corrected by disrupting what is usually a fibrous ankylosis of the subtalar joint and everting the heel. The position can be maintained by the compression device with the distal pins placed through the calcaneus.

The compression clamps can then be loosely attached to the distal pins. The proximal clamps are then aligned with the distal tibia while holding the foot and leg in the desired 90° position for fusion. The tibial pins are placed in a similar manner from medial to lateral so that the centrally threaded pins will not pass through the anterior compartment muscle fibres. Usually it is necessary to predrill the tibial holes if dense cortical bone is present. The tibial pins should be placed along the midlateral axis of the bone (see Fig. 60.10b). Should the pins be inserted just under the subcutaneous anterior cortex of the tibia, pin track infection or drainage are more likely to occur.

The two compression clamps are then attached to all the pins with about 2 cm of clearance between the skin and the compression devices. The pins are cut

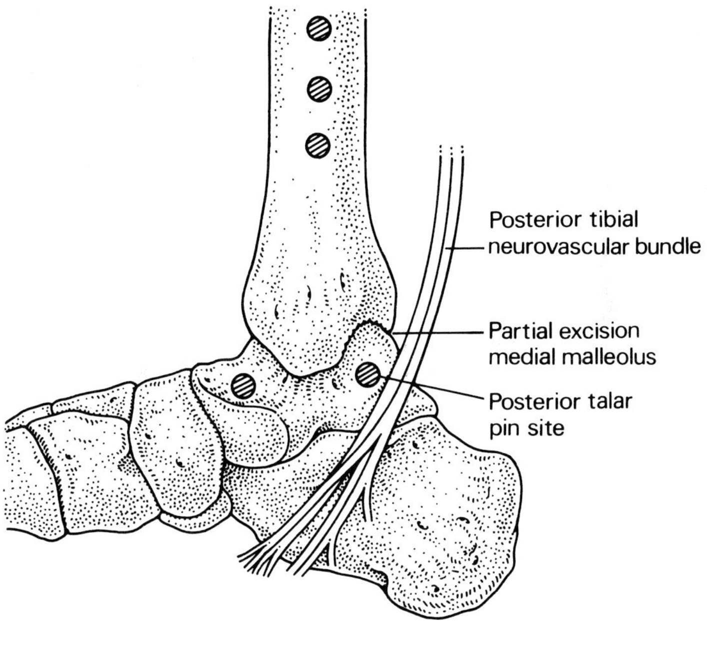

Fig. 60.10a A medial view showing the posterior tibial neurovascular bundle and the position of the pins for compression arthrodesis of the ankle. The pins should be placed in the talus and the distal tibia if the hindfoot is mobile. Care must be taken to protect the neurovascular bundle. It may be necessary to excise a small amount of the posterior portion of the medial malleolus

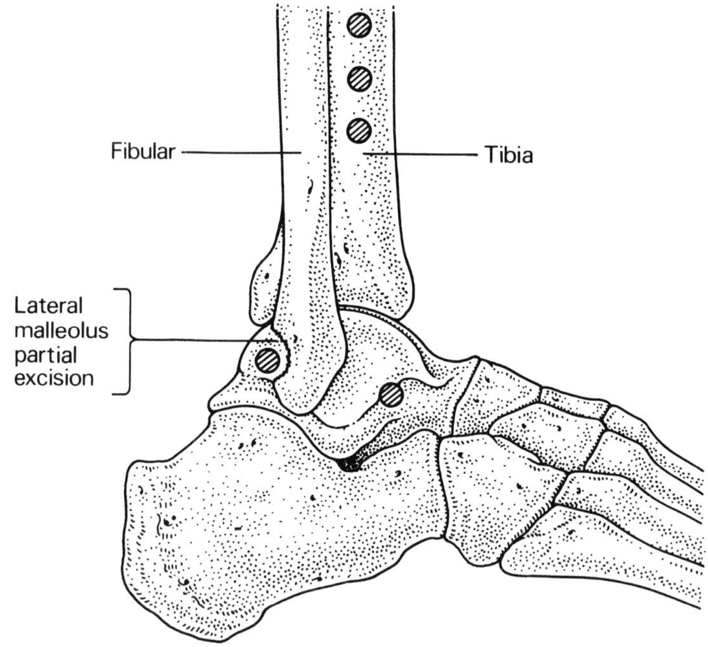

Fig. 60.10b A lateral view of the pin tracts in the distal tibia and the position of the pins in the talus with one being just posterior to the lateral malleolus so the pin will hold enough talus and not abut against the fibula in compression. The second pin is in the neck of the talus

and the compression clamp moved out slightly so that the cut pin ends are just inside the holes in the vertical and transverse bars (Fig. 60.10c). The pins are then secured to the bars with locking screws. Compression must not be a substitute for excellent preparation of the bony surfaces. The final position for arthrodesis must align the foot with the leg at a 90° angle and position the talus posteriorly on the surface of the tibia. Only then can the bolts be tightened until there is a moderate degree of bow in the pins. The talus should be rigidly held to the tibia and the compression device must be securely locked in place.

To assess the position of the foot to the tibia more accurately, remove all drapes from the distal half of the leg. Observation alone may not be sufficient, especially if other pathology exists and radiographs are often necessary (Figs. 60.11a, b).

Another additional benefit of the external fixator is that adjustments in position can be made postoperatively should an incorrect position be observed.

Other variations of applying external fixation have been reported. The Hoffman external fixation device has been utilized (Stazzeri et al 1984, Newman 1980). A triangular double frame has been constructed with pins in the tibia, calcaneus (or the talus) and in the base of the metatarsals (Newman 1980). Half pins are suggested if the frame extends to the metatarsals to minimize soft tissue injury. Such pin placement may be necessary if other foot deformities exist such as severe equinus or varus of the midfoot or the forefoot.

Postoperative care

An external fixation device must be kept in place for several weeks if a successful fusion is to be achieved. For this to occur, particular care must be given to the pin sites. The skin around the pins must not be under any tension. Should any skin tension exist it must be relieved by incising the tense skin with a scalpel. Circumferential gauze dressings are then placed around the set of pins in the foot and the tibia so that they pass between the skin and the compression clamp. Sufficient gauze is used to minimize motion of the skin about the pins and reduce oedema. It is essential that these gauze packs be changed daily and the area cleansed and encrustations about the pins removed. This essential task is not difficult and can

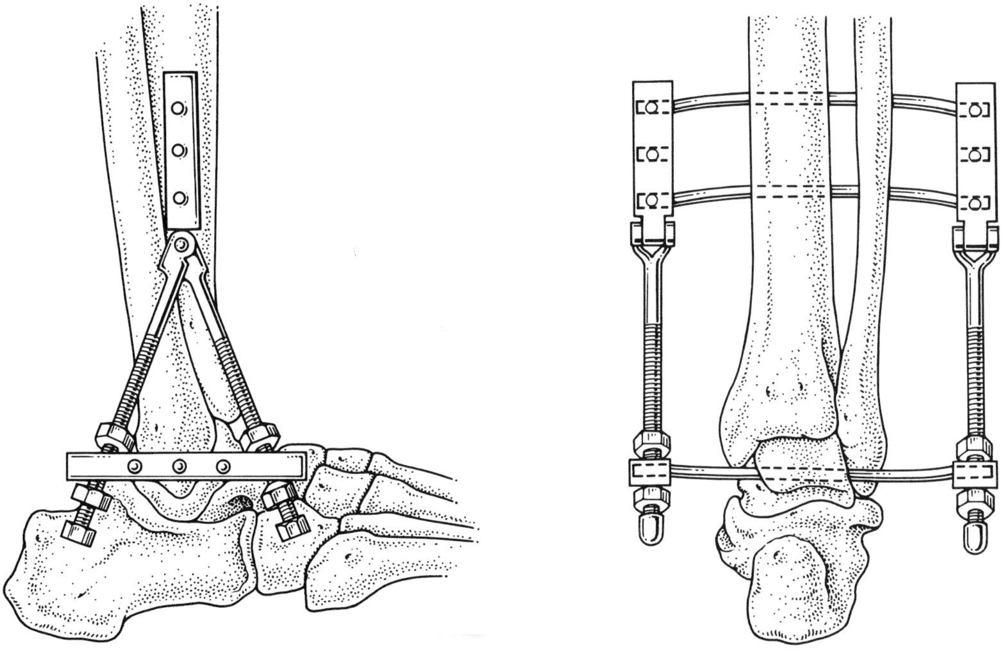

Fig. 60.10c The triangular compression device in place with three pins in the talus and three in the tibia

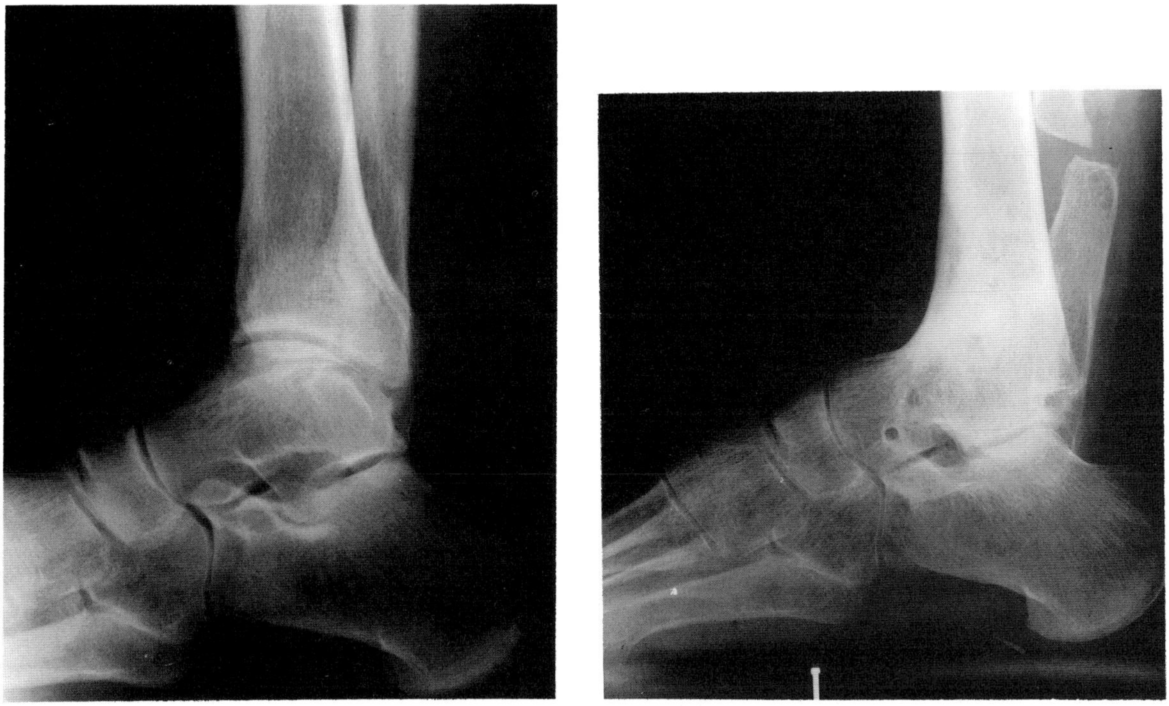

a b

Fig. 60.11 a, A 52-year-old Caucasian male with a negative history but whose lateral radiograph shows evidence of a probable distal tibial epiphyseal plate injury. The ankle mortise was grossly malaligned and the ankle was painful and arthritic; b, A solid ankle arthrodesis with the pin tracts in the talus and the tibia. There is nonunion of an osteotomy of the distal fibula performed at a previous operation. The talus could have been positioned slightly more posteriorly under the tibia. The patient has an excellent result usually be done by a family member who should be trained in the proper technique by the nursing staff.

The length of time for which the pins remain in place varies. One or more pins may need to be removed for local wound problems. However, the external fixator should remain in place for at least six weeks. Charnley (1951) initially recommended that the pins be removed after four weeks and a walking cast applied for another four weeks. However, others report removal of the external fixator between six and 14 weeks (Stazzeri et al 1984, Ratliff 1959, Newman 1980, Rothacker & Cabanella 1983). This is usually followed by a short-leg walking cast for up to 10 additional weeks (Stazzeri et al 1984, Rothacker & Cabanella 1983) although not everyone (Newman 1980) advocates a postfixator cast. The fixator can easily be removed in the office usually with the aid of an intravenous analgesic and hypnotic agent. The time required for a solid arthrodesis varies widely from an average of 12 weeks (Markus et al 1983) to 18 weeks (Rothacker & Cabanella 1983) and is probably related to the particular pathology. In some patients union occurs very slowly and some patients who are destined to unite require the use of a brace for 6–12 months postoperatively (Lance et al 1979). Some patients, however, are more comfortable in their brace despite having a solid bony ankylosis. This is usually due to pain from an arthritic subtalar joint, which can usually be verified clinically and radiographically. Swelling of the foot and ankle usually occurs and must be controlled by external support.

Once the arthrodesis is well healed, some consideration must be given to shoewear. Satisfactory transverse tarsal motion will allow use of a regular shoe. Initially the patient's shoe should be modified by adding a SACH heel and a rocker sole which makes walking much easier.

The transfibular approach. The lateral, transfibular approach gives the widest possible view of the articular surfaces. By using a high speed power burr, only the articular surfaces are removed and this may reduce the amount of shortening of the leg.

The posterior approach. This is highly recommended when multiple procedures have been previously performed through an anterior approach or when the anterior skin is poor. The prone position allows free access to the leg and ankle. Bone grafts can easily be removed from the posterior iliac crest if needed. Through this approach the grafts have a fresh new bed and are covered in part by muscle fibres which may improve the vascularity of the area and enhance arthrodesis.

Medial approach. A standard medial incision may also be utilized for compression arthrodesis. This has the relative advantage of exposing the medial malleolus and removing a small amount of bone posteriorly and inferiorly to avoid impingement with the posterior medial pin. The neurovascular bundle can also be retracted avoiding any potential damage from the distal posterior talar pin. The medial approach of Thomas (1969) offers excellent exposure and also adds a most needed osteotomy of the fibula. After gaining exposure he denudes the articular surfaces, including the subchondral bone, and if necessary the gouges resect the articular surfaces to correct angular deformities. Thomas utilized the Charnley clamp for compression. Postoperatively the pins were removed at four weeks and a short leg walking cast applied for an additional four weeks. The ankle was then supported with a compression bandage for an additional three weeks. He reported 19 successful fusions and one failure (Fig. 60.12).

Arthrodesis using internal fixation

The use of internal fixation utilizing a compression technique with cancellous screws or compression plate fixation offers some potential advantages for ankle arthrodesis (Scranton 1985, Morgan et al 1985). Scranton (1985) utilized the anterior two-thirds of the medial malleolus that had been previously osteotomized to gain medial exposure as a bone graft. His technique described resecting the articular surfaces perpendicular to the longitudinal axis of the tibia. Then a specially designed T-plate fitted easily against the medial border of the talus and the distal tibia with 4.5 mm cortical A-O screws. Care was taken not to penetrate the subtalar joints with the screws. The foot was held in the desired position, basically neutral, and the compression screws attached the plate to the tibia (Fig. 60.13). 24 ankles all fused within 12 weeks. Another had a delayed union which fused at six months (Scranton 1985).

The use of screws as internal fixation for ankle arthrodesis has been described by Morgan et al (1985). They reported a 95% fusion rate over a

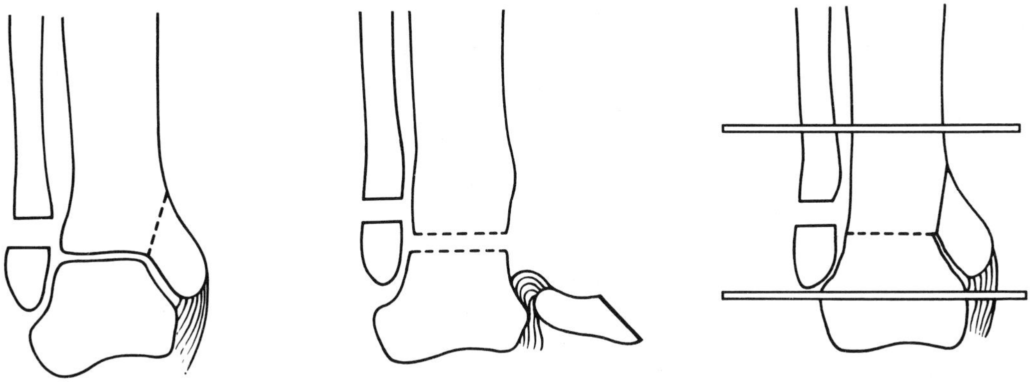

Fig. 60.12 The arthrodesis technique of Thomas (1969)

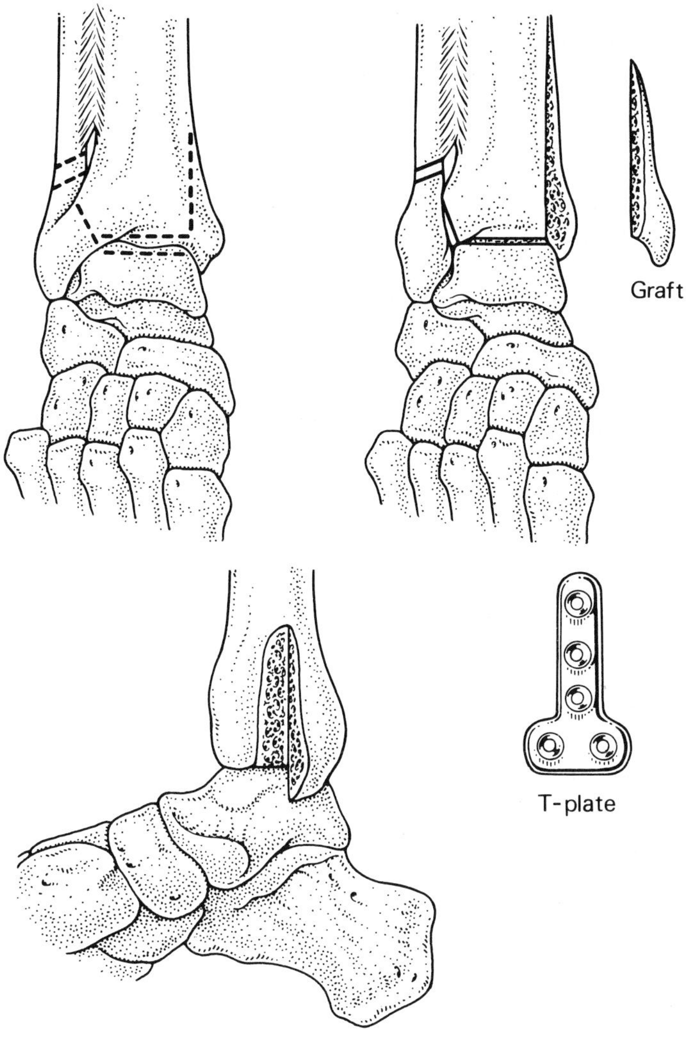

Fig. 60.13 The medial and lateral approach as described by Scranton (1985). The anterior two-thirds of the medial malleolus is transected and is utilized as a bone graft. The posterior one-third protects the neurovascular bundle. A special T-plate is in place, first on the talus and held by screws and then compressed to the distal tibia being held in place by screws

25 year period. Patients with pseudoarthrosis all had a sensory defect. An anterolateral approach was used to expose the ankle and the articular surfaces were resected maintaining the original bone contours of the distal tibia and the talar dome. The talus was positioned as close to the medial malleolus as possible and posteriorly along the longitudinal axis of the tibia. Screws were placed from the distal tibia and fibula into the talus and angulated anteriorly about 40° to gain maximum purchase (Fig. 60.14). Only two screws were used and in more recent cases cancellous grafts were also used. Also a smooth Steinman pin was used to transfix the ankle joint during the application of the screws and then frequently removed. Morgan et al (1985) found tarsal hypermobility in all patients, but this did not correlate with function or degenerative joint changes in the hindfoot joints.

With the use of compression screw fixation, both Scranton (1985) and Morgan et al (1985) advocate the use of intraoperative radiographs to be certain that the desired position for arthrodesis has been achieved.

Should a lateral approach be used then it should be possible to place an additional screw through the posterior malleolus either through the same exposure or a short posterior ancillary incision (Fig. 60.15). Also, if the distal tibia were wide enough, the lateral screw could also be placed from the lateral and distal tibia into the talus. If indicated an additional third screw could be used through the distal fibula and into the talus. However, the talus is always of smaller size than the tibia and fibula and it can only accommodate a limited amount of internal devices (Fig. 60.15). However, in a large adult with good bone stock the current practice is to place at least two and possibly three 6.5 mm cancellous screws across the tibia into the talus. The anterolateral incision offers the best exposure for this procedure with a short curved ancillary incision needed over the medial malleolus for placing the medial tibotalar screw and removing part or all of the malleolus if necessary. Additionally the fibula should be osteotomized obliquely about 10 cm above its tip and retracted laterally, to aid in the exposure. After the tibia has been solidly secured to the talus, the adjacent surfaces of the fibula and talus are prepared so that the fibula can be used as a strut graft. The

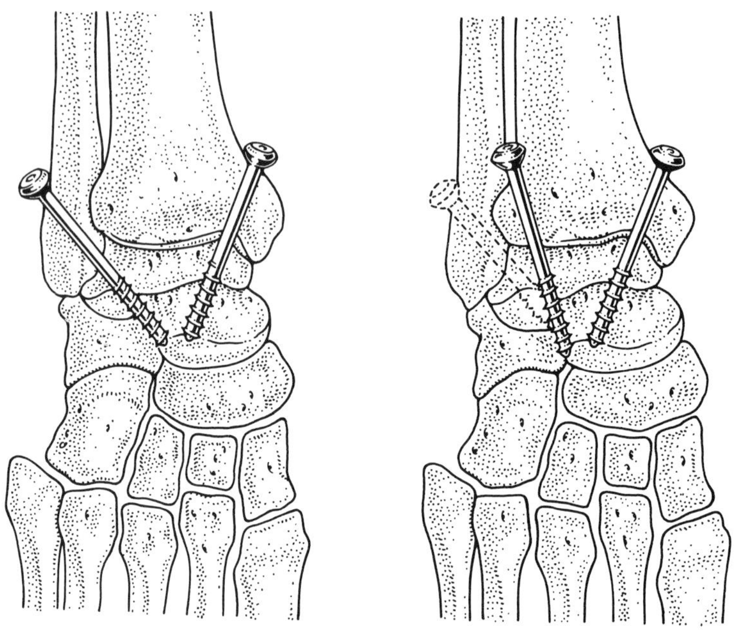

Fig. 60.14 The use of cancellous screws for ankle arthrodesis. On the left the screws have been placed into the distal fibula and the tibia directed into the talus. On the right the screws have been placed either through the distal tibia and into the talus with or without supplementation of a third screw or through the distal fibula and into the talus. It is important that those screws be angulated anteriorly to gain maximum purchase and also to properly position the talus well underneath the tibia and so avoid anterior malposition of the foot and ankle

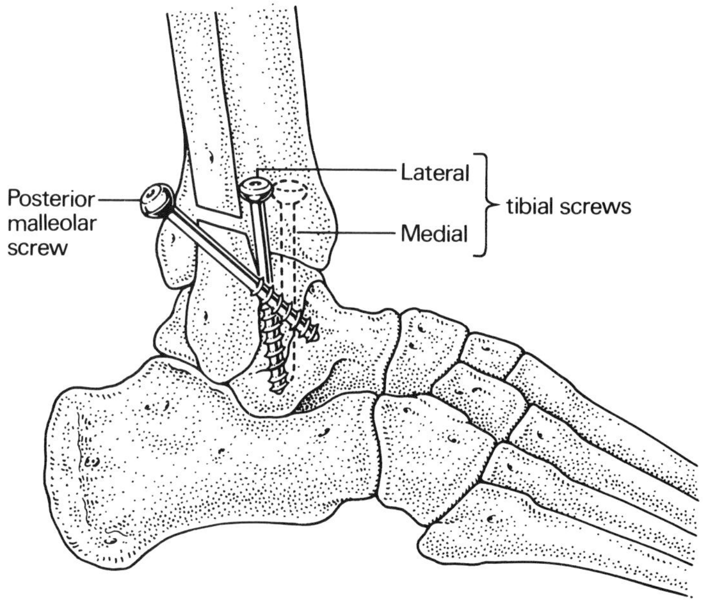

Fig. 60.15 If a lateral approach is used then an additional screw can be placed through the posterior malleolus angulated well into the anterior portion of the talus. This can be supplemented with medial and lateral screws and it is important to use more than one screw for this type of arthrodesis technique

fibula is displaced medially and secured to the talus with a short 6.5 mm cancellous screw. An additional screw just under the osteotomy site fixes the fibula proximally to the tibia, thus completing the strut graft.

The malleoli in ankle arthrodesis

The medial and lateral malleoli can pose a problem in ankle arthrodesis:

1. If there has been significant bone loss from the dome of the talus or the distal tibia, the malleoli become quite prominent and widen the posterior portion of the foot. This can present significant problems with shoe fit as these prominences will rub on the counters of the shoe. Such patients also have a poor cosmetic result.

2. The inner surfaces of the malleoli usually do not significantly contribute to the arthrodesis. Resecting the adjacent articular surfaces of the malleoli and talus leaves a gap which can only be filled with bone graft. Bimalleolar incisions have been reported in ankle arthrodesis, resecting one or both of the malleoli (Markus et al 1983, Anderson 1945), which can be used as bone grafts and held in place with screws. Additional internal fixation can be used to promote arthrodesis. Markus et al (1983) and Stewart et al (1983) described the use of compression arthrodesis while narrowing the malleoli and fixing them with screws. Improved cosmesis and shoewear are an advantage of this technique.

Complications of arthrodesis

Local complications

These include problems with wound healing and failure of fusion. Arthrodesis procedures are usually secondary or revision operations so that the skin and soft tissues may be compromised leading to difficulties with healing. Sepsis, shortening and malalignment can also occur. Neurovascular damage is a possible consequence particularly if internal or external fixation is used. Oedema may persist and fractures may occur through a tibial donor site or a pin track.

Two large reviews report a significant percentage of complications from ankle arthrodesis, from 48–60% (Johnson & Boseker 1969, Morrey & Weideman 1980). White's review of the literature lists almost every conceivable complication from an uncosmetic scar to a below-knee amputation for intractable pain. Morrey & Weideman (1980) cite infection (23%) and nonunion (23%) as the most frequent complications. Inadequate surgical alignment or early loss of position (15%), malunion (12%) and delayed union (7%) were the next most common complications.

Systemic complications

No specific systemic complications are attributable to arthrodesis procedures. However, any systemic complication is possible such as pulmonary embolus, myocardial infarction or cerebral vascular accident. These are all major operations and require some period of immobilization and bed rest. Therefore all patients must be advised of these potential complications although they rarely occur.

Results of ankle arthrodesis

The results of ankle arthrodesis have improved as proper techniques have evolved. Lance et al (1979) have shown that the highest rate of union occurred after compression arthrodesis (94%). Their anterior arthrodesis oeperation resulted in 84% fusion, the distraction-compression procedure gave a 74% fusion rate and the transfibular technique was the least successful (64%). The rate of successful bony arthrodesis has varied between 78% and 94% (Morrey & Weideman 1980, Lance et al 1979, Charnley 1951, Campbell et al 1974, Stewart et al 1983, Rothacker & Cabanella 1983, Markus et al 1983, Ratliff 1959). Evidence of the improved ability to gain ankle arthrodesis is particularly evident in the success reported in fusing all cases of failed total ankle arthroplasty (Strazzeri et al 1984, Rothacker & Cabanella 1983) (see Figs. 60.9a and b).

However, one of the problems with ankle arthrodesis relates to the overall success of the operation, which involves more than a successful union between the talus and the tibia. After reviewing four types of arthrodesis techniques, Lance et al (1979) reported more patients with an unsatisfactory result than the nonunion rate in each group. Despite solid bony fusion at the ankle, 17 patients had an unsatisfactory result due to pain. The degree of prefusion pathology, especially in the adjacent joints and the patient's perception of the result frequently alter the final success ratings. Obviously a fused ankle will never have as good a result as one with near normal motion. The cosmetic result is at best acceptable as there is always a supramalleolar thickness on the fused side. Shoes must frequently be modified and women need to accept some limitation in their fashion. For all these reasons the overall success rate of ankle arthrodesis is usually lower than the reported percentage of bony arthrodesis.

Fortunately ankle arthrodesis is usually an operation which *must* be performed. It is frequently the only solution to a painful and deformed ankle. Careful surgical technique and proper patient management should result in a high rate of success (Figs. 60.16a–d).

Hindfoot arthrodesis

Clinical findings

Hindfoot pathology frequently involves all three of the hindfoot joints, subtalar, talonavicular and calcaneocuboid. Such involvement is most commonly seen in systemic arthritic diseases such as rheumatoid arthritis or in developmental conditions as in residual clubfoot deformities. Isolated pathology of the subtalar joint is usually seen following fracture of the calcaneus which involves that joint. Traumatic arthritis of the remaining joints is also possible but much less frequent. Patients usually perceive hindfoot pain as ankle pain as they are unaware of the hindfoot complex, but of course are very familiar with the ankle joint. Therefore pain in that general area will always initially be perceived by the patient as coming from the ankle.

At times it can be very difficult to determine the origin of the pain particularly if ankle arthritis is also present. This combination of pathology is seen most frequently with a systemic arthritis, but can also be present following severe trauma involving the ankle and hindfoot.

The primary source of pain can be distinguished in the usual fashion by a careful history and physical examination. If radiographs show pathology in both areas, more sophisticated studies such as radionucleide scanning or computer assisted tomography or plain tomography may be of value in selected cases. The technique of differential injections is also very helpful. Most of the time there is complete separation of the synovial cavity of the ankle from that of the hindfoot. An intra-articular injection of a

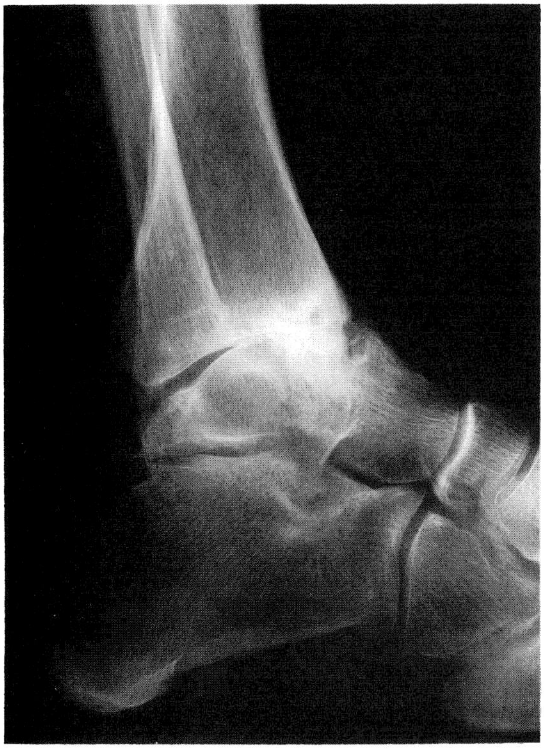

Fig. 60.16a Lateral radiograph of a 26-year-old Caucasian male with Reiter's syndrome showing advanced arthritic changes in the tibiotalar joint

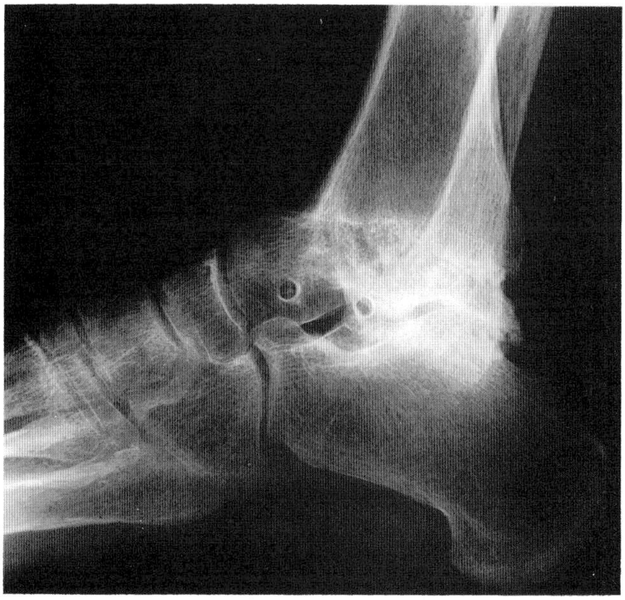

Fig. 60.16c The postoperative radiograph showing the pin tracts in the talus and not in the calcaneus

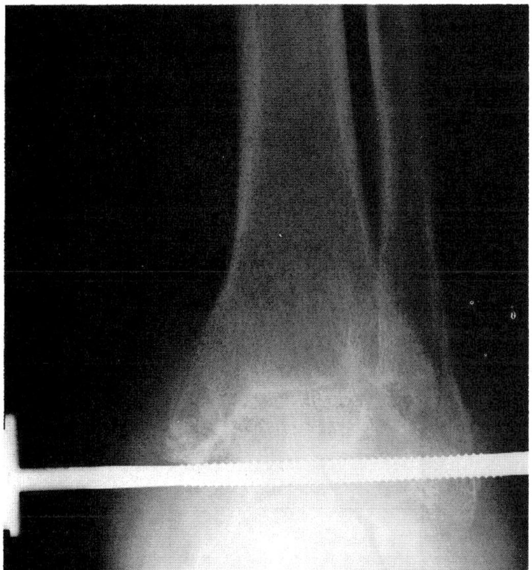

Fig. 60.16b The patient underwent arthrodesis of the ankle and the centrally threaded pin is shown in the talus

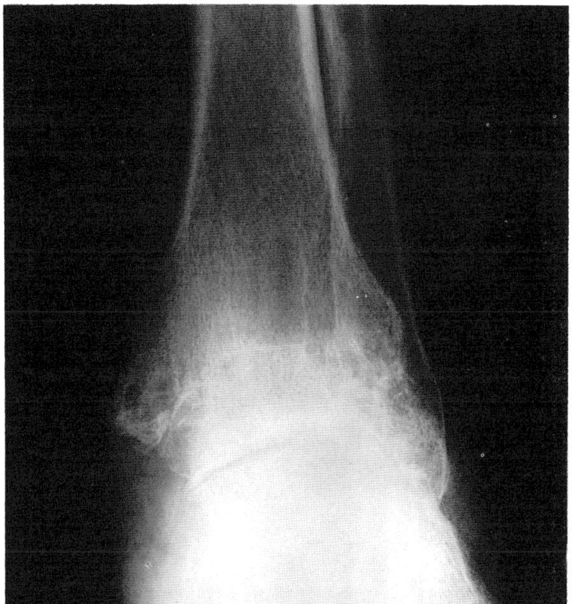

Fig. 60.16d Solid arthrodesis at the tibiotalar joint

local anaesthetic with or without a corticosteroid preparation into the ankle from an anteromedial approach might isolate the ankle joint from the hindfoot complex. Likewise an injection of the same material through the sinus tarsi will usually cause relief of pain in some patients with hindfoot pathology. Following the injection the patient should be allowed to ambulate and then report any changes in their pain. A positive finding should be confirmed by a second injection done at another time. Should there be some doubt as to this technique, a small amount of contrast media can be placed with the medications and followed radiographically to determine whether the anaesthetic agent is localized to the ankle or the hindfoot. Most patients will have more pain from one or another area if both are involved.

At times the hindfoot deformity causes these symptoms and not the joint pathology. This is most frequently seen in cases of advanced hindfoot valgus where the majority of the pain comes from an abutment between the calcaneus and the distal fibula. Peroneal spasm is also another cause of pain in the area. Other patients with a pronounced cavus deformity may present with symptoms of plantar fasciitis. A rupture of the posterior tibialis tendon should not be overlooked. Such patients classically develop a unilateral flatfoot and have discomfort in the hindfoot area as well.

Evaluation of patients with hindfoot pain should also include weight-bearing radiographs. A series of three films is most helpful. An anteroposterior and a lateral view of the foot as well as a weight-bearing anteroposterior view of the ankle will clearly show the degree of deformity and involvement in the key areas of consideration. The ankle view is most important when a valgus deformity is being evaluated as the valgus deformity could be at the tibiotalar joint.

Nonoperative care of the hindfoot pain is difficult. Injections can be attempted with some success. Shoe modifications, especially early in the pathology, may be of considerable aid (Cracchiolo 1982). A longitudinal arch support may provide a more contoured surface for greater skin contact with the plantar surface of the foot and possibly distribute some of the weight bearing more evenly. The counters of the shoe may be strengthened by laminating them with fibreglass and this helps support the hindfoot. A widening of the heel of the shoe also reduces hindfoot motion. In some patients a foot/ankle orthosis made of fibreglass will reduce motion and give relief. This usually results in reduced ankle motion as well and such patients might require additional shoe modifications with the use of the SACH heel and rocker bottom sole.

Persistent pain and loss of function, however, in a patient with malaligned arthritic joints will inevitably lead to the need for an arthrodesis.

Hindfoot arthrodesis techniques

Careful preoperative analysis both clinically and radiographically allows a division of patients with hindfoot pathology into three preoperative groups: (1) Those with no malalignment; (2) those with varus malalignment who usually have a cavus component to their deformity at the midfoot and (3) those with a valgus hindfoot who usually have an associated pronation deformity. In this latter group with the valgus deformity, some may also have a valgus deformity at the ankle particularly if the pathology is rheumatoid arthritis. Such patients may be the most difficult to fuse and they should be encouraged to have the procedure early rather than late.

The ultimate aim of a successful hindfoot arthrodesis is to: (1) have the foot in a plantigrade position, (2) the ankle at 90°, (3) the hindfoot in neutral to 5° of valgus and most importantly (4) the metatarsals should all be level (Jahss et al 1980). Any residual forefoot varus usually leads to a painful callus under the fifth ray as all the compensatory motions of the hindfoot no longer exist.

Triple arthrodesis in patients with a valgus hindfoot

Valgus deformities of the hindfoot with associated pronation deformities may be a very difficult and challenging problem. Frequently, a considerable amount of the patient's pain comes from the abutment of the talus and calcaneus against the fibula. One goal of the operation is to restore the normal alignment of the foot and bring the heel to neutral. Usually a bone grafting technique is necessary (Fig. 60.17a). The basic concepts are: (1) to reduce the talonavicular joint which is

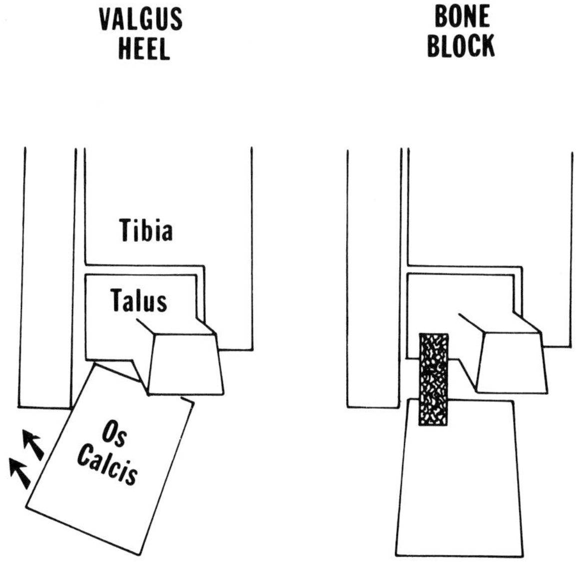

Fig. 60.17a The valgus heel results in a deformity of the subtalar joint with abutment of the calcaneus against the distal fibula. Usually these types of deformities, if severe, require bone grafting to restore the anatomy and allow correction of the deformity

frequently subluxated laterally; (2) to reduce and hold the subtalar joint in a normal neutral position by the use of a bone graft placed through the sinus tarsi and into the posterior facet of the subtalar joint; (3) to fuse the talonavicular and calcaneocuboid joints and (4) to immobilize the foot for a sufficient time to allow solid arthrodesis.

Traditionally triple arthrodesis was performed by excising the joint surfaces and removing appropriate wedges of bone. It is difficult to remove a medial wedge of the subtalar joint through a lateral incision. The use of the medial incision is contraindicated due to anatomical structures and vascular supply to the talus. Frequently these bones are also osteoporotic. Excision of joints in the hindfoot also results in a smaller foot. Should pathology only be on one side this will be a problem for the patient particularly in purchasing shoes.

Operative technique for correction of valgus hindfoot

Patient position. The patient should be positioned on the operating table so that both the lateral and medial sides of the foot are easily accessible. Because of the normal external rotation of the hip, with the patient supine it is essential to place a support or a towel roll under the ipsilateral buttock to internally rotate the hip and keep the foot in neutral or some degree of internal rotation (see Fig. 60.3).

Lateral and medial incisions are by far the best to correct the deformity and obtain solid arthrodesis in an adult patient with a valgus deformity. The lateral longitudinal incision is preferred. It may be necessary to Z-lengthen the peroneal tendons and they should be repaired postoperatively. The sural nerve should always be protected. It is always best to attempt to correct deformities to a normal or neutral alignment prior to proceeding with an arthrodesis. Frequently it is necessary to free the lateral side of the calcaneus and sometimes the talus from the lateral malleolus. Release of the calcaneofibular ligament may be necessary and this should be done by subperiosteal elevation of the calcaneal attachment. This will subsequently heal in normal position.

It is necessary also to proceed with the medial longitudinal incision centred over the talonavicular joint as the talonavicular joint may be the key to reducing the deformity. Periosteal elevators can be used to free all three joints but usually the calcaneocuboid joint is relatively uninvolved. It should be possible to correct the deformity by soft tissue releases. However, at times it is necessary to resect a small amount of the head of the talus to reduce the talonavicular joint. At this point inspection of the subtalar joint will show the amount of joint surface and subchondral bone loss which can be corrected by subsequent bone grafting techniques (Fig. 60.18 and see Figs. 60.7a and b).

Any technique which employs bone grafts across the joints is preferable to ensure correction of the deformity and maintain a normal foot size.

Triple arthrodesis in patients with a neutral hindfoot or a valgus hindfoot can be performed using the same techniques. The only variation is in dealing with the subtalar joint and in correcting the pronation deformity.

Exposure is through the medial and lateral incisions as previously described. On the lateral side the sinus tarsi is cleared of its fatty tissue and the origin of the extensor digitorum brevis is reflected distally to expose the calcaneocuboid joint and the important area between the head of the talus, the lateral portion of the talonavicular joint and the calcaneocuboid joint. Medially care is taken to identify the talonavicular joint which may pose some difficulties for the inexperienced surgeon. However, the wide tuberosity of the navicular is an excellent landmark. Following correction of any deformity and reestablishing the normal alignment of the hindfoot it is essential to determine the method to achieve arthrodesis. Three fusion techniques should be considered, and all have the advantage of maintaining the normal size of the hindfoot.

1. Inlay grafting, where slots are cut across the joints (particularly the talonavicular and calcaneocuboid joints) and autogenous grafts from a local or iliac crest site are impacted across the joints (Kilfoyle & Byrne 1976). Frequently these need to be held with some internal fixation device like a staple. Such a graft is also suitable for the subtalar joint even when there is loss of articular surface and bone (Thomas 1967) (see Fig. 60.7b). A tricortical graft from the iliac crest can be cut to the appropriate length and slotted across the posterior facet of the subtalar joint allowing correction of some of the valgus deformity. In a neutral hindfoot one must take care not to produce a varus deformity of the heel. Usually there is enough compression of this graft that internal fixation is unnecessary.

2. Rotating a dowel of bone 90° to the normal axis of the joint is also an effective method to promote arthrodesis (Cracchiolo 1984, Adam & Ranawat 1976). Each half of the dowel contains one of the adjacent joint surfaces. A Cloward dowel cutter should be selected which will remove enough bone on each side of the joint (Fig. 60.19). A staple or large Kirschner wire can also be used for internal fixation if necessary depending on the postoperative stability. A dowel can also be rotated across the posterior facet of the subtalar joint. However, if the bone quality is poor, the deformity can be corrected using a solid dowel of an appropriate diameter which is removed from the iliac crest through a very small incision and inserted into a prepared hole in the posterior facet created by one of the Cloward drills (Cracchiolo 1984) (Fig. 60.20). This will make up for the loss of articular surface and bone in the subtalar joint and correct some of the valgus deformity of the calcaneus. Internal fixation is usually not required.

3. Internal fixation using 6.5 mm cancellous screws may also be performed in obtaining a triple arthrodesis in skeletally mature feet. This technique should be considered when a valgus deformity can be passively corrected without need for grafting the subtalar joint. Such large screws used across a graft in the subtalar joint might interfere with the placement of the bone graft. However this type of cancellous screw, usually 50 mm long, can stabilize the talonavicular joint and hold it in normal alignment. A shorter, 35 mm long screw can also be placed across the calcaneocuboid joint and this will hold well. The articular surfaces should be debrided of any remaining articular or fibrocartilage and this is accomplished using sharp curettes and periosteal elevators. The surfaces can be further roughened with a gouge prior to placement of the screw. Should a screw be selected to stabilize the subtalar joint, it is placed just anterior to the cartilage of the ankle joint and the head can be counter sunk if good bone stock is present. Usually a 65 mm long screw is sufficient. It may be necessary to remove this screw post-fusion as it can cause some ankle irritation when the patient returns to unrestricted ambulation. The screw across the talonavicular joint also frequently requires removal as it is quite subcutaneous in position and gives some skin irritation when shoes are worn. This screw can easily be removed in a clinic setting. Washers should also be used if the bone is osteoporotic (Figs. 60.17b,c,d).

The wounds must be carefully closed in layers if possible. There is frequently a problem with the lateral wound especially in patients in whom a valgus deformity has been corrected. That portion of the wound which is over or near the sinus tarsi has no underlying subcutaneous support or cover. The sinus tarsi area should be thoroughly drained as it is a dead space for accumulation of blood and other tissue fluids. Skin staples or interrupted sutures are satisfactory for the skin.

A soft compressive dressing is sufficient for the first few days postoperatively. Prior to discharge a short leg plaster cast is applied. If there has been correction of a valgus deformity some degree of equinus of the ankle will be present. This equinus is simply from tightening of the triceps surae as a result of correcting the deformity. No attempt should be made to correct this equinus. When the patient returns 14 to 21 days later for suture removal it is usually quite easy to place the second cast with the ankle in a neutral position. The second cast can be made of a fibreglass material and the patient is kept

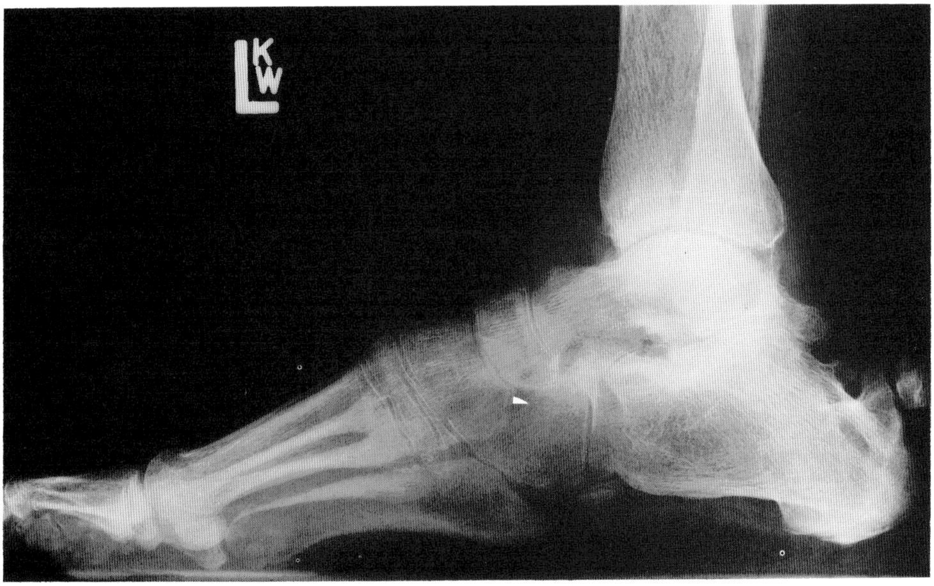

Fig. 60.17b A 62-year-old woman with a diagnosis of rheumatoid arthritis who also had signs of secondary degenerative arthritis in the upper and lower extremities. Her main complaint was a painful left hindfoot of several years duration

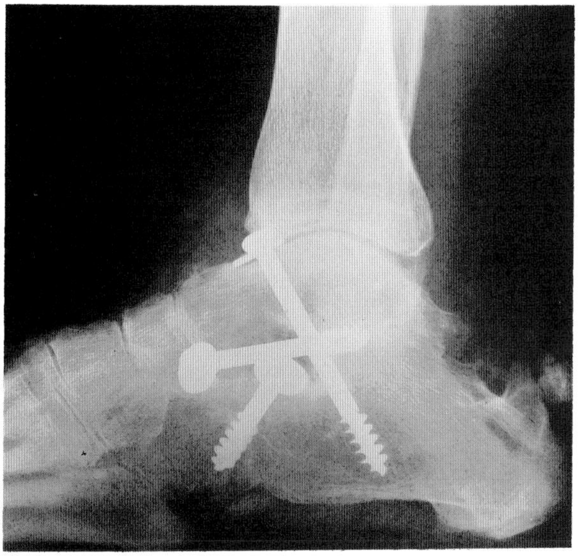

Fig. 60.17c Triple arthrodesis was performed through lateral and medial incisions by removing all remaining fibrocartilage from the talonavicular, calcaneocuboid and subtalar joints. The surfaces were then roughened and all three joints were stabilized using 6.5 cancellous screws. A 65 mm long screw was placed just anterior to the articular cartilage of the ankle joint using the lateral incision and directed posteriorly and laterally into the calcaneus. The talonavicular joint was approached through the medial incision and stabilized using a 50 mm long screw and then through the lateral incision again a 35 mm long screw was placed across the calcaneocuboid joint, directing the screw just at the base of the anterior process plantarward and distally. Because of the osteoporotic bone, washers were required and fixation was quite solid

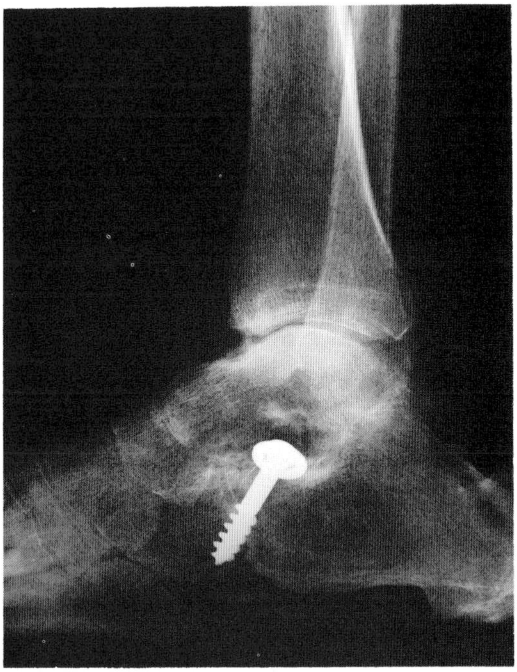

Fig. 60.17d One year postoperatively the patient has a clinical and radiographic solid triple arthrodesis. The screws stabilizing the subtalar joint and the talonavicular joint were removed because of their position and they gave some moderate discomfort

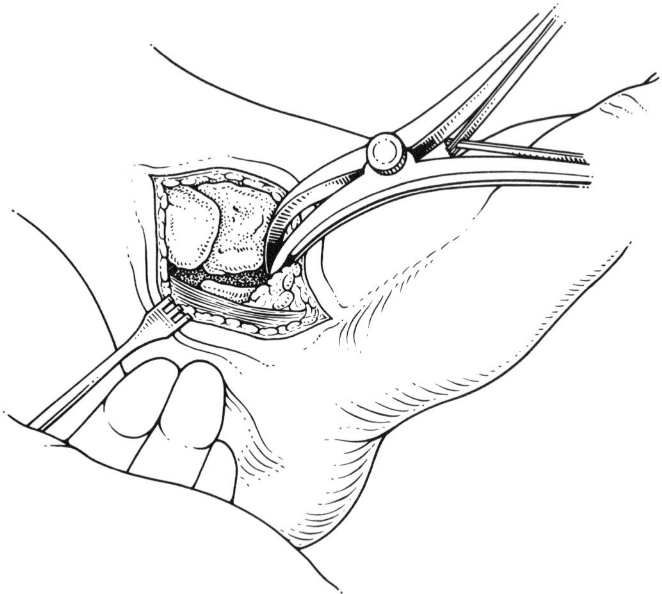

Fig. 60.18 A small laminar spreader in the sinus tarsi distracting the talus from the calcaneus. There has been a loss of articular cartilage and bone from the subtalar joint. Using this method of distraction, it is possible to determine the approximate amount of bone that needs to be placed across the subtalar joint to achieve correction of the valgus hindfoot

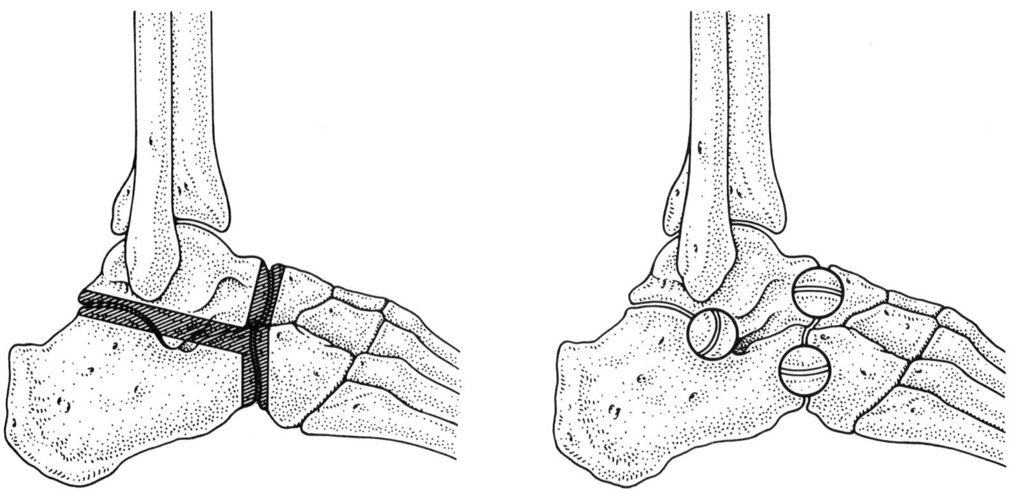

Fig. 60.19 Comparison of a dowel fusion technique on the right which should be considered in a neutral or valgus hindfoot. The conventional resectional Reyerson's arthrodesis on the left is indicated in varus deformity. Wedges of bone can be removed to correct deformities

non-weightbearing for a total of six weeks. At that point the patient can be instructed to begin weight bearing on the cast. Usually immobilization is necessary for approximately 10 to 12 weeks. Depending upon the condition of the joints and the amount of bone grafting necessary, time to fusion may vary between 10 to 16 weeks. One of the best guides to discontinuing external support is when the patient can walk fully weight bearing in the short leg cast without pain. Following removal of the cast

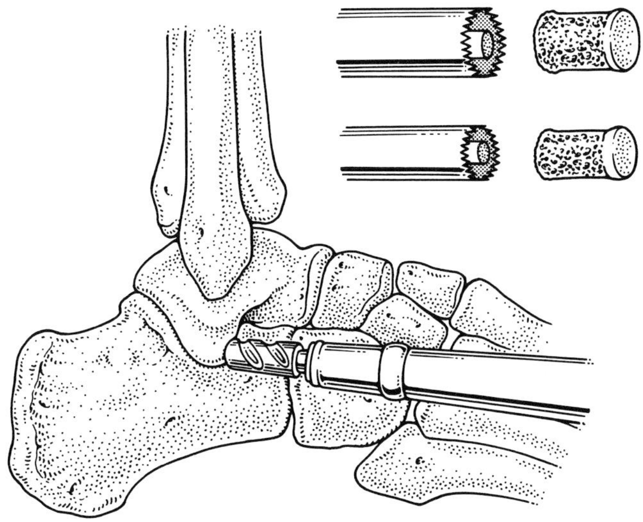

Fig. 60.20 When the quality of bone in the subtalar joint area is poor, a Cloward drill is used to open a hole across the posterior facet. Then a larger Cloward dowel cutter is used to obtain a full thickness graft from the iliac crest. This graft is placed into the preprepared hole. A wider diameter graft will correct some of the hindfoot valgus

swelling can be anticipated and external support to the skin is helpful. No particular type of shoewear is necessary following successful triple arthrodesis.

Varus deformities of the hindfoot

Varus deformities of the hindfoot are usually also associated with cavus deformities. These most often occur in children and are frequently associated with some type of muscle imbalance or paralysis. Such patients have a paralytic equinocavovarus while others may have the same deformity as a residuum of clubfoot. These deformities are markedly different from the previously described valgus deformities. Frequently there is hypertrophy of bone usually on the anterolateral aspect of the calcaneus, cuboid and head and neck of the talus. In viewing the foot dorsally both clinically and radiographically, the head of the talus lies lateral to the midline of the foot. The metatarsal shafts are in varus and directed plantarward. Correction of deformity, if possible, should be the goal of any operative technique. In the varus foot, the talus should be realigned slightly to the medial side of the midportion of the foot. Depending on the degree of deformity triple arthrodesis to correct varus or cavovarus or equinocavovarus deformities usually requires resection of the joints or other portions of the hindfoot bones.

Operative procedure

Many techniques have been blended into a general operative approach for the above deformities (Campbell 1980).

Incision. An oblique incision over the sinus tarsi is satisfactory to expose the hindfoot articulations. One need not worry as much about subsequent closure because swinging the foot out of the varus and into at least a neutral position or some valgus should provide sufficient laxity of the skin about the lateral incision.

Exposure. The contents of the sinus tarsi are carefully divided retaining as much of the subcutaneous tissues as possible, and the extensor digitorum brevis is reflected distally giving wide exposure to the subtalar, calcaneocuboid and the lateral side of the talonavicular joints. The anterior process of the calcaneus frequently requires removal parallel to the floor of the sinus tarsi. This bone can be utilized later for bone graft material. Resection of the calcaneocuboid and talonavicular joints should be done using parallel cuts on all joint surfaces. The posterior facet of the subtalar joint is then exposed and the interosseous membrane between the talus and calcaneus is divided. Likewise, if possible, parallel surfaces should be removed. At this point, one can assess the degree of correction obtained and make decisions whether wedges of bone based laterally need to be removed for appropriate correction. Prior to removing more bone, an assessment of soft tissue contractures should be made. It may be necessary to release the plantar structures from the medial tubercle of the os calcis. Contractures about the talonavicular or naviculo-cuneiform joint may require release as well as possible attention to lengthening the posterior tibialis tendon or releasing a portion of its wide insertion.

In most adult feet and in some children with severe deformity it is wise to approach the talonavicular joint through a separate longitudinal dorsomedial incision. This allows access to soft tissue release, better preparation of the convex and concave surfaces of this joint and also allows resection of the tuberosity of the navicular for better correction and for subsequent use as bone graft if necessary.

Once satisfactory correction has been obtained, any bone available can be placed in the joints as small fragments of graft. It may be desirable to use staples or large Kirschner wires to transfix the joints. Cancellous type screws are also helpful for internal fixation. After-treatment is similar to that previously described triple arthrodesis.

Many variations of triple arthrodesis are described and should be used depending upon the particular pathology. In certain conditions where there is muscle imbalance of the foot and ankle, it is desirable posteriorly to displace the foot. This transfers the fulcrum of the ankle anteriorly to a position nearer the centre of the foot and lengthens the posterior lever arm which may be a particular advantage if there is triceps surae weakness. The Hoke or Dunn triple arthrodesis procedures are then advised (Campbell 1980). The Hoke procedures resect a varying amount of the head and neck of the talus or, in the Dunn, resect a significant portion of the navicular. Sufficient other bone must be excised to permit the resected surfaces to fit together.

A severe fixed equinus deformity also may require a special type of triple arthrodesis. The Lambrinudi operation appears to be the standard procedure for correcting such a deformity. Obviously, it cannot correct a dropfoot unless muscles are available for transfer. The Lambrinudi operation is performed by resecting a predetermined wedge of the plantar and distal portions of the neck and body of the talus. A trough is cut into the inferior portion of the proximal navicular and the calcaneocuboid joint is resected to correct any lateral deformity.

Careful preplanning for a difficult arthrodesis is essential. Proper lateral radiographs are important and tracings of the film should be a part of the preoperative operation. The tracings are cut into pieces along the outlines of the subtalar and midtarsal joints and rearranged providing the desired arthrodesis. Then an estimate can be made of the approximate amount of bone which needs to be resected to correct the deformity.

Two of the feared complications following extensive triple arthrodesis are:

1. possible osteonecrosis of the body of the talus. This complication may be more frequent in adult patients. The lateral approach, however, does spare the most important medial extraosseous vascular supply to the talus. The talus has a rich vascular supply through three major regional arteries which enter the five nonarticulating surfaces of the bone (Gelberman & Mortensen 1983). The major blood supply to the body of the talus is provided by the artery of the tarsal canal. The deltoid and sinus tarsi vessels provide significant minor sources of vascular supply. An intraosseous blood supply with various internal anastomoses is also present. Care should be taken to avoid any damage to the artery of the tarsal canal. This may be especially prone to damage when resecting the posterior facet of the subtalar joint. Major resection should be confined to the articular surfaces if possible.

2. A stable ankle is an obvious prerequisite to long term success following triple arthrodesis. Probably any instability of the ankle or likewise any significant arthritic involvement of the ankle will lead to further ankle pathology following successful triple arthrodesis.

Thus a good result following arthrodesis of the hindfoot should meet the following requirements (Campbell 1980): (1) the foot should look natural in shoes; (2) it should not require a brace; (3) it should appear natural without shoes or at least not be grossly deformed; (4) weight bearing should be evenly distributed over the plantar surface during standing and gait; (5) the axis of the ankle should be forward and at a right angle to the long axis of the foot; (6) the patient should be able to control ankle motion and (7) there should be no pain.

Isolated arthrodesis of hindfoot joints

The subtalar joint is the hindfoot joint most frequently requiring an isolated arthrodesis. Since this joint is commonly involved in intra-articular fractures of the calcaneus, a painful traumatic arthritis frequently ensues. However, one must carefully evaluate such patients as other pathology may be present which is not amenable to surgical correction such as weakness of the tendo Achillis caused by residual deformity of the calcaneus, an injured heel pad and peroneal tenosynovitis. Widening of the os calcis is also a problem but if impingement of the calcaneus occurs on the lateral malleolus this can also be relieved operatively. Johansson et al (1982) studied 21 patients with 23 painful traumatic arthritic subtalar joints following intra-articular fracture of the calcaneus. He recommended waiting at least one year after injury before considering subtalar arthrodesis. The reason for waiting is that his original group consisted of 360 patients with these types of fractures and only 30% had painful feet at one year or longer. Most of the patients were men with an average age of 43 years. Average follow-up was 4.3 years and patients returned to work an average of 6.2 months following the fusion. All fusions were solid clinically and radiographically. Both the patient and the surgeons rated the results as 44% good, 52% satisfactory and only 4% unsatisfactory. 86% of the patients returned to full activity and the remainder changed to lighter work.

Operative procedure

A modification of the basic Grice (1952) arthrodesis provides stability to the subtalar joint and an extremely high rate of fusion while also allowing correction of some deformity (Thomas 1967, Johansson et al 1982). Through a standard oblique incision the sinus tarsi is cleared. A half inch osteotome cuts a trough through the sinus tarsi and across a portion of the posterior facet of the subtalar joint to the medial side of the talus and calcaneus, but not through the medial cortex. The tunnel measures about an inch in height and is as wide as the thickness of the iliac crest. A full thickness graft is taken from the iliac crest and it must be of sufficient size to occupy the entire width of the tunnel and sinus tarsi. The graft is oriented with the inner and outer tables at right angles to the plane of the subtalar joint thus being able to resist vertical compression. The unbroken cortex of the graft lies laterally. The subtalar joint should be completely locked when the graft is tapped into place. Any gaps should be packed with cancellous bone from the ilium (Thomas 1967).

Postoperatively, a short leg non-weightbearing cast is in place for four weeks and then replaced with a walking short leg cast for four additional weeks. A skin support is then utilized to control oedema.

Kalamchi & Evans (1977) described a modification of the posterior fusion of the subtalar joint as originally described by Gallie (1943). They stressed that the operation should only be done when the midtarsal joints are functional. The posterior subtalar fusion of Gallie does not allow correction of varus or valgus position of the calcaneus or any other deformity of the foot (Fig. 60.21). The Gallie fusion is not suitable when the hindfoot is in varus and should be reserved for patients who have a neutral hindfoot.

Both operations are done with the patient prone. An 8 cm long incision is made lateral to the Achilles tendon extending to its insertion (Kalamchi & Evans 1977). The flexor hallucis longus tendon is retracted medially to protect the neurovascular bundle. The subtalar joint is exposed and a trapezoidal slot 2 x 1 cm is made, removing the articular cartilage and subchondral bone of the posterior facet of the subtalar joint (Fig. 60.22). This extends into the sinus tarsi. A rectangular block of bone measuring 1 x 2 cm is removed from the lateral half of the calcaneus keeping the outer cortex intact. After removing the graft the lateral cortex is fractured and displaced medially narrowing the heel. The calcaneofibular ligament is then released allowing the heel to come out of valgus and the peroneal tendons are freed of adhesions. Correcting the valgus transposes the trapezoidal slot to a rectangular one and the bone graft is inserted (Fig. 60.22). All fusions were solid by three months and there was no instability from release of the calcaneofibular ligament.

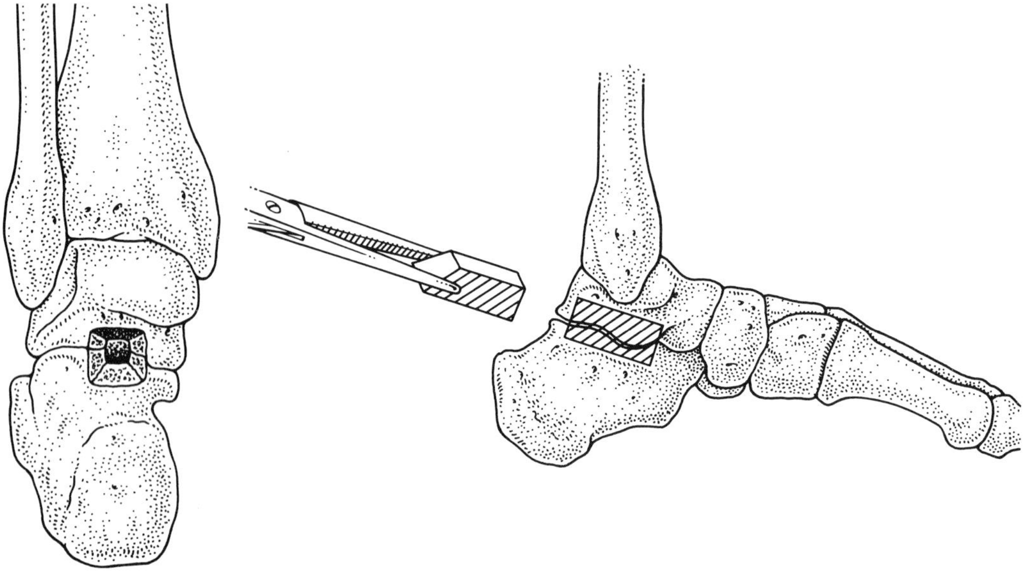

Fig. 60.21 The Gallie subtalar arthrodesis using a separate bone graft into a slot created through the posterior aspect of the subtalar joint. This technique fuses the subtalar joint but is limited in the amount of correction it affords any varus or valgus deformity

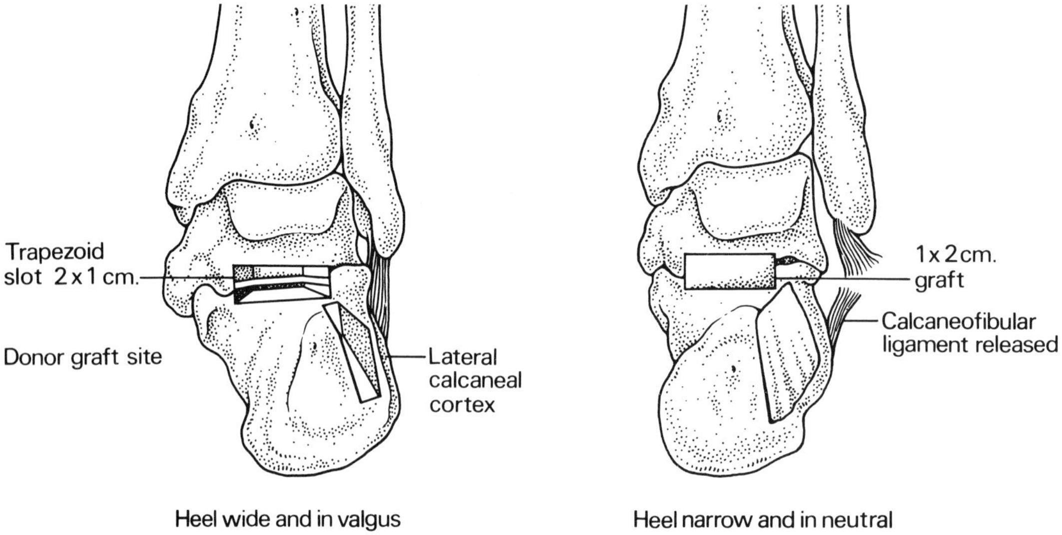

Fig. 60.22 The technique of Kalamchi & Evans (1977) for arthrodesis of the subtalar joint showing the correction of the valgus deformity. Following insertion of the graft the lateral calcaneal cortex is fractured to narrow the heel. Release of the calcaneal fibular ligament is also necessary

Therefore it is unnecessary to perform a triple arthrodesis if only the subtalar joint is involved.

Isolated hindfoot arthrodesis in arthritic patients

Although Thomas (1967) reported arthrodesis of the subtalar joints in six patients with arthritis most had osteoarthritic changes. In rheumatoid arthritis, it is most unusual to be able to arthrodese only the subtalar joint. Selective arthrodesis of rheumatoid hindfoot joints usually involves the talonavicular joint (Ruff & Turner 1984, Elbaor et al 1976). The talonavicular joint seems particularly prone to destructive changes and these can be seen relatively early in the disease. Should such involvement be noted, arthrodesis of the talonavicular joint should be performed promptly and usually prevents the valgus hindfoot deformities from occurring (Elbaor et al 1976).

Operative technique

The talonavicular joint is easily exposed through a dorsomedial longitudinal incision. Any remaining articular surfaces are removed by a curette. The tuberosity of the navicular can be utilized as a source of bone graft. The bone graft is then placed in a prepared slot made across the talonavicular joint. Internal fixation using a staple or a Kirschner wire is necessary in most cases (see Fig. 60.7a).

Postoperatively, immobilization and a non-weightbearing short leg cast for six weeks is followed by six weeks in a weight-bearing cast. It is difficult at times to see a solid arthrodesis radiographically especially following removal of the weight-bearing cast. Painless weight bearing should be a good indication of fusion.

SYNOVECTOMY OF THE ANKLE AND HINDFOOT

Experience with excising the synovium from the ankle and hindfoot has been limited. Usually synovectomy is only considered in patients with rheumatoid arthritis. Such patients frequently have major complaints in other joints, usually major weight-bearing joints which receive first consideration for treatment. Synovitis may be prominent about the ankle and hindfoot. It is important to distinguish the synovitis about the tendons, particularly the anterior tibialis and long toe extensors, from synovitis involving the joints. Synovitis about the posterior tibial tendon has also remained a neglected area of treatment (Cracchiolo 1984). Rupture of the posterior tibialis tendon frequently adds to the hindfoot deformities seen in such patients. Although rupture of the tendons is infrequent, the large amount of synovium may produce pain and is unsightly. Inflamed bursae are seen, particularly about the insertion of the tendo Achillis where there is frequently one superficial to the tendon and one deep to the tendon. Conservative care, rest and injections may be of some help early in the disease. However, once a mass of proliferative synovium has been established, it should be excised. Benjamin & Helal (1980) report ankle synovectomy in only two patients, both with an unsatisfactory result. Mohing et al (1982) report a large series of 123 ankle synovectomies in 99 patients. 81 of these ankles were followed for an average of four years. Only 10 joints had early synovitis with minimal articular damage and results were good in that group. Despite varying degrees of advanced joint pathology in the other patients only 19% reported pain as unchanged or worse on postoperative evaluation. 14% of their ankles had full motion and in 37% there was a significant improvement following synovectomy.

Operative procedure

The ankle was approached through anterior longitudinal medial and lateral incisions at the anterior edges of the malleoli. The anterior ankle is then easily exposed from the inferior tibiofibular joint across to the medial malleolus. Extensor tendons can also be visualized and synovium about these tendons can easily be excised. All synovium that can be seen is excised as well as any osteophytes. A separate posterior incision may be indicated to excise synovium about the posterior tibialis tendon and the peroneal tendon can also be approached through a separate incision posterior to the fibula.

Postoperatively, it is essential to establish early range of motion. If simultaneous procedures have been performed such as an osteotomy or a localized arthrodesis this should be stabilized internally and external immobilization, if necessary, should be delayed until a full range of ankle motion has been obtained.

Synovectomy of the ankle has probably been overlooked because such patients usually have involvement of their hips and knees which disable them to a greater extent. Usually such patients have limited walking and have less stress on their ankles. Conservative care is also helpful in reducing ankle pain and maintaining some function so that these joints do not immediately come to attention and require synovectomy. However, now with the advent of arthroscopy it may be possible to explore these joints at an earlier time in the disease.

OSTEOTOMY OF THE ANKLE, HINDFOOT AND MIDFOOT

Osteotomies are useful in correcting angular deformities about the ankle and foot. Although infrequently performed, they must be considered when the adjacent joints are normal or salvageable.

Ankle osteotomy

Indications

The main indications are malunion of an ankle fracture or malalignment due to growth arrest of the epiphyseal plate. Disability due to malunion, particularly in an adult, usually requires operative treatment. If the condition is left unresolved, traumatic arthritis may rapidly occur. An abnormal position of the talus within the mortise for over three months may result in a traumatic arthritis and osteotomy would be of no value (Campbell 1980). Irreversible changes within the articular cartilage usually do not allow subsequent painless motion of the joint.

Types of osteotomies and technique

Osteotomy through the fracture site

If the lateral malleolus only has been fractured and there is malalignment then one must suspect injury to the deltoid ligament as well. The lateral malleolus is exposed through a long incision over the fracture site. An oblique osteotomy is performed through the fracture site. Through a longitudinal medial incision, the medial malleolus is exposed. Excision of scar tissue between the malleolus and the talus is necessary in order to allow reduction of the talus and subsequent fixation of the fibular osteotomy either with screws or a small semitubular plate.

Malalignment secondary to a bimalleolar fracture also requires exposure of the medial malleolar fracture. An osteotomy is performed through the fracture site. Usually the medial malleolus is fixed first with cancellous screws. Depending upon the time following the fracture, bone grafting with local cancellous bone may be important to achieve union. The lateral malleolus can then be fixed.

A few factors should be considered and emphasized regarding this treatment. (1) The ankle joint should be assessed as being as near normal as possible and this can be done through the usual radiographic techniques assisted perhaps by the use of computer assisted tomography (CAT scan). (2) Radiographic control should be utilized during the osteotomies and following fixation so that as near perfect alignment as possible is restored. (3) Early postoperative motion is most helpful if it can be tolerated by the clinical situation.

Supramalleolar osteotomy

Indications. The presence of the talus within a normal anatomical mortise in a patient with significant malalignment is an ideal candidate for supramalleolar osteotomy. In such conditions, the ankle joint may have a much higher incidence of being normal. Such deformities are seen in distal tibiofibular fractures but are probably more commonly seen in injuries of the distal tibial epiphysis or epiphyseal plate. Separation of the distal tibial epiphyseal plate may lead to complete growth arrest of the plate. Continued fibular growth then produces a varus deformity. Incomplete growth arrest of the distal tibial epiphysis may produce a varus or a valgus deformity. Growth arrest of the distal fibula should be considered if appropriate. In a young child, a significant malalignment may be closely followed for as long as possible, so that repeated osteotomies are not necessary.

Operative technique. An incision beginning at the ankle joint and coursing proximally along the anterior edge of the fibula is used to expose the anteromedial aspect of the fibula and anterolateral aspect of the tibia. The fibula is osteotomized obliquely usually at the fracture site if one exists. If the osteotomy is being performed in a child, a greenstick technique can be utilized by osteotomizing the tibia through 80% of its cortex and then manipulating the medial cortex into a greenstick fracture. A wedge of proximal tibia can then be used as a graft inserted laterally in the tibial osteotomy. The reverse procedure should be performed if there is a varus deformity. At times two longitudinal incisions are made, one along the anterior fibula and the other along the medial portion of the distal tibia.

An essential aspect in supramalleolar osteotomy for adults is to utilize internal fixation. If the osteotomy can be made sufficiently proximal to the ankle joint, a compression plate may be used for internal fixation. Otherwise if there is not enough room in the distal fragment, an external fixator can be used to provide stable fixation for the osteotomy. One must not rely upon more inadequate fixation such as staples to hold the osteotomy sites in adults. A greenstick technique is inappropriate and plaster cast fixation is inadequate in adult patients. The use of a well positioned compression plate or external fixator will ensure anatomic reduction and allow early motion postoperatively.

Occasionally, supramalleolar osteotomy can be considered for the management of deformities secondary to arthritis involving the ankle. Heywood (1983) has utilized this technique in selected patients with rheumatoid arthritis. This was done simply to improve alignment and to correct significant equinus deformities. Most of these patients had ankle arthritis and two developed a fibrous ankylosis preoperatively. At final follow-up several had progressed to spontaneous bony fusion and the remainder had reduced ankle motion. However, their severe preoperative malalignment remained corrected.

Osteotomies of the hindfoot

Most osteotomies performed to correct hindfoot deformities are directed towards the calcaneus. They represent an attempt to correct either varus or valgus deformities which may have associated midfoot and forefoot deformities. Most have been reported in children but there has been an increasing interest in these realignment operations for skeletally mature adolescents and adults. Some deformities such as cavus, cavovarus or calcaneocavus deformities are often related to neuromuscular disorders that result in muscle imbalances (Samilson & Dillin 1983). Thus soft tissue procedures such as plantar release and tendon transfers are often as important as the osteotomy in obtaining correction of deformity and improved function.

Calcaneal osteotomies have been done mostly through the lateral approach due to the ease of exposure. Dwyer (1959) first popularized calcaneal osteotomy through the lateral approach in the correction of patients with cavus and cavovarus deformities.

Technique (Dwyer)

After dividing the plantar fascia the lateral aspect of the calcaneus is exposed through the usual incision parallel to the peroneal tendons. The calcaneus is exposed in a line with the peroneus longus and the periosteum is divided from the superior, lateral and inferior surfaces. A lateral wedge of bone is removed, but the medial cortex of the calcaneus is manipulated closing the lateral gap. The varus deformity should be corrected and, depending upon the age of the patient, internal fixation may be necessary. The wound is closed and a short-leg cast immobilizes the foot until healing has occurred. Since the calcaneus is composed mostly of cancellous bone, healing is usually inevitable.

However, Dwyer (1959) also reported an osteotomy of the calcaneus for relapsed clubfoot in which an opening wedge osteotomy was made on the medial side of the os calcis. This procedure has been associated with sloughing of the tight skin along the incision over the calcaneus, as correcting a varus deformity places extensive tension on the medial heel incision.

Evans (1975) rationalized that varus and valgus deformities are opposite deformities and related these to the relative lengths of the medial and lateral columns of the foot. A long lateral column was associated with varus deformities of the tarsus including a varus heel and possibly equinus. A short lateral column was associated with a valgus deformity of the tarsus including a valgus heel and possibly a calcaneus deformity. He had shown that it was possible to improve calcaneovalgus deformities by lengthening the lateral border of the foot and to perform this through an opening wedge osteotomy of the anterior portion of the calcaneus parallel to and about 1.5 cm behind the calcaneocuboid joint.

Technique (Evans)

The calcaneus is exposed through an incision over its lateral surface parallel to and above the peroneal tendons. The sural nerve is protected. The calcaneocuboid joint is identified and the anterior portion of the calcaneus proximal to the joint is cleared. The osteotomy is performed through the narrow part of the calcaneus in front of the peroneal tubercle in line with, parallel to and about 1.5 cm behind the calcaneocuboid joint. The osteotomy is prised apart by means of a special spreader and a cortical graft is inserted to separate the calcaneal osteotomy. The foot must be inspected to determine the degree of forefoot adduction and heel varus which has occurred. A relative equinus position is also noted. Evans recommended a plaster cast for about four months to allow consolidation of the calcaneal osteotomy, but permitted weight bearing at four weeks.

Phillips (1983) reported a long term follow-up of Evans' patients. 20 patients (23 flat feet) whose average age at operation was 15 years (range 9–42 years) were followed an average of 13 years (7–20 years). Only three feet in three patients were classified as poor. 17 feet were classified as either very good or good results, indicating that this procedure had been effective. It is interesting that 15 of these patients had suffered from severe idiopathic flat foot.

A medial displacement osteotomy of the calcaneus performed in the same area as Dwyer's osteotomy has also been reported for the treatment of mobile flat foot (Koutsogiannis 1971). The osteotomy is made parallel and a little behind and inferior to the peroneal tendons. Once completed, the posterior fragment of the calcaneus is displaced medially until the medial cortex lies in line with the sustentaculum tali. This usually requires a displacement of between one-third to one-half the width of the calcaneus. The displacement is held by two Kirschner wires. Only two patients were over the age of 17 at the time of operation, one being 39 and the other 55. Two of 19 patients were judged to have failed.

Samilson & Dillin (1983) divided cavus deformities into the areas of the foot where the apex of the deformity was found. Thus they separated the deformity into an anterior or forefoot cavus, a midfoot cavus and a hindfoot cavus or calcaneocavus deformity. The latter deformity is characterized as having a more vertical position of the calcaneus with a calcaneal 'pitch' of 30° or more. This is an angle measured on a standard lateral radiograph of the foot between the horizontal and a line drawn on the plantar surface of the os calcis from the posterior to the anterior tuberosity. This calcaneal deformity involving the hindfoot is corrected by an osteotomy through the os calcis in combination with plantar release. Samilson & Dillin (1983) described a crescentic osteotomy performed posterior to the posterior facet of the subtalar joint. The posterior calcaneal fragment is moved posterosuperiorly to correct the calcaneocavus and fixed with a pin for six weeks. A posterior displacement osteotomy of the calcaneus was also described by Mitchell (1977) and by Bradley & Coleman (1981). This osteotomy is also preceded by an extensive plantar release performed through a short horizontal medial incision. It may also be necessary to divide the calcaneocuboid and talonavicular joint capsules to obtain as much correction of the cavus deformity as possible before osteotomy. The lateral aspect of the calcaneus is exposed through a curved lateral incision and the osteotomy is performed obliquely just posterior to the peroneal tendons. The posterior fragment is displaced upwards and held by a Steinman pin. Any resistance to this displacement is usually a result of an inadequate plantar release. The pin remains in place for three to four weeks, then is removed and the patient placed in a walking cast. Subsequent tendon transfers can be performed.

Osteotomy for pes cavus

Pes cavus may be associated with hindfoot abnormalities or with a normal hindfoot. A careful evaluation of pes cavus deformities may also indicate that they are associated with a variety of neurological disorders which initially may be obscure. Other causes of pes cavus are (1) residual clubfoot deformity, (2) poliomyelitis, (3) compartment syndromes and (4) the idiopathic pes cavus (Jahss et al 1980). In most cases, operations such as triple arthrodesis and arthrodesis of Chopart's joints will not correct fixed deformities of the midfoot and forefoot. Triple arthrodesis in such patients should only be considered when stabilization of the hindfoot is necessary because of a neurological abnormality. However, whenever possible, subtalar and transtarsal motion should be preserved to avoid excessive stress on the ankle joint which may be already abnormal. Jahss et al (1980) have proposed a truncated-wedge arthrodesis of the tarsometatarsal joints to correct pes cavus and equinovarus deformity of the forefoot. He prefers this to multiple, basilar, dorsal-wedge metatarsal osteotomies which are difficult to stabilize and may result in nonunion or incomplete correction. The contraindications to performing these operations and considering a more proximal procedure are:

1. A painful subtalar joint or a stiff hindfoot complex; such feet can have their forefoot corrected by a triple arthrodesis.

2. A subtalar joint previously fused in varus, which is causing a similar varus deformity of the forefoot. Correction of the varus hindfoot is necessary with refusion in a more normal valgus alignment. Calcaneal osteotomy should also be considered if the hindfoot joints are mobile.

3. Should plantar callosities be seen more proximally, as under the cuboid, then a midtarsal or triple arthrodesis or an osteotomy should be considered.

Operative technique (Jahss et al 1980). The tarsometatarsal truncated-wedge arthrodesis is performed without the use of a tourniquet. The area is exposed sequentially through three vertical incisions about 4 cm long which are centred on the arthrodesis site. The first incision is medial to the extensor hallucis longus exposing the underlying first metatarsal-medial cuneiform joint. The second incision is between the bases of the second and third metatarsals exposing the second and third metatarsal cuneiform joints. The third incision is made medial to the base of the fifth metatarsal exposing the fourth and fifth metatarsocuboid joints. Care is taken not to retract these incisions excessively so that subsequent skin problems will not develop. A distal osteotomy through the base of the first metatarsal is done first using a thin, flat, sharp osteotome. Next the proximal osteotomy of the medial cuneiform is performed so that a dorsal truncated-wedge can be removed. The importance of removing a truncated rather than a triangular wedge of bone is to prevent tightening of the plantar fascia when the osteotomy is closed and to permit closure of the osteotomy. The truncated wedge does not shorten the overall length of the foot but only lowers the height of the foot allowing shoewear to be more comfortable.

Through the second vertical incision a dorsal truncated wedge is then removed from the second metatarsal-intermediate cuneiform joint and, working laterally through the same incision, the third metatarsal-lateral cuneiform joint is similarly exposed and resected. Through the third vertical incision similar wedges are resected from the fourth and fifth metatarsal cuboid joints.

The forefoot is then dorsiflexed to close the dorsal wedges. Each metatarsal head is palpated on the plantar surface to ensure proper elevation of the metatarsal heads while keeping the ankle in maximum dorsiflexion. Rotational or adduction deformities can also be corrected. This is a very precise operation and care must be taken to preserve blood supply to the skin as well as ensuring complete correction. It is important carefully to guard against excessive bone resection so that a rocker-bottom deformity is not created. Internal fixation is not used and the foot is encased in the corrected position in a short leg cast.

Haglund's disease

The posterior superior tuberosity of the calcaneus has various shapes that can lead to a very pronounced posterior prominence of the calcaneus. The development of painful posterior lesions of the heel is also related to the angle made between the posterior surface and the plantar surface of the calcaneus. The condition was attributed to Haglund (1928) who first described the relationship between the shape of the calcaneus and the appearance of a posterior mass, a tendo Achillis bursitis, a retrocalcaneal bursitis or a small spur at the attachment of the tendo Achillis. In addition to the term Haglund's disease the condition is also called 'pump bump' to describe the mass which occurs as the result of wearing low back shoes. Pavlov et al (1982) and Fowler & Philip (1945) did measure the angle between the posterior surface and the plantar surface of the calcaneus finding a normal range of between 44° and 69°. It was felt that abnormal pressures were likely to occur in the area of the posterior superior calcaneus with angles above 75° (Fig. 60.23). Pavlov et al (1982) described the parallel pitch lines as a measurement of the os calcis. A positive parallel pitch line was present in all of their patients with Haglund's disease. They also noted that a pump bump might occur in association with certain systemic inflammatory articular disorders such as Reiter's syndrome.

The treatment is to resect the prominent posterior superior portion of the calcaneus. This is usually performed through a longitudinal lateral incision being careful to avoid damage to the sural nerve or the tendo Achillis. A significant wedge of bone must

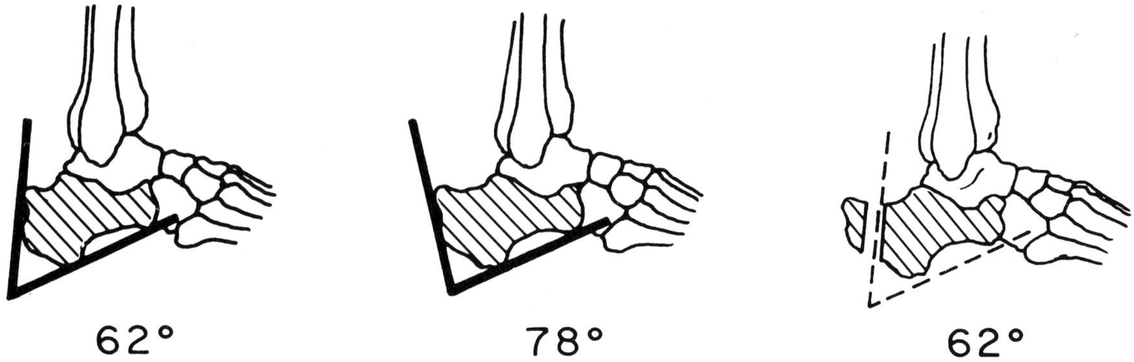

Fig. 60.23 The angles as measured in Haglund's disease; an angle between the posterior surface and the plantar surface of the calcaneus. A significant portion of the posterior surface requires resection properly to remove the posterior prominence and correct this condition

be removed from the posterior superior angle of the calcaneus. Removing an offending bursa alone is of little value and will result in recurrent symptoms of pain with or without significant recurring deformity.

In a young vigorous patient it is wise to place the ankle in 15° of plantar flexion and encase it in a non-weightbearing plaster cast for four to six weeks. This allows soft tissue healing to occur without incident and avoids any possible complication which might result in a rupture of the tendo Achillis.

TOTAL ANKLE ARTHROPLASTY

Recent clinical evaluations of patients with total ankle arthroplasty have been disappointing at best (Demottaz et al 1979, Newton 1982, Stauffer & Segal 1981). Currently the indications for prosthetic ankle arthroplasty are not clear and most orthopaedic surgeons who have used these components in the past have ceased to perform the operation.

Definite contraindications to ankle arthroplasty seem to include: (1) patients with severe malalignment and unstable ankles with grossly distorted anatomy, particularly loss of bone stock from the talus, (2) recent sepsis, (3) failed arthrodesis and (4) severe osteonecrosis of the talus.

Most reports have presented their results based in part on the patient's diagnosis. The most favourable current indications have been put forth by Newton (1982) whose results indicate that probably a patient with osteoarthritis having the following criteria would be a suitable risk for ankle arthroplasty: (1) an ankle with good stability, (2) reasonable normal anatomy, and (3) no significant varus or valgus instability especially if there is any involvement of the subtalar or midtarsal joints. Unfortunately most patients with arthritic ankles cannot be included within these strict indications. Therefore the availability of patients on whom one could perform ankle arthroplasty would be very low indeed. Stauffer has included patients over the age of 60 who have post-traumatic arthritis of the ankle as also being suitable for ankle arthroplasty. In his series this group attained a 77% satisfactory result and a 23% unsatisfactory result.

In rheumatoid patients satisfactory results of 88% have been reported (Stauffer & Segal 1981) and no clinical failures were reported in 15 ankle replacements reported by Lachiewicz et al (1984). However even this latter report gave an average follow-up of only 39 months, contained five patients who had some residual pain in the ankle and showed significant radiolucent lines in 73% and subsidence of six implants (2 tibial and 4 talar implants) all of which were disturbing prospects for possible future failure. In addition Newton's results indicate that rheumatoid patients are not good candidates for this operation particularly if they have had long term steroid use or if they have erosions. Complications in rheumatoid patients have been as high as 23% (Stauffer & Segal 1981) and six of 10 ankles failed in Newton's (1982) study, all with rheumatoid arthritis. Demottaz et al (1979) reviewed 21 ankle replacements in 19 patients, 14 of whom were rheumatoid with an average follow-up of only 15 months. Using a very strict grading system they could rate only two as having a good result; in 81%

there was not complete relief of pain. Thus when these arthroplasties are compared to hip and knee arthroplasties the results look even worse as there is a great difference in the degree of pain relief obtained. Moreover Demottaz et al (1979) also reported 88% progressive radiolucencies and 10% late loosenings.

Younger patients in Stauffer & Segal's (1981) series, having post-traumatic osteoarthritis, also had a complication rate of 54%. The most frequent complication was talofibular bone impingement. An overall loosening in this study was 7% and deep sepsis 3%.

Problems in technique also seemed to contribute to failure of total ankle arthroplasty. Proper placement and alignment of the implants have not been stressed. Whereas in knee replacement the implants are carefully aligned with the patient's hip and ankle the converse has not been attempted with ankle replacement. Also many of these patients have abnormal subtalar and transtarsal joints. What effect this might have upon a successful implant is speculative. However, it is well known that the modulating effect of the hindfoot joints probably act in concert with normal ankle motion for a smooth gait. Any disruption of these factors should cause increased stresses about the ankle implants. Impingement of the talus on either the medial or lateral malleolus has also led to failure (Samuelson et al 1982). Problems with skin healing have been seen frequently. Following the operation it is unusual to be able to suture the ankle capsule. Thus, unlike other joint replacements, the ankle implants are very superficial and close to the skin incisions. Perhaps this is responsible for the somewhat higher incidence of sepsis as compared to other joint replacements. Immobilization of the ankle joint (Cracchiolo 1984) in a short-leg cast postoperatively for 2 to 6 weeks was found to protect against delayed wound healing and reduce oedema, while not restricting ankle motion.

Thus it is difficult to select the best patients for this procedure. An ideal patient for an ankle replacement would come along very rarely. If one waited simply for these patients, technical skills would soon regress and any possible clinical series would be very small. Also, if elderly patients can be shown to have better results they are also patients in whom the risk of reoperation would be higher should failure occur. Arthrodesis of a failed ankle replacement is a more extensive operation than primary fusion, usually requiring extensive bone grafting and the application of an external fixator.

There are probably many reasons for the poor clinical results seen following ankle replacement. The implants seem to have been underdesigned. Larger implants with better fixation which might not loosen as frequently would also take up more room thus sacrificing more bone stock. If larger implants did loosen, obtaining a secondary arthrodesis might not be possible resulting in a flail ankle or, worse yet, a below knee amputation. Also the surface area available for ankle replacement is very small. Transmitting such loads across such small surfaces is difficult and leads to loosening and other complications. The very close relationship between the ankle and the hindfoot joints is unlike the anatomy of the knee and hip, where one is dealing with a single joint which is not as influenced by other adjacent joints. It appears at this time that ankle replacement has a limited role if any in arthritic reconstructive operations. Ankle arthrodesis remains the current treatment of choice in patients with ankle deformities. This is particularly true if some degree of transtarsal motion remains in the calcaneocuboid and talonavicular joints as frequently these patients can walk without a detectable limp.

REFERENCES

Adam W, Ranawat C 1976 Arthrodesis of the Hindfoot in Rheumatoid Arthritis. Orthop Clin N Am 7: 827

Anderson R 1945 Concentric Arthrodesis of the Ankle Joint. J Bone Joint Surg 27: 37–48

Benjamin A, Helal B 1980 Surgical Repair and Reconstruction in Rheumatoid Disease. The MacMillan Press Ltd, London. p 224

Bordelon R L 1980 Correction of Hypermobile Flatfoot in Children by Molded Insert. Foot Ankle 1: 143–150

Bradley G W, Coleman S S 1981 Treatment of the Calcaneocavus Foot Deformity. J Bone Joint Surg 63A: 1159–1166

Buck P G, Stauffer R N, Laeghman R K, Chao E Y 1982 Influence of Position of Ankle Arthrodesis on Ankle and Knee. Orthop Transactions p 129

Calandruccio R 1984 Personal Communication

Campbell C J, Rinehart W T, Kalenak A 1974 Arthrodesis of the Ankle. J Bone Joint Surg 56A: 63–70

Campbell 1980 In: Edmonson A S, Crenshaw A H (eds) Campbell's Operative Orthopaedics. C. V. Mosby Co., St. Louis

Charnley J 1951 Compression Arthrodesis of the Ankle and the Shoulder. J Bone Joint Surg 33: 180–191

Chuinard E G, Peterson R E 1963 Distraction Compression Bone Graft Arthrodesis of the Ankle. J Bone Joint Surg 4A: 481–490
Cracchiolo A 1982 Office Practice. Footwear and Orthotic Therapy. Foot Ankle 2: 242–248
Cracchiolo A 1984 Foot Abnormalities in Rheumatoid Arthritis. AAOS Instructional Course Lectures Vol. 33: 386–404. C. V. Mosby Co., St. Louis
Demottaz J D, Mazur J M, Thomas W H, Sledge C B, Simon S R 1979 Clinical Study of Total Ankle Replacement with Gait Analysis. J Bone Joint Surg 61A: 976–988
Drobocky I Z 1986 Radiographic Examination of the Normal Foot. Surgery of the Foot, Fifth Edition C. V. Mosby Company, St. Louis, pp 50–64
Dwyer F C 1959 Osteotomy of the Calcaneum for Pes Cavus. J Bone Joint Surg 41B: 80–86
Elbaor J E, Thomas W K, Weinfeld M S, Potter T A 1976 Talonavicular Arthrodesis for Rheumatoid Arthritis of the Hindfoot. Orthop Clin N Am 7: 827
Evans D 1975 Calcaneo-Valgus Deformity. J Bone Joint Surg 57B: 270–278
Fowler A, Philip J F 1945 Abnormality of the Calcaneus as a Cause of Painful Heel. Br J Surg 32: 494–498
Gallie W E 1943 Subastragalar Arthrodesis in Fractures of the Os Calcis. J Bone Joint Surg 25: 731–736
Gamble F O, Yale I 1966 Clinical Foot Roentgenology. Williams and Wilkins, Baltimore
Gatellier J, Chastane 1924 Access to Fractured Malleolus with Piece Chipped Off at Back. J Chir 24: 513
Gelberman R H, Mortensen W W 1983 The Arterial Anatomy of the Talus. Foot Ankle 4: 64–72
Gould N 1982 Technique Tips: Footing. Foot Ankle 3(3): 184
Grice D S 1952 An Extra-Articular Arthrodesis of the Subtalar Joint for Correction of Paralytic Flat Feet in Children. J Bone Joint Surg 34A: 927
Haglund P 1928 Beitrag zur Klinik der Achillessehne. Z Orthop Chir 49: 49
Heywood A W B 1983 Supramalleolar Osteotomy in the Management of the Rheumatoid Hindfoot. Clin Orthop 177: 76–81
Hoppenfeld S, de Boer P 1984 Surgical Exposure in Orthopaedics. J. B. Lippincott Co, Philadelphia
Jackson A, Glasgow M 1979 Tarsal Hypermobility after Ankle Fusion. J Bone Joint Surg 61B: 470–473
Jahss M H 1980 Tarsometatarsal Truncated-Wedge Arthrodesis for Pes Cavus and Equinovarus Deformity of the Fore Part of the Foot. J Bone Joint Surg 62A: 713–722
Jahss M H, Godsick P A, Leven H 1980 Quadruple arthrodesis with iliac bone graft. In: Bateman J E, Trott A W (eds) The Foot and Ankle. Brian C Decker, New York, pp 93–102
Johansson J E, Harrison J, Greenwood F A H 1982 Sub-talar Arthrodesis for Adult Traumatic Arthritis. Foot Ankle 2: 294–297
Johnson E W, Boseker E H 1968 Arthrodesis of the Ankle. Arch Surg 97: 766
Kalamchi A, Evans J G 1977 Posterior Subtalar Fusion. J Bone Joint Surg 59B: 287–289
Kilfoyle R M, Byrne D P 1976 Nonexcisional Triple Arthrodesis of the Foot. Orthop Clin N Am 7: 841–850
King H A, Watkins T B, Samuelson K M 1980 Analysis of Foot Position in Ankle Arthrodesis and Its Influence in Gait. Foot Ankle 1: 44–49
Koutsogiannis E 1971 Treatment of Mobile Flat Foot by Displacement Osteotomy of the Calcaneus. J Bone Joint Surg 53B: 96–100
Lachiewicz P F, Inglis A E, Ranawat C S 1984 Total Ankle Replacement in Rheumatoid Arthritis. J Bone Joint Surg 66A: 340–343
Lance E M, Paval A, Fries I, Larsen I, Patterson R L 1979 Arthrodesis of the Ankle Joint. Clin Orthop 142: 146–158
Lionberger D R, Bishop J O, Tullos H S 1982 The Modified Blair Fusion. Foot Ankle 3: 60–62
Markus R E, Balourdas G M, Heiple K G 1983 Ankle Arthrodesis by Chevron Fusion with Internal Fixation and Bone Grafting. J Bone Joint Surg 65A: 833–838
Mazur J M, Schwartz E, Simon S R 1979 Ankle Arthrodesis. J Bone Joint Surg 61: 964–975
Mitchell G P 1977 Posterior Displacement Osteotomy of the Calcaneus. J Bone Joint Surg 59B: 233–235
Mohin W, Kohler G, Coldewey J 1982 Synovectomy of the Ankle Joint. Int Orthop 5: 117–121
Morgan C D, Henke J A, Bailey R W, Kaufer H 1985 Long Term Results of Tibiotalar Arthrodesis. J Bone Joint Surg 67A: 546–550
Morrey B F, Wiedeman G P 1980 Complications and Long Term Results of Ankle Arthrodesis following Trauma. J Bone Joint Surg 62: 777–784
Newman A 1980 Ankle Fusion with the Hoffman External Fixation Device. Foot Ankle 1: 102–108
Newton S 1982 Total Ankle Arthroplasty. J Bone Joint Surg 64A: 104–111
Pavlov H, Heneghan M A, Hersh A, Goldman A B, Vigorita V 1982 The Haglund Syndrome: Initial and Differential Diagnosis. Radiology 144: 83–88
Penneau K, Lutter L D, Winter R D 1982 Pes Planus: Radiographic Changes with Foot Orthosis and Shoes. Foot Ankle 2: 299–303
Phillips G E 1983 A Review of Elongation of Os Calcis for Flat Feet. J Bone Joint Surg 65B: 15–18
Ratliff A H C 1959 Compression Arthrodesis of the Ankle. J Bone Joint Surg 41B: 524–534
Rothacker J W, Cabanella M E 1983 External Fixation for Arthrodesis of the Knee and Ankle. Clin Orthop 180: 101–108
Ruff M E, Turner R H 1984 Selective Hindfoot Arthrodesis in Rheumatoid Arthritis. Orthopaedics 7: 49–54
Samilson R L, Dillin W 1983 Cavus, Cavovarus and Calcaneocavus: An Update. Clin Orthop 177: 125–132
Samuelson K M, Freeman M A R, Tuke M A 1982 Development and Evaluation of the ICLH Ankle Replacement. Foot Ankle 3: 32–36
Scranton P E 1985 Use of Internal Compression Arthrodesis of the Ankle. J Bone Joint Surg 67A: 550–555
Stauffer R N, Segal N M 1981 Total Ankle Arthroplasty: Four Years Experience. Clin Orthop 160: 217–221
Stazzeri J C, Prietio M P, Anzel S H, McMaster W C 1984 Compression Arthrodesis of the Ankle Following Failed Ankle Arthroplasty using Hoffmann External Fixation. Orthopaedics 7: 993–995
Steel M W, Johnson K A, DeWitz M A, Ilstrup D M 1980 Radiographic Measurements of the Normal Adult Foot. Foot Ankle 1: 151–158
Stewart M J, Beeler T C, McConnell J C 1983 Compression Arthrodesis of the Ankle. J Bone Joint Surg 65A: 219–225
Thomas F B 1967 Arthrodesis of the Subtalar Joint. J Bone Joint Surg 49B: 93–97
Thomas F B 1969 Arthrodesis of the Ankle. J Bone Joint Surg 51B: 53–59
White A A 1974 A Precision Posterior Ankle Fusion. Clin. Orthop 98: 239–250

B. G. Andrews

Amputations

Amputations of a single toe usually cause little disturbance to stance or gait. Amputation of the little toe does not result in any functional loss and in congenital elevation of the toe, is often preferred to plastic reconstructive procedures which have a variable end result. Similarly, amputation of the second, third or fourth toes has negligible functional loss, but in the case of the second toe may predispose to an increased valgus deformity of the great toe.

Amputation of the great toe through the metatarsophalangeal joint does not significantly affect standing or walking at a moderate pace, but when hurrying or attempting to run, a limp develops because of the loss of push-off normally provided by the big toe.

Amputation of all the toes whilst not noticeably affecting standing or slow walking, results in considerable loss of spring and resilience and the patient generally is limited to a steady, rather plodding gait.

The more proximal the amputation through the metatarsals, the greater is the loss of agility because of the diminished power of push-off due to the shortened lever arm of the foot.

Amputations through the tarsometatarsal joint and the midtarsal region have largely been abolished. Symes's amputation of the ankle joint and its variants result in a considerable functional loss, although it often provides full end bearing sufficient for the unprotected stump to accept body weight. A satisfactory gait can only be achieved by the use of a prosthesis up to the area of the patellar tendon.

AMPUTATION THROUGH A TOE

A long plantar flap and a short dorsal flap are required. The skin incision begins at the intended level of the bone section at the midpoint on the medial side curving slightly forwards over the dorsum of the toe to a similar point on the lateral side. A similar flap is now fashioned on the plantar surface, but extending distally well beyond the level of bone section. The skin flaps are dissected proximally to the level of the bone section. The flexor and extensor tendons and the digital nerves and vessels are sectioned and allowed to retract into the depths of the wound. The bone is sectioned and if necessary smoothed with a file. Only the skin is sutured with nonabsorbable material, after trimming the flaps so that the terminal aspect of the stump is covered by plantar skin with the suture line lying anterodorsally.

The same technique may be used for disarticulation at the interphalangeal joints but it is sometimes necessary to trim with bone nibblers the flare of the distal end of the phalanx in order to improve skin cover.

Disarticulation of the metatarsophalangeal joint

Disarticulation of the second, third or fourth toes should be performed by making incisions to either side of the toe at its base beginning on the plantar surface and curving slightly forwards up onto the base of the shaft of the toe in the web of the foot to meet on the dorsal surface. The toe is vigorously plantar flexed and the extensor tendon and dorsal capsule divided. Further flexion of the toe is now possible and the remains of the joint capsule and ligaments are exposed and divided. Division of the flexor tendon and vessels and nerves complete the amputation. The vessels, nerves and tendon are allowed to retract into the depths of the wound. The skin is sutured with nonabsorbable material so that the suture line is vertical and it subsequently sinks into the cleft on the anterodorsal aspect of the foot.

Disarticulation of the fifth toe

This is best performed through a racquet incision beginning in the cleft between the fourth and fifth toes and extending dorsally across the toe to a point 1 cm behind and lateral to the metatarsophalangeal joint. The plantar incision curves forwards over the base of the proximal phalanx and then backwards to join the dorsal incision laterally. The toe is flexed and the extensor tendons and capsule divided and with further flexion all the other structures are divided and allowed to retract. The metatarsal head if left intact may be excessively prominent on the side of the foot and subject to painful pressure in footwear, and the lateral third of the metatarsal head should therefore be removed, carefully smoothing the bone surface with a file to produce an even junction with the metatarsal shaft. Nonabsorbable sutures are used having trimmed the flaps if necessary so that the suture line lies anterodorsally with the tough plantar skin protecting the anterior and lateral bone surfaces.

Disarticulation of the great toe

As with the little toe the purpose is to protect the exposed metatarsal head with thick plantar skin. Begin the incision over the middle of the medial side of the great toe 1.5 cm proximal to the metatarsophalangeal joint, curving the incision forwards over the medial and plantar surface of the toe producing a long medial plantar flap. Dorsally the incision passes gently convex forwards from the medial border to the web of the toe. The extensor tendon and capsule are divided; the digital nerves cut and allowed to retract; the vessels divided and ligated. The flexor tendon is divided and sutured to the extensor tendon in order to stabilize the position of the sesamoids. If the medial side of the metatarsal head is at all prominent it should be trimmed with bone nibblers and smoothed with a file. The skin is sutured with nonabsorbable material having trimmed the skin flaps so that the suture line lies on the anteromedial border of the stump.

AMPUTATION OF ALL THE TOES

Whilst this procedure may be necessary for trauma to the toes, the usual indication is for long-standing progressive painful deformity of the toes. In the late stages of deformity associated with a very severe hallux valgus and possibly dislocation and/or subluxation of the other toes, reconstructive surgery may not be possible and amputation is to be preferred. Similarly, with severe deformities of the toes associated with rheumatoid arthritis and particularly if most of the disability is due to dorsal dislocation and deformity of the toes, amputation through the metatarsal necks may be a more satisfactory end result than forefoot arthroplasty.

Fashions in foot operations vary somewhat as do fashions in shoes and amputation of the toes is less commonly performed now than 15 years ago. Nevertheless many patients are happy with the outcome; they stand and walk well although they have some difficulty in hurrying. They can often wear shoes of their choice, the space for the toes being filled with a toe blocker of Plastazote® or similar material. Persuading patients to agree to this operation isn't easy and they are often helped in their decision, as with other amputations, by talking to patients who have already undergone the procedure.

Technique

No specific preoperative measures are required apart from the elimination of local infection and a careful assessment of the blood supply of the foot. General anaesthesia is preferred and a tourniquet, which should be pneumatic, applied above the knee makes the operation simpler and quicker.

Parallel incisions are made on the plantar and dorsal surfaces of the foot commencing at the first metatarsophalangeal joint and passing laterally rising up a little onto the plantar surface of the toes and not quite meeting in the clefts. The incisions are deepened dividing all of the structures down to the capsules of the metatarsophalangeal joints. After division of the capsules the toes can be removed strung together by the bridges of skin.

The metatarsal heads are generally very prominent in the sole of the foot covered often only by thick skin and painful bursae. The heads should be completely excised, sectioning the neck of the metatarsal just behind the head, so that the plantar surface of the bone is smooth and not unduly prominent when palpated through the plantar skin. The metatarsals must be carefully cut so that they form a gentle arc convex distally with the second metatarsal neck at the apex. This is most important for if a metatarsal head remains prominent it will be subject to excessive pressure on weight bearing and a further painful callosity will develop and despite further bony excisions it can be difficult to restore the correct balance and alignment.

The sesamoids in the flexor tendons must be excised and all the tendons pulled down and sectioned so that the cut ends retract deeply into the wound.

The digital nerves can be difficult to find, lying between the metatarsal necks. They too should be gently drawn into the wound and sectioned as far back as possible with a sharp knife so that they retract deeply into the wound and the inevitable neuroma that develops on the cut nerve ends will not be subjected to pressure or pinched between the ends of the metatarsals. The digital vessels are coagulated or ligated and haemostasis fully secured after release of the tourniquet. Drainage is only required if there is a risk of infection. The skin and subcutaneous tissues are sutured in one layer after trimming the skin edges so that the durable plantar skin protects both the plantar and anterior aspect of the stump, the suture line being drawn up onto the anterodorsal surface of the foot.

A firm crepe bandage is applied over a large quantity of wool covering the ankle as well as the foot. It should be elevated for 48 hours and only very limited weight bearing on the heel allowed with the aid of crutches until the sutures are removed at the 14th day. In patients with rheumatoid arthritis or on steroids or those in which the blood supply is in any doubt, sutures should be retained for three weeks. After the wound has healed the patient can progress quickly to full weight bearing using a stiffener in the shoe. No special supports are required.

Almost any type of shoe can be worn with a sponge or Plastazote® filler in the toe space. A normal gait should be possible and although hurrying may be difficult, there is generally functional gain on the preoperative state because of the absence of painful, deformed and useless toes.

AMPUTATION OF A SINGLE METATARSAL

On rare occasions ischaemic changes and gangrene may be limited to a single toe with evidence of ischaemia extending proximally along an individual ray of the foot. Providing the blood flow is adequate, healing may be obtained by amputation of the toe combined with excision of its metatarsal ray. It is important that all the infected and necrotic material is excised and sufficient bone must be excised so that the skin flaps can be sutured without any tension. For single second, third, fourth toes and rays, a wedge of tissue with its apex proximally placed at the base of the metatarsal is excised and this closes well leaving a symmetrical foot. The function and gait are better than with a transmetatarsal amputation. As the wounds in metatarsal ray excision are generally infected, irrigation using antibiotic solution facilitates healing.

TRANSMETATARSAL AMPUTATION

This amputation is performed at a level a little more proximal than the operation described for amputation of all the toes. It may be used in gangrene due to diabetes and arteriosclerosis and other ischaemic conditions such as Buerger's disease and frostbite. McKittrick et al (1949) and Pedersen & Day (1954) outlined the indications for transmetatarsal amputation in the diabetic patient in 1949. Gangrene must be limited to the toes and should not involve the web space. The infection should be controlled and the incision should not extend through infected or hypoaesthetic areas. Palpable foot pulses are not necessary, but there should be no dependant rubor. Numerous techniques for assessing the blood flow in the foot are now available and they include measuring segmental blood pressure, skin blood pressure, clearance of xenon, transcutaneous $Po2$ etc., but the proper use of these tests will continue to require clinical judgement.

The technique is similar to that described for amputation of all the toes. The skin incisions however are more proximally placed. The dorsal incision is slightly curved and is made across the foot at a level just proximal to the metatarsal necks. The plantar incision is curved dorsally and placed just behind the creases at the base of the toes. The metatarsals are sectioned at the level of the dorsal skin incision and their edges carefully bevelled. The skin flaps are sutured so that the cut metatarsal ends are covered by thick plantar skin and its thick subcutaneous tissue. Mobilization can begin in a walking plaster of Paris cast at 10 days.

AMPUTATIONS THROUGH THE MIDDLE OF THE FOOT

These are largely of historical interest only. They include the Lisfranc amputation through the tarsometatarsal joints, Chopart's amputation through the midtarsal joint and Pirogoff's amputation in which part of the os calcis is fused to the lower end of the tibia. Lisfranc's amputation has been discarded because a severe equinus deformity generally develops as a result of muscle imbalance. Consequently there is excessive pressure and friction on the anteroinferior aspect of the stump producing painful callosities and in a diabetic or ischaemic foot skin breakdown will follow.

Similar complications occur also with Chopart's amputation very frequently and in most surgical clinics the use of these two procedures has been abandoned.

To salvage these operations Burgess (1966) recommends division of the tendo Achillis a short distance proximal to its insertion and manipulating the ankle and hindfoot into a plantigrade position maintaining it in a walking below-knee cast for two weeks. He states that recurrence of the deformity has not been a problem and an appropriate partial boot prosthesis can be used subsequently.

While the use of these midfoot amputations is to be discouraged in vascular, ischaemic and diabetic feet, they may occasionally be of value in cases of severe trauma confined to the forepart of the foot.

Lisfranc's operation

The operation is easier using a tourniquet. A distally convex incision in the plantar skin is made commencing laterally just proximal to the prominent base of the fifth metatarsal and ending medially 2.5 cm distal to the tubercle of the navicular. The curve of the plantar flap distally lies parallel to the metatarsal heads. A thick plantar flap is dissected off the shafts of the metatarsals and elevated until the tarsometatarsal joints are reached. The anterior part of the foot is plantarflexed and a dorsal incision made to curve parallel and just distal to the line of the tarsometatarsal joints. This flap is elevated proximally to expose the tarsometatarsal joints. Three lateral metatarsals are detached from the cuboid and lateral cuneiform by sharp dissection and the first metatarsal similarly detached from the medial cuneiform. The second metatarsal has its base wedged between the medial and lateral cuneiforms and is sawn across flush with the line of the disarticulations. Haemostasis is secured and the flaps sutured after any necessary trimming of the plantar flap so that the suture line is close to the anterior dorsal edge of the stump. Suction drainage should be used and the stump is protected by a padded below-knee plaster of Paris cast with the heel in a neutral position for three weeks.

Walking can then commence in a modified boot. The control of the position of the stump and the gait are greatly improved if a stabilizing polypropylene orthosis extending to the midcalf is used. The operation and prosthesis are well accepted by men. The result is generally cosmetically unacceptable for women.

Chopart's amputation

The operation is easier using a tourniquet. The incision is commenced on the plantar surface of the foot beginning medially just behind the tubercle of the navicular, curved generously forwards towards the head of the first metatarsal then curving laterally across the shafts of the metatarsals before turning back on the lateral side to a point between the styloid process of the fifth metatarsal and the lateral malleolus. The ends of this incision are then linked by a dorsal incision gently curved convexly forwards. The plantar flap is elevated carefully from the bony and ligamentous structures preserving the fatty tissue as much as possible until the talonavicular and calcaneocuboid joints are reached. The dorsal flap should require only minimal elevation. By sharp dissection the talonavicular joint can be entered on the medial side and the ligaments and capsule divided. The tibialis anterior tendon is detached at its insertion into the navicular. By a forcible manipulation of the foot the capsule and ligaments of the calcaneocuboid joint can be exposed and divided completing the disarticulation. The tendency for an equinus deformity to develop can be minimized by firmly anchoring the tendon of the tibialis anterior in a vertical hole drilled in the neck of the talus with a pull-through suture. The posterior tibial and anterior tibial nerves should be gently drawn down and sectioned with a sharp knife so that any neuroma formation will not be in an area subject to pressure. The posterior tibial and dorsalis pedis vessels should be ligated and haemostasis secured after releasing the tourniquet. The flaps are sutured in a single layer after trimming them so that the suture line is placed anterodorsally on the stump. A suction drain is used for 48 hours and a padded below-knee plaster of Paris cast applied so that the tension is taken off the tibialis anterior tendon for four weeks. Wound healing at the end of this time should be sufficient to allow fitting a prosthesis and partial weight bearing can be commenced. A simple boot with an above-ankle extension may be sufficient as a prosthesis but a stiffened orthotic extension of the boot to the midcalf posteriorly, greatly improves function. The prosthesis is ugly and is generally unacceptable to women.

Syme's amputation

James Syme was Professor of Surgery in Edinburgh from 1833 to 1869. He first performed the amputation as a disarticulation at the ankle joint in 1842 and subsequently modified the technique which has stood the test of time (Syme 1843). Numerous attempts to modify the technique since then have generally ended in failure. Harris in 1961 reviewed the history and described the technique of the operation which has not been improved upon.

The advantage of the Syme's amputation is that in the ideal stump full body weight can be carried on the end of the stump which is stable and durable. There are many cases recorded of trouble-free use in excess of 40 years. However, the conventional prosthesis is bulky, particularly over the flare of the malleoli and is therefore unacceptable cosmetically for most women as it results in noticeable asymmetry of the ankles and calves.

Syme's amputations are either successes or failures. There is no middle ground. If the heel pad fails to become adherent and stable under the cut tibial surface and tends instead to migrate, then the stump ceases to be end bearing and the body weight has to be borne at the level of the patella tendon, losing all the advantages of the Syme's amputation whilst retaining its cosmetic disadvantages. In addition, once the heel pad has become unstable, attempts to revise the amputation are seldom successful.

Opportunities to use the amputation are now relatively uncommon and as a method of choice it is often forgotten. It may however be the best level of amputation in cases of severe trauma to the foot providing the heel pad is intact. It may be suitable for paralytic and congenital deformities of the foot requiring ablation, particularly those associated with trophic ulceration, such as spina bifida or leprosy. Preferably protective sensation should be present in the heel pad, but frequent long-lasting success has been achieved even in the total absence of heel sensation providing the heel pad is in a stable plantigrade position.

In congenital deformities of the leg particularly associated with severe shortening and deformity such as congenital shortening of the femur or absence of the fibula, Syme's amputation or ankle disarticulation may be of great benefit both from a functional and cosmetic point of view in prosthetic management. The end-bearing quality of the Syme's amputation in these circumstances is less important and in children there is generally migration of the heel pad posteriorly associated with growth.

The amputation has a definite place in the management of the diabetic foot particularly where infection is the predominant factor and in this situation Wagner (1977) recommends the use of a staged Syme's procedure.

There are some references to its successful use in patients with peripheral vascular disease and Whitfield claims a 50% success rate in dysvascular patients where a temperature gradient can be detected by the examining hand distal to the heel. Dale in 1961 has demonstrated that even in the absence of peripheral ankle pulses this level may be justifiable in peripheral vascular disease.

Technique

No specific preoperative measures are required except eradication of infection. An above-knee pneumatic tourniquet should be used except in cases of peripheral vascular disease. General anaesthesia is used and the patient lies supine with the foot just projecting over the end of the operating table and the calves suitably protected.

Two points (the first 1 cm below the tip of the lateral malleolus and the second 2 cm below the tip of the medial malleolus) are joined by a horizontal skin incision. From the ends of the incision, vertical incisions are made to join each other across the sole of the foot, the line of the incision curving slightly forwards. The vertical incisions are deepened, dividing all of the structures in the line of the skin incision until the calcaneum is exposed on all three sides. The dorsal incision is deepened, dividing all the structures at the front of the ankle joint and opening the ankle joint to expose the neck of the talus. The foot is now forcibly plantarflexed and the talus pulled firmly forwards and downwards with the aid of a bone hook. The capsular attachments and the medial lateral ligaments of the ankle are divided and the talus gradually pulled forwards out of the mortice. The superior and posterior aspects of the calcaneum gradually come into view. The Achilles tendon is divided close to its insertion into the calcaneum. Great care must be taken to keep the dissection virtually subperiosteal in order to minimize the risk of perforating the posterior heel skin which is thin and closely adherent to the bone. Pulling the foot further forwards and downwards the dissection is continued along the inferior aspect of the calcaneum peeling the bone out of the soft tissue, remaining close to the bone and carefully preserving the integrity of the plantar skin and its specialized subcutaneous fatty compartments and the underlying short muscle origins. The vertical incision is finally reached and the foot removed after dividing any residual long tendons on the medial and lateral sides.

Attention is now turned to the lower ends of the tibia and fibula and by a little dissection and periosteal stripping they can be easily exposed. A transverse cut is made in the tibia and fibula as close to the dome of the ankle mortice as possible exposing cancellous bone to which the heel flap will more readily adhere than articular cartilage. It is essential that the saw cut is exactly at right angles to the axis of the leg in both planes so that the bone surface is horizontal in relation to the ground when the patient is standing, otherwise the heel pad will become unstable and displace on weight bearing.

The anterior and posterior tibial vessels and the long saphenous vein are identified and ligated, care being taken to preserve the calcaneal branches on which the vascularity of the heel flap in part depends. The anterior and posterior tibial nerves are gently pulled down and sectioned with a sharp knife and allowed to retract away from the wound. All the tendons are treated in a similar manner. At this stage the tourniquet should be released and haemostasis secured. The long heel flap should be brought up to the anterior flap and the bone ends palpated through the flap and any sharp or irregular bony ridges smoothed down with bone nibblers. A suction drain is brought out through the lateral aspect of the calf. The subcutaneous tissues are approximated with catgut and the skin with nylon. The final stump always looks untidy with large 'dog ears' as two flaps of unequal length and shape have been brought together. The temptation to trim dog ears *must be resisted* as essential elements of the blood supply to the heel pad are contained within them. Skin shrinkage gradually occurs and they always disappear.

The heel pad forms a bulbous mass over the lower end of the tibia. Since success in Syme's amputation depends upon this pad becoming stable and adherent to the cut surface of the tibia it must be carefully held in position in the postoperative phase. A narrow strip of gauze dressing is applied to the suture line and the heel pad is firmly held in place by broad strips of nonstretch strapping which are applied to the upper posterior aspect of the calf and carried downwards and forwards holding the heel pad close against the cut surface of the tibia and fibula and then carried upwards to be attached to the shin. If for some reason strapping cannot be used, an alternative, but less satisfactory method, is to transfix the heel flap to the bone with three transfixing wires of the Kirschner type, the ends of which must be left projecting and protected with corks. Orthopaedic wool and a plaster of Paris cast are applied extending up to the tibial tubercle. The leg should be kept elevated for 48 hours and the suction drain removed at the end of this time. After this the patient may be mobilized non-weightbearing with crutches but prolonged dependency must be avoided.

The sutures are generally removed on the 14th postoperative day but in dysvascular cases they should be retained for 21 days. The strapping and a plaster cast are reapplied and should be retained for a total of four weeks.

The two-stage Syme's amputation

Because the Syme's amputation frequently failed in the infected and dysvascular limb, a two-stage operation has occasionally been used in which the infected forefoot was removed through disarticulation of the ankle and the definitive amputation performed six to eight weeks later. A much higher success rate was thus achieved. Wagner (1977) performs the operation in dysvascular patients who have infection or gangrene in the forefoot that has failed to respond to medical treatment or distal surgical care and who are not suitable for a transmetatarsal amputation. The patient should be a prosthetic candidate. The heel pad should be intact. There should be no gross pus at the amputation site. The ischaemic index, he states, should be 0.45 or higher in the diabetic and 0.35 in others. The ischaemic index is determined using transcutaneous ultrasound, coupled with the Doppler effect, with the normal systemic flow in the arm representing 1.0 in the index.

Technique

The initial technique of amputation of the foot does not differ in any significant feature from the method already described except that in order to give slightly longer flaps the incisions are begun both 1 cm below and 1 cm anterior to the tips of the malleoli.

The disarticulation of the foot is performed with the aid of a tourniquet. On its release the time for the onset of bleeding from the distal skin is accurately assessed. If the most distal skin does not bleed within three minutes serious consideration is given to amputating at the higher level. If there is no bleeding in the flap distally at five minutes then the Syme procedure should be abandoned and the amputation carried out at the below-knee level. Having determined that the blood flow is adequate, a drain is inserted and is retained in the cavity of the ankle and drawn out through a stab wound 10 cm above the ankle joint. Irrigation is commenced with 1 l of Ringer's lactate solution containing 50 000 units of bacitracin and 500 000 units of polymyxin per 24 hours.

Closure

The heel pad should be trimmed allowing it to be sutured without tension. Deep fascia over the anterior tibia is sutured to the deep fascia of the sole. A few subcutaneous sutures level the skin edges and the skin is closed with nylon. A dressing of wool and crepe is applied. Drainage from the tube is collected and the tube is clamped every two to three hours to distend the cavity with irrigating fluid. Irrigation is continued for 72 hours but may be continued longer if there is fever or signs of local infection. Systemic antibiotics are continued according to preoperative cultures for one week.

Following removal of the tubing the stump is wrapped in plaster of Paris, care being taken not to fold the dog ears and create pressure areas. Thick pieces of felt with holes cut in them for the malleoli work well to protect them. When the patient is clinically stable, ambulation is allowed and weight bearing is permitted if the stump appears satisfactory.

Healing is usually secure enough at six weeks to perform the definitive amputation. An occasional patient will remain infected and require further debridement and if healing does not occur rapidly after this, a below-knee amputation should be performed.

At the second stage two elliptical incisions are made over the malleoli to remove the dog ears. The amount of tissue removed should be equal to the volume of the malleolus. Care must be taken not to damage the neurovascular bundle on the posterior-medial aspect. After subperiosteal dissection the malleoli are cut flush with the joint surface. The fat pad is generally partially adherent to the central cartilage which is left intact. The malleoli are dissected subperiosteally to approximately 3 cm above the joint line and the flare removed parallel with the shaft. This leaves the anterior and posterior flares for suspension and moderate narrowing and flattening of the sides of the stump. Closure is important. Soft tissue must be removed from the ellipses until the pad is tight against the under surface of the tibia. It is then sutured through two drill holes in the tibia and fibula as well as to the periosteum. Following skin suture soft dressings are used for a few days and then replaced with plaster. Weight bearing is begun at two weeks. A weight-bearing cast is retained for six weeks being changed at two-weekly intervals or before if there is any loosening of the fit. At eight weeks the first prosthesis can be applied.

Modification of Syme's amputation

Because of the bulkiness of the prosthesis used in the Syme's amputation, attempts have been made to reduce the bulbous shape of the stump and thus allow the use of a more cosmetic prosthesis. Sarmiento et al (1966) advise transection of the tibia and fibula 1.3 cm proximal to the ankle joint and excising the flare of the malleoli. This produces a stump only slightly larger in circumference than the diaphyseal portion of the leg allowing the use of a slimmer prosthesis. However, diminishing the surface area of end bearing increases the pressure in kg/cm^2 on the heel pad to a level that may critically diminish the weight-bearing capacity of the stump and more weight bearing will then have to be taken at the level of the patellar tendon and tibial flare, to a large extent eliminating the prime advantage of the Syme's amputation.

Pirogoff (in Harris 1961) described a modification in which part of the calcaneum was arthrodesed to the cut lower surface of the tibia. The calcaneum is sectioned vertically and the anterior half is removed. The remaining posterior part of the heel flap is rotated upwards through 90° so that the raw surface of the calcaneum meets and fuses with the raw surface of the tibia. This amputation is more difficult than the Boyd operation and has no advantages.

Boyd amputation

Boyd in 1939 described an operation that produces an excellent end-bearing stump and eliminates the problem of migration of the heel pad which occasionally occurs with Syme's amputation. Following the same initial technique of the Syme's amputation a talectomy is performed but the bulk of the calcaneum is retained in the heel pad and drawn forwards under the cut section of the tibia and arthrodesis of the rawed upper surface of the calcaneum and tibia achieved. It is therefore more difficult than the Syme's amputation and the stump considerably more bulbous. Whilst a satisfactory prosthesis has been designed for this stump it is not cosmetically readily acceptable. If a sound arthrodesis is achieved however, the end-bearing qualities of the stump are excellent and it is probably most suitable for use in third world countries where shoe wearing is less common and prostheses of any kind less readily available.

REFERENCES

Boyd H B 1939 Amputation of the foot with calcaneo tibial arthrodesis. J Bone Joint Surg 21: 997

Burgess E M 1966 Prevention and correction of fixed equinus deformity in mid foot amputations. Inter-Clin. Inform. Bull 6: 20

Dale G M 1961 Syme's amputation for gangrene from peripheral vascular disease. Artif Limbs 6: 44

Flint M, Sweetman R 1960 Amputation of all toes. J Bone Joint Surg 42B: 90

Harris R I 1961 The history and development of Syme's amputation. Artif Limbs 6: 4–43

Hunter G A 1975 Results of minor foot amputations for ischemia of the lower extremity in diabetics and non-diabetics. Can J Surg 18: 273

Lindquist C, Riska E B 1966 Chopart, Pirogoff and Syme amputations. A survey of twenty-one cases. Acta Orthop Scand 37: 110

McKittrick L J, McKittrick J B, Risley T S 1949 Transmetatarsal amputation for infection and gangrene in patients with diabetes mellitus. Ann Surg 130: 826–842

Pedersen H E, Day A J 1954 The transmetatarsal amputation in peripheral vascular disease. J Bone Joint Surg 36A: 1190

Sarmiento A, Gilmer R E, Finnieston A 1966 A new surgical-prosthetic approach to the Syme's amputation. A preliminary report. Artif Limbs 10 (1): 52

Spittler A W, Brennan J J, Payne J W 1954 Syme's amputation performed in two stages. J Bone Joint Surg 36A: 37

Syme J 1843 Amputation at the ankle joint. London Edinburgh Monthly J Med Sci 2: 93

Wagner F W Jr 1977 Amputation of the foot and ankle: current status. Clin Orthop 122: 62

Plastic surgery

PRINCIPLES OF SKIN REPLACEMENT AND ITS USE AS A DONOR SITE FOR MICROVASCULAR TISSUE TRANSFER

The importance of the foot is perhaps underestimated particularly in view of the present day interest in the hand. Primitive man would have probably been more concerned with the condition of his feet to provide him with the swiftness and mobility to outmanoeuvre an aggressor. In the hand, movement of the digits and cutaneous sensation are vital to function. Cutaneous sensation in this context provides tactile gnosis which augments vision by ascertaining texture. Painful sensation protects the delicate structure of the hand from damage.

The foot, unlike the hand, bears weight. The skin of the sole is specially thickened for protection and the more harshly it is exposed the thicker it becomes. The sensation of the sole is primarily designed to monitor pressure. Unconsciously, constant adjustments are made to the weight-bearing area to avoid overlong pressure which would lead ultimately to skin necrosis. Sensory sole skin is probably the single most important structural unit in the foot, indeed if either the sensation is absent or there is extensive loss of the skin, amputation will have to be seriously considered.

Sommerlad & McGrowther (1978) have elegantly demonstrated the importance of these factors in their examination of patients who had suffered skin loss on the sole and undergone replacement with distant flaps. They found that those patients who avoided ulceration in the area of the flap were in fact not bearing weight on it, but instead taking the pressure through an intact area of undamaged sole skin.

Recent surgical endeavour has therefore been directed to replacing damaged weight-bearing sole skin with skin from non-weightbearing areas and preserving the cutaneous sensation. The donor sites can then be replaced with less sophisticated skin.

The primary area of concern is the heel, where 80% of the body weight is borne on standing, the remaining 20% is taken along the lateral side of the foot and across the metatarsal heads.

The further advantage of replacing 'like with like' relates to the subcutaneous structure of sole skin. Fibrous septa attaching the skin to the deep longitudinal ligament break up the intervening fat into compartments; this arrangement prevents shear and provides the feeling of stability. Where the subcutaneous architecture is lost as occurs in extensive abdominal flap replacements, the patient will comment on the 'feeling of walking on a bar of soap'.

Sole skin naturally forms a thick layer of keratin to protect the basement cells from damage. In people accustomed to not wearing shoes this layer is thicker than in the habitually shod. The keratin layer may become pathologically exuberant where an incision is made into the sole skin or at the interface between a flap or skin graft. Unfortunately, this hyperkeratosis does not improve with time and requires repeated paring to control discomfort.

Clearly the sole skin is of primary significance in respect of the fact that unsatisfactory replacement can precipitate amputation but the skin of the dorsum of the foot and over the Achilles tendon are also important. The skin over the dorsum is thin and freely mobile but when the toes are plantarflexed the skin becomes taut, so that functionally there is little to spare. In major skin loss of the dorsum, particularly in burns or abrasion injuries, inadequate skin replacement tends to cause hyperextension of the toes at the metatarsophalangeal joints and difficulty with the wearing of shoes. The latter may be intensified in children who develop hypertrophic scars.

Providing the paratenon is intact skin grafts may prove sufficient to resurface the dorsum. Skin grafts, however, do tend to contract and although they are an easily available source of skin in quantity, they do not always provide good quality cover. The skin grafts tend to adhere to underlying structures and are therefore liable to breakdown. Stabilization and mobility do occur with time, but dermal overgrafting as recommended by Hynes (1957) may prove necessary. Where the dorsum of the foot is particularly liable to trauma by wearers of specialized heavy boots such as mountaineers, then flap cover may have to be provided.

Finally, the Achilles tendon area is liable to skin loss either by serious abrasion injury, pressure or iatrogenically as a result of surgical repair of a ruptured Achilles tendon. Skin grafts do not take well over the Achilles tendon particularly where this structure has been damaged. Flap cover is not easily available locally and may indeed be rendered impossible by unsuitable incisions in the area. Distant flaps may be essential particularly where the Achilles tendon requires lengthening as in equinus deformities. The grave disadvantage of a distant flap in this site, however, is their bulk which makes the wearing of shoes difficult.

Causes of skin loss

The causes of skin loss are protean but they do fall into several recognizable categories:

Congenital: Epidermolysis bullosa

Acquired: Injury — laceration
- abrasion
- run over, degloving
- burn
- iatrogenic, harvesting microvascular flaps
- pressure — (secondary to sensory loss)

Infection — cellulitis
- secondary to diabetic arteriopathy

Vascular — ischaemic — arterial disease
- secondary to deep vein thrombosis
- embolic — meningococcal septicaemia
- subacute bacterial endocarditis

Conditions requiring surgical excision:
- benign verruca
- Dupuytren's disease

Malignant — melanoma
- squamous cell carcinoma
- other rare tumours

Standard methods of replacement

When the surgeon is faced with a problem of skin loss or intended skin loss on the foot he must have in his mind a number of methods available whereby the skin loss may be replaced. It may well be that the first method chosen may fail and a secondary means may then prove necessary. In any method of reconstruction a period of at least 10 days will be required before the patient is permitted dependency of the limb. Attempts to skin graft the lower leg and foot with immediate mobilization have occasional dramatic results and in the elderly would be desirable but in general have a higher failure rate than is acceptable.

Sole of foot

Full thickness skin grafts

Injuries in which skin has been clearly excised or in degloving injuries, where the proximal part of a distally-based flap is not going to survive as determined either clinically or by fluorescein injection studies, there is a place for replacing the skin as a full thickness graft. In order to achieve a successful outcome to this manoeuvre meticulous defatting of the skin must be carried out. The fibrous septa make this defatting procedure less than easy. The recipient bed on to which the graft is to be applied should be carefully irrigated free of dirt and necrotic tissue as survival of the graft will be hampered by infection or tissue breakdown beneath it. Examples of excellent takes of these full thickness grafts have been reported and are worth the attempt as they at least provide specialized sole skin even if insensitive. It must be accepted, however, that full thickness grafts are prone to failure particularly in circumstances where the skin itself is damaged as in degloving injury. The recipient area is usually the rather avascular longitudinal ligament which forms the plane of shear.

Once it is clear that the full thickness grafts have failed then the next course of action may be invoked.

Split thickness skin grafts

Providing there is a vascularized bed, split thickness skin grafts (SSG) should take without difficulty. They enable rapid reepithelialization of the area of skin loss and protect underlying structures from further damage. Long term cover by SSG is acceptable in non-weightbearing areas such as the medial area of the sole but is unlikely to withstand heavy duty wear on a weight-bearing area. SSG if used in such areas should be considered interim cover before proceeding to a more durable replacement. SSG do not have sufficient dermis to provide movement over the immobile recipient site. The dermis can be augmented by dermal overgrafting (Hynes 1957), which constitutes removing the epidermal layer from the SSG and placing a thick SSG on top; this process can be repeated. By this means mobility of the epidermal layer can be achieved and the skin made more resilient to ulceration. If skin grafts are to be used on the sole, suitably adapted footwear will be required to protect the grafts from injury.

Flaps

Flaps constitute an area of skin and underlying fat with an intact vascular network sufficient to maintain their viability.

They may be divided into random and axial pattern types. Random pattern flaps have no specific vascular pedicle enclosed within them and are supplied by perforating vessels; in consequence they have constraints regarding length to breadth ratios. Axial pattern flaps are created around known vascular pedicles and providing the pedicle is not damaged their length may be unrelated to the breadth of the skin base. Free flaps are extensions of the axial pattern flaps whereby the whole flap may be disconnected from the donor site and placed into a recipient site with viability restored by microvascular anastomotic techniques (Fig. 62.1).

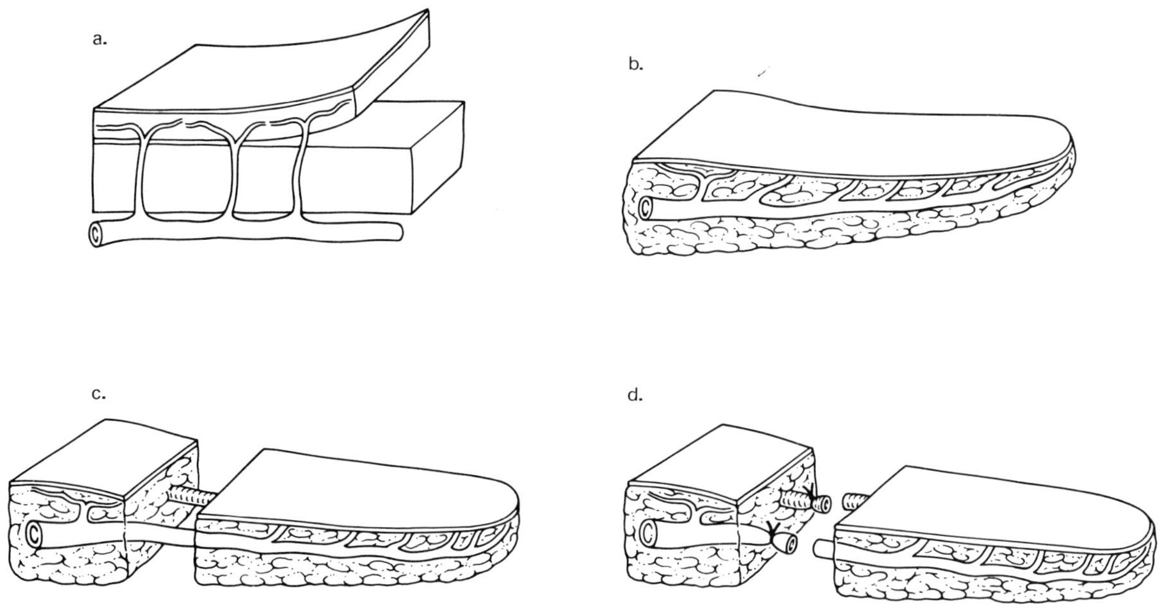

Fig. 62.1 Vascular patterns of flaps in descending order, a = random, b = axial, c = island and d = free flaps

Flaps may be distant or local depending on the proximity of the donor site to the recipient. They may be sensory or insensitive depending on the inclusion of a cutaneous nerve.

Local random pattern flaps

These flaps have been the mainstay of treatment for major skin loss in the weight-bearing sole in past times and do have occasional application, but have been largely superseded by one-stage reliable axial pattern flaps.

The most commonly employed are transposition flaps (Fig. 62.2), which require a skin graft to close the donor site and are usually medially based (Maisels 1961). Laterally based flaps do have the benefit of a donor site which can be placed in the non-weightbearing medial sole (Curtin 1977). For larger transposition flaps, a delay procedure is advisable to ensure survival of the terminal part of the flap but this does make the flap more rigid.

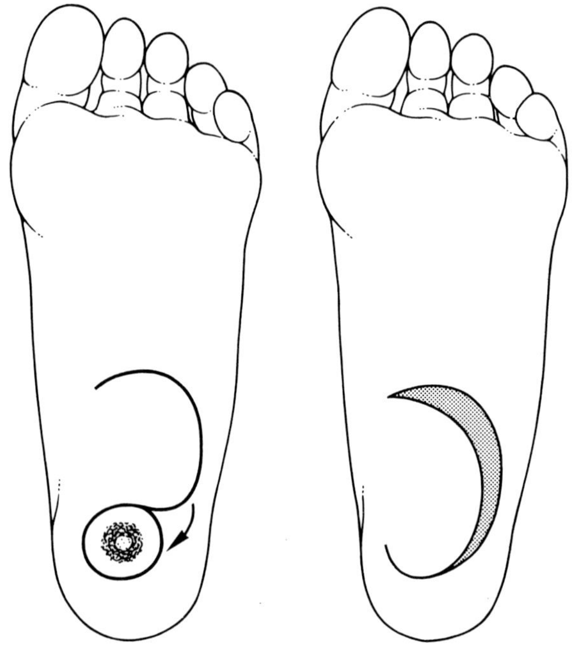

Fig. 62.2 Medially based transposition flap to resurface a heel defect. Cross-hatched donor site is skin grafted

Transposition flaps from the distal sole area (Fig. 62.3) are ideal for resurfacing excised plantar warts or callosities over the metatarsal heads. There is a relative redundancy of skin present between the metatarsal heads and the proximal phalangeal crease; therefore a transversely orientated flap may be raised and transposed longitudinally into the defect over the head. The flap is reliable and may be carried out in one stage. Rotation flaps are relatively uncommon as it is unusual to close the donor site of the flap because of the inelastic quality of sole skin.

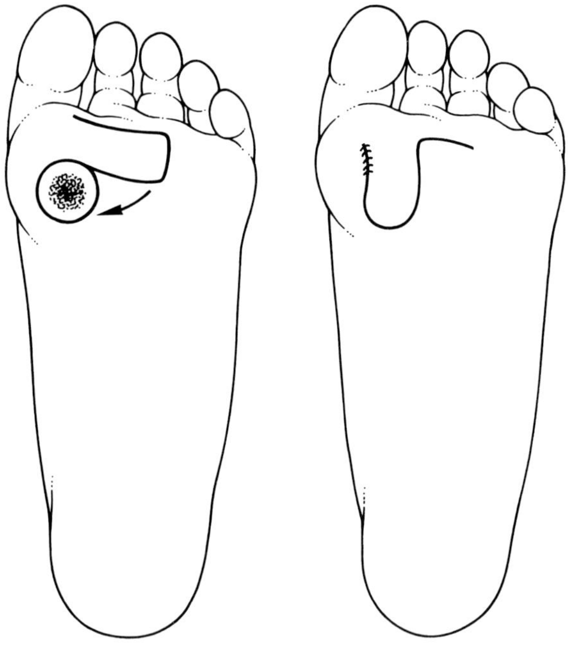

Fig. 62.3 Transposition flap from distal sole to resurface an excised defect over the 1st metatarsal head

All transposition flaps of the foot are insensitive.

Axial pattern local flaps

These flaps are based on a known vascular pedicle and are therefore more flexible than the previously described transposition flaps and are generally more reliable. They also have the advantage of incorporating a cutaneous sensation.

Filletted toes

The big toe (Kaplan 1969) or the second and third toes (Snyder & Edgerton 1965) may be filletted, in respect of removing skeletal support, and the skin transferred to resurface defects in the distal weight-bearing sole or the heel area if required. The digital nerves to the toes are preserved and therefore perfect sensation is retained.

Filletted toes are safe and are used to resurface areas over the metatarsal heads where it is unnecessary to divide the dorsal skin and therefore the veins are left intact. If a single toe such as the second is employed then a minimal cosmetic deformity is apparent. (Fig. 62.4).

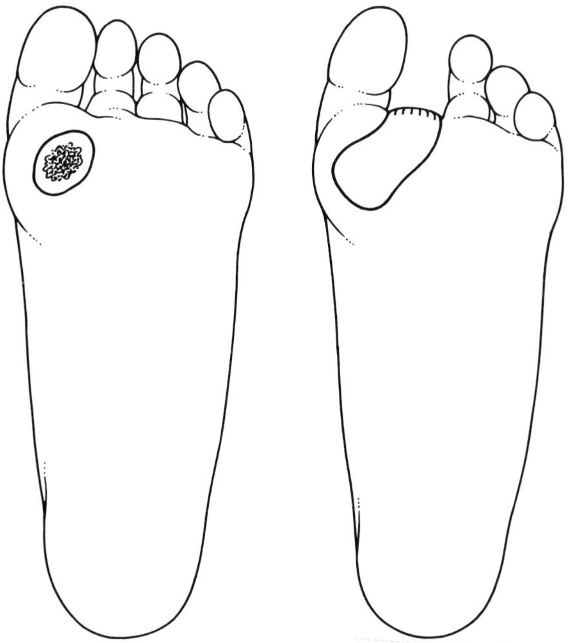

Fig. 62.4 To resurface a more extensive defect over the first metatarsal head the second toe may be filleted to provide sensory skin cover

Filletted toes can be used to resurface the heel area; these are neurovascular island flaps and detailed knowledge of the vascular pattern of the individual foot is required before proceeding.

The arterial supply to the toes on their plantar aspect is derived from three main sources. 81% of 361 feet dissected by Vann (1943) were found to have the deep plantar branch of the dorsalis pedis artery playing the major role in the formation of the plantar arterial arch. Except for the deep plantar branch of the dorsalis pedis the plantar arterial circulation is formed by the lateral plantar branch of the posterior tibial artery. The medial plantar artery plays only a minor role. The deep arteries of the foot do have accompanying venae comitantes, thus the medial and lateral plantar veins drain into the posterior tibial vein and so into the deep venous system.

Whereas there is no superficial arterial arch as in the hand, there is a superficial venous arch at the level of the metatarsal heads which drains into the long saphenous vein.

The foot is extremely variable in its blood supply and this may be intensified by pre-existing vascular impairment. Arteriography is therefore virtually mandatory if a toe fillet is to be used to resurface a heel. Variation such as no medial plantar or dorsalis pedis artery may occur or alternatively the dorsalis pedis artery may be the only source of the plantar metatarsal arch. Both of these anatomical situations may render toe fillets difficult. Generally the lateral plantar artery (or medial plantar) is the desirable vessel on which to base the toe.

The surgery is carried out under tourniquet. The whole toe may be filletted or alternatively just the plantar aspects of the toes may be used preserving the dorsal skin. The neurovascular pedicle is then dissected out as far as the proximal sole.

The area of skin available from one or more toes is not great and therefore the procedure has limitations in proximal sole resurfacing. It is probably the method of choice, however, in distal sole resurfacing where loss of a toe is of minimal functional importance and it provides rapidly available sensory flap tissue.

Medial plantar island flap (instep island flap)

Shanahan & Gingras (1979) transposed a medial plantar sensory flap for coverage of heel defects. This flap was based on the medial plantar artery and the cutaneous nerves, but retained a skin bridge and because of a delay took two stages to reach the recipient site. As the flap was axial pattern based on the medial plantar artery, there was no advantage in the skin bridge and therefore the medial plantar island flap (Harrison & Morgan 1981) was described shortly afterwards. A flap measuring 10 cm long by 7 cm broad may be taken from the medial plantar area of the foot without invading the weight-bearing area (Fig. 62.5). A larger flap can be taken and will be supplied by the medial plantar artery but will then pass on to the weight-bearing area. The flap is based on the medial plantar artery and the cutaneous nerves and may be raised as an island flap without a

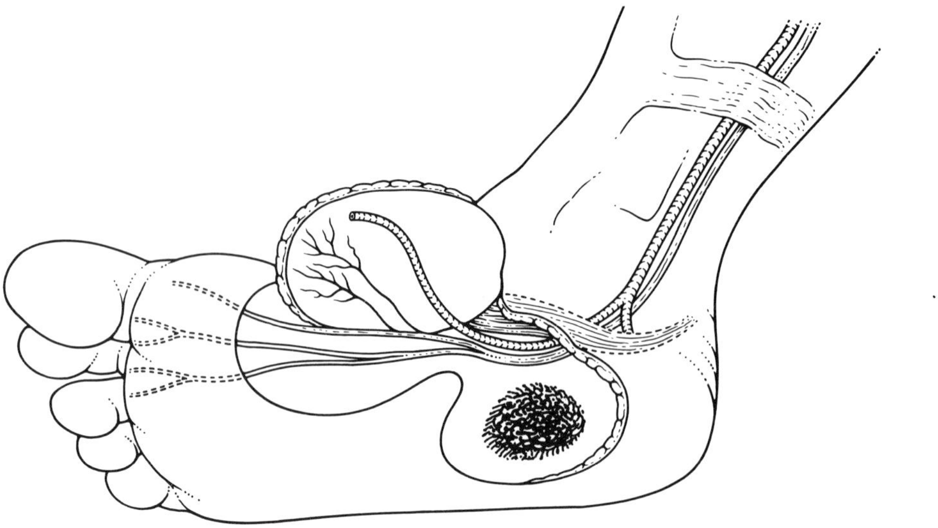

Fig. 62.5 The medial plantar island flap elevated, based on the medial plantar artery and vena comitans and the cutaneous branches of the medial plantar nerves, prior to transfer

delay. This provides a large area of sole skin which is freely mobile on a neurovascular pedicle, retains normal sensation and is ideally suited for resurfacing the vital area over the heel.

Surgical anatomy. The nerve supply to the medial two-thirds of the sole of the foot comes from the cutaneous branches of the medial plantar nerve. The lateral one-third of the sole is supplied by the cutaneous branches from the lateral plantar nerve. These cutaneous branches emanate from the common digital branches of the plantar nerves usually in fine fascicles piercing the plantar fascia. The neurovascular bundles pass along the intermuscular septum between the abductor hallucis and the flexor digitorum brevis on the medial side and between the flexor digitorum brevis and the abductor digiti minimi on the lateral side. It is thus unnecessary to raise the medial plantar flap with included muscle, as it is not myocutaneous but dependent on perforating vessels passing through the intermuscular septum. It is possible to raise the medial plantar flap either on the medial plantar neurovascular bundle or on the lateral plantar neurovascular bundle, but the former is easier, quicker and does not invade a weight-bearing surface (Figs. 62.6, 7 and 8).

The flap is raised distally by marking out the area of skin required and then deepening the distal incision in the cleft between the abductor hallucis and the flexor digitorum brevis, where the medial plantar neurovascular bundle is easily found.

The vessels are divided and the plane of dissection is between the medial plantar vessels and the medial plantar nerve. As the dissection proceeds proximally great care must be taken to avoid damaging the cutaneous nerves which emanate from the medial plantar nerve. Magnification is certainly desirable for this procedure. As the cutaneous fascicles are defined they can be split off the medial plantar nerve by intraneural dissection to provide increased mobility of the flap. The medial plantar neurovascular bundle is traced as far as the lateral border of the abductor hallucis beneath which it passes. It is usually unnecessary to dissect proximal to the abductor hallucis as the pedicle thus formed is usually sufficient for transposition to the heel area.

Normal two point discrimination of the heel skin is about 20 mm and therefore the sensitivity required for this area is not high grade. In the early postoperative period following transfer of the medial plantar flap, sensation is often quite poor and may well reflect neuropraxia of the fine cutaneous fascicles. Over the course of the succeeding few weeks the sensation recovers. In a series of 10 flaps none have proceeded to ulceration and all have withstood normal weight bearing.

Morrison et al (1983) have suggested that it would be desirable to resurface the whole calcaneal area as a

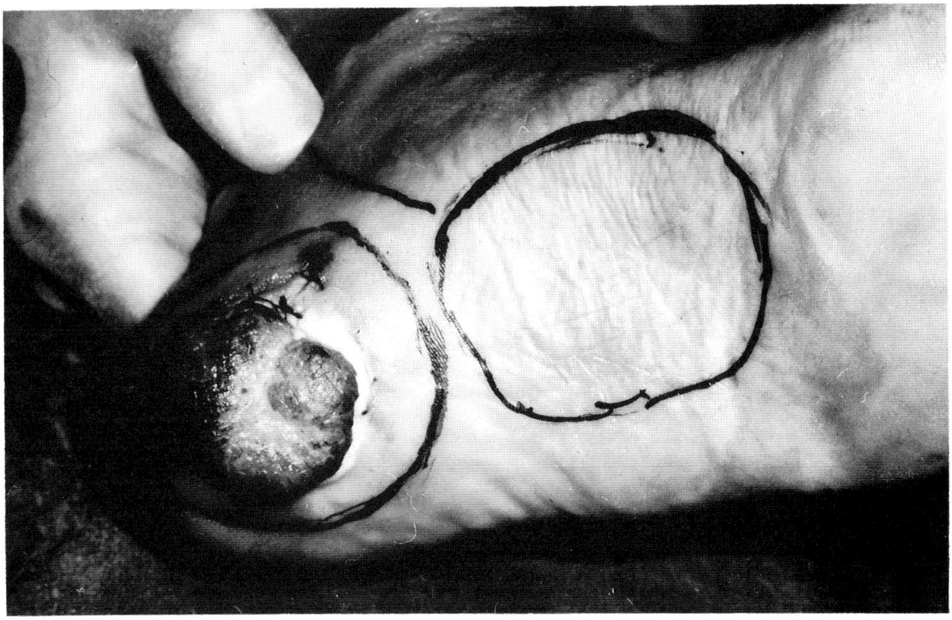

Fig. 62.6 A large malignant growth on the heel area to be excised and replaced with a medial plantar island flap

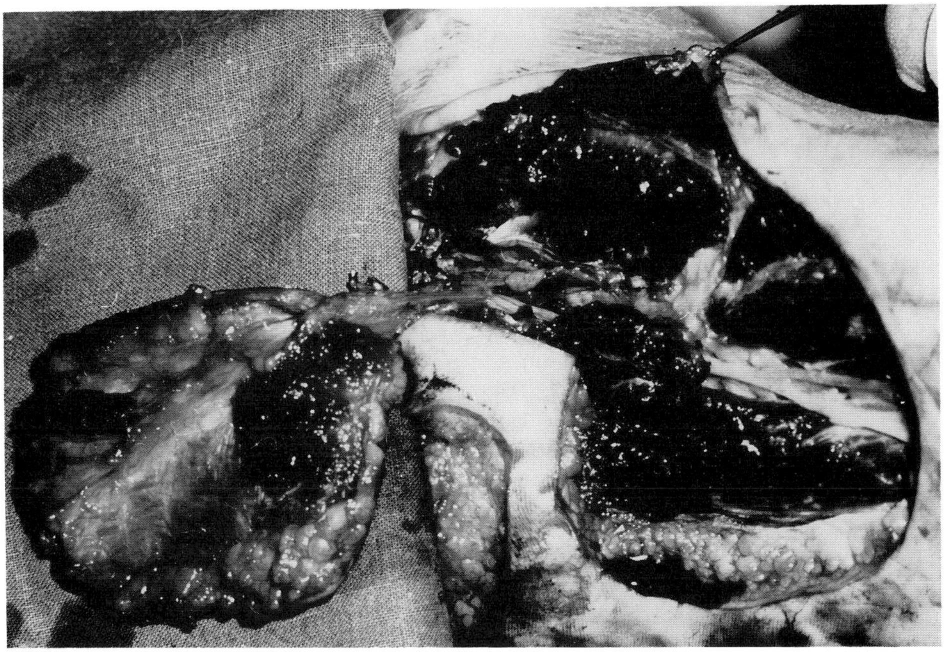

Fig. 62.7 Medial plantar flap elevated to show the vascular pedicle

unit rather than just the ulcerated area in order to avoid scars passing across the weight-bearing sole. Hyperkeratosis along the suture lines can occur and is not easily treated. Unfortunately, this can occur in scars even along the lateral border of the foot which is apparently non-weightbearing, but may be so in certain phases of gait. The medial plantar flap may be used as a free vascularized transfer and the

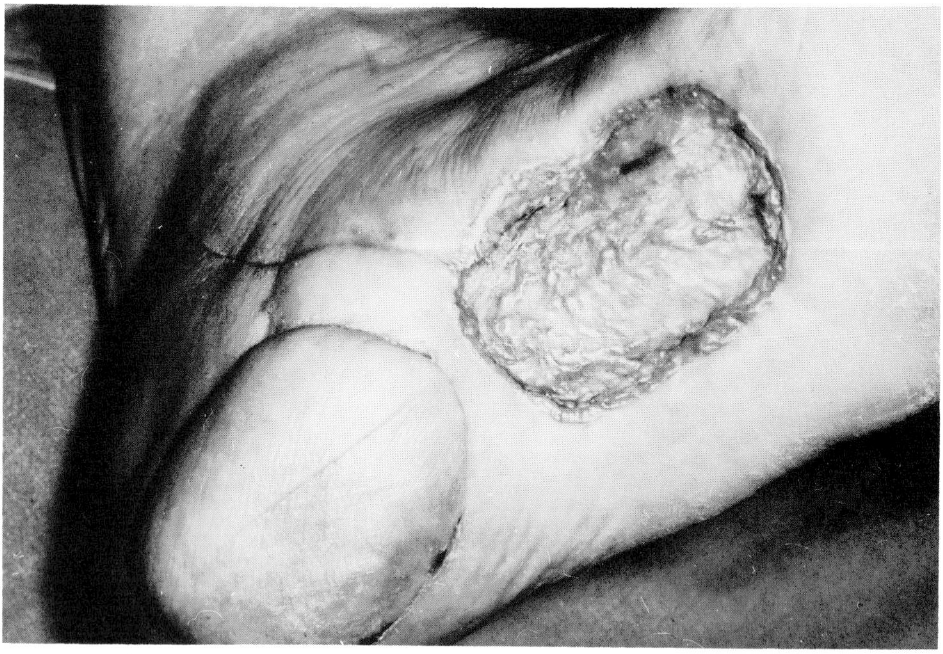

Fig. 62.8 Flap inset into the defect and the donor site successfully skin grafted

cutaneous nerves may also be repaired providing a sensory free flap.

Innervated skin grafts to provide sensation to the reconstructed heel

In circumstances where the calcaneal area has been resurfaced with a distant flap sensation may remain poor over the weight-bearing area and therefore susceptible to recurrent ulceration. Lister (1978) described a case in which a crossed thigh flap had been used to resurface skin loss over the calcaneum. Five months later the sural nerve on the same foot was blocked with local anaesthetic just above the ankle delineating an area of sensory loss over the lateral aspect of the dorsum of the foot. At surgery the sural nerve was then dissected behind the lateral malleolus and traced along the lateral aspect of the foot. A full thickness innervated skin graft was then raised from the lateral aspect of the dorsum of the foot. This skin graft based on the sural nerve was then transposed to the central area of the flap overlying the calcaneum. The donor site was then skin grafted using a split thickness graft. The innervated skin graft then took and provided sensation to this previously insensitive area.

Providing the surgical technique is meticulously carried out and a good take of the graft achieved this is a useful method of introducing sensory tissue into the weight-bearing area of an insensitive flap.

Distant flaps

Distant flaps are introduced into the recipient foot from an unconnected donor site. Again they may be divided into random pattern flaps or axial pattern flaps. Random pattern flaps as previously described are not based on a known vascular pedicle and depend for their blood supply on perforating vessels. They are in general less reliable than axial pattern flaps and as the pedicle of such flaps is relatively short the positioning and fixation between the recipient and donor sites are much more critical.

The art of raising these flaps, insetting them and achieving a satisfactory outcome requires a high degree of skill. They are mentioned here for two reasons; first historical and, second, because modern and sophisticated methods occasionally do go wrong and a secondary method may prove necessary.

Cross leg flaps

This group of flaps may be divided into three.

1. The medial calf cross leg flap. This flap was

possibly the most commonly used flap for resurfacing the anterior part of the lower tibia before the advent of the axial pattern flap. It can be used for the heel area, but is not ideally suited for this and is better used for resurfacing the dorsum of the foot when this is necessary (Fig. 62.9). The flap is based on the cutaneous markings of the long saphenous vein. The length/breadth ratio is important and the flap should not be raised longer than its width. The plane of elevation of the flap is immediately above the fascia. The flap can be raised deep to the fascia on the premise that it increases the viability, this is doubtfully true as the fascial vessels run longitudinally down the limb. If the fascia is included with the flap it is stiffer and less easy to inset and also skin grafts which are required for the donor site of the flap will then be placed directly on

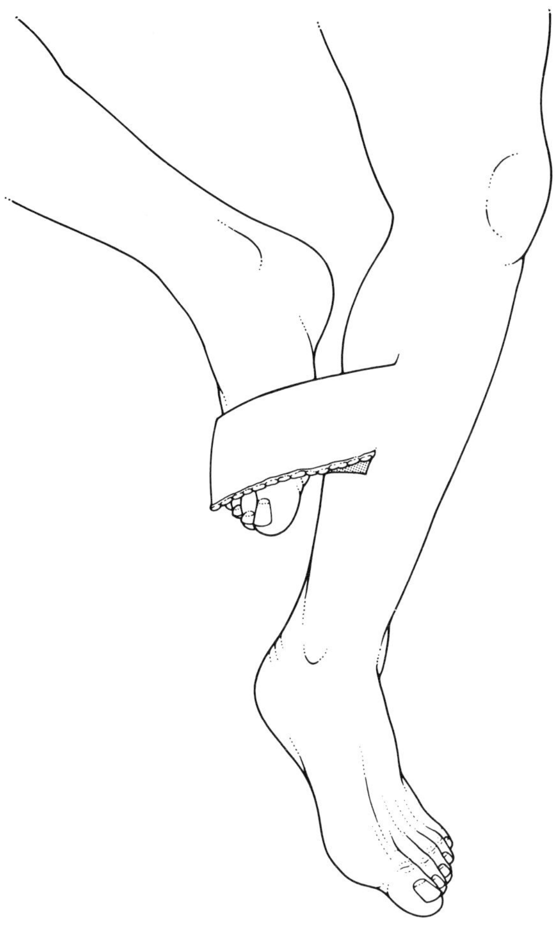

Fig. 62.9 Medial calf cross leg flap inset into the dorsum of the foot

to the muscle causing discomfort particularly in the early postoperative period. Having raised the flap it is inset into the recipient area and must be retained in this position for some three weeks before division. Maintaining this often uncomfortable position for three weeks can be achieved in a number of different ways but perhaps the commonest are the use of heavily padded plaster of Paris or an adapted orthopaedic external fixation device. Whatever the method, considerable care has to be taken to avoid pressure sores on exposed bony points.

2. *Cross thigh flap*. The principle is similar to the previously described medial calf cross leg flap but the cross thigh flap is more suitable for resurfacing the heel area because of the direction of its raw surface. It is however only acceptable in patients with very flexible knees as to hold the position of 90° of knee flexion for three weeks is likely to be extremely uncomfortable, particularly in a rather stiff jointed Caucasian. The more flexibly jointed Eastern races are at a distinct advantage if this flap is to be used. The flap is raised on a superiorly orientated base and again its length/breadth ratio should not exceed 1 : 1. Preoperative planning is of considerable importance in the siting of the flap. The donor site is skin grafted and the recipient foot placed into association with the flap. Following insetting the flap it is important to avoid pressure between the recipient foot and the underlying quadriceps muscle otherwise the pressure of the foot itself can cause necrosis of the underlying muscle. The flap is divided at three weeks and then inset.

3. *Cross foot flap*. Mir y Mir in 1954 described the transfer of a laterally based flap from the sole of the opposite foot. Its principle was to provide skin from the medial plantar area of the opposite foot to resurface the heel area of the recipient foot. A double pedicle flap was prepared from the non-weightbearing part of the sole of the donor foot and a thick graft was applied immediately to the raw surface beneath it. In the second stage two weeks after the delay the bridge flap on the medial side was detached and then inset into the recipient heel. The standard position was the sole of the donor foot placed against the inner side of the recipient foot and then the flap laid into position (Fig. 62.10). A single plaster bandage is usually sufficient to secure absolute immobilization of the operative site. The flap was divided at three weeks. The advantage of

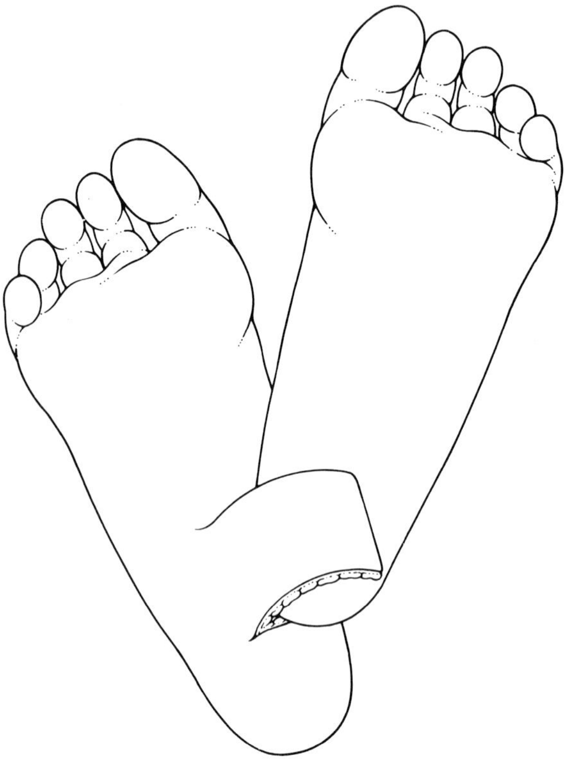

Fig. 62.10 Cross foot flap inset into the heel of the recipient foot. The donor site is the medial plantar area which is non-weightbearing

this flap was to provide specially adapted sole skin to resurface the important heel area. The skin used from the medial plantar area does not interfere with the physiology of the donor foot. A modern adaptation of this flap is to carry out the surgery in one stage dissecting out the cutaneous nerve supply to the medial plantar skin. The flap is then transferred to the recipient foot and the cutaneous nerves are sutured to suitable nerves in the recipient foot, thus restoring sensation to the flap in its new site.

Abdominal tube pedicles

The abdominal tube pedicle described by Gillies (1920) had been the mainstay of major reconstruction on the sole of the foot before the advent of the axial pattern flaps. It constitutes the use of two conjointed random pattern flaps of abdominal skin. The flap is usually designed 18 cm long and 9 cm in breadth. It is based over the groin area and the lateral flank. It has been appreciated in recent years that the survival of these flaps probably depends on incorporating the epigastric artery and vein inferiorly and the lateral branches of the intercostal vessels laterally. The flap requires delays and has to be taken down to the foot on a wrist carrier. On average the surgery takes some 5.8 months to achieve its termination and some five operations (Stranc et al 1975). The position required of the patient where the hand has to be in close association with the foot is again highly uncomfortable and usually is only tolerated in young people.

Axial pattern flaps

The distant axial pattern flaps which may be of value in resurfacing the foot form three categories: musculocutaneous, fascial and free flaps (see Fig. 62.1).

Musculocutaneous. The two musculocutaneous flaps which may be of particular use in resurfacing parts of the foot are the medial gastrocnemius musculocutaneous flap (McCraw 1977) and the tensor fascia lata flap (Nahai 1980). There are a number of areas on the body surface where the blood supply to the skin is largely supplied by the perforating vessels from the underlying muscle. It is therefore possible to elevate skin and the underlying muscle as a unit and providing the hilar vessels of the muscle are not divided this unit may be transferred to another area and the skin expected to survive.

The medial gastrocnemius flap constitutes a musculocutaneous unit 10 cm broad and 23 cm long based on the medial gastrocnemius muscle of the contralateral calf. The muscle itself is 8 by 15 cm in size, so clearly the distal part of the cutaneous blood supply relies on a fascial plexus. The hilar vasculature to the muscle originates close to its origin and therefore the flap is freely mobile. The distal end of the flap can be taken to within 8 cm of the medial malleolus. Following inset of the flap on to the recipient area on the damaged foot it is left connected to the recipient area for three weeks before division. It is a highly reliable flap but because it contains muscle it is rather thick. Its further disadvantage is that it does cause an unsightly defect on the donor leg and oedema of the ankle may be slow to settle. It is insensitive.

The dominant vascular pedicle of the tensor fascia

lata flap is the terminal branch of the lateral circumflex femoral artery and its vena comitans. The skin territory supplied by the tensor fascia lata muscle is the skin overlying it and most of its tendon. The skin of the lateral thigh therefore can be raised with the tensor fascia lata and its muscle included, and provides a very safe flap for covering defects. To use the flap, much as with the random cross thigh flap, does require the patient to have flexible knees. The lateral cutaneous nerve of the thigh may be incorporated with the tensor fascia lata flap and at the time of division of the pedicle the nerve may be further dissected proximally and then taken with the flap across to the recipient foot. If there is a suitable cutaneous nerve into which to inset the divided distal part of the lateral cutaneous nerve the flap may be rendered sensory.

Fasciocutaneous flaps. The fasciocutaneous flap includes skin, the subcutaneous fat and the deep fascia but not the muscle. The most useful of these flaps was described by Ponten in 1981 using skin on the medial side of the calf measuring some 18 cm in length by 8 cm broad. The vascular anatomy of the flap has been well described by Haertsch (1981a, b) who showed that there are axial vessels running just superficial to the deep fascia forming a network to supply the overlying skin. The axial feeding vessel is the saphenous artery which arises as a common trunk with the descending genicular vessel running deep to sartorius and entering the leg between the tendons of the sartorious and the gracilis muscle. The flap is planned with the base sited proximally. The incision is carried through the skin, subcutaneous tissue and fascia but the underlying muscle is left intact. Inclusion of the saphenous vein is important in order to provide good venous drainage. Although the free flap transfers are probably the treatment of choice for distant flap cover the fasciocutaneous flap does have special advantages. The flap itself is easy to raise and it is safe (Barclay et al 1982). The pedicle may be long and therefore rigid plaster of Paris fixation between the donor and recipient site is probably not necessary. The flap is thin, which may not be so in free flap transfers. The time in hospital required for a fasciocutaneous flap differs only moderately from that for free flap transfer (Barclay et al 1983). The operating time is considerably shorter and the expertise required to raise the flap and inset it is much less than for a free flap transfer. These flaps are suitable for covering dorsal or plantar surfaces of the foot.

Free flap transfers. Free flaps constitute a flap of skin with fat and sometimes muscle based on a known artery which is transferred from one part of the body to another and its circulation reestablished by the use of microvascular anastomotic techniques. There are a considerable number of these flaps which have been described and perhaps the most commonly known are the groin flap and the latissumus dorsi flap (O'Brien & Shanmugan 1973, Serafin et al 1980, Taylor & Daniel 1975). It would be a needless waste of space to describe every microvascular free flap that would be suitable for resurfacing the sole, heel, or dorsum of the foot. The surgeon has merely to consider the clinical problem and choose a suitable transfer. These techniques have revolutionized the ability with which flaps may be transferred to the foot. The surgery is time consuming but essentially the flap reaches it recipient area in one operation dispensing with the previous 5.8 months (Stranc et al 1975) required by the tube pedicle and also it is more comfortable for the patient, avoiding a lengthy period in a fixed position. Before contemplating a free flap transfer to the foot an arteriogram is often valuable. As previously mentioned the variation in anatomy of the foot can be marked and although assessment with a Doppler ultrasound may well provide most of the information, errors can be made.

Every flap has advantages and disadvantages and these must be understood by the surgeon before embarking on the technique. A few factors of particular importance in flap choice is firstly the thickness of the flap. When importing a flap to the foot it is desirable to have it fairly thin. This is particularly relevant on the dorsum and in the area over the Achilles tendon. If the flap is introduced too thick then thinning procedures may have to be carried out in order to enable the patient to wear shoes satisfactorily. On the sole of the foot the thickness is possibly of not quite so much importance. Conflicting arguments exist as to the importance of a thick flap on the sole. If the flap is thick then patients can describe walking on the flap as similar to being on a 'pad of butter'. If, however, the flap is thin then it is possibly more vulnerable to ulceration as the pressure is not distributed so evenly. A thick flap such as the latissimus dorsi musculocutaneous free flap certainly undergoes considerable muscular degeneration, but nevertheless does remain thick.

It is possible now to introduce sensation into the recipient area on the sole of the foot. The tensor fascia lata flap previously described is suitable as it has a reliable vascular pedicle and the lateral cutaneous nerve of the thigh supplies sensation to the cutaneous area. It is therefore possible to take the flap down to the sole of the foot and provide sensation to the skin by neurorrhaphy with either a divided cutaneous nerve present in the recipient area or to the medial or lateral plantar nerve according to availability. Morrison et al (1983) have extended the value of the medial plantar flap by elevating this flap from the contralateral foot on the medial plantar artery and its cutaneous nerves and transferring it to the heel area on the injured side. In some respects it has similarities to the crossed foot flap described by Mir y Mir (1954) but the procedure is carried out in one stage and restoring the continuity of the cutaneous nerve pathways should be of real benefit to the patient.

An additional possibility is the introduction of vascularized bone grafts. In some circumstances with severe injuries to the foot, continuity of the bony skeleton may be lost and the stability of the foot may be improved by restoring the lost bone. A deep circumflex iliac artery osteocutaneous flap is of particular value in this reconstruction (Taylor 1983). The bone is viable and therefore will withstand infection without being sequestrated and because of its vascularization it does not have to be reconstituted by 'creeping substitition' as the osteocytes remain viable within the Haversian systems. Should the bone graft fracture it will unite in a similar way to a long bone.

A young man had a severe injury to the lateral part of his foot with a comminuted compound injury to his fourth and fifth metatarsals with actual bone loss (Fig. 62.11 and 12). Because of the bone loss and infection the lateral side of his foot was unstable. The dead metatarsals were therefore excised and the bony continuity restored with a deep circumflex iliac artery osteocutaneous flap, which supplied not only stability to the lateral side of his foot but also skin cover. He is now able to walk satisfactorily (Fig. 62.13, 14 and 15).

In circumstances where there has been complete loss of tendon continuity on the dorsum of the foot, both of the long and short extensors, and there is foot drop, vascularized tendon grafts can be used. The simplest method of achieving this is the use of a radial artery free flap (Song et al 1982). Thin skin from the volar aspect of the forearm is provided, incorporating within the flap the flexor carpi radialis and also the palmaris longus. These tendons may be used to restore the continuity of the lost tendons. The surgery can then be carried out in one stage rather than two.

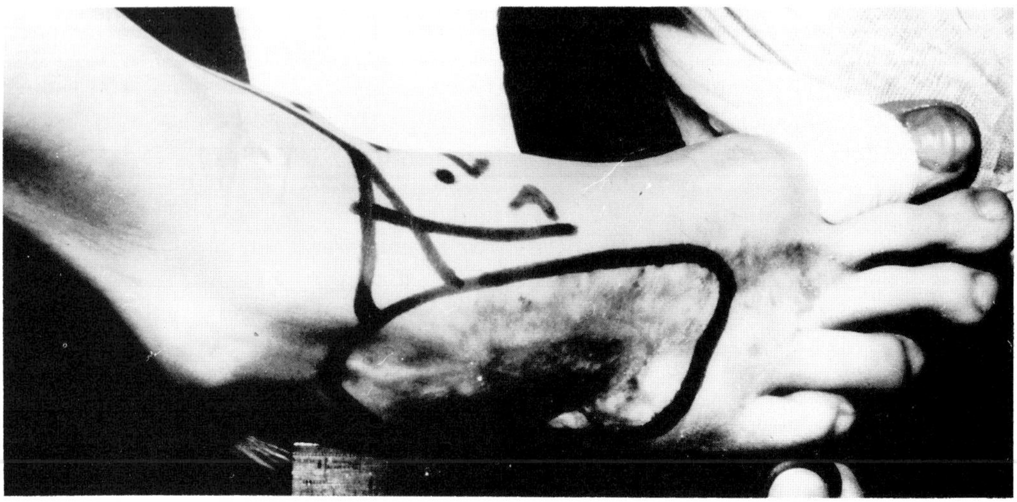

Fig. 62.11 Injury to the lateral side of foot with infected exposed metatarsals excised and skin grafted to eradicate infection

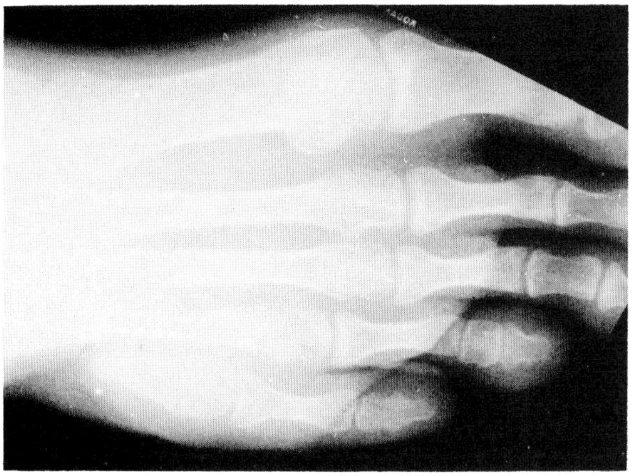

Fig. 62.12 Radiograph to show bone loss and instability of lateral side of foot

PLAN OF RECONSTRUCTION FOR SPECIFIC AREAS APART FROM THE SOLE

Dorsum of the foot

The dorsum of the foot in urban living does not have to withstand heavy wear. In consequence skin grafts are usually sufficiently stable. For the first six months after the skin has been applied minor ulcerations will occur and require treatment, but after this time the skin graft becomes more mobile on the underlying structures and ulceration becomes less frequent. The area over the base of the first and second metatarsals receives most wear and therefore is more liable to ulceration. A dermal overgraft may be sufficient to correct this and avoid the need to proceed to flap cover. If the patient is recurrently ulcerating the area then flap cover may be required and may either be a free microvascular transfer or alternatively a cross leg fasciocutaneous flap. The choice between these two will depend on the requirements of the recipient area, the desire of the patient and the technical skill of the surgeon. The decision to introduce a vascularized bone graft with the free flap or vascularized tendon grafts is more relevant in resurfacing the dorsum of the foot.

The Achilles tendon area

The skin overlying the Achilles tendon may be damaged directly by trauma. It may be necrosed by

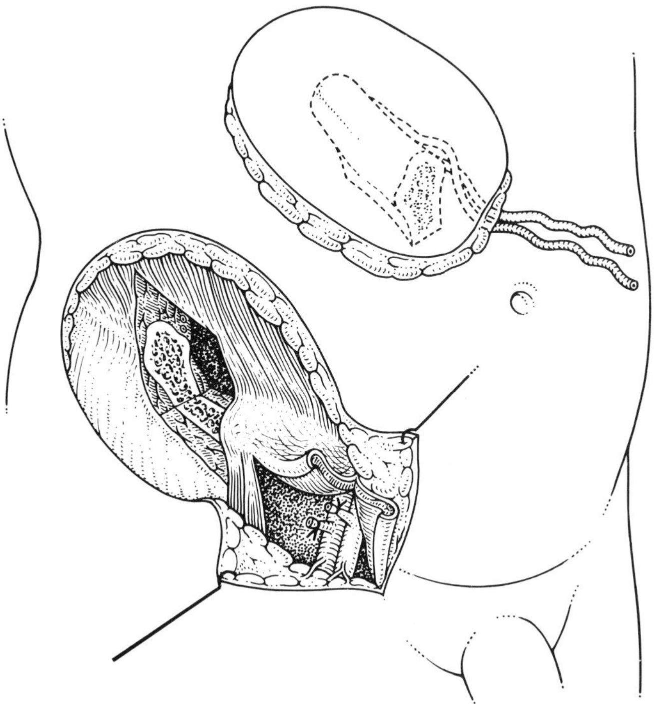

Fig. 62.13 The deep circumflex iliac artery supplies the iliac crest and an area of overlying groin skin. An osteocutaneous flap may therefore be elevated based on this vessel

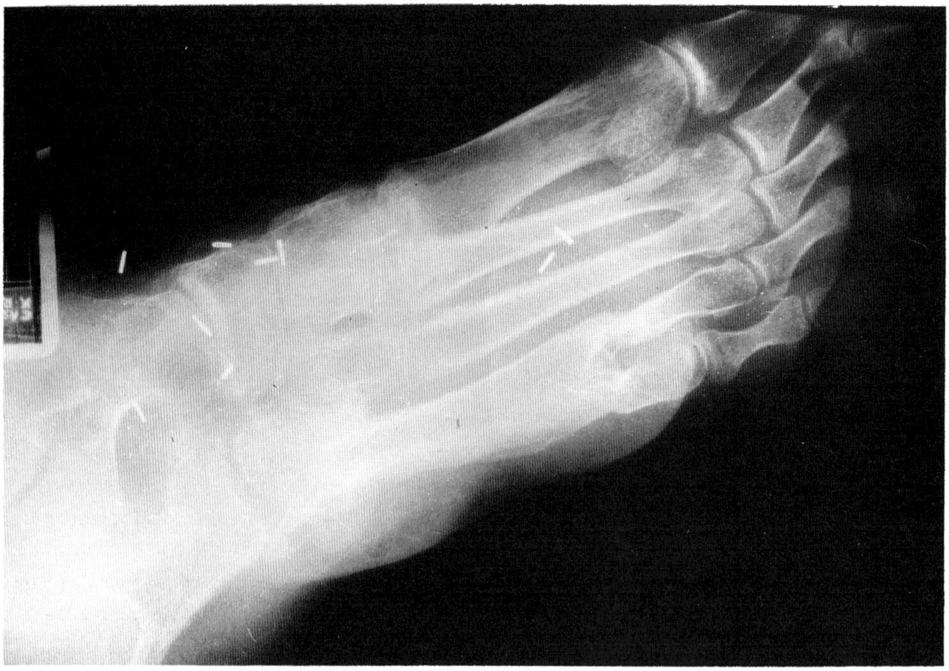

Fig. 62.14 Radiograph showing solid bone union bridging the defect between the proximal and distal ends of the fourth and fifth metatarsals

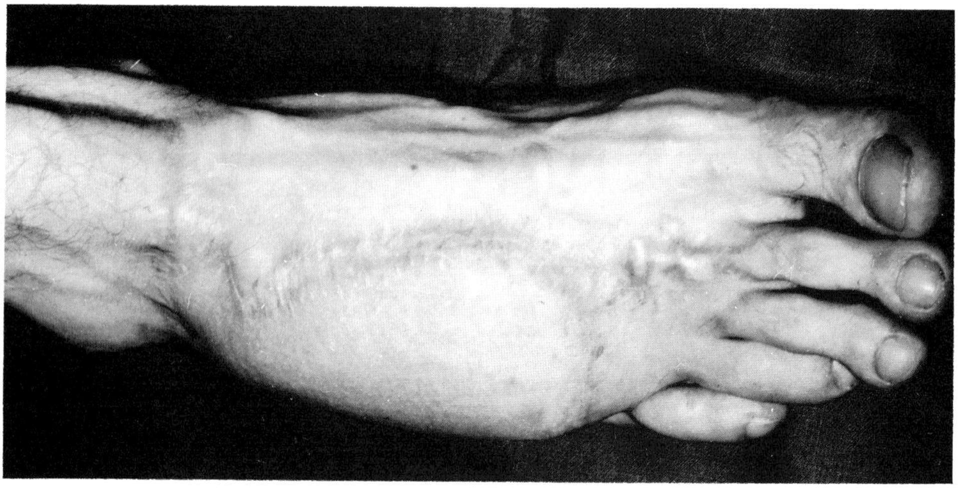

Fig. 62.15 Healed osteocutaneous flap on the dorsum of the foot

pressure exposing the Achilles tendon in the base of an ulcer. It may be damaged iatrogenically in an attempt to repair the Achilles tendon surgically and skin replacement may be required when the Achilles tendon is lengthened in equinus deformity. The overriding problem in reconstruction is to provide stable reepithelialization without a thick fatty layer, unfortunately this is not always possible.

Skin grafts

Shaving of the exposed Achilles tendon and splitting of the tendinous fibres longitudinally commonly permits granulation tissue to penetrate through tendon fibres. If this can be achieved then a skin graft can be expected to take on the tendon itself. The Achilles tendon is thick just above its insertion into the calcaneum and therefore considerable shaving of its fibres can be carried out without disrupting its continuity. If this fails then flap cover must be considered.

Transposition flaps

The most useful of these flaps is a flap based proximally extending between the lateral malleolus and the defect almost to the sole skin. The axial vessel which is incorporated within the flap is the terminal branches of the peroneal artery which emanates from beneath the flexor hallucis longus muscle. The donor site will require a skin graft (Fig. 62.16).

The turn over flap

A flap may be raised based on the edge of the ulcerated area, deepithelialized and then turned over to resurface the Achilles tendon. The raw surface which then presents externally may be skin grafted (Thake 1981).

Axial pattern flap

The dorsalis pedis artery flap to be described below will reach the heel, but the transfer is tight. Considerable dissection needs to be carried out to achieve this transfer. The medial plantar flap may also be used but the abductor hallucis muscle has to be divided to achieve sufficient freedom for the vascular pedicle.

Muscle flaps

The abductor hallucis muscle originates from the medial part of the calcaneum and inserts into the base of the proximal phalanx of the first toe. Its innervation and blood supply emanate from the medial plantar neurovascular bundle. In order to elevate the flap an incision is made along the non-weightbearing surface and the tendon divided distally. The muscle is then separated from the fibres of the flexor hallucis brevis. The muscle is turned over on itself and elevated up to its pedicle. In order to resurface defects on the posterior heel however it will be necessary to divide the medial plantar artery distally and elevate the artery with the flap up to its bifurcation with the posterior tibial artery. The muscle may then be transposed to the area of the Achilles tendon and skin grafted. The procedure is

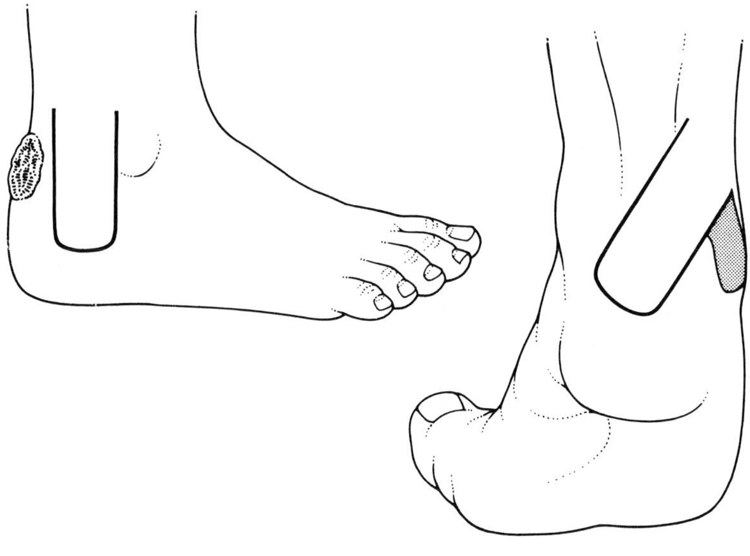

Fig. 62.16 Transposition flap for resurfacing the Achilles tendon area. It is designed to include the terminal branches of the peroneal artery and the sural nerve. The donor site is skin grafted

satisfactory but depends on the size of the abductor hallucis muscle. In general it is probably easier to take a medial plantar flap as the dissection is similar.

Free flap transfers

When circumstances demand, a free flap transfer may be used to resurface the area over the Achilles tendon. Particularly this may be necessary where the Achilles tendon is to be lengthened in equinus deformities (Figs. 62.17, 18 and 19). A thin flap is desirable and therefore flaps such as the radial artery forearm flap may be particularly relevant. If the area to be resurfaced is extensive, as may occur in injury, then a groin flap or a tensor fascia lata flap may be more suitable.

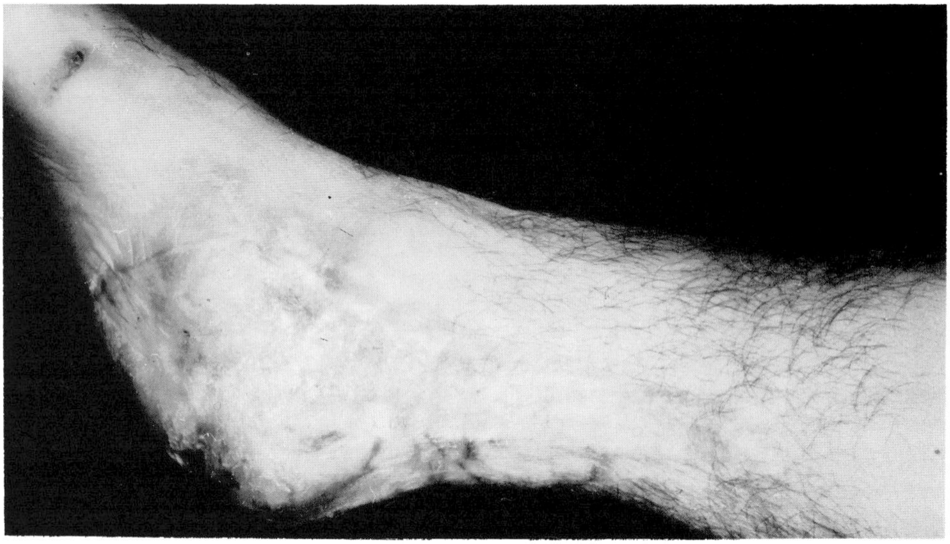

Fig. 62.17 Severe injury to heel skin and area over the Achilles tendon which has epithelialized but is unstable and has an equinus deformity

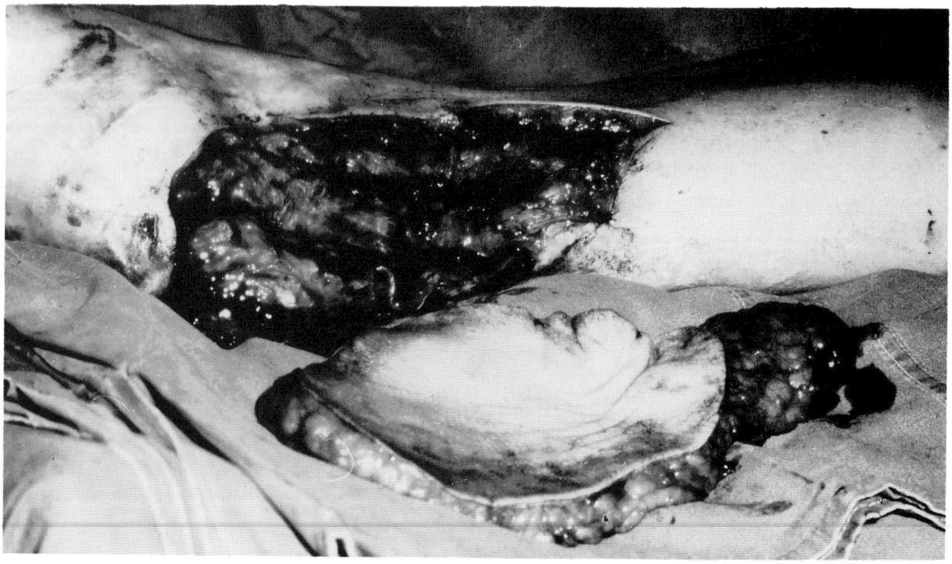

Fig. 62.18 The unstable skin excised, Achilles tendon lengthened and a 15 cm × 21 cm groin flap has been harvested

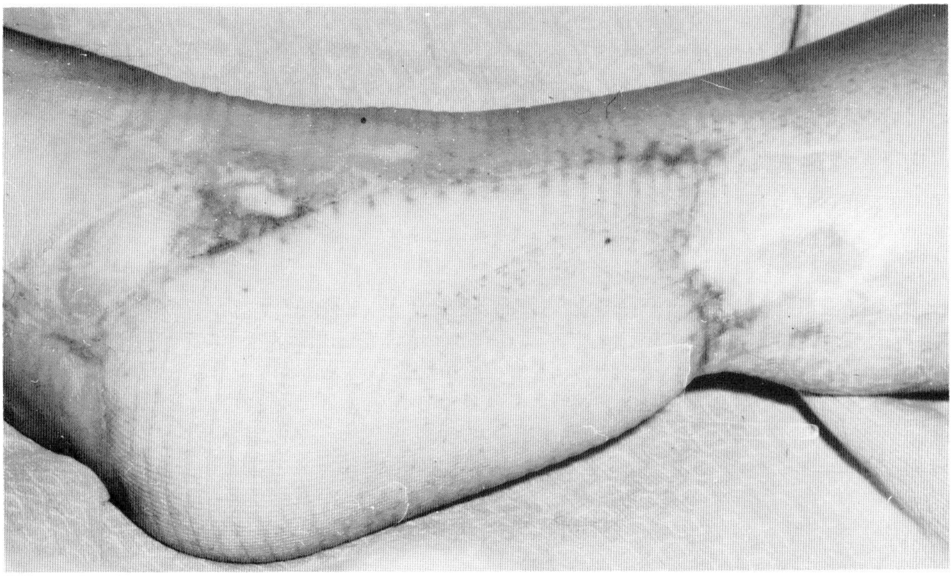

Fig. 62.19 Free groin flap has been successfully revascularized and provides stable skin cover

In an effort to try and produce the thinnest possible reepithelialization of this area, a recent innovation is the use of vascularized fascial grafts.

Vascularized fascial grafts

The most commonly used donor sites for vascularized fascia are the radial artery fascial flap which constitutes taking the radial artery and an expanse of the deep fascia on the forearm but retaining the overlying skin intact. The radial artery and the fascia may be then transferred to the lower leg where the radial artery is anastomosed to the posterior tibial artery and vein and the fascia used to cover the area over the exposed Achilles tendon. The vascularized fascia may then be skin grafted and in consequence the area reepithelialized. A further suitable donor site for vascularized fascia is the galeal flap. The hair bearing scalp may be elevated over an extensive area of the lateral side of the scalp and the galea beneath raised on the superficial temporal artery and vein. Following removal of the galea the scalp may be closed directly. The galea may then be transferred to the ankle region and revascularized by microvascular anastomosis and skin grafted.

In conclusion, there are many methods of resurfacing the sole of the foot, the dorsum of the foot and Achilles tendon. It is highly desirable, if possible, to try and provide sensory flap tissue to resurface the sole and the medial plantar flap and filletted toes are particularly useful to achieve this aim. Where a distant flap has to be introduced, the most useful of which are innervated free flap transfers, a period of at least nine months non-weightbearing on the flap is probably essential to avoid pressure ulceration due to insensitivity.

THE FOOT AS A DONOR SITE FOR COMPOSITE TISSUE MICROVASCULAR TRANSFERS

Over the course of the last few years the foot has proved a most useful conservatory for the harvesting of free flaps and for reconstructing thumbs or fingers using toes or parts of toes. Some of these methods will be described.

The dorsalis pedis free flap

The dorsalis pedis flap was first described by O'Brien & Shanmugan in 1973. It is based on the dorsalis pedis artery and two venae comitantes. It also includes part of the long saphenous vein and its connecting dorsal venous arch. The flap is particularly valuable because of its thinness, but is limited in its size. It should not be used unless the posterior tibial artery is intact. The flap may be incorporated with a great or second toe transfer. The palpable dorsalis pedis artery may come from the anterior tibial artery or a perforating branch of the peroneal artery.

Flap design

The flap is centred over the dorsalis pedis artery pulsation and may be taken medially just beyond the extensor hallucis longus tendon incorporating the visible and palpable long saphenous vein (Fig. 62.20). Laterally it is taken to within 2 cm of the sole skin interface. The distal extent of the flap is controversial. The safe distal end of the flap is the cleft between the first and second metatarsals through which the dorsalis pedis artery enters the plantar surface. If the flap is extended as far as the metatarsophalangeal joints some 1.5 cm distal to the point where the dorsalis pedis exits from the dorsum of the foot then the survival of the flap is less reliable. If it is essential to retain this 1.5 cm extension of the flap then a delay procedure is advisable. If the first dorsal metatarsal artery can be incorporated within the flap then the survival of this distal 1.5 cm is more certain. The proximal margin of the flap is at the level of the extensor retinaculum. The flap is elevated in the plane just above the paratenon and special care has to be taken as the extensor hallucis longus tendon is approached. The dorsalis pedis artery often lies closely adjacent to this tendon and is liable to damage. The dorsalis pedis artery is divided as it passes down to the first dorsal interosseous muscle. Following division, the plane of dissection of the flap remains at the paratenon level and also deep to the dorsalis pedis artery. As the dissection proceeds proximally the tendon of the extensor hallucis brevis is divided as it passes superficial to the artery. The long saphenous vein and its dorsal venous arch is incorporated within the flap to enhance venous drainage. If a long pedicle is required the extensor retinaculum may be divided and the anterior tibial artery dissected proximally. The donor site of the flap is then skin grafted following confirmatory evidence of the flap survival on release of the tourniquet.

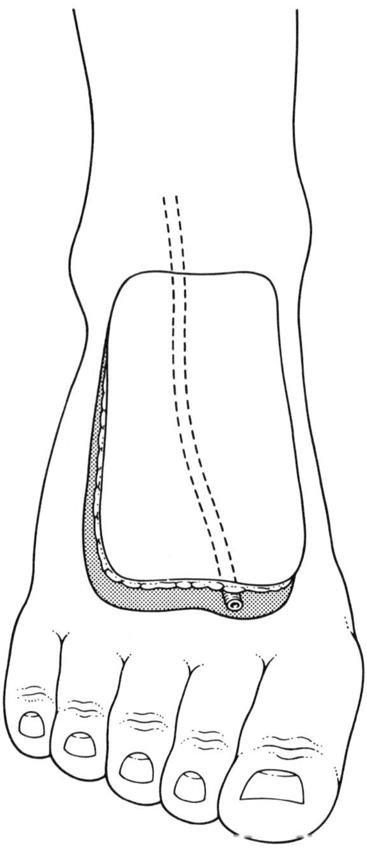

Fig. 62.20 The dorsalis pedis artery flap marked out on the dorsum of the foot

Use of the flap

The dorsalis pedis flap is useful where a small thin flap is required with a long pedicle, indications for its use are in repairing large palatal fistulae, reconstruction of the floor of the mouth in oral carcinoma and resurfacing the hand (Figs. 62.21 and 22).

The second metatarsal may be incorporated with the flap if bony support is required to reconstruct the mandible. The donor site may be slow to heal where bone is taken but usually epithelializes satisfactorily.

First web space flap

The dorsalis pedis artery as it enters the first dorsal interosseous muscle gives off the first dorsal metatarsal branch in over 80% of cases. This small artery may lie superficial to the interosseous muscle or may pass through its substance (Fig. 62.23). It passes distally and bifurcates to supply the adjacent

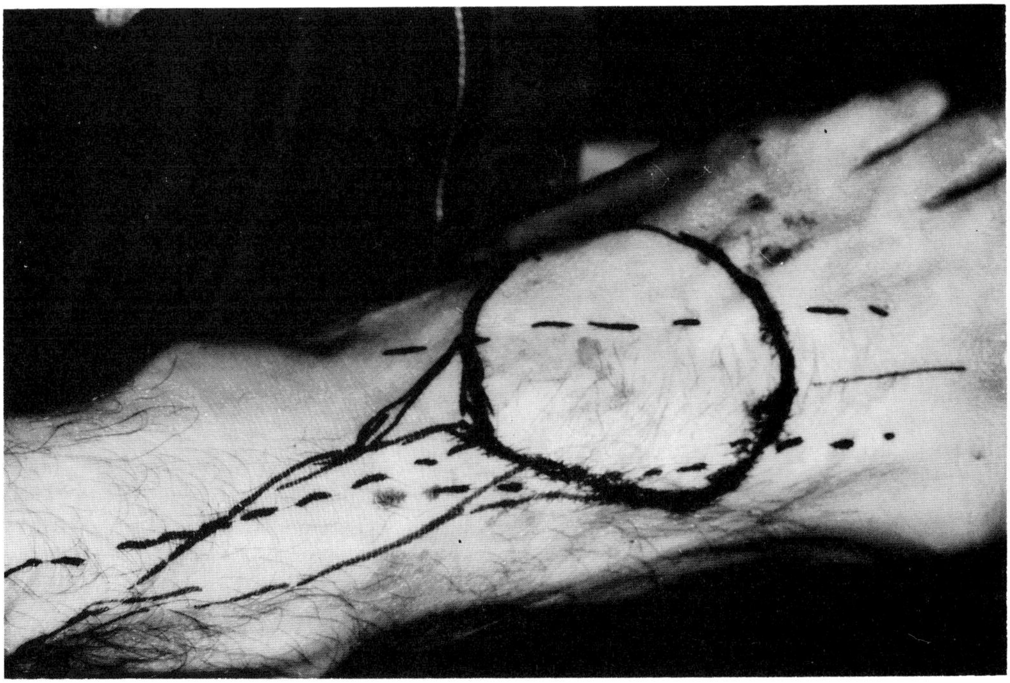

Fig. 62.21 Small dorsalis pedis flap marked out in this case for transfer to the palate

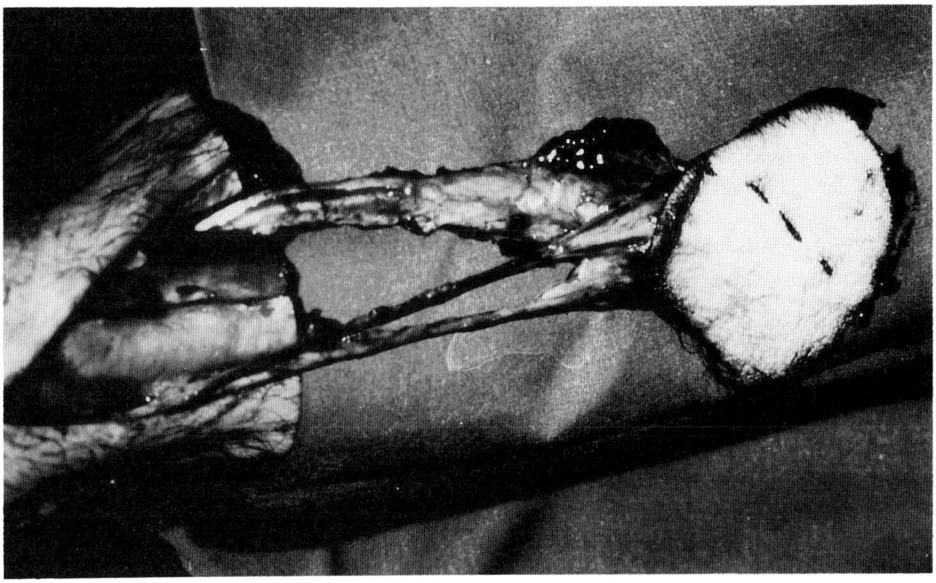

Fig. 62.22 Dorsalis pedis flap elevated to show the length of its vascular pedicle

surfaces of the first and second toes. The venous drainage is provided by the long saphenous vein and its dorsal venous arch. This flap is reliable and provides an area of skin from the adjacent halves of both of these toes and is therefore suitable for resurfacing the first cleft in the hand when an adduction contracture is released (Gilbert et al 1975). The adjacent plantar digital nerves can be

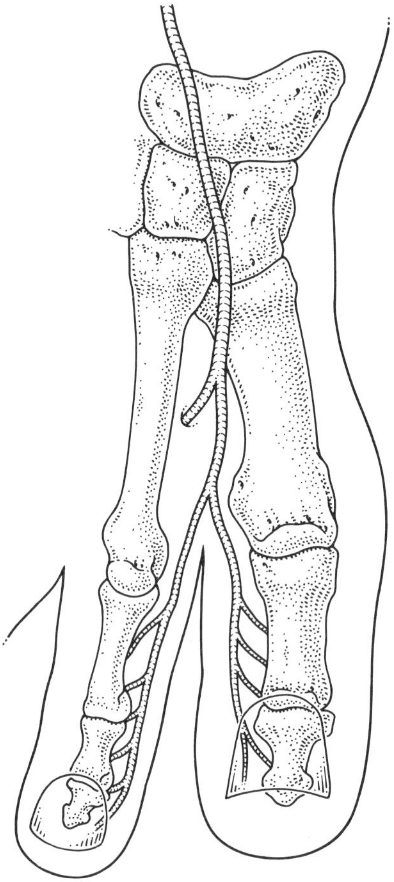

Fig. 62.23 Dorsalis pedis artery exiting to the plantar area and giving off the first dorsal metatarsal artery which supplies the adjacent sides of the first cleft

incorporated with the flap as can the anterior tibial nerve which provides sensation to the first cleft. A neurorrhaphy at the recipient site with a suitable cutaneous nerve can provide a neurovascular flap. The dissection of the first dorsal metatarsal artery which is the crucial part of the safe harvesting of the flap paved the way to toe transfers.

One staged toe to hand transfers

The big toe has been employed to reconstruct the thumb since 1900 when Nicaladoni first described it. This procedure required two stages and was very uncomfortable for the patient (Clarkson 1962). With the advent of microvascular surgery, free toe transfers to the hand became possible. Experimentally this was successfully achieved by Buncke et al in 1966 when they transferred the big and second toes to the hand of a rhesus monkey. Cobbett in 1969 carried out the first human big toe transfer.

Toe dissection

Essentially, whether a big toe or a second toe, multiple toes or a wrap around flap are used, the vascular supply of the transfer depends on the first dorsal metatarsal artery and its proximal extension, the dorsalis pedis artery. The distal branches of the long saphenous vein augment the venous drainage.

Occasionally the dorsalis pedis artery is absent or the first dorsal metatarsal artery is very small and then consideration may be given to using the medial plantar or lateral plantar vascular arch.

The designated toe or toes are marked out incorporating whatever extra flap cover may be required on the hand. The dorsalis pedis artery is then dissected out through a longitudinal incision, usually sited just medial to the artery. The long saphenous vein and its branches are also preserved. The first dorsal metatarsal artery is then dissected and the plantar extension of the dorsal pedis artery is divided in the cleft between the interossei. The first dorsal metatarsal artery is preserved distally until it is clearly seen entering the chosen toe. If the second toe is to be transferred then the branch to the great toe is divided. The cleft between the toes is then deepened protecting the first dorsal metatarsal artery. The extensor tendon to the toe is divided at a suitable length for its repair in the hand. The plantar aspect of the toe is then approached and both plantar digital nerves are dissected free retaining as much length as possible for their repair in the hand. The long flexor to the toe is divided (Fig. 62.24).

The length of the transfer required will have been assessed preoperatively and a suitable osteotomy of the toe is carried out usually through the neck of the metatarsal. The toe is then elevated from the foot based on its vascular pedicle. Having divided these vessels the toe may be taken as a transfer to the hand. Essentially this procedure remains the same for the big toe except that it is advisable not to divide the toe proximal to the head of the metatarsal as it is valuable in maintaining stability of the foot.

If two toes are to be taken essentially the dissection is the same but a longer dorsal venous arch is required. The donor site is then closed and providing

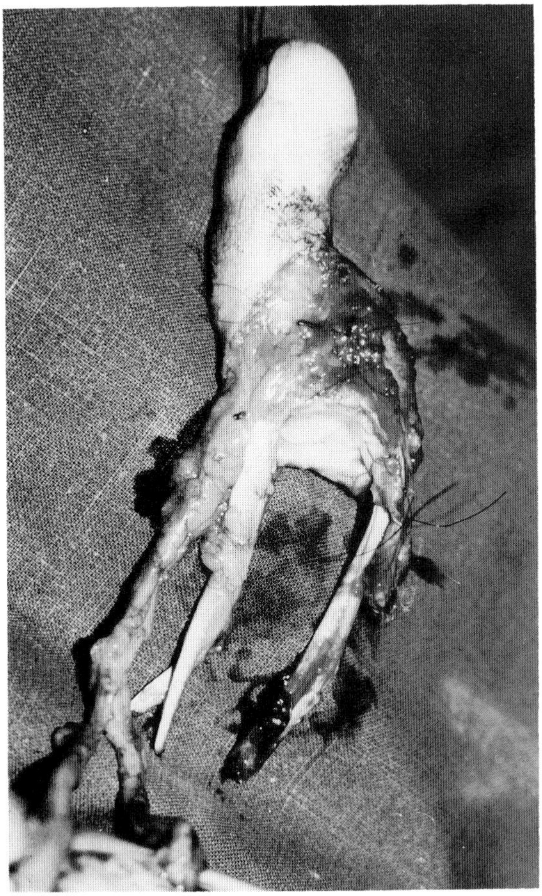

Fig. 62.24 A second toe elevated from the foot but with the vascular pedicle still intact. The tendons and nerves have been preserved

sufficient of the proximal metatarsal is removed the closure is carried out directly. Clearly if a dorsalis pedis flap has been taken with the toes this will require resurfacing with a skin graft. A second toe transfer produces very little cosmetic deformity and indeed if two toes, the second and third are taken it can be surprisingly acceptable. Controversy exists as to the advisability of removing two toes from the same foot, but in our experience it does not appear to compromise walking or running.

Choice of toes

The choice of toe transfer to produce the best aesthetic and functional result is open to discussion.

Essentially the second toe is rather small, it commonly flexes at the interphalangeal joint and certainly does not look cosmetically like a thumb. Its advantages, however, are that it leaves a minimally deformed donor site. The big toe is really too large, does not have a good range of movement at the interphalangeal joint, and leaves an unsightly donor site which may even lead to functional problems. There has therefore been the advent of other methods of thumb reconstruction depending on composite use of tissue from the toes again based on the first dorsal metatarsal artery and the long saphenous vein.

The wrap around flap

In order to improve the cosmetic appearance of the reconstructed thumb Morrison et al (1980) described a cosmetically very acceptable method of achieving a thumb reconstruction. The method is particularly applicable where the base of the proximal phalanx of the thumb remains intact.

In order to increase the length of the thumb a bone graft is taken from the hip between 5 and 6 cm long. The bone graft is modelled and fixed to the base of the proximal phalanx either with interosseous wires or crossed Kirschner wires. It is important to maintain the metacarpophalangeal joint intact, as clearly the bone graft is not capable of flexion at the interphalangeal joint area and flexion therefore is dependent on metacarpophalangeal joint movement. The bone graft is then resurfaced using a flap of tissue from the great toe. Rather similar to the first web space flap, it is dependent on the first dorsal metatarsal artery which is an extension of the dorsalis pedis artery. Most of the circumference of the big toe is degloved including the toe nail. A medial strip of the toe however is left intact. Having degloved the great toe based on its vascular pedicle it is then taken up to the hand, wrapped around the bone graft and sutured into place without tension. The flap is then revascularized by microvascular anastomotic techniques to the radial artery in the 'snuff box'. The degloved toe is reconstructed using a crossed toe flap and skin grafts. The results produced by Morrison are excellent and are probably the best cosmetic results in thumb reconstruction. The problem of this procedure is that flexion of the new thumb is achieved at the metacarpophalangeal joint and therefore inter-phalangeal joint movement which permits conversion of fine pinch to pulp-to-pulp pinch is not available. The bone graft is not vascularized and must be reconstituted by 'creeping substitution'. It is therefore likely to become osteoporotic and liable to fracture. It is however an excellent technique for resurfacing degloved fingers or thumbs.

Free joint transfers

The metatarsophalangeal joint of the second toe may be used to reconstruct a damaged joint. The first dorsal metatarsal artery supplies the distal part of the second metatarsal and the proximal phalanx of the second toe. It is therefore possible to elevate a composite transfer on the artery and transfer it to the hand (Foucher et al 1980). The overlying skin can be taken as well and will act as confirmatory evidence of the survival of the underlying bone. It will be noted that the metatarsophalangeal joints are often hyperextended in the normal and have a relatively limited range of flexion. It may therefore be desirable to put the joint transfer in upside down, thus hyperextension of the toe joint will produce flexion of the finger. The indication for this transfer is not common but may be suitable for a severely damaged joint in a young person.

Pulp flaps

If restoration of sensation and skin cover is required at the finger tips a small pulp flap, usually taken from the lateral side of the great toe, is useful in providing skin for resurfacing; also the digital nerve may be incorporated with the flap and, following a neurorrhaphy at the recipient site, provide a neurocutaneous flap.

SUMMARY

The advent of microvascular anastomotic techniques and improving knowledge of the small vessel anatomy, has made possible the reconstruction of complex injuries of the hand by the use of suitably designed flaps of bone, soft tissue and nerves from the foot.

The variety of transfers is numerous and exact requirements will depend on the injury itself. It is an exciting area of surgical endeavour merely requiring educated imagination and some skill.

CONGENITAL DEFORMITIES OF THE FOOT

Introduction

The surgery of congenital deformities either of foot or hand should be designed to correct functional deficits simply and quickly. Functional deficits in the foot generally relate to the wearing of shoes and this may be prevented by such conditions as polydactyly, gross clinodactyly of the pre or postaxial digits or macrodactyly.

Complex multiple stage operations are generally less successful than simple procedures. The earlier the surgery is carried out the more easily the child adapts to the change and makes use of it.

The classification of congenital deformities of the hand prepared by the American Society for Surgery of the Hand is equally applicable to the foot, thus:

1. Failure of formation of parts (developmental arrest)
2. Failure of differentiation or separation of parts
3. Duplication
4. Overgrowth (gigantism)
5. Undergrowth (hypoplasia)
6. Congenital constriction bands
7. Generalized skeletal abnormalities

Failure of formation of parts

Arrest of development may be transverse or longitudinal. Transverse arrest produces congenital amputations and can occur at any level. Congenital ring constriction can also produce amputation of the terminal digits and should be differentiated from a true arrest. Longitudinal arrest includes central or pre and postaxial failures of development (Fig. 62.25).

There is little that need or indeed can be done for most of these conditions but a central deficit may produce spreading of the lateral segments as in lobster claw deformities. In the latter, wearing shoes may prove difficult because of the width of the foot.

Correction is directed to trying to narrow the foot and may necessitate osteotomies of the lateral metatarsals to permit them to fall into the central defects, suitable excisions of central skin and usually the maintenance of the position by a wire or fascial loop around the necks of the metatarsals.

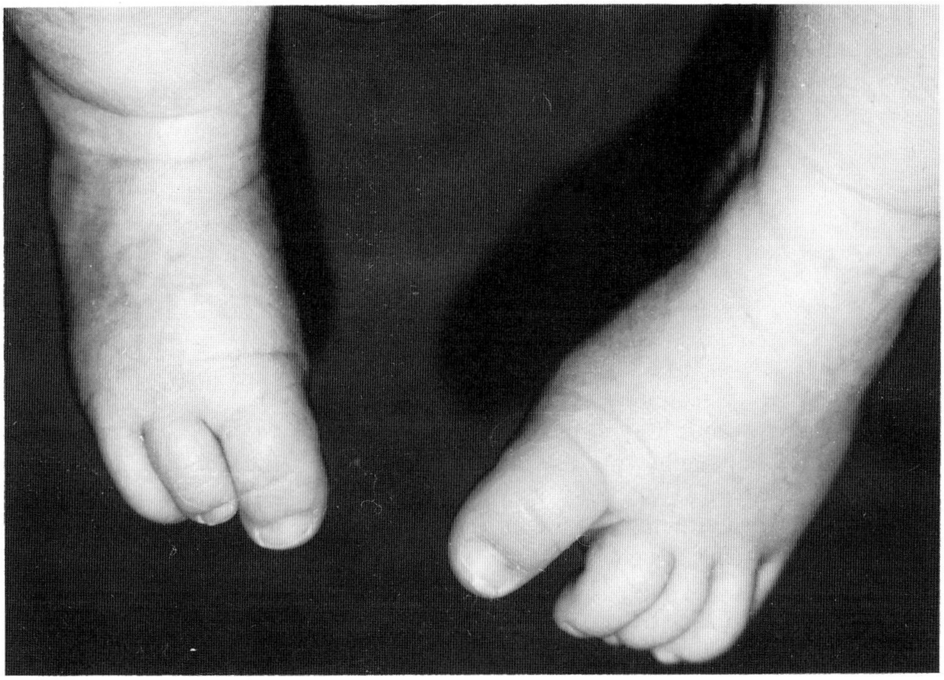

Fig. 62.25 An example of postaxial longitudinal arrest

Failure of differentiation (or separation) of parts

Syndactyly of the toes is one of the most common congenital deformities (Fig. 62.26). Functionally it produces no deficit and its correction is a purely cosmetic exercise; advice should therefore be given against separation.

Modern techniques of desyndactylization emphasize a long dorsal flap into the base of the cleft to prevent distal creep, zigzag design of interdigitating skin flaps along the adjacent sides of the cleft and full thickness grafts in areas where the skin flaps do not meet. Scarring on the dorsum of the foot is therefore inevitable and draws attention to a deformity which prior to surgery would probably not have been apparent to any but the most careful observers. Scarring along the sides of the cleft from incisions and skin grafts will lead to clinodactyly towards the cleft. Finally, scars on the plantar surface of the foot are undesirable as they may become hyperkeratotic and therefore painful.

Exceptions to this rule are 'fenestrated syndactyly' (acrosyndactyly), often associated with the ring constriction syndrome where cleaning the cleft between the toes may be troublesome and separation of the toes is particularly easy as the base of the cleft is well formed. The other indication for surgical correction is the syndactylized nail where difficulty may be experienced in trimming. Separation of the distal phalangeal segment only is recommended and

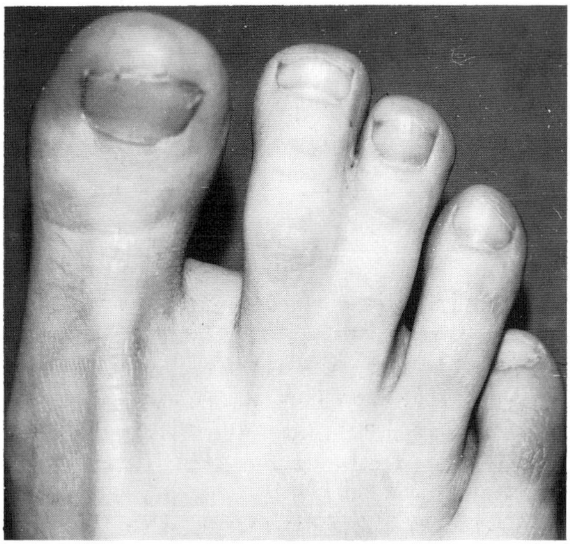

Fig. 62.26 Syndactyly of 2nd and 3rd toes

is usually achieved by turning a flap from the pulp of one of the toes into the cleft and placing a full thickness graft onto the donor site of the other toe.

Polydactyly

This is probably the most common congenital deformity of the foot. It is commoner in black races and is more frequently seen in females.

It is often associated with polydactyly of the fingers.

An extra digit is normally seen on the postaxial side of the foot and may be connected with the foot by a narrow stalk or alternatively a fully formed toe may be attached to the foot at metatarsophalangeal or interphalangeal joint level.

Correction is directed to narrowing the foot to enable the wearing of shoes and is usually simply achieved.

Preaxial polydactyly can be associated with medial deviation of the big toe (Fig. 62.27). The accessory digit can be removed, but the deviation is caused by an inclination of the metatarsal head and in order to straighten the toe to permit the wearing of shoes a lateral wedge osteotomy at the metatarsal neck may be required.

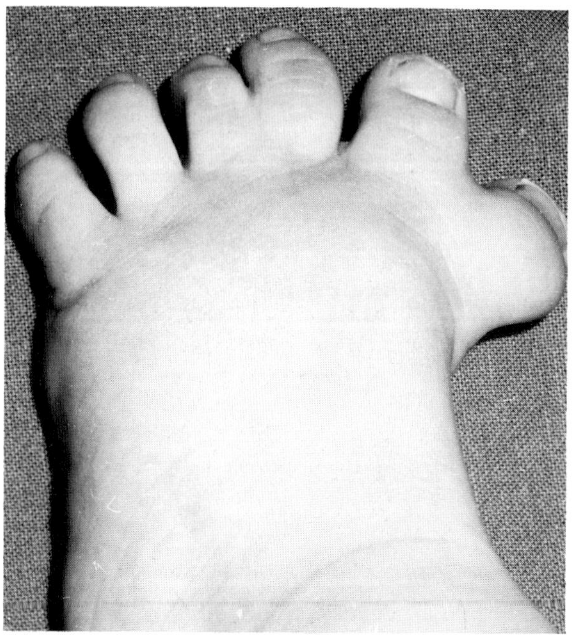

Fig. 62.27 Polydactyly on the preaxial side

Macrodactyly

This is a congenital pathological enlargement of soft tissue and associated skeletal enlargement. Fortunately it is rare and usually affects one digit, but if more than one is involved they are adjacent.

The digital nerves in macrodactyly are commonly enlarged with fatty tissue and the condition may be associated with neurofibromatosis.

The enlargement may be stable, in the respect that the digit remains in proportion, or progressive, in which the digit increases out of proportion to the rest of the foot. The surgical treatment is either conservative or ablative. Conservative methods constitute reducing the bulk of the digit by thinning soft tissue and controlling excessive growth by shortening bone and preventing epiphyseal growth.

Thinning of soft tissue has to be carried out with care to avoid skin necrosis. The results of conservative surgery are usually poor with a stiff, enlarged digit commonly the outcome. Amputation of the digit is usually the best method of treatment and permits the wearing of shoes (Figs. 62.28, 29 and 30).

Congenital constriction rings

Ring constrictions consist of deep grooves in the lower leg running transversely to the long axis. The depth varies and may be sufficient to cause autoamputations.

Commonly the groove passes down to the deep fascia and deep structures are unaffected. The constriction rings produce obstructions to the superficial lymphatics and therefore distal lymphoedema.

Constriction rings are often multiple and autoamputation of digits or fenestrated syndactyly may be found in association.

The aetiology is debatable and may be due to the fetus pushing its foot into the amniotic sac with subsequent development of a tight band around it, filamentous strands from the amnion wrapping around the limb or a local dysplasia of the mesoderm.

Treatment is undertaken early in order to prevent the distal lymphoedema becoming chronic with irreversible skin changes.

Excision of the constriction ring is carried out to its full depth, if necessary including deep fascia and repaired with multiple Z-plasties. In view of the fact

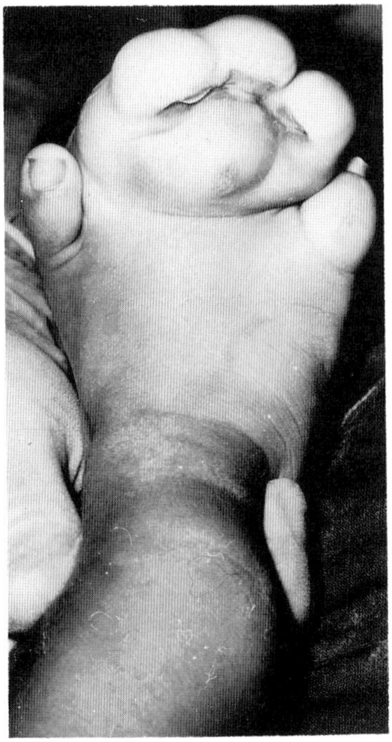

Fig. 62.28 Klippel–Trenaunay syndrome with macrodactyly of 2nd, 3rd and 4th toes

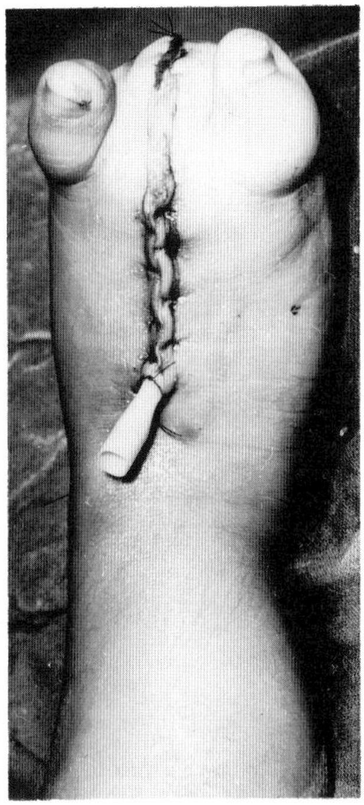

Fig. 62.30 Early postoperative result to show a foot of normal width

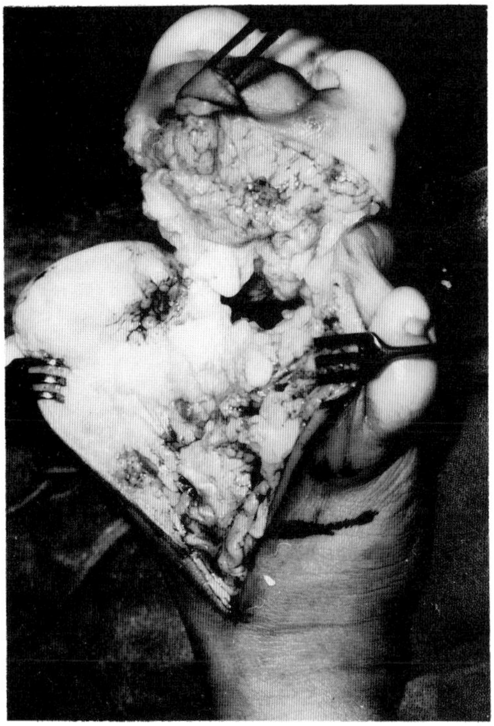

Fig. 62.29 Removal of the central three toes in order to permit the wearing of shoes

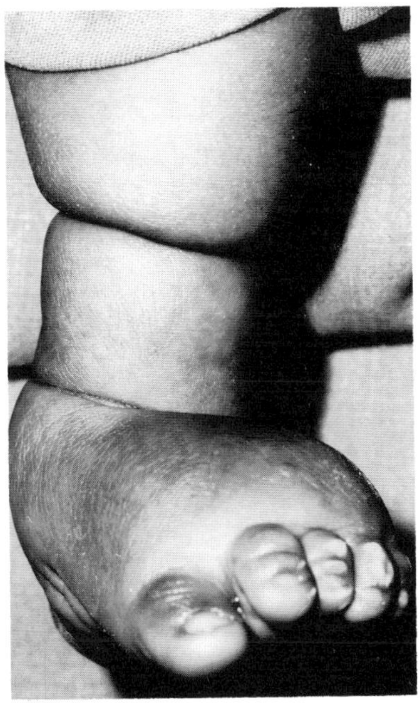

Fig. 62.31 Ring constriction deformity of the lower leg with distal lymphoedema

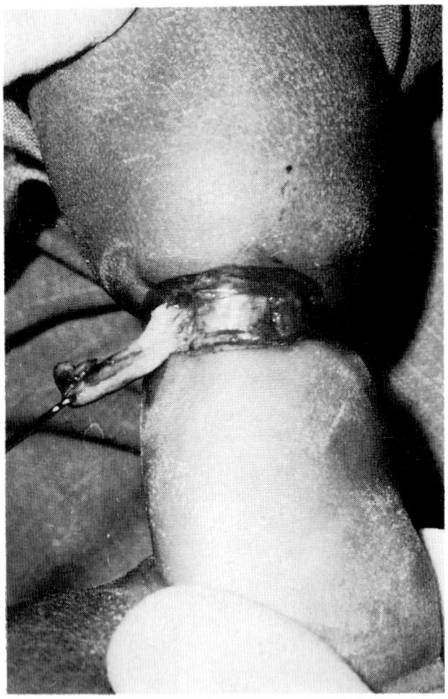

Fig. 62.32 Excision of the constriction ring including the deep fascia

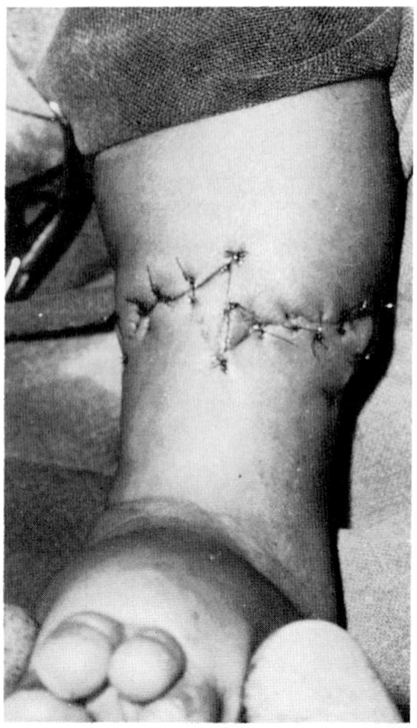

Fig. 62.33 Closed with the incorporation of a series of Z-plasties

that a circumferential excision will be necessary there is a risk to the distal viability of the limb and it may be advisable, particularly where there is suspected deep involvement, to carry out the correction in two stages doing half the circumference of the limb at a time (Figs. 62.31, 32 and 33).

Following surgery the distal lymphoedema usually disperses completely.

REFERENCES

Barclay T L, Cordoso E, Sharpe D T, Crockett D J 1982 Repair of lower leg injuries with fasciocutaneous flap. Br J Plast Surg 35: 127–132

Barclay T L, Sharpe D T, Chisholm E M 1983 Cross-leg fasciocutaneous flaps. Plast Reconstr Surg 72: 843–846

Buncke H J, Buncke C M, Shutz W P 1966 Immediate Nicalodoni procedure in the Rhesus monkey or hallux-to-hand transplantation, utilizing micro-miniature vascular anastomosis. Br J Plast Surg 19: 332–337

Clarkson P 1962 On making thumbs. Plast Reconstr Surg 29: 325–331

Cobbett J R 1969 Free digital transfer: Report of a case of transfer of a great toe to replace an amputated thumb. J Bone Joint Surg 51B: 677–679

Curtin J W 1977 Functional surgery for intractable conditions of the sole of the foot. Plast Reconstr Surg 59: 806–811

Foucher G, Merle M, Marcaud M, Miebou J 1980 Microsurgical free partial toe transfer in hand reconstruction, a report of 12 cases. Plast Reconstr Surg 65: 616–626

Gilbert A, Morrison W A, Tubiana R 1975 Transfert sur la main d'un lambeau libre sensible. Chirurgie 101: 691–694

Gillies H D 1920 The tubed pedicle in plastic surgery. NY Med J III: 1

Haertsch P A 1981a The surgical plane in the leg. Br J Plast Surg 34: 464–469

Haertsch P A 1981b The blood supply to the skin of the leg: a post mortem investigation. Br J Plast Surg 34: 470–477

Harrison D H, Morgan B D G 1981 The instep island flap to resurface plantar defects. Br J Plast Surg 34: 315–318

Hynes W 1957 The treatment of scars by shaving and skin graft. Br J Plast Surg 10: 1

Kaplan I 1969 Neurovascular island flap in the treatment of trophic ulceration of the heel. Br J Plast Surg 22: 143–148

Lister G D 1978 Use of an innervated skin graft to provide sensation to the reconstructed heel. Plast Reconstr Surg 62: 151–161

McCraw J B 1977 In Converse J M (ed) Reconstructive Plastic Surgery, Vol. 7, Saunders, Philadelphia, p 3563

Maisels D O 1961 Repairs of the heel. Br J Plast Surg 14: 117–125

Mir y Mir L 1954 Functional graft of the heel. Plast Reconstr Surg 14: 444–450

Morrison W A, O'Brien B McC, McLeod A M 1980 Thumb reconstruction with a free neurovascular wrap-around flap from the big toe. J Hand Surg 5: 515–583

Morrison W A, Crabb D McK, O'Brien B McC, Jenkins A 1983 The instep of the foot as a fasciocutaneous island and as a free flap for heel defects. Plast Reconstr Surg 72: 56–63

Nahai F 1980 The tensor fascia lata flap. Clin Plast Surg 7: 51

Nicoladoni C 1900 Dannenplastik und argmerscher Ersatz der Finger Spitze. Archiv fur Klinische Chirurgie 61: 606–614

O'Brien B McC, Shanmugan M 1973 Experimental transfer of composite free flaps with microvascular anastomosis. Aust NZ J Surg 43: 285–288

Ponten B 1981 The fasciocutaneous flap: its use in soft tissue defects of the lower leg. Br J Plast Surg 34: 215–220
Serafin D, Sabatier R F, Morris R L, Gengicide N G 1980 Reconstruction of the extremity with vascularised composite tissue: Improved tissue survival and specific indications. Plast Reconstr Surg 66: 230–241
Shanahan R E, Gingrass R P 1979 Medial plantar sensory flap for coverage of heel defects. Plast Reconstr Surg 64: 295–298
Snyder G B, Edgerton M T 1965 The principle of the neurovascular flap in the management of ulcerated anaesthetic weight-bearing areas of the lower extremity. Plast Reconstr Surg 36: 518–528
Somerlad B C, McGrowther D A 1978 Resurfacing the sole: long term follow-up and comparison of techniques. Br J Plast Surg 31: 107–116
Song R, Gao Y, Song Y, Yu Y, Song Y 1982 The forearm flap. Chir Plast Surg 9: 21–26
Stranc M F, Labandter H, Roy A 1975 A review of 196 tubed pedicles. Br J Plast Surg 28: 54–58
Taylor G I 1983 Current status of free vascularised bone grafts. Clin Plast Surg 10: 185–209
Taylor G I, Daniel R K 1975 Anatomy of several free flap donor sites. Plast Reconstr Surg 56: 243
Thake R L 1981 Random pattern de-epithelialised 'turn-over' flaps to replace skin loss in the upper third of the leg. Br J Plast Surg 34: 312–314
Vann H M 1943 A note on the formation of the plantar arterial arch of the human foot. Anat Rec 85: 269

Index

Vol 1 pp 1–580 Vol 2 pp 581–1279